Health Care Needs Assessment

The epidemiologically based needs assessment reviews

Third Series

Edited by

Andrew Stevens
Professor of Public Health
Department of Public Health and Epidemiology
University of Birmingham

James Raftery
Professor of Health Technology Assessment
School of Medicine
University of Southampton

Jonathan Mant
Senior Clinical Lecturer
Department of Primary Care and General Practice
University of Birmingham

and

Sue Simpson
Research Fellow
Department of Public Health and Epidemiology
University of Birmingham

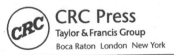

CRC Press
Taylor & Francis Group
Boca Raton London New York

CRC Press is an imprint of the
Taylor & Francis Group, an **informa** business

First published 2007 by Radcliffe Publishing

Published 2018 by CRC Press
Taylor & Francis Group
6000 Broken Sound Parkway NW, Suite 300
Boca Raton, FL 33487-2742

© 2007 by Andrew Stevens, James Raftery, Jonathan Mant and Sue Simpson
CRC Press is an imprint of Taylor & Francis Group, an Informa business

First issued in paperback 2019

No claim to original U.S. Government works

ISBN 13: 978-0-367-44635-2 (pbk)
ISBN 13: 978-1-84619-063-6 (hbk)

Visit the Taylor & Francis Web site at
http://www.taylorandfrancis.com

and the CRC Press Web site at
http://www.crcpress.com

British Library Cataloguing in Publication Data

A catalogue record for this book is available from the British Library.

Typeset by Advance Typesetting Ltd, Oxford

Contents

Preface

This book is the third series of the Health Care Needs Assessment reviews. Although in recent years needs assessment has been made more achievable by the increased provision of, and improved access to, data made possible by the Internet, this is often in disparate and disconnected chunks. Policy makers, planners and purchasers of health care continue to need a perspective on entire disease areas. These reviews bring together the plethora of data in an established structured approach.

The first series (second edition) published in 2004 comprises reviews of 19 diseases, interventions or services selected for their importance to purchasers (now Primary Care Trusts in the main) of health care: Diabetes Mellitus; Renal Disease; Stroke; Lower Respiratory Disease; Coronary Heart Disease; Colorectal Cancer; Cancer of the Lung; Osteoarthritis affecting the Hip and Knee; Cataract Surgery; Groin Hernia; Varicose Veins and Venous Ulcers; Benign Prostatic Hyperplasia; Severe Mental Illness; Alzheimer's Disease and Other Dementias; Alcohol Misuse; Drug Misuse; Learning Disabilities; Community Child Health Services; and Contraception, Induced Abortion and Fertility Services.

The second series published in 1996 extended the topic range to include: Accident and Emergency Departments; Child and Adolescent Mental Health; Low Back Pain; Palliative and Terminal Care; Dermatology; Breast Cancer; Genitourinary Medicine Services; and Gynaecology.

This third series now completes the collection of needs assessments and covers: Adult Critical Care; Continence; Dyspepsia; Black and Minority Ethnic Groups; Hypertension; Obesity; Chronic Pain; Mental Ill Health in Primary Care; Peripheral Vascular Disease; Pregnancy and Childbirth; and Health Care in Prisons.

In all three series the chapters have been selected for their importance in health care commissioning and their coherence as topics. The same protocol incorporating the three main elements of epidemiological needs assessment (prevalence and incidence; current services available; and effectiveness and cost-effectiveness) has been used throughout for each chapter. This comprises:

- statement of the problem
- sub-categories
- prevalence and incidence
- services available and their costs
- effectiveness and cost-effectiveness
- quantified models of care and recommendations
- outcome measures, audit methods and targets
- information and research requirements.

Consistency has therefore been a priority in putting the series together. We hope that readers find it easy to access key data and that they will in addition be able to understand key diseases and service areas as an entity. The editors wish to acknowledge with gratitude the immense effort put in by individual authors and groups of authors, as well as our numerous chapter reviewers and others who helped to contribute to the value of the Health Care Needs Assessment Series.

Andrew Stevens
James Raftery
Jonathan Mant
Sue Simpson
January 2007

List of contributors

Raj S Bhopal
Bruce and John Usher Professor of Public Health
Public Health Sciences Section, Division of Community Health Sciences
University of Edinburgh

Jean Chapple
Consultant in Public Health Medicine
Westminster PCT

Eugenia Cronin
Head of Healthier Communities
Greenwich Council

Leslie L Davidson
Professor of Clinical Epidemiology
Mailman School of Public Health
Columbia University, NY

Brendan C Delaney
Professor of Primary Care
Department of Primary Care and General Practice
University of Birmingham

Madeleine Donaldson
Research Fellow in Epidemiology
Department of Health Sciences
University of Leicester

Nigel Edwards
Director of Policy, NHS Confederation
Honorary Visiting Professor
London School of Hygiene and Tropical Medicine

Gerald Fowkes
Professor of Epidemiology
Director, Wolfson Unit for Prevention of Peripheral Vascular Diseases
Public Health Sciences
University of Edinburgh

Jo Garcia
Senior Research Officer
Social Science Research Unit
The Institute of Education, University of London

John Garrow
Retired Professor

Paramjit S Gill
Clinical Senior Lecturer
Department of Primary Care and General Practice
University of Birmingham

Jane Henderson
Researcher in Health Economics
National Perinatal Epidemiology Unit, University of Oxford

Joe Kai
Professor of Primary Care
University of Nottingham
Graduate Medical School
Derby City General Hospital

Tony Kendrick
Professor of Primary Medical Care
Community Clinical Sciences
School of Medicine, University of Southampton

Paul Lelliott
Director, College Research and Training Unit
Royal College of Psychiatrists

Jonathan Mant
Senior Clinical Lecturer
Department of Primary Care and General Practice
University of Birmingham

Tom Marshall
Senior Lecturer
Department of Public Health and Epidemiology
University of Birmingham

Catherine W McGrother
Senior Lecturer in Epidemiology
Department of Health Sciences
University of Leicester

Richard J McManus
Senior Lecturer
Department of Primary Care and General Practice
University of Birmingham

Henry J McQuay
Professor of Pain Relief
University of Oxford Pain Relief Unit

Paul Moayyedi
Professor of Gastroenterology
McMaster University
Hamilton, Ontario

R Andrew Moore
Honorary Professor
School of Health Sciences
University of Wales, Swansea

Mick Nielsen
Consultant in Critical Care
Southampton University Hospitals NHS Trust

Jo Paton
Honorary Lecturer
Institute of Psychiatry, King's College London

Stavros Petrou
Health Economist
National Perinatal Epidemiology Unit, University of Oxford

Siân Rees
Senior Policy Adviser
Department of Health

Sue Simpson
Research Fellow
Department of Public Health and Epidemiology
University of Birmingham

Lesley A Smith
Pain Research
Nuffield Department of Anaesthetics
University of Oxford

Andrew Stevens
Professor of Public Health
Department of Public Health and Epidemiology
University of Birmingham

Carolyn Summerbell
Professor of Human Nutrition
School of Health and Social Care
University of Teesside

Sarah Wild
Lecturer in Public Health Medicine
Health Care Research Unit
University of Southampton

Date of acceptance for publication

Chapter	Date accepted for publication
Adult Critical Care	December 2000
Continence	September 2002
Dyspepsia	January 2002
Black and Minority Ethnic Groups	August 2001 + update 2003
Hypertension	March 2004
Obesity	January 2000 + update 2004
Chronic Pain	June 2004
Mental Ill Health in Primary Care	October 2004
Peripheral Vascular Disease	December 1998
Pregnancy and Childbirth	February 2002
Health Care in Prisons	September 2005

1 Adult Critical Care

Eugenia Cronin, Mick Nielsen, Martin Spollen and Nigel Edwards

1 Summary

Introduction

Adult critical care is an important, high-profile and high-cost area of modern healthcare provision. This chapter aims to provide an objective synthesis of evidence available from published and other sources that can inform debate on the planning of critical care services.

Definition of critical care

The term *critical care* has been defined as:

> care for patients who have potentially recoverable conditions who can benefit from more detailed observation (with or without invasive treatment) than can be provided safely in an ordinary ward.[1]

Background to the development of critical care services

Critical care services are atypical in the wide heterogeneity of their patients. This is in part a reflection of the way in which these services have evolved.

The progress of intensive care in the UK has been described as 'haphazard', consisting of 'largely unplanned and unevaluated' developments that occurred in reaction to changes in surgical and medical practice.

There has been debate about the configuration of critical care services, fuelled by a perception that there are not enough beds in some parts of the country and that existing beds are not in the right places.

During the late 1990s, the NHS Executive established a National Expert Group to review adult critical care services in the UK and to produce a national Framework for future organisation and care delivery. As a result, in May 2000 a critical care modernisation plan was announced.

Scope of this chapter

Throughout this chapter, we present and discuss both UK and international research findings on adult critical care services. Data on the profile of service provision, utilisation and associated costs relate to England and Wales unless otherwise stated.

Critical care services have previously been differentiated into intensive care and high-dependency care. The critical care modernisation plan announced in May 2000 introduced the notion that adult acute care should be seen as a spectrum, classified across four levels, much as paediatric critical care is organised. The four levels are:

- Level 0 – normal acute ward care
- Level 1 – acute ward care, with additional advice and support from the critical care team
- Level 2 – more detailed observation or intervention
- Level 3 – advanced respiratory support alone, or basic respiratory support together with support of at least two organ systems.

Sub-categories

In contrast with needs assessments for disease groups, where disease classification is central to the discussion and is relatively straightforward, in critical care practice it is difficult to classify and group clinical data into defined categories or hierarchies. Healthcare Resource Groups (HRGs) or Diagnosis Related Groups (DRGs) are used to categorise patients on the basis of diagnosis; but this approach is not applicable in critical care, where there is wide heterogeneity within diagnostic groups.[7]

Patients can be categorised by severity of illness; on the basis of demographic characteristics; on more precise measures of severity of illness; or according to the organ systems needing monitoring or support.

Epidemiology of critical care

Age and gender

There is evidence that critical care patients are mostly males and that a high proportion are elderly.

Intensive Care National Audit and Research Centre (ICNARC) data show that 4.8% of admissions are in the age range 0–17, and that 46.5% of admissions are of people aged 65 years or over. The mean age of patients is 57.3 years.

Types of admission

Intensive care

There is evidence that the greatest proportion of admissions to ICUs are for medical emergencies (41%), followed by planned admissions from elective surgery (25%) and emergency surgical admissions (18%). There are more recent data suggesting that the proportion of non-surgical admissions to ICUs is increasing.

The most common source of admission to intensive care is theatre or recovery in the same hospital (44.1%), followed by a ward in the same hospital (22.3%) and A&E in the same hospital (17.1%).

High-dependency care

There is little information available on the types of admission and diagnostic categories of patients in HDUs in the UK, but the Augmented Care Period (ACP) dataset, introduced in 1997, will go some way towards addressing this.

Several studies have examined the potential for using HDU beds to alleviate some of the demand on ICU beds, by differentiating between those patients requiring high-dependency care and those requiring intensive care.

The reclassification of critical care into three levels, announced in the critical care modernisation plan in May 2000, will lead to a better reflection of severity in activity data.

Indications for admission

One study reported that over 70% of admissions to ICUs were in the cardiovascular or respiratory categories. Other data show that the ten most frequent reasons for admission are:

- Aortic or iliac dissection or aneurysm – surgical
- Acute myocardial infarction – non-surgical
- Pneumonia, with no organism isolated – non-surgical
- Bacterial pneumonia – non-surgical
- Septic shock – non-surgical
- Primary brain injury – non-surgical
- Large bowel tumour – surgical
- Left ventricular failure – non-surgical
- Asthma attack in a new or known asthmatic – non-surgical
- Non-traumatic large bowel perforation or rupture – surgical.

The most common condition admitted made up only 6.5% of admissions, and the top ten conditions made up only 26.8% of admissions.

The ten conditions that use the greatest number of bed-days are as follows:

- Bacterial pneumonia – non-surgical
- Pneumonia, with no organism isolated – non-surgical
- Aortic or iliac dissection or aneurysm – surgical
- Septic shock – non-surgical
- Primary brain injury – non-surgical
- Non-traumatic large bowel perforation or rupture – surgical
- Acute myocardial infarction – non-surgical
- Exacerbation of chronic obstructive airways disease – non-surgical
- Inhalation pneumonitis (gastrointestinal contents) – non-surgical
- Non-cardiogenic pulmonary oedema (ARDS) – non-surgical.

These conditions made up 32.8% of bed-days.

Severity of illness

Patients are usually admitted to intensive care because of the severity of their illness, rather than solely on the underlying diagnosis. Studies of ICUs have shown a considerable range in the mean APACHE II score for patients admitted.

The critical care modernisation plan introduced an approach to the classification of critical care that reflects the variable severity of illness.

Length of stay

It is essential that the length of stay in critical care be defined in terms of fractions of days rather than whole days, because many patients are admitted for periods of only a few hours. One study reported the median length of stay in ICUs as 1.6 days, while another dataset indicates an overall median length of stay of 2 days, and an average of 5.02. Mean length of stay is consistently higher than median length of stay, indicating that outlying lengthy periods have skewed the average.

Population demand for critical care

The need for intensive care is related to the severity of the patient's clinical condition and the need for invasive monitoring and treatment. Establishing the need for critical care beds is therefore problematic, and one is restricted to establishing some measure of demand for beds.

A mismatch between the continuum of health needs and the management of illness in hospitals may inflate the demand for critical care services. General advances in medicine and surgery and changes in surgical practice may also increase the demand on facilities.

Numbers of admissions to ICUs and HDUs

One estimate of admission rates to ICUs is 92.8 per 100 000 population. Another estimate, using data for the North West region, identified 154 admissions per 100 000, but noted several possible sources of bias.

Although information is available about the demand for critical care, until recently there was none relating to population need. A prospective assessment of the need for both intensive care and high-dependency care beds has recently been published. It concluded that to meet the needs of a population of 500 000 on 95% of occasions would require 30 intensive care beds and 55 high-dependency care beds if these were provided in a single unit; and if they were provided in three separate units, the number of beds would increase by 10%.

Occupancy levels

Occupancy is often used as a measure of health service activity, indicating the activity of an inpatient unit in terms of its maximum capacity. There are several different methods of calculating bed occupancy, and the choice of method can have a significant impact.

One study reported the median average occupancy to be 83% in ICUs, 81% in combined ICU/HDUs and 74% in HDUs. Another study of London ICUs found 86% occupancy, with some as high as 95%.

These levels of occupancy seem inappropriately high for a service expected to respond to unpredictable emergencies.

Unmet demand

One study found a wide variation across trusts in the proportion of patients refused intensive care admission owing to lack of beds. There is evidence that refusal rates are influenced by type of unit, type of hospital and staffing, and that patients who are refused admission to intensive care have worse outcomes.

Substantial numbers of transfers occur because of bed shortages. Such transfers indicate bed shortage in the originating unit and may not reflect shortages across an entire system.

There is evidence from transfers data that shows markedly increased demand during the winter.

There is research to suggest that the most common indications for transfers are referrals for neurosurgical care, lack of beds in ICU and lack of renal support services.

For a patient needing intensive care following major elective surgery, the lack of a bed will often cause the operation to be cancelled at the last minute, since only then will the bed situation be known with certainty. One study suggested that a lack of intensive care beds had caused 124 out of 256 units (48%) to cancel operations in an eight-week period.

In some instances, a bed may be created by prematurely discharging a patient not previously deemed ready to leave the ICU. Data suggest that over 7% of intensive care survivors are discharged early because of a shortage of unit beds.

Limitations of the data

It should be noted that the data discussed above probably underestimate the shortfall of supply.

Estimating need from data on bed occupancy, refusals and transfers is complicated by the variations in admissions and discharge criteria.

The Augmented Care Period (ACP) dataset was introduced in 1997 to collect data on intensive and high-dependency care activity for patients other than neonates, enabling the level of care that patients receive to be identified.

Early analyses of limited ACP datasets suggest that a significant number of days of intensive or high-dependency care may be provided in inappropriate locations.

International comparisons

There is some evidence that smaller bed numbers in the United Kingdom mean that only the most severely ill patients are admitted.

In the USA, up to about 20% of patients receive care in an ICU or CCU at some time during their stay in hospital, but the use of intensive care is much less common in Europe. However, without case-mix data it is questionable whether such international comparisons are helpful.

Future demand

Indications are that the demand for critical care in the future will grow. Increasingly aggressive surgery is likely to escalate the demand for high-dependency and intensive care. If the current shortage in donor organs is corrected, more frequent transplant activity will also increase the pressure on critical care.

Services available and their costs

Service provision in England and Wales

The haphazard development of critical care has led to a marked variability in the provision of these services across the country. Until the announcement of the critical care modernisation programme in May 2000 there had been no national or even regional strategy for critical care. As a consequence, the number of intensive care beds and the spending on intensive care per head of population, in relation to population figures, have varied considerably.

There is currently a substantial debate about the configuration of intensive care services, fuelled by a perception that there are not enough beds in some parts of the country and that existing beds may not be in the right places. Surveys have confirmed substantial variation in the provision of critical care beds.

Little routine statistical information has previously been available for critical care. The ACP dataset should go some way to meeting this need, and additional information is now available through the Audit Commission and through initiatives such as ICNARC.

The critical care modernisation plan calls for a data-collecting culture, promoting an evidence base, and requires NHS trusts to comply with the ACP dataset.

A recent study found 521 critical care units in operation in England and Wales. There is evidence for great variability in configuration of critical care facilities within trusts, and there are many combinations of generalist and specialist ICUs, HDUs and combined ICU/HDUs.

One study reported data on bed numbers in individual units. The median numbers of available beds were as follows:

- 5.3 in ICUs
- 6 in combined ICU/HDUs
- 4 in HDUs.

Pattern of care provided in critical care

Data from ICNARC indicate that 54% of admissions are mechanically ventilated and 42.3% are not. Another dataset shows that the average proportion of admissions who receive ventilation is 57.8%. Evidence suggests wide variation between ICUs in the levels of dependency of their patients.

Admission guidelines

Identifying those patients most likely to benefit from critical care is one of the key challenges in providing the service.

The admission guidelines developed by a Department of Health working party in 1996 described the characteristics of intensive care and high-dependency care. These guidelines were superseded in 2000 by a new approach to categorising critical care based on three levels.

Discharge guidelines

The decision to discharge a patient from intensive care or high-dependency care will depend partly on the level of care available in the unit or ward to which the patient is to be discharged. Assessment of the continuing appropriateness of intensive care should be made at regular intervals.

The availability of step-down care within the hospital has an important influence on the decision to discharge from critical care.

Staffing

Intensive care should be a consultant-led service with considerable direct consultant input into decisions on admission, care and discharge.

Intensive care and high-dependency units are critically dependent on adequate numbers of appropriately trained nurses. One recent study found wide variations in the numbers of nurses employed.

Difficulties with recruitment and retention of nurses is one of the reasons for discrepancies between the numbers of funded and available beds. Support workers may be employed to help trained nursing staff, potentially reducing the need for nurses to perform non-nursing tasks.

A central focus of the modernisation programme for critical care was workforce development. This includes the recruitment, training and retention of medical and nursing staff, and requires a balanced skill-mix so that professional staff are able to delegate less skilled and non-clinical tasks. The programme also injected additional resources into NHS trusts for the recruitment and retention of critical care nurses.

Clinical management

Critical care units generally follow one of two different patterns of clinical management: 'closed' (in which a critical care consultant has complete responsibility for a patient) or 'open' units (in which responsibility remains with the patient's admitting consultant}.

The modernisation programme for critical care required that admission to Levels 2 and 3 of critical care should be by agreement between consultants only.

Costs

Intensive care provides care at a high cost to a small number of patients. Annual spending on intensive care in the UK has been estimated at £675 million, representing about 2% of the hospital budget. It appears that at least 50% of ICU patient costs are incurred by staffing.

Cost accounting in critical care is underdeveloped, even though critical care is an increasingly expensive speciality in the UK.

One study found a median cost per patient day of £1064 in 1994/5 and £1087 in 1995/6, and wide variation between trusts on annual costs.

Another study found the average daily patient-related cost of care to be £592 and overhead costs to be £560, resulting in a total average cost of £1152. This study found a strong, highly significant statistical correlation between (1) the Therapeutic Intervention Scoring System (TISS) and the cost of care for each calendar day, and (2) the APACHE II score and cost of the first 24-hour period.

There is evidence of high variability in the daily cost of individual critical care patients, and so top-down costing approaches that average out daily costs may be misleading. Bottom-up methodologies are more useful.

Effectiveness of services and interventions

Perceptions of constraints in supply cause questions to be raised about the appropriate use of intensive care, and, more fundamentally, about the need to determine which types of patient actually benefit from critical care.

Evidence of the effectiveness of specific interventions

For a few conditions, the benefits of intensive care are indisputable. For the majority of conditions, however, its effectiveness remains unproven. Indeed, the role of intensive care in preventing death has yet to be properly investigated.

Given the enormous heterogeneity of the case-mix, any trials in intensive care will require huge numbers of patients if these questions are to be answered.

Where such evidence exists, it clearly needs to be widely publicised. Even then, whether such strategies are adopted in practice depends on factors such as the magnitude and precision of estimates of benefit and harm, as well as access, availability and costs.

Cost effectiveness

Recent data suggest that 22% of ICU patients die before leaving the unit, a further 8% die before leaving hospital and 7% die in the first six months at home. The relatively high mortality rates in critical care patients mean that large sums of money are spent on patients who, ultimately, do not survive. Evidence from one study suggests that the 15% of ICU patients who died consumed 37% of the ICU budget.

Other research has estimated the total hospital cost per quality adjusted life year (QALY) at £7500. When the cost-per-QALY comparisons are made with other healthcare interventions, intensive care is found to lie between heart transplantation and home dialysis.

Models of care

Possible models of care

The modernisation programme for critical care called for a strategic change to modernise services, and injected additional resources into NHS trusts for the recruitment and retention of critical care nurses.

Four main elements of the programme required action by NHS trusts. These were:

- a hospital-wide approach to critical care, with services that extend beyond the physical boundaries of intensive care and high-dependency units, making optimum use of available resources, including beds
- a networked service across those NHS trusts that together serve one or more local health economies, meeting the critical care needs of those within the network, and minimising the need for transfer outside
- workforce development, including the recruitment, training and retention of medical and nursing staff, and the creation of a balanced skill-mix so that professional staff are able to delegate less skilled and non-clinical tasks
- better information, with all critical care services collecting reliable management information, and participating in outcome-focused clinical audit.

A new approach to classifying critical care was also introduced, as described earlier.

There have been suggestions that critical care services should be more centralised. This would lead to units becoming larger, a concept familiar in other countries. An inevitable consequence of centralisation or stratification is an increased need to transfer patients between hospitals.

Specialist weaning units have been proposed to address 'bed blocking' by patients dependent on ventilation and to concentrate expertise in weaning such patients.

Several recent studies have suggested that earlier recognition and intervention of seriously ill patients on general wards is likely to reduce their need for critical care, and have proposed the development of 'outreach' services from critical care specialists to support ward staff in managing patients at risk.

The role of intermediate care

Some commentators see the existence of intermediate care as a way of managing illness that matches the continuum of health needs. It has been argued that grouping patients by level of need can enable the best use to be made of available technical resources and staffing.

The critical care modernisation programme introduced a new approach to classifying critical care services across four levels, thereby matching more closely the continuum of health needs.

The focus on high-dependency care as an alternative to intensive care was made somewhat redundant by the announcement of the modernisation programme. The following discussion of high-dependency care makes some general points about having a stratified system, reflecting severity of illness.

Several studies have examined the impact of opening a high-dependency unit, finding that:

- the occupancy of intensive care beds by patients needing only high-dependency care was reduced
- the occupancy by patients needing intensive care was increased

- a significant decrease was seen in re-admissions
- ICU patients' initial severity of illness was lower and their length of stay reduced, but there was no reduction in demand for intensive care
- admissions to the ICU decreased initially as would be expected, but this was followed by an increase over the pre-HDU level of ICU admissions
- there was a significant reduction in the cancellation of elective surgery and in the number of patients transferred out of the ICU because of demand for beds.

The impact of opening an HDU in a given hospital will depend on the case-load and case-mix that it sees, plus the extent to which existing facilities meet that demand.

How many beds are needed?

There is no fixed formula for the number of critical care beds needed by a trust, and it is important that the number is tailored to the workload and case-mix that the hospital treats.

The following have been put forward as factors to be considered when estimating the size of an ICU:

- number of acute beds in hospital or catchment area
- type of acute bed
- previously calculated occupancies of wards, HDUs and ICUs
- history of refusals
- location of other high-care areas
- number of operating theatres
- surgical specialities services and case-mix
- medical specialities
- A&E department
- sub-regional or regional services
- ability to transfer patients to an off-site ICU
- paediatric care
- location.

There is no firm guidance as to the optimum size for an ICU.

The number of beds needed will in part depend on how they are configured. One researcher has calculated that, to meet needs on 95% of occasions for a population of 500 000 would require 30 intensive care beds and 55 high-dependency beds if these were all in a single unit. For three separate units to meet an identical need on 95% of occasions, 10% more beds would be needed.

Detailed mathematical models have an established place in providing quantitative information about healthcare resource needs; but, to be helpful, they must be able to deal with complexity, uncertainty, variability and, sometimes, inadequate data.

Appropriate use of critical care beds

It is important that the use of critical care facilities is reserved for appropriate patients, as far as possible. This will depend in part on the facilities available, but also on the presence of experienced, suitably trained, senior clinicians able to make timely decisions on admission, on discharge and on withholding or withdrawing treatment.

Configuration and provision of critical care services

Recurring crises because of shortages of intensive care beds suggest that the present configuration of critical care services is failing, and have led to the belief that more such beds are required. However, there are data to suggest that some intensive care beds are used for patients needing only high-dependency care. Reliable information is urgently required to illuminate this area.

In the absence of adequate information, it is impossible to make explicit recommendations regarding the centralisation or stratification of critical care services. Nonetheless, given the shortcomings in the current service configuration, greater collaboration between trusts would seem desirable.

These issues were recognised in the report of the National Expert Group set up in 1999 by the NHS Executive to review adult critical care services in the UK. This resulted in a critical care modernisation plan that injected extra resources for additional staff, beds and services, and introduced a new approach to the classification of critical care services.

The notion of outreach medical emergency teams was also acknowledged in the report and resulted in a call for the establishment of such teams.

Recommendations

Provision and configuration at trust level

The provision of critical care beds must be sufficient to meet the needs of emergency referrals on at least 95% of occasions, while at the same time allowing major elective surgery to be undertaken without frequent cancellations. The numbers and types of critical care beds should be tailored to the workload and case-mix of each individual trust.

When assessing the need for critical care services in a trust, the numbers of refused admissions, premature discharges, transfers, cancelled operations and the numbers of patients being managed on general wards who would benefit from critical care should all be considered.

The configuration of the service in terms of the geographical, operational and management relationship between different levels of critical care beds needs also to be considered.

Outreach services should be developed so that seriously ill patients elsewhere in the trust can benefit from the expertise and skills of the intensive care staff, both medical and nursing.

Operational policies at inter-trust level

With a scarce, expensive resource such as critical care, trusts and their patients would benefit from a more collaborative approach than currently exists. A possible model would be one based on centralisation, along the lines of that adopted for paediatric intensive care.

Coping with pressure

Trusts should plan for an escalating response to escalating pressure, defining how and under what circumstances other resources will be called upon. Similar strategies should be agreed between trusts.

Appropriate use of resources

Critical care beds should be used for appropriate patients, and decisions on withholding and withdrawing treatment should be made in a timely manner. This requires input from appropriately trained and experienced consultants. Units should have clear guidelines covering issues such as admission, discharge, clinical care and patient transfers.

There should be sufficient numbers of general ward beds to ensure the prompt discharge of patients no longer needing critical care.

The allocation of nurses to patients should be tailored to individual patient need rather than according to rigid ratios.

Data requirements

Information on the need for, the use of, and the outcome from critical care is urgently needed to inform strategic planning.

Universal and accurate completion of the ACP dataset should be encouraged and will provide valuable data on the use of critical care facilities. All intensive care units should participate in ICNARC's Case Mix Programme.

Hospital survival after intensive care has been over-emphasised as a measure of performance. While many patients survive to leave hospital, not enough is currently known about their longer-term outcome and quality of life.

In the absence of current measures of process for critical care services, performance indicators should be defined and introduced.

Staffing needs

Trusts should review the number of consultant sessions they allocate to intensive care, to ensure that decisions on admission, discharge, transfers and withholding or withdrawing treatment are made by appropriate clinicians.

Trusts should also ensure that critical care nursing staff are being used optimally, with nurse:patient ratios tailored as far as possible to individual patient need. Consideration should be given to employing other staff to take over any non-nursing roles.

Outreach services are likely to need additional staff.

Commissioning for critical care services

At present, very few critical care units deal directly with commissioners and, for the majority, costs are theoretically built into block contracts for the major clinical specialities. The development of HRGs for critical care will help to make critical care activity and costs more explicit.

The call, in May 2000, for NHS trusts to establish Critical Care Delivery Groups, with the involvement of both medical and nursing critical care clinicians, may provide an avenue for clinicians to become more involved in contracting.

Critical care services should be specifically identified in discussions with commissioners, and intensive care clinicians should be involved in that exercise.

It may be appropriate for critical care to be considered outside the remit of PCGs except where it occurs as a planned episode following major elective surgery.

A suitable currency for critical care services remains to be defined.

Information requirements, outcome measures, targets and research priorities

Information requirements

Information is required on the need for, the use of and the outcome from critical care in order to inform strategic planning at trust, regional and national level. The paucity of such data has plagued previous attempts to review adult critical care services.

The introduction of the mandatory Augmented Care Period (ACP) dataset has given responsibility for critical care data collection to acute trusts. This requirement was reinforced by the critical care modernisation programme, announced in May 2000.

A twice-yearly national census of adult intensive care and high-dependency beds was also introduced because of a lack of basic information in this area.

In 1994, the Intensive Care National Audit and Research Centre (ICNARC) was established, offering a national Case Mix Programme for intensive care units. While at present only about 60% of units in England and Wales participate, the critical care modernisation programme called for all trusts to join ICNARC.

Outcome measures

Traditionally, the most commonly used outcome measure from critical care has been patient survival. The APACHE II method allows a case-mix-adjusted probability of hospital death to be calculated for each adult patient, enabling a standardised mortality ratio (SMR) to be derived.

Even with case-mix-adjustment, the importance of hospital survival has been somewhat over-emphasised and would not be considered adequate for other life-threatening pathologies.

Similarly, not enough is known about restoration of function and quality of life in survivors of critical illness. Patients should be evaluated in terms of their ongoing health and the extent to which they are restored to their previous lifestyle. One measure of the quality of life that may be appropriate for use with survivors is the Short Form 36.

Targets

There is an urgent need for performance indicators to be agreed and introduced for critical care services.

Research priorities

A major criticism of intensive care practice is that, despite its rapid development, it is not sufficiently underpinned by a firm basis of research. This is partly because of the ethical questions surrounding doing research in this area and the large size of samples needed.

In 1997, a joint Medical Research Council/Department of Health working party on intensive and high-dependency care highlighted the need for research and specifically identified five priority areas.

A study exploring clinicians' views of research priorities in critical care found that the priority was felt to be in the organisation and delivery of critical care.

2 Introduction and statement of the problem

Adult critical care is an important, high-profile and high-cost area of modern hospital healthcare provision. This chapter provides a comprehensive review of up-to-date research findings, and is set out under eight key headings:

- introduction to the services reviewed
- sub-categories
- epidemiology of critical care
- services available and their cost
- effectiveness of services and interventions
- models of care
- recommendations
- information requirements, outcome measures, targets and research priorities.

Our aim is to provide an objective synthesis of evidence available from published and other sources that can inform debate on the planning of critical care services.

Definition of critical care

The term *intensive care* has been defined by the Intensive Care Society (ICS)[1] as:

> *a service for patients who have potentially recoverable conditions, who can benefit from more detailed observation and invasive treatment than can be provided safely in an ordinary ward or high-dependency area. It is usually reserved for patients with threatened or established organ failure, often arising as a result or complication of an acute illness or trauma, or as a predictable phase in a planned treatment programme.*

In 1996, the Department of Health defined *high-dependency care* as providing a level of care between that of a general ward and intensive care.

The term *critical care* has emerged in light of the development of high-dependency care, and has been defined as:

> *care for patients who have potentially recoverable conditions who can benefit from more detailed observation (with or without invasive treatment) than can be provided safely in an ordinary ward.*[2]

Critical care, therefore, encapsulates intensive care, high-dependency care and any other care with higher observational requirements than those available on a general ward. Throughout this chapter, the term 'critical care' will be used to refer collectively to both intensive care and high-dependency care.

There are some aspects of critical care that are outside the scope of this chapter. These are highlighted later in this section.

Background to the development of critical care services

Intensive care and high-dependency services are characterised by wide heterogeneity among the patients. This is in part a reflection of the way in which these services have evolved.

Critical care evolved from the need to care for post-operative patients away from the general ward. This was recognised by Florence Nightingale in her observation of recovery areas near the operating theatre in many country hospitals.[3] In 1923, what could be claimed as the first intensive care unit (ICU) – a small facility for post-operative neurosurgical patients – was opened at the Johns Hopkins Hospital in Baltimore, USA. However, many of the procedures and treatments that are routine in ICUs today were developed during the Second World War, and subsequently in the rapid evacuation and care of those wounded in the Korean and Vietnam wars.[4]

The modern concept of the intensive care unit has largely evolved from the work of Larsen[5] in the polio epidemic in Copenhagen in 1952. He showed that deaths from respiratory failure decreased from 87% to 40% with the change from cuirasse ventilation (the 'iron lung') to manual positive pressure ventilation through a cuffed tracheostomy tube.

As new procedures and equipment were developed for the treatment of critically ill patients, there was a growth in intensive care provision during the 1960s.[6] The progress of intensive care in the UK has been described as 'haphazard',[7] consisting of 'largely unplanned and unevaluated' developments that occurred in reaction to changes in surgical and medical practice. Such developments often resulted more from local enthusiasm than from any evidence of benefit.

A paucity of information about critical care services was largely responsible for the abandonment of an attempted review by the King's Fund in 1989;[8] to a great extent, this position still applies over ten years later.

There is currently debate about the configuration of critical care services, fuelled by a perception that there are not enough beds in some parts of the country and that existing beds are not in the right places. There is certainly evidence suggesting that, at least in some places, levels of bed provision are failing to meet demand, and that many intensive care units run at occupancy levels too high for a service expected to respond to unpredictable emergencies. A widely reported case in March 1995 involved a patient being transferred from Kent to Yorkshire because of a lack of specialist neurosurgical facilities.[9] A small proportion of such cases draw the attention of the media and, by their very nature, attract considerable publicity.

In a recent initiative, the NHS Executive established a National Expert Group to review adult critical care services in the UK and to produce a national Framework for future organisation and care delivery. As a result of the report of the Group,[10] in May 2000 a critical care modernisation plan was announced,[11] which injected extra resources for additional staff, beds and services, and introduced a new approach to the classification of critical care services.

Scope of this chapter

Throughout this chapter, we present and discuss both UK and international research findings on adult critical care services. Data on the profile of service provision, utilisation and associated costs relate to England and Wales unless otherwise stated.

In this chapter, we have excluded consideration of:

- specialised units that restrict their intake to certain specialities (e.g. neurosurgical units)
- units that restrict their intake to certain patient groups (e.g. coronary care)
- services for children (i.e. paediatric intensive care).

However, our review of provision in England and Wales does include units where combined general and coronary care work is undertaken.

General intensive care units

Most ICUs are general and take both medical and surgical patients with a range of underlying diseases. Many units have a number of designated high-dependency beds, while others (usually in the absence of other high-dependency facilities) will admit high-dependency patients into intensive care beds. In much the same way, coronary care beds are sometimes provided in the same unit.[12,13] Audit Commission data[14] show that 32% of trusts have general adult ICUs and 28% have combined ICU/HDUs.

An ICU should be able to manage all the common organ system failures and hence provide respiratory support (including mechanical ventilation), circulatory support and renal support and provide the full range of invasive monitoring required for such activity[1] (*see* Figure 1).

The Department of Health[15] categorised organ system monitoring and support as follows:

1. **Advanced respiratory support**

   - mechanical ventilatory support (excluding mask continuous positive airways pressure (CPAP) or non-invasive, e.g. mask ventilation);
   - the possibility of a sudden, precipitous deterioration in respiratory function requiring immediate endotracheal intubation and mechanical ventilation.

2. **Basic respiratory monitoring and support**

   - the need for more than 40% oxygen via a fixed performance mask;
   - the possibility of progressive deterioration to the point of needing advanced respiratory support;
   - the need for physiotherapy to clear secretions at least two-hourly, whether via a tracheostomy or mini-tracheostomy or in the absence of an artificial airway;
   - patients recently extubated after a prolonged period of intubation and mechanical ventilation;
   - the need for mask CPAP or non-invasive ventilation;
   - patients who are intubated to protect the airway but need no ventilatory support and are otherwise stable.

3. **Circulatory support**

   - the need for vasoactive drugs to support arterial pressure or cardiac output;
   - support for circulatory instability owing to hypovolaemia from any cause and which is unresponsive to modest volume replacement. This will include, but not be limited to, post-surgical or gastrointestinal haemorrhage or haemorrhage related to a coagulopathy;
   - patients resuscitated following cardiac arrest where intensive or high-dependency care is considered clinically appropriate.

4. **Neurological monitoring and support**

   - central nervous system depression from whatever cause, sufficient to prejudice the airway and protective reflexes;
   - invasive neurological monitoring.

5. **Renal support**

   - the need for acute renal replacement therapy (haemodialysis, haemofiltration or haemodiafiltration).

Figure 1: ICU organ monitoring and support.

High-dependency units

The role of the HDU is to provide an intermediate 'step-up' or 'step-down' facility between the ICU and the general ward. High-dependency units deserve particular attention, as their role has been the subject of debate in recent years. In some hospitals there are separate high-dependency units. Such units can be separate entities or form part of a general ward or ICU.[16] Recent Audit Commission data indicate that 39% of acute trusts have separate HDUs,[17] while 28% have high-dependency beds in combined ICU/HDU units.

Table 1 sets out typical attributes of both care settings.[12]

Table 1: Attributes of intensive and high-dependency care.

Intensive care should provide:	High-dependency care should provide:
a designated area where such care is provided	
a clear operational policy based on a background of multidisciplinary care and effective communication	
a designated consultant as director, supported by consultants with allocated intensive care sessions sufficient to provide continuous (non-resident) availability	a designated consultant as director, with continuous cover from either the admitting speciality or intensive care
a minimum nurse:patient ratio of 1:1 throughout the 24 hours of the day, together with a nurse-in-charge plus additional nurses according to patient needs, the total number of beds and geographical arrangements within the unit. The skill-mix of nurses should reflect the physiological instability of the patient	an average nurse:patient ratio of 1:2 throughout the 24 hours of the day, together with a nurse-in-charge plus additional nurses according to patient needs, the total number of beds and geographical arrangements within the unit. The skill-mix of nurses should reflect the possibility that patients may be physiologically unstable
24-hour dedicated cover by resident trainee medical staff	continuous availability of trainee medical staff either from the admitting speciality or from intensive care
the ability to support common organ system failures – in particular, ventilatory, circulatory and renal failure	appropriate monitoring and other equipment
a sufficient case-load to maintain skills and expertise	
administrative, technical and secretarial support	
continuing education, training and audit	

Specialised units

Specialised units also exist. These include cardiothoracic surgical units, neurological and neurosurgical units as well as burns units, liver units and spinal injury units. These may operate at an intensive care level, at a high-dependency level or as combined units. Because they deal with specific disease categories, it is more appropriate to consider these units in chapters that deal with specific diseases.

Coronary care units

Coronary care unit (CCU) patients often require close patient monitoring and observation rather than intensive care.[16] Coronary care units are excluded from this chapter, as they are not considered to be a sub-category of ICUs. This also reflects the approach taken by the Department of Health in its *Guidelines on admission to and discharge from intensive care and high-dependency units.*[15]

The critical care modernisation plan, announced in May 2000,[11] introduced the notion that adult acute care should be seen as a spectrum across four levels, much as paediatric care is organised. The four levels are:

- Level 0 – normal acute ward care
- Level 1 – acute ward care, with additional advice and support from the critical care team, e.g. patients who are at risk of deterioration, or who are recovering after requiring higher levels of care
- Level 2 – more detailed observation or intervention; e.g. patients with a single failing organ system, or post-operative patients, or patients stepping down from higher levels of care
- Level 3 – advanced respiratory support alone, or basic respiratory support together with support of at least two organ systems.

Paediatric units

Paediatric units are facilities designed, staffed and equipped for the management of critically ill children. Our focus will exclude intensive care and high-dependency services for children, although any consideration of adult intensive care services should take account of the fact that children are sometimes treated in adult general or specialised ICUs, often before transfer to a specialised paediatric ICU.

3 Sub-categories

In contrast to needs assessments for disease groups, where disease classification is central to the discussion and relatively straightforward, it is difficult in critical care practice to classify and group clinical data into defined categories or hierarchies. Healthcare Resource Groups (HRGs) or Diagnosis Related Groups (DRGs) are used to categorise patients on the basis of diagnosis, but this approach is not applicable in critical care, where there is wide heterogeneity within diagnostic groups.[18]

Patients can be categorised by severity of illness, as discussed earlier. Alternatively, categories can be based on demographic characteristics, on more precise measures of severity of illness or according to the organ systems needing monitoring or support. In this section a variety of approaches to sub-categorisation have been used, according to available datasets. Data are frequently broken down into surgical and non-surgical, often with further classification below this level such as emergency and elective. Other methods of sub-categorisation are based on clinical condition, but usually encompass only the most common conditions and are therefore not exhaustive.

4 Prevalence and incidence

This section is in two parts: the first focuses on the characteristics of patients admitted to critical care services, and the second discusses the demand for critical care. It has been split in this way because data on the need for critical care are not available. We can only report the types of cases and the numbers presenting.

Characteristics of patients admitted to critical care

Age and gender

Dragsted and Qvist[13] concluded that there is little systematic information about the characteristics of ICU patients; but the available data showed a consistent predominance of males and a high proportion of elderly patients.

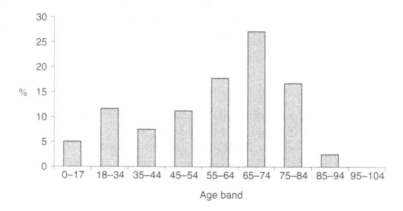

Source: ICNARC

Figure 2: Admissions to intensive care units by age, 12/95–4/98.

Figure 2 shows the age distribution across the Case Mix Programme Database (n=22 058) of the Intensive Care National Audit and Research Centre (ICNARC) for the period December 1995 to April 1998. The 62 units covered by the database are all adult units and have contributed data for varying periods.

These ICNARC data show that 4.8% of admissions were in the age range 0–17, and that 46.5% of admissions were of people aged 65 or over. The mean age of patients in this dataset is 57.3 years.

In comparison, the percentage of overall hospital admissions by age band over the period 1995 to 1998, as extracted from Hospital Episode Statistics (HES) datasets, is:

- under 18 years – 11.0%
- over 55 years – 43.2%
- over 65 years – 31.7%.

Elderly patients are likely to need more intensive care than their proportion in the hospital or general population indicates. Bull[19] suggested that the high proportion of patients aged 65 or over reflects a substantial change in clinical policy towards actively treating and resuscitating critically ill patients irrespective of age. It may also reflect more aggressive policies of medical and surgical treatment in the elderly.

Data from individual ICUs in the UK indicate that at least 50% of patients admitted in the early 1990s were aged 55 years or over.[20,21,22] The ICNARC data reflected in Figure 2 show that over 64% of admissions are now of people aged 55 or over. This may indicate that greater numbers of elderly people are being admitted to intensive care.

These data indicate a mean age of 57.3 years. As this dataset and that used by Rowan[23] included large samples, it appears that critical care patients are getting increasingly elderly. However, changes in paediatric intensive care policy following the report of the National Co-ordinating Group in 1997[24] may have resulted in fewer children being admitted to adult units, thereby causing an increase in mean age.

Data from a survey by a working party of the British Paediatric Association (BPA) indicated that in 1991 at least 20% of children receiving intensive care were admitted to adult ICUs.[25] Even very young children were being cared for in adult units: about 23% of children admitted to adult ICUs were aged under 1 year, and almost 5% were under 1 month old.[26] In the Study of Intensive Care in England[12] it was reported that 79% of general adult ICUs treated at least one child during 1992. Paediatric intensive care services have since been reorganised, but data from the Audit Commission indicate that small numbers of children are still being treated in adult units.

Our analysis of Audit Commission data[17] indicates that adult units continue to treat small numbers of children even though there has been rationalisation and improvement of paediatric critical care services.[23] Data from the Audit Commission give the median percentage of admissions under 16 years old to adult units as 1.22 for all units, 1.97 for ICUs, 1.18 for combined units and none for HDUs. It is likely that these admissions are for short periods pending transfer; however, information on length of stay is not available.

In the ICS study,[27] 60% of the patients were male, a proportion similar to that on the intensive care census day in England in 1992 (58%).[12]

Types of admission

Intensive care

Metcalfe and McPherson[12] looked at the proportions of types of admission to general ICUs in England in 1992. These are shown in Table 2. Overall, the greatest proportion of admissions were for medical emergencies (41%), followed by planned admissions from elective surgery (25%), and emergency surgical admissions (18%). However, in each category there were wide ranges in the numbers of admissions per ICU.

Table 2: Types of admission to general ICUs in England in 1992.

Type of admission	No. of ICUs	Range	Admissions	%
Elective, after elective surgery	117	1–998	11,128	25
Unplanned, after elective surgery	102	0–120	2,906	7
Emergency surgical	114	2–224	8,123	18
Emergency medical	129	0–937	18,102	41
Other	123	0–443	4,086	9
Total			44,345	100

Proportions are approximate (incomplete because the breakdowns are from different numbers of hospitals; data cover 73% of all 60,761 admissions recorded for 1992). Data from Metcalfe and McPherson.[12]

Table 3 shows types of admission reported to ICNARC's Case Mix Programme Database (n=22 058) for the period December 1995 to April 1998 compared with data from the Intensive Care Society's APACHE II study in Britain and Ireland.[27] The 62 units covered by the ICNARC's Case Mix Programme Database are all adult units and have contributed data for varying periods. Patients under 16 years old have been excluded.

Table 3 shows a marked increase in non-surgical admissions to intensive care units. Although this may reflect a true change in case-mix, several factors complicate the comparison. For example, the earlier dataset was from fewer hospitals, of which a far higher proportion were university hospitals (62% compared to 31%).

Table 3: Types of admission reported via APACHE II and ICNARC, 12/95–4/98.

APACHE II Study (1993)		ICNARC (1995–98)	
Type	*%*	*Type*	*%*
Surgical	52.3	Surgical	44.5
Emergency & Urgent	23.9	Emergency*	9.9
		Urgent**	9.0
Elective & Scheduled	28.3	Scheduled	10.0
		Elective	15.3
Non-surgical	47.7	Non-surgical	55.4
Total	100.0	Total	100.0

*Refers to immediate surgery where resuscitation is simultaneous with surgical treatment.
**Refers to surgery as soon as possible after resuscitation.

The Audit Commission[14] has calculated that surgical admissions to ICUs amount to 48%, while admissions to ICUs and HDUs overall amount to 47%, indicating a less pronounced decrease in surgical admissions than is shown in Table 3.

Figure 3 shows admissions to intensive care by source of admission. Data are taken from ICNARC's Case Mix Programme Database for the period December 1995 to April 1998 (n=22 058). The 62 units covered by the database have contributed data for varying periods.

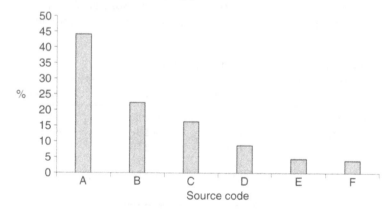

Source code	Source
A	Theatre/recovery, same hospital
B	Ward, same hospital
C	A&E, same hospital
D	Other hospital
E	Other sources
F	Other critical care units

Source: ICNARC

Figure 3: Admissions to intensive care by source, 12/95–4/98.

The most common source of admission is theatre or recovery in the same hospital (44.1%), followed by a ward in the same hospital (22.3%) and A&E in the same hospital (17.1%).

High-dependency care

Little information is available on the types of admission and diagnostic categories of patients in HDUs in the UK, but the Augmented Care Period (ACP) dataset, introduced in 1997, will go some way towards addressing this. In the survey by Thompson and Singer of 28 HDUs in 26 hospitals in the UK and Northern Ireland,[28] information on patient admissions was available for 22 of the units, as shown in Figure 4.

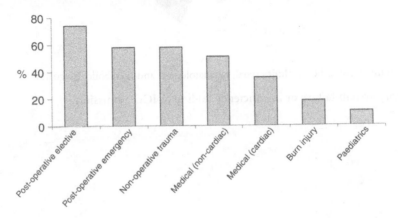

Figure 4: Patient admissions in 28 HDUs.

Unfortunately, data from the Audit Commission[14] do not describe case-mix or severity separately for high-dependency care. However, several studies[29,30,31,32,33,34] have examined the potential for HDU beds to alleviate some of the demand on ICU beds by differentiating between patients requiring high-dependency and patients requiring intensive care.

The reclassification of critical care into three levels, announced in the critical care modernisation plan in May 2000,[11] will result in a better reflection of severity within the activity data.

Indications for admission

In the three-month prospective audit of six general ICUs in the Study of Intensive Care in England,[12] seven diagnostic categories were used to indicate the primary system failure or insufficiency that made it necessary to admit the patient to the ICU. Over 70% of the 483 admissions were in the cardiovascular and respiratory categories (Figure 5).

The ICU is characterised by the presence of a wide variety of underlying diseases, and there is no generally accepted classification system that describes the clinical characteristics of ICU patients.[11]

ICNARC's Case Mix Programme Database provides data on the primary reason for admission. The ten most frequent conditions admitted to ICUs during the period December 1995 to April 1998 are shown in Figure 6. The 62 units covered by the database have contributed data for varying periods.

It can be seen that the most common condition admitted made up only 6.5% of admissions, and that the top ten conditions made up only 26.8% of admissions. This indicates the high variability of reasons for admission to intensive care units.

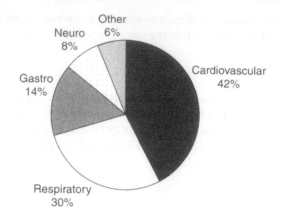

Data are for 483 admissions; 'other' includes renal, haematological and metabolic categories.

Figure 5: Primary system failure or insufficiency leading to ICU admission.

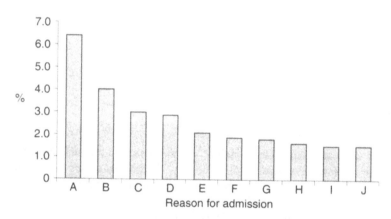

Reason code	Primary reason
A	Aortic or iliac dissection or aneurysm – surgical
B	Acute myocardial infarction – non-surgical
C	Pneumonia, no organism isolated – non-surgical
D	Bacterial pneumonia – non-surgical
E	Septic shock – non-surgical
F	Primary brain injury – non-surgical
G	Large bowel tumour – surgical
H	Left ventricular failure – non-surgical
I	Asthma attack in new or known asthmatic – non-surgical
J	Non-traumatic large bowel perforation or rupture – surgical

Source: ICNARC

Figure 6: Most frequent reasons for admission.

Figure 7 shows reason for admission (using the coding above) by average age of patient. Not surprisingly, primary brain injury and asthma are seen in a significantly younger population.

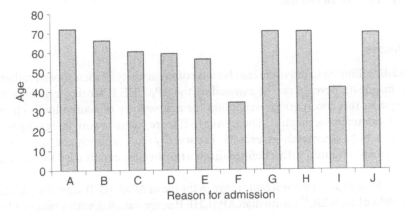

N.B. For codes giving the primary reason for admission, *see* Figure 6.

Figure 7: Reason for admission by average age.

The ten conditions that used the greatest number of bed-days for the period December 1995 to April 1998 are shown in Figure 8. These conditions made up 32.8% of bed-days. The 62 units covered by the database have contributed data for varying periods.

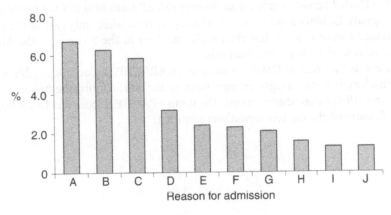

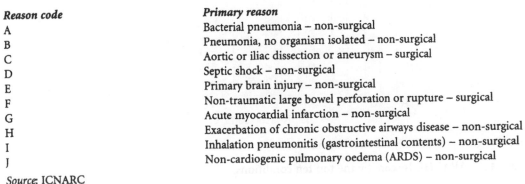

Reason code	Primary reason
A	Bacterial pneumonia – non-surgical
B	Pneumonia, no organism isolated – non-surgical
C	Aortic or iliac dissection or aneurysm – surgical
D	Septic shock – non-surgical
E	Primary brain injury – non-surgical
F	Non-traumatic large bowel perforation or rupture – surgical
G	Acute myocardial infarction – non-surgical
H	Exacerbation of chronic obstructive airways disease – non-surgical
I	Inhalation pneumonitis (gastrointestinal contents) – non-surgical
J	Non-cardiogenic pulmonary oedema (ARDS) – non-surgical

Source: ICNARC

Figure 8: The ten conditions using the greatest number of bed-days.

The primary reason for admission is very variable, with the greatest user of bed-days, bacterial pneumonia, making up only 6.7% of the total, and the ten conditions which consume the greatest number of bed-days making up only 32.8% of all bed-days.

Severity of illness

Patients are usually admitted to intensive care because of the severity of their illness, rather than solely on the underlying diagnosis. Severity can be assessed by the APACHE II scoring system, a physiologically-based scoring system that incorporates weightings for age, severity of acute illness, chronic illness and operative status (*see* later in the chapter). The APACHE II score increases with increasing severity of illness: the maximum is 71, but a score rarely exceeds 55. The severity score is closely correlated with risk of death in hospital, and, when combined with a defined diagnostic category, can be used to derive a probability of death in hospital.

Studies of ICUs have shown a considerable range in the mean APACHE II score for patients admitted. In a three-month audit of six ICUs,[12] the median APACHE II score was 19.0, with a range of 1.0–54.0 (a score of 20 indicates a severely ill patient). Rowan *et al.*[23] reported an overall mean APACHE II score of 17.9 for the 26 ICUs studied; the range of means was 14.8–22.6, but the highest and lowest scores over all units ranged between 0 and 51.

There is evidence that case-mix severity in this country may be higher than in the United States. One study[35] compiled the APACHE II risk-of-death score of a group of 12 762 admissions to 15 ICUs in the North Thames region between January 1992 and May 1996. The authors found an average risk of death of 0.286, which agrees approximately with the 0.272 found by Rowan *et al.*[36] in another British study in 1993. Research from the United States[37] reported an average risk of death of 0.188 for teaching and 0.151 for non-teaching hospitals. Goldhill and Summer[35] also report that, while only two of the 15 ICUs in their study had an average risk of death of less than 0.25, only four of the 37 units in the American study[37] reported an average risk of death greater than this.

ICNARC's Case Mix Programme Database includes an APACHE II score for eligible patients (aged 16 years or over with a length of stay of eight or more hours in the unit). During the period December 1995 to April 1998 there were 19 421 eligible admissions. The mean APACHE II score was 16.29. Figure 9 shows the mean APACHE II score by the top ten conditions admitted.

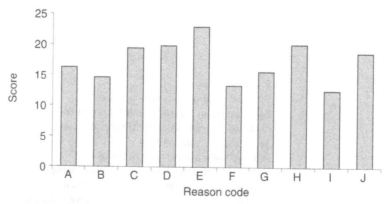

N.B. For codes giving the primary reason for admission, *see* Figure 6.

Figure 9: Mean APACHE II score by the top ten conditions.

The critical care modernisation plan[11] introduced an approach to the classification of critical care that reflects variable severity of illness.

Length of stay

In the three-month audit,[12] the median length of stay over the six ICUs was 1.6 days. However, the range was very large, from less than one hour to 64.3 days.

It is essential that the length of stay in critical care be defined in terms of fractions of days rather than whole days, because many patients are admitted for periods of only a few hours. A system whose minimum unit is 1 day will fail to consider a significant proportion of patients. The use of whole days also makes occupancy figures difficult to interpret. Ridley and Rowan[38] advocate measuring length of stay in hourly units, because the duration of admission to intensive care is generally short but highly variable, and throughput is high.

ICNARC's Case Mix Programme Database provides length-of-stay data by primary reason for admission. Figure 10 shows the median and mean length of stay for the ten most frequent conditions admitted to intensive care units during the period December 1995 to April 1998.

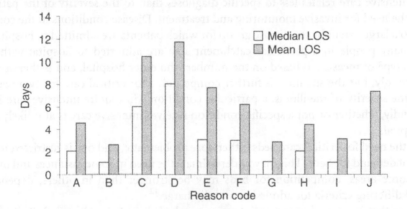

N.B. For codes giving the primary reason for admission, *see* Figure 6.

Figure 10: Length of stay (LOS) for the top ten conditions.

ICNARC's dataset provides an overall median length of stay of 2 days, and an average of 5.02. Figure 10 also shows that the mean length of stay is consistently higher than the median length of stay, indicating that outlying lengthy periods have skewed the average.

Data for 148 non-specialist ICUs from the Royal College of Anaesthetists' national audit of intensive care in 1992/93[39] are shown in Table 4 and clearly illustrate the skewed pattern for length of stay.

Table 4: Statistics on length of stay in 148 non-specialist ICUs.

Time in ICU	Percentage of patients*	
	Mean ± SD	Range
< 24 hrs	29.93 ± 15.87	3–73
24–48 hrs	26.77 ± 11.41	10–72
2–7 days	29.77 ± 14.09	5–80
> 7 days	13.13 ± 7.40	2–55

*Proportions of all patients in all 148 ICUs, and ranges of means of patients per ICU over 148 ICUs.

Needs assessment for critical care

Population demand for critical care

The need for intensive care relates less to specific diagnoses than to the severity of the patient's clinical condition and the need for invasive monitoring and treatment. Disease conditions in the community can be monitored to a large extent by the disease group for which patients are admitted to hospital. HRGs can indicate how many people in a particular catchment area are admitted to hospital with a particular condition. This type of measure is based on the number who enter hospital, and is therefore dependent somewhat on supply; but the situation is further compounded for critical care for two reasons. Firstly, depending on the severity of the illness, a particular condition will require intensive care in only some instances. Secondly, whether or not a specific condition receives intensive care is also likely to vary from hospital to hospital.

Establishing the need for critical care beds is therefore problematic, and one is restricted to establishing some measure of demand for beds. This may underestimate the need in some instances and overestimate it in others. In some areas, competition for beds may be stronger than in others, depending on bed availability and differing criteria for admission and discharge.[12]

Various factors that increase demand on intensive care beds have been identified. Ridley[40] perceives a mismatch between the continuum of health needs and the management of illness in hospitals – the latter traditionally has been divided into specialist areas. In many hospitals, a gulf between care available in ICUs and that available in general wards has developed, and may have contributed to problems with ICU bed availability. There may be a reluctance to return to general wards those patients who, while no longer needing intensive care, might not receive there the level of care they do require. This perceived gulf supports the notion of graduated care.[41]

General advances in medicine and surgery, such as improvements in outcome following perioperative intensive care of high-risk surgical patients[42,43,44] and changes in surgical practice, may also increase the demand on intensive care facilities. There may further be a growing tendency, following the implementation of the internal market, for NHS trusts to introduce additional major surgery without investing concurrently in ICU, HDU and anaesthetic services to support such activity.[45]

In the past, any spare capacity in an ICU has been used for patients who may have been considered 'borderline'. This 'open door' policy[39] may establish a pattern whereby, in time, all such cases are admitted even though their severity of illness might not strictly justify it. Any lack of high-dependency facilities reinforces this pattern.

Numbers of admissions to ICUs and HDUs

The Audit Commission's 1998 study[14] received data on admissions from 113 of 128 ICUs in England and Wales. The total number of admissions for 1997/98 was 42 640. If this figure is extrapolated to estimate the number of admissions for all 128 units, assuming that missing data follow a similar pattern, the total number of admissions was 48 300. This gives a rate of admission to an ICU per 100 000 population (based on mid-1996 population data) of 92.8.

A separate exercise to identify the demand for intensive care beds has also been attempted, using the North West NHS region to illustrate a population rate. Table 5 shows the rate of admission to intensive care per 100 000 admissions to hospital. Hospital Episodes Statistics (HES) for 1996/97 have been used to establish general rates of hospital admission, and ICNARC data for the North West, to establish rates of intensive care use. ICBIS (the Intensive Care Bed Information Service) for the North West provided data for 1996/97 relating to transfers out of the North West.

The advantages of using the North West region were that all units there are registered with ICNARC and that it has a comprehensive intensive care bed register allowing identification of transfers out of the system.

Unfortunately ICNARC does not collect data on HDUs, so population rates of demand for high-dependency beds were not available.

Data were available from 33 intensive care units in the North West. Data covered different periods of time and were therefore scaled up to a standard period (three years). Data relating to patients under 15 years of age were removed. There were only 28 transfers out of the North West during the period.

Table 5: Rate of admission to intensive care per 100,000 admissions to hospital.

Health authority	ICU patients per 100,000 admissions: 15 years and over	Hospitalisation rate per 100,000 population per year: 15 years and over	ICU admits – age standardised rate per 100,000 pop. per year: 15 years and over	Conversion rate: hospitalisations to ICU admissions
Morecambe Bay	940	25,326	242	1.0%
South Lancashire	550	28,618	161	0.6%
St Helen & Knowsley	570	29,296	173	0.6%
NW Lancashire	810	24,014	188	0.8%
West Pennine	560	26,842	148	0.6%
Manchester	510	26,972	139	0.5%
East Lancashire	640	24,400	151	0.6%
Wirral	500	26,997	135	0.5%
Salford & Trafford	590	27,978	167	0.6%
Liverpool	460	27,975	129	0.5%
Stockport	680	26,603	180	0.7%
Sefton	570	21,979	124	0.6%
South Cheshire	630	28,092	176	0.6%
North Cheshire	630	26,431	163	0.6%
Bury & Rochdale	440	26,449	118	0.4%
Wigan & Bolton	510	25,890	130	0.5%
Average	**590**	**26,373**	**154**	**0.6%**

The hospitalisation rate given in Table 5 may appear high. This is because a large segment of the population with a proportionally lower number of episodes (i.e. those under 15 years of age) has been removed.

Two main assumptions have been made in this analysis. The first concerns missing postcode information from the ICNARC data: the pattern of postcode distribution in the data was used, assuming that there was no systematic reason for the data to be missing. Secondly, one unit gave no information on length of stay, so the overall rate was used.

The overall North West ICU admission rate is higher than that calculated from the Audit Commission data: 154 admissions per 100 000, compared with 92.8. There are several possible sources of bias: (a) Audit Commission data have been extrapolated because only 88% of units responded to this question; (b) scaling up the ICNARC data may have overestimated admissions if, for instance, there had been bed-closures during the three-year period. More information is needed from other parts of the country, and overall, about population rates of admission to intensive care.

Although information is available regarding demand for critical care, until recently there was none relating to population need. Lyons et al.[46] have recently published the results of a prospective assessment of need for both intensive care and high-dependency beds for a population of 500 000. They concluded that to meet the need on 95% of occasions would require 30 intensive care beds and 55 high-dependency beds if these were provided in a single unit. They suggested that if there were three separate units for the same population with equal demand, the total number of beds required to meet the need on 95% of occasions would increase by 10%.

Occupancy levels

Occupancy is often used as a measure of health service activity, indicating the activity of an inpatient unit in terms of its maximum capacity. There are several different methods of calculating bed occupancy, and the choice of method can have a significant impact. Ridley and Rowan[38] report that the impact of methodological differences in calculating the occupancy will tend to be greatest in specialised areas such as critical care, where the duration of admission is generally short but highly variable, and throughput is high.

An interpretation of occupancy calculations rests fundamentally on how accurately the length of stay is measured. If it is measured in whole numbers of days, critical care units can show an occupancy of greater than 100%, as more than one patient may use a particular bed on a given day.

The Audit Commission[15] in its 1998 survey reported the median average occupancy to be 83% in ICUs, 81% in combined ICU/HDUs and 74% in HDUs. However, occupancy was not defined in the survey.

St George's Hospital in South London conducted two one-day telephone surveys of 34 London-area intensive care units and 56 from a nationwide sample during January 1995.[29] The researchers concluded that most ICUs were running at about 86% occupancy, with some as high as 95%. The first survey, of 34 ICUs within the London M25 area, suggested that only eight intensive care beds were available in London on the day of the survey.

These levels of occupancy are high for a service expected to respond to unpredictable emergencies.

The Audit Commission[15] in its 1998 survey asked units to report on how many days there had been no spare bed with available staffing; how many patients had been refused admission because the unit was full; and how many cancelled operations there had been. These data were analysed to provide both the proportion of the year when the unit has a spare bed, and a 'refused-access rate' – the proportion of admissions refused and operations cancelled. The results are shown in Table 6.

One conclusion drawn from the telephone surveys undertaken by St George's Hospital in 1995[29] was that the number of patients in London requiring intensive care was greater than the number of beds available, with occupancy levels in ICUs ranging from 86% to 95%.

Table 6: How often an ICU has a spare bed, and the refused-access rate.

		Proportion of year with a spare bed	Refused-access rate
ICUs	– median	0.63	0.13
	– average	0.60	0.14
Combined ICU/HDUs	– median	0.67	0.10
	– average	0.59	0.12
HDUs	– median	0.43	0.07
	– average	0.44	0.25

Unmet demand

Evidence of shortfall: refusals

One of the aims of the study of the provision of intensive care in England[12] was to assess demand relative to supply by examining requests for admission, particularly those that had to be refused. It emerged that the provision of intensive care, based on the number of staffed beds, was unequal between regional health authorities, and that reported refusal rates also varied.

Part of the study prospectively examined a three-month period in six ICUs, chosen to provide a span of high, average and low bed-provision in relation to population; the overall mean refusal rate for appropriately referred patients was 18%. Although the most powerful determinant of the refusal rate was the provision of staffed beds per 100 000 population, the refusal rate was also determined by a number of other factors.

The results of multiple regression analysis demonstrated that the following factors influenced refusal rates:

- type of unit – 'unmixed' ICUs (i.e. those without high-dependency or coronary care beds) were associated with high refusal rates
- type of hospital – high refusal rates were associated with referral centres, hospitals with large numbers of other critical care beds, and district general hospitals with undergraduate teaching responsibilities
- staffing – ICUs with an exclusive director and those with high nurse staffing levels were associated with high refusal rates, and so were units in which ICU-allocated consultant sessions were shared with other duties (e.g. anaesthetics).

Metcalfe et al.[47] note that the number of refusals they found in their study is probably an underestimate, as some patients, not referred because hospital or ambulance staff knew that a unit was already full, may have been omitted from data collection.

In its 1998 survey, the Audit Commission[2] found a wide variation in the proportion of patients who were refused admission to intensive care because there was no bed. It ranged from none to almost 50% of requests, with a median value of 8%. Some of these patients will have been transferred to units with spare capacity.

Evidence of shortfall: transfers

Substantial numbers of transfers occur because of bed shortages. Such transfers indicate a bed shortage in the originating unit and may not reflect shortages across an entire system. Nevertheless, such transfers suggest at least deficiencies in the distribution of beds or units.

When no bed is available and none can be created, there are significant implications for the patient and relatives. One option is to transfer the patient to an alternative ICU where there is a vacant bed. This may be many miles away and entails moving a critically ill patient, with the associated risks. It also means transferring care for the patient, who may often have many and complex problems, to a team previously unfamiliar with the case. Such transfers also involve significant upheaval for the relatives, who thereafter may have to travel long distances in order to visit the patient. In some instances a bed may not be available anywhere, and it is likely that deaths have occurred in such situations.

The Emergency Bed Service (EBS), which covers London, Anglia and Oxford, South and West, South East, West Midlands and Trent Regions, records transfers and transfer enquiries. It should be noted that some transfers result from independent negotiation between consultants, and these may be missed by EBS. Therefore the data presented in Figure 11 may underestimate activity; however, the markedly increased demand during winter is clear.

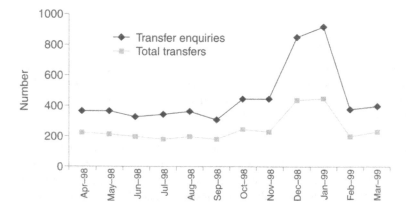

Figure 11: Emergency Bed Service – transfers and enquiries.

ICBIS monitors bed availability by telephoning each unit in the region four times a day. Figure 12 provides information on bed availability and number of transfers. The bed availability figure is an average of the four daily figures, averaged over the month. It should be noted that bed availability information reflects only the ability and willingness of units to accept patients from other hospitals, but nonetheless it represents availability from an operational perspective.

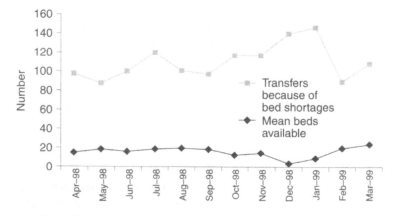

Figure 12: Beds available and transfers in the North West Region, 1998/99.

The shortage of beds experienced in December and the simultaneous increase in transfers are clear from the diagram.

Data from 198 general and mixed intensive care units in the UK, collected in 1994,[48] provided a mean annual number of admissions of 353 (range 40–1540) and a mean of 19 patients transported from each unit per year. The most common indications for these transfers were referrals for neurosurgical care (109; 55%), lack of beds in ICU (87; 44%) and lack of renal support services (54; 27%). These indications were not mutually exclusive. Only 12 ICUs transferred more than 40 patients a year to another hospital.

The authors estimate that the number of critically ill patients requiring secondary transport to adult intensive care units in Britain that year exceeded 11 000. In a large proportion of these patients, transfer was necessary for non-clinical reasons, primarily relating to a lack of intensive care beds in the originating hospital.

A national postal survey conducted by the Royal College of Anaesthetists in 1992/93[39] asked about patient transfers in the eight weeks preceding the questionnaire. Figure 13 provides information on units and numbers of patients transferred. Figure 14 shows the principal reasons for transfer.

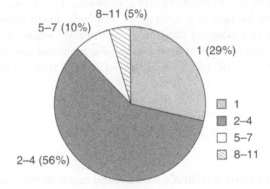

Figure 13: Transfers out in the preceding 8 weeks.

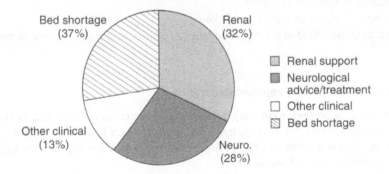

Figure 14: Reasons for transfer.

Evidence of shortfall: cancelled operations

For a patient needing intensive care following major elective surgery, the lack of a bed will entail cancellation of the operation – often at the last minute, since only then will the bed situation be known with certainty. Apart from the distress for the patient, such episodes waste the theatre resources allocated to the case.

The national postal survey conducted by the Royal College of Anaesthetists in 1992/93[39] revealed that lack of intensive care beds had caused 124 out of 256 units (48%) to cancel operations in the eight weeks preceding the questionnaire.

Evidence of shortfall: early discharge

In some instances, a bed may be created by prematurely discharging a patient not previously deemed ready to leave the ICU. In the absence of a designated HDU, such patients are likely to be returned to a general ward where, inevitably, they receive a lower level of observation and care. Data from ICNARC's Case Mix Programme, covering a total of 22 059 intensive care admissions, suggest that over 7% of intensive care survivors are discharged early because of a shortage of unit beds. Furthermore, recent data also from ICNARC[49] suggest that case-mix-adjusted outcome is significantly worse in patients discharged from ICUs at night, most often because of a lack of beds. Discharge at night was associated with a 33% increased risk of ultimate hospital mortality (OR: 1.33; 95% CL: 1.06–1.65) and seems to be increasing, from 2.7% in 1988–90 to 6% in 1995–98.

Limitations of the data

Unidentified demand

It should be noted that, although data on refusals, transfers and cancelled operations provide an indication of unmet demand, they probably underestimate it, because:

- referrals stop when units are full
- refusal information is difficult to collect
- units may not be told about cancelled operations
- intensive care may be provided in places outside the unit: for example, in recovery, in resuscitation and on the ward.[30,50]

Evidence of patients managed in inappropriate areas

Estimating need from data on bed occupancy, refusals and transfers is complicated by the variations in admission and discharge criteria. There is evidence that intensive care beds are sometimes used for high-dependency cases and vice versa, but also that patients meriting both high-dependency and intensive care are sometimes managed on general wards.

The Augmented Care Period (ACP) dataset[51] was introduced in 1997. Data on intensive and high-dependency care activity for patients other than neonates are collected in the form of an ACP dataset. These periods should be recorded wherever they occur, with the exception of general wards, A&E, radiology departments, labour wards and special care baby units. The dataset will enable the level of care that patients receive to be identified in the areas covered.

A very preliminary analysis has been performed on the first six months' data from the national ACP dataset (October 1997–March 1998).[51] This included information from an estimated 102 acute trusts, which, when cleaned to remove obviously illogical or incomplete data, left details relating to a total of

75 trusts and 22 140 patients. Analysis was performed at the level of individual ACPs, and ratios were averaged. The data suggest that approximately 25% of bed-days on general ICUs are accounted for by patients requiring only high-dependency care. Similarly, it appears that around 11% of bed-days on general HDUs are taken up by patients actually needing intensive care. These figures should be interpreted with caution, given that they represent the first six months of input to a new dataset.

An audit[30] conducted over seven months at the Royal Cornwall Hospital applied ACP definitions to patients in all hospital inpatient areas, including general wards. The ACP dataset identifies successive periods of augmented care (intensive or high-dependency care), should a patient require more than one within a single hospital episode. Tables 7a, 7b and 7c summarise the findings for patients receiving up to three ACPs.

Table 7a: Data relating to first ACPs.

Location	ICU days	HDU days	Total ACP days
General ICU/HDU	1,035	366	1,401
CCU	165	120	285
Recovery	13	4	17
General wards	74	100	174

Table 7b: Data relating to second ACPs.

Location	ICU days	HDU days	Total ACP days
General ICU/HDU	57	36	93
CCU	3	1	4
General wards	6	17	23

Table 7c: Data relating to third ACPs.

Location	ICU days	HDU days	Total ACP days
General ICU/HDU	44	0	44

It is evident from the data that a significant number of days of intensive or high-dependency care were provided in inappropriate locations – most notably, for patients receiving a first ACP, 74 days and 100 days respectively on general wards.

Another study[31] used three different methods to identify potential HDU admissions: an APACHE III score of 10 or less; low risk monitor rating in the Wagner risk stratification method; or not requiring advanced respiratory support. The study found that between 20.8% and 51.2% of ICU patients might be more appropriately managed in an HDU. The authors suggest that the perceived national shortage in intensive care beds might be improved by the development of more HDUs.

In a survey of ICUs in six hospitals, Crosby and Rees[32] reported that more than 50% of patients who required high-dependency care were placed in ICUs.

The study by Metcalfe et al.[47] examining data from six intensive care units over a three-month period suggested that 65% of patients admitted inappropriately could have been treated in HDUs, and 13% could have been treated in coronary care units.

Ryan et al.[33] examined admissions to Freeman Hospital's ICU over a two-month period, classifying each admission through criteria for either intensive or high-dependency care. They found that 23% of bed-days were occupied by patients thus classified as high-dependency, and that 12% of discharges were delayed because of the absence of a high-dependency unit. The authors estimated that, over the study period, 22 additional patients could have been cared for if a high-dependency unit had existed.

A similar study was conducted in Leicester,[34] using the more recent 1996 guidelines for admission to intensive care and high-dependency units[15] to classify patients being admitted to an ICU over a two-month period. High-dependency patients accounted for 1914 bed hours (21.6%) out of the potential available 8880 hours.

However, in a survey[52] of admissions to intensive care in three acute hospitals where high-dependency care was provided, only 2.4% of patients were found to have been placed inappropriately, as assessed by clinical guidelines drawn up by an multidisciplinary group.

Crosby and Rees carried out a 'snapshot' two-day survey to assess the clinical dependency of patients on acute surgical wards in eight hospitals in England and Wales.[32] Using slightly different criteria, they found an average requirement for high-dependency care of 6.8% in terms of bed-days for patients on these wards. (High-dependency care was defined as continuous monitoring with appropriately trained nurses constantly present, and a nurse-to-patient ratio of about 1:2.5.)

The Audit Commission's 1998 survey examined admissions receiving high-dependency care, and reported[14] the median number of admissions receiving high-dependency care as a percentage of admissions to various units, as shown in Table 8.

Table 8: Median percentage of admissions receiving high-dependency care, of total admissions to unit.

ICUs	Combined ICU/HDU units	HDUs
26%	47%	84%

The Commission also looked at the use made of available beds across ICUs, combined units and HDUs, reporting the results shown in Table 9.

Table 9: Use made of available beds.

The percentage of available beds used for:	ICUs	Combined ICU/HDU units	HDUs
Only intensive care patients	54%	19%	6%
Either intensive or high-dependency care patients	46%	61%	23%
Only high-dependency care patients	0%	20%	71%

International comparisons

There is some evidence that the smaller bed numbers in the United Kingdom mean that only the most severely ill patients are admitted. Comparisons between the UK[35] and US[37] have already been reported. The EURICUS[53] study found severity of illness (measured by the Simplified Acute Physiology Score II) to be higher in the UK than in any of the other 11 countries or areas. The overall score for the UK was 38.5, while other scores ranged from 28.5 in Germany to 37.5 in Portugal.

Table 10: Numbers of critical care beds in European countries.

Country	Critical care beds per 100,000 population
England and Wales (1)	4.8
Finland (2)	6.0
Denmark (3)	6.5
Italy (4)	9.0
Belgium (5)	21.3
Luxembourg (6)	21.8

1 *Source:*[14] Based on available beds, and mid-1996 population census information. Bed numbers include specialist critical care beds but exclude coronary care.

2 *Source:*[54]

3 *Source:*[55]

4 *Source:*[56]

5 *Source:*[57]

6 *Source:*[58] Author states these beds are available.

These comparisons should be treated with some caution. In the case of Italy, Denmark, Finland, Luxembourg and Belgium, it is not clear whether high-dependency, coronary care or specialist units have been included (though it is unlikely). Neither is it clear for any of these countries except Luxembourg whether bed numbers refer to beds that are actually available, or to those that would be, given staff and/or equipment. The figure for England and Wales, which is relatively low, does include high-dependency beds and specialist beds. This suggests that the number of beds per 100 000 population in England and Wales is actually significantly lower than that of the comparison group.

There is little information available on admission rates to ICUs as a proportion of the hospital or general population. In the USA, up to about 20% of patients receive care in an ICU or CCU at some time during their stay in hospital, but the use of intensive care is much less common in Europe.[13] In a Danish university hospital, 1.6% of patients were admitted to the ICU, while a Norwegian study reported that 1.7% of a hospital's patients were admitted to an ICU;[13] but another European author cites 5% as the percentage of hospital patients requiring intensive care.[59]

A comparison of ICUs in 13 hospitals in the USA and two hospitals in New Zealand revealed that the US hospitals designated 5.6% (range: 2.6%–10.3%) of their total beds as adult intensive care, compared with 1.7% (0.8%–2.6%) in the two New Zealand hospitals.[60]

However, without case-mix data it is questionable whether such international comparisons are helpful.

Future demand

The NHS reforms in 1990 led to greater emphasis on assessing the benefit of costly technological advances and to more focus on effective clinical practice.[61]

Even in this changing climate, indications are that demand for critical care in the future will increase.

Two recent studies on optimising treatment for high-risk surgical patients[42,43] illustrate a trend towards greater critical care intervention preoperatively. They showed improved outcomes for high-risk patients and may herald further demand on intensive care facilities.

5 Services available and their costs

Service provision in England and Wales

Introduction

The haphazard development of critical care has resulted in markedly variable provision of these services across the country. Until the announcement of the critical care modernisation programme in May 2000[11] there had been no national or even regional strategy for critical care. As a consequence, the number of intensive care beds and spending on intensive care, in relation to population figures, has varied considerably.[62]

There is currently substantial debate about the configuration of intensive care services, fuelled by a perception that there are not enough beds in some parts of the country and that existing beds may not be in the right places. Ryan, basing his findings on eight units, argued that there is an uneven distribution of ICU beds in the UK, and placed provision at a level between 1.8 and 3 beds per 100 000 population.[63] Our analysis of more recent Audit Commission data, however, suggests that this figure is at the lower end of the range, with 1.8 adult ICU beds per 100 000 and 3.6 beds if combined ICU/HDU units are included. If beds in HDUs are included, however, the data indicate 4.8 beds per 100 000. These figures are still significantly lower than those for other European countries, but do not include coronary care beds.

A survey conducted for the Department of Health in 1993[12] showed similar variations in intensive care bed provision. The numbers across the then 14 regional health authorities varied between 1.8 and 3.0 intensive care beds per 100 000 population (mean value 2.2), with evidence of clustering around London.

Critical care differs from other acute services in that it crosses speciality boundaries and therefore spans all hospital services. This has implications for contracting and budgeting, as resources for critical care are usually top-sliced, reducing direct accountability and control in the funding.

A fundamental challenge for critical care is that episodes of care have not until recently been easily identifiable from centrally held datasets such as HES. This has resulted in little routine statistical information being available for critical care. The recently introduced mandatory ACP dataset should go some way to meeting this need, and additional information is available through the Audit Commission and through initiatives such as ICNARC.

The critical care modernisation plan[11] calls for a data-collecting culture that promotes an evidence base, and requires NHS trusts to comply with the ACP dataset.

Critical care units

The Audit Commission undertook a study of critical care services across England and Wales during 1998, basing it on two questionnaires.[14] One covered the number of critical care units and beds for all specialities in a trust; the other asked more detailed questions about general adult critical care units. Every acute trust gave information about the critical care facilities in their hospital(s). Detailed information on general adult ICUs and HDUs was provided for 94% of units.

As Table 11 shows, there were 521 critical care units in operation in England and Wales. 32% were described as ICUs, 39% as HDUs and 28% as combined ICU/HDUs.

Table 11: Critical care facilities in England and Wales.

	Number of Trusts reporting presence of unit:			
	ICU	Combined ICU/HDU	HDU	Total (% of all units)
General or mixed speciality	128	83	25	236 (45%)
Surgical	2	3	26	31 (6%)
Medical	0	1	8	9 (2%)
Cardiac or coronary care	16	16	101	133 (26%)
Cardiothoracic	9	14	8	31 (6%)
Combined general and coronary care	8	10	1	19 (4%)
Neurological/surgical	5	8	11	24 (5%)
Short-term critical care	0	2	3	5 (1%)
Burns	1	4	6	11 (2%)
Trauma	0	1	1	2 (0%)
Liver	0	3	1	4 (1%)
Renal	0	1	10	11 (2%)
Spinal	0	1	4	5 (1%)
Total units	**169 (32%)**	**147 (28%)**	**205 (39%)**	**521**

A survey of HDUs in UK hospitals published in 1995[28] found that most (80%) of the units were geographically separate from the ICU within the hospital; about 40% were part of an acute ward. Some hospitals provide high-dependency and intensive care beds in the same unit,[12,28] an arrangement that may be more flexible and have advantages for staff deployment and morale. However, the HDU is sometimes adjacent to the ICU, and nurse staffing may be common to both units.[12] Formal rotations for staff in a separate HDU can avoid problems of staff isolation, and maintain expertise.[15]

Thompson and Singer[28] found that 71% of the HDUs acted as a 'step-down' facility for patients discharged from an ICU and 75% used the HDU as a 'step-up' for patients from general ward areas.

In some hospitals, ICUs and/or HDUs may specialise in the care of certain groups of patients – for example, post-operative thoracic or neurosurgical patients.[52]

The Audit Commission[17] data were also examined to identify the configuration of critical care services at the individual hospital level. Adult general/mixed speciality units and combined general/coronary care were included. There was great variability in configuration, and many combinations of generalist and specialist ICUs, HDUs and combined ICU/HDUs. The most prevalent configurations are shown in Table 12. The large number of trusts with 'some other combination' in each of the categories reflects the high variability between units, which makes summary difficult.

Table 12: Critical care configurations in NHS trusts.

Trusts with:	Critical care configuration
1 hospital (135 trusts)	26 (19%) had a combined ICU/HDU only 22 (16%) had an ICU only 33 (24%) had an ICU and an HDU 2 (2%) had a combined ICU/HDU that admitted coronary care patients 52 (39%) had some other combination
2 hospitals (44 trusts)	5 had a combined ICU/HDU only 2 had an ICU only 10 had an ICU and an HDU on the same site 27 had some other combination
3 hospitals (28 trusts)	5 had a combined ICU/HDU only 5 had an ICU and an HDU 18 had some other combination
4 hospitals (10 trusts)	4 had a combined ICU/HDU 5 had an ICU only 1 had some other combination
5 hospitals (5 trusts)	3 had an ICU only 2 had some other configuration

Total trusts: 222 (*excludes those that did not provide acute care for adults*)

Critical care beds

Data on bed numbers across England and Wales in Table 13 have been taken from the Audit Commission's survey,[17] which used the following definitions[2] for bed status:

- *equipped*: the beds exist now and have the necessary equipment to allow them to be used;
- *funded*: the budget exists for the nursing and other staff to allow the bed to be used;
- *available*: the staff are in post and the bed is generally available to admit patients into.

The Audit Commission[17] also reported data on bed numbers in individual units. Table 14 shows the median number of available beds by type of unit.

Numbers of beds were also reported on a trust basis. The median numbers of available critical beds per 500 acute beds are shown in Table 15.

Variability in units

As already noted, there is marked variability in the organisation and operation of critical care units in the UK. Ridley *et al.*[64] reviewed activity and organisation of eight intensive care units in the former Anglia NHS region and found considerable heterogeneity. Table 16 provides some comparisons on staffing and activity indicators for 1994. Some of these variations may be explained by hospital size and type, but the authors did not provide this information.

Significant variations between units were also noted for the mean age of patients (range approximately 55–60), APACHE scores (range approximately 11–16), length of stay (range approximately 1–1.7)

Table 13: Numbers of critical care beds across England and Wales.

Critical care beds	Equipped	Funded	Available
General or mixed speciality	1,564	1,412	1,421
Surgical	137	127	136
Medical	39	34	35
Cardiac or coronary care	799	795	817
Cardiothoracic	289	245	241
Combined general & coronary care	153	142	147
Neurological/surgical	154	142	130
Short-term critical care	33	23	22
Burns/plastics	54	52	51
Trauma	4	4	4
Liver	25	25	12
Renal	103	103	106
Spinal injury	26	26	25
Other types – not specified	172	140	135
Total	**3,552**	**3,270**	**3,311**

Table 14: Median number of available beds by type of unit.

	ICUs	Combined ICU/HDUs	HDUs
Median number of available beds	5.3	6.0	4.0

Table 15: Median number of available beds per trust.

Size of trust	Median number of critical care beds per 500 acute beds
Small trusts (less than 500 beds)	12.4
Medium trusts (between 500 and 750 beds)	7.9
Large trusts (over 750 beds)	9.8

Table 16: Staffing and activity indicators (1994).

ICU	Total consultant sessions	Nursing WTEs	Staffed beds (WTE/bed)	Number of admissions (1994)	Admits per bed	Refused admits
Cambridge	10	52.8	8 (6.6)	483	60.4	no record
Ipswich	9	32	6 (5.3)	393	65.5	no record
King's Lynn	9	24	4 (6.0)	261	65.3	22
Norwich	10	43	6 (7.1)	675	112.5	61
Peterborough	10	31	5 (6.2)	339	67.8	34
Bury St Edmunds	5.5	25	4.25 (5.9)	266	62.6	14
Yarmouth	10	27	4 (6.75)	274	68.5	no record
Hinchinbrooke	10	25	3 (8.3)	295	98.3	no record

and occupancy (range 56%–76%). Occupancy was calculated by summing all lengths of stay and dividing by the maximum number of available bed days.

Pattern of care provided in critical care

ICNARC's Case Mix Programme Database provides information on whether patients in intensive care units were mechanically ventilated or not. Of 17 712 admissions during the period December 1995 to April 1998, 54% were mechanically ventilated and 42.3% were not. Data regarding mechanical ventilation were missing for the remainder.

Audit Commission figures[17] indicate that the average percentage of admissions receiving ventilation is 57.8%. This agrees with the Study of Intensive Care Provision in England,[12] which reported that mechanical ventilation was required in 57% of patients admitted on the day of a census. The initial support required at admission on the census day is shown in Figure 15.

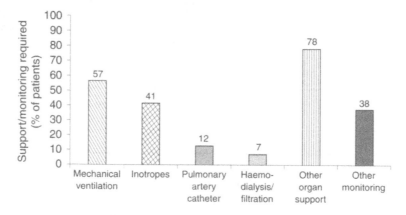

Figure 15: Initial support required at admission (SICP census day).

At midnight on the census day 646 beds were occupied in 162 ICUs in England. The types of support/ monitoring provided to these patients during the census day are shown in Table 17.

Table 17: Types of support/monitoring provided (SICP census day).

Support/monitoring	No. (%) of patients*	No. (%) of ICUs
Mechanical ventilation	417 (65)	136 (85)
Invasive haemodynamic monitoring (excluding PAC)	470 (73)	134 (84)
Enteral feeding	235 (36)	115 (72)
Parenteral feeding	140 (22)	81 (51)
Pulmonary artery catheter (PAC)	118 (18)	68 (43)
Renal replacement therapy	57 (9)	39 (24)
TOTAL	646 (100)	162 (100)

*Some patients were receiving more than one type of support/monitoring.

In 15% of units, no patient was receiving mechanical ventilation.

There is recent evidence to suggest that the type of support required may be changing. Parker *et al.*,[65] in their study of admissions to one critical care unit over a four-year period, found that the proportion of patients requiring respiratory support decreased consistently, from 65% of patients in 1993 to 32% in 1996. They also observed that the median duration of respiratory support decreased from 20 hours in 1993 to 16 hours in 1996.

The authors also noted a decrease in the proportion of patients undergoing pulmonary artery catheterisation, from 20% in 1995 to 13% in 1996. The percentage of patients having inotropic support showed a consistent fall over the period, with 52% receiving vasoactive drugs in 1993, 44% in 1994, 35% in 1995 and a projected 22% in 1996.

The pattern that emerges is one of wide variation between ICUs in the levels of dependency of their patients. It is likely that significant numbers of intensive care beds are occupied by patients requiring only high-dependency care.

Admission guidelines

Identifying those patients most likely to benefit from critical care is one of the key challenges in providing the service.

The Admission Guidelines developed by a Department of Health working party[15] described the characteristics of intensive care and high-dependency care, as shown in Table 18.

Table 18: Characteristics of intensive and high-dependency care.

Intensive care is appropriate for:	High-dependency care is appropriate for:
patients requiring or likely to require advanced respiratory support alone	patients requiring support for a single failing organ system, but excluding those needing advanced respiratory support
patients requiring support of two or more organ systems	patients who can benefit from more detailed observation or monitoring than can safely be provided on a general ward
patients with chronic impairment of one or more organ systems sufficient to restrict daily activities (co-morbidity) and who require support for an acute reversible failure of another organ system	patients no longer needing intensive care, but who are not yet well enough to be returned to a general ward
	post-operative patients who need close monitoring for longer than a few hours

Thompson and Spiers[34] report that measurement of Therapeutic Intervention Scoring System (TISS) points and APACHE II scores confirmed that categorising patients according to these guidelines produced significantly different populations of patients. Mean TISS points for intensive-care-status patients were 38.7 (standard deviation 10.4) compared to 21.66 points (standard deviation 5.98) for high-dependency-status patients. The median APACHE II score for intensive-care-status patients was 16 (range 1–45) compared to 11 (range 1–27) for high-dependency-status patients. The authors commented that the criteria appear to differentiate well between ICU and HDU patients.

Classification of critical care is to be based on three levels following the announcement of the critical care modernisation programme.[11] These levels are:

- Level 1: acute ward care, with additional advice and support from the critical care team; e.g. patients who are at risk of deterioration, or who are recovering after requiring higher levels of care
- Level 2: more detailed observation or intervention; e.g. patients with a single failing organ system, or post-operative patients, or patients stepping down from higher levels of care
- Level 3: advanced respiratory support alone, or basic respiratory support together with support of at least two organ systems.

Discharge guidelines

The Department of Health guidelines[15] state that a patient should be discharged from intensive care when the condition that led to admission has been adequately treated and reversed, or when the patient can no longer benefit from the treatment available. The guidelines go on to say that stringent discharge criteria need to be developed and applied locally to ensure that other patients are not denied admission.

The decision to discharge a patient from intensive care or high-dependency care will depend partly on the level of care available in the unit or ward to which the patient is to be discharged.

The availability of an HDU within the hospital has an important influence on the decision to discharge. In the absence of step-down care, many patients stay on an ICU longer than necessary.[12]

It has been suggested that the continuing appropriateness of intensive care should be assessed at regular intervals. A decision to limit further treatment should be made only after discussion amongst the intensive care team and the referring team, and should have the full acceptance and understanding of the patient and his/her family/partner.[12]

A recent UK study[66] looked at the frequency with which treatment was withdrawn from intensive care patients and the primary reason for the decision. The authors examined 1745 admissions to an intensive care unit in Bristol, of whom 338 (19.4%) died in ICU. Of these, 220 deaths followed the withdrawal of treatment (12.6% of all ICU admissions). The primary reason for withdrawal of treatment was imminent death in 45% of cases, qualitative considerations in 50% and lethal conditions in 5%. The authors report that the reason varied significantly depending on the patient's age.

A King's Fund Panel[8] recognised that, when death is inevitable, discharge from the ICU can generate a sense of rejection in patients and family and that death in the ICU can be more humanitarian. Conversely, in some circumstances, the atmosphere of another ward may be more appropriate for terminal care. Inevitably, competing pressures for beds will affect these decisions.

Where a patient needs to be transferred to a specialist unit, close collaboration between the senior medical staff of both units is required to ensure appropriate timing of the transfer.[12]

As with discharge from intensive care, it is important that policies are in place to expedite timely discharge from high-dependency care to general wards.[12]

Staffing

Medical staff

It has been recommended that every critical care unit have a designated consultant with administrative responsibility.[1,12] Of 220 trusts responding to the Audit Commission's recent survey,[17] 41% reported that they had one consultant with overall responsibility for critical care services, and 53% reported that they did not. The remainder did not respond.

The Intensive Care Society[1] recommends a minimum allocation of 15 consultant sessions for an ICU of four or more beds and recognises that large, busy units may need as many as 30 allocated sessions.

Evidence suggests that a high level of consultant input produces better patient outcomes. A retrospective study suggested that the appointment of a full-time intensive care specialist had a significant impact on both unit and hospital mortality in a Canadian teaching hospital[67] and followed similar findings in both teaching[68] and community hospitals[69] in the United States.

The study by Metcalfe and McPherson[12] commented on the level of consultant input to intensive care in England in 1993. Their one-day census of all ICUs revealed that in almost 40% of units no consultant was present at all during the 24-hour period surveyed. This fits with the findings of the Royal College of Anaesthetists' national audit of intensive care,[39] which also examined the allocation of consultant sessions. This found that 57% of ICUs had six or fewer sessions per week and that 15 units had no sessions allocated at all.

A central focus of the modernisation programme for critical care[11] was workforce development, including the recruitment, training and retention of medical and nursing staff, with a balanced skill-mix so that professional staff are able to delegate less skilled and non-clinical tasks.

The Intensive Care Society recommends that trainee medical staff should have no responsibilities other than intensive care and related activities, such as cardiac arrest or major trauma teams.[1]

Nursing staff

Intensive care is synonymous with a 1:1 nurse:patient ratio. Busy units may also have additional, supervising or supernumerary nurses. Such staffing requires at least 6.3 whole-time equivalents (WTEs) per bed,[1] a figure that allows for annual and professional leave but does not take into account sickness or maternity leave.

High-dependency patients are generally considered to require an average of one nurse to two patients.[13] On occasions, however, a confused, restless patient on the HDU may require more nursing input than does one who is stable, sedated and ventilated on the ICU. A seven-month study of nursing workload on an adult general HDU concluded that a nurse:patient ratio of 1:2 may be insufficient, and recommended a ratio of 2:3.[70]

The Audit Commission found wide variations in the number of nurses employed in terms of the usual number on duty or in relation to patient workload. Although the average number of nursing WTEs employed per intensive care bed had increased from 5.2 in 1993[12] to 7.6 in 1998,[17] many units still fail to meet the Intensive Care Society standards.

Difficulties with recruitment and retention of nurses is one of the reasons for discrepancies between the numbers of funded and available beds. Figures reported by the Audit Commission[17] indicated that 53% of ICUs, 49% of combined ICU/HDUs and 48% of HDUs blamed recruitment difficulties for differences between the funded establishment and staff in post. Turnover rates for qualified nurses during 1997/98 were 12.2% in ICUs, 11% in combined units and 8.3% in HDUs. Sickness absence rates for qualified nurses during 1997/98 were 4.6%, 4.3% and 5% respectively.

Support workers such as auxiliary nurses and healthcare assistants may be employed to assist the trained nursing staff. Such personnel may reduce the need for nurses to perform non-nursing tasks and allow them to concentrate on direct patient care.

The modernisation programme for critical care[11] injected additional resources into NHS trusts for the recruitment and retention of critical care nurses, and called for a balanced skill-mix so that professional staff are able to delegate less skilled and non-clinical tasks. The programme requirements were based on a report by a Department of Health Expert Group,[10] which included an in-depth review of adult critical care nursing.

Other staff

Technicians, physiotherapists, pharmacists, radiographers and dieticians all have important roles in the critical care unit, and appropriate clerical support is also essential.[1]

Clinical management

Intensive care units generally follow one of two different patterns of clinical management: 'closed' or 'open' units.[1] In a 'closed' unit, the intensive care consultant(s) have complete responsibility for the care of patients admitted to the unit, and the referring team are involved only when their specialist input is needed.

Patients are admitted to 'open' units under the care of their admitting consultants and remain so throughout their stay.

Current evidence favours the 'closed' system[71,72,73] that seems to operate in the majority of ICUs in the United Kingdom. In HDUs, on the other hand, the 'open' model predominates.

The modernisation programme for critical care[11] required that admission to Levels 2 and 3 of critical care should be by consultant-to-consultant agreement only.

Costs

Intensive care provides care at high cost to a small number of patients. Annual spending on intensive care in the UK has been estimated at £675 million, representing about 2% of the hospital budget.[74] Costs of intensive care elsewhere in Europe have been estimated to represent up to 20% of a hospital's budget.[75]

It has been estimated that about 1% of the USA's GNP is spent on ICU services. While few of the constraints on critical care experienced in the UK would apply or be acceptable in the US, the available clinical data suggest that ICU clinical performance is similar in the two countries.[61]

Because of the high cost of intensive care, there is considerable interest in information regarding costs and effectiveness, but cost accounting in intensive care is underdeveloped.[76] A study of a non-random sample of intensive care units in twelve European countries[77] found that only 14 out of 88 (in five countries) had cost-accounting within the unit, and only 38 out of 88 ICU directors indicated that there was an awareness of cost per bed per day in their units.

Costs in the UK

Singer et al.[78] noted that intensive care is an increasingly expensive speciality in the UK, the costs for which are rising over and above general inflation.

A national working group led by the Medical Economics and Research Centre based in Sheffield has been looking at ICU costs, using both top-down and bottom-up approaches.

Top-down approach

The top-down approach defines a total cost for the service and derives from that an average cost per bed-day. Work by the Sheffield group has identified six 'cost blocks' as follows:[79]

1   Current cost of using equipment
2   Estates
3   Non-clinical support services
4   Clinical support services
5   Consumables
6   Staff

This cost classification was applied to 11 units in 1994/5 and 1995/6 (5 district general hospitals and 6 university hospitals). The first three cost blocks were related to overheads, and consistently constituted 15% of total ICU costs. Cost block 4 accounted for 9% of total costs in 1994/5 and 6% in 1995/6, whereas cost blocks 5 and 6 accounted for 22% and 53% of the total costs in 1994/5 and 24% and 55% in 1995/6. This study found a median cost per patient day of £1064 in 1994/5 and £1087 in 1995/6. Table 19 shows staff costs as a proportion of median cost per bed.

Table 19: Staff costs as a proportion of median cost per bed.

% of median cost per bed:	1994/95	1995/96
Consultants	5%	5%
Other medical	4%	5%
Total medical	10%	9%
Senior nurses	14%	14%
Junior nurses	24%	29%
Total nurses	38%	43%
Total medical/nursing staff	48%	52%

One of the authors' major findings was of a wide variation in annual costs between trusts but similar proportional contributions for each cost block.

Singer et al.,[78] also using a top-down method, examined changes in the costs of critical care in one trust between two periods: April 1988–February 1989 and January–July 1991. For the more recent of these periods, they found similar intensive care costs at £1149 per patient day. The corresponding cost for high-dependency care was £438 per patient day.

The authors noted that 'hidden' costs such as infrastructure maintenance, capital assets and diagnostic services accounted for nearly a quarter of total expenditure, and that staff costs accounted for over 50%.

Bottom-up approach

The bottom-up approach ascribes a cost to individual patients on the basis of the resources they use. Although more accurate than the top-down method, it is complex and costly to implement.

Edbrooke et al.[74] used a bottom-up method to identify ICU patient costs. This activity-based costings methodology, operational in the ICU of the Royal Hallamshire Hospital since 1995, uses a computerised data management system to record actual costs of nursing, medical ward rounds, drug treatments, disposables, equipment use and clinical support services such as physiotherapy, radiology and laboratory services. The authors report the average daily patient-related cost of care to be £592 and overhead costs to be £560, resulting in a total average cost of £1152 (standard deviation £243). They found a strong, highly significant statistical correlation between (1) the Therapeutic Intervention Scoring System (TISS) and the cost of care for each calendar day, and (2) the APACHE II score and cost of the first 24-hour period. They note that patient-related costs of care are high initially and then fall rapidly to a constant level.

Another survey using a bottom-up approach showed that caring for ventilated patients costs twice as much as caring for those breathing spontaneously.[80] Patients with severe sepsis or early septic shock are also significantly more expensive to treat than are non-septic patients.[81]

These average daily costs may appear to be comparable with those reported by Singer et al. (£1148 per patient day).[78] However, Edbrooke et al.[74] caution that the distribution of costs is non-gaussian and therefore that the mean is an insufficient descriptor of average costs of care. They also point out that the effects of case-mix on these figures is unknown.

There is evidence of high variability in the daily cost of individual ICU patients. It has been suggested that the cost of individual patients per day ranges from £100 to £8000.[82] For this reason, top-down costing approaches that average out daily costs may be misleading. Bottom-up methodologies are clearly more useful in intensive care but may not be practicable for the majority of units.

The Audit Commission has also collected information relating to service contracts, staff budgets and expenditure that is useful in showing the variability between units.

Cost drivers

A consistent finding has been that at least 50% of ICU patient costs are incurred by staffing. Havill et al.[83] tested the hypothesis that nursing hours may predict cost, and found a very strong correlation between direct nursing hours and cost.

This is important where health authorities or trusts may be considering providing more critical care beds. While the average or median cost per day may be approximately £1150, each new bed will not cost this amount, as some 25% of costs relate to fixed overheads.

An economic analysis that examined the daily costs of 90 critically ill patients[84] found a wide variation in costs between patients and diagnoses; a strong relationship between the cost of the first day of management and the APACHE II score; and higher daily costs of treatment in patients who died in intensive care. Table 20 provides descriptive statistics for daily costs of treatment.

Table 20: Daily costs of patients.

	Died in ICU	Died after ICU	Survivors
Number of patients	21	13	56
Patient days	122	57	262
Overall mean cost per patient (£)	816	508	550
Standard errors of mean	80	33	25
95% CL of mean	649–982	435–580	498–601
Range of mean costs (£) between patients	349–1238	377–750	262–1017

Table 21 shows the distribution of mean daily costs for each diagnostic category.

Table 21: Mean daily cost per patient for each diagnostic category.

Diagnosis	n	ICU mortality (n)	Mean daily cost (£)	95% CI
Respiratory				
Chronic obstructive airways disease	5	1	597	461–773
Pneumonia	4	3	760	370–1149
Post-op. respiratory failure	2	1	385	246–524
Pulmonary neoplasm	3	1	484	318–649
Post-respiratory arrest	1	0	609	
Respiratory observation	24	0	479	380–577
Cardiovascular				
Aortic aneurysm repair	6	0	525	437–612
Septic shock	7	4	911	768–1053
Cardiac disease	10	5	573	410–735
Shock	6	2	569	226–912
Gastro-intestinal bleeding	1	0	438	
Perforation/obstruction	6	0	619	585–654
Other	3	2	816	416–1217
Trauma	3	0	500	258-743
Neurological	2	0	509	148–870
Renal failure	2	0	691	517–864
Metabolic	4	3	944	710–1177
Total	89			

While APACHE II score and cost of first-day care are related, severity of illness is only an indirect measure of overall costs because the healthcare costs depend more upon the intensity of observation, nature of interventions required and care actually delivered.

6 Effectiveness of services and interventions

Perceptions of constraints in supply raise questions about the appropriate use of intensive care and, more fundamentally, the need to determine which types of patient actually benefit from critical care. This is especially important given the high costs involved.

It is beyond the scope of this chapter to provide a systematic review of the effectiveness of all the interventions used in critical care. We have, however, identified some important recent studies to illustrate general points.

Evidence for the effectiveness of specific interventions

For a few conditions, the benefits of intensive care are indisputable. In patients with an acute reversible polyneuropathy such as Guillain-Barré syndrome, mechanical ventilation is undeniably life-saving at the point where respiratory failure becomes life-threatening. For the majority of conditions, however, the effectiveness of intensive care remains unproven. Indeed, the role of intensive care in preventing death has yet to be properly investigated.[47] The main problem with establishing the effectiveness of intensive care is the common view that, because its use for various conditions is considered standard for good medical practice, prospective randomised controlled trials of the benefits are deemed ethically unacceptable.[59] However, given the wide variation in practice and genuine doubt as to which practices are best, others are not convinced that such trials would be unethical.[85]

Given the enormous heterogeneity of case-mix, any trials in intensive care would require huge numbers of patients if questions are to be answered. These difficulties have meant that very few satisfactory trials have been carried out in intensive care settings. As a result, there remain large areas of practice that lack evidence about risks and benefits – for example, optimum fluid balance strategies and the use of pulmonary artery catheters (PACs).[86] Given the paucity of evidence in critical care, decisions tend to be based on the clinician's experience and judgement and on individual patient circumstances, which may result in treatments being used despite evidence that they are ineffective – for example, low-dose dopamine infusions in preventing renal failure, or albumin infusion in hypoalbuminaemia. It may also result in withholding interventions such as PAC to guide haemodynamic management in the high-risk surgical patient, despite evidence of effectiveness.

Examples of areas where evidence exists to guide critical care practice are as follows:

- ventilator circuit and secretion management strategies in the prevention of ventilator-associated pneumonia[87]
- strategies to prevent upper gastrointestinal bleeding in ventilated patients[88]
- the use of formal protocol-driven strategies for weaning patients from mechanical ventilation[89,90]
- the use of selective decontamination of the digestive tract in critically ill adults[91]
- the optimisation of high-risk patients before major surgery[42,43]
- the increased mortality associated with growth hormone treatment in critically ill adults[92]
- mechanical ventilation with lower total volumes, which decreases mortality in patients with acute lung injury and acute respiratory distress syndrome.[93]

Where such evidence exists, it clearly needs to be widely publicised. Even then, whether such strategies are adopted in practice depends on factors such as the magnitude and precision of estimates of benefit and harm, as well as access, availability and costs.[91]

Cost effectiveness

Recent data suggest that, on average, 22% of ICU patients die before leaving the unit, a further 8% die before leaving hospital and 7% die in the first six months at home. Nine percent are left with severe limitations to daily living, 38% have some limitation but are able to live independently, and only 16% are left in good health with no limitations. For combined ICU/HDUs, 16% of patients die before leaving the unit and a further 20% before leaving hospital. For HDUs, the corresponding figures are 6% and 9% respectively.[17]

The relatively high mortality rates for intensive care patients mean that large sums of money are spent on patients who, ultimately, do not survive. Although current methods of predicting outcome can fairly accurately predict mortality rates for groups of patients, they cannot as yet do so for individuals with sufficient accuracy for non-survivors to be confidently identified at the time of intensive care admission.

A group at Guy's Hospital surveyed 3600 adult ICU admissions. The 15% who died consumed 37% of the ICU budget.[94] Ridley *et al.* [84] reported that in 1989 the mean daily cost per patient for non-survivors was £816 (95% CL £649–£982), while for survivors it was £550 (95% CL £498–£601).

An effective cost per survivor can be derived by dividing the total ICU budget by the number of patients surviving. A series of 523 intensive care patients studied at Guy's Hospital gave an effective cost per survivor of £4916. However, when considered separately, the figure for patients staying in the ICU for more than 72 hours was £24 925.[95] Gilbertson et al.[96] studied a series of 156 patients, of whom 29% had severe respiratory conditions as well as renal failure. The effective cost per survivor was almost £12 000.

Ridley et al.[97] performed a cost-utility analysis by looking at both costs and quality of life in 56 survivors one year after their admission to the ICU in 1989. They estimated the total hospital cost per quality adjusted life year (QALY) at £7500. When the cost-per-QALY comparisons are made with other healthcare interventions (all adjusted to 1989 costs), intensive care was found to lie between heart transplantation (£6070) and home dialysis (£13 070). If the costs of non-survivors were built into the calculation, however, the cost per QALY for intensive care would increase considerably.

Stockwell[98] estimates the cost of every extra survivor produced by intensive care to be approximately £45 000. Comparing this with corresponding costs for statins used to treat men with hypercholesterolaemia (£226 560) and enalapril to control hypertension (£36 300), he contests that intensive care does not compare unfavourably on a cost basis with other treatments.

Developments in costing

For the reasons outlined earlier, DRGs are inappropriate in the ICU, and work is currently in hand to develop and validate HRGs for intensive care. The ACP dataset, introduced throughout the NHS in October 1997, may provide a basis for HRGs. While there are no published studies at present, preliminary work suggests a reasonably good correlation between some ACP parameters and intensive care costs.[62]

7 Models of care and recommendations

Possible models of care

The modernisation programme for critical care[11] called for strategic change to modernise services, and injected additional resources into NHS trusts for the recruitment and retention of critical care nurses.
 Four main elements of the programme required action by NHS trusts. These were:

- a hospital-wide approach to critical care, with services that extend beyond the physical boundaries of intensive care and high-dependency units, making optimum use of available resources, including beds
- a networked service across those NHS trusts that together serve one or more local health economies, meeting the critical care needs of those within the network and minimising the need for transfer outside
- workforce development, including the recruitment, training and retention of medical and nursing staff, and a balanced skill-mix so that professional staff are able to delegate less skilled and non-clinical tasks
- better information, with all critical care services collecting reliable management information and participating in outcome-focused clinical audit.

A new approach to classifying critical care was also introduced, with a spectrum of three levels of critical care (where Level 0 denotes normal acute ward care) as follows:

- Level 1 – acute ward care, with additional advice and support from the critical care team; e.g. patients who are at risk of deterioration, or who are recovering after requiring higher levels of care
- Level 2 – more detailed observation or intervention; e.g. patients with a single failing organ system, or post-operative patients, or patients stepping down from higher levels of care

- Level 3 – advanced respiratory support alone, or basic respiratory support together with support of at least two organ systems.

A regional approach

In 1989, a King's Fund panel, considering intensive care services, suggested that there may be a case for concentrating intensive care provision in a smaller number of units, each of which would have a workload large enough to enable it to develop appropriate expertise.[8] The Intensive Care Society noted in 1990[1] that centralising the intensive care service would force units to become larger, a concept familiar in other countries of Europe, in Australia and in the US – certainly, large units are less vulnerable to fluctuation in demand.

To some extent, the National Intensive Care Bed register is already encouraging a more regional approach to critical care by having a wider perspective and by facilitating transfers accordingly. However, this is not a desirable way in which to move towards centralisation; transferring patients to locations where beds happen to be available does not guarantee that the appropriate expertise will be there as well.

An inevitable consequence of centralisation or stratification is the increased need to transfer patients between hospitals, and it needs to be ensured that this is accomplished safely. Wallace and Lawler[99] argue that transfer teams must be fully equipped and skilled, and note that dedicated teams are common in Europe, the US and Australia. They suggest that intensive care transfer teams should be established on a regional basis and should provide skilled attendants and appropriate equipment in order to ensure a safer service and to avoid the necessity for on-call staff in referring hospitals to accompany patients.

Paediatric critical care model

The new classification approach[11] mirrors the recent reorganisation of paediatric critical care services to some extent.

In July 1997, the National Co-ordinating Group on Paediatric Intensive Care reported on the future provision of that service.[24] The report identified three levels of high-dependency or intensive care, as shown in Table 22.

Table 22: Levels of high-dependency or intensive care.

Level	Distinction
Level 1	• Requirement for closer observation and monitoring than is available on a standard ward • Single-organ support, but excluding advanced respiratory support • Step-down from intensive care • Following major surgery: cardiac, neuro, spinal, etc. • Advanced analgesic techniques • Non-intubated children with moderately severe croup, bronchiolitis, etc. • The recently extubated child
Level 2	• Advanced respiratory support OR • Two or more organ systems requiring support OR • One acute organ failure receiving support, plus one chronic failure
Level 3	• Two or more organ systems requiring technological support, including advanced respiratory support of one of these systems; e.g. renal support or haemofiltration plus mechanical ventilation

The report recommended that within any defined geographical area there should be a service that provides care for each critically ill child in a facility that is best able to meet his or her needs. The system that is needed to care for critically ill children will involve accident and emergency departments and the ambulance service as well as hospitals.

Specialist weaning units

Although patients stay in intensive care usually for only one or two days, a small proportion remain for much longer. Many of them have suffered with very severe acute respiratory distress syndrome (ARDS) or sepsis complicated by multiple organ failure. Often, the major problem for the latter phases of these prolonged intensive care stays is continuing dependence on mechanical ventilation, with difficulty in weaning that support. One such patient on a unit will have a significant effect on its effective capacity by 'blocking' a bed for the duration of his/her stay. Specialist weaning units have been proposed to address this situation and to concentrate expertise in weaning such challenging patients.

Several such units in the United States have reported their experiences[100,101,102,103] and claim a high success rate in weaning from ventilation. It has also been suggested that they may represent a cost-saving alternative to intensive care units, and possibly that they may reduce mortality in such cases.[101]

In 1998, a survey was undertaken of 70 ICUs in the London area to see whether they would use a specialist weaning service if one were provided for such patients.[104] Intensive care units in district hospitals, teaching hospitals and specialist hospitals were included and a 71% response rate was obtained. The results showed that 68% of units would refer to a specialist weaning unit for advice, diagnosis and support, and that 74% would refer patients for long-term ventilator management.

At present, such specialist facilities are not widely available in this country, but the results of this survey suggest that there may be a case for reviewing this situation.

Other models

In recent years, several studies have suggested that earlier recognition and intervention of seriously ill patients on general wards is likely to reduce their need for intensive care and, more importantly, improve outcome.[105,106,107,108,109] 'Medical emergency teams'[105] or 'patient-at-risk teams'[108,109] have been proposed to address this problem, operating as outreach services from the intensive care unit. The Audit Commission, in its report on critical care services in acute hospitals,[14] identified as one of its highest priority recommendations the need to 'improve services for patients on wards who are at risk of deterioration into a need for critical care'. The mainstay of this approach was to 'develop an "outreach" service from critical care specialists to support ward staff in managing patients at risk'.

Mercer et al.[110] support this view, but warn that once severely ill patients are identified, there must be provision to monitor them closely; so medical emergency teams must be coupled with adequate high-dependency facilities. Fletcher and Flabouris also stressed this point.[109]

The role of intermediate care

Ridley[40] sees high-dependency care as a system of managing illness that matches the continuum of health needs. Developing intermediate care has been seen as a means of alleviating both the perceived lack of intensive care facilities and the increased burden of ill patients on general wards. There is evidence to suggest that the provision of high-dependency care may address some of the shortages created by a lack of intensive care beds.[111,112,113]

The critical care modernisation programme[11] introduced a new approach to classifying critical care services, using a spectrum of four levels, thereby matching more closely the continuum of health needs.

Wallis et al.[114] reviewed the outcome of 1700 patients admitted to an intensive care unit over a five-year period in a hospital with an HDU. Twenty percent died on the ICU, but a further 9% died after return to the general wards. When they were discharged from the ICU, of those dying on the wards, 25.5% were expected to die, 54.2% were considered at risk of death, but 20.3% were expected to survive. The authors felt that some of these deaths would have been preventable, given adequate care, and suggested that HDUs could have a key role in providing a level of care between the ICU and the general wards for compromised patients.

The rationale underlying the HDU is 'progressive patient care', a system in which patients are grouped together on the basis of their dependency or degree of illness, rather than their speciality or diagnosis. It is argued that grouping patients by level of need can enable the best use to be made of available technical resources and staffing.[15] This was a concept endorsed by the Royal College of Anaesthetists and the Royal College of Surgeons of England in their report on graduated patient care.[115]

The Intensive Care Society[1] recommended that there should be an HDU in each district general hospital with clear lines of communication to a central ICU. They argued that the HDU should not manage patients with multi-organ failure but should provide monitoring and support to patients at risk of developing organ system failure.

The Association of Anaesthetists[16] suggested that the type of unit developed should depend on local requirements and constraints. Planning for high-dependency care needed to take into consideration the size and case-mix of admissions to the hospital, the needs of particular sub-specialities and the numbers and skills of available medical, nursing and support staff. It was suggested that the number of beds should be ascertained by an audit of the numbers of patients who might have been admitted to such a unit over a six-month period.

The focus on high-dependency care was made somewhat redundant by the announcement of the modernisation programme for critical care,[11] which called for strategic change to modernise services and introduced a new approach to classifying critical care according to a spectrum of four levels of care. The following discussion of high-dependency care makes some general points about having a stratified system that reflects severity of illness.

High-dependency care has traditionally been provided in a dedicated area, either as part of a general ward or adjacent to an ICU. There are advantages in having the facilities and skills of the ICU close at hand if a patient suddenly deteriorates. Such a system may also make management easier. In some hospitals, the ICU and HDU are integrated to the extent that they share the same area, with beds to a degree being interchangeable. The advantages and disadvantages of this arrangement are summarised in Table 23.

Table 23: Advantages and disadvantages of mixing or separating ICU and HDU.

Advantages	Disadvantages
Separate units	
Protected step-down bed availability	No extra flexible intensive care capacity
Patients/relatives with lesser illness are not mixed with very anxious or bereaved relatives of intensive care patients	Less continuity of care for patients, and the anxiety of moving to a new and unfamiliar environment.
Mixed units	
If a patient has a crisis on the HDU, ICU doctors and nurses are nearby to help out	
Cost-efficiency for staffing, less duplication of equipment	In times of bed stress, high-dependency beds are lost because they are used for intensive care
A larger pool of nurses with specialist qualifications to draw upon	Some nurses may have less experience in either high-dependency or intensive care

Several studies have examined the impact on the ICU of opening a high-dependency unit. Fox et al.[116] found that the use of intensive care beds became more appropriate; the occupancy of intensive care beds by patients needing only high-dependency care was reduced; and the occupancy by patients needing intensive care was increased. There was also a significant decrease in re-admissions, suggesting that the presence of an HDU reduced the number of patients discharged prematurely to general wards.

Dhond et al.[117] found, following the opening of an adjacent HDU, that the ICU patients' initial severity of illness was lower and their length of stay reduced. Also, fewer ICU patients were admitted directly from the general wards. They found no reduction in demand for intensive care – indeed, the HDU appeared to have generated new demand for critical care services overall. In their experience, the HDU was unlikely to relieve pressure on intensive care beds per se or to reduce the overall cost of critical care. There is other evidence that opening a high-dependency unit may reveal significant underlying demand. Parker et al.[118] studied the admissions to one critical care unit over a four-year period. The number of ICU beds was increased from 7 to 12, and then a 6-bed HDU was opened. Despite total capacity more than doubling from 7 to 18 critical care beds, overall occupancy decreased by only 16%, suggesting that demand was increasing to fill capacity.

The impact of opening an HDU in a given hospital will depend on the case-load and case-mix that it sees, as well as on the extent to which existing facilities meet that demand.

Peacock and Edbrooke,[119] reporting the effect of opening a high-dependency unit on numbers of cancellations of elective surgery and emergency transfers, also presented data that suggested some supply-induced demand, as shown in Table 24.

Table 24: The effect of opening a high-dependency unit.

	1992/3	1993/4	1994/5
Admissions to HDU	0	219	315
Cancellations	15	1	0
Admissions to ICU	310	268	346
Transfers out of ICU	19	2	0

With the opening of the HDU, admissions to the ICU decreased in 1993/4 as would be expected. However, the following year saw an increase over the pre-HDU level of ICU admissions. The authors also noted a significant reduction in the cancellation of elective surgery and in the number of patients transferred out of the ICU because of bed pressures.

How many beds are needed?

Previous recommendations

Hospital Building Note 27, published in 1970 and revised in 1974,[120] recommended that the number of beds in an ICU should be about 1%–2% of total acute beds, with additional allocation for any specialist services on site.

The more recent Health Building Note 27 avoids a specific formula, suggesting instead an occupancy of 65% as appropriate. Occupancy in units admitting a high proportion of elective cases and a low proportion of emergencies can safely be significantly higher.

The Royal College of Anaesthetists[121] states that the number of beds provided must be such that no elective patient is cancelled more than once because of the lack of critical care beds, and that immediate availability of beds for emergency admissions must be satisfied for more than 95% of requests.

Clearly, there is no fixed formula for the number of critical care beds needed by a trust, and it is important that the number is tailored to the workload and case-mix that the hospital treats.

The Intensive Care Society lists the factors to be considered when estimating the size of an ICU.[1] These are:

- number of acute beds in the hospital or catchment area
- type of acute bed (adult, paediatric)
- previously calculated occupancies of wards, HDUs and ICUs
- history of refusals
- location of other high-care areas (other ICUs or HDUs in hospital, other hospitals)
- number of operating theatres
- surgical specialities services and case-mix (e.g. vascular, cardiac, thoracic, emergency, urgent, elective)
- medical specialities (e.g. respiratory, cardiology)
- A&E department
- sub-regional or regional services (e.g. neurosurgery, maxillo-facial surgery, complex orthopaedic, renal services, oncology, etc.)
- ability to transfer patients to an off-site ICU (staff, equipment, transport)
- paediatric care
- location – motorways, holiday resort, mainline transport terminal (rail, coach, etc.).

There is no firm guidance as to the optimum size for an ICU. Units that are too small may not benefit from economies of scale, whereas units with more than eight beds may present problems of clinical management.

The number of beds needed will in part depend on how they are configured. Lyons *et al.*[122] calculated that to meet needs on 95% of occasions for a population of 500 000 would require 30 intensive care beds and 55 high-dependency beds if these were all in a single unit. For three separate units to meet an identical need on 95% of occasions, 10% more beds would be needed.

Modelling bed availability

Detailed mathematical models have an established place in providing quantitative information about healthcare resource needs and, to be helpful, must be able to deal with complexity, uncertainty, variability and, sometimes, inadequate data.[123] Critical care involves all these features, with a complicated mix of planned and emergency patients, complex arrival patterns, variable lengths of stay, uncertain outcomes, high mortality and scarce resources, and with considerable variation in all these factors between hospitals. Despite these difficulties, operational models can be developed which, as well as predicting need, can also take account of the resources needed for treatment.[124]

Constructing a model requires enough information to describe the natural history of patients or categories of patients in terms of their requirements for critical care. It also requires information about the resources available to manage them and the operating rules that govern the way those resources are used. Average lengths of stay are inadequate for developing such a model and, if used, will seriously underestimate bed requirements.[125] Instead, within a unit's case-mix, clinically meaningful and statistically homogenous groups of patients can be identified from relatively basic information.[18] Rather than taking mean lengths of stay for each of these groups, the statistical distributions of actual lengths of stay are used to inform the model.

Having developed the model, simulations can be performed and used to estimate the following, for example:

- the number of intensive care and/or high-dependency beds needed to cope with a particular case-mix, or to achieve a given level of occupancy

- what the effect would be of changing operating rules
- what impact on critical care would result from the introduction of new medical or surgical services at the trust
- how, if similar models were available for critical care units in adjacent trusts, a collaborative service might best be developed and managed.

Appropriate use of critical care beds

It is important that the use of critical care facilities is limited, as far as possible, to appropriate patients. This will depend in part on the facilities available, but also on the presence of experienced, suitably trained, senior clinicians able to make timely decisions on admission and discharge and on withholding or withdrawing treatment, should this be indicated.

The modernisation programme for critical care[11] called for NHS trusts to ensure that admission to critical care Levels 2 and 3 should be by consultant-to-consultant agreement only.

It is likely that, despite attempts to define firm admission and discharge criteria for intensive care units, patients are still admitted who are too ill to benefit. Resisting such referrals is often difficult and can be done only by someone with the authority that comes from appropriate training and experience. There are currently too few consultant sessions allocated to intensive care for this important gatekeeping role to be fulfilled around the clock. Commissioners should discuss with trusts the need for additional consultant sessions which, as well as meeting this need, might be used to set up medical emergency teams as discussed earlier.

Configuration and provision of critical care services

Recurring crises because of the shortage of intensive care beds suggest that the present configuration of critical care services is failing, and have led to the belief that more intensive care beds are required. There are considerable data, on the other hand, to suggest that a large proportion of intensive care beds are used for patients needing only high-dependency care, although the extent to which this applies varies greatly from trust to trust. Against this background and in the absence of reliable information, it is impossible to generalise on the need for additional beds or on the split between intensive care and high dependency. Some trusts will need more intensive care beds, some will need more high-dependency beds and others will need more of both. Reliable information is urgently required to inform this area.

The frequent use of intensive care beds by high-dependency patients suggests an underprovision of high-dependency facilities, and this is reinforced by studies showing shortcomings in the ward care of such patients. A lack of high-dependency or even of general ward beds makes it hard to use an intensive care unit efficiently and difficult to discharge patients when they would otherwise be ready.

In the absence of adequate information, it is impossible to make explicit recommendations regarding the centralisation or stratification of intensive care services. Nonetheless, given shortcomings in current service configuration, greater collaboration between trusts would seem desirable.

These issues were recognised in the report of the National Expert Group to review adult critical care services in the UK,[10] established in 1999 by the NHS Executive. As a result of the report, in May 2000 a critical care modernisation plan was announced,[11] which injected extra resources for additional staff, beds and services, and introduced a new approach to the classification of critical care services.

Individual trusts should also have an operational policy, discussed and agreed in advance, to put into practice at times of pressure: perhaps a recurring winter crisis or an unexpected local emergency. This strategy should replace the crisis-management approach that more often applies at present. Such a policy could take into account:

- cancellation of major elective surgery
- flexible use of other, specialist intensive care beds where present
- flexible use of high-dependency facilities
- transfers to adjacent hospitals, given appropriate transport arrangements.

At present, on general wards, some patients deteriorate in an unrecognised manner, to the point where intensive care becomes necessary. If these patients were identified earlier, it is likely that the need for intensive care might be avoided by earlier intervention either on the ward or in a high-dependency unit. One solution is the wider introduction of 'medical emergency teams' based on the intensive care unit, but which could be called whenever patients met defined criteria that identified them as being at risk. Consultant appointments will be needed to establish such teams, but the costs might be offset by a reduced need for intensive care.

This notion was also acknowledged in the report of the National Expert Group[10] and resulted in a call for the establishment of outreach teams.[11]

Commissioners should be involved in decisions on the allocation of resources to intensive and high-dependency care, but, as with other high-cost, low-volume services, it is probably appropriate for critical services to be specifically identified and considered outside the remit of PCGs. The current regional reviews of these services may address this. The only exception to this might be for episodes of intensive or high-dependency care following major elective surgery. In these instances, the level and duration of such care is usually fairly predictable and thus easily costed and built into overall contractual costs for these procedures.

A suitable currency for clinical care services remains to be defined, although work is currently underway on HRGs, and progress in this area would be welcomed.

Recommendations

Provision and configuration at trust level

The provision of critical care beds must be sufficient to meet the needs of emergency referrals on at least 95% of occasions, while at the same time allowing major elective surgery to be undertaken without frequent cancellations. It is not possible to generalise, and so fixed recommendations relating numbers of critical care beds to total hospital bed numbers are unhelpful. The numbers and types of critical care beds should be tailored to the workload and case-mix of each individual trust. To achieve this, some trusts will need more Level 1 and 2 beds, some will need more Level 3 beds, and some will need more of all levels. For some trusts, it might be appropriate for a proportion of Level 3 beds to be replaced by Level 1 and 2 beds.

When assessing the need for critical care services in a trust, as well as considering refused admissions, premature discharges, transfers and cancelled operations, the numbers of patients being managed on general wards who would benefit from critical care also need to be taken into account. This information can be obtained by conducting repeated, one-day snapshots using, for example, the ACP dataset or something similar to identify patients for whom critical care admission would be appropriate. Mathematical modelling can be used to provide a more accurate picture of need, as it can take into account the various uncertainties and complexities associated with critical care.

Once need has been defined, the next thing to consider is the configuration of the service in terms of the geographical, operational and management relationships between different levels of critical care beds. The integration of critical care beds, or at least the positioning of units next to one another, seems to offer advantages of flexibility and ease of management. Where a new unit is being developed in an existing building, however, limitations on space may make this difficult.

Outreach services should be developed so that seriously ill patients elsewhere in the trust can benefit from the expertise and skills of the intensive care staff, both medical and nursing. There should be agreed and widely publicised criteria which, when met by a patient, would trigger referral to a 'medical emergency team' or a 'patient-at-risk team' based on the intensive care unit. The aim would be to recognise seriously ill patients early, and certainly before they deteriorate to the point of suffering cardiorespiratory arrest. For some of these patients, early recognition and prompt appropriate treatment might avoid the need for subsequent critical care. For others, however, critical care facilities will be needed and must be available if outreach services are properly to achieve their aims.

To embrace all of these areas, there needs to be a process of strategic planning for critical care services in the trust, ideally conducted at board level.

Operational policies at inter-trust level

Since critical care is a scarce, expensive resource, trusts and their patients would benefit from a more collaborative approach than currently exists, particularly at times of pressure. Where appropriate, operational policies should be developed between trusts to ensure that resources are used to the greatest overall benefit. This will require strategic planning by a regional critical care group, with the whole exercise overseen by some corresponding national body. In the same way in which mathematical modelling can help with planning at trust level, it can also help to define optimal working relationships over wider geographical areas. It is at this level that data are helpful on population needs for critical care.

A possible model would be one based on centralisation, along the lines of that adopted for paediatric intensive care. This provides a clear operational structure and concentrates skills and expertise where they will be used, although there is no evidence that such a model would produce better patient outcomes. It must also be remembered that the scale of need for adult critical care services is far greater than that for children.

By implication, greater collaboration between trusts will entail more frequent patient transfers. If so, it must be ensured that these are conducted safely, according to agreed policies and guidelines, and that they are properly audited. Funding arrangements will also need to be in place to ensure that receiving trusts are not penalised.

Coping with pressure

It is unrealistic to assume that trusts will have enough critical care beds to cope with every peak of demand. Rather than relying on crisis management, therefore, strategies for coping with pressure should be agreed beforehand. At trust level, a plan needs to be formulated to escalate response to meet escalating pressure, defining how and under what circumstances other resources will be called into play – for example, other specialist critical care beds where present, or theatre recovery areas.

Similar strategies should be agreed between trusts for occasions when demand exceeds local provision. If bed availability is continuously monitored across a group of trusts, pressure can often be seen developing and therefore can be anticipated before the situation reaches crisis point.

Appropriate use of resources

It needs to be ensured that available beds are used for appropriate patients and that, where necessary, decisions on withholding and withdrawing treatment are made in a timely manner. This, in turn, requires input from appropriately trained and experienced consultants with sufficient sessional allocation for the task. Trusts should therefore review their allocation of consultant sessions to critical care to ensure that this need is being met.

The number of beds and the balance of provision should ensure that, as far as possible, critical care beds are occupied by appropriate patients. This also requires enough general ward beds to ensure that patients no longer needing critical care can be discharged promptly.

Given the paucity of suitably trained nurses, it is essential that those in post are used appropriately. To this end, the allocation of nurses to patients should be tailored to individual patient need rather than according to rigid 1:1 or 1:2 ratios.

Finally, units should have clear policies and guidelines covering issues such as admission, discharge, clinical care and patient transfers.

Data requirements

Information on critical care activity is urgently needed to inform strategic planning at trust, regional and national level. This must include data on the need for, the use of and the outcome from critical care.

The needs assessment should take into account patients currently managed on general wards who would benefit from critical care services. This exercise will require trust-wide surveys using, for example, the ACP dataset or similar criteria to identify such patients. In order to keep pace with changing activities and workloads, these surveys will need to be repeated at regular intervals.

Universal and accurate completion of the ACP dataset should be encouraged and will provide valuable data on the use of critical care facilities.

Reliable, case-mix-adjusted hospital outcome data should be available for all intensive care units through participation in ICNARC's Case Mix Programme. The same information will also be necessary for clinical governance purposes. While obviously important, hospital survival after intensive care has been perhaps over-emphasised as a measure of performance. For other life-threatening illnesses such as cancer and AIDS, long-term survival is the prime consideration, and more information of this sort is urgently needed in the intensive care setting. This is particularly important given that intensive care units seem to be admitting an increasingly elderly population of patients. While many of these patients survive to leave hospital, not enough is currently known about their longer-term outcome and quality of life.

In the absence of any current measures of process for critical care services, performance indicators should be defined and introduced. For intensive care units, these might include details of delayed or refused admissions, transfers to other units for non-clinical reasons, premature discharges because of pressure on beds, and readmission rates.

To be of value, data collection must be reliable and robust, and staff should be identified for the purpose. This will require appropriate funding and should be recognised as a priority by commissioners.

Staffing needs

The allocation of consultant sessions to intensive care should be reviewed in all trusts to ensure that decisions on admission, discharge, transfers and withholding or withdrawing treatment are made by experienced, appropriately trained senior clinicians. Any increase in the numbers of such consultants will clearly have implications for workforce planning and training.

Trusts should also ensure that critical care nursing staff are being used optimally, with nurse:patient ratios tailored, as far as possible, to individual patient need. The issues of nursing recruitment and retention should receive active attention, with consideration given to employing other staff to take over any non-nursing roles.

Outreach services, or any other expansion of clinical responsibilities outside the critical care unit, are likely to need additional staff, both medical and nursing.

Commissioning for critical care services

At present, for the majority of critical care units, costs are theoretically built into block contracts for the major clinical specialities. As a result, intensive care clinicians rarely deal directly with commissioners, and negotiations are conducted on their behalf by clinicians who may have little understanding of the service. This system may be appropriate if the need for intensive care is regular and predictable as, for example, following elective cardiac surgery. It is unsatisfactory when the need is unpredictable and comprises mainly emergencies – the pattern of work for most ICUs. When block contracts are being negotiated, intensive care needs and costs are frequently underestimated or forgotten. Current arrangements also fail to recognise the impact of specialities that use intensive care only rarely and so make no allowance for it in negotiating contracts. Cumulatively, however, such patients account for a significant proportion of intensive care admissions. As a result of these anomalies, the service is inevitably underfunded.

A Department of Health working group[15] recommended that commissioners should be involved in decisions about the allocation of resources to critical care and contracting for these services. It is clearly important for clinicians actually involved in providing such services also to be closely involved in these discussions. The development of HRGs for critical care would greatly facilitate this process.

The call in May 2000[11] for NHS trusts to establish Critical Care Delivery Groups with the involvement of both medical and nursing critical care clinicians may provide an avenue for clinicians to become more involved in contracting.

Critical care services should be specifically identified in discussions with commissioners, and intensive care clinicians should be involved in that exercise. As with other high-cost, low-volume services, it may be appropriate for critical care to be considered outside the remit of PCGs except where it occurs as a planned episode following major elective surgery. In these instances, the level and duration of such care is usually fairly predictable and thus easily costed and built into overall contractual costs for these procedures.

A suitable currency for critical care services remains to be defined, although work is currently underway on HRGs, and progress in this area would be welcomed.

8 Outcome measures

Traditionally, the most commonly used outcome measure has been patient survival, both from the intensive care unit and, more especially, from hospital. The APACHE II method has been validated on a British population and allows a case-mix-adjusted probability of hospital death to be calculated for each adult patient. From that, the number of deaths expected in a group of patients can also be calculated. If this is compared with the actual number of hospital deaths, a standardised mortality ratio (SMR) can be derived and, with some reservations, be used as a basis for comparisons between units. Such comparisons rely on a robust process for data collection and analysis and it is therefore important to ensure that all units participate in the ICNARC Case Mix Programme (*see* above).

Even with case-mix adjustment, the importance of hospital survival has been somewhat overemphasised and would not be considered adequate for other life-threatening pathologies. In cancer and AIDS, for example, it is considered more helpful to examine long-term survival over periods of months and years, and similar data should be collected routinely for intensive care patients.

Similarly, not enough is known about restoration of function and quality of life in survivors of critical illness. Patients should be evaluated in terms of their ongoing health and the extent to which they are restored to their previous lifestyle. It has been suggested that, six months after hospital discharge, 9% of patients admitted to intensive care have severe limitations to daily living, 38% have some limitations but are able to live independently, and only 16% enjoy good health with no limitations.[17]

Given that intensive care units are admitting an increasingly elderly population of patients, more information on long-term survival and quality of life is urgently needed. While many elderly patients survive to leave hospital, not enough is currently known about their prognosis thereafter. Djaiani and Ridley[126] followed 474 patients aged over 70 years and admitted to intensive care, and found their survival at one year to be significantly poorer than that of an age- and sex-matched normal population.

Many of the considerable number of quality-of-life measures available are disease-specific, and few have been formally assessed in the critical care setting for acceptability, reliability and validity. The Sickness Impact Profile[127] has been validated in 3655 Dutch intensive care patients six months after hospital discharge,[128] and the Short Form 36 (SF-36)[129] was found to be a robust tool when assessed in a smaller population of British adult intensive care patients.[130] Using SF-36, Ridley et al.[131] found that the pre-morbid quality of life of patients admitted to intensive care was not the same as in a normal population. They showed that patients who were previously fit and with a normal quality of life suffered significant decreases following their illness, while those with pre-existing ill health showed some improvement in quality of life six months after intensive care admission. Increasing severity of illness and length of intensive care stay were associated with decreases in quality of life after critical illness.

Targets

There is an urgent need for performance indicators to be agreed and introduced for critical care services. For intensive care patients, these should include the routine collection of data on:

- refused or delayed admissions
- transfers for non-clinical reasons
- premature discharges because of pressure on beds
- re-admissions following discharge to ward areas.

The National Intensive Care Bed Register collects data on bed availability, enquiries about possible transfers and transfers actually undertaken, but unfortunately the data are not robust enough to be of great value.

9 Information and research requirements

Information requirements

Information is required on the need for, the use of and the outcome from critical care in order to inform strategic planning at trust, regional and national level. It was noted earlier in this chapter that a paucity of such data had plagued previous attempts to review adult critical care services and that it still makes planning difficult. In part, this is because the need for critical care relates primarily to severity of illness rather than specific diagnoses (see Section 1) and so, until recently, was not captured in the diagnostic and activity-related information routinely collected by trusts. With the introduction of the mandatory Augmented Care Period (ACP) dataset[132] in October 1997, this situation has changed and a responsibility for critical care data collection now rests firmly with acute trusts. This was reinforced by the critical care modernisation programme,[11] which noted that only 63% of NHS trusts were complying with the ACP data collection and called for all trusts to do so.

The ACP dataset was introduced as an extension to the NHS Contract Minimum Dataset. Its function is to provide standardised data on intensive and high-dependency care activity to support contracting, internal management, national statistical analysis and policy development. Having been only recently introduced, there are currently concerns about the quality of the data and, despite being mandatory, it is still not universally collected. Also, because the dataset focuses on defined critical care areas and excludes general wards, it records only activity and not need. There needs to be a concerted effort to ensure that the ACP dataset is collected accurately and universally, as intended.

In March 1999, a twice-yearly national census of adult intensive care and high-dependency beds was introduced because of a lack of basic information in this area. This, the KH03a data, should provide further valuable information for policy and planning purposes.

Historically, most intensive care units have collected data on their activity for local use and, as well as basic demographics, this has usually included information about numbers and sources of admissions, interventions, length of stay and outcome. Some measure of severity of illness was usually included, most often using the APACHE II method. Unfortunately, since definitions were not standardised and data were collected by untrained, often very busy staff, the results were not comparable with those from other units and sometimes were of doubtful value even in-house.

In January 1994, the Intensive Care National Audit and Research Centre (ICNARC) was established, offering as its main audit activity a national Case Mix Programme for intensive care units. Under this Programme, data are collected by trained staff using standardised definitions, and with external validation. The result is a high-quality, comparative audit exercise providing valuable information on activity, case-mix and case-mix-adjusted outcome. At present, participation in the Case Mix Programme is not mandatory, and units have to pay an annual registration fee to take part – only about 60% of units in England and Wales participate.[11] It is important to ensure that, in the future, all units are registered with ICNARC and participate in the Case Mix Programme. This was reflected in the circular announcing the critical care modernisation programme,[11] which called for all trusts to join ICNARC.

To be of value, any data collected must be reliable and robust, and staff should be specifically identified for the purpose. This will require appropriate funding and should be recognised as a priority by commissioners.

Research priorities

A major criticism of intensive care practice is that, despite its rapid development over the past 50 years, it is not sufficiently underpinned by a firm basis of research. In 1996, a Department of Health working group[15] identified several areas requiring further work. It recommended that further research be undertaken to evaluate the outcome of intensive and high-dependency care. One of the difficulties, however, is that patients are perceived inevitably to have a poor outcome if denied intensive care. As a result, it is not considered ethical to conduct randomised controlled trials allocating patients arbitrarily to intensive care or to an alternative level of care in order to compare outcomes.

The group also recommended that work should be done to examine the role of nurses and other members of the multi-disciplinary team in intensive care and, in particular, to look at the relationship between patient dependency and the use of nursing resources.

In 1997, a joint Medical Research Council/Department of Health working party on intensive and high-dependency care highlighted the need for high-quality research and specifically identified five priority areas:

- the development and validation of risk-adjusted methods for adult, paediatric and neonatal intensive care and high-dependency care in order to be able validly to compare different models of care and to compare the performance of similar models of care
- the development of models for costing adult, paediatric and neonatal intensive and high-dependency care

- the evaluation and comparison of new and existing forms of care for adult, paediatric and neonatal intensive and high-dependency care
- the development of methods of needs assessment to identify the need for and appropriate targeting of adult, paediatric and neonatal intensive and high-dependency care and
- health technology assessment of specific interventions commonly used in adult, paediatric and neonatal intensive and high-dependency care.

Vella et al.[133] recently explored clinicians' views of research priorities in critical care, and reported that topics related to research into the organisation and delivery of critical care predominated, with less support for evaluation of specific healthcare technologies.

ICNARC has a key role in identifying and co-ordinating research needs and is currently involved in work relating to a number of the above points. This includes research into both adult and paediatric risk adjustment, and randomised controlled trials into the benefits of high-dependency care and the use of pulmonary artery catheters.

References

1 Intensive Care Society. Standards for intensive care units. London: Intensive Care Society, 1997.
2 Audit Commission. Questionnaire – Critical care services across the trust as a whole. London: Audit Commission, 1998.
3 Nightingale F. *Notes on hospitals.* (3e) London: Longman, Roberts and Green, 1863.
4 Sibbald W, Inman K. Problems in assessing the technology of intensive care. *Int J Technol Assess Health Care* 1992; **8**: 419–43.
5 Larsen H. A preliminary report on the 1952 epidemic of poliomyelitis in Copenhagen with special reference to the treatment of acute respiratory insufficiency. *The Lancet* 1953; **ii**: 37–41.
6 Bone R, McElwee N, Eubanks D, Gluck E. Analysis of indications for intensive care unit admission. Clinical efficacy project: American College of Physicians. *Chest* 1993; **104**: 1806–11.
7 Association of Anaesthetists of Great Britain and Ireland. Intensive care services – provision for the future. London: Association of Anaesthetists of Great Britain and Ireland, 1988.
8 King's Fund Panel. Intensive care in the United Kingdom: report from the King's Fund Panel. *Anaesthesia.* London: The King's Fund, 1989.
9 Wells W. Investigation into the neurosurgery patient transfers. London: South Thames Regional Health Authority, 1995.
10 Department of Health, 2000. Comprehensive critical care. Report of an Expert Group.
11 NHS Executive, 2000. Modernising critical care services, Health Service Circular 2000/017.
12 Metcalfe A, McPherson K. Study of provision of intensive care in England, 1993 – Revised report for Department of Health. London: London School of Hygiene and Tropical Medicine, 1995.
13 Dragsted L, Qvist J. Epidemiology of intensive care. *Int J Technol Assess Health Care* 1992; **8**: 395–407.
14 Audit Commission. *Critical to Success.* London: Audit Commission, 1999.
15 Department of Health. Guidelines on admission to and discharge from Intensive Care and High-dependency Units, 1996.
16 Association of Anaesthetists of Great Britain and Ireland. The high-dependency unit – acute care in the future. London: Association of Anaesthetists of Great Britain and Ireland, 1991.
17 Audit Commission. The provision of critical care services in England and Wales: survey results. London: Audit Commission, 1999.

18 Ridley S, Jones S, Shahani A, Brampton W, Nielsen M, Rowan K. Classification trees: a possible method for iso-resource grouping in intensive care. *Anaesthesia* 1998; **53(9)**: 833–40.

19 Bull A. Rationing intensive care. *BMJ* 1995; **310**: 1010.

20 Kilpatrick A, Ridley S, Plenderleith L. A changing role for intensive therapy: is there a case for high-dependency care? *Anaesthesia* 1994; **49**: 666–70.

21 Ridley B, Jackson R, Findlay J, Wallace P. Long term survival after intensive care. *BMJ* 1990; **301**: 1127–30

22 North Derbyshire HA. ITU Provision – discussion paper.

23 Rowan K, Kerr J, Major E, McPherson K, Short A, Vessey M. Intensive Care Society's APACHE II study in Britain and Ireland – I: variations in casemix of adult admissions to general intensive care units and impact on outcome. *BMJ* 1993; **307**: 972–77.

24 Department of Health. Paediatric Intensive Care: a framework for the future. London: National Co-ordinating Group on Paediatric Intensive Care, 1997.

25 Randolph A. Personal communication on the Internet *(Sent by Dr Jack Leach of West Yorkshire Health Authority)*, 1996.

26 British Paediatric Association. The care of critically ill children. Report of the multidisciplinary working party convened by the British Paediatric Association. London: British Paediatric Association, 1993.

27 Rowan K, Kerr J, Major E, McPherson K, Short A, Vessey M. Intensive Care Society's APACHE II study in Britain and Ireland – I: variations in casemix of adult admissions to general intensive care units and impact on outcome. *BMJ* 1993; **307**: 972–77.

28 Thompson F, Singer M. High-dependency units in the UK: variable size, variable character, few in number. *Postgrad Med J* 1995; **71**: 217–21.

29 St George's Healthcare. Doctors at St George's call for more intensive care beds and nurses: Press release, 1995.

30 Morgan G. Audit of use of Royal Cornwall Hospital ICU, using ACP definitions, 1999. Personal communication.

31 Pappachan J, Millar B, Barrett D, Smith G. Analysis of intensive care populations to select possible candidates for high-dependency care. *Accid Emerg Med* 1998; 15.

32 Crosby D, Rees G. Provision of postoperative care in UK hospitals. *Ann R Col Surg Engl* 1994; **76**: 14–18.

33 Ryan D, Bayly P, Weldon O, Jingree M. A prospective two-month audit of the lack of provision of a high-dependency unit and its impact on intensive care. *Anaesthesia* 1997; **52**: 265–75.

34 Thompson H, Spiers P. Occupancy of a teaching hospital adult intensive care unit by high-dependency patients. *Anaesthesia* 1998; **53**: 589–603.

35 Goldhill D, Summer A. Outcome of intensive care patients in a group of British intensive care units. *Crit Care Med* 1998; **26(8)**: 1337–45.

36 Rowan K, Kerr J, Major E, McPherson K, Short A, Vessey M. Intensive Care Society's APACHE II study in Britain and Ireland – II: outcome comparisons of intensive care units after adjustment for case mix by the American APACHE II method. *BMJ* 1993; **307**: 977–81.

37 Zimmerman J, Shortell S, Knaus W *et al.* Value and cost of teaching hospitals: a prospective, multicenter inception cohort study. *Critical Care Medicine* 1993; **21**: 1432–42.

38 Ridley S, Rowan K. Be wary of occupancy figures. *Health Trends* 1997; **29(4)**: 100–05.

39 Stoddart J. National ITU Audit 1992/1993: Royal College of Anaesthetists, 1993.

40 Ridley S. Intermediate care: possibilities, requirements and solutions. *Anaesthesia* 1998; **53**: 654–64.

41 Royal College of Anaesthetists, England RCoSo. Report of the Joint Working Party on Graduated Patient Care. London, 1996.

42 Boyd O, Grounds R, Bennett E. A randomised clinical trial of the effect of deliberate perioperative increase of oxygen delivery on mortality in high-risk surgical patients. *JAMA* 1993; **270**: 2699–707.

43 Wilson J, Woods I, Fawcett J, Whall R, Dibb W, Morris C *et al.* Reducing the risk of major elective surgery: randomised controlled trial of preoperative optimisation of oxygen delivery. *BMJ* 1999; **318**: 1099–103.

44 Treasure T, Bennett D. Reducing the risk of major elective surgery: optimising oxygen delivery before surgery does work; now we have to implement it. *BMJ* 1999; **318**: 1087–88.

45 Tzabar Y. Cancellation of major surgery due to lack of ITU beds. *Anaesthesia* 1998; **53**: 407.

46 Lyons RA, Wareham K, Hutchings H A, Major E, Ferguson B. Population requirement for adult critical-care beds: a prospective quantitative and qualitative study. *The Lancet* 2000; **355**: 595–98.

47 Metcalfe M, Sloggett A, McPherson K. Mortality among appropriately referred patients refused admission to intensive care units. *The Lancet* 1997; **350**: 7–11.

48 Mackenzie P, Smith E, Wallace P. Transfer of adults between intensive care units in the United Kingdom: postal survey. *BMJ* 1997; **314**: 1455–56.

49 Goldfrad C, Rowan K. Consequences of discharges from intensive care at night. *The Lancet* 2000; **355**: 1138–42.

50 Department of Health. Hospital Episode Statistics, 1999.

51 NHS Executive. Executive Letter: Introduction of the Augmented Care Period dataset. Leeds, 1997.

52 Donnelly P, Sandifer Q, O'Brien D, Thomas E. A pilot study of the use of clinical guidelines to determine appropriateness of patient placement on intensive and high-dependency care units. *J Public Health Med* 1995; **17**(3): 305–10.

53 Miranda DR, Ryan DW, Schaufeli WB, Fidler V (eds). *Organisation and management of intensive care.* Berlin: Springer-Verlag, 1998.

54 Niskanen M. Intensive care medicine in Finland. In: Miranda DR, Ryan DW, Schaufeli WB, Fidler V (eds). *Organisation and management of intensive care: a prospective study in 12 European countries.* Berlin: Springer-Verlag, 1998.

55 Strom J. Intensive care medicine in Denmark. In: Miranda DR, Ryan DW, Schaufeli WB, Fidler V (eds). *Organisation and management of intensive care: a prospective study in 12 European countries.* Berlin: Springer-Verlag, 1998.

56 Japichino G. Intensive care medicine in Italy. In: Miranda DR, Ryan DW, Schaufeli WB, Fidler V (eds). *Organisation and management of intensive care: a prospective study in 12 European countries.* Berlin: Springer-Verlag, 1998.

57 Alexander J. Intensive care medicine in Belgium. In: Miranda DR, Ryan DW, Schaufeli WB, Fidler V (eds). *Organisation and management of intensive care: a prospective study in 12 European countries.* Berlin: Springer-Verlag, 1998.

58 Hemmer M. Intensive care medicine in Luxembourg. In: Miranda DR, Ryan DW, Schaufeli WB, Fidler V (eds). *Organisation and management of intensive care: a prospective study in 12 European countries.* Berlin: Springer-Verlag, 1998.

59 Miranda D. Critically examining intensive care. *Int J Technol Assess Health Care* 1992; **8**: 444–56.

60 Zimmerman J, Knaus W, Judson J *et al.* Patient selection for intensive care: a comparison of New Zealand and United States hospitals. *Crit Care Med* 1988; **16**: 318–26.

61 Osborne M, Evans T. Allocation of resources in intensive care: a transatlantic perspective. *The Lancet* 1994; **343**: 778–80.

62 Edbrooke D, Hibbert C, Jacobs P. Health Economics in Intensive Care, 1998.

63 Ryan D. Intensive care medicine in the United Kingdom. In: Miranda DR, Ryan DW, Schaufeli WB, Fidler V (eds). *Organisation and management of intensive care: a prospective study in 12 European countries.* Berlin: Springer-Verlag, 1998.

64 Ridley S, Burchett K, Gunning K, Burns A, Kong A, Wright M *et al.* Heterogeneity in intensive care units: fact or fiction? *Anaesthesia* 1997; **52**: 531–37.

65 Parker A, Wyatt R, Ridley S. Intensive care services; a crisis of increased expressed demand. *Anaesthesia* 1998; **53**: 113–20.

66 Manara A, Pittman J, Braddon F. Reasons for withdrawing treatment in patients receiving intensive care. *Anaesthesia* 1998; **53**: 523–28.

67 Brown JJ, Sullivan G. Effect on ICU mortality of a full-time critical care specialist. *Chest* 1989; **96**: 127–29.

68 Reynolds HN, Haup MT, Thill-Baharozian MC, Carlson RW. Impact on critical care physician staffing on patients with septic shock in a university hospital medical intensive care unit. *JAMA* 1998; **260**: 3446–50.

69 Li TCM, Phillips MC, Shaw L, Cook EF, Natanson C, Goldman L. On-site physician staffing in the community hospital intensive care unit: Impact on test and procedure use and on patient outcome *JAMA* 1984; **252**: 2023–27.

70 Garfield M, Jeffrey R, Ridley S. An assessment of the staffing levels required for a high-dependency unit. *Anaesthesia* 2000; **55**: 137–43.

71 Ghorra S, Reinert SE, Cioffi W, Buczko G, Simms HH. Analysis of the effect of conversion from open to closed surgical intensive care unit. *Annals of Surgery* 1999; **229**: 163–71.

72 Hanson CW, Deutschmann CS, Anderson HL, Reilly PM, Behringer EC, Schwab CW, Price J. Effects of an organised critical care service on outcomes and resource utilisation: a cohort study. *Critical Care Medicine* 1999; **27**: 270–74.

73 Carson SS, Stocking C, Podsadecki T, Christenson J, Pohlman A, MacRae S, Jordan J, Humphrey H, Seigler M, Hall J. Effects of organisational change in the medical intensive care unit of a teaching hospital: a comparison of 'open' and 'closed' formats. *JAMA* 1996; **276**: 322–28.

74 Edbrooke D, Stevens V, Hibbert C, Mann A, Wilson A. A new method of accurately identifying costs of individual patients in intensive care: the initial results. *Intensive Care Med* 1997; **23**: 645–50.

75 Mennitz P. Patient data management systems in intensive care – the situation in Europe. *Intensive Care Medicine* 1995; **21**: 703–15.

76 Jegers M. Cost accounting in ICUs: beneficial for management and research. *Intensive Care Med* 1997; **23**: 618–19.

77 Jegers M. Finances. In: Miranda D, Ryan D, Schaufeli W, Fidler V (eds). *Organisation and management of intensive care: a prospective study in 12 European countries*. Berlin: Springer-Verlag, 1998.

78 Singer M, Myers S, Hall G, Cohen S, Armstrong R. The cost of intensive care: a comparison on one unit between 1988 and 1991. *Intensive Care Med* 1994; **20**: 542–49.

79 Edbrooke D, Hibbert C, Ridley S, Long T, Dickie H. The development of a method for comparative costing of individual intensive care units. *Anaesthesia* 1998; **54**: 110–20.

80 Ridley S, Biggam M, Stone P. Cost of intensive therapy. A description of methodology and initial results. *Anaesthesia* 1991; **46**: 523–30.

81 Edbrooke D, Hibbert C, Kingsley J, Smith S, Bright N, Quinn J. The patient-related costs of care for sepsis patients in a UK adult general intensive care unit. *Crit Care Med* 1999; **27**: 1760–7.

82 Edbrooke D. Personal communication, 1998.

83 Havill J. Charging for intensive care using direct nursing hours as the cost marker. *Anaesth intensive Care* 1997; **24(4)**: 372–77.

84 Ridley S, Biggam M, Stone P. A cost-benefit analysis of intensive therapy. *Anaesthesia* 1993; **48**:14–19.

85 Williams A. Foreword. In: Miranda D, Ryan D, Schaufeli W, Fidler V (eds). *Organisation and management of intensive care*. Berlin: Springer-Verlag, 1998.

86 Wijetunge A, Baldock G. Evidence-based intensive care medicine. *Anaesthesia* 1998; **53**: 419–21.

87 Cook D, De Jonghe B, Brochard L, Brun-Buisson C. Influence of airway management on ventilator-associated pneumonia. Evidence from randomised trials. *JAMA* 1998: 781–87.

88 Cook D, Guyatt G, Marshall J, Leasa D, Fuller H, Hall R, Peters S, Rutledge F, Griffith L, McLellan A, Wood G, Kirby A. Canadian Critical Care Trials Group. A comparison of sucralfate and ranitidine for the prevention of upper gastrointestinal bleeding in patients requiring mechanical ventilation. *NEJM* 1998; **338**: 791–97.

89 Kollef M, Shapiro S, Silver P *et al.* A randomised controlled trial of protocol-directed versus physician-directed weaning from mechanical ventilation. *Crit Care Med* 1997; **25**: 56–74.

90 Ely E, Baker A, Dunagan D *et al.* Effect on the duration of mechanical ventilation of identifying patients capable of breathing spontaneously. *NEJM* 1996; **335**: 1864–69.

91 D'Amico R, Pifferi S, Leonetti C, Torri V, Tinazzi A, Liberati A. Effectiveness of antibiotic prophylaxis in critically ill adult patients: Systematic review of randomised controlled trials. *BMJ* 1998; **316**: 1275–85.

92 Takala J, Ruokonen E, Webster NR, Neilsen MS, Zandstra DF, Vundelinckx G, Hinds CJ. Increased mortality associated with growth hormone treatment in critically ill adults. *NEJM* 1999; **341**: 785–92.

93 The Acute Respiratory Distress Syndrome Network. Ventilation with lower tidal volumes as compared with traditional tidal volumes for acute lung injury and the acute respiratory distress syndrome. *NEJM* 2000 (in press).

94 Atkinson S, Bihari D, Smithies M, Daly K, Mason R, McColl I. Identification of futility in intensive care. *The Lancet* 1994; **344**: 1203–06.

95 Daly K, Smithies M, Everington R, Bihari D. Presentation at ICS Scientific meeting, Dublin, 1994.

96 Gilbertson AA, Smith JM, Mostafa SM. The cost of an intensive care unit: a prospective study. *Intensive Care Medicine* 1991; **17**: 204–08.

97 Ridley S, Biggam M, Stone P. A cost-utility analysis of intensive therapy II: Quality of life in survivors. *Anaesthesia* 1994; **49**: 192–96.

98 Stockwell M. Intensive care is not expensive compared with other treatments. *BMJ* 1999; **319**: 516.

99 Wallace P, Lawler P. Regional intensive care unit transfer teams are needed. *BMJ* 1997; **314**: 369.

100 Scheinhorn DJ, Artinian BM, Catlin JL. Weaning from prolonged mechanical ventilation. The experience of a regional weaning center. *Chest* 1994; **105**: 534–39.

101 Gracey DR, Naessens JM, Viggiano RW, Koenig GE, Silverstein MD, Hubmayr RD. Outcome of patients cared for in a ventilator-dependent unit in a general hospital. *Chest* 1995; **107**: 494–99.

102 Scheinhorn DJ, Chao DC, Stearn-Hassenpflug M, LaBree LD, Heltsley DJ. Post-ICU mechanical ventilation. Treatment of 1123 patients at a regional weaning center. *Chest* 1997; **111**: 1654–59.

103 Dasgupta A, Rice R, Mascha E, Litaker D, Stoller JK. Four-year experience with a unit for long-term ventilation (respiratory special care unit) at the Cleveland Clinic Foundation. *Chest* 1999; **116**: 447–55.

104 Field D, Goldstone JC. Personal communication.

105 Lee A, Bishop G, Hillman KM, Daffurn K. The medical emergency team. *Anaesth Intensive Care* 1995; **23**: 183–86.

106 McGloin H, Adam SK, Singer M. Unexpected deaths and referrals to intensive care of patients on general wards. Are some cases potentially avoidable? *J R Coll Physicians* London 1999; **33**: 255–259.

107 Goldhill DR, Mulcahy AJ, Tarling MM, Worthington LM, Singh SR, White SA, Sumner A. Patients admitted to the ICU from the wards: effect of the patient at risk team. *Brit J Anaesth* 1998; **81**: 812P–13P

108 Goldhill DR, Worthington L, Mulcahy A, Tarling, M, Sumner A. The patient-at-risk team: identifying and managing seriously ill ward patients. *Anaesthesia* 1999; **54**: 853–60.

109 Fletcher SJ, Flabouris A. The patient-at-risk team. *Anaesthesia* 2000; **55**: 198.

110 Mercer M, Fletcher SJ, Bishop GF. Suboptimal ward care of critically ill patients. Medical emergency teams improve care. *BMJ* 1992; **318(7175)**: 54–55.

111 Bion J. Cost containment: Europe. The United Kingdom. *New Horizons* 1994; **2**: 341–44.

112 Leeson-Payne C, Aitkenhead A. A prospective study to assess the demand for a high-dependency unit. *Anaesthesia* 1995; **50**: 383–87.

113 Ryan D. Rationing intensive care. High-dependency units may be the answer. *BMJ* 1995; **310**: 1010–11.

114 Wallis C, Davies H, Shearer A. Why do patients die on general wards after discharge from intensive care units? *Anaesthesia* 1997; **52**: 9–14.

115 Royal College of Anaesthetists, England RCoSo. Report of the Joint Working Party on Graduated Patient Care. London, 1996.

116 Fox AJ, Owen-Smith O, Spiers P. The immediate impact of opening an adult high-dependency unit on intensive care occupancy. *Anaesthesia* 1999; **54**: 280–83.

117 Dhond G, Ridley S, Palmer M. The impact of a high-dependency unit on the workload of an intensive care unit. *Anaesthesia* 1998; **53**: 841–47.

118 Parker A, Wyatt R, Ridley S. Intensive care services; a crisis of increased expressed demand. *Anaesthesia* 1998; **53**: 113–20.

119 Peacock J, Edbrooke D. Rationing intensive care. Data from one high-dependency unit supports their effectiveness. *BMJ* 1995; **310**: 1413.

120 Department of Health and Social Security. Hospital building note (HBN) 27 – intensive therapy unit. London, 1970.

121 The Royal College of Anaesthetists. Guidelines for the provision of anaesthetic services. London, 1999.

122 Lyons RA, Wareham K, Hutchings HA, Major E. Ferguson B. Population requirement for adult critical care beds: a prospective quantitative and qualitative study. *Lancet* 2000 Feb 19; **355(9204)**: 595–98.

123 Shahani AK, Brailsford SC, Roy RB. HIV and AIDS patient care. Operational models for resource planning. In: Kaplan EH, Brandeau ML (eds). *Modelling the AIDS epidemic: planning policy and prediction*. New York: Raven Press Ltd, 1994.

124 Ridge J, Jones S, Nielsen M, Shahani A. Capacity planning for intensive care units. *Eur J Operational Res* 1998; **105**: 346–55.

125 Shahani AK. Reasonable averages that give wrong answers. Teaching statistics 1981; **3**: 50–54.

126 Djaiani G, Ridley S. Outcome of intensive care in the elderly. *Anaesthesia* 1997; **52**: 1130–36.

127 Bergner M, Bobbitt RA, Kressel S, Pollard WE, Gilson BS, Morris JR. The sickness impact profile: development and final revision of a health status measure. *Med Care* 1981; **19**: 787–805.

128 Tian ZM, Miranda DR. Quality of life after intensive care with the sickness impact profile. *Intensive Care Medicine* 1995; **21**: 422–28.

129 Ware JE. SF-36 health survey manual and interpretation guide. Boston: The Medical Outcomes Trust, 1993.

130 Chrispin PS, Scotton H, Rogers J, Lloyd D, Ridley SA. Short Form 36 in the intensive care unit: assessment of acceptability, reliability and validity of the questionnaire. *Anaesthesia* 1997; **52**: 15–23.

131 Ridley S, Chrispin P, Scotton H, Rogers J, Lloyd D. Changes in quality of life after intensive care: comparison with normal data. *Anaesthesia* 1997; **52**: 195–202.

132 Intensive and high-dependency care data collection. Department of Health, London. March 1997.

133 Vella K, Goldfrad C, Rowan K, Bron J, Black N. Use of consensus development to establish national research priorities in critical care. *BMJ* 2000; **320**: 976–80.

Acknowledgements

The authors would like to thank the following for their help in the preparation of this chapter:

- Nuffield Trust
- Lucy McCullough and Sam Jackson, *Audit Commission*
- Claire O'Connor, *ICBIS North West Region*
- Emergency Bed Service
- David Edbrooke and Claire Hibbert, *Medical Economics and Research Centre, Sheffield*
- Giles Morgan, *Royal Cornwall Hospital Trust*
- Val Chishty, *Department of Health*
- Caroline Goldfrad and Kathy Rowan, *ICNARC*
- Paul Lawlor, President, *Intensive Care S*

2 Continence

Catherine W McGrother and Madeleine Donaldson*

1 Summary

Statement of the problem

Urinary incontinence is the main symptom of disordered storage of urine as distinct from disordered voiding. It represents several underlying conditions within a classification of diseases of the bladder which needs further development. The two main disorders featuring incontinence are overactive bladder, involving urge incontinence, and sphincter incompetence, involving stress incontinence. However, there are substantial overlaps with conditions such as dementia and stroke, particularly in elderly people, and for those with discrete neurological disorders and long-term disabilities including MS, and learning disability.

The two most important recent issues in relation to service provision have been (i) the extent of need related to incontinence, in view of symptom prevalence reports ranging up to two-thirds of the population in women and (ii) the effectiveness of a nurse-led service crossing the primary/secondary care interface. These issues have been comprehensively addressed over the last few years by a research programme funded by the MRC with DoH support. This review includes insights from this research which is still ongoing.

The role of the GP in assessment and management of the underlying condition is hampered by a lack of information, training and experience and the lack of an integrated specialist service. Further issues, where more information is needed to develop policy, concern the best management of people with overlapping conditions, e.g. stroke, MS and learning disability, who already receive specialist input of various kinds. One of the longer-term issues concerns the merits of extending an integrated incontinence services to include all disorders of the bladder and its outlet, in view of the extensive overlap between storage and voiding symptoms and the uncertainty about the distinctions between underlying conditions and about the management of prostatic enlargement.

* The following people also contributed to this chapter:
RP Assassa, Consultant Urogynaecologist, Mid-Yorkshire Hospital NHS Trust and Honorary Senior Lecturer, Department of Epidemiology and Public Health, University of Leicester; TA Hayward, Research Assistant, Department of Epidemiology and Public Health, University of Leicester; G Matharu, Specialist Registrar in Obstetrics and Gynaecology, Leicester General Hospital; DA Turner, Research Associate in Health Economics, Trent Institute for Health Services Research, Department of Epidemiology and Public Health, University of Leicester; A Wagg, Consultant in Geriatrics, Care of the Elderly Department, University College Hospital, London; J Warsame, Specialist Registrar in Public Health Medicine, Department of Epidemiology and Public Health, University of Leicester; JM Watson, Research Associate, Department of Epidemiology and Public Health, University of Leicester; KS Williams, Senior Nursing Research Fellow, Department of Epidemiology and Public Health, University of Leicester.

Sub-categories

Storage disorder signifies the totality of clinically recognised abnormal storage symptoms including incontinence, urgency, frequency and nocturia. Incontinence serves as the main epidemiological indicator and has two commonly recognised levels of severity – any and moderate/monthly. At primary care level the syndrome of *overactive bladder* is commonly represented by the symptoms of urgency, including urge incontinence, often occurring in association with frequency and nocturia. Similarly, *sphincter incompetence* is commonly represented by the symptom of *stress incontinence*.

The ICD-10 codes (*see* **Table 2**) encompass all the conditions associated with incontinence but the sub-categories lack coherence. The International Continence Society reflects current thinking in re-organising the main sub-categories as *detrusor overactivity* (DO) with idiopathic and neurogenic components, and *urodynamic stress incontinence* (USI). Less common categories involving incontinence in men include chronic retention of urine with overflow, mostly due to prostatic enlargement and post-micturition dribble due to abnormal relaxation of the external sphincter.

Health care need is defined in terms of objectively defined abnormal storage symptoms and impact on life. *Felt need* is defined more subjectively in terms of apparent motivation to obtain help indicated by either using services or wanting help. *Health care requirement* represents felt need within the context of the defined health care need.

Prevalence and incidence

The results of a systematic review of UK studies suggest that bladder malfunction is very common, often distressing for the individual and represents a major public health problem in the UK that may be increasing over time. Incontinence and other storage symptoms should be conceptualised as disorder of the bladder on a par with and indeed related to other organ systems of the body and deserve similar consideration for research and service development.

Across a range of UK studies, the prevalence of any incontinence averages out at around 40% for women and 10% for men. Incontinence with impact on life is estimated around 30% for women. For those aged 40 or more, storage disorder as a whole affects around 39% of women and 29% of men. This represents considerably more men than are affected by incontinence alone (**Table 1**). These results are consistent with findings from around the world and the current MRC programme of research. There were no published UK studies available that estimated the full extent of felt need in relation to storage disorder. We estimate this at 25% in women and 18% in men within the previous year, indicating the level of health care requirement. These levels cannot be ascribed to measurement error or uncertainty over thresholds. They appear high in relation to other individual conditions partly because incontinence/storage disorder represents several common conditions affecting the bladder. There is an overall increase in prevalence of symptoms with age in both women and men but the latter start from a lower base after childhood, increasing to similar levels in old age. Women experience a peak of prevalence around menopause, due to stress incontinence. The rise seen in elderly people is related to urge incontinence. These two types of incontinence place very different demands on services, especially with regard to surgery. Overall, the prevalence of need increases with age and the major problem is apparent in old age, equally among men and women.

Table 1: Urinary incontinence and storage disorder: prevalence, impact and use of services from UK studies – 1960–2001.

	Average prevalence % (range in studies)[a]	
	Women	Men
Storage disorder[d]	39 (–)	29 (–)
Incontinence (minor)[d]	40 (16–69)	10 (8–25)
Incontinence (monthly)	12 (8–23)	5 (3–9)
Nocturia (2+)	15 (14–26)	15 (14–20)
Frequency (hourly)	9 (–)	5 (–)
Urgency (difficulty)	9 (6–9)	5 (3–5)
Impact – any[d]	30 (17–44)	12[b] (11–12)
– more than a little	8 (8–30)	4 (3–6)
Consultation	6 (2–11)	3 (1–7)
Want help/uptake on offer[c]	5 (4–9)	4 (3–4)

[a] Estimated from graphs.
[b] Elderly ages only.
[c] Indicator of unmet need.
[d] Indicator of health care need.

The prevalence of incontinence is 2–3 times higher in residential care and hospitals and among people with severe disabilities of various kinds than in the general population. Incontinence probably operates as a selection factor but it could deteriorate as a result of institutional care.

The incidence of incontinence suggests three distinct peaks in women – early reproductive age, menopause and old age with rates ranging between 6–22% for women and half this for men. The natural history suggests a marked tendency to fluctuation with elements of both remission and progression. There are clear associations with pregnancy/parity, obesity and cognitive impairment, and fairly consistent relationships with stroke and depression.

Services available and their costs

Division of care between professionals is complex, with varied models of service around the country. Patients may present to GPs or go directly (or indirectly) to continence nurses in the community. They may be treated extensively within primary care with behavioural and medical therapies or be referred at an early stage to specialists, including neurologists, geriatricians, urologists and gynaecologists. In relation to health service pathways for incontinence, most younger women are referred to gynaecologists whereas most older men and women are referred to physicians for the elderly; whilst for voiding problems most men are referred to urologists. Continence nurses of various kinds play a considerable role in managing the problem but the nature and extent of provision is very variable across the country. Community nurses are often the first port of call for patients with incontinence. They may make the initial in-depth assessment and are often involved in providing some degree of behavioural therapy for the common disorders and long-term aids for intractable conditions.

Primary care

The key issues in the provision of appropriate services to date have been the level of interest in continence on the part of the health care provider, the fragmented approach to provision of specialised services in secondary care and the variable nature of provision. This variation in service delivery affects patient outcomes. Interventions available in primary care include giving general advice, behavioural and lifestyle changes, pelvic floor muscle training, bladder training and drug treatment, all of which form the mainstay of the conservative management of urinary incontinence. Pelvic floor muscle training is usually reserved for individuals with stress incontinence and occasionally urge incontinence. The latter is more commonly treated with bladder training or drug therapy.

Secondary care

The interventions in primary care may also be introduced in the secondary care setting, where assessment and treatment may be provided by any one of a number of clinical specialists with or without specialist nursing or physiotherapist support. It is in secondary care that facilities such as urodynamic investigation are available to diagnose the underlying abnormality, as well as a more multidisciplinary approach to care.

Surgery is clearly within the remit of secondary care and plays a major part in the treatment of urodynamic stress incontinence. Over 100 operative techniques have been described to treat this condition. Colposuspension is currently regarded as the gold standard procedure. Surgery is generally performed in those cases where conservative measures, such as pelvic floor muscle training have failed. However, surgical therapies for urodynamic stress incontinence are relatively expensive and not without complications.

Health care utilisation

Official statistics indicate that 36/10 000 of the population per annum consult a GP for incontinence; however, this represents only 7% of adults who self-report such consultations. The corresponding level of hospital episodes is 14/10 000 p.a. and the level of surgery is 2/10 000 p.a. In primary care the pattern of recognised consultation reflects that in the community in relation to age and sex. However, hospital episode rates are disproportionately high for elderly men compared to women. Hospital episode rates remained stable overall in recent years but within this there has been a substantial increase in the rates for elderly people. Whether this reflects trends in admission or more people developing incontinence during a hospital episode is unknown. The majority of surgery is carried out on women mostly around the time of menopause. This pattern reflects the high peak in mild/moderate incontinence in the community. However, surgical rates are too small to account for much of the sharp decline in prevalence following menopause. There has been a steady increase in the number of prescriptions for drugs used exclusively for incontinence in recent years. An estimated 1.6 million such prescriptions are dispensed per year. The MRC Incontinence Study estimates 6.2% of people aged 40+ are using incontinence aids of some kind.

Costs

The overall annual cost to the UK of urinary incontinence was estimated in 1998 by the Continence Foundation to be £353.6 million. This does not include patient-borne financial costs and estimates from elsewhere in the world would suggest considerably higher levels. However, one study has estimated NHS and patient-borne costs in women to be £37 (1995) for a three-month period. Patients also bear other types of costs such as discomfort and embarrassment, disruptions to usual activities and disruption of social life. These costs are difficult to quantify but the concept of 'Willingness to Pay' in relation to urinary incontinence provides some indication. Estimates in the region of £18 per month for a reduction in symptoms indicate the level of importance to the individual.

Effectiveness of services and interventions

There is clear evidence in the literature showing the benefit of pelvic floor exercises and bladder training, both in primary and secondary care. Drug treatment, which is mainly aimed at patients with detrusor overactivity, is also effective but has been hampered by unacceptable side effects. The introduction of newer, more effective drugs is addressing this problem, but they are much more expensive. As with many other areas of health care, there is very limited evidence of the cost-effectiveness of any interventions in primary care.

Surgery provides differing cure/improvement rates for urodynamic stress incontinence. Despite the large number of studies published, the quality of trials comparing different techniques has been criticised. Surgery is expensive and is associated with morbidity and mortality. It is therefore essential that treatments are evaluated properly before being introduced into everyday practice. Furthermore, outcome is related to the experience of the surgeon. Once again, there is little evidence of the cost-effectiveness of surgery for incontinence.

Quantified models of care/recommendations

As outlined in the previous two sections, there are considerable inconsistencies in current continence care available to the population. What is lacking is co-ordination of continence care. Continence nurse practitioners can not only provide this co-ordination, but also deliver these services in primary care with effect and high levels of patient satisfaction. A new model of care is proposed based on current research. The new ideal service would span the primary and secondary care interface, with Continence Nurse Practitioners (CNPs) bridging the gap and leading and co-ordinating the service. The CNPs would provide much of the care in the community with an emphasis on conservative interventions, e.g. bladder retraining and pelvic floor muscle exercises, thereby reducing referrals to secondary care. They would be part of a multidisciplinary team along with other health care professionals, such as GPs, surgical specialists and physicians. The service would be structured around evidence-based protocols, regular audit and quality assurance systems, in order to ensure the delivery of high quality care.

Within this context there is considerable consensus about the main issues that need to be addressed in order to improve services including:

- raising public awareness to remediable symptoms of bladder disorder and overcoming the lack of knowledge and reticence of patients, particularly elderly women, with this highly stigmatising and neglected condition
- employing standard identification and assessment procedures in primary care to assist professionals in identifying and not discouraging appropriate people who need to access services, including those in residential care
- training and expansion of the primary care workforce to provide first line therapy including bladder training, pelvic floor exercises and behavioural interventions in accordance with evidence-based best practice
- developing an integrated service including specialist continence nurses, urology, uro-gynaecology and gerontology that bridges the primary/secondary interface to minimise confusion over referral pathways and to rationalise the use of expertise.

Patient outcomes, audit tools, information and future research

Urinary incontinence is associated with significant psychological distress and poor quality of life. It is therefore necessary to assess symptoms and impact on patients' lives to establish the need for services and to evaluate outcomes. A variety of questionnaires exist which variously assess urinary incontinence symptoms, lower urinary tract symptoms and impact on quality of life, with some designed specifically for use in clinical trials.

Evidence-based audit tools have been developed to promote the quality of incontinence services in primary and secondary services.

The Working Group on Outcome Indicators for Urinary Incontinence has identified indicators that are routinely available from health care data or periodic surveys and some which require further development.

Until very recently, research concerning the bladder received very little investment in the UK or around the world. Consequently the levels of understanding and conceptual development are at an early stage. There is a lack of any long-term infrastructure to maximise contributions from around the country in building a coherent evidence base for innovative forms of management and prevention.

Future research needs to focus on providing an evidence base for preventive action; investigating mechanisms for dual diagnoses, e.g. depression as a basis for innovative therapeutic development; improving access and equality in the use of services; development and evaluation of services, especially those for elderly and disabled people; plus the development of a comprehensive classification and related non-invasive assessment and diagnostic tools.

2 Introduction and statement of the problem

This chapter contains an interpretation of the evidence concerning appropriate levels of NHS provision and treatment for urinary incontinence and related symptoms in adults. The broad questions addressed include:

- What is the level of need for services?
- What are the roles of primary and secondary services?
- How effective are the medical and surgical treatments available?
- What are the costs of treatment?
- What overall level of provision should be commissioned for urinary incontinence among adults?

Urinary incontinence has been defined as the involuntary loss of urine.[1] This concept has served to highlight a substantial but neglected, indeed taboo, subject and stimulated varied development of services across the country. In itself, however, incontinence is only one symptom of disordered storage of urine. It indicates a number of underlying conditions which are themselves only partially conceptualised at present. Nevertheless, abnormal symptoms may be useful markers of the pattern of disease in the population.

The bladder is a relatively complex system of the body because, although it operates largely autonomously, we are obliged to learn and maintain voluntary control of its functioning. Thus a wide range of neurological and mental disorders make considerable contributions to the nature of bladder dysfunction. The lower urinary tract differs markedly between females and males and is subject to the different risks of childbirth and prostatic enlargement. Physical disability and acute disorders have additional implications for maintenance of continence, even when the bladder functions within normal limits, because of the necessity of accessing a toilet and adjusting clothing.

The manner in which lower urinary tract (LUT) disorder tends to be subdivided in relation to service provision is necessarily complex. It owes something to the specific underlying conditions in so far as they are perceived and to the range of client groups involved. Classifications abound, suggesting that none integrate all the various dimensions and few capture the difference in perspective between primary and secondary care. **Figure 1** represents a system based on underlying condition but arranged to illustrate the main health service orientations. All the disorders may present as incontinence and other storage symptoms. Common general conditions such as immobility and acute confusion also impinge on the overall functioning of the bladder/nervous system, particularly in old age. Currently the commonest disorders of the LUT are conceptualised in terms of function or structure rather than the inter-related pathology. This represents a relatively early stage of development compared with other systems of the body.[2]

NERVOUS SYSTEM	BLADDER	GENERAL HEALTH
– dementia – stroke *(elderly)*	overactive bladder *(elderly/urology)*	frailty *(elderly)*
– Parkinson's disease – multiple sclerosis – spinal injury *(neurology)*	sphincter incompetence *(gynaecology)*	urinary tract infection *(primary care)*
– diabetes + neuropathy *(general medicine)*	prostatic enlargement *(urology)*	long-term disability *(e.g. learning disability/ psychiatry)*

Figure 1: Lower urinary tract disorder – a public health classification (*main service orientation*).

The difficulty faced by commissioners in the case of incontinence is defining what level of severity is significant and the appropriate boundaries for an integrated service. The challenges for service planning and delivery also include:

1 determining the extent of need, taking into account significant symptoms, the impact on people's lives and personal goals, the attendant stigma and low expectations;
2 getting people to come forward with their problem; and primary care recognising and responding appropriately to the problem;
3 identifying the appropriate structured care pathways for patients to make use of available resources;
4 determining the roles of the parties involved in providing care, including general practitioners (GPs), nurses and consultants and the corresponding levels of expertise and degrees of specialisation required;
5 organising secondary care teams and clinics to provide essential multidisciplinary advice and avoid duplication of costly resources such as cystometry;
6 determining the effectiveness of modern treatments;
7 deciding on the indications for surgery, what type of specialist should do it and what procedures should be used;
8 developing approaches to prevention/early intervention;
9 addressing priorities in terms of how far to treat those most able to benefit, those most liable to deteriorate and those in the worst state of health.

Available evidence from epidemiological research, evaluative studies and economic analysis will be presented in this chapter. This information, together with guidance on best practice, will be considered and analysed as a basis for advice on commissioning services. However, it is important to acknowledge that although a considerable amount of research has been carried out, its contribution is limited by the lack of development of appropriate conceptual frameworks (including diagnostic classification and thresholds for symptom severity and need) and well designed studies and trials. Hopefully this review will help to reduce the uncertainty, but there is still along way to go to obtain a clear picture of disorders of the bladder and appropriate services.

3 Sub-categories

Urinary incontinence as a whole does not have a specific code in the International Classification of Diseases (ICD). Details of the diagnostic codes of all relevant underlying conditions are shown in **Table 2**.

Table 2: Relevant diagnostic ICD-10 codes.[3]

Code	Diagnosis
N31.0	Uninhibited neuropathic bladder, not elsewhere classified
N31.1	Reflex neuropathic bladder, not elsewhere classified
N31.2	Flaccid neuropathic bladder, not elsewhere classified
	Neuropathic bladder: atonic (motor, sensory)
	autonomous
	non-reflex
N31.8	Other neuromuscular dysfunction of the bladder
N31.9	Neuromuscular dysfunction of the bladder, unspecified
N32.2	Vesical fistula, not elsewhere classified (excludes fistula between bladder and female genital tract)
N39.3	Stress incontinence
N39.4	Overflow, reflex, urge incontinence
N82.0	Vesico-vaginal fistula
N82.1	Cervico-vaginal, uretero-vaginal, urethro-vaginal fistulae
R32	Unspecified urinary incontinence
	Enuresis not otherwise specified
R39	Extravasation of urine*
F98.0	Non-organic enuresis

From the perspective of clinical management, particularly in primary care, LUT disorders are currently thought of as either a problem of storage or voiding (*see* Appendix 1). Here the notion of storage disorder includes incontinence but also the other commonly associated symptoms of urgency, frequency and nocturia.[1] Storage disorder includes the predominant sub-groups of patients with sphincter incompetence and overactive bladder. To a fair extent, these relate to the underlying categories of urodynamic stress incontinence (USI) and detrusor overactivity (DO), respectively. (The notion of voiding disorder includes bladder outlet obstruction with symptoms of hesitancy, straining, slow stream, spraying, terminal dribble and intermittency. It includes primarily the underlying condition of prostatic enlargement.) The division between storage and voiding is useful, but not entirely coherent because, for example, chronic obstruction with retention of urine leads to overflow incontinence.

Storage symptoms represent an objectively defined element of normative need, as perceived by professionals.[4] However, there is variation in symptom severity and in the concept of normality in the general population. In this context especially, the definition of need for health care must take account of the impact on the individual. Impact is a concept we will define in two main ways: (i) overall or *general impact* using global terms such as 'problematic'; (ii) disabling or *specific* impact using *interference* with important area of life, including activities, feelings/well-being, quality of life and relationships. Symptoms and impact are indicators of the *health care need*[5] for therapeutic services, and may be applied to incontinence or storage symptoms as a whole. The unusual degree of stigma and coping attached to incontinence may lead this to be an underestimate of the true extent of health care need. The *felt need* for help is used here to indicate the likely motivation to use services assuming basic awareness of their existence.[4] It is indicated by the individual reporting that they sought or want help. In relation to symptoms and impact it represents the priority or extent of *health care requirement* for therapeutic services.[6]

Operation codes for procedures that may be carried out for conditions involving incontinence are shown in **Table 3**.

Table 3: OPCS operation codes: relevant OPCS operation codes, 4th revision (April 1988 onwards).[7]

Code	Procedure
M51.1	Abdominoperineal suspension of urethra
M51.2	Endoscopic suspension of bladder neck
M52.1	Suprapubic sling operation
M52.2	Retropubic suspension of bladder neck
M52.3	Colposuspension
M53.1	Vaginal buttressing of urethra
M53.8	Tension-free vaginal tape insertion
M55.2	Artificial urethral sphincter insertion (female)
M56.3	Periurethral collagen injection
M64.2	Artificial urethral sphincter insertion (male)
M65.1	Endoscopic resection of prostate using electrotome
M65.2	Endoscopic resection of prostate using punch
M65.3	Endoscopic resection of prostate
P25.1	Repair of vesicovaginal fistula
P25.4	Repair of ureterovaginal fistula
A70.1	Implantation of neurostimulator into peripheral nerve (sacral nerve implant)

4 Prevalence and incidence

A literature search was carried out to identify all papers on the prevalence of urinary incontinence and related storage symptoms in the UK published since 1960. The electronic sources were Medline and Embase. Keywords employed were 'urinary disorders', 'epidemiology', 'prevalence' and 'UK' or 'Great Britain'. The search was limited to English language papers. Index medicus was searched for relevant publications between 1960 and 1966 using 'urinary disorders' and 'urinary incontinence' headings.

References from located publications were examined for further prevalence papers and an author search was also undertaken.

Thresholds for incontinence are based on a general consensus present in the UK literature. In essence this distinguishes minor or any leakage from moderate or monthly leakage whilst major leakage denotes a more severe level. Variations are grouped under these thresholds on the basis of either similar terminology (any, ever, yearly) or a notional average frequency × volume (**Table 4**).

Table 4: Standardised incontinence thresholds (ratings) based on the UK literature.

Minor (1)	Moderate (2)	Major (3)
any × leakage	monthly × leakage	monthly × damp/wet/soaked
ever × leakage	any × damp/wet/soaked	weekly × leakage/damp/wet/soaked
yearly × leakage	ever × damp/wet/soaked	daily × leakage/damp/wet/soaked
	yearly × damp/wet/soaked	

Estimates for minor leakage for all adults average out at around 40% for women and 10% for men; for moderate incontinence at around 12% for women and 5% for men; and for major leakage at around 5% for women and 3% for men (**Figure 2**). Moderate incontinence shows an overall increase with age affecting around 5% in younger women and 20% in old age, compared to around 2% in younger men and 10% in old age. Major incontinence shows a similar but lower prevalence pattern. However, in women the pattern for minor leakage shows substantial increases across the reproductive period to a high peak around the time of menopause. This has no parallel with minor incontinence in men, which follows the same age-related pattern of moderate and major incontinence. The majority of studies in the UK show an increase in moderate incontinence after the age of 70, affecting around 17% of women and 12% of men. However, the prevalence in older people is probably underestimated in many cases because of exclusion of those in care homes and non-response bias.

The main methodological features of all UK studies are summarised in order of prevalence in **Table A2.1(a)**. It is most apparent that higher prevalence is associated with milder severity of incontinence both between and within studies. The average female to male ratio of prevalence for all studies was 1.9 but was higher in studies involving younger subjects (2.5) compared to those confined to old age (1.5). In order to identify methodological and other factors associated with the prevalence of urinary incontinence, univariate and multivariate meta-regression models were generated in relation to age, date, response rate, number of prompts and type of study, with prevalence weighted for study size. Models were generated separately in men and women for each severity rating using $p < 0.05$ to indicate significance.

In addition to gender, severity and age, meta-regression identified significant associations with number of prompts and response rate. The length of time since the study was published was also significant for increasing prevalence. There was little apparent relationship with study region or sample type. In the early stages of research development, some learning and therefore increase in prevalence is to be expected. However, controlling for the number of questions or prompts on incontinence should take account of this to a large extent. Therefore, it is possible that a genuine increase has occurred over time. This would be consistent with known increases occurring to recognised co-morbidities for incontinence, e.g. obesity.

Recently, the focus has moved to include other significant storage symptoms (nocturia, urgency, frequency and bladder pain) within overall prevalence estimates. The effect is illustrated in a recent MRC study where monthly incontinence in women affected 20% whilst storage symptoms affected 39%. The prevalence also doubled for men from 9% to 20%.[8] Studies of storage disorder in older people suggest the prevalence is similar in men and women and doubles between 70 and over 809. Increasingly in the future, services are likely to be oriented towards levels of storage symptoms as a whole.

The results of this review are consistent with studies of urinary incontinence from around the world. The prevalence of any incontinence across a variety of ages ranged from 10–71.9% for women and 3.4–19.6% for men. For moderate incontinence, the range was 6.5–46% for women and 8.5–15% for men (*see* Appendix 2).

Relatively few studies have included the other individual storage symptoms of nocturia, frequency and urgency.[8,10–13] Overall, there is some comparability between studies for each symptom but only nocturia is consistently defined across several studies (**Table A2.2**). Nocturia at the level of twice a night is reported consistently between studies and averages out at around 15% for men and women. It increases markedly between young and old, around four-fold in women and ten-fold in men. However, at age 75+ the prevalence of nocturia (twice a night) averages out similarly for men and women at around 35–40%.

Frequency was captured in several ways, length of interval between micturitions, number of micturitions in a day, as well as on the basis of change in pattern and without specification. Estimates for specified frequency suggest a slight overall increase with age in both men and women. There is inconsistency between studies as to whether the prevalence is higher in men or women. However, the largest and most recent study suggests slightly higher rates in women.[8]

Urgency was also defined in a variety of ways. Those that included expressions of 'difficulty' or 'inability' were grouped as more severe than those described in terms of 'hurrying' or 'having control'. Estimates for specified urgency suggest an increase with age, particularly old age, and slightly higher levels in women.

Prevalence among elderly people in institutional care

In the UK, the prevalence of urinary incontinence is 2–3 times higher in populations in institutional care than elsewhere in the community[9,14,15] in line with studies from elsewhere in Europe.[16,17] In Britain, recent evidence suggests an overall prevalence of regular incontinence in institutional settings of around 40%, with estimates of 15–30% for those in residential homes, 30–60% for those in nursing homes and 30–70% for those on geriatric and psycho-geriatric wards.[15] The higher prevalence of urinary incontinence in institutional care is probably largely due to the selection of frail, incontinent individuals into this type of accommodation. Prevalence estimates are likely to vary between and within institutions over time due to differences in admission and management policies and as residents age. The threshold for defining incontinence tends to be higher in institutions because it relies on observations from carers rather than on self-reported incontinence. There is a strong correlation between the prevalence of incontinence and the level of dependency plus a suggestion of an excess observed prevalence associated with incontinence among psycho-geriatric patients (**Table 5**).

In institutions, almost half of those with urinary incontinence also experience faecal incontinence. This is a far higher proportion than in the general population, where only 1% of women aged 65 or over have regular faecal or double incontinence compared with 12% who have regular urinary incontinence.[18–20]

Incontinence is associated with dementia, stroke and problems of mobility and dexterity.[21,22] This may contribute to a tendency for staff to be more reluctant to treat incontinence as vigorously in older people as they would in younger people. It is worth noting that among all people aged 75 or more, only 20% of those with troublesome incontinence are reported as being cognitively impaired. Incontinence in older people is often a remediable condition and this age group is likely to benefit considerably from appropriate treatment. Furthermore, it has been suggested that dementia is no bar to achieving continence in elderly people.[23]

Among elderly people in residential and nursing homes it has been estimated that 87% of residents needed changes in the management of their condition and 57% of homes requested more help from the specialist services.[24]

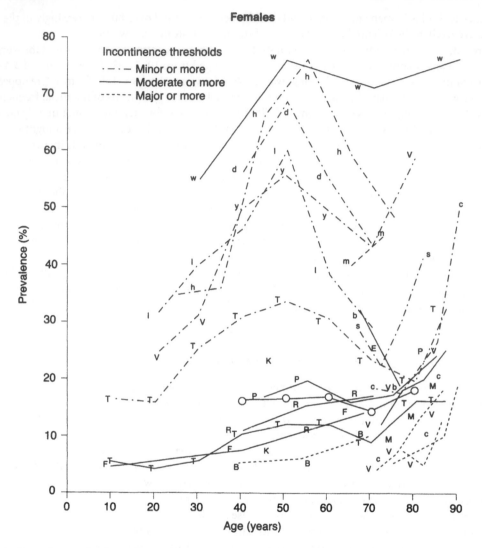

Figure 2: Prevalence of urinary incontinence by age, sex and severity (UK, 1960–2001).

Prevalence in people with disabilities

The OPCS surveys of disability in Great Britain[25] estimate that 14.2% of all adults have a limiting and longstanding disability, which may relate to physical, sensory, intellectual and/or social functioning. The study looks at 10 main areas of disability, including continence. Among adults with any disability, 17% of those living in private households and 44% of those resident in institutions have a disabling problem with urinary and/or faecal incontinence.

The researchers calculated a severity score of overall disability for each adult in the survey with one or more disabilities and described a positive relationship between the prevalence of incontinence and the overall severity of disability score (**Figure 3**). As people age, the prevalence of incontinence rises and multiple disabilities also become more common, with a corresponding increase in the overall severity score. It is only among people within the most severe category of disability (score 9–10) that there is a

Males

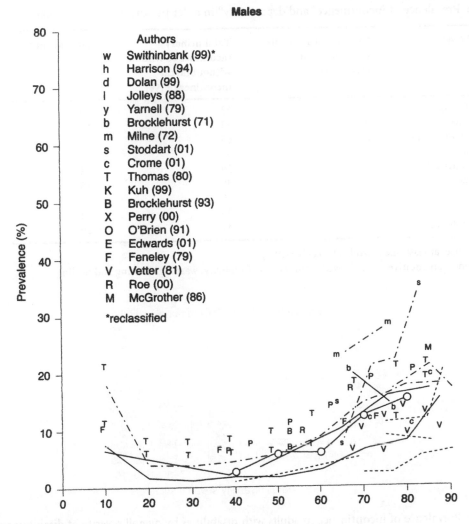

Authors

w	Swithinbank (99)*
h	Harrison (94)
d	Dolan (99)
l	Jolleys (88)
y	Yarnell (79)
b	Brocklehurst (71)
m	Milne (72)
s	Stoddart (01)
c	Crome (01)
T	Thomas (80)
K	Kuh (99)
B	Brocklehurst (93)
X	Perry (00)
O	O'Brien (91)
E	Edwards (01)
F	Feneley (79)
V	Vetter (81)
R	Roe (00)
M	McGrother (86)

*reclassified

Figure 2: Continued

significant difference in the prevalence of incontinence between those living in their own households and in institutions (56% and 72% respectively).

There is a paucity of information about incontinence in people with specific disabilities. A community-based study found that survivors of stroke living in the community had double the prevalence of urinary symptoms of the non-stroke population (64% v 32%).[22] The prevalence among women with severe learning disability resembles that of older people in residential care more than the general population[26] (**Table 6**). Data from the Leicestershire Learning Disability Register shows that 23% of women and 16% of men with learning disability are wet at least once a week.[26]

Table 5: Prevalence of incontinence[a] and dependency[b] in older persons in residential care.[15]

Type of home	Urinary incontinence without faecal incontinence (%)	Total urinary incontinence with or without faecal incontinence (%)	Dependent (%)
Private nursing	30	63	70
NHS geriatric	31	58	61
NHS psycho-geriatric	28	65	47
NHS acute	21	30	35
Private residential	19	29	32
Local authority	21	35	26
Voluntary	6	10	17
Other	15	23	24
All types of home	23	41	39

[a] Incontinence: at least one episode of weekly wetting.
[b] Dependency: an additive score derived from ratings of mobility, washing/dressing and feeding.

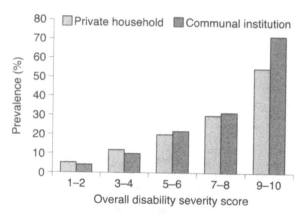

Figure 3: Prevalence of incontinence in adults with disabilities by overall severity of disability and place of residence.

Table 6: Prevalence of urinary incontinence in women with learning disabilities compared with older people and the general population.

Study	Sandvik 1993[27]	Peet 1995[15]	McGrother 1996[26]
Subgroup Definition	General population >drops weekly	Institutional care leakage weekly	Learning disability wet weekly
Age group		**Prevalence %**	
40–49	3	–	16
50–59	12	–	14
60–69	6	22	27
70–79	9	30	22
80+	18	32	44

Health care need and requirement

In the UK, need for services is an important domain that relies on quality of life for disorders like urinary incontinence and other storage symptoms. This review suggests health care need should be defined in terms of the recognised *storage symptoms* having an *impact* on life. There is a large degree of consistency in the literature suggesting 'any' or 'minor' incontinence represents the lower threshold of abnormality. Impact includes general 'problems' and specific 'interference' with life. There is a fair degree of consistency in the literature suggesting 'mild' or 'little' impact represents the lower threshold of abnormality. Although impact is more subjectively defined than symptoms, it still represents an external norm rather than a felt need in Bradshaw's original sense of wanting help. Indicators of felt need identified in this review are any reported use of a relevant service, reported need for help or take-up of services when offered and represents the health care requirement or priority in the context of the overall health care need.

Urinary incontinence may interfere with activities of daily living, social activities, relationships, feelings, self-perception, general health and overall quality of life in a variety of ways.[28–36] Activities most commonly affected are shopping, visiting friends and sport. Travel becomes problematic, with initial avoidance of long journeys and eventually also of short journeys. Relationships may be affected, particularly sexual relationships since incontinence can occur during coitus.[30] Disturbance of sexual relations due to incontinence has been reported in 1.1%[32] and 0.1%[33] of community populations, i.e. in approximately 1–4% of those with incontinence. In clinic populations this proportion can be as high as 40%.[35,36] Incontinence tends to be more restrictive than stress incontinence.[32] Interference with activities, feelings and relationships is commonly reported in 1–5% of the population.[8,28–31,37]

Women tend to experience more bother or social restriction than men, but the prevalence shows only a slight increase with age. However, care is needed in interpreting studies of very elderly people, especially women, since non-response and admission to residential care lead to underestimation of the problem. Some people are able to modify their lifestyle to cope fairly successfully with incontinence, though the coping strategies may contribute to their becoming socially isolated.[33] Others experience shame, embarrassment, loss of self-esteem, anxiety and depression.[35]

Twelve UK studies[8,9,18,28,37–44] have addressed some aspects of the extent of need and are profiled in **Table A2.3**. Although there are variations in the definitions of need they are similar enough to allow some comparison. A minority of studies relate to storage disorder as a whole but most relate to incontinence. *General impact* was defined as a 'problem', 'a difficulty' or 'a bother'. Precise thresholds used had a marked effect on prevalence estimates. Four studies covering a range of ages identified a *problem* for 8–30% in women and 3.8–6.2% in men.[8,40,42,45] In old age, one comparable study estimated *difficulty* in control of micturition affected 12% of men and women aged 75+.[9] Three studies explicitly included a relatively mild problem/bother with incontinence which affected more people (17–44% of women of all ages and 17% of elderly women and 12% of elderly men).[41–43]

Estimates of *specific interference* with life also varied depending on the threshold used. Five studies across a *range of ages* estimated <2%–8.6% of women and <1%–2.9% of men experienced interference with their daily lives.[8,18,28,37,40] In *older* people similar interference was estimated to affect 5% of men and women.[9] However, a *little* interference with life affected substantially more people, 18% of women and 12.2% of elderly men.[43]

Reported consultation in primary care was estimated across a *range of ages* at 2.1–11.4% for women and 1.3–6.7% for men[28,37,39,40,44] and for *older people* at 5.1–6.2%.[9,38] More broadly defined use of health services was estimated at the higher level of 14% of women and 9.2% of men aged 65+.[43] Reported consultation confined to the last year was relatively low but was more prevalent than incontinence recorded by services.[37,18] *Uptake* of services offered was estimated across a range of ages at 6.1–9.2% of women and 3.4% in men and 4.4% for *elderly* men and women.[9,28,39] The levels of currently *wanting help* across a range of ages was 3.8% in women and in men at 4.4%.[8]

An association between the level of incontinence and level of impact or use of services has been demonstrated within the UK studies.[18,37,38,41] Amongst women, 69% of those with severe incontinence regard it as a problem compared with 55% with moderate and 27% with mild incontinence. In men the relationship was stronger: 86%, 65% and 27% respectively.[43] A similar relationship occurs with specific interference with life. The gender difference may suggest women adapt their lifestyle more than men.

Reports in the UK are consistent with studies elsewhere in the western world in terms of overall impact,[27,46–48] consultation rates,[29,31,46,48–52] and relationship between symptoms and impact.[29,31,53]

Consultation reported directly by an individual is a far better measure than consultation recorded by a professional, which forms the basis of routine statistics. Reported rates vary considerably depending on the sample and the definition of incontinence. Between 9% and 32% of women with incontinence (2% to 7% of the total population) have spoken to their doctor about it.[28,29,31,37,48,52] Younger sufferers and those in full-time work are most likely to seek help.[30] Consultation rates increase with increasing severity and impact of incontinence but the association is not strong. In Reker's study,[31] 44% of women experiencing incontinence at least once a week sought help compared with 22% with less frequent incontinence. Even among women reporting worry about their symptoms, only a third had spoken to a doctor and among women reporting more severe restriction to their social life, only half had consulted a health professional. The relationship is stronger for use of aids: 73% of elderly people with severe incontinence used aids compared to 17% with milder incontinence.[54]

A major reason for not seeking professional help is a misconception of the aetiology and natural history of the condition. Many women view incontinence as the inevitable result of childbearing and ageing and consider that seeking medical attention is an inappropriate use of consulting time.[55] There is a general lack of awareness of the range and efficacy of treatments.[28,48] Some do not consult a doctor because they fear surgery.[55] Unfortunately, these views are often reinforced by health professionals.[56]

Table 7: Estimated prevalence of impact and felt need in relation to storage disorder/incontinence from UK studies 1960–2001.

Condition	(rating)	Definition	Prevalence %			
			Women		Men	
			all ages	elderly	all ages	elderly
Impact	(>mild)	problem/bother/ difficulty	8–30	12	3.8–6.2	12
		interference with life	<2–8.6	5	<1–2.9	5
	(mild)	mild problem	17–44	17	–	12
		a little interference	–	18	–	12.2
Felt need	('met')	primary care consultation	2.1–11.4	6.1–6.2	1.3–6.7	5.1–6.2
		use of any health service	–	14	–	9.2
		consultation in last year	2.1	–	–	–
		routine statistics of use	<2	–	<1	–
	(unmet)	uptake on offer	6.1–9.2	4.4	3.4	4.4
		currently want help	3.8	–	3.8	–

The prevalences of significant impact and unmet felt need increase with age, in men and women[8,57] (*see* **Figure 4**). A higher proportion of men with bothersome symptoms complain of interference with life compared to women. However, the proportion reporting an unmet need is slightly greater in women.

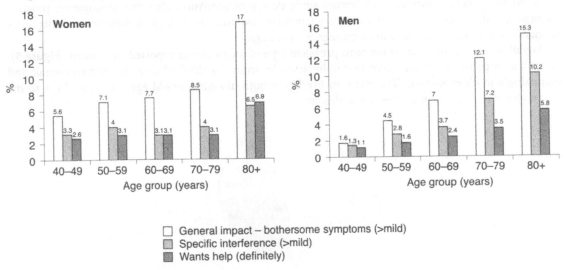

General impact – bothersome symptoms (>mild)
Specific interference (>mild)
Wants help (definitely)

Figure 4: Prevalence of significant impact and unmet felt need in adults by age (storage symptoms).

There is limited information concerning the prevalence of incontinence among ethnic minorities in the UK. It has been suggested that white women are at greater risk[58] but others have found no difference between ethnic groups.[59] One small study in London found that fewer than 50% of women with incontinence from a range of ethnic minority groups sought help.[60] However, only Muslim women had a strong preference for female doctors. In general it is recognised that South Asians within the UK make greater use of GP services and less use of specialist care than the general population.[61–64]

In the USA prevalence rates for Caucasian women appear consistently higher than Afro-American women,[65–68] but consultation rates are lower.

Prevalence by type of incontinence

In women, the most common conditions underlying incontinence are detrusor overactivity and urethral sphincter incompetence. Several studies have shown a relationship between these disorders and the symptoms of urge incontinence (leakage associated with a strong urge to void) and symptoms of stress incontinence (leakage during coughing, laughing, exercise or other physical exertion) respectively. Studies relying on standardised questions have shown moderate validity.[69,70] In Lagro-Janssen's study,[69] for example, the sensitivity and specificity of pure urge incontinence for detrusor overactivity diagnosed by cystometry are 61% and 95% respectively; and 78% and 84% of pure stress incontinence for urodynamic stress incontinence. Although symptoms of urge and stress incontinence are not sufficiently accurate predictors to be clinically diagnostic for surgical interventions, they provide markers with which to examine the different epidemiological patterns of the two leading bladder disorders.

A range of studies report on the symptomatic diagnosis of incontinence in women (**Table A2.4**). Again, the prevalence values are wide-ranging and depend on the precise definition used and the age of the population studied.

The prevalence of stress incontinence increases gradually through the reproductive years to a slight peak around the time of the menopause, followed by a possible decline. In contrast, the prevalence of urge incontinence steadily increases with age and is most pronounced in old age. These studies suggest that, to some extent, stress incontinence undergoes some degree of remission after the menopause, possibly through genuine recovery and/or through adaptation and treatment. Urge incontinence contributes primarily to the overall increase in incontinence in old age.

Overall, stress incontinence is the most prevalent type of incontinence reported by women (**Figure 5**). Stress and urge incontinence occur in combination in around a third of cases in women overall and increasingly in older women. The extent of overlap of both disorders in old age may contribute to the preponderance of severe incontinence at this stage.

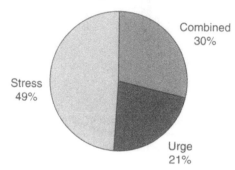

Figure 5: The overall pattern of incontinence by type of incontinence in women.[37]

The predominant type of urinary incontinence in men is urge incontinence. The most common condition underlying this is detrusor overactivity, with or without prostatic enlargement. Urge incontinence accounts for most of the overall increase of incontinence with age in men.

Incidence and natural history

The *incidence rate* represents the number of new cases developed in a disease-free population in a year.* In order to estimate the incidence rates and natural history of a condition it is necessary to conduct repeated surveys on the same large random sample of the population over several years. For this reason, very few prospective studies are available. Retrospective studies are subject to problems with recall. Episodes of incontinence may be forgotten or there may be difficulty recalling the correct year of onset, especially in the distant past. These reports are therefore likely to underestimate the true incidence, especially among older persons who may have memory defects. The only advantage of retrospective studies is that they readily provide a perspective on the pattern of incidence over a lifetime (**Figure 6**). The overall incidence of incontinence mirrors the pattern of prevalence in younger women. It highlights two distinct peaks in incidence, one in the early reproductive years and another around menopause. There is also a third peak in old age.

Table A2.5 summarises three key prospective studies of the incidence of urinary incontinence in adults living in the community, each carried out using sound methodology on a large and representative study population.[72–74] Like prevalence, incidence is very dependent on the definition and severity of the

* Incontinence incidence rate = number of new cases of incontinence at the current assessment/number of respondents who were continent at the previous assessment (non-cases).

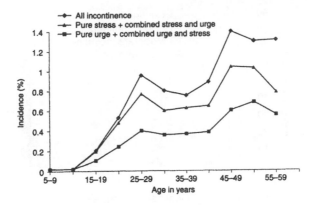

Figure 6: Incidence of urinary incontinence in women by age.[71]

symptom being studied, making comparison between studies difficult. Broadly, however, these studies indicate that 6–22% of middle-aged and older women who are previously continent develop incontinence each year. The incidence rates are higher where the study population is older and when the definition of symptoms studied is milder. The incidence rates in men are about half those in women, which is consistent with men's lower prevalence rates.

The *remission rate* denotes the number of cases remitted from a diseased population in a year and is not directly comparable with incidence rate.* Results from the prospective studies[72–74] show remission rates in women ranging between 9% p.a. and 42% p.a. The remission rates are lower where the population is older and incontinence more severe, thus contributing to the cumulative effect of incontinence with age. Remission rates in men are higher than in women, estimated in one study at 30% compared to 12% in women.[72] The MRC programme estimates incidence rates for storage disorder at 15.4% p.a. for women and 12.7% p.a. for men and remission rates at 23.1% p.a. for women and 30.4% p.a. for men aged 40 and over.[72]

When continent people first become incontinent, they are most likely to develop a mild form of incontinence. **Figure 7** shows the changes in continence and severity of incontinence for 726 women during the first year of study[72] (**Table A2.6**). A large proportion of mild and moderate incontinence appears to fluctuate in severity but severe incontinence is relatively persistent. The pattern in men is similar, with higher remission rates.

Associated factors

Incontinence is more common in pregnancy.[75] Although the problem is generally self-limiting, it may predispose women towards incontinence later in their lives, such as during a subsequent pregnancy or as they age.[76] Several studies have shown that nulliparous women are less likely to develop incontinence than parous women and that increasing parity is a risk. However, the precise relationship between pregnancy, parity, childbirth and incontinence needs further investigation. Similarly, there are inconsistent findings in the literature about the role of oestrogen loss around the menopause and hysterectomy in the development of incontinence and other urinary symptoms.

---

* Incontinence remission rate = number of recovered cases of incontinence at the current assessment/number of respondents who were incontinent at the previous assessment (cases).

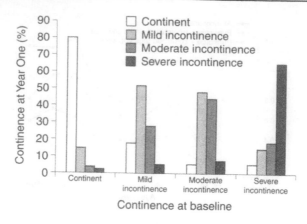

Figure 7: Changes in self-reported incontinence after one year of follow-up in women.[72]

There is stronger evidence for the association of incontinence with obesity and with cognitive and functional impairment, especially mobility problems. Prostatectomy is an established iatrogenic cause of male stress incontinence. Comorbidities identified in a review of the literature[42,74,77–85] are shown in **Figure 8**.

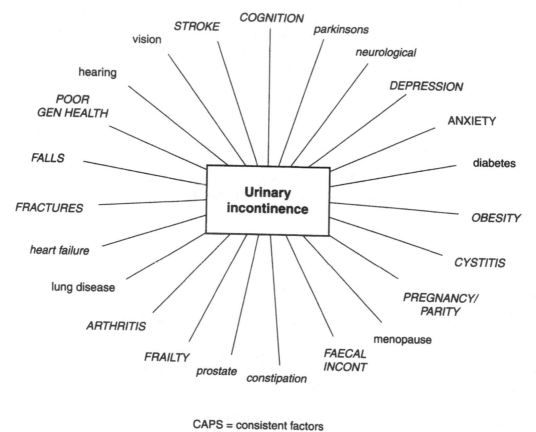

Figure 8: Co-morbidities for urinary incontinence.

Well-controlled analyses of potential lifestyle risk factors for the development of urinary incontinence are limited.[77] Most of the data have been derived from cross-sectional studies of volunteers and clinical subjects. Early indications from the population-based cohort study within the current MRC programme suggest adherence to a healthy diet may offer protection.

5 Services available and their costs

Primary care

The organisation of continence services affects patient outcomes and thus the mode of delivery in continence provision is an important factor in delivering positive outcomes.[86] At present, primary continence care provision shows great variation across the country and is often fragmented. There are wide variations in nursing input and a lack of continuity of care. Care may be provided by one or more health care professional, with referral from one to another, but there are no consistent care pathways. When individuals first present with incontinence or lower urinary tract symptoms, they tend to see a GP, despite the fact that continence advisors have been in existence for over 20 years in many areas. Primary care may then be provided by a continence advisor, continence link nurse, practice nurse, district nurse or health visitor.

Continence care pathway in primary care

The two key continence service providers are described below in terms of role, access to provider, training and reasons for variation in care provision and costs (**Figure 9**).

General practitioners

General practitioners (GPs) are the most likely first point of contact when patients seek formal help for their incontinence.[40,87] The GP usually carries out the clinical assessment, screening, giving advice, prescribing medication and arranging referral to secondary care. As with other aspects of general practice, GPs have a gate-keeping role in continence provision. They may refer their patients to other health professionals in primary care, such as a continence advisor, practice nurse or district nurse or, more commonly, to a specialist in secondary care. GPs provide this service without having undergone essential specialist training in the management of patients with urinary symptoms, as this is not available. Access to GPs is usually through self-referral.

The estimated cost of a GP consultation is £18.[88]

Inadequacies in incontinence care have been acknowledged for some time. In 1983, the Incontinence Action Group published a report[89] which identified 'the huge gap which exists between available knowledge of the causes and methods of management and that which is actually known to practising nurse and doctors.' In their review of the evaluation and treatment of women with urinary incontinence in the primary care setting, Walters and Realini found that urinary incontinence can be diagnosed accurately by family physicians using basic tests.[90] A later study found that outpatient geriatric assessment units were better than physicians in community based practices at identifying patients with both mild and severe incontinence.[91] There is evidence that there is a need for further education of health care professionals.[92] Brocklehurst found that less than 25% of patients with urinary incontinence were given a full examination by their GPs.[40] Deficits in the knowledge of GPs about urinary incontinence were found by Jolleys and

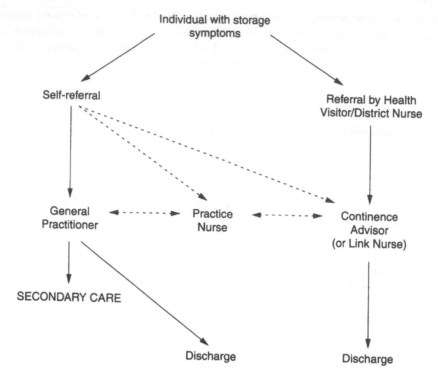

Figure 9: Flow diagram of typical care pathways for individuals with storage symptoms.

Wilson in a survey of 1284 GPs.[93] They also found that GPs lacked confidence in their abilities to diagnose and manage urinary incontinence, although this lack of confidence was not related to length of practice as a GP. In an analysis of incontinence in the community, the action taken by many GPs was found be suboptimal, with considerable geographical variation.[94] Fewer than 5% of those who consulted a doctor in this survey were referred to a nurse or incontinence clinic. It also suggested that medication was often prescribed without clinical examination and probably without a diagnosis being made. In Briggs' study[95] 42 of 101 general practitioners surveyed never used the service of a continence advisor for older patients although the service was available to them.

Nurses involved in continence care provision

A common model of care provision comprises a service led by a team of continence advisors, which, in turn, has a team of link nurses, largely drawn from the pool of district nurses. Some health care trusts, often covering a large geographical area, rely on a single continence advisor, with no link nurse system. Other trusts have teams of continence advisors offering expertise in the care of individuals who have, for example, learning disabilities or mental health problems as well as urinary symptoms.[96,97] However, continence advisors often work in isolation without expert medical support.[96] The majority of health authorities now have the services of a continence advisor.

Continence advisors are trained to carry out clinical examinations and complex holistic assessments to initiate treatment for individuals with urinary symptoms. The link nurse may also be able to perform some or all of these duties. A few continence advisors also perform urodynamic investigations. The specific role of each link nurse shows considerable variation throughout the country. Some continence advisors have a limited clinical remit, leaving all, apart from the most complex, clinical care to the nurse link team. Apart from clinical practice, the role of the continence advisor is to provide management, advice and education, research and audit, to co-ordinate the service and support the link nurses. Some may also have the responsibility of holding the continence budget. The amount of time spent in each activity varies enormously between continence advisors. Geographical variations in the time spent in core activities and in the type of service offered result in inconsistencies in care provision.

Training of the continence advisor includes completing an ENB 978 course. Various continence modules are available in addition, but there are geographical inconsistencies. Access to the continence advisor may be via the GP, district nurse, link nurse, practice nurse, health visitor or through self-referral.

Cost of a continence advisor – Grade F (£22 302–£27 039), G (£24 903–£28 854) and occasionally H (£27 819–£32 326).

The lack of knowledge amongst medical staff regarding urinary incontinence outlined above is mirrored within the nursing profession. In her study of nurses' attitudes towards incontinence, Cheater found that there was a need for increased education of nurses in relation to preventative care and the therapeutic and rehabilitation aspects of continence promotion.[98] The same author also found that qualified nurses lacked the knowledge to complete an adequate assessment of incontinent patients.[99] Health visitors wanted more information in a training needs analysis by Burnet et al.[100]

Secondary care

The following groups currently provide secondary care:

- core medical professionals
- nurses
- allied health care professionals (physiotherapists/occupational therapists)
- allied diagnostic specialist professionals.

The role of each of these groups will be briefly outlined in terms of professionals involved, variation in care provision and costs.

Core medical professionals

In the UK the vast majority of secondary care is provided from acute hospitals by consultant-led services. Most of these operate a traditional referral pathway directly from the GP and some allow referral from specialist nursing services. Unfortunately, many specialist nursing services are located in community trusts whereas hospital specialists became based in acute trusts when these were formed. This led to the further fragmentation of continence care. The formation of Primary Care Trusts may lead to further isolation of community services from those in secondary care. Consultant-to-consultant referral may also occur where the skills needed to deal with patients do not exist within a consultant's own service. Such tertiary referrals previously required GP approval, but the need for this appears to have reduced. There are direct referral pathways to urologists or gynaecological oncologists from specialties when life-threatening conditions such as renal or genital tract cancer are discovered. There are also facilities for frail elderly individuals to be specifically referred to physicians for the care of the elderly; such referrals may originate from other secondary care specialists dealing with urinary incontinence. The trend for increasing sub-specialisation is evident in gynaecology. There are at present six recognised sub-specialty training rotations in uro-gynaecology, to which more are likely to be added in the near future. Such sub-specialisation has been recognised as desirable following the publication of data concerning the results of operations conducted by general gynaecologists when compared with the published results of interventions from research studies.[101] Urologists have also begun to recognise the need to develop their input into female urology.

Services have often been developed because of the interest of individual practitioners, with little strategic overview in any location, rather than in response to an identified need of the local population. Continence services led by physicians for the care of the elderly in particular have a large regional variation. Geriatrician membership of the International Continence Society, UK, for example, numbers approximately 20 of a total consultant population of over 700. Each of these medical specialties tends to work in isolation and care pathways vary similarly between specialties. Some regions may have clear linkage and referral pathways. There is also great variation within each medical specialty in terms of services and interventions provided. All specialists provide access to diagnostic services, behavioural therapies, medical interventions (including drugs) and surgery. There is little appreciation of the desires or needs of users in the design or delivery of secondary care services. With the advent of national service frameworks and the NHS Plan this is likely to change, with user and carer involvement becoming central to future service planning and delivery.

The percentage time that each specialty devotes to incontinence management may be calculated indirectly and hence cost calculations can be made. The Continence Foundation has estimated the cost of both urinary and faecal incontinence to an average primary care group (PCG) of 102 000 people to be approximately £737 000 per year. Similarly, the cost to the NHS in England has been estimated at £353 595 000 per year; and a total of £423 467 000 per year for the UK. This takes into account the time and services of both primary and secondary care resources but only the salary costs of staff.[102]

Nurses

The Royal College of Nurses sees clinical nurse specialists in continence care as an essential part of continence services, able to give cost-effective expert care, advice and treatment. As first line referral for people with incontinence, their services compare favourably to hospital consultants.[103] Hospital continence nurse specialists may originate from any of the incontinence-based backgrounds, notably from urology or gynaecology. They are, however, an ill-defined entity throughout the specialties. Within certain specialties such as urology, they may have a limited remit in continence care. Often they have a combined role in performing urodynamic studies and providing a service to the patients under the care of their department. Some specialist nurses within hospital have a remit to serve the entire hospital. There is a wide variation in the degree of collaboration between nurses from the different specialties and between hospital- and community-based specialist nurses. However, a recent survey of continence nurses suggested that the majority had both hospital and community responsibilities.[104] The referral pathway to these nurses is through any of the consultants from the incontinence-based specialties and, for those with a hospital-wide remit, from nursing or medical staff within the institution. The services tend to be consultant-led with the nurses providing the majority of continence care.

The differences between continence nurse specialists and continence advisors are ill-defined. Historically, providers of continence care in secondary care are involved in staff education and training, providing expert advice to staff and direct care to patients, often with involvement from an interested medical consultant. The role of the continence nurse specialists is currently variable and has been outlined in the previous section. The type of services provided includes patient assessment, diagnosis and conservative intervention such as bladder re-education and pelvic floor re-education therapies. Depending upon the role of the nurse within each department and the wider educational and training role, such nurses may be of varying grade. Nurse specialists are most often employed as a G grade (£24 903–£28 854); others may be either F (£22 302–£27 039) or even E (£18 212–£22 387). The lower grade nurses tend to have a role limited to their host department and may spend a limited amount of time in continence care delivery.

Other allied health care professionals

Physiotherapists

Although continence care in the community is largely provided by nurses, the situation is different in secondary care. In this setting, care may be provided by either nurses or physiotherapists. Both may receive referrals from the community or hospital clinicians. Traditionally, assessment and conservative treatments used to be administered by physiotherapists, who may or may not have had a particular interest in the pelvic floor. They have been superseded by physiotherapists who do have a special interest in the pelvic floor and incontinence. More recently, the role of the physiotherapist in secondary care has been supplemented by the continence nurse, who has been trained in the management of incontinence and pelvic floor problems. One of the reasons for this is that the only remit for the nurses is incontinence and so they can be based in the relevant clinical department. This encourages a closer working relationship, especially between clinician and nurse. This is more likely to happen in the larger units where there is a greater workload. The vast majority of physiotherapists have a more general role so tend to be based in their own departments. The result is a variation in the continence service, largely determined by local circumstances. National average salary, senior 1 grade: £26 148.

Occupational therapists

Occupational therapists may be involved in continence care provision by advising on techniques to improve function, or aids to maximise an individuals ability in self-toileting, thereby avoiding incontinence. They may recommend modification to clothing or alternatives to the toilet that will help to maintain continence. National average salary, senior 1 grade: £26 148.

Allied diagnostic specialist professionals

Certain services may have access to specialists in other disciplines who are involved in the delivery of continence care, for example, uro-radiology, neuro-urology and rehabilitation physicians. Often these people exist in specialist centres and their services have evolved in an unplanned fashion, rather than as a result of any coherent plan for a continence service. In some areas, the services provided by such professionals may be provided by core specialists within urology or gynaecology.

Summary

Division of care between professionals is complex, with varied models of service around the country. Patients may present to GPs or go directly (or indirectly) to continence nurses in the community. They may be treated extensively within primary care with behavioural and medical therapies or be referred at an early stage to specialists, including neurologists, geriatricians, urologists and gynaecologists. In relation to health service pathways for incontinence, most younger women are referred to gynaecologists whereas most older men and women are referred to physicians for the elderly; whilst for voiding problems most men are referred to urologists.

Continence nurses of various kinds play a considerable role in managing the problem but the nature and extent of provision is very variable across the country. Community nurses are often the first port of call for patients with incontinence. They may make the initial in-depth assessment and are often involved in providing some degree of behavioural therapy for the common disorders and long-term aids for intractable conditions. The role of the GP in assessment and management of the underlying condition is hampered by lack of information concerning the long-term natural history of bladder problems and the lack of an integrated specialist service.

Treatment in primary care

Treatment for urinary incontinence in both primary and secondary care has been the subject of a number of World Health Organization sponsored international conferences. The available data concerning treatments has been reviewed by a number of committees and recommendations published.

Conservative therapies

Pelvic floor muscle training

Pelvic floor muscle training (PFMT) is the most commonly recommended physical therapy treatment for women with stress incontinence. It is also used in the treatment of women with mixed incontinence, and less commonly for urge incontinence. PFMT involves the voluntary contraction and relaxation of the levator ani muscle, which supports the vagina, bladder and urethra and which contributes to the skeletal muscle component of the urethral sphincteric mechanism. The goal of these exercises is to increase the strength and endurance of the levator, thereby enhancing the force of urethral closure under certain conditions, such as with a sudden increase in abdominal pressure.

Although the use of PFMT is the main non-surgical treatment for women with mild to moderate stress incontinence, there has been little research into how pelvic floor exercises should be taught and there is wide variation in the elements of teaching such as frequency of training, number of repetitions, duration and quality of contractions and exercise period reported in studies.[105] Prior to PFMT, a woman should be assessed by a person with skills in the assessment and training of pelvic floor muscles to ensure that a correct pelvic floor muscle contraction is being performed, and to determine if any facilitation techniques or adaptations are required to the recommended training programme.[106] On the basis of extrapolation from exercise science literature, PFMT programmes should include three sets of 8 to 12 slow velocity maximal voluntary pelvic floor muscle contractions sustained for six to eight seconds each, performed three to four times a week and continued for at least 15 to 20 weeks.[106]

Not all women are able to perform pelvic floor exercises correctly and so may require instruction and supervision from a nurse or physiotherapist. Adjuncts such as biofeedback and electrical stimulation are also commonly used with PFMT. Biofeedback is most commonly employed when using a perineometer to measure pelvic floor muscle strength. The use of electrical stimulation in the treatment of incontinence is described in detail by Laycock.[107] Use of this mode of treatment has increased in recent years, partly due to the introduction of portable equipment. The technique has been used in both neurologically and non-neurologically impaired individuals to manage both bladder and urethral dysfunction. Electrical stimulation is usually given to mimic a normal pelvic floor muscle contraction and is a treatment option for patients who are unable to produce a voluntary contraction or only a weak contraction. Such electrical stimulation recruits muscle fibres. Having been made aware of the specific pelvic floor muscle activity by means of electrical stimulation, the patient then tries to join in and reproduce the contraction. Naturally, these adjunctive treatments do require nursing or physiotherapy input.

More recently, vaginal cones have been used as an alternative form of PFMT. The use of weighted vaginal cones to assess and train pelvic floor muscles was first reported by Plevnik.[108] The cones are the same size but are of different weights, usually five. When a cone of the appropriate weight is inserted into the vagina, it tends to slip out. This feeling of 'losing the cone' provides a sensory feedback which makes the pelvic floor contract around the cone retaining it. This principle can be used to exercise the pelvic floor muscles correctly.

Therapies to strengthen the pelvic floor have the advantage over other therapies in that they have no physical side effects or morbidity. Rational use of these therapies may offer treatment to women who would or could not undergo more invasive treatments.

Bladder retraining

Bladder retraining is the most commonly used behavioural treatment for patients with overactive bladder symptoms. Bladder retraining can successfully be taught and monitored in a primary care setting, but has also been employed as part of an in-patient programme for urinary incontinence. It relies on three basic concepts: (1) education, (2) voiding schedule and (3) positive reinforcements.[109]

Education emphasises the voluntary control over motor and sensory impulses. Distraction techniques to control urinary urgency are also incorporated. The voiding schedule includes mandatory voiding at specific intervals. These intervals are gradually extended until a reasonable time between voids is established.

Caffeine restriction

Dietary advice regarding the restriction of caffeine is often given. There is evidence that theoretically supports its association with bladder overactivity.[110]

Fluid advice

Drinking excessive amounts of fluid, especially at night, may contribute to a patient's symptoms of frequency and nocturia. It may be appropriate in such circumstances to advise some sort of fluid restriction.

Weight reduction

There are no data on the relationship between urinary incontinence and obesity in males. In females, however, there is good evidence for a positive association of stress urinary incontinence and body mass.[111,112] Obese women should, therefore, be advised to lose weight.

Relief of constipation

Subjects who report urinary incontinence are more likely to report constipation. Faecal impaction can lead to urinary retention, and there have been conflicting reports of an association between incontinence and constipation.[7,113] It would seem sensible to advise all patients, not just those with constipation, to eat a high fibre diet.

Smoking

An association of bladder problems with cigarette smoking has been identified for both men and women.[114–117] However, there are clearly many more convincing arguments for not smoking.

Drug therapy

Drug therapy for urinary symptoms is mainly aimed at patients with detrusor overactivity (DO). Bladder contractions are mediated by the release of acetylcholine to act on muscarinic receptors in the bladder. Most drugs for detrusor overactivity work at least in part by blocking these receptors. The most commonly used drugs today are oxybutynin and tolterodine. Other drugs include trospium chloride, flavoxate hydrochloride, propiverine hydrochloride, imipramine, desmopressin and oestrogens. All of the currently available drug therapies have side effects that limit their use. At present most secondary care sites do not have the resources to provide effective behavioural therapies and so there is a reliance on drug therapy alone. The vast majority of drug prescribing occurs in the community.

All of the above interventions can be delivered in primary care, but need time and positive reinforcement.

Continence aids

A wide variety of continence products are available in the UK, from the NHS, over the counter and by mail order,[118–121] but accessibility still remains a problem. Continence aids may be divided into (1) containment devices such as absorbent pads, penile sheaths and bed sheets; (2) conduction devices such as catheters; (3) occlusive devices such as clamps and urethral plugs; and (4) intravaginal devices which support the bladder neck. These aids may be used in individuals with intractable incontinence, in cases where other treatments have failed, when alternative treatments such as surgery are inappropriate or for patient preference. The product used should be tailored to the individual and all of these products are used for both the long and short term. Absorbent pads and pants are probably the most commonly used aids and are, for many, the first method of control. There are a large variety of types available. Occlusive devices and devices to support the bladder neck tend to be used the least.

In an evaluation of health interventions by primary health care teams and continence advisory services, Roe et al.[122] reported that the majority of people with incontinence felt that health services for sufferers could be improved by the supply of continence products. The most recent Department of Health Guidelines[119] recommend that the initial assessment of a person's continence needs at primary care level should include assessment of the need for appropriate continence products. There should be a range of pads available in all categories, consideration should be given to patient choice, there should be periodic re-assessment of those receiving long-term supplies, the provision of pads should be available equally to anyone in the geographical area, regardless of where they live, and pads should be provided in quantities appropriate to the individual's continence needs.

Treatments in secondary care

Initial treatment of bladder problems, following an assessment in secondary care, is little different from that offered in the primary care setting. Secondary care may offer greater experience in terms of adjustment and experience with drug therapy and combinations of conservative techniques. Surgical intervention is clearly the role of secondary and, in the case of certain specialist areas, tertiary care. In secondary care the treatment of symptom clusters such as frequency, urgency, nocturia and urge and stress incontinence often gives way to treatment of underlying pathophysiology. The common conditions being diagnosed are urodynamic stress incontinence (USI), detrusor overactivity and bladder outflow obstruction. These are diagnosed using a series of invasive techniques termed urodynamic investigations based on definitions from the International Continence Society.[123] Symptoms have not been found to predict the underlying diagnosis accurately,[124–131] hence the need for investigation. Not all patients require urodynamic investigation in order to make a diagnosis or before implementing treatment, but there is a consensus of opinion that such investigation should be performed prior to surgery. The main argument for urodynamic investigation is that it avoids unnecessary surgery in a woman complaining of stress incontinence, where the cause of urine leakage is due to detrusor overactivity and not bladder neck descent or urethral sphincter incompetence.[132–134]

Surgery for incontinence

The vast majority of surgery performed in the UK is for urodynamic stress incontinence, a condition in which the bladder sphincter mechanism has failed. After behavioural and pelvic floor therapies have been tried in either primary or secondary care, the next line of treatment is often surgery. The aim of surgery is to increase closure pressure within the urethra and so prevent urinary leakage when the pressure within the bladder rises (such as when the patient coughs or exercises). The commonly performed operations include colposuspension, needle suspension, bladder sling, anterior repair and urethral buttress, Marshall-Marchetti-Krantz (MMK), all of which are usually performed under general anaesthesia, and injection of collagen or synthetic material into the bladder neck, which can be performed under general, regional or local anaesthesia. The aim of these injectables is to bulk up the junction between bladder neck and urethra, increasing pressure transmission and causing a partial obstruction. This technique is particularly useful in frail or elderly patients where more major operations are not possible. Colposuspension is still widely regarded as the gold standard surgical procedure, although tension-free vaginal tape (TVT) insertion, a new sling procedure, is rapidly gaining popularity and has the advantages of being performed under regional or local anaesthesia. There is still some uncertainty over the mechanisms of cure for some of these surgical procedures. Colposuspension, needle suspension and the MMK procedure aim to stabilise the bladder neck, so that abdominal pressure is equally transmitted to bladder and proximal urethra, and also to increase the urethrovesical angle. The older sling procedures also elevate the bladder neck, whilst the TVT insertion is thought to cause kinking of the urethra during an increase in abdominal pressure. The anterior colporrhaphy is no longer recommended as a sole procedure for the treatment of stress urinary incontinence.[135]

Men may also suffer with stress incontinence, although far fewer than women. Some may require insertion of an artificial urethral sphincter to treat their problem. Rarely, women may also need an artificial sphincter. A small number of surgical procedures are performed for other types of incontinence. Severe cases of detrusor overactivity in both men and women can be treated with a sacral nerve implant, which is expensive. Very occasionally there are cases of detrusor overactivity which fail to respond to all conservative interventions and surgery may become necessary. Techniques include urinary diversion, augmentation cystoplasty and detrusor myomectomy. These are complex surgical procedures, associated with not insignificant morbidity and should only be considered as a last resort.

Health care utilisation

Consultation

The most recent available data for urinary incontinence consultation in primary care was obtained from the Fourth National General Practice Morbidity Survey 1991–1992[136] on the basis of the ICD-9 codes listed in **Table 8**. The survey involved a representative cross-section of practices in England and Wales. The consultation rates were calculated using denominator data from the 1991 census. The numerator for *consultation rates* was the number of consultations for urinary incontinence during 1991/92. The number of *patients* forms the numerator for *patient rates* consulting with urinary incontinence during the same period.

Table 8: ICD-9 codes for urinary incontinence included in the National General Practice Morbidity Survey 1991–1992.

Diagnosis code from ICD-9	Description
788.3	Male and neurogenic urinary incontinence
625.6	Female stress urinary incontinence
307.6	Non-organic incontinence

The recognised level of patients presenting to primary care with urinary incontinence in 1991–1992 was 36/10 000.[136] For people aged 40 or more, these rates are considerably lower than estimates based on consultations reported by patients themselves 600/10 000 (40+) (610/10 000 for men and 650/10 000 for women) identified by the MRC Incontinence Study. The difference may be due to urinary incontinence not registering as a presenting complaint. The sex and age pattern of distribution of urinary incontinence in primary care is consistent with that in population studies, with the rate being appreciably higher in women than men and increasing with age in both sexes (**Figure 10**).

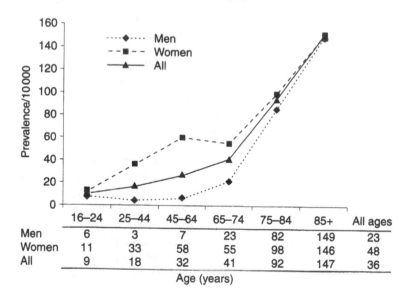

	16–24	25–44	45–64	65–74	75–84	85+	All ages
Men	6	3	7	23	82	149	23
Women	11	33	58	55	98	146	48
All	9	18	32	41	92	147	36

Figure 10: Patient rates consulting for urinary incontinence per 10 000 population by age and sex in general practice in England and Wales 1991–1992.[136]

The total consultation rate for urinary incontinence in general practice was 54 per 10 000 population, with women consulting almost twice as often as men (**Table 9**). Among these patients, the average number of consultations per incontinent patient was 1.5, with similar levels in men and women, young and old.

In a typical Primary Care Trust with 150 000 population, 25 900 patients aged 40 and over with storage symptoms would be expected to be present at any one time, based on population studies. In the course of a year 6700 people will develop a condition worthy of assessment, whilst 5154 prevalent cases are likely

Table 9: Consultation rates for urinary incontinence per 10,000 population by age and sex in general practice 1991–1992.[136]

Sex	Age (years)						All ages
	16–24	25–44	45–64	65–74	75–84	85+	
Men	8.4	6.1	10.8	40.8	153.4	202.0	36.9
Women	16.0	44.1	84.9	86.3	160.8	216.8	70.2
All	12.2	25.1	47.5	65.9	158.0	213.1	53.9

to remit. Self-reported annual patient consultation rates suggest 4014 will visit the GP and mention incontinence. However, official patient consultation rates suggest only around 300 (i.e. 7%) will actually be recorded by the GP; this may be due to patients reporting an incontinence problem whilst consulting for a more 'serious' medical problem.

For secondary care service utilisation, urinary incontinence data for England in the period 1999–2000 was obtained from Hospital Episode Statistics (HES). The data were based on the ICD-10 codes given in **Table 2**. Rates were calculated using the corresponding population estimates.

In that year, the overall rate of admission to hospital of patients with urinary incontinence was 13.9 per 10 000 population. These patients were not necessarily admitted because of their urinary incontinence, but a diagnosis of UI was recorded during the hospital stay.

The rate of *hospital episodes* is approximately one third of patients consulting in primary care (**Figure 11**). The rate of admissions was higher in women than men and increased steadily with age for both sexes, with a slight peak for women at age 45–64 years. In old age, the admission rates in males overtook those in women, apparently.

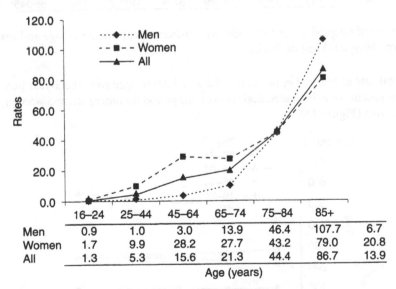

	16–24	25–44	45–64	65–74	75–84	85+	
Men	0.9	1.0	3.0	13.9	46.4	107.7	6.7
Women	1.7	9.9	28.2	27.7	43.2	79.0	20.8
All	1.3	5.3	15.6	21.3	44.4	86.7	13.9

Figure 11: Hospital in-patient episode rates for urinary incontinence per 10 000 by age and sex in England, 1999/2000.

The overall pattern of use of secondary care is similar to that in primary care. However, there appears to be a disproportionate rate of hospital episodes for older men compared with older women. This may reflect a disproportionate tendency to refer elderly men rather than women, possibly related to overlapping concerns about prostate enlargement, and the development of incontinence *de novo* in hospital among men, among other factors.

It appears that 56 045 patients with urinary incontinence were admitted to hospital in England in 1999/2000 (**Figure 12**). Numerically, more women than men attend hospital at every age. There is a peak in women in the age group 45–64 years, suggesting an increased service use in this age group.

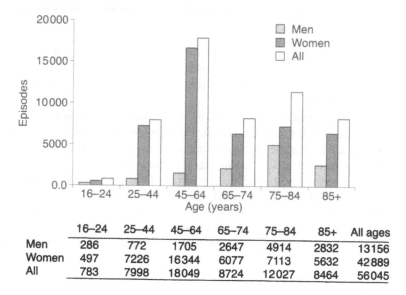

	16–24	25–44	45–64	65–74	75–84	85+	All ages
Men	286	772	1705	2647	4914	2832	13156
Women	497	7226	16344	6077	7113	5632	42889
All	783	7998	18049	8724	12027	8464	56045

Figure 12: Number of hospital patient episodes with urinary incontinence by age and sex in England 1999/2000. *Source*: Hospital Episode Statistics.

The overall annual rate of hospital episodes has remained unchanged over the 5-year period 1995–2000. However, the age-specific rates increased slightly over this period for older men and women, particularly at age 75 years and over (**Figure 13**).

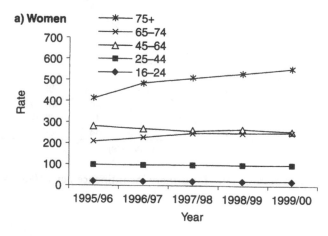

Figure 13: Hospital episode rates for urinary incontinence per 10 000 population by age and sex in England and Wales 1995–2000.

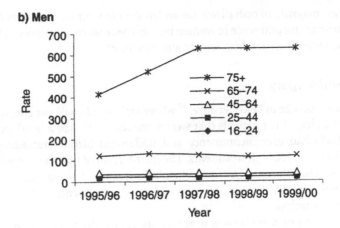

b) Men

Figure 13: Continued.

The data in **Figure 14** was obtained from Hospital Episode Statistics, Department of Health, and represents surgical activity for urinary incontinence performed during 1999/2000 in England & Wales. The Office for National Statistics' Surgical Classification codes (OPCS4) for urinary incontinence were used to extract data on surgical activity for this condition (**Table 3**) (*see* **Table A3.1** for actual numbers of surgical procedures).

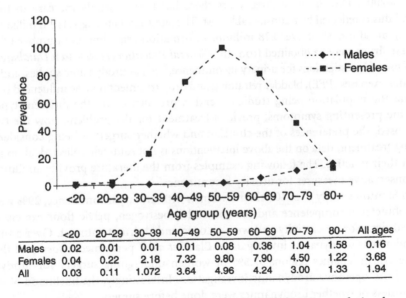

	<20	20–29	30–39	40–49	50–59	60–69	70–79	80+	All ages
Males	0.02	0.01	0.01	0.01	0.08	0.36	1.04	1.58	0.16
Females	0.04	0.22	2.18	7.32	9.80	7.90	4.50	1.22	3.68
All	0.03	0.11	1.072	3.64	4.96	4.24	3.00	1.33	1.94

Figure 14: Surgical procedures rates for urinary incontinence per 10 000 population by age and sex in England and Wales 1999/2000.

The overall rate of surgical procedures for urinary incontinence was 1.94 per 10 000 population in 1999/2000 (**Figure 14**). For women the rate was 3.68 compared with 0.16 per 10 000 population for men. The number of surgical operations was minimal below age 20 for both women and men but thereafter, for women, the rate starts to rise rapidly to a peak of 9.8 operations per 10 000 at 50–59 years. Thereafter the frequency declines for women and rises steadily for men, arriving at comparable levels at age 80 and over.

Numerically, the vast majority of operations are undertaken in women. This is not only because of the higher prevalence of urinary incontinence in women but also because most surgery in the UK is performed for urodynamic stress incontinence, which largely affects women.

Use of therapies and surgery

In a nurse-led continence service in Leicestershire[137] where male and female patients were seen and treated by nurses in the community, of 101 patients that were assessed, 37.6% had a 'weak pelvic floor' and were treated with PFE. 21.8% had urge incontinence and underwent bladder retraining. 12.9% had both conditions and therefore received both treatments. The distribution of the diagnostic groups was different in a later study carried out in Somerset.[39] Of those eligible for treatment, stress incontinence was diagnosed in 55%, urge incontinence in 10% and mixed stress and urge incontinence in 31%. All patients received both PFE and bladder retraining.

Among the different forms of incontinence, urge incontinence is the one most often treated with drugs, most commonly with anticholinergic drugs. Pharmacological treatment may or may not be combined with bladder retraining. These drugs may also be used to treat urinary urgency and frequency, when not accompanied by urge incontinence. Detrusor overactivity, which is a urodynamic diagnosis, is treated similarly. These drugs are increasingly being used in both primary and secondary care settings and the number of such drugs available on the market is increasing. The more modern drugs are more effective and have fewer side effects, which will lead to increased utilisation. **Table A4.2** indicates the numbers of prescriptions dispensed and the cost of four types of drug dispensed in the community in England for the three years 1998–2000. During these three years there has been a steady increase in the number of prescriptions and this is reflected by a considerable cost. The latest estimate suggests 1.6 million prescriptions dispensed each year, at a cost of over £28 million. Information regarding the number of people being treated with these drugs may be obtained from the *General Practitioners Research Database*.

The extent of use of investigations for urinary incontinence, such as urodynamic studies, and interventions such as pelvic floor exercises (PFE), bladder retraining and drug treatment may be influenced by a number of factors including the population being studied (gender, prevalence and the different types of urinary incontinence), the presenting symptoms, previous treatment for the problem, how the type of incontinence is diagnosed, the preferences of the clinician and whether surgery is being considered. With the exception of drug treatment, data on the above interventions is not routinely collected, although individual units may audit their practice. The following examples from the literature provide an illustration of the utilisation of conservative measures for urinary incontinence.

In Hilton and Stanton's study[138] of 100 elderly women with urinary incontinence, 29% were diagnosed with urethral sphincter incompetence and recommended oestrogen, pelvic floor exercises or surgery, whereas 56% had detrusor overactivity and were recommended drug treatment. Over a third (39%) of their sample underwent urodynamic investigation. Black et al.[139] performed a survey of the practice of clinicians in the North Thames region. 57.5% of women undergoing surgery for urodynamic stress incontinence had pre-operative urodynamic investigation. Interestingly, the likelihood of improvement was similar regardless of whether urodynamics were done before surgery.

Use of continence aids

A wide variety of continence products such as pads, sheaths, catheters, urinals and bed sheets are available in the UK, from the NHS, over the counter and by mail order[118,119] but there is limited epidemiological data on their use. The MRC Incontinence Study estimates 6.2% (women 10.1%, men 1.7%) of the population are using incontinence aids of some kind. The study by Roe et al. in 1996[122] revealed that only a minority of people who were incontinent, both in a health authority with and in a health authority without a continence service, used NHS aids or appliances to manage their incontinence. The majority of incontinent people (83%) bought their own aids or appliances. This may be due to sufferers being unaware that these products are available, not knowing how to obtain them, difficulties obtaining them or some individuals having to pay for their products. In the United States, Herzog[72] reported that 66% of the men and women with urinary incontinence aged 60 or over living in the community used one or more aid to control leakage and 47% of these used absorbent pads.

Hellström's study[16] of an 85-year-old population in Sweden found that among incontinent people living in the community significantly more women (68%) used continence aids during the day than men (43%). At night, 77% of women and 62% of men used aids, the major difference during the night being the increased use of disposable sheets. Nearly half of the men living at home who had daily incontinence did not use any form of continence aid. This may be due to different attitudes towards and/or awareness of the products available between men and women. Among those incontinent people living in an institution, 92% of women and 86% of men used continence aids. Pads were the commonest form of aid used both by those living in the community and those in an institution. Indwelling catheters were used by 2% of the 85-year-old population living in an institution.[16] In other studies, a figure of up to 28% is cited as the proportion of patients with long-term urinary catheters in residential long-term care.[140] There has been a suggestion that the over-use of catheters to manage incontinence, other than for short-term periods, is a potential sign of suboptimal care and an indication that further assessment and alternative treatment could be offered.[141]

Among adults with a learning disability within the UK, women are more likely to use continence aids than men (**Table 10**).

Table 10: Prevalence of incontinence and use and need for incontinence aids in adults with learning disability living in Leicestershire (Leicestershire Learning Disability Register 1994–1999).

Age group	Prevalence of weekly wetting[a] (%)		Using continence aids (%)		Total felt need for aids (% – met and unmet need)	
	Men	Women	Men	Women	Men	Women
20–29	20	34	3	34	7	39
30–39	15	20	1	23	2	25
40–49	15	15	16	21	16.5	22
50–59	10	23	15	27	15	29
60–69	20	16	23	34	26	39
70–79	25	31	36	39	36	42
80+	14	44	14	33	14	33
All ages	16	23	19	27	20	30

[a] Wetting on one or more days/nights a week.

Overall estimates of the cost of urinary incontinence

Cost of illness studies aim to estimate the total amount of societies' resources involved with the care or treatment of a condition, or that arise because of that condition. There are a number of cost of illness studies which deal with urinary incontinence. Probably the most comprehensive estimate of the cost of urinary incontinence (urinary incontinence) was made for the USA,[142] subsequently updated to 1995 US dollars,[143] and the later study estimated the cost of urinary incontinence to be $26.3 billion in 1995 US dollars, of which $704 million were indirect costs. These estimates were derived for the over-65s and included costs associated with extended hospital stays, urinary incontinence as a reason for admission to nursing homes and residential care, and indirect costs relating to loss of earning due to urinary incontinence. Wilson and colleagues also estimated the direct cost of urinary incontinence for the USA, this was £16.3 billion in 1995 US dollars.[144] Doran and colleagues estimated the cost of urinary incontinence for Australian women aged over 18 to be $710.44 million Australian dollars in 1998[145] (equivalent to $439.76 million US dollars) equating to $387 dollars per person with incontinence. An estimate of the cost of urinary incontinence to Italy in 1998[146] was based on a survey of 229 Italian women over 40 years of age. Focusing only on direct expenditure for the health service, i.e. costs associated with diagnosis, hospitalisation for detrusor overactivity, diapers and drugs, and excluding the cost of GP visits, the cost in 1998 was 351 800 billion lira, equivalent to 255 519 lira ($158 1998 US dollars) per person. An estimate was also made for Sweden that suggested that urinary incontinence costs comprised 2% of the total health care costs in 1993.[147]

There have been a number of estimates of cost for urinary incontinence in the UK. The most recent was made for the year 1998.[102] This included drugs and prescription appliances, containment products, the proportions of time spent by various staff on urinary incontinence and surgery. The estimated cost for the UK was £353.6 million. There were also two earlier estimates that focused on equipment, pads and appliances.[102,148] An estimate of the cost of urinary incontinence to health authorities was produced as part of an study carried out by the Social Policy Research Unit, York University.[149] The authors produced estimates of the costs of continence services to two health authorities, labelled as area 2 and area 3. The cost for area 2 was £2.72 per person and for area 3 £4.71 per person (1993/4 UK pounds). Both areas included urodynamic investigations, a continence advisory service, issue of products, drugs, and urinary appliances and stoma appliances, but area 2 also included the involvement of health care professionals in continence management while area 3 included outpatient clinic and social services.

Work has also been carried out to estimate the costs of urinary incontinence on an individual basis. Clayton and colleagues[150] surveyed 118 women, of whom 28 were disabled. The costs of NHS and patient-borne costs for a three-month period had a mean value of £37 in 1995 prices. An earlier study estimated the cost for people with multiple sclerosis as £1.53 per week in 1977/8 prices.[151] This author also found that mothers of severely handicapped children spent 10 hours a week on incontinence care. Utilisation of services due to urinary incontinence was examined by Roe and colleagues.[122] The authors found that those with incontinence were more likely to have contacted their GP and also any other health care providers compared with individuals without urinary incontinence.

One common feature of these studies is that they are limited to financial costs of urinary incontinence. They typically look at health service or provider costs. Some studies also consider financial costs borne by individuals such as purchases of pads. None of these studies estimate the non-resource-related costs of urinary incontinence. Examples of these types of cost would be discomfort and embarrassment of urinary incontinence, disruptions to usual activities and disruption of social life. These costs are not easily quantifiable but they represent a burden of urinary incontinence to individuals and society. Wagner and Hu recognised the lack of any estimate of these costs in their work but at the time of publication they felt there was no way to quantify these costs.[143] However, one tool that could be used to estimate these non-financial costs is willingness to pay (WTP). In this method a respondent is asked how much they would be prepared to pay for a defined change in their health. For example, a change in an individual's continence level would be defined and that individual may be asked to identify how much they would pay a month for this change. Alternatively, they might be given a series of amounts and asked to say whether they would pay these amounts, a technique used in the field of urinary incontinence.[152] In a study using this technique, respondents were asked about their willingness to pay for a reduction in their urinary symptoms. Responses were consistent with prior expectations in that they increased with severity of symptoms and with the ability to pay of the respondent. The mean willingness to pay for a respondent in the middle of their severity range was 530 Swedish krona per month (1996 prices). This equates to approximately £35 per month (UK pounds with an exchange rate of 15 krona to £1). In an evaluation of these results Kobelt[153] found that willingness to pay was correlated with improvements in health, urinary incontinence symptoms and income. A similar method was used on a sample of US respondents[154] where 257 respondents completed a WTP survey in 1997. The mean WTP was US$87.7 for a 25% reduction in micturitions and leakages. These results show that the non-financial part of the burden of urinary incontinence is potentially very important to those with the condition.

These studies are very mixed in that they use varying methodologies on different populations from different countries and in different time periods, but as a whole demonstrate that urinary incontinence has large resource implications, both to societies and to individuals. Any planned change in services for urinary incontinence should consider the wider costs associated with any change in level of function, as they are likely to be important.

6 Effectiveness of services and interventions

Primary care

Overall rates of cure and improvement resulting from primary care services are estimated at around 44%.[122] The presence of a Continence Advisory Service appeared to have little effect on the condition but a marked difference on levels of satisfaction with services.

Pelvic floor muscle training

Although therapies designed to strengthen the pelvic floor muscles and enhance closure of the bladder under stress have been extensively investigated, studies report markedly different results. These differences may be the result of different methods in applying the interventions, differences in the patients undergoing them, differences in compliance or differences in measuring the effects of treatment. Most studies have investigated small numbers of patients and few have used any form of satisfactory control group.

There is some evidence to support the effectiveness of bladder re-education, pelvic floor exercises and drug therapies in primary care. Hall[137] set up a team of trained district nurses supervised by a continence advisor in Leicestershire and found that 59–65% of patients were cured or improved. Short and longer term cure/improvement rates vary from 65–74%.[39,94,155,156] In a review of the literature by Williams et al.,[157] the authors concluded that studies varied in their design, the exercise programmes implemented, the person undertaking the training programme and the measures used to test effectiveness. This is reflected in the cure/improvement rates of 25–84% in the studies reviewed. A recent Cochrane review of the literature[121] showed that PFMT appeared to be an effective treatment for adult women with stress or mixed incontinence. PFMT was better than no treatment or placebo treatments. 'Intensive' appeared to be better than 'standard' PFMT programmes for women with stress incontinence and postnatal women with symptoms of urine leakage. There is insufficient evidence to determine if: PFMT is better or worse than other treatments; e.g. electrical stimulation or weighted cones in women with stress incontinence; or whether adding PFMT to other treatments for women with SI (e.g. electrical stimulation or behavioural therapy) is effective. Evidence of the effect of adding other adjunctive treatments to PFMT (e.g. vaginal cones, intravaginal resistance devices) is equally limited. On the basis of the evidence available, there does not appear to be any benefit of biofeedback-assisted PFMT over PFMT alone.

There have been very few trials comparing PFMT with pharmacological therapy or surgery. In a recent review of the literature, in women with stress and mixed incontinence, there may be no difference between PFMT and phenylpropanolamine (an alpha-adrenergic antagonist), but in women with detrusor overactivity, with or without stress incontinence, PFMT may be better than oxybutynin. In women with urodynamic stress incontinence, PFMT may be better than topical oestrogens, but surgery may be better than PFMT.[106]

Long-term outcomes of PFMT are unclear. Most studies have reported a follow-up of no longer than 12 months. The best quality and most complete data comes from the follow-up study by Lagro-Janssen and Van Weel.[158] The number of continent women (25%) was the same after five years, but a significant number of women reported their condition had worsened. Women with urge or mixed incontinence were less likely to be satisfied with the outcome of treatment at five years, although two-thirds of all the women followed up remained satisfied with the outcome of treatment and did not want any further intervention. Nearly half (43%) of the women who had received PFMT were no longer training at all. For women with stress incontinence, continued training was the only significant predictor of outcome at five years. Five years after an intensive exercise program, Bø and Talseth[159] found that 70% of women were satisfied with treatment and did not want further treatment, despite a significant increase in urine loss over this period. This may reflect the fact that women became more empowered over their condition and accepted greater urine loss. O'Brien[160] evaluated non-specialist nurse continence classes using pelvic floor exercises and bladder retraining and showed that 68% of patients were improved or cured, compared with 5% in the GP control group. When the treated group was followed up four years later[161] 69% had either maintained their original improvement or cure or had improved further.

The role of PFMT for women with urge incontinence alone remains unclear.[121] There is level 1 evidence that PFMT is better than placebo treatments for women with urge incontinence.[106] In their review of the literature of pelvic floor exercises for the treatment of overactive bladder, Bø and Berghmans found that because of the lack of evidence, no firm conclusion can be drawn on the effect of pelvic floor muscle exercise on the overactive bladder.[162] In a review of 15 randomised controlled trials to assess the efficacy of physical therapies for first line use in the treatment of urge urinary incontinence in women, Berghmans *et al.* concluded that although almost all studies included reported positive results in favour of physical therapies, there were too few studies to evaluate the effect of pelvic floor muscle exercise with or without biofeedback in this group of women.[163]

Electrical stimulation (ES)

Electrical stimulation for the treatment of urinary incontinence in women is currently the subject of a Cochrane review.[164] A previous review of the literature by Wilson *et al.*[106] found that due to a lack of good quality trials, there is insufficient evidence to judge whether ES is better than no treatment for women with urodynamic stress incontinence or detrusor overactivity. With regard to ES versus placebo ES, the findings of two good quality trials are contradictory.[165,166] For women with detrusor overactivity, there is a trend in favour of active stimulation over placebo stimulation.[106] When reviewing ES trials in general, and trials comparing ES protocols in particular, it appears that some ES protocols may be more effective than others and/or some populations of women receive more benefit from ES than others. Both these variables require further investigation.[106] With only single small trials comparing ES with medication, there is insufficient evidence to determine if ES is better than vaginal oestrogens in women with urodynamic stress incontinence, or better than anticholinergic therapy in women with detrusor overactivity.[106]

Weighted vaginal cones

A Cochrane review has provided some evidence that weighted vaginal cones are better than no active treatment in women with stress incontinence and may be of similar effectiveness to PFMT and ES.[167] The authors suggest that this conclusion must remain tentative until further larger, high quality studies are carried out using comparable and relevant outcome measures. Some women treated with cones, PFMT or

ES drop out of treatment early. Therefore, cones should be offered as one option so that if women find them unacceptable there are other treatments available.

Behavioural and lifestyle changes

Bladder retraining

Evidence for the efficacy of lifestyle changes in the management of urinary incontinence is lacking. Much of current practice is based upon expert opinion and a 'common sense' approach. Such measures include advice relevant to the maintenance of general health and therefore should not be neglected. It appears that, when taken as a whole, the basket of interventions is effective in reducing the subjective severity of bladder problems as assessed by sufferers. The evidence for bladder retraining is a little more robust and data suggest that, in certain groups, bladder retraining can gain as much improvement as drug therapy. When employed as part of a package of measures, bladder retraining appears to be as effectively delivered on an outpatient as an in-patient basis,[168,169] but remote delivery, by telephone, does not work.[170] This suggests that the therapeutic relationship and direct contact with their clinician or therapist is important in achieving success. In many studies the technique is used as part of a package of other lifestyle measures (diet and fluid advice, caffeine restriction) with or without pelvic floor therapy and medication.[171,172] Studies of bladder retraining alone indicate that among incontinent women successfully undertaking a bladder retraining programme 60–80% will be improved in terms of urine loss and urinary frequency.[173–176]

A number of trials of this technique, which aims to control urinary frequency and increase functional bladder capacity, have been performed and have recently been the subject of a Cochrane Review. This noted that many of the available studies were flawed and that limitations on the available data led the reviewers to issue a guarded positive recommendation based upon the available evidence.[177] Where the patient is confused and unable to participate in bladder retraining then there are other toileting regimens which have been found useful in care homes in the US. These techniques have also been the subject of a Cochrane review.[178]

Effect of caffeine restriction

There has been a short-term, urodynamic study using oral caffeine, which has shown minimal effect on the bladder while retrospective analyses have found an association between high caffeine intake and a diagnosis of detrusor overactivity.[110,179] Clinical trials, most of which assessed fluid intake and caffeine, have found no sustained benefit,[81] although a recent trial of caffeine reduction in a predominantly elderly group of women reported that reduction in caffeine intake with maintenance of total fluid intake led to a reduction in urinary frequency.[180] However, the practicality of meaningful caffeine reduction and the achieved magnitude of resolution of symptoms may not result in this being a worthwhile option for most patients.

Fluid advice

Limiting or reducing overall fluid intake is not effective for managing incontinence and may lead to adverse effects especially in the elderly, who are likely to be taking other medication, who have a decreased total body water and are more susceptible to volume depletion. There are no randomised trials of fluid intake adjustment alone on which to base management. Retrospective studies have shown that nurse intervention is useful in achieving appreciation of fluid requirements[181] and a study examining the association of caffeine and fluid intake resulted in improvements in continence status.[180]

Weight reduction

There are no data on the relationship between urinary incontinence and obesity in males. In females, however, there is good evidence for a positive association of stress urinary incontinence and body mass.[111,112] In community surveys a greater number of women with incontinence reported themselves as obese, or being too heavy for their height.[59]

There is also evidence that being obese is associated with a poorer result from operation for stress incontinence.[182] However, the evidence that weight reduction might be able to correct some of this disadvantage is limited to two studies of women who had undergone surgery for their obesity with consequent massive weight reduction.[183,184] The latter study reported that, in women losing at least 50% of their excess weight, the prevalence of urinary incontinence was reduced by 50%. An association of obesity with types of incontinence other than stress incontinence is seldom reported[185] and the single report which did, did not control for age.[186] It seems that the weight loss achieved by advice from physicians is unlikely to have a significant impact upon urinary incontinence.

Relief of constipation

There has been one community-based study in women of 60 years and older which has examined the relationship between self-reported urinary incontinence and constipation. Subjects who reported urinary incontinence were more likely to report constipation. A relationship between straining and impaired function of rectal emptying is hypothesised but there are no studies which systematically evaluate the effect of relieving constipation on urinary incontinence.[187] Faecal impaction can lead to urinary retention, and there have been conflicting reports of an association between incontinence and constipation.[113]

Smoking

An association of bladder problems with cigarette smoking has been identified for both men and women.[114,116] The odds ratio of men suffering lower urinary tract symptoms was 1.47 for current smokers and 1.38 for former smokers when compared with men who had never smoked.[114] For women, smokers were 1.9 times more likely to suffer from incontinence.[115] However, studies in other populations have found no association.[66,84] As with other adverse effects of smoking, this association weakened following cessation of smoking and appeared to reach baseline after 40 years of abstinence. In men, the association of smoking appeared to be strongest with the occurrence of detrusor overactivity. An association with both stress and urge incontinence is found in women, smoking-related cough thought to be a precipitating factor in the development of stress incontinence.[188]

There are no prospective intervention trials of smoking cessation on improving bladder symptoms. However, there is little doubt that smoking should be discouraged in view of the cardiovascular risk, regardless of its effect upon lower urinary tract function.

Lifestyle interventions for the treatment of urinary incontinence have been a subject of the Cochrane review process.[189]

Drug therapy

Drug therapy for urinary symptoms is mainly aimed at patients with detrusor overactivity. All of the currently available drug therapies have side effects that limit their use. At present the most effective drug therapies with the most favourable side effect profiles are controlled release oxybutynin and tolterodine. These drugs, although of proven efficacy, have limited clinical effects (about 50% reduction in urinary frequency and incontinence episodes) and should not be started without ensuring that simple behavioural therapies have been started. The costs of the drugs vary with the compound and dose used (**Table A4.1**).

Details of the individual drug studies and the evidence of benefit may be found in Appendix 4.

Economic evidence

To be considered an economic evaluation a study must consider both the costs of any intervention and also some measure of benefits produced. These must be combined; for example, cost per quality adjusted life year, cost per case cured etc.

Although there is some evidence for the effectiveness of primary care interventions for lower urinary tract symptoms, there is very little evidence of the cost-effectiveness of interventions. One study investigated the use of tolterodine for overactive bladder[190] and estimated quality of life using a rating scale; this was used to generate quality-adjusted life years (QALYs). Costs measured related to drug costs, pad usage and visits to a GP. Costs in the tolterodine arm were SEK (Swedish Krona) 5309 higher than in the control arm. The improvement in quality of life was 0.025 equating to a cost per QALY of SEK 213 000, which equates to US$28 000 or UK£14 200. There are also two studies which consider the costs of urinary incontinence interventions in primary care,[191,192] but neither of these studies combined an estimate of costs with any measure of whether the interventions studied were effective.

Secondary care

Drug therapy

The main indication for pharmacological therapy is detrusor overactivity, whether idiopathic or secondary to a neurological cause. Whatever the indication, drug therapy appears to maximally improve or cure approximately 50% of patients in terms of urinary frequency or urgency, with a lesser effect on the number of incontinence episodes. The main limitation of antimuscarinic drugs for this indication has been the relatively high incidence of side effects, notably dry mouth, leading to withdrawal from medication. The newer, once daily, formulations of both oxybutynin and tolterodine are an attempt to minimise the effect of these and to maximise the effective dose of medication. Although drug therapies are in common use in secondary care many patients will not have undergone behavioural therapies before starting medication. There is little evidence that drug therapy is superior to behavioural therapies[172] but some suggestion that a combination of drug therapy with behavioural therapy is advantageous.[193] In fact most studies investigating the efficacy of drug therapy in secondary care do not allow any of the patients to receive concurrent behavioural therapies. It therefore seems appropriate to make sure that behavioural therapies have been applied appropriately before starting medication. The evidence supporting the use of anti-muscarinic medication has been subject to recent Cochrane reviews.[194–196]

Oxybutynin

Oxybutynin is the most established antimuscarinic drug in use today. Trials comparing oxybutynin to placebo have consistently shown a reduction in symptoms and urodynamic parameters with the active drug (**Table A4.5**). Oxybutynin is thus the drug against which all new preparations are compared. Drug-related unwanted side effects occur in the majority of patients taking standard doses of oxybutynin and these can result in about 1 in 4 patients discontinuing treatment.[197,198] It has been suggested that oxybutynin should be started at a low dose and gradually increased, titrating the dose against side-effects and efficacy. Inevitably this will lead to more hospital appointments with associated cost.[199]

Recently controlled-release oxybutynin has been studied. This modified release, once daily preparation avoids large peaks in plasma levels of the drug and its active metabolite.[200] Trials seem to show an improved side effect profile with this preparation (**Table A4.6**).

Tolterodine

Tolterodine has functional selectivity for muscarinic receptors in the bladder compared to the salivary gland. Given in a dose of 2 mg twice per day, there seems to be similar efficacy between oxybutynin and tolterodine, but tolterodine had a more favourable side effect profile in terms of unwanted dry mouth and gastrointestinal effects resulting in less patients needing to stop therapy. Controlled-release tolterodine may have less adverse side effects (**Table A4.7**).

Trospium chloride

There is limited evidence that trospium chloride is useful in the treatment of detrusor overactivity. Randomised controlled trials have shown improvements in urodynamic parameters and subjective symptomatic improvement.[201,202] Trospium (20 mg bd) seems to be better tolerated than oxybutynin (5 mg tds) and as the compound does not cross the blood-brain barrier, very few CNS side effects have been reported.

Flavoxate

This tertiary amine has not been shown to have any clear advantages over placebo in double blind controlled studies.[203,204]

Imipramine

Imipramine is a tricyclic antidepressant with anticholinergic side effects. It may also have some bladder anaesthetic and adrenergic properties that may aid bladder filling. There is some evidence that imipramine may be useful in children with nocturnal enuresis,[205] but the only double blind controlled trial in adults was small and inconclusive.[206]

Propiverine

This drug, with combined antimuscarinic and calcium channel blocking properties, has been shown to be superior to placebo in controlled clinical trials. It appears to be as effective as oxybutynin in the treatment of detrusor overactivity. There are no data comparing the drug to behavioural intervention. Approximately 20% of users develop some adverse side effect but dry mouth is less common and milder than with oxybutynin.

Desmopressin

This synthetic vasopressin analogue can be used to suppress diuresis overnight. It has been shown to be useful in nocturnal enuresis in children[205] and in reducing nocturnal frequency in adults.[207] There are potential problems in producing worsening daytime frequency due to increased daytime diuresis and fluid overload may be a problem, particularly the elderly.

Oestrogens

Although oestrogen therapy has been advocated for the treatment of urinary frequency and incontinence in randomised controlled trials, no beneficial effect was shown on bladder function.[208,209] The only symptom that appears to be reduced with oestrogen therapy is urinary urgency.[210]

Alpha-adrenergic agents

Alpha-adrenergic receptor agonists have been used for the treatment of stress incontinence. Where the urethral sphincter is incompetent, they are thought to increase the intrinsic tone of the sphincter and so prevent incontinence on pressure. Currently there is no recommended indication for this type of drug in stress incontinence.[211]

Surgery

As might be expected when there are such a large number of operations for one condition (**Table A4.8**), there is variable efficacy and morbidity associated with each. Until recently there were few trials comparing these procedures and evidence for efficacy of recent techniques, such as the tension-free vaginal tape (TVT), is still being generated. Evaluation of the efficacy of this operation in particular is part of the 6th work program of the National Institute for Clinical Excellence.

Jarvis, in 1994, completed a systematic review of surgery for urodynamic stress incontinence.[212] This showed that some procedures had only limited efficacy (which is usually unacceptable when considering major surgery for a non-life threatening disease). Others, although efficacious, had high levels of morbidity associated with them.

Anterior repair with bladder buttress has been evaluated in a recent Cochrane review.[213] This procedure, when done for stress incontinence alone, was shown to have low initial cure rates with high recurrence and repeat operation rates compared to colposuspension. Although morbidity is low with this operation, it is significantly higher than the minimally invasive procedures that are now available. No such procedures should now performed for significant incontinence in the absence of prolapse.

Marshall-Marchetti-Krantz procedures have generally been abandoned as there is a high incidence of osteitis pubis (2.5%) following the procedure. When this occurs the patient has severe pain, often necessitating further surgery. All other rates of efficacy and morbidity are similar to colposuspension.

Many different types of needle suspension have been described. All involve minimal access surgery inserting (with the use of needles) stitches between the abdominal wall and the anterior vaginal wall. Although associated with minimal short-term morbidity, long-term success rates have been disappointing and fewer numbers of these procedures are performed. Bladder neck needle suspension surgery is probably not as good as open abdominal retropubic suspension for the treatment of primary stress urinary incontinence in terms of lower cure rates and higher morbidity.[214]

Traditional suburethral sling procedures were originally designed for recurrent stress incontinence but have recently been used for patients with severe primary disease. A recent systematic review showed no increased efficacy over colposuspension but there was a longer in-patient stay.[215] Suburethral sling procedures are usually associated with high rates (37%) of postoperative voiding disorder and subsequent repeat operation (28%) to release the sling. They involve a relatively large abdominal incision resulting in moderate short-term morbidity.

The tension-free vaginal tape (TVT) for primary treatment of stress incontinence has become fashionable. It is based on the suburethral sling but this is sited at the mid-urethra under no tension. Using angled needles, a specially developed sling (polypropylene tape) can be inserted with minimal dissection. The tape should be inserted without tension so that minimal obstruction of the urethra occurs. Large case series seem to show that this operation has reduced short- and long-term morbidity compared to a colposuspension.[216] In particular the in-patient stay is dramatically reduced. There is comparable reduction in symptoms for up to five years compared to a colposuspension. A randomised controlled trial has been conducted comparing TVT with colposuspension. The unpublished results of this trial in the short term seem to be encouraging. The major disadvantage of this operation is the cost of the tape. However, this is more than outweighed by the reduced costs of hospitalisation.

Any decision about which operation to perform will usually take into account the chance of cure, the likelihood of surgical complications, the severity of the patients' condition, medical comorbidities and what previous therapies have been tried. The ideal surgery should be effective, have few risks and be long-lasting. At present the gold standard operation is the colposuspension despite a failure rate of 10% in the short term and 20% in the long term. The operation is also associated with a 10% incidence of genitourinary prolapse, a 10% incidence of voiding disorder and a 10% incidence of *de novo* detrusor overactivity. This 'gold standard' is far from ideal.[217] Colposuspension may be performed either as an open operation or using a laparoscope. Currently there are exponents of each technique and no clear consensus as to whether one is superior in terms of cure or improvement. The long-term performance of colposuspension is uncertain. Currently available evidence suggests that laparoscopic colposuspension may be poorer than open colposuspension. Like other laparoscopically performed operations, laparoscopic colposuspension leads to a quicker recovery, but takes longer to perform and may be associated with more surgical complications. These matters should hopefully be answered in the near future as the results of a randomised controlled trial sponsored by the MRC become available. If laparoscopic colposuspension is performed, two paravaginal sutures appear to be more effective than one.[218]

There is conflicting evidence from trial data of effectiveness versus the real-life experience of women undergoing these operations, the results seldom reaching those attained in clinical trials.[101,219]

Injection of various different materials into the bladder neck has been described.[220] The aim of these procedures is to bulk up the junction between bladder neck and urethra, increasing pressure transmission and, although unclear, probably causing a partial obstruction. The operation is minimally invasive and can be performed under local anaesthetic. There is little associated morbidity and most patients will be treated as day cases. This has the advantage of allowing frail elderly patients to receive treatment where more major operations are not possible. The short-term success rate is acceptable but may fall to as low as 40% by four years. There is no strong evidence that any agent has a marked increased success rate but they vary considerably in their cost.

Surgical therapies for urodynamic stress incontinence are relatively expensive in terms of health service usage. Most have significant associated morbidity and mortality. Effectiveness will depend on patient selection and the skill and experience of the surgeon.[101] It seems reasonable that surgery should only usually take place where conservative measures, in particular pelvic floor therapies, have already been tried and failed. In view of the possible adverse consequences of surgery, all patients should undergo a detailed expert assessment to confirm the diagnosis and assess the severity of disease. Where surgery is necessary it should ideally be performed by a small team of experienced surgeons in each locality. This will allow development of expert local expertise and allow local figures for success and complication rates to be quoted.

Urinary incontinence after prostatectomy is a common problem. Conservative management of this condition includes pelvic floor muscle training, biofeedback, electrical stimulation using a rectal electrode, transcutaneous electrical nerve stimulation, or a combination of methods. Conservative management is often combined with lifestyle adjustments including: decreased intake or elimination of caffeine, physical exercise, cessation of smoking, and bladder retraining. A Cochrane review of six randomised trials, each evaluating different treatments, concluded that the value of the various approaches to manage this particular problem remains uncertain.[221]

Economic evidence

There is very limited evidence relating to the economic evaluation for surgery for lower urinary tract symptoms. Two studies were found which could be categorised as economic evaluations. Open and laparoscopic colposuspension were evaluated by Kohli in a cost-minimisation study, using intra-operative complications, postoperative haematocrit change and estimated blood loss as the outcome measures.[222] The authors found no statistically significant differences in outcome between the groups, although the total hospital charges were found to be higher for the laparoscopic group, $4960 versus $4079. In Canada, Kung[223] carried out a cost-effectiveness analysis of laparoscopic Burch procedures compared to an abdominal Burch procedure. This time the measure of effectiveness used was the percentage cure rate for the surgical procedure. The costs of the surgical procedure were also estimated. The hospital costs *per case cured* were $3029 for laparoscopy and $6325 for Burch and open surgery.

Although there have also been a number of studies that have considered costs relating to surgery, they were not combined with a measurement of outcomes,[224–229] therefore these studies are of limited use as decisions cannot be made on the basis of cost only. For example, if an intervention is more expensive than an alternative it may still be preferable if it is also more effective. Whether it is indeed preferable will depend on the degree of extra cost and extra effectiveness.

7 Models of care and recommendations

Minimal evidence exists on the effectiveness of current UK service provision. Such evidence as does exist has tended to have been generated by the more motivated, specialist centres and probably does not reflect the more general experience. As noted above, there are large inconsistencies in care provision, with many areas either having a consultant-led or a continence nurse-led service. Considerable scope for improvement lies in supplementing primary care teams with special expertise and resources. However, there are a number of problems in comparing the merits of the different models of service provision using the results of existing studies. First, it is probable that, due to selection factors, the severity and type of condition treated varies substantially between hospital clinics, district nurse clinics and GP sessions. Second, the age distribution of patients is different. For example, attendance at non-specialist nurse clinics declines with age. Third, no standard definition of cure or improvement has been applied. Finally, the number of patients seen and the levels of improvement achieved have not been related to the resources used.

Rhodes *et al.* carried out a two-phased feasibility study which aimed (i) to examine continence services in three district health authorities (to reflect different approaches to continence management), (ii) to examine costs to the health and social services, (iii) to determine policy and provision and (iv) to explore professionals' perceptions of quality in service delivery.[230] The different services ranged from a very limited community continence service to an integrated continence service covering both the acute and community sectors. However, problems were identified in each service, with all three exemplifying many of the problems in providing a truly integrated service. In none of the three areas had GPs shown any real enthusiasm or interest in continence services. Two of the districts had little in the way of community physiotherapy provision and access of the service was controlled by GPs. Even in the most well-established continence service, the service was integrated more in name than in practice. Hospital and community services operated virtually autonomously, largely as a result of management structures. Consultants seemed to know very little about the community service. Continence advisors and the nursing management saw integration as a potential loss of autonomy. Furthermore, there seemed to be little incentive for co-operation, with different hospital departments and community services competing for business from GPs. Other concerns raised included insufficient medical input to the service, routes of referral from primary to secondary sector and varying paths of clinical decision making. One solution proposed by medical staff would be for all patients to be channelled through a hospital department, the route of referral being from GP to hospital consultant. A single gateway service may avoid loops in the system but would swamp hospital clinics.

The researchers were also unable to report any interprofessional consensus on best practice issues or the structure of a continence service. They suggested that in defining a good quality service it is necessary, first, to identify various professionals and services which make a contribution and, second, to extricate a continence service from other services. Should continence promotion and continence care be an integral part of all health professionals or should there be a separately defined continence service?

There were clear difficulties in identifying the costs of providing continence services at local levels. Identifying the input of health care professionals in the community was particularly difficult. Variations between individual health authorities were exposed in terms of the allocation of resources between the acute and community sectors.

The second phase of the study looked at the costs of incontinence to individuals and to services, and users' perceptions of quality and effectiveness of services.[231] On the whole patients did not find it easy to describe their referral route through the service. Patients also had difficulty in identifying the links between assessment, intervention and review and in describing the outcomes they might expect from service contact. The most common difficulty for patients was recognition of the role and responsibility of the professionals they met. Members of the continence advisory service in one area were frequently praised for their patience, understanding and support but were not readily recognised as part of that service. As a result the authors suggested that a 'care management' (multi-referral) model may be more effective in meeting the needs of incontinence sufferers. Continence advisors or specialists could act as sole 'care managers' where they assess a patient, directing and monitoring the appropriate path(s) of care. This may involve referral to GPs for drug treatment or to other professionals for assessment for continence aids, to physiotherapists for pelvic floor exercises or other specialists for urodynamics. The continence care manager would then be responsible for case review to ensure that the patient is successfully moved through the system with outcomes which can be readily evaluated. Where no continence advisor is in post, the team model would be applied, with one individual (a key worker) taking overall responsibility for the management of care of that individual, ensuring progress through the system. The study concluded that district-wide comparative studies of the cost-effectiveness of different service models are not feasible, given the current rate of change of service structures and the fact that continence services are made of many disparate elements which may not be related in the coherent way that the word 'model' suggests. They proposed that it would be more valuable to study the cost-effectiveness of particular interventions or specific service innovations.

Another study of continence services[122] compared the health needs and use of health services by people who suffered from incontinence compared to a background population who were not incontinent. Comparisons were also made between individuals who were incontinent within two health authorities to provide an evaluation of their health interventions and patient outcomes in relation to a health authority with a continence advisory service and one without. There was some evidence that people in the health authority with a continence service received more appropriate treatment and care for their incontinence than those in the health authority without a continence service. Despite significant differences between the health interventions undertaken in the two health authorities, these findings did not transfer through to people's perceptions of their continence status. Only 44% of incontinent people in the health authority with a continence service felt that their incontinence was cured, improved or better managed, compared to 43% in the health authority without a service. However, the difference in health interventions did follow through to satisfaction with services and health care, with significantly more incontinent people in the authority with the continence service reporting that they were satisfied compared to those in the authority without a service.

The researchers also felt that type and severity of incontinence are important factors that should be considered when evaluating health care and services in relation to their outcomes. Using The Short Form 36 as a measure of health status, people who were incontinent had a significantly lower health status than those who were not incontinent. Women who were incontinent tended to have a better health status than men who were incontinent. Using the Incontinence Impact Questionnaire (IIQ) as a measure of the impact of incontinence, there were no significant differences between the IIQ scores of people whose incontinence was effectively or ineffectively managed. People who were incontinent in the health authority without the continence service had significantly lower mean scores for their self-esteem than those in the authority with a continence service. Furthermore, people whose incontinence was successfully managed tended to have a higher self-esteem than those whose incontinence was not successfully managed.

People who sought help early for their incontinence were considered to be successfully managed and the vast majority of sufferers who sought help early lived in the health authority with the continence service. Establishing management techniques that suited individuals and evaluating their health gains and outcomes were important indicators identified by the authors as contributing to the successful management of incontinence. People who had participated in decisions taken about the management of their incontinence were generally considered as being successfully managed.

There was some evidence that multiple referral to members of the multidisciplinary team which focused and targeted their particular health intervention skills was associated with incontinence being successfully managed. Greater flexibility of services was considered as being important by a number of sufferers, and related to the acceptability and appropriateness of health services. A person's incontinence was considered successfully managed when their views were considered and their expectations were met.

In 1997, a report of a working group to the Department of Health highlighted a number of aims that a continence service should strive for, including:

- given the possibility of cure or improvement, a continence service should not have provision of products as its primary focus;
- acute and community services need careful co-ordination across trust boundaries and across the primary care/hospital interface.

The group concluded that given the paucity of research evidence, any care which provides a systematic approach to the management of incontinence may improve outcomes.

The Leicestershire MRC Incontinence Pilot Study has evaluated a new nurse-led continence service.[232] This involves specially trained continence nurse practitioners delivering pre-defined, evidence-based treatment interventions. The service was shown to be effective in reducing urinary symptoms (60% reported cure or improvement), with high levels of patient satisfaction (99%). This service is currently being evaluated in a comparison with care provided by GPs in a randomised controlled trial. Further work from the Leicester team showed that an informal, friendly approach by nurses with good communication skills relieved patients' embarrassment and anxiety, giving them confidence and trust in the nurses, thus facilitating information exchange and effectiveness of care.[233] Good communication skills conveyed the nurses' specialist technical skills and knowledge, encouraging patient compliance with treatments. An RCT of the new service is now published.*

The following model of care describes an ideal service that may overcome some of the variability in continence care available to the population. This proposal is based on analysis of available evidence and consensus within the main groups concerned. The principles underlying an integrated continence.service have been outlined in a Department of Health document *Good Practice in Continence Services* (March 2000), which has recommended an evolutionary approach to service development from the existing local

---

* Williams KS *et al.* Clinical and cost-effectiveness of a new nurse-led continence service: a RCT. *Brit J Gen Prac* 2005; **55**: 696–703.

provision. The ideal new service for continence care would span both primary and secondary care and would comprise a large volume, community-provided service which would include a number of key elements:

- All patients with bladder symptoms would be eligible to enter the service.
- There should be a defined method of entry into the service regardless of the original source of the referral.
- Service co-ordination would be provided by a multidisciplinary team.
- The service, whilst provided by a multidisciplinary team, is likely to be led by the specialist continence practitioners.
- The service would be structured around evidence-based protocols.
- There would be clear patterns of referral to specialist secondary care providers.
- The service would have access to medical and surgical consultants with a special interest in continence.
- Secondary care provision would be provided by trained specialist professionals.
- Nurse prescribing of limited medications would be implemented using a patient group directive following appropriate training.
- Continence specialist clinicians (either nursing or physiotherapy background) would take part in secondary care clinical sessions to ensure continuity and consistency of approach throughout the service.
- Regular user satisfaction surveys and analysis of performance indicators.
- Well defined and regular audit and quality assurance systems.
- The service would undertake training of other health care professionals and would promote continence awareness.
- The service would involve consumers in its evaluation.

A comprehensive list of elements of an ideal continence service follows:

- There should be a defined method of entry to the service regardless of the original source of the referral, whether this be from medical or nursing practitioners or by self-referral.
- Service co-ordination would be provided by an interdisciplinary team: a specialist continence nurse or physiotherapist with specialist continence training and a consultant.
- The service, whilst provided by an interdisciplinary team, is likely to be led by the specialist continence practitioners within primary care, whether they have a nursing or physiotherapy background.
- Effective liaison with GPs would be essential.
- User and carer involvement would be invited, not only as a part of clinical governance of the service, but as an integral part of service planning, development and delivery.
- Regular user satisfaction surveys and analysis of performance indicators would be necessary for the effective governance of the service.
- There would be well defined and regular audit and quality assurance systems.
- All patients with bladder problems, SS or VS would be eligible to enter the service.
- Assessment and screening procedures would be in place to enable case-finding exercises to be a core element of activity, regardless of where a potential patient might have contact with a health professional.
- The service would be based on evidence-based protocols, and timed elements of care provision would be built into the protocols.
- There would be clear patterns of referral to specialist secondary care providers where when the initial assessment led to specified diagnoses (for example, significant prolapse would be referred to a uro-gynaecologist).
- The service would have access to medical and surgical consultants with a special interest in continence; these might exist as a virtual continence centre with clear pathways of referral between specialists.
- The service would clearly define successful or unsuccessful treatment rooted in subjective and objective outcome measures.

- Diagnostic urodynamic investigation would be available at a defined point in treatment provision. This would require central organisation of primary and secondary care to avoid duplication of testing and the avoidance of unnecessary tests.
- Secondary care provision would be provided by trained specialist professionals who would undertake intensive physiotherapy and provide treatment for bladder overactivity based on an evidence-based protocol.
- Nurse prescribing of limited medications including antibiotics, relevant antimuscarinic medication and topical oestrogen would be implemented using a patient group directive following appropriate training.
- The service would target high risk groups and people with special needs.
- The service would undertake training of other health care professionals and would provide general health promotion information and advice.
- Specialist continence practitioners (as defined above) would take part in secondary care clinical sessions to ensure continuity and consistency of approach throughout the service.
- Specific groups would be targeted for health promotion.
- The service would participate in general continence awareness promotion.
- The service would have an integrated multidisciplinary record, which is freely accessible to all members of the team. All members would be expected to record care interactions cumulatively.
- The team database would form the basis for audit and research.

The document recommends that continence services should be organised as integrated continence services. This will include a locally provided service comprising continence nurse specialists as well as medical and surgical specialists. Furthermore, each primary care and community team should have available professionals trained to carry out initial assessments and care, and arrangements that ensure that patients are identified, assessed and reviewed. There is no research evidence regarding the optimal way to provide a primary care continence service, but three distinct approaches have emerged:

- creating posts which include the specific responsibility and time provision for the delivery of continence services (continence co-ordinators) and giving them appropriate training;
- providing a basic level of training to many members of a primary care team who provide continence services as part of their job;
- referring all patients with continence problems to a specialist continence service for initial assessment and treatment as well as more complex problems.

The ideal service would incorporate all three elements. The result would be a continence nurse practitioner who would become the leading health care professional responsible for the provision of primary continence care. The continence nurse practitioner will accept referrals from other primary care health professionals and be responsible for patient education and advice, clinical assessment, investigation (e.g. urodynamic investigation) diagnosis and conservative treatment (e.g. pelvic floor exercises, behavioural therapy) as a member of an expert clinical team, based in secondary care. The continence nurse practitioner will also help develop and maintain care pathways to and from primary care and specialist services. A nurse practitioner would also be able to provide continuity of care, which is currently lacking. By taking part in secondary care clinical sessions, this continuity and consistency can be ensured. The continence nurse specialists will therefore play a vital role in the new service as they span the interface between primary and secondary care.

Referral mechanisms would incorporate the following features:

- A core consultant team including a nominated urologist, gynaecologist and gerontologist would meet regularly with the remit of accepting direct referrals from the primary care portion of the continence service. The core team would implement an evidence-based protocol for failures of secondary care, specifying where joint management needs to be implemented for continuing care.

- Patients who were found to be obstructed would be referred directly to the core consultant team urologist.
- Patients who failed conservative treatment for urodynamic stress incontinence would be referred directly to the core consultant team gynaecologist or urologist. All surgical interventions would be evidence-based and regularly audited. Rare conditions, e.g. fistulae would be referred to designated specialist centres.
- Patients who failed treatment for detrusor overactivity would be referred directly to the core consultant team.
- Patients with prolapse would be referred directly to the core consultant team for pelvis floor assessment and management.
- Patients with complex medical needs or chronic comorbidity with an impact upon continence status would be referred directly to the core consultant team physician/elderly care physician for initial assessment and management.
- All patients would have clear pathways of care back into the community team for the long-term monitoring of management.

Quantitative comparison of two models of care

The main difference between the recommended model and the existing model of care is that in the new model there is an emphasis in primary care on PFE and bladder training managed by continence nurse practitioners (CNPs). This results in a reduction in the number of patients who go through to secondary care. The service in secondary care remains similar to the current service.

Future service configuration and associated costs

The Leicestershire MRC Incontinence Study has evaluated a new nurse-led continence service,[232] which may be the principle upon which continence services will be based in the future. **Figure 15** shows the structure of part of the study and patient flow through the service. An economic evaluation of this new service will be compared to that of an existing continence service.

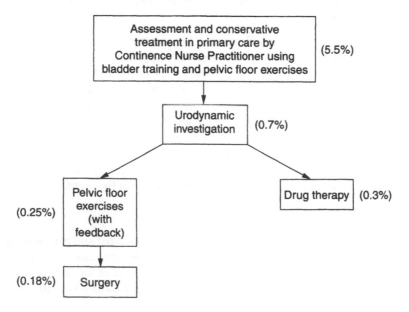

Figure 15: New model of care based upon a nurse-led continence service (prevalence).

The prevalence of individuals eligible for assessment and treatment in primary care for this model was based upon screening the local population through a postal questionnaire and home interview to establish severity of symptoms. In the new model, management in primary care would be provided in the main by CNPs with support from the GP in the first instance and referral to secondary care as appropriate.

All costs for these services are based on costing work carried out as part of the evaluation of the nurse-led continence services. These evaluations of the nurse-led continence services are ongoing, so the published costs may be revised in subsequent publications. All costs are in UK pounds for the year 2000. Although it is proposed that these costs should provide an estimate of the costs of this type of service, there are a number of caveats that need to be considered. The services evaluated were set up as part of a research project so workload and patterns of working may differ from those to be found in normal practice. Also, although the entry criteria for these services were based on symptoms relating to urinary incontinence, some of those admitted to the services would also have symptoms that related to voiding problems. Therefore, not all the resource used necessarily relates to urinary incontinence. In addition, these services were aimed at those over 40 years of age and so do not address the needs of those below this age.

All patients were seen by the CNP over an eight-week treatment period, with three planned visits, together with additional visits depending on the interventions provided and the degree of support deemed necessary by the nurse. Each patient underwent a one-hour assessment visit, which included taking a clinical history, physical examination, urinalysis, a mid-stream specimen of urine (MSU), a bladder scan to estimate post-void residual volume of urine, blood pressure, weight, height and, in women, vaginal examination. All patients were instructed in how to complete a urinary diary and pad test. Patients were seen one week after provision of the diary and pad test, which were then reviewed and a treatment regime was begun. A battery of clinical interventions could be implemented by the nurses, including bladder re-education for frequency, urgency and urge incontinence, Canesten for vaginal candida, pelvic floor awareness for stress incontinence, antibiotics for urinary tract infection, topical oestrogen for atrophic vaginitis, medication change for symptoms caused by loop diuretics, and advice on diet and fluid intake. Each CNP had a maximum caseload of 60 patients. Up to three visits could be scheduled over the subsequent five weeks, before a final assessment. Preliminary results of the costs for these services for older adults are given in **Table 11**.

Table 11: Costs* for the new model of care as developed in the Leicestershire MRC Incontinence Study for people aged 40 or over.

	Total number of contacts (% of study population)	Unit cost	Cost per 1000 people in Leicestershire over 40
Treatment in primary care	7,147 (5.5%)	£163	£9,008
Urodynamics	906 (0.7%)	£154	£1,076
Pelvic floor	329 (0.25%)	£293	£745
Drug therapy (oxybutynin)	390 (0.3%)	£418	£1,261
Surgery**	237 (0.18%)	£1,966	£3,602
Total			£15,691

* For the year 2000 (preliminary results subject to revisions); **This value is taken from HRG and OPCS data.

The total cost for the new service is estimated at £15 691 per 1000 per annum. This is likely to be an overestimate for several reasons:

- The services evaluated were set up as part of a research project, so workload and patterns of working may differ from those to be found in normal practice.
- Although the entry criteria for these services were based on symptoms relating to urinary incontinence, some of those admitted to the services would also have symptoms that related to voiding problems and this is likely to result in an *overestimate* of resource use.

Estimate of current service costs

Costs for the conventional incontinence service were estimated from a survey carried out as part of the Leicestershire MRC Incontinence Study. Respondents were asked for details of services they had used in the last year. The survey was carried out on 29 268 community residents over the age of 40. The percentages of respondents who used each category of service are given in **Table 12**. Since this was a snapshot of patients' experiences in just one year, none reported any surgery therefore an estimate of this was made using average rates and cost for surgery for the over 40s in the UK, calculated using OPCS statistics. Preliminary results of the costs for these services for older adults are given in **Table 12**.

Table 12: Estimate of costs[a] with conventional pattern of care based on survey of service contacts of 29,268 community dwelling adults aged 40 and over.

	Proportion using this service	Unit cost	Average cost per 1000
Any health care professional	11.2%		
GP	8.7%	£18[88]	£1,566
Hospital doctor	2.9%	£61[234]	£1,769
Physiotherapist	1.5%	£16[88]	£240
Specialist continence nurse	1.2%	£17[88]	£200
Other nurse	1.2%	£17[88]	£200
Antibiotics	4.0%	£2[234]	£91
Other medications	2.2%	£60[235]	£1,323
Surgery[b]			£975
Pelvic floor exercises urinary diary	1.5%	£293[236]	£4,493
Total			£10,856

[a] For the year 2000 (preliminary results subject to revision).
[b] This value is taken from HRG and OPCS data.

The total cost for existing services is estimated at £10 856 per 1000 per annum. This is likely to be an *underestimate* for several reasons:

- Costs are based on just the previous year's experience of a sample of respondents.
- Costs were used for a single contact as there is no data on the numbers of times respondents contacted a service.
- Costs for urodynamics are not included, as only values for consultations with a hospital doctor were available.

8 Outcome measures

This section summarises the results of a review of the literature in relation to outcome from the patient's perspective, audit tools and the information that is relevant for monitoring the effectiveness of intervention and care for urinary incontinence and an outline of future research.

Patient outcome

Urinary incontinence is associated with serious psychological suffering and poor quality of life.[237] It is therefore necessary to measure symptoms of urinary incontinence and the impact on patients' lives as part of the process of establishing the need for services and evaluating outcomes.[238,239,240] Symptom assessment helps determine the type, frequency and quantity of urinary leakage, and the extent of psychological and social disruption caused by these.

A wide range of questionnaires has been developed and used for symptom assessment. Most of these are designed either for men (often secondary to benign prostatic hyperplasia and surgical treatment of it) or for women, with very few for both. There are variations in the length and content of these questionnaires depending on whether they are developed for clinical or research purposes.

Some of these questionnaires were recommended in the First International Consultation on Incontinence[241] and elsewhere;[242,243] commonly used examples include the King's Health Questionnaire, the Bristol Female Lower Urinary Tract Symptoms Questionnaire (BFLUTS), the ICS male Questionnaire and the Quality of Life in Persons with Urinary Incontinence (I-QOL). Further details of these and other questionnaires are given in **Table A5.1**.

The King's Health Questionnaire and the BFLUTS were developed in the UK for assessing urinary incontinence symptoms in women. The former is also used to measure the impact on the quality of life. For men, the ICS male Questionnaire is used to assess lower urinary tract symptoms. It contains five questions concerning incontinence symptoms including urge and stress.

The Quality of Life in Persons with Urinary Incontinence (I-QOL) is designed for use in clinical trials to measure the impact of urinary incontinence on men and women. It contains 22 items and is scored on a four-point categorical scale.

A new questionnaire, the ICIQ-SF, has been launched in the second edition of the International Consultation on Incontinence, published in 2002.[244] The ICIQ-SF is aimed to provide a brief and robust tool for measuring frequency, severity and impact on quality of life of incontinence symptoms in all patient groups: 'men and women, young and old, in the developed and developing'. Preliminary data on its scores suggest that it is valid, reliable and responsive to change.

Audit tools

A number of audit tools have been published to promote the quality of urinary incontinence services in the UK. These are briefly described below.

The Royal College of Physicians has produced a clinical audit scheme for collecting information in relation to urinary and faecal incontinence in primary and secondary care settings.[245] The purposes of the scheme are to educate staff and to identify areas that need change and improvement. It offers three instruments for three types of audit: single patient audit, multiple patient audit and facility audit.

Single patient audit comprises a comprehensive checklist of good practice for one or two patients. It is intended that a completed questionnaire should provide the basis for discussion and decision making for improved management of incontinence.

Multiple patient audit was developed from a review of standards of good practice among larger groups of incontinent patients. The aim is to give an overview of current practice and the extent to which standards of good practice are being achieved. Facility audit covers policy, procedures and staff education in relation to incontinence management.

Cheater et al.[246] have developed an evidence-based audit protocol for primary health care teams. The protocol proposes two levels of audit. Audit-one comprises a set of minimum criteria or must-do criteria (**Table 13**). The authors propose that each practice needs to undertake audit-one because there is strong research evidence in support of that.

Audit-two comprises the must-do criteria in audit-one and should-do criteria in relation to additional risk factors that are modifiable such as obesity and smoking. For the should-do criteria there is some research evidence of their importance but the impact on outcome is less certain. The protocol includes instructions and advice regarding the organisation of the audit, collection of data and implementation of change.

Table 13: Urinary incontinence: summary of audit criteria.

'MUST DO' CRITERIA
These are the minimum criteria that practices need to audit, as there is firm research evidence to justify their inclusion. Every practice must include these criteria in the audit.

1 The records show that a patient with urinary incontinence has had an initial assessment that includes a history and/or completion of a continence chart and physical examination.
2 The records show that a patient with urinary incontinence has had a urine dipstick examination or microscopy or a mid-stream specimen of urine for culture and sensitivities.
3 The records show that there has been an estimation of the post-void residual (PVR) urine volume when indicated by the history/continence chart or physical examination.
4 The records show that the type of incontinence has been identified as either stress incontinence, urge incontinence, mixed incontinence, overflow incontinence (voiding disorder) or if the type of incontinence is unclear, appropriate specialist referral has been made.
5 The records show that at presentation a medication review has been undertaken to identify drugs which can cause or contribute to urinary incontinence; and in post-menopausal women an examination has been made for atrophic vaginitis/urethritis.

'SHOULD DO' CRITERIA
These are additional criteria for which there is some research evidence of their importance but where the impact on outcome is less certain.

The records show that at presentation modifiable risk factors of obesity, chronic constipation and smoking have been sought and appropriate action taken if indication

---

Source: Cheater et al.[246]

The Royal College of Obstetricians and Gynaecologists has produced a report on effective procedures in gynaecology that are suitable for audit.[247] Section 10 of the report deals with auditable procedures in urogynaecology that are relevant for female urinary incontinence. The section presents seven evidence-based statements of audit standards. For each statement a suggestion for audit is made, followed by a list of the research studies or reports on which the standard was based.

9 Information and research requirements

Information

This section summarises the health outcome indicators from the report of the Working Group on Outcome Indicators for Urinary Incontinence.[141] An outcome indicator is an aggregated statistical measure that can be used to describe a group of people or a population in terms of a change in health, health-related status or risk factors to health. The change may be the result of intervention or the lack of it.

The group's report was based on a health outcome model. There were 18 indicators recommended in it. The aim of the group was to develop a set of ideal indicators that could be used for gathering information from the patient, doctor and population perspectives by a variety of professionals. An ideal indicator refers to what should be known or could realistically be known about an outcome of prevention and care of incontinence. **Table A5.2** gives a complete list of these indicators, their characteristics and implementation.

For a number of the indicators, information can be obtained from existing sources such as routine health care data or periodic surveys at national or local levels. For the other indicators, the availability of information depends on further developments in relation to the indicator or to other aspects such as information technology.

The indicators that depend on routine sources of information are:

- percentage of anterior repair procedures undertaken in a population of women undergoing surgery for stress incontinence
- rate of re-operation in a population (provided by a hospital provider unit) within two years following surgical treatment for urinary incontinence
- rate of emergency re-admission (for urinary-related condition and/or specific post-operation complication) within 30 days of discharge for a hospital provider unit population which has undergone surgery for urinary incontinence.

Those that depend on further development before information for deriving them is available are numbered 5, 9, 10, 16, 17 and 18 in **Table A5.2**.

Future research

The level of knowledge about urinary incontinence and related conditions is very limited compared with, for example, the cardiovascular system. Recent investment in the MRC Incontinence Programme is addressing the essential epidemiology, including associated dietary and lifestyle factors, together with the cost of illness and the effectiveness and cost of a nurse-led service including behavioural and drug therapies. These results have established the extent of health care need and requirement and suggest a significant effect from treatment in primary care. However, considerable further investment is needed to reach a firm foundation for the development of future services as a whole. The priorities for further research include:

1 the natural history and prognosis relating to incontinence and other lower urinary tract symptoms
2 environmental and occupational factors along with diet and lifestyle determinants as a basis for prevention
3 investigation of disease mechanisms and management particularly relating to dual diagnosis e.g. depression, MS, diabetes and hormonal determinants

4 the association with pregnancy, particularly the mode of childbirth
5 development of the genetic basis of incontinence
6 evaluation of innovative approaches to improving access to appropriate services, especially in primary care
7 evaluating the long-term outcomes of treatment and support services in the community
8 evaluation of services for frail and elderly people with incontinence in and out of care homes
9 extent of incontinence, need and services for children and teenagers
10 development of a standard classification of urinary disorders based on an improved understanding of structure in relation to function and natural history
11 development of appropriate assessment and categorisation tools.

Appendix 1: Lexicon for the definition and classification of lower urinary tract function in adults

The following functional classification is largely derived from work produced by the Urodynamic Society[248] and the International Continence Society Standardisation Committee[123] as applied in practice.[249,250]

The lower urinary tract (LUT) comprises the bladder and urethra. These form a functional unit and their interaction cannot be ignored. For simplicity, however, the functions of the bladder (to store and to void) and those of the urethra (to control and to convey) may be considered separately. Similarly, since the bladder and urethra may behave differently during the storing and voiding phases of *micturition* (a term for the whole process), these phases should also be considered separately. Thus, LUT function may be classified using a dichotomy of anatomical site by phase of micturition (Figure A1.1).

		Bladder	Urethra
Storage phase	Detrusor activity	• normal • overactive: neurogenic idiopathic	Urethral closure • competent • incompetent
	Bladder sensation	• normal • increased • reduced • absent • non-specific	
	Bladder compliance		
	Bladder capacity	• normal • low [4.1]*	[4.2]*
Voiding phase	Detrusor activity	• normal • underactive • acontractile [4.3]*	Urethral opening • normal • obstructive: overactive mechanical [4.4]*

*reference to the relevant sections of this appendix

Figure A1.1: Factors affecting LUT function.

LUT function may be described in terms of symptoms, syndromes, signs, urodynamic observations and conditions:

1	Symptoms	the subjective indicators of a disease or change in condition as perceived by the individual, carer or partner that may lead him/her to seek help from health care professionals
2	Syndromes	constellations or varying combinations of symptoms that form functional abnormalities for which a precise cause has not been defined (after routine assessment has excluded obvious local causes)
3	Signs	observations by the physician including simple means to verify symptoms and quantify them
4	Urodynamic observations	the observations made during urodynamic studies
5	Conditions	the presence of urodynamic observations associated with characteristic symptoms or signs and/or non-urodynamic evidence of relevant pathological processes

1 Lower Urinary Tract Symptoms (LUTS)

LUTS may be volunteered or elicited during history taking. They are usually qualitative; and can seldom be used to make a definitive diagnosis. LUTS may indicate pathologies other than LUT dysfunction such as urinary infection. LUTS are grouped into storage, voiding and post-micturition symptoms.

1.1 Storage symptoms

These are symptoms experienced during the storage phase of the bladder:

- **Increased daytime frequency (pollakisuria):** The complaint by the individual who considers that he/she voids too often by day.
- **Nocturia:** The complaint that the individual has to wake at night one or more times to void.
- **Night-time frequency:** Differs from *nocturia* in that it includes voids which occur after the individual has gone to bed, but before he/she has gone to sleep; and voids which occur in the early morning that prevent the individual from getting back to sleep as he/she wishes.
- **Urgency:** The complaint of a sudden compelling desire to pass urine which is difficult to defer.
- **Urinary incontinence:** The complaint of any involuntary leakage of urine; this should be further described by specifying relevant factors such as the type, frequency, severity, precipitating factors, social impact, effect on hygiene and quality of life, the measures used to contain the leakage and whether or not the individual seeks or desires help because of urinary incontinence.
- **Stress urinary incontinence:** The complaint of involuntary leakage on effort or exertion or on sneezing or coughing.
- **Urge urinary incontinence:** The complaint of involuntary leakage accompanied by or immediately preceded by urgency; may present as frequent small losses between micturitions or as a catastrophic leak with complete bladder emptying.
- **Mixed urinary incontinence:** The complaint of involuntary leakage associated with urgency and also with effort or exertion or with sneezing or coughing.
- **Enuresis:** Any involuntary loss of urine.
- **Nocturnal enuresis:** The complaint of loss of urine occurring during sleep.
- **Continuous urinary incontinence:** The complaint of continuous leakage.
- **Situational urinary incontinence:** Such as during giggling or sexual intercourse.
- **Bladder sensation:** Defined during history taking by five categories:
  - normal
  - increased
  - reduced
  - absent
  - non-specific.

1.2 Voiding symptoms

These are symptoms experienced during the voiding phase of the bladder:

- **Slow stream:** The individual's perception of reduced urine flow, usually compared with previous performance or in comparison with others.
- **Splitting or spraying:** The individual's report of splitting or spraying of the urine stream.
- **Intermittent stream (intermittency):** The individual describes urine flow which stops and starts, on one or more occasions, during micturition.

- **Hesitancy:** The individual describes difficulty in initiating micturition, resulting in a delay in the onset of voiding after the individual is ready to pass urine.
- **Straining:** Straining to void describes the muscular effort used to initiate, maintain or improve the urinary stream (suprapubic pressure may be needed to initiate or maintain urine flow).
- **Terminal dribble:** The individual describes a prolonged final part of micturition, when the flow has slowed to a trickle/dribble.

1.3 Post-micturition and other symptoms

Post-micturition symptoms are those experienced immediately after micturition; other symptoms may occur at varying times during the micturition cycle:

- **Feeling of incomplete emptying:** A feeling of incomplete emptying experienced by the individual after passing urine.
- **Post-micturition dribble:** The involuntary loss of urine immediately after he/she has finished passing urine, usually after leaving the toilet in men or after rising from the toilet in women.
- **Symptoms associated with pelvic organ prolapse:** These include feeling a lump ('something coming down'), low backache, heaviness, dragging sensation and the need to replace the prolapse digitally in order to defaecate or micturate.
- **Symptoms associated with sexual intercourse:** In women, symptoms include dyspareunia, vaginal dryness and incontinence during or after sexual intercourse; these should be described as fully as possible, defining whether leakage of urine occurs during penetration, during intercourse or at orgasm.
- **Genital and LUT pain:** Pain, discomfort or pressure; should be characterised by type, frequency, duration, precipitating and relieving factors and by location as defined below:
  - bladder pain
  - urethral pain
  - vulval pain
  - vaginal pain
  - scrotal pain
  - perineal pain
  - pelvic pain.

2 Syndromes suggestive of LUT dysfunction

These are grouped into genito-urinary pain syndromes and symptom syndromes. In all cases, it is presumed that routine assessment (history taking, physical examination and other appropriate investigations) has excluded obvious local pathologies such as those that are infective, neoplastic, metabolic or hormonal in nature.

2.1 Genito-urinary pain syndromes

These are all chronic in nature. Pain is the major complaint but concomitant complaints are of a LUT, bowel, sexual or gynaecological nature:

- **Painful bladder syndrome:** Suprapubic pain related to bladder filling, accompanied by other symptoms such as increased daytime and night-time frequency, in the absence of proven urinary infection or other pathology such as carcinoma-in-situ and endometriosis.

- **Urethral pain syndrome:** Recurrent episodic urethral pain, usually on voiding, with daytime frequency and nocturia, in the absence of proven infection or other obvious pathology.
- **Vulval pain syndrome:** Persistent or recurrent episodic vulval pain, which is either related to the micturition cycle or associated with symptoms suggestive of urinary tract or sexual dysfunction; no proven infection or other obvious pathology.
- **Vaginal pain syndrome:** Persistent or recurrent episodic vaginal pain which is associated with symptoms suggestive of urinary tract or sexual dysfunction; no proven vaginal infection or other obvious pathology.
- **Scrotal pain syndrome:** Persistent or recurrent episodic scrotal pain which is associated with symptoms suggestive of urinary tract or sexual dysfunction; no proven epididimo-orchitis or other obvious pathology.
- **Perineal pain syndrome:** Persistent or recurrent episodic perineal pain which is either related to the micturition cycle or associated with symptoms suggestive of urinary tract or sexual dysfunction; no proven infection or other obvious pathology.
- **Pelvic pain:** Persistent or recurrent episodic pelvic pain associated with symptoms suggestive of LUT, sexual, bowel or gynaecological dysfunction; no proven infection or other obvious pathology.

2.2 Symptom syndromes

In clinical practice, empirical diagnoses are often used as the basis for initial management after assessing the individual's LUT symptoms, physical findings and the results of urinalysis and other indicated investigations.

- **Overactive bladder syndrome (urge syndrome) (urgency-frequency syndrome):** Urgency with or without urge incontinence, usually with frequency and nocturia; no proven infection or other obvious pathology.
- **LUTS suggestive of bladder outlet obstruction:** In men, predominately voiding symptoms in the absence of infection or obvious pathology other than possible causes of outlet obstruction.

Overactive bladder syndrome is suggestive of urodynamically demonstrable detrusor overactivity but can be due to other forms of urethro-vesical dysfunction. In women, voiding symptoms usually suggest detrusor under-activity rather than bladder outlet obstruction.

3 Signs suggestive of LUT malfunction

3.1 Measuring the frequency, severity and impact of LUTS

Asking the patient to record micturitions and symptoms for a period of days provides invaluable information. Validated questionnaires are useful for recording symptoms; their frequency, severity and bother; and the impact of LUTS on the quality of life. The instrument used should be specified. The recording of micturition events can be in three main forms:

- **Micturition time chart:** Records only the times of micturitions, day and night, for at least 24 hours.
- **Frequency volume chart (FVC):** Records the volumes voided as well as the time of each micturition, day and night, for at least 24 hours.
- **Bladder diary:** Records the times of micturitions and voided volumes, episodes of incontinence, pad usage and other information such as fluid intake (allowing for eating significant quantities of

water-containing foods such as fruit or vegetables), diuretic use, the degree of urgency and the degree of incontinence.

The following measurements can be abstracted from frequency volume charts and bladder diaries:

- **Daytime frequency:** The number of voids recorded during waking hours, including the last void before sleep and the first void after waking and rising in the morning.
- **Nocturia:** The number of voids recorded during a night's sleep; each void is preceded and followed by sleep.
- **24-hour frequency:** The total number of daytime voids and episodes of nocturia during a specified 24-hour period.
- **24-hour production:** Measured by collecting all urine for 24 hours; usually begun *after* the first void produced after rising in the morning and completed by *including* the first void on rising the following morning.
- **Polyuria:** The measured production of more than 2.8 litres of urine (based on a 70 kg adult voiding >40 ml/kg), usually in 24 hours, though it may be useful to look at output over shorter time frames.
- **Nocturnal urine volume:** The total volume of urine passed between the time the individual goes to bed with the intention of sleeping and the time of waking with the intention of rising (this excludes the last void before going to bed but includes the first void after rising in the morning).
- **Nocturnal polyuria:** Present when an increased proportion of the 24-hour output occurs at night, normally during the eight hours whilst the patient is in bed (the night-time urine output *excludes* the last void before sleep but *includes* the first void of the morning); values vary with age, from >20% in young adults to >33% in those aged over 65 years.
- **Maximum voided volume:** The largest volume of urine voided during a single micturition as determined from the frequency volume chart or bladder diary.
- **Minimum voided volume:** The smallest volume of urine voided during a single micturition as determined from the frequency volume chart or bladder diary.
- **Mean voided volume:** The average volume of urine voided during a single micturition as determined from the frequency volume chart or bladder diary.

3.2 Physical examination

Physical examination is essential in the assessment of all patients with LUT dysfunction. It should include abdominal, pelvic, perineal and a focused neurological examination. For patients with possible neurogenic LUTS, a more extensive neurological examination is needed.

Abdominal examination

The bladder may be felt by abdominal palpation or by suprapubic percussion. Pressure suprapubically or during bimanual vaginal examination may induce a desire to pass urine.

Perineal/genital inspection

This allows the description of the skin, for example the presence of atrophy or excoriation; any abnormal anatomical features; and the observation of incontinence:

- **Urinary incontinence (sign):** Urine leakage seen during examination; this may be urethral or extraurethral.
- **Stress urinary incontinence (sign):** The observation of involuntary leakage from the urethra, synchronous with effort or exertion or with sneezing or coughing; stress leakage presumed to be due to raised abdominal pressure.

- **Extra-urethral incontinence (sign):** The observation of urine leakage through channels other than the urethra.
- **Uncategorised incontinence (sign):** The observation of involuntary leakage that cannot be classified into one of the above categories on the basis of signs and symptoms.

Vaginal examination

This allows the description of observed and palpable anatomical abnormalities and the assessment of pelvic floor muscle function:

- **Pelvic organ prolapse:** The descent of one or more of the anterior vaginal wall; the posterior vaginal wall; the apex of the vagina (cervix/uterus) or vault (cuff) after hysterectomy; absence of prolapse is stage 0 support; prolapse can be staged from stage I to stage IV.
- **Anterior vaginal wall prolapse:** Descent of the anterior vagina so that the urethro-vesical junction (a point 3 cm proximal to the external urinary meatus) or any anterior point proximal to this is less than 3 cm above the plane of the hymen.
- **Prolapse of the apical segment of the vagina:** Any descent of the vaginal cuff scar (after hysterectomy) or cervix, below a point which is 2 cm less than the total vaginal length above the plane of the hymen.
- **Posterior vaginal wall prolapse:** Any descent of the posterior vaginal wall so that a midline point on the posterior vaginal wall 3 cm above the level of the hymen or any posterior point proximal to this is less than 3 cm above the plane of the hymen.
- **Pelvic floor muscle function:** Can be qualitatively defined by the tone at rest and the strength of a voluntary or reflex contraction as strong, weak or absent or by a validated grading system (such as Oxford 1–5); a pelvic muscle contraction may be assessed by visual inspection, palpation, electromyography or perineometry, noting factors such as strength, duration, displacement and repeatability.

Rectal examination

This allows the description of observed and palpable anatomical abnormalities and is the easiest method of assessing pelvic floor muscle function in men.

3.3 Pad testing

Pad testing may be used to quantify the amount of urine lost during incontinence episodes. The methods range from a short provocative test to a 24-hour pad test.

4 Urodynamic observations

In general, a urodynamic observation may have a number of possible underlying causes and does not represent a definite diagnosis of a disease or condition. There are two main techniques:

- **Conventional urodynamic studies:** usually take place in the urodynamic laboratory and involve artificial bladder filling:
  - **Artificial bladder filling:** Filling the bladder via a catheter with a specified liquid at a specified rate.
  - **Provocative manoeuvres:** Techniques used during urodynamics in an effort to provoke detrusor overactivity, for example rapid filling, use of cooled or acid medium, postural changes and hand washing.

- **Ambulatory urodynamic studies:** A functional test of the LUT using natural filling and reproducing the subject's everyday activities; monitoring usually takes place outside the urodynamic laboratory.
- **Natural filling:** The bladder is filled by the production of urine rather than by an artificial medium.

Both filling cystometry and pressure flow studies of voiding require the following measurements:

- **Intravesical pressure:** The pressure within the bladder.
- **Abdominal pressure:** The pressure surrounding the bladder; in current practice, estimated from rectal, vaginal or, less commonly, from extraperitoneal pressure or a bowel stoma; the simultaneous measurement of abdominal pressure is essential for the interpretation of the intravesical pressure.
- **Detrusor pressure:** That component of intravesical pressure that is created by forces in the bladder wall (passive and active); estimated by subtracting abdominal pressure from intravesical pressure.

Storage phase

Filling cystometry is the method by which the pressure/volume relationship of the bladder is measured during bladder filling. The storage phase begins when filling starts and ends when the patient and urodynamicist decide that 'permission to void' has been given. During filling, bladder and urethral function need to be defined separately (Figure A1.1). The rate at which the bladder is filled is divided into:

- **Physiological filling rate:** a filling rate less than the predicted maximum, where the predicted maximum is the body weight in kg divided by 4 expressed as ml/min.
- **Non-physiological filling rate:** a filling rate greater than the predicted maximum filling rate as defined above.

4.1 Bladder storage function

Bladder storage function should be described according to detrusor activity, bladder sensation, bladder compliance and bladder capacity.

Detrusor activity may be normal or overactive; and the latter may be associated with incontinence:

- **Normal detrusor function:** Allows bladder filling with little or no change in pressure; no involuntary *phasic* (wave form) contractions occur despite provocation.
- **Detrusor overactivity:** Characterised by involuntary detrusor contractions during the filling phase which may be spontaneous or provoked; certain patterns and causes may be noted:
  - **Phasic detrusor overactivity:** Defined by a characteristic wave form; may or may not lead to urinary incontinence.
  - **Terminal detrusor overactivity:** Defined as a single involuntary detrusor contraction occurring at cystometric capacity that cannot be suppressed and results in incontinence, usually due to bladder emptying.
  - **Detrusor overactivity incontinence:** Incontinence due to an involuntary detrusor contraction; in a patient with normal sensation, urgency is likely to be experienced just before the leakage occurs.
  - **Neurogenic detrusor overactivity:** The cause is a relevant neurological condition.
  - **Idiopathic detrusor overactivity:** There is no defined cause.

Bladder sensation assessed by filling cystometry is a subjective process. It is not possible to quantify measures such as *low bladder volume*. The assumption that this technique measures sensation from the bladder alone without urethral or pelvic components may be false. Bladder sensation may be categorised as follows:

- **Normal bladder sensation:** Can be judged by three defined points noted during filling cystometry and evaluated in relation to the bladder volume at that moment and in relation to the patient's symptomatic complaints.

- **First sensation of bladder filling:** The feeling the patient has during filling cystometry when he/she first becomes aware of the bladder filling.
- **First desire to void:** The feeling during filling cystometry that would lead the patient to pass urine at the next convenient moment, but voiding can be delayed if necessary.
- **Strong desire to void:** During filling cystometry, a persistent desire to void without the fear of leakage.
- **Increased bladder sensation:** During filling cystometry, an early first sensation of bladder filling (or an early desire to void) and/or an early strong desire to void, which occurs at low bladder volume and which persists.
- **Reduced bladder sensation:** During filling cystometry, diminished sensation throughout bladder filling.
- **Absent bladder sensation:** During filling cystometry, the individual has no bladder sensation.
- **Non-specific bladder sensations:** During filling cystometry, these may make the individual aware of bladder filling, for example abdominal fullness or vegetative symptoms.
- **Bladder pain:** Pain during filling cystometry; always an abnormal finding.
- **Urgency:** During filling cystometry, a sudden compelling desire to void (motor urgency and sensory urgency have little intuitive meaning and are no longer used).
- **Vesical/urethral sensory threshold:** The least current which consistently produces a sensation perceived by the subject during stimulation at the site under investigation.

Bladder compliance describes the relationship between change in bladder volume and change in detrusor pressure. It is calculated by dividing the volume change (ΔV) by the change in detrusor pressure (Δpdet) during that change in bladder volume (C= V.Δpdet); and expressed in ml/cm H_2O.

Bladder compliance may be measured in various ways, but should include at least two standard points:

- the detrusor pressure at the start of bladder filling and the corresponding bladder volume (usually zero)
- the detrusor pressure and corresponding bladder volume at cystometric capacity or immediately before the start of any detrusor contraction that causes significant leakage.

Bladder capacity measured during filling cystometry may be normal or reduced:

- **Cystometric capacity:**
  - in patients with normal sensation, the bladder volume at the end of the filling cystometrogram, when 'permission to void' is usually given
  - if there is uncontrolled voiding, the volume at which the voiding begins
  - in the absence of normal sensation, the volume at which the clinician decides to terminate filling in all cases, the end point and reason(s) for terminating filling should be specified (such as a high detrusor filling pressure, large infused volume or pain):
  cystometric capacity = urine voided + any residual urine
- **Maximum cystometric capacity:** In patients with normal sensation, the volume at which the patient feels he/she can no longer delay micturition (has a strong desire to void).
- **Maximum anaesthetic bladder capacity:** The volume to which the bladder can be filled under deep general or spinal anaesthetic; this should be qualified according to the type of anaesthesia used and the speed, length of time and pressure at which the bladder is filled.

4.2 Urethral closure mechanism

The urethral closure mechanism during the storage phase may be competent or incompetent; and an incompetent mechanism may result in incontinence:

- **Normal urethral closure mechanism:** Maintains a positive urethral closure pressure during bladder filling even in the presence of increased abdominal pressure, although it may be overcome by detrusor overactivity.

- **Incompetent urethral closure mechanism:** Allows leakage of urine in the absence of a detrusor contraction.
- **Urethral relaxation incontinence:** Leakage due to urethral relaxation in the absence of raised abdominal pressure or detrusor overactivity.
- **Urodynamic stress incontinence:** The involuntary leakage of urine during increased abdominal pressure, in the absence of a detrusor contraction.

In patients with stress incontinence, there is a spectrum of urethral characteristics ranging from a highly mobile urethra with good intrinsic function to an immobile urethra with poor intrinsic function. Any delineation into categories such as *urethral hypermobility* and *intrinsic sphincter deficiency* may be simplistic and arbitrary, and requires further research.

The assessment of urethral function may include the following measurements:

- **Urethral pressure:** The fluid pressure needed to just open a closed urethra.
- **Urethral pressure profile:** A graph of the intraluminal pressure along the length of the urethra.
- **Urethral closure pressure profile:** The urethral pressure minus the intravesical pressure.
- **Maximum urethral pressure:** The maximum pressure of the measured profile.
- **Maximum urethral closure pressure:** The maximum difference between the urethral pressure and the intravesical pressure.
- **Functional profile length:** In women, the length of the urethra along which the urethral pressure exceeds intravesical pressure.
- **Pressure 'transmission' ratio:** The increment in urethral pressure on stress as a percentage of the simultaneously recorded increment in intravesical pressure.
- **Abnormal leak point pressure:** The intravesical pressure at which urine leakage occurs due to increased abdominal pressure in the absence of a detrusor contraction; this should be qualified according to the site of pressure measurement (rectal, vaginal or intravesical) and the method by which the pressure is generated (cough or valsalva).
- **Detrusor leak point pressure:** The lowest detrusor pressure at which urine leakage occurs in the absence of either a detrusor contraction or increased abdominal pressure.

Voiding phase

Voiding is described in terms of detrusor and urethral function and assessed by measuring urine flow rate and voiding pressures. The voiding phase begins when 'permission to void' is given or when uncontrollable voiding starts, and ends when the patient considers voiding has finished.

Urine flow is defined either as *continuous* (without interruption) or *intermittent* (an individual states that the flow stops and starts during a single visit to the bathroom in order to void). The continuous flow curve is defined as a smooth arc-shaped curve or, when there are multiple peaks during a period of continuous urine flow, fluctuating. The precise shape of the flow curve is determined by detrusor contractility, the presence of any abdominal straining and by the bladder outlet. Measurements are made of:

- **Flow rate:** The volume of fluid expelled via the urethra per unit time (ml/s).
- **Voided volume:** The total volume expelled via the urethra.
- **Maximum flow rate:** The maximum measured value of the flow rate after correction for artefacts.
- **Voiding time:** Total duration of micturition, including interruptions.
- **Flow time:** The time over which measurable flow actually occurs.
- **Average flow rate:** Voided volume divided by flow time.

- **Time to maximum flow:** The elapsed time from onset of flow to maximum flow.

Pressure flow studies of voiding are the method by which the relationship between pressure in the bladder and urine flow rate is measured during bladder emptying. Pressure measurements may be made for intravesical, abdominal and detrusor pressures as follows:

- **Pre-micturition pressure:** The pressure recorded immediately before the initial isovolumetric contraction.
- **Opening pressure:** The pressure recorded at the onset of urine flow (consider time delay).
- **Opening time:** Elapsed time from initial rise in detrusor pressure to onset of flow.
- **Maximum pressure:** The maximum value of the measured pressure.
- **Pressure at maximum flow:** The lowest pressure recorded at maximum measured flow rate.
- **Closing pressure:** The pressure measured at the end of measured flow.
- **Minimum voiding pressure:** The minimum pressure during measurable flow; not necessarily equal to either the opening or closing pressures.
- **Flow delay:** Time delay between a change in bladder pressure and corresponding change in measured flow rate.

4.3 Detrusor function during voiding

Detrusor activity may be normal or underactive. A normal detrusor contraction will be recorded as *high pressure* if urethral resistance is high; *normal pressure* if it is normal; or *low pressure* if it is low.

- **Normal detrusor function:** Achieved by a voluntarily initiated continuous detrusor contraction that leads to complete bladder emptying within a normal time span and in the absence of obstruction; for a given detrusor contraction, the magnitude of the recorded pressure rise will depend on the degree of outlet resistance.
- **Detrusor underactivity:** A contraction of reduced strength and/or duration, resulting in prolonged bladder emptying and/or a failure to achieve complete bladder emptying within a normal time span.
- **Acontractile detrusor:** A detrusor that cannot be demonstrated to contract during urodynamic studies.
- **Post-void residual:** The volume of urine left in the bladder at the end of micturition.

4.4 Urethral function during voiding

Urethral functioning may be normal or obstructive:

- **Normal urethra function:** A urethra that opens and is continuously relaxed to allow the bladder to be emptied at a normal pressure.
- **Abnormal urethra function:** May result from obstruction due to urethral overactivity or from the urethra being unable to open due to anatomical abnormality such as an enlarged prostate or a urethral stricture.
- **Bladder outlet obstruction:** In men, generic term for obstruction during voiding characterised by increased detrusor pressure and reduced urine flow rate; usually diagnosed by studying the synchronous values of flow rate and detrusor pressure in women, not yet adequately defined.
- **Dysfunctional voiding:** Characterised by an intermittent and/or fluctuating flow rate due to involuntary intermittent contractions of the periurethral striated muscle during voiding in neurologically normal individuals.

- **Detrusor sphincter dyssynergia:** A detrusor contraction concurrent with an involuntary contraction of the urethral and/or periurethral striated muscle; occasionally flow may be prevented altogether.
- **Non-relaxing urethral sphincter obstruction:** Characterised by a non-relaxing, obstructing urethra resulting in reduced urine flow; usually related to a neurological lesion.

5 Conditions

In the absence of inflammation, infection and neoplasia, LUT dysfunction may be caused by:

- a disturbance of the pertinent nervous or psychological control system
- disorders of muscle function
- structural abnormalities:
  - congenital lesions (such as epispadias, ectopic ureter, spina bifida)
  - fistulae (vesico-vaginal, uretero-vaginal, urethro-vaginal)
  - urethral diverticula.

The underlying conditions may be presumed or definite. Presumed conditions are documented clinically. Definite conditions are documented by urodynamic techniques. When reporting results, it should be clearly stated whether the conditions causing urinary incontinence are definite or presumed; and the techniques by which the conditions are documented should be specified.

The following conditions are specifically defined for LUT dysfunction:

- **Acute retention of urine:** A painful (usually), palpable or percussable bladder, when the patient is unable to pass any urine.
- **Chronic retention of urine:** A non-painful bladder, which remains palpable or percussable after the patient has passed urine; but excluding transient voiding difficulty, for example after surgery for stress incontinence; the patient may be incontinent.
- **Benign prostatic obstruction:** A form of *bladder outlet obstruction*, which may be diagnosed when the cause of outlet obstruction is known to be benign prostatic enlargement, due to histological benign prostatic hyperplasia.
- **Benign prostatic hyperplasia:** A term used (and reserved for) the typical histological pattern which defines the disease.
- **Benign prostatic enlargement:** Prostatic enlargement due to histological benign prostatic hyperplasia; the term *prostatic enlargement* should be used in the absence of prostatic histology.

Functional incontinence may result from difficulties with mobility, environmental impediments (such as the location and accessibility of toilet facilities), sedation, confusion, depression or other psychiatric problems. Other related factors such as poor manual dexterity, impaired eyesight and unsuitable clothing and footwear may also predispose to incontinence.[248]

Other conditions related to LUT dysfunction include:

- **Faecal incontinence:** Involuntary or inappropriate passage of faeces.
- **Double incontinence:** Urinary and faecal incontinence occurring together.
- **Encopresis:** The repeated passage of faeces into inappropriate places (such as in clothing or on the floor), whether involuntary or intentional.

Appendix 2: Prevalence and incidence

Population prevalence

Prevalence studies with a rigorous methodology carried out on a total population are summarised in **Table A2.1**. The precise prevalence depends upon the definition of incontinence, the study population, the sampling procedure and the research instruments, which may or may not include an objective validation of reported symptoms. Variations due to study design are confounded by problems of differential reporting and a scarcity of validated scales. Incontinence is clearly a common problem but the precise prevalence depends upon the definition used.

Table A2.1(a): Prevalence of incontinence, UK Studies 1960–2001: Summary of methodological features in relation to ranked overall prevalence of incontinence.

Author/Year	Location	Sample	Response	Study type	Prompts	Age	Respondents	Thresholds and (ratings)†	Prevalence %	
									Female	Male
Swithinbank[251,252] 1999, 2000	Bristol	GP – total	[a]80%	Postal Q	++++	19+	F: 2,075	Ever <damp (1) / *Reclassified – from monthly <damp (2)*	69	
Harrison[28] 1994	Bristol	GP – random	[a]83%	Postal Q (2 stage)	++	20+	F: 314	Any <damp (1)	53.2	
Kuh[42] 1999	Britain	Birth cohort	[o]93%	Postal Q	++	48	F: 1,378	Yearly <damp (1) / Monthly <damp (2) / Monthly × damp (3)	55 / 23 / 8	
Yarnell[37] 1981	S Wales	Electoral register	[a]95%	Interview	++	18+	F: 1,000	Yearly <damp (1)	45	
Milne[13,253] 1972 1971	Edinburgh	GP – random	[a]65%	Interview + exam	++	62–90	F: 272 M: 215	Ever <damp (1)	42	25
Jolleys[55] 1988	Leicestershire	GP – random	[u]89%	Postal Q	+++	25+	F: 833	Any <damp (1)	41	
Dolan[44] 1999	N Ireland	GP – random	[a]66%	Postal Q	+++	35–74	F: 689	Any <damp (1) / Monthly <damp (2)	33.5 / 23.4	
Stoddart[43] 2001	Bristol	GP – stratified	79%	Postal Q	++	65+	F: 740 M: 781	Any <damp (1)	31.6	23
Thomas[18] 1980	London/ S Wales	GP – random	[a]89%	Postal Q	++	5+	F: 9,323 M: 8,761	Ever <damp (1) / Monthly <damp (2)	25.1 / 8.5	8.7 / 3.3
Brocklehurst[10] 1971	SE England	GP – total	[u]85%	Interview	+	65+	F: 375 M: 182	Ever wet (2)	25	16
Edwards[254] 2001	UK	Population – random	94%	Interview	++	65+	F: 1,695 M 1,099	Ever wet (2)	24.2	8.6
Crome[255] 2001	Wales	Population – random	76.9%	Interview	+	70+	F: 1,010 M: 598	Occasionally (1) / Frequently (3)	21.6 / 8.0	17.2 / 8.5
Perry[8] 2000	Leicestershire	GP – random (excl. residential)	[a]70%	Postal Q	++++	40+	F: 5,544 M: 4,682	Monthly <damp (2)	20.2	8.9

Table A2.1(a): Continued.

Author/Year	Location	Sample	Response	Study type	Prompts	Age	Respondents	Thresholds and (ratings)†	Prevalence % Female	Prevalence % Male
Vetter[38] 1981	S Wales	GP – random	?95%	Interview	++	70+	F/M 1,280	Ever × damp (2); Daily × damp (3)	18.1; 6.7	7.3; 2.5
Yarnell[45] 1979	S Wales	GP + total (incl. residential)	a98%	Interview	+	65+ *	F: 219 M: 169	Yearly <damp (1)	17	11
O'Brien[39] 1991	Somerset	GP – random	a79%	Postal Q	+	35+	F: 3,165 M: 2,496	Monthly <damp (2)	16.4	7.4
Brocklehurst[40] 1993	Britain	Electoral stratified, random (MORI poll)	[not reported]	Interview (highly structured)	+	30+	F: 2,124 M: 1,883	Ever damp (2); Yearly damp (2); Monthly damp (3); Weekly damp (3)	14.0; 9.3; 7.5; 5.7	6.6; 3.8; 2.8; 2.2
McGrother[9,22,256,257] 1986, 1987, 1987, 1990	Melton Mowbray	GP – total (incl. residential)	a95%	Interview	+	75+	F: 820 M: 381	Monthly × damp (3)	12	12
Roe[258] 2000	England	GP – random	a53%	Postal Q	+++	18+	F: 2,699 M: 3,409	Monthly × damp (3)	11.3	5.3
Feneley[259] 1979	Bristol	GP – total	?93%	Postal Q	++	5+	F/M: 6,510	Monthly <damp (2)	8	3.3
Akhtar[260,261] 1973, 1972	Scotland	Population (3 samples)	70–80%	Interview + exam	+	65+	F: 490 M: 318	Monthly × wet (3)	1.6	2.2

Denominator: a adjusted for ineligibles and u unadjusted.
° Overestimate of true response rate.
? Unknown.
† (1) minor, (2) moderate, (3) major.
* Selected ages 65/66 and 75+.

Table A2.1(b): Summary of population studies of the prevalence of urinary incontinence from around the world.

Author/Year	Location	Sample	Response	Study type	Age	Respondents (N)	Thresholds and (ratings)	Prevalence % Female	Prevalence % Male
MacLennan[262] 2000	Australia	Population – random	73.3%	Home interview	15–97	F: 1,546 M: 1,464	Yearly <damp (1)	35.3	4.4
Simeonova[56] 1990	Sweden	Visitors to GP/ nurse	82%	Questionnaire	18+	F: 451	Ever <damp (1)	44	
Lara[263] 1994	New Z.	Electoral – random	54%	Postal Q	18+	F: 556	Yearly <damp (1) 2 × month <damp (2) daily <damp (3) continuously	34.0 25.2 12.6 3.0	
Chiarelli[185] 1999	Australia	Health database – random	47%	Questionnaire	18–23, 45–50, 70–75	F: 41,724	Yearly <damp (1)	27.5	
Hagglund[264] 1999	Sweden	Total population	88%	Postal Q	18–70	F: 3,076	Monthly <damp (2)	25.6	
Samuelsson[265] 2000	Sweden	Women having health check	77%	Postal Q	20–59	F: 382 (who received follow-up)	Any <damp (1) Monthly <damp (2) weekly <damp (3) daily <damp (3)	23.6 6.5 4.1 1.0	
Samuelsson[48] 1997	Sweden	Women scheduled for gynae exam	77%	Postal Q	20–59	F: 491	Any <damp (1) Monthly <damp (2) weekly <damp (3) daily <damp (3)	27.7 12.5 8.4 3.5	
Sommer[57] 1990	Denmark	National register random	69%	Postal Q	20–79	F: 414	Any <damp (1)	40	
Peyrat[266] 2002	France	Hospital employees	61%	Questionnaire	22–62	F: 1,700	Any <damp (1) Daily <damp (3)	27.5 2.2	
Makinen[50] 1992	Finland	Total population	71%	Questionnaire	25–55, cohort	F: 5,247	Any <damp (1) daily <damp (3)	20.1 3.5	
Vinker[267] 2001	Israel	GP list	84%	Questionnaire	30–75	F: 418	Any <damp (1) weekly <damp (3) daily <damp (3)	36.0 18.7 13.3	

Table A2.1(b): Continued.

Author/Year	Location	Sample	Response	Study type	Age	Respondents (N)	Thresholds and (ratings)	Prevalence % Female	Male
Fultz[268] 2000	USA	Population sample	58%	Postal Q	40+	F: 930	Yearly <damp (1)	12.2s 23.6l	
Bortolotti[84] 2000	Italy	GP random	~100%	Telephone interview	40+ F, 50+ M	F: 2,767 M: 2,721	Yearly <damp (1)	11.4	3.4
Moller[75] 2000	Denmark	Population – random	71.7%	Postal Q	40–60, cohort	F: 2,860	Any <damp (1) weekly <damp (3) daily <damp (3)	71.9 16.1 5.3	
Ueda[269] 2000	Japan	Population – random	52.5%	Postal Q	40–80	F: 968 M: 818	Ever <damp (1)	53.7	10.5
Muscatello[270] 2001	Italy	Telephone list random – area stratified	97%	Telephone interview	41+	F: 262 M: 232	Monthly <damp (2)	46.0	15.0
Hording[271] 1986	Denmark	Total population	84%	Interview	45	F: 515	Ever <damp (1)	22.1	
Malmsten[272] 1997	Sweden	Population – random	74%	Postal Q	45+, cohort	M: 7,763	Monthly <damp (2) weekly <damp (3) daily <damp (3)		9.2 7.9 5.9
Sherburn[78] 2001	Australia	Telephone numbers – random	94.8% (not clear)	Telephone interview	45–55	F: 1,897	Monthly <damp (2)	15.3	
Milsom[273] 1993	Sweden	Population – random	74.6%	Postal Q	46–86, cohorts	F: 7,459	Ever <damp (1) Any <damp (1)	21.1 14.8	
Holtedahl[274] 1998	Norway	Population – random	72.6%	Gynae exam	50–74	F: 507	Any <damp (1) 2+ × month <damp (2)	47.3 30.6	
Kok[275] 1992	N'lands	Electoral – random	69%	Postal Q	60+	F: 719	2 × week <damp (2) daily <damp (3)	23.5* 13.4	
Iosif[276] 1984	Sweden	Population random	75%	Postal Q	61	F: 902	Any <damp (1)	29.2	

	Country	Population	Response	Method	Age	N	Definition	%	%
Bogren[277] 1997	Sweden	Total population	91%	Postal Q	65	F: 220 M: 238	Any <damp (1)	28.0	9.0
Damian[46] 1998	Spain	Population – representative sample	71.2%	Home interview	65+, stratified	F/M: 589	Monthly <damp (2)	16.1	14.5
Tseng[278] 2000	Taiwan	Residents – random	80%	Home interview	65+	F: 256 M: 248	Ever <damp (1)	27.7	15.0
Maggi[279] 2001	Italy	Population random	73.3%	Home interview	65+, stratified	F: 1,531 M: 867	Yearly <damp (1) Monthly <damp (2) weekly <damp (3) daily <damp (3)	21.6 14.4 11.4 7.3	11.5 8.5 6.8 5.2
Brown[81] 1996	USA	Population-based listings	95%	Questionnaire	65+	F: 7,949	Monthly <damp (2) daily <damp (3)	41.3 14.2	
Harris[280] 1986	USA	Total population	95%	Home interview	65+	F: 3,346 M: 2,291	Any <damp (1) daily <damp (3)	10.0 7.3	7.0 5.3
Tilvis[281] 1995	Finland	Population register	81.6%	Postal Q + exam	75–85, cohort	F: 478 M: 171	Any <damp (1)	20.3	16.3
Lagaay[17] 1992	N'lands	Total population	94%	Home interview	85+	F/M: 937	Any <damp (1)	27.9	19.6

*Weighted mean.

s = short questionnaire, l = long questionnaire.

Table A2.2: Definitions and prevalence of nocturia, frequency and urgency in the UK: studies 1960–2001.

Author	Nocturia	Prevalence	Frequency	Prevalence	Urgency	Prevalence
Brocklehurst[10] 1971 (ages 65+)	Do you get up at night to pass urine?	Females: 28% Males: 33%	Can you go longer than 2 hours in the day time without having to pass urine?	Females: 9% Males: 14%	Do you have to go to pass urine in a hurry?	Females: 32% Males: 28%
Milne[13] 1972 (ages 62+)	Do you rise to pass urine at night (2 or more times)?	Females: 26% Males: 19%	Has there been a change in how often you pass urine in a day?	Females: 23% Males: 33%	Do you have control of your bladder if unable to go to the lavatory as soon as you need to pass urine?	Females: 21% Males: 21%
McGrother[9,257]* 1986, 87 (ages 75+)	Do you feel the need to get up during the night to pass urine (2 or more times)? (+ difficulty in control)	Females: 4.8% Males: 5.6%	How often do you go to the toilet to pass urine in the day usually (more than once every 2 hours)? (+difficulty in control)	Females: 4.3% Males: 5.0%	How long can you hold your water once you feel the urge to go (unable to wait for an occupied toilet)? (+ difficulty in control)	Females: 6.2% Males: 3.3%
Hunter[11]*** 1994 (ages 55+)			Frequency** – (level unspecified) more than half the time	Males: 9%	Urgency – (level unspecified) more than half the time	Males: 8%
Jolleys[282] 1994 (ages 40+)	Nocturia at least twice a night	Males: 14%	Frequency at least 9 times a day	Males: 12%	Urgency unspecified	Males: 48%
Kuh[42] 1999 (age 48)	How often passed urine during the night (2 or more times)	Females: 14.6%	How often passed urine during the day (more than once very 2 hours)	Females: 9.9%		
Swithinbank[12] 2000 (ages 18+)	Night-time voiding (2 or more times)	Females: 18%	Frequency unspecified	Females: 15%	Urgency – unspecified	Females: 61%
Perry[8] (ages 40+)	How often do you feel the need to get up at night to pass urine usually (2 or more times)?	Females: 21% Males: 20%	How often do you go to the toilet to pass urine usually (hourly or more)?	Females: 9.1% Males: 6.1%	Do you have difficulty holding urine once you have the urge to go, usually (most of the time or urge overwhelming)?	Females: 8.8% Males: 5.4%

* Threshold question (difficulty in control) applies to all symptom estimates; these estimates exclude residential care; two-stage study with 2% prevalence (of difficulty in control) drop-out between stages.

** AUA symptom index, modified for UK population (Barry MJ, Fowler FJ et al. J Urol 1992; **148**: 1549–57).

*** Random sample from eight GP practices in NW Thames Region. 1905 male respondents. Postal questionnaire, response 78% adjusted, minimal bias.

Table A2.3: Definitions and prevalences of need associated with urinary incontinence and related symptoms in UK studies 1960–2001.

Author	Group	General impact	Specific interference	Consultation/Uptake
Thomas[18] 1980	Males/Females, age 15+		Moderate or severe incontinence with some restriction of activities. 22% of those with regular incontinence, i.e. <2% prev in females and <1% prev in males	Recognised incontinence known to health and social services in 1 year. *Females: 15–64: 0.2%* *65+: 2.5%* *Males: 15–64: 0.1%* *65+: 1.3%*
Vetter[38] 1981	Males and females, age 70+			Seen GP in past month. Males and females: 6.2%
Yarnell[37] 1981	Females, age 18+	Problem with 'waterworks' and incontinent. *Females: 9.4%*	Interferes with social or domestic life: *Females: 3.5%* Causes continual embarrassment *Females: 1.3%*	Consulted a GP in last 12 months. *Females: 2.1%*
McGrother[9,256] 1986, 87	Males and females, age 75+	Difficulty in controlling water. *Females: 12%* *Males: 12%*	Interference with one or more social activity including daily, social life, relationships, feelings and quality of life. *Males and females: 3.6% ?*	Communicated the problem to GP or nurse. *Males and females: 5.1%* Took up offer of service *Males and females: 4.4%*
O'Brien[39] 1991	Males and females, age 35+			Discussed with GP or district nurse at some time. *Females: 2.8%* *Males: 1%* Took up treatment when offered *Females: 9.2%* *Males: 3.4%*
Brocklehurst[40] 1993	Males and females, age 30+	Bladder problems e.g. leaking, wet pants, damp pants, in the previous 2 months. *Females: 9.3%* *Males: 3.8%*	Effect on life style. Any effect – 77% cases (M&F); prevalence: *Females: 7.2%* *Males: 2.9%* A fair amount/great deal of effect – 34% F cases and 45% M cases; prevalence: *Females: 3.2.%* *Males: 1.7%* Concerned or worried = 60% of cases	Consulted GP. 80% of cases (M>F). Prevalence: *6.7% for males and females combined*

Table A2.3: Continued.

Author	Group	General impact	Specific interference	Consultation/Uptake
Harrison[28] 1994	Females, age 20+		Worry or affects social life and activities *Females: 8.6%*	Spoken to GP *Females: 3.2%* Took up offer of advice and treatment *Females: 6.1%*
Swithinbank[41] 1999	Females, age 19+	A bit or more of a problem with incontinence *Females: 40%*		
Dolan[44] 1999	Females, age 35–74			Consulted their GP *Females: 11.4%*
Kuh[42] 1999	Females, age 48	Bothered by incontinence in everyday life. *A little: 43.9%* *A lot: 29.9%*		
Perry[8] 2000	Males and females, age 40+	Incontinence and related symptoms described as a lot of bother or a moderate or severe problem *Females: 8%* *Males: 6.2%*	Interferes a lot: with daily activities, social life, relationships or quality of life or upsets or distress *Females: 3.2%* *Males: 2.2%*	Want help (not offered) *Females: 3.8%* *Males: 3.8%*
Stoddart[43] 2001	Males and females, age 65+	A little or more of a problem with incontinence *Females: 16.7%* *Males: 11.7%*	A little or more interference with life *Females: 18%* *Males: 12.2%*	Used health services *Females: 14%* *Males: 9.2%*

Table A2.4: Summary of population studies of the prevalence of stress and urge incontinence.

Study Population prevalence	Study sample	Definition of types of incontinence studied	
Maclennan 2000[262] Australia	1,544 women, 15–97	Stress: lost urine when coughed, laughed or sneezed	20.8%
		Urge: felt urge to go to toilet but accidentally wet themselves before reaching the toilet	2.9%
		Mixed: stress and urge combined	11.6%
Yarnell 1981[37] South Wales	1,060 women, 18+	Stress: loss of urine without urgency at any time	22.0%
		Urge: loss of urine with urgency at any time	9.0%
		Mixed: both types combined	14.0%
Holst 1988[49] New Zealand	851 women, 18+	Stress: not specifically stated	16.5%
		Urge: not specifically stated	7.7%
		Mixed: both types combined	7.2%
Lara 1994[263] New Zealand	556 women, 18+	Stress: loss when performing manoeuvres which increased intra-abdominal pressure e.g. coughing, exercising	16.3%
		Urge: sudden involuntary loss	9.2%
		Mixed: stress and urge combined	7.1%
		Other: not specified	1.4%
Simeonova 1990[56] Sweden	451 women, 18+	Stress: voided into clothes when coughing or laughing	16.2%
		Urge: could not avoid leakage when feeling urge to void	12.2%
		Mixed: stress and urge combined	15.5%
Samuelsson 1997[48] Sweden	487 women, 20–59	Stress: leakage during effort	15.8%
		Urge: leakage with a sense of urge	2.1%
		Mixed: both types combined	5.3%
		Other: leakage, not during effort or with sense of urge	4.7%
Samuelsson 2000[265] Sweden	382 women, 20–59	Stress: leakage during effort	14.7%
		Urge: leakage with sense of urge	1.6%
		Mixed: stress and urge combined	2.1%
		Other: non-specific	5.2%
Peyrat 2002[266] France	1,588 women, 20–62	Stress: involuntary urethral loss associated with coughing laughing, sneezing or physical exercise	12.5%
		Urge: involuntary urethral loss preceded by a sensation of urgency or by rapid uncontrollable voiding with little or no warning	1.5%
		Mixed: stress and urge combined	13.4%
Sommer 1990[57] Denmark	414 women, 20–79	Stress: not defined	15.3%
		Urge: not defined	13.3%
		Mixed: stress and urge combined	11.5%

Table A2.4: Continued.

Study Population prevalence	Study sample	Definition of types of incontinence studied	
Temml 2000[47] Austria	1,262 women, 20+	Stress: how often does urine leak when you are physically active, cough or sneeze?	10.5%
		Urge: how often does urine leak before you can get to the toilet?	1.8%
		Mixed: not specifically defined	12.6%[c]
		Other: nocturnal incontinence	0.1%
Harrison 1994[28] UK	314 women, 20+	Stress: leak when cough, laugh or exercise	24.5%
		Urge: not defined	4.5%
		Mixed: stress and urge combined	22.6%
Hannestad 2000[283] Norway	27,936 women, 20+	Stress: leak when coughing, sneezing, laughing, lifting heavy items	12.5%
		Urge: leakage accompanied by sudden and strong urge to void	2.8%
		Mixed: stress and urge combined	9.0%
		Other: not classified	0.7%
Makinen 1992[50] Finland	5,247 women 25–55	Stress: involuntary loss occurring during physical activity, such as coughing, heavy lifting, walking	14.7%
		Urge: such a very strong urge to pass water that you cannot hold on until you reach a toilet	0.8%
		Mixed: stress and urge combined	4.1%
		Other: other types of incontinence	0.5%
Elving 1989[71] Denmark	2,631 women 30–59	Stress: ICS	5.7%
		Urge: ICS	0.9%
		Mixed: both types combined	6.1%
Moller 2000[75] Denmark	2,860 women 40–60	Stress: ICS	13.0%
		Urge: ICS	7.2%
		Other: continuous, nightly or sexual	5.8%[a]
Ueda 2000[269] Japan	968 women, 40–80	Stress: do you ever leak urine when you cough, sneeze or laugh?	33.9%
		Urge: do you have difficulty holding your urine until you can get to the toilet?	6.9%
		Mixed: stress and urge combined	12.9%
Muscatello 2001[270] Australia	262 women, 40+	Stress: in the last month, how often did urine leak when you were physically active, exerted yourself, coughed or sneezed, during the day or night?	17.0%
		Urge: in the last month how often did urine leak before you could get to the toilet, during the day or night?	11.0%
		Mixed: stress and urge combined	18.0%
Burgio 1991[66] USA	486 women, 42–50	Stress: leakage with physical activity	28.0%
		Urge: loss associated with running water, urge to void, and being able to reach a toilet in time	6.8%
		Mixed: stress and urge combined	21.0%
Hørding 1986[271] Denmark	515 women, 45 only	Stress: loss of urine on coughing, running etc (ICS)	16.5%
		Urge: loss of urine after strong desire to void (ICS)	2.4%
		Mixed: both types combined	3.1%

Roberts 1998[51] USA	756 women, 50+	Stress: leakage of urine when coughed or sneezed in last year	6.4%
		Urge: in last year, when leakage occurred, were you aware of the need to urinate before the leakage occurred?	2.6%
		Mixed: stress and urge combined	37.9%
		Other: neither stress or urge	1.7%
Diokno 1986[83] USA	1,150 women, 60+	Stress: loss at time of physical exertion	10.0%
		Urge: loss after urge to void or uncontrollable voiding with little or no warning	3.4%
		Mixed: stress and urge combined	20.9%
Iosif 1984[276] Sweden	902 women, 61 only	Stress: involuntary loss of urine when coughing, laughing, lifting heavy objects, climbing/descending stairs or in rapid movement on level ground	11.7%
		Urge: usually get such a very strong urge that you cannot hold back until you reach a toilet	8.0%
		Mixed: stress and urge combined	9.5%
Bogren 1997[277] Sweden	225 women, 65 only	Stress: loss of urine due to physical exertion	9.2%[a]
		Urge: loss preceded by an urge to void	18.4%[a]
Damian 1998[46] Spain	589 men + women, 65+	Stress: escapes connected with exertion movements	2.0%[b]
		Urge: escapes connected with specific triggering situations	2.2%[b]
		Mixed: stress and urge combined	9.9%[b]
		Other: neither stress or urge	2.0%[b]
Koyama 1998[284] Japan	1,448 women, 65+	Stress: loss caused by coughing, sneezing, exercise	6.5%
		Urge: loss with urgency	6.8%
		Other: including abdominal pressure, during sleep	5.9%
Nygaard 1996[74] USA	2,025 women, 65+	Stress: leak when cough, sneeze or laugh	41.4%[a]
		Urge: how often have difficulty holding urine until reach a toilet	37.1%[a]
Tseng 2000[278] Taiwan	256 women, 65+	Stress: loss associated with physical exertion	10.9%
		Urge: loss because of inability to delay voiding following a micturition urge	6.6%
		Mixed: stress and urge combined	6.3%
		Other: undetermined	3.9%
Stoddart 2001[43] UK	740 women, 65+	Stress: leak after cough or sneezing	15.0%
		Urge: 'before I can get to the toilet'	16.0%
Liu 2002[285] Australia	2,272 men + women, 70+	Stress: accidentally pass urine	29.0%[a,b]
		Urge: have any difficulty holding urine until get to the toilet	41.4%[a,b]
Hellstrom 1990[16] Sweden	658 women, 85 only	Stress: involuntary loss precipitated by coughing, sneezing or physical exertion, etc	9.0%
		Urge: involuntary loss preceded by the urge to void or uncontrollable voiding with little or no warning	19.9%
		Mixed: stress and urge combined	14.2%

[a] Fixures may include mixed incontinence; [b] Women only; [c] Approximately.

Table A2.5: Summary of key prospective studies of the incidence of lower urinary tract symptoms (LUTS) in adults living in the community.

Study	Study population/ sample size/ (response rate)	Methodology	Definitions of symptoms studied	Prevalence at baseline (95% CI)	Incidence rate (95% CI)	Remission rate of cases (95% CI)
Møller 2000[73] Denmark	Women, 40–60 Random sample from civil registers in 1 urban and 1 rural county Sample: 4,000 Baseline: 2,860 (72%) Year 1: 2,284 (80%)	Postal questionnaire at baseline (1996) and year 1	Stress incontinence: leakage caused by exertion	13.1 (11.7–14.4) %	4.0 (3.2–4.9) %	41.4 (39.2–43.6) %
			Urge incontinence: leakage associated with urgency	7.3 (6.3–8.4) %	2.7 (2.2–3.4) %	42.0 (39.8–44.1) %
			Any urinary incontinence	16.4 (14.9–17.9) %	5.8 (4.7–6.8) %	37.7 (35.5–39.9) %
			Any LUTS ... occurring weekly or more	28.5 (26.7–30.4) %	10.0 (8.5–1.4) %	27.8 (25.6–30.0) %
Nygaard 1996[74] Iowa, USA – part of EPESE project (Establishment of Populations for Epidemiologic Studies of the Elderly)	Women, 65+ (65–104) total population of non-institutionalised women in 2 rural counties Sample: 2,541 Baseline: 2,025 (80%) of which SI 1,714 (68%) UI 1900 (75%) Year 3: 1,861 alive of which SI 1,550 (83%) UI 1,736 (9,3%)	Annual home interviews for 6 years; incontinence at baseline (1981/2), year 3 and year 6. 6 year results omitted here (do not correct for effects of ageing) Rates corrected for deaths	Stress incontinence (SI): leaking urine when cough, sneeze or laugh Urge incontinence (UI): difficulty holding urine until get to a toilet – occurring at least some of the time	41.4% 37.1%	3-year rates: baseline-year 3: 22.9% [7.6% pa] 19.6% [6.5% pa]	3-year rates: baseline-year 3: 27.0% [9.0% pa] 30.0% [10.0% pa]
Herzog 1990[72] Michigan, USA – part of MESA project (Medical, Epidemiologic and Social Aspects of Aging	Persons 60+ selected by multistage stratified area probability sampling of non-institutionalised residents in Washtenaw Sample: 2,968 Baseline: 1,956 (66%) Year 1: 1,333 (69%) Year 3: 662 (72%)	Annual home interviews for 2 years (baseline 1983/4); clinical evaluation + stress test in a subset persons at baseline Rates omit non-•responders from denominator	Any uncontrolled urine loss in the past 12 months	women: 37.7% men: 18.9%	women: year 1: 22.4% year 2: 22.2% men: year 1: 9.0% year 2: 10.6% Adjusted for remissions: women: 19% men: 8%	women year 1: 11.2% year 2: 13.3% men year 1: 26.7% year 2: 32.3%

Table A2.6: Changes in self-reported continence and severity of incontinence during one year.[286]

Baseline status	Baseline total	Year 1 status			
		Continent	Mild incontinence	Moderate incontinence	Severe incontinence
Women					
Continent	470	374	68	18	10
Mild incontinence	117	21	60	31	5
Moderate incontinence	85	3	41	36	5
Severe incontinence	54	2	7	10	35
Total	726	400	176	95	55
Men					
Continent	438	402	29	7	0
Mild incontinence	55	6	32	7	0
Moderate incontinence	21	6	6	7	2
Severe incontinence	9	2	1	2	4
Total	523	43	72	26	9

Appendix 3

Table A3.1: Actual numbers of operations by age group and sex for 1999–2000 (*Source*: Hospital Episode Statistics, Department of Health).

Age	under 20 M	under 20 F	20-24 M	20-24 F	25-29 M	25-29 F	30-34 M	30-34 F	35-39 M	35-39 F	40-44 M	40-44 F	45-49 M	45-49 F	50-54 M	50-54 F	55-59 M	55-59 F	60-64 M	60-64 F	65-69 M	65-69 F	70-74 M	70-74 F	75-79 M	75-79 F	80+ M	80+ F	All M	All F	All
A701	0	0	0	0	0	0	0	0	0	0	0	2	0	1	0	0	0	0	0	2	0	1	0	2	0	0	0	0	0	8	8
M511	0	0	0	1	0	3	0	21	0	47	0	75	0	84	0	120	0	98	0	97	0	65	0	52	0	41	0	11	0	715	715
M512	0	0	0	0	0	2	0	4	0	9	0	12	0	43	0	33	0	40	0	19	0	21	0	36	0	11	0	13	0	243	243
M521	0	2	0	2	0	3	0	10	0	20	0	33	0	67	0	67	0	60	0	61	0	52	0	24	0	15	0	12	0	428	428
M522	0	3	0	0	0	0	0	0	0	6	0	16	0	8	0	9	0	11	0	8	0	2	0	5	0	3	0	1	0	72	72
M523	0	6	0	3	0	35	0	137	0	435	0	745	0	908	0	1,085	0	796	0	597	0	378	0	201	0	85	0	27	0	5,438	5,438
M531	0	0	0	0	0	2	0	8	0	26	0	41	0	68	0	91	0	82	0	68	0	62	0	54	0	26	0	8	0	536	536
M538	0	0	0	1	0	2	0	21	0	46	0	82	0	106	0	133	0	121	0	81	0	77	0	56	0	51	0	20	0	797	797
M552	0	1	0	0	0	3	0	2	0	2	0	3	0	0	0	1	0	1	0	0	0	0	0	0	0	0	0	0	0	13	13
M563	0	11	0	3	0	8	0	34	0	45	0	86	0	129	0	203	0	198	1	178	2	184	0	174	1	137	0	81	4	1,471	1,475
M642	12	0	0	0	4	0	5	0	0	0	2	0	0	0	1	0	1	0	10	0	8	0	13	0	7	0	1	0	64	0	64
M651	1	0	0	0	0	0	0	0	0	0	0	0	2	0	4	0	9	0	7	0	17	0	39	0	30	0	41	0	150	0	150
M652	0	0	0	0	0	0	0	0	0	0	0	0	0	0	0	0	0	0	0	0	0	0	0	0	0	0	1	0	1	0	1
M653	0	0	0	0	0	0	0	0	1	0	0	0	0	0	1	0	10	0	18	0	22	0	34	0	52	0	64	0	202	2	204
P251	0	2	0	1	0	3	0	8	0	21	0	16	0	14	0	16	0	2	0	7	0	2	0	13	0	3	0	4	0	112	112
Total	13	25	0	11	4	61	5	245	1	657	2	1,111	2	1,428	6	1,758	20	1,409	36	1,119	49	845	86	617	90	372	107	177	421	9,835	10,256

Appendix 4: Treatments in primary and secondary care

Table A4.1: Drug treatment.

Drug	Dose	Cost per month (28 days)*
Oxybutynin	2.5–5 mg tds	£8.48–£18.43
Oxybutynin XL	5–10 mg once daily	£8.86–£17.71
Tolterodine	2 mg bd	£30.56
Trospium	20 mg bd	£23.33
Propiverine	15 mg bd – qds	£30.56–£61.12

* BNF 41

Table A4.2: Drugs, numbers of prescriptions dispensed in the community and cost for 1998–2000 (figures are rounded to the nearest 100 or £100).

1998

Drug name	Prescription items dispensed	Net cost (£)	Cost per item dispensed (£)
Flavoxate hydrochloride	77,700	765,300	9.85
Oxybutynin hydrochloride	1,015,800	12,291,000	12.10
Propiverine hydrochloride	1,000	31,400	30.13
Tolterodine tartrate	1,141	3,862,100	33.83
Total	1,208,700	16,950,000	

1999

Drug name	Prescription items dispensed	Net cost (£)	Cost per item dispensed (£)
Flavoxate hydrochloride	71,200	717,800	10.09
Oxybutynin hydrochloride	1,004,900	11,658,300	11.60
Propiverine hydrochloride	18,300	602,600	32.98
Tolterodine tartrate	329,300	11,189,200	33.98
Total	1,423,700	24,168,600	

2000

Drug name	Prescription items dispensed	Net cost (£)	Cost per item dispensed (£)
Flavoxate hydrochloride	64,900	681,200	10.49
Oxybutynin hydrochloride	1,003,400	9,397,300	9.37
Propiverine hydrochloride	40,400	1,402,700	34.71
Tolterodine tartrate	516,200	16,789,000	32.53
Total	1,624,900	28,270,200	

Source: Prescription Cost Analysis (Department of Health website: www.doh.gov.uk).

Table A4.3: Trials comparing bladder re-education to drug therapy.

	Type of study and size	Condition studied	Interventions	Incontinence reduction	Patient subjective cure	Further treatment needed
Burgio [172] 1998	RCT N=197	Detrusor overactivity in fit elderly	Behavioural	80.7%	74.1%	14%
			vs			
			oxybutynin	68.5%	50.9%	75.5%
			vs			
			placebo	39.4%	26.9%	75.5%
				Number of patients cured		
Burgio [193] 2000	Crossover from failed treatment in 1998 trial: N=8+27	Detrusor overactivity resistant to previous therapy	Addition of oxybutynin to failed behavioural therapy (8 patients)	4/8		
			Addition of behavioural to failed oxybutynin (27 patients)	13/27		

Table A4.4: Trials comparing combinations of behaviour and drug therapies.

	Type of study and size	Condition studied	Interventions	Reduction in episodes of incontinence per week	Patient subjective cure	Reduction in micturition frequency
Szonyi[287] 1995	RCT, N=57	Detrusor overactivity in fit elderly	Behavioural + oxybutynin vs Behavioural + placebo	4.75 4.75	86% 55%	1.9/day 0.4/day
				Reduction in incontinence episodes		
Ouslander[288] 1995	RCT, N=75	Urge incontinence in institutionalised elderly	Prompted voiding + oxybutynin vs Prompted voiding + placebo	2.8% 6.3%		
				Cure rate		
Castleden[206] 1986	RCT, N=33	Detrusor overactivity elderly clinic attenders	Bladder retraining + imipramine vs Bladder retraining + placebo	14/19 6/15		
				Continence	**No symptoms**	
Jarvis[289] 1981	RCT, N=50	Detrusor overactivity	In-patient bladder retraining vs Flavoxate 200 mg tds + imipramine 25 mg tds	84% 56%	76% 48%	

Table A4.5: Trials comparing oxybutynin with placebo.

	Type of study and size	Population	Intervention	Increase in maximum urodynamic capacity	Increase in volume at first desire to void
Madersbacher[290] 1999	Multi-centre (32) RCT, N=366	Secondary and tertiary centres	Propiverine 15 mg tds vs Oxybutynin 2.5 mg bd vs placebo	89 ml 96 ml 52 ml	67 ml 71 ml 27 ml
Thuroff[291] 1991	Multi-centre RCT, N=169	Secondary and tertiary centres	Propantheline 15 mg tds vs Oxybutynin 5 mg tds vs placebo	**Subjective improvement** 44.7% 58.2% 43.4%	
Moore[292] 1990	RCT, N=53	Secondary centre	Oxybutynin 3 mg tds vs placebo	**Symptoms improved** 60% 2.3%	**Reduction in frequency** 35% 9%
Tapp[293] 1990	RCT with crossover, N=37	Tertiary centre	Oxybutynin 5 mg qds vs placebo	**Stable urodynamics** 62% 42%	**Reduction of incontinence** 40% 25%
Zorzitto[294] 1989	RCT with crossover, N=24	Elderly institutionalised	Oxybutynin 5 mg bd vs placebo	**Incontinence profile reduction** 24% 27%	

Table A4.6: Controlled release oxybutynin.

	Type of study and size	Population	Intervention	Daytime continence	Side effects
Birns[200] 2000	RCT multicentre, N=130	Patients already stabilised on oxybutynin. Secondary and tertiary centres	Oxybutynin 5 mg bd vs Oxybutynin CR 10 mg om	58% 53%	Less with controlled release tablets
				Reduction of urge incontinence	
Versi[199] 2000	RCT multicentre, N=226	Patients responsive to oxybutynin. Tertiary centres	Oxybutynin vs Oxybutynin CR (dose titrated against side effects and efficacy)	83% 76%	In efficacious doses there was no difference in side effect profiles
				Reduction of urge incontinence	
Anderson[295] 1999	RCT multicentre, N=105	Secondary and tertiary centres	Oxybutynin vs Oxybutynin controlled release (variable dose)	88% 84%	Slight reduction in dry mouth with CR oxybutynin

Table A4.7: Controlled release tolterodine.

	Type of study and size	Population	Intervention	Reduction in voids per day	Reduction in incontinent episodes per 24 hours
Millard[296] 1999	RCT, multicentre, N=316	Tertiary centres	Tolterodine 2 mg bd vs Tolterodine 1 mg bd vs placebo	2.3 2.3 1.4	1.7 NS 1.7 NS 1.3
Larson[297] 1999	Pooled phase II efficacy data, N=319	Tertiary centres	Tolterodine 4 mg bd vs Tolterodine 2 mg bd vs Tolterodine 1 mg bd vs Tolterodine 0.5 mg bd vs placebo	1.4 1.5 1.0 0.8 0.5 $p=0.043$	1.7 1.6 0.8 1.2 1.4 $p=0.18$
Abrams[298] 1998	RCT, multicentre, N=293	Tertiary and secondary centres	Tolterodine 2 mg bd vs Oxybutynin 5 mg tds vs placebo	2.7 $p=0.002$ 2.3 $p=0.06$	1.3 $p=0.22$ 1.7 $p=0.023$
Appell[299] 1997	Pooled phase III efficacy data, N=1,120	Tertiary and secondary centres	placebo Tolterodine 2 mg bd vs Tolterodine 1 mg bd vs Oxybutynin 5 mg tds vs	1.6 2.25 $p<0.05$ 2.10 $p<0.05$ 1.95 $p<0.05$	0.9 1.55 $p<0.05$ 1.65 $p<0.05$ 1.75 $p<0.05$
Appell[197] 2001	RCT, multicentre, N=378	Tertiary and secondary centres	placebo Oxybutynin 10 mg Controlled release vs Tolterodine 2 mg bd	1.35 3.5 $p<0.05$ 2.9	1.05 3.1 $p<0.05$ 2.5
Kerrebroeck[300] 2001	RCT, multicentre, N=1,529	Tertiary and secondary centres	Tolterodine 2 mg bd vs Tolterodine Controlled release 4 mg om vs placebo	3.3 $p<0.005$ 3.5 $p<0.005$ 2.2	1.5 $p<0.05$ 1.7 $p<0.05$ 1.0

Table A4.8: (adapted from Jarvis 1994[212]).

Procedure	Cure (%)
Anterior repair and urethral buttress	67.8
Marshal-Marchetti-Krantz (MMK)	89.5
Colposuspension	89.9
Needle suspension	70–86.7
Bladder sling	93.9
Bladder neck injection	45.5
TVT	84.7

Appendix 5

Table A5.1: Recommended questionnaires for the assessment of urinary incontinence symptoms and impact on the quality of life of patients.

Questionnaire	Items developed from	Sample	Content
York Incontinence Perceptions Scale (YIPS)	Open-ended questions	Female, community sample, all types of urinary incontinence, age range 29–98 years	8 items; control, acceptance, coping, knowledge, sleep, QOL, family
Incontinence Impact Questionnaire (IIQ)	Literature, qualitative interviews, experts (modification of previous scale)	Female, community sample, USI, DO, >44 years	30 items; activities, feelings relationships
Quality of Life of Persons with Urinary Incontinence (I-QOL)		Male and female, community sample, mixed UI	28 items; worry, emotions, self-image
Incontinence Stress Index	Literature review	Female nursing home residents, mean age 85.3 years	41 items; agitated depressive symptoms, retarded depressive symptoms, feeling of abandonment, somatic concerns and activities
ICS male Questionnaire	Interviews with men with lower urinary tract symptoms, discussion experts	Men, community and clinic samples, lower urinary tract symptoms	22 items; urge, stress, nocturnal incontinence, post-micturition dribble, degree of impact of symptoms
Incontinence Impact Questionnaire	Literature, qualitative interviews, experts (modification of previous scale)	Female, community sample, USI, DO, >44 years	30 items; activities, feelings relationships
Urogenital Distress Inventory	Literature review, qualitative interviews, experts	Female, community sample, USI, DO, >44 years	19 symptoms and related bother
Kings Health Questionnaire	Literature review, experts	Female, community sample, mixed UI	Role limitations (2 items), physical/social limitations (4 items), personal relations (3 items), emotions (3 items), sleep/energy (2 items)
Bristol Female LUTS	Discussion with patients, experts, literature review	Female	Sex (4 items), activities (7 items)
Urge Incontinence Impact Scale (URIS-24)	Focus groups with older people with urge incontinence	Male and female, community sample, mean age 74 years, urge incontinence	24 items; self-image, emotions, worry
ICIQ-SF (developmental)	Literature review, experts, patient interviews	All ages, males, females	10 items covering frequency, severity and impact on quality of life of incontinence symptoms in all patient groups

USI = urodynamic stress incontinence, DO = detrusor overactivity, UI = urinary incontinence

Table A5.2: Summary of outcome indicators for urinary incontinence recommended by the NCHOD Working Group reporting for the Department of Health.

Indicators (grouped by the aims of intervention to which they relate)	Characteristics	Recommendation for implementation
Avoidance or reduction of the risk of urinary incontinence		
1 Incidence and prevalence of urinary incontinence	Specificity: generic Perspective: population Time frame: cross-sectional Relation to outcome: direct	To be further developed either because the link with effectiveness is not clear or because the indicator specification is not complete
2 Prevalence of urinary incontinence in long-term care	Specificity: condition-specific Perspective: population Time frame: cross-sectional Relation to outcome: direct	To be implemented generally by periodic survey
3 Incidence of urinary incontinence among women following pregnancy	Specificity: condition-specific Perspective: population Time frame: cross-sectional Relation to outcome: direct	To be implemented where local circumstances allow by periodic surveys
4 Rate of pelvic floor exercise training among pregnant women	Specificity: condition-specific Perspective: clinical Time frame: cross-sectional Relation to outcome: indirect	To be further developed either because the link with effectiveness is not clear or because the indicator specification is not complete
Avoidance or reduction of adverse effects of delayed diagnosis or treatment		
5 Delay to presentation with urinary incontinence	Specificity: condition-specific Perspective: clinical Time frame: cross-sectional Relation to outcome: indirect	To be further developed either because the link with effectiveness is not clear or because the indicator specification is not complete
6 Clinical assessment rates following presentation with urinary incontinence within a GP population	Specificity: condition-specific Perspective: clinical Time frame: cross-sectional Relation to outcome: indirect	To be implemented where local circumstances allow by periodic surveys
7 Rate of referral following presentation with urinary incontinence within a GP population	Specificity: condition-specific Perspective: clinical Time frame: cross-sectional Relation to outcome: indirect	To be implemented where local circumstances allow by periodic surveys

Table A5.2: Continued.

Indicators (grouped by the aims of intervention to which they relate)	Characteristics	Recommendation for implementation
8 Clinical assessment rates for those with urinary incontinence in long-term care	Specificity: condition-specific Perspective: clinical Time frame: cross-sectional Relation to outcome: indirect	To be implemented generally by periodic survey
Treating underlying mechanisms and causes and avoiding adverse consequences		
9 Rate of pre-operative cystometry in women undergoing surgery for urinary incontinence	Specificity: condition-specific Perspective: clinical Time frame: cross-sectional Relation to outcome: indirect	To be implemented following IT development on a routine basis
10 Rate of one-to-one training in pelvic floor exercises among women with stress incontinence	Specificity: condition-specific Perspective: clinical Time frame: cross-sectional Relation to outcome: indirect	To be further developed either because the link with effectiveness is not clear or because the indicator specification is not complete
11 Percentage of anterior repair procedures undertaken in a population of women undergoing surgery for stress incontinence	Specificity: condition-specific Perspective: clinical Time frame: cross-sectional Relation to outcome: indirect	To be implemented generally on a routine basis
12 Rate of re-operation in a hospital provider unit population within two years following surgical treatment for urinary incontinence	Specificity: generic Perspective: clinical Time frame: cross-sectional Relation to outcome: direct	To be implemented where local circumstances allow on a routine basis
13 Rate of emergency re-admission (for urinary-related condition and/or specific post-operation complication) within 30 days of discharge, for a hospital provider unit population which has undergone surgery for urinary incontinence	Specificity: generic Perspective: clinical Time frame: cross-sectional Relation to outcome: indirect	To be implemented where local circumstances allow on a routine basis
14 Changes in urinary symptoms from before treatment to six months afterwards within a provider unit population receiving treatment for urinary incontinence	Specificity: condition-specific Perspective: clinical Time frame: longitudinal Relation to outcome: direct	To be implemented where local circumstances allow by periodic surveys

Reducing impact of urinary incontinence on general well-being

15 Use of indwelling catheters in long-term care	Specificity: condition-specific Perspective: clinical Time frame: cross-sectional Relation to outcome: indirect	To be implemented generally by periodic survey
16 Changes in health-related quality of life as assessed before treatment to six months afterwards within a provider unit population receiving treatment for urinary incontinence	Specificity: generic Perspective: patient Time frame: longitudinal Relation to outcome: direct	To be further developed either because the link with effectiveness is not clear or because the indicator specification is not complete
17 A measure of patient satisfaction at six months within a hospital provider unit population which has undergone surgery for urinary incontinence	Specificity: surgery-specific Perspective: patient Time frame: cross-sectional Relation to outcome: direct	To be further developed either because the link with effectiveness is not clear or because the indicator specification is not complete
18 A measure of attainment of patient-specified outcome goals, within a population receiving treatment for urinary incontinence	Specificity: generic Perspective: patient Time frame: longitudinal Relation to outcome: direct	To be further developed either because the link with effectiveness is not clear or because the indicator specification is not complete

References

1 Bates P, Bradley WE, Glen E, Melchior H, Rowan D, Sterling A *et al.* First report on the standardisation of terminology of lower urinary tract function. *Br J Urol* 1976; **48**: 39–42.

2 Mattiasson A. Characterisation of lower urinary tract disorders: a new view. *Neurourol Urodyn* 2001; **20**: 601–21.

3 World Health Organization. *The ICD-10 classification of disease.* Geneva: WHO, 1992.

4 Bradshaw J. A taxonomy of social need. In: Mclachlan G (ed.). *Problems and progress in medical care.* London: Oxford University Press, 1972; 71–82.

5 Stevens A, Gabbay J. Needs assessment needs assessment.... *Health Trends* 1991; **23**: 20–3.

6 Frankel S. Health needs, health-care requirements, and the myth of infinite demand. *The Lancet* 1991; **337**: 1588–90.

7 Office of Population Censuses and Surveys. *Classification of surgical operations and procedures.* 4th revision. London: OPCS, 1987.

8 Perry S, Shaw C, Assassa P, Dallosso H, Williams K, Brittain KR *et al.* An epidemiological study to establish the prevalence of urinary symptoms and felt need in the community: the Leicestershire MRC Incontinence Study. *J Public Health Med* 2000; **22**: 427–34.

9 McGrother CW, Castleden CM, Duffin H, Clarke M. Provision of services, for incontinent elderly people at home. *J Epidemiol Community Health* 1986; **40**: 134–8.

10 Brocklehurst JC, Fry J, Griffiths LL, Kalton G. Dysuria in old age. *JAMA* 1971; **19**: 582–92.

11 Hunter DJW, McKee CM, Black NA, Sanderson CFB. Urinary symptoms: prevalence and severity in British men aged 55 and over. *J Epidemiol Community Health* 1994; **48**: 569–75.

12 Swithinbank LV, Abrams P. A detailed description, by age, of lower urinary tract symptoms in a group of community-dwelling women. *BJU Int* 2000; **82**: 19–24.

13 Milne JS, Williamson J, Maule MM, Wallace ET. Urinary symptoms in older people. *Modern Geriatrics* 1972; **2**: 198–210.

14 The Royal College of Physicians. Incontinence – causes, management and provision of services. *J R Coll Physicians Lond* 1995; **29**: 272–4.

15 Peet SM, Castleden CM, McGrother CW. Prevalence of urinary and fecal incontinence in hospitals and residential and nursing-homes for older-people. *BMJ* 1995; **311**: 1063–4.

16 Hellstrom L, Ekelund P, Milsom I, Mellstrom D. The prevalence of urinary incontinence and use of incontinence aids in 85-year-old men and women. *Age and Ageing* 1990; **19**: 383–9.

17 Lagaay AM, Vanasperen IA, Hijmans W. The prevalence of morbidity in the oldest old, aged 85 and over – a population-based survey in Leiden, the Netherlands. *Arch Gerontol Geriatr* 1992; **15**: 115–31.

18 Thomas TM, Plymat KR, Blannin J, Meade TW. Prevalence of urinary incontinence. *BMJ* 1980; **281**: 1243–5.

19 Thomas TM, Egan M, Walgrove A, Meade TW. The prevalence of faecal and double incontinence. *Community Med* 1984; **6**: 216–20.

20 Nakanishi N, Tatara K, Naramura H, Fujiwara H, Takashima Y, Fukuda H. Urinary and fecal incontinence in a community-residing older population in Japan. *J Am Geriatr Soc* 1997; **45**: 215–9.

21 Brittain KR, Perry SI, Peet SM, Shaw C, Dallosso H, Assassa RP *et al.* Prevalence and impact of urinary symptoms among community-dwelling stroke survivors. *Stroke* 2000; **31**: 886–91.

22 McGrother CW, Jagger C, Clarke M, Castleden CM. Handicaps associated with incontinence – implications for management. *J Epidemiol Community Health* 1990; **44**: 246–8.

23 Resnick NM. Urinary incontinence. *The Lancet* 1995; **346**: 94–9.

24 Peet SM, Castleden CM, McGrother CW, and Duffin HM. The management of urinary incontinence in residential and nursing homes for older people. *Age and Ageing* 25: 139–43.

25 Martin J, Melzer H, Elliot D. *The prevalence of disability among adults.* OPCS surveys of disability in Great Britain. London: HMSO, 1988.

26 McGrother CW, Hauck A, Bhaumik S, Thorp C, Taub N. Community care for adults with learning disability and their carers: needs and outcomes from the Leicestershire Register. *Journal of Intellectual Disability Research* 1996; **40**: 183–90.

27 Sandvik H, Hunskaar S, Seim A, Hermstad R, Vanvik A, Bratt H. Validation of a severity index in female urinary incontinence and its implementation in an epidemiologic survey. *J Epidemiol Community Health* 1993; **47**: 497–9.

28 Harrison GL, Memel DS. Urinary incontinence in women – its prevalence and its management in a health promotion clinic. *Br J Gen Pract* 1994; **44**: 149–52.

29 Lagro-Janssen TLM, Smits AJA, Vanweel C. Women with urinary incontinence – self-perceived worries and general-practitioners knowledge of problem. *Br J Gen Pract* 1990; **40**: 331–4.

30 Lam GW, Foldspang A, Elving LB, Mommsen S. Social-context, social abstention, and problem recognition correlated with adult female urinary incontinence. *Dan Med Bull* 1992; **39**: 565–70.

31 Rekers H, Drogendijk AC, Valkenburg H, Riphagen F. Urinary incontinence in women from 35 to 79 years of age – prevalence and consequences. *European Journal of Obstetrics Gynecology and Reproductive Biology* 1992; **43**: 229–34.

32 Sandvik H, Kveine E, Hunskaar S. Female urinary incontinence: psychosocial impact, self care, and consultations. *Scandinavian Journal of Caring in Science* 1993; **7**: 53–6.

33 Mitteness LS. The management of urinary incontinence by community-living elderly. *Gerontologist* 1987; **27**: 185–93.

34 Macaulay AJ, Stern RS, Stanton SL. Psychological-aspects of 211 female-patients attending a urodynamic unit. *Journal of Psychosomatic Research* 1991; **35**: 1–10.

35 Norton PA, Macdonald LD, Sedgwick PM, Stanton SL. Distress and delay associated with urinary incontinence, frequency, and urgency in women. *BMJ* 1988; **297**: 1187–9.

36 Sutherst JR. Sexual dysfunction and urinary incontinence. *Br J Obstet Gynaecol* 1979; **86**: 387–88.

37 Yarnell JWG, Voyle GJ, Richards CJ, Stephenson TP. The prevalence and severity of urinary incontinence in women. *J Epidemiol Community Health* 1981; **35**: 71–4.

38 Vetter NJ, Jones DA, Victor CR. Urinary incontinence in the elderly at home. *The Lancet* 1981; **2**: 1275–7.

39 O'Brien J, Austin M, Sethi P, Oboyle P. Urinary incontinence – prevalence, need for treatment, and effectiveness of intervention by nurse. *BMJ* 1991; **303**: 1308–12.

40 Brocklehurst JC. Urinary incontinence in the community – analysis of a MORI poll. *BMJ* 1993; **306**: 832–4.

41 Swithinbank LV, Donovan JL, Du Heaume JC, Rogers CA, James MC, Yang QA *et al.* Urinary symptoms and incontinence in women: Relationships between occurrence, age, and perceived impact. *Br J Gen Pract* 1999; **49**: 897–900.

42 Kuh D, Cardozo L, Hardy R. Urinary incontinence in middle aged women: childhood enuresis and other lifetime risk factors in a British prospective cohort. *J Epidemiol Community Health* 1999; **53**: 453–8.

43 Stoddart H, Donovan J, Whitley E, Sharp D, Harvey I. Urinary incontinence in older people in the community: a neglected problem? *Br J Gen Pract* 2001; **51**: 548–52.

44 Dolan LM, Casson K, Mcdonald P, Ashe RG. Urinary incontinence in Northern Ireland: a prevalence study. *BJU Int* 1999; **83**: 760–6.

45 Yarnell JWG, St Leger AS. The prevalence, severity and factors associated with urinary incontinence in a random sample of the elderly. *Age and Ageing* 1979; **8(2)**: 81–5.

46 Damian J, Martin-Moreno JM, Lobo F, Bonache J, Cervino J, Redondo-Marquez L *et al.* Prevalence of urinary incontinence among Spanish older people living at home. *European Urology* 1998; **34**: 333–8.

47 Temml C, Haidinger G, Schmidbauer J, Schatzl G, Madersbacher S. Urinary incontinence in both sexes: Prevalence rates and impact on quality of life and sexual life. *Neurourol Urodyn* 2000; **19**: 259–71.

48 Samuelsson E, Victor A, Tibblin G. A population study of urinary incontinence and nocturia among women aged 20–59 years – prevalence, well-being and wish for treatment. *Acta Obstet Gynecol Scand* 1997; **76**: 74–80.

49 Holst K, Wilson PD. The prevalence of female urinary incontinence and reasons for not seeking treatment. *New Zealand Medical Journal* 1988; **101**: 756–8.

50 Makinen JI, Gronroos M, Kiiholma PJA, Tenho TT, Pirhonen JP, Erkkola RU. The prevalence of urinary incontinence in a randomized population of 5247 adult Finnish women. *Int Urogynecol J* 1992; **3**: 110–3.

51 Roberts RO, Jacobsen SJ, Rhodes T, Reilly WT, Girman CJ, Talley NJ, Lieber MM. Urinary incontinence in a community-based cohort: prevalence and healthcare-seeking. *JAGS* 1998; **46**: 467–72.

52 Seim A, Sandvik H, Hermstad R, Hunskaar S. Female urinary incontinence – consultation behavior and patient experiences – an epidemiologic survey in a Norwegian community. *Fam Pract* 1995; **12**: 18–21.

53 Gavira Iglesias FJ, Ocerin JMCy, Martin JPdM, Gama EV, Perez ML, Lopez MR *et al.* Prevalence and psychosocial impact of urinary incontinence in older people of a Spanish rural population. *Journals of Gerontology Series a – Biological Sciences and Medical Sciences* 2000; **55**: M207–M214.

54 McGrother CW, Castleden CM, Duffin H, Clarke M. Do the elderly need better incontinence services? *Community Medicine* 1987; **9(1)**: 62–7.

55 Jolleys JV. Reported prevalence of urinary incontinence in women in a general-practice. *BMJ* 1988; **296**: 1300–2.

56 Simeonova Z, Bengtsson C. Prevalence of urinary incontinence among women at a Swedish primary health care centre. *Scand J Prim Health Care* 1990; **8**: 203–6.

57 Sommer P, Bauer T, Nielsen KK, Kristensen ES, Hermann GG, Steven K *et al.* Voiding patterns and prevalence of incontinence in women – a questionnaire survey. *Br J Urol* 1990; **66**: 12–15.

58 MacArthur C, Lewis M, Knox G. *Health after childbirth.* London: HMSO, 1991.

59 Roe B, Doll H. Lifestyle factors and continence status: comparison of self-report data from a postal survey in England. *Journal of Wound Ostomy Continence Nurse* 1999; **26**: 312–9.

60 Chaliha C, Stanton SL. The ethnic cultural and social aspects of incontinence – a pilot study. *International Urogynecology Journal* 1999; **10**: 166–70.

61 Gillam S, Jarman B, White P, and Law R. Ethnic differences in consultation rates in urban general practice. *BMJ* 1989; **299**: 953–7.

62 Balarajan R, Yuen P, Raleigh VS. Ethnic-differences in general-practitioner consultations. *BMJ* 1989; **299**: 958–60.

63 Modood T, Berthoud B, Blakey J, Nazroo J, Smit P, Virdee S *et al. Ethnic minorities in Britain: diversity and disadvantage.* London: Policy Studies Institute, 1997.

64 Lee B, Syed Q, Bellis M. *Improving the health of black and ethnic minority communities: a north west of England perspective.* Liverpool: Sexual Health and Environmental Epidemiology Unit, 1998.

65 Fultz NH, Herzog AR, Raghunathan TE, Wallace RB, Diokno AC. Prevalence and severity of urinary incontinence in older African American and caucasian women. *Journals of Gerontology Series a – Biological Sciences and Medical Sciences* 1999; **54**: M299–M303.

66 Burgio KL, Matthews KA, Engel BT. Prevalence, incidence and correlates of urinary incontinence in healthy, middle-aged women. *J Urol* 1991; **146**: 1255–9.

67 Burgio KL, Locher JL, Zyczynski H, Hardin JM, and Singh K. Urinary incontinence during pregnancy in a racially mixed sample: characteristics and predisposing factors. *Int Urogynecol J Pelvic Floor Dysfunct* 1996; **7**(2): 69–73.

68 Thom DH, Van den Eeden SK, and Brown JS. Evaluation of parturition and other reproductive variables as risk factors for urinary incontinence in later life. *Obstet Gynecol* 1997; **90**(6): 983–9.

69 Lagro-Janssen ALM, Debruyne FMJ, Vanweel C. Value of the patient's case-history in diagnosing urinary- incontinence in general-practice. *Br J Urol* 1991; **67**: 569–72.

70 Versi E, Cardozo L, Anand D, Cooper D. Symptoms analysis for the diagnosis of genuine stress-incontinence. *Br J Obstet Gynaecol* 1991; **98**: 815–9.

71 Elving LB, Foldspang A, Lam GW, Mommsen S. Descriptive epidemiology of urinary incontinence in 3,100 women age 30–59. *Scand J Urol Nephrol Suppl* 1989; **125**: 37–43.

72 Herzog AR, Diokno AC, Brown MB, Normolle DP, Brock BM. Two-year incidence, remission, and change patterns of urinary incontinence in noninstitutionalized older adults. *Journal of Gerontology* 1990; **45**: M67–74.

73 Moller LA, Lose G, Jorgensen T. Incidence and remission rates of lower urinary tract symptoms at one year in women aged 40–60: longitudinal study. *BMJ* 2000; **320**: 1429–32.

74 Nygaard IE, Lemke JH. Urinary incontinence in rural older women: prevalence, incidence and remission. *J Am Geriatr Soc* 1996; **44**: 1049–54.

75 Moller LA, Lose G, Jorgensen T. The prevalence and bothersomeness of lower urinary tract symptoms in women 40–60 years of age. *Acta Obstet Gynecol Scand* 2000; **79**: 298–305.

76 Foldspang A, Mommsen S, Djurhuus JC. Prevalent urinary incontinence as a correlate of pregnancy, vaginal childbirth, and obstetric techniques. *Am J Public Health* 1999; **89**: 209–12.

77 Moller LA, Lose G, Jorgensen T. Risk factors for lower urinary tract symptoms in women 40 to 60 years of age. *Obstet Gynecol* 2000; **96**: 446–51.

78 Sherburn M, Guthrie J, Dudley EOH, Dennerstein L. Is incontinence associated with menopause? *Obstet Gynecol* 2001; **98**: 628–33.

79 Thom DH, Haan MN, Vandeneeden SK. Medically recognized urinary incontinence and risks of hospitalization, nursing home admission and mortality. *Age and Ageing* 1997; **26**: 367–74.

80 Tinetti ME, Inouye SK, Gill TM, Doucette JT. Shared risk-factors for falls, incontinence, and functional dependence – unifying the approach to geriatric syndromes. *JAMA* 1995; **273**: 1348–53.

81 Brown JS, Seeley DG, Fong J, Black DM, Ensrud KE, Grady D. Urinary incontinence in older women: who is at risk? *Obstet Gynecol* 1996; **87**: 715–21.

82 Ouslander JG, Palmer MH, Rovner BW, German PS. Urinary incontinence in nursing homes – incidence, remission and associated factors. *J Am Geriatr Soc* 1993; **41**: 1083–9.

83 Diokno AC, Brock BM, Brown MB, Herzog AR. Prevalence of urinary incontinence and other urological symptoms in the noninstitutionalized elderly. *J Urol* 1986; **136**: 1022–5.

84 Bortolotti A, Bernardini B, Colli E, Di Benedetto P, Nacci GG, Landoni M *et al.* Prevalence and risk factors for urinary incontinence in Italy. *European Urology* 2000; **37**: 30–5.

85 Brown JS, Vittinghoff E, Wyman JF, Stone KL, Nevitt MC, Ensrud KE *et al.* Urinary incontinence: does it increase risk for falls and fractures? *J Am Geriatr Soc* 2000; **48**: 721–5.

86 Anon. Treating urinary incontinence with timed schedules and exercises. *Nursing* 1995; **25**: 32C-D.

87 Pearson M, Richmond D, Cullum N, Hutton J, Abbott S, and Nelson C. The development of methodologies to identify urinary incontinence and set targets for health gain. Liverpool: Health and Community Care Research Unit, University of Liverpool, 1995.

88 Netten A, Curtis L. *Unit costs of health and social care.* Canterbury: University of Kent, Personal Social Services Research Unit, 2000.

89 King's Fund. *Action on incontinence: report of a working group.* London: King's Fund, 1983.

90 Walters MD and Realini JP. The evaluation and treatment of urinary incontinence in women: a primary care approach. *JABFP* 1992; **5(3)**: 289–301.

91 McDowell BJ, Silverman M, Martin D, Musa D, Keane C. Identification and intervention for urinary incontinence by community physicians and geriatric assessment teams. *Journal of the American Geriatric Society* 1994; **42**: 501–5.

92 Sandvik H, Hunskaar S, and Eriksen BC. Management of urinary incontinence in women in general practice: actions taken at the first consultation. *Scandinavian Journal of Primary Health Care* 1990; **8**: 3–8.

93 Jolleys JV, Wilson JV. Urinary incontinence. GPs lack confidence. *BMJ* 1993; **306**: 1344.

94 Henalla SM, Hutchins CJ, Robinson P, Macvicar J. Non-operative methods in the treatment of female genuine stress-incontinence of urine. *Journal of Obstetrics and Gynaecology* 1989; **9**: 222–5.

95 Briggs M, Williams ES. Urinary incontinence. *BMJ* 1992; **304**: 255.

96 Rhodes P and Parker G. The role of continence advisors in England and Wales. York: Social Policy Research Unit, University of York, 1996.

97 Rhodes P. A postal survey of continence advisers in England and Wales. *J Adv Nurs (H3L)* 1995; **21**: 286–94.

98 Cheater F. Attitudes towards urinary incontinence. *Nursing Standard* 1991a; **20**: 23–7.

99 Cheater F. The aetiology of urinary incontinence. In Roe BH (ed.) *Clinical nursing practice. The promotion and management of incontinence.* London: Prentice Hall, 1992.

100 Burnet C, Carter H, and Gorman D. Urinary incontinence: a survey of knowledge, working practice and training needs of nursing staff in Fife. *Health Bulletin* 1992; **50(6)**: 448–52.

101 Black NA, Downs SH. The effectiveness of surgery for stress incontinence in women: a systematic review. *Br J Urol* 1996; **78**: 497–510.

102 The Continence Foundation. *Making the case for investment in an integrated continence service. A source book for continence services.* London: The Continence Foundation, 2000.

103 Royal College of Nursing. *Commisioning Continence Advisory Services: an RCN guide.* London: Royal College of Nursing, 2000.

104 Wells M. The role of the nurse in urinary incontinence. *Best Practice & Research in Clinical Obstetrics & Gynaecology* 2000; **14**: 335–54.

105 Wells M. Stress incontinence and pelvic floor exercises. *Professional Nurse* 1990a; **6**: 4–6.

106 Wilson PD, Bo K, Hay-Smith J, Nygaard I, Statskin D, Wyman J, and Bourcier A. Conservative treatment in women. In Abrams P, Cardozo L, Khoury S, and Wein A. *Incontinence: 2nd International Consultation on Incontinence.* 573–626. Plymouth: Health Publication Ltd, 2002.

107 Laycock J. Pelvic floor re-education for the promotion of incontinence. In Roe BH (ed.). *Clinical nursing practice,* London: Prentice Hall, 1992.

108 Plevnik S. *New method for testing and strengthening of pelvic floor muscles.* London: Proceedings of the 15th Annual Meeting of The International Continence Society, 1985.

109 Fantl JA. Behavioural therapies in the management of urinary stress incontinence in women. Cardozo L and Staskin D. *Textbook of female urology and urogynaecology.* 343–349. 2001. London: Isis Medical Media.

110 Creighton SM, Stanton SL. Caffeine – does it affect your bladder? *Br J Urol* 1990; **66**: 613–4.

111 Mommsen S, Foldspang A. Body mass index and adult female urinary incontinence. *World J Urol* 1994; **12**: 319–22.

112 Kolbl H, Riss P. Obesity and stress urinary incontinence: significance of indices of relative weight. *Urology International* 1988; **43**: 7–10.

113 Diokno AC, Brock BM, Herzog AR, Bromberg J. Medical correlates of urinary incontinence in the elderly. *Urology* 1990; **36**: 129–38.

114 Koskimaki J, Hakama M, Huhtala H, Tammela TLJ. Association of smoking with lower urinary tract symptoms. *J Urol* 1998; **159**: 1580–2.

115 Samuelsson E, Victor A, Svardsudd K. Determinants of urinary incontinence in a population of young and middle-aged women. *Acta Obstet Gynecol Scand* 2000; **79**: 208–15.

116 Nusbaum ML, Gordon M, Nusbaum D, McCarthy MA, Vasilakis D. Smoke alarm: a review of the clinical impact of smoking on women. *Prim Care Update Ob Gyns* 2000; 7: 207–14.

117 McHorney CA, Kosinski M, Ware JE. Comparisons of the costs and quality of norms for the SF-36 health survey collected by mail versus telephone interview: results from a national survey. *Medical Care* 1994; **32**: 551–67.

118 White H. Continence products: a national resource. *Elderly Care* 1997; **9**: 18, 20.

119 Department of Health. *Good practice in continence services.* London: Department of Health, 2000.

120 Abrams P, Cardozo L, Khoury S, Wein A. *Incontinence: 2nd International Consultation on Incontinence.* 2nd ed. Plymouth: Health Publication Limited, 2002.

121 Button D, Roe B, Webb C, Frith T, Thome DC, Gardener L. *Continence – promotion and management by the primary health care team. Consensus guidelines.* London: Whurr Publishers Ltd., 1998.

122 Roe B, Wilson K, Doll H, Brooks P. *An evaluation of health interventions by primary health care teams and continence advisory services on patient outcomes related to incontinence.* Volume 1: Main report, 30–59. Oxford: Health Services Research Unit – Dept of Public Health and Primary Care, University of Oxford, 1996.

123 Abrams P, Cardozo L, Fall M, Griffiths D, Rosier P, Ulmsten U *et al.* The standardisation of terminology of lower urinary tract function: report from the Standardisation Sub-committee of the International Continence Society. *Neurourol Urodyn* 2002; **21**: 167–78.

124 Cardozo LD, Stanton SL. Genuine stress incontinence and detrusor instability – a review of 200 patients. *Br J Obstet Gynaecol* 1980; **87**: 184–90.

125 Jarvis GJ, Hall S, Stamp S, Millar DR, Johnson A. An assessment of urodynamic examination in incontinent women. *Br J Obstet Gynaecol* 1980; **87**: 893–6.

126 Eastwood HDH, Warrell R. Urinary incontinence in the elderly female – prediction in diagnosis and outcome of management. *Age and Ageing* 1984; **13**: 230–4.

127 Kirschner-Hermanns R, Scherr PA, Branch LG, Wetle T, Resnick NM. Accuracy of survey questions for geriatric urinary incontinence. *J Urol* 1998; **159**: 1903–8.

128 Ramsay N, Ali HM, Heslington K, Hilton P. Can scoring the severity of symptoms help to predict the urodynamic diagnosis? *Int Urogynecol J* 1995; **6**: 267–70.

129 Haeusler G, Hanzal E, Joura E, Sam C, Koelbl H. Differential-diagnosis of detrusor instability and stress incontinence by patient history – the Gaudenz Incontinence Questionnaire revisited. *Acta Obstet Gynecol Scand* 1995; **74**: 635–7.

130 Amundsen C, Lau M, English SF, McGuire EJ. Do urinary symptoms correlate with urodynamic findings? *J Urol* 1999; **161**: 1871–4.

131 Fitzgerald MP, Brubaker L. Urinary incontinence symptom scores and urodynamic diagnoses. *Neurourol Urodyn* 2002; **21**: 30–5.

132 Bent AE, Richardson DA, Ostergard DR. Diagnosis of lower urinary tract disorders in post-menopausal patients. *Am J Obstet Gynecol* 1983; **145**: 218–22.

133 Versi E. The significance of an open bladder neck in women. *Br J Urol* 68, 42–43. 91.

134 Clarke B. The role of urodynamic assessment in the diagnosis of lower urinary tract disorders. *Int Urogynecol J* 1997; **8**: 196–2000.

135 Glazener GMA, Cooper K. Anterior vaginal repair for urinary incontinence in women. *The Cochrane Library.* Oxford: Update Software, 2000.

136 McCormick A, Fleming D, Charlton J. *Morbidity statistics from general practice: a study carried out by the Royal College of General Practitioners, the OPCS and the Department of Health. Fourth national study 1991–1992.* London: HMSO, 1995.

137 Hall C, Castleden CM, Grove GJ. 56 continence advisors, one peripatetic teacher. *BMJ* 1988; **297**: 1181–2.

138 Hilton P, Stanton SL. Algorithmic method for assessing urinary incontinence in elderly women. *BMJ* 1981; **282**: 940–2.

139 Black N, Griffiths J, Pope C, Bowling A, Abel P. Impact of surgery for stress incontinence on morbidity: cohort study. *BMJ* 1997; **315**: 1493–8.

140 Getliffe K. Long-term catheter use in the community. *Elderly Care* 1995; **7**: 19–22.

141 Brocklehurst J, Amess M, Goldacre M, Mason A, Wilkinson E, Eastwood A, Coles J. *Health outcome indicators: urinary incontinence. Report of a working group to the Department of Health.* Reports in the series on Health Outcomes Development. Oxford: National Centre for Health Outcomes Development, Department of Health, 1999.

142 Hu TW. The economic impact of urinary incontinence. *Clin Geriatr Med* 1986; **2**: 673–87.

143 Wagner TH, Hu TW. Economic costs of urinary incontinence in 1995. *Urology* 1998; **51**: 355–60.

144 Wilson L, Brown JS, Shin GP, Luc KO, Subak LL. Annual direct cost of urinary incontinence. *Obstet Gynecol* 2001; **98**: 398–406.

145 Doran CM, Chiarelli P, Cockburn J. Economic costs of urinary incontinence in community-dwelling Australian women. *Medical Journal of Australia* 2001; **174**: 456–8.

146 Tediosi F, Parazzini F, Bortolotti A, Garattini L. The cost of urinary incontinence in Italian women – a cross-sectional study. *Pharmacoeconomics* 2000; **17**: 71–6.

147 Ekelund P, Grimby A, Milsom I. Urinary incontinence – social and financial costs high. *BMJ* 1993; **306**: 1344.

148 Smith JP. *The problem of promoting continence. An account of 16 regional study days convened by the Royal College of Nursing of the United Kingdom in association with Squibb Surgicare Ltd.* London: Squibb Surgicare Ltd, 1982.

149 Clayton J. Summary of: Rhodes P, Jones C, Qureshi H, Wright K. *Stage one: feasibility study of costs, service and quality of continence services.* York: University of York, SPRU, 1995. DH 1321 3.95.

150 Clayton J, Smith K, Qureshi H, Ferguson B. Collecting patients' views and perceptions of continence services: the development of research instruments. *Journal of Advanced Nursing* 1998; **28**: 353–61.

151 Townsend J, Heng L. Costs of incontinence to families with severely handicapped children. *Community Med* 1981; **3**: 119–22.

152 Johannesson M, O'Conor RM, Kobelt-Nguyen G, Mattiasson A. Willingness to pay for reduced incontinence symptoms. *Br J Urol* 1997; **80**: 557–62.

153 Kobelt G. Economic considerations and outcome measurement in urge incontinence. *Urology* 1997; **50**: 100–7.

154 O'Conor RM, Johannesson M, Hass SL, Kobelt-Nguyen G. Urge incontinence – quality of life and patients' valuation of symptom reduction. *Pharmacoeconomics* 1998; **14**: 531–9.

155 Burns PA, Pranikoff K, Nochajski TH, Hadley EC, Levy KJ, Ory MG. A comparison of effectiveness of biofeedback and pelvic muscle exercise treatment of stress incontinence in older community-dwelling women. *Journals of Gerontology* 1993; **48**: M167–M174.

156 Lagro-Janssen ALM, Debruyne FMJ, Smits AJA, Vanweel C. The effects of treatment of urinary incontinence in general practice. *Fam Pract* 1992; **9**: 284–9.

157 Williams K, Roe B, Sindhu F. *An evaluation of nursing developments in continence care.* Oxford: University of Oxford, National Institute for Nursing, 1995.

158 Lagro-Janssen T, Van Weel C. Long-term effect of treatment of female incontinence in general practice. *Br J Gen Pract* 1998; **48**: 1735–8.

159 Bø K, Talseth T. Long-term effect of pelvic floor muscle exercise 5 years after cessation of organized training. *Obstet Gynecol* 1996; **87**: 261–5.

160 O'Brien J. Evaluating primary care interventions for incontinence. *Nursing Standard* 1996; **10**: 40–3.

161 O'Brien J, Long H. Urinary incontinence – long-term effectiveness of nursing intervention in primary care. *BMJ* 1995; **311**: 1208.

162 Bø K, Berghmans LC. Non-pharmacologic treatments for overactive bladder – pelvic floor exercises. *Urology* 2000; **55**: 7–11.

163 Berghmans LC, Hendriks HJ, De Bie RA, van Waalwijk van Doorn ES, Bø K. Conservative treatment of urge urinary incontinence in women: a systematic review of randomized clinical trials. *BJU Int* 2000; **85**: 254–63.

164 Hunskaar S, Emery S, Jeyaseelan S. Electrical stimulation for urinary incontinence (Cochrane review). *The Cochrane Library.* Oxford: Update Software, 2002.

165 Luber KM, Wolde-Tsadik G. Efficacy of functional electrical stimulation in treating stress incontinence: a randomized controlled trial. *Neurology and Urodynamics* 1997; **16**: 543–51.

166 Sand PK, Richardson DA, Staskin DR, Swift SE, Appel RA, Al AE. Pelvic floor electrical stimulation in the treatment of genuine stress incontinence: a multicentre placebo-controlled trial. *Am J Obstet Gynecol* 1995; **173**: 72–9.

167 Herbison P, Plevnik S, Mantle J. Weighted vaginal cones for urinary incontinence. *The Cochrane Database of Systematic Reviews* 2000; 24 + 28 graphics pages.

168 Davies JA, Hosker G, Lord J, Smith ARB. An evaluation of the efficacy of in-patient bladder retraining. *Int Urogynecol J Pelvic Floor Dysfunct* 2000; **11**: 271–6.

169 Ramsay IN, Ali HM, Hunter M, Stark D, McKenzie S, Donaldson K et al. A prospective, randomized controlled trial of inpatient versus outpatient continence programs in the treatment of urinary incontinence in the female. *Int Urogynecol J Pelvic Floor Dysfunct* 1996; **7**: 260–3.

170 Visco AG, Weidner AC, Cundiff GW, Bump RC. Observed patient compliance with a structured outpatient bladder retraining program. *Am J Obstet Gynecol* 1999; **181**: 1392–4.

171 Svigos JM, Matthews CD. Assessment and treatment of female urinary incontinence by cystometrogram and bladder training programs. *Obstet Gynecol* 1977; **50**: 9–12.

172 Burgio KL, Locher JL, Goode PS, Hardin JM, McDowell BJ, Dombrowski M et al. Behavioral vs drug treatment for urge urinary incontinence in older women – a randomized controlled trial. *JAMA* 1998; **280**: 1995–2000.

173 Weinberger MW, Goodman BM, Carnes M. Long-term efficacy of nonsurgical urinary incontinence treatment in elderly women. *Journals of Gerontology Series a – Biological Sciences and Medical Sciences* 1999; **54**: M117–M121.

174 Fantl JA. Behavioral intervention for community-dwelling individuals with urinary incontinence. *Urology* 1998; **51**: 30–4.

175 Wyman JF, Fantl JA. Bladder training in ambulatory care management of urinary incontinence. *Urologic Nursing* 1991; **11**: 11–7.

176 Fantl JA, Wyman JF, McClish DK, Harkins SW, Elswick RK, Taylor JR et al. Efficacy of bladder training in older women with urinary incontinence. *JAMA* 1991; **265**: 609–13.

177 Roe B, Williams K, Palmer M. Bladder training for urinary incontinence in adults. *The Cochrane Database of Systematic Reviews* 2000.

178 Ostaszkiewicz J, Johnson L, Roe B. Habit retraining for the management of urinary incontinence in adults. *Cochrane Database of Systematic Reviews* 2002.

179 Arya LA, Myers DL, Jackson ND. Dietary caffeine intake and the risk for detrusor instability: a case-control study. *Obstet Gynecol* 2000; **96**: 85–9.

180 Tomlinson BU, Dougherty MC, Pendergast JF, Boyington AR, Coffman MA, Pickens SA. Dietary caffeine, fluid intake and urinary incontinence in older rural women. *Int Urogynecol J Pelvic Floor Dysfunct* 1999; **10**: 22–8.

181 Dowd TT, Campbell JM, Jones JA. Fluid intake and urinary incontinence in older community-dwelling women. *Journal of Community Health Nursing* 1996; **13**: 179–86.

182 Brieger G, Korda A. The effect of obesity on the outcome of successful surgery for genuine stress incontinence. *Australian & New Zealand Journal of Obstetrics & Gynaecology* 1992; **32**: 71–2.

183 Bump RC, Sugerman HJ, Fantl JA, McClish DK. Obesity and lower urinary-tract function in women – effect of surgically induced weight-loss. *Am J Obstet Gynecol* 1992; **167**: 392–9.

184 Deitel M, Stone E, Kassam HA, Wilk EJ, Sutherland DJA. Gynecologic obstetric changes after loss of massive excess weight following bariatric surgery. *Journal of the American College of Nutrition* 1988; **7**: 147–53.

185 Chiarelli P, Brown WJ. Leaking urine in Australian women: prevalence and associated conditions. *Women & Health* 1999; **29**: 1–13.

186 Dwyer PL, Lee ETC, Hay DM. Obesity and urinary incontinence in women. *Br J Obstet Gynaecol* 1988; **95**: 91–6.

187 Lubowski DZ, Swash M, Nicholls RJ, Henry MM. Increase in pudendal nerve-terminal motor latency with defecation straining. *Br J Surg* 1988; **75**: 1095–7.

188 Bump RC, McClish DK. Cigarette smoking and urinary incontinence in women. *Am J Obstet Gynecol* 1992; **167**: 1213–8.

189 Nygaard I, Bryant C, Dowell C, Wilson PD. Cochrane incontinence group lifestyle interventions for the treatment of urinary incontinence in adults. *Cochrane Database of Systematic Reviews.* 2002.

190 Kobelt G, Jonsson L, Mattiasson A. Cost-effectiveness of new treatments for overactive bladder: the example of tolterodine, a new muscarinic agent: a Markov Model. *Neurourol Urodyn* 1998; **17**: 599–611.

191 McGhee M, O'Neill K, Major K. Evaluation of a nurse-led continence service in the south-west of Glasgow, Scotland. *Journal of Advanced Nursing* 1997; **26**: 723–8.

192 Simons AM, Dowell CJ, Bryant CM, Prashar S, Moore KH. Use of the Dowell Bryant Incontinence Cost Index as a post-treatment outcome measure after non-surgical therapy. *Neurourol Urodyn* 2001; **20**: 85–93.

193 Burgio KL, Locher JL, Goode PS. Combined behavioral and drug therapy for urge incontinence in older women. *J Am Geriatr Soc* 2000; **48**: 370–4.

194 Ellis G, Hay-Smith J, Herbison P. Anticholinergic drugs versus non-drug active therapies for urinary urge incontinence in older women. *Cochrane Database of Systematic Reviews.* 2002.

195 Ellis G, Hay-Smith J, Herbison P. Anticholinergic drugs versus other medications for urinary incontinence in adults. *Cochrane Database of Systematic Reviews.* 2002.

196 Ellis G, Hay-Smith J, Herbison P. Anticholinergic drugs versus placebo for urinary incontinence. *Cochrane Database of Systematic Reviews.* 2002.

197 Appell RA, Abrams P, Drutz HP, Van Kerrebroeck P, Millard R, Wein A. Treatment of overactive bladder: long-term tolerability and efficacy of tolterodine. *World J Urol* 2001; **19**: 141–7.

198 Kelleher CJ, Cardozo LD, Khullar V, and Salvatore S. A medium-term analysis of the subjective efficacy of treatment for women with detrusor instability and low bladder compliance. *Br J Obstet Gynaecol* 1997; **104(9)**: 988–93.

199 Versi E, Appell R, Mobley D, Patton W, Saltzstein D. Dry mouth with conventional and controlled-release oxybutynin in urinary incontinence. *Obstet Gynecol* 2000; **95**: 718–21.

200 Birns J, Lukkari E, Malone-Lee JG. A randomized controlled trial comparing the efficacy of controlled-release oxybutynin tablets (10 mg once daily) with conventional oxybutynin tablets

(5 mg twice daily) in patients whose symptoms were stabilized on 5 mg twice daily of oxybutynin. *BJU Int* 2000; **85**: 793–8.

201 Cardozo L, Chapple CR, Toozs-Hobson P, Grosse-Freese M, Bulitta M, Lehmacher W *et al*. Efficacy of trospium chloride in patients with detrusor instability: a placebo-controlled, randomized, double-blind, multicentre clinical trial. *BJU Int* 2000; **85**: 659–64.

202 Madersbacher H, Stohrer M, Richter R, Burgdorfer H, Hachen HJ, Murtz G. Trospium chloride versus oxybutynin – a randomized, double-blind, multicenter trial in the treatment of detrusor hyper-reflexia. *Br J Urol* 1995; **75**: 452–6.

203 Milani R, Scalambrino S, Milia R, Sambruni I, Riva D, Pulici D *et al*. Double blind cross-over comparison of flixovate and oxybutynin in women affected by urinary urge syndrome. *Int Urogynecol J Pelvic Floor Dysfunct* 1993; **4**: 3–8.

204 Chapple CR, Parkhouse H, Gardener C, Milroy EJG. Double-blind, placebo-controlled, cross-over study of flavoxate in the treatment of idiopathic detrusor instability. *Br J Urol* 1990; **66**: 491–4.

205 Glazener CMA, Evans JHC. Tricyclic and related drugs for nocturnal enuresis in children. *Cochrane Database of Systematic Reviews*. 2002.

206 Castleden CM, Duffin HM, Gulati RS. Double blind study of imipramine and placebo for incontinence due to bladder instability. *Age and Ageing* 1986; **15**: 299–303.

207 Hilton P, Stanton SL. The use of desmopressin (DDAVP) in nocturnal urinary frequency in the female. *Br J Urol* 1982; **54**: 252–5.

208 Fantl JA, Bump RC, Robinson D, McClish DK, Wyman JF, Elser DM *et al*. Efficacy of estrogen supplementation in the treatment of urinary incontinence. *Obstet Gynecol* 1996; **88**: 745–9.

209 Jackson S, Shepherd A, Abrams P. The effect of oestradiol on objective urinary leakage in post-menopausal stress incontinence; a double blind placebo controlled trial. *Neurourol Urodyn* 1996; **15**: 322–23.

210 Fantl JA, Cardozo L, McClish DK. Estrogen therapy in the management of urinary incontinence in postmenopausal women – a meta-analysis – first report of the Hormones and Urogenital Therapy Committee. *Obstet Gynecol* 1994; **83**: 12–8.

211 Radley SC, Azam U, Collin PG, Richmond DH, Chapple CR. Alpha adrenergic drugs for urinary incontinence in women. *Cochrane Database of Systematic Reviews* 2002.

212 Jarvis GJ. Surgery for genuine stress incontinence. *Br J Obstet Gynaecol* 1994; **101**: 371–4.

213 Glazener CMA, Cooper K. Anterior vaginal repair for urinary incontinence in women (Cochrane Review). *The Cochrane Library* 2001; **4**.

214 Glazener CMA, Cooper K. Bladder neck needle suspension for the treatment of primary stress urinary incontinence in terms of lower cure rates and higher morbidity. *Cochrane Database of Systematic Reviews*. 2002.

215 Nilsson CG, Kuuva N. The tension-free vaginal tape procedure is successful in the majority of women with indications for surgical treatment of urinary stress incontinence. *Br J Obstet Gynaecol* 2001; **108**: 414–9.

216 Rezapour M, Ulmsten U. Tension-free vaginal tape (TVT) in women with recurrent stress urinary incontinence – a long-term follow up. *Int Urogynecol J Pelvic Floor Dysfunct* 2001; **12**: S9–S11.

217 Feyereisl J, Dreher E, Haenggi W, Zikmund J, Schneider H. Long-term results after Burch colposuspension. *Am J Obstet Gynecol* 1994; **171**: 647–52.

218 Moehrer B, Ellis G, Cary M, Wilson PD. Laparoscopic colposuspension for urinary incontinence in women. *Cochrane Database of Sytematic Reviews*. 2002.

219 Hutchings A, Griffiths J, Black NA. Surgery for stress incontinence: factors associated with a successful outcome. *Br J Urol* 1998; **82**: 634–41.

220 Monga AK, Robinson D, Stanton SL. Periurethral collagen injections for genuine stress incontinence: a 2 year follow-up. *Br J Urol* 1995; **76**: 156–60.

221 Moore KN, Cody DJ, and Glazener CM. Conservative management for post prostatectomy urinary incontinence (Cochrane review). *The Cochrane Library*. Oxford: Update Software, 2002.

222 Kohli N, Jacobs PA, Sze EHM, Roat TW, Karram MM. Open compared with laparoscopic approach to Burch colposuspension: a cost analysis. *Obstet Gynecol* 1997; **90**: 411–5.

223 Kung RC, Lie K, Lee P, Drutz HP. The cost-effectiveness of laparoscopic versus abdominal Burch procedures in women with urinary stress incontinence. *Journal of the American Association of Gynecologic Laparoscopists* 1996; **3**: 537–44.

224 Brown JA, Elliott DS, Barrett DM. Postprostatectomy urinary incontinence: a comparison of the cost of conservative versus surgical management. *Urology* 1998; **51**: 715–20.

225 Sanchez-Ortiz RF, Broderick GA, Chaikin DC, Malkowicz SB, Vanarsdalen K, Blander DS *et al*. Collagen injection therapy for post-radical, retropubic prostatectomy incontinence: role of valsalva leak point pressure. *Journal of Urology* 1997; **158**: 2132–6.

226 Gomes CM, Broderick GA, Sanchez-Ortiz RF, Preate D, Rovner ES, Wein AJ. Artificial urinary sphincter for post-prostatectomy incontinence: impact of prior collagen injection on cost and clinical outcome. *J Urol* 2000; **163**: 87–90.

227 Berman CJ, Kreder KJ. Comparative cost analysis of collagen injection and fascia lata sling cystourethropexy for the treatment of type III incontinence in women. *J Urol* 1997; **157**: 122–4.

228 Curtis MR, Gormley EA, Latini JM, Halsted AC, Heaney JA. Prospective development of a cost-efficient program for the pubovaginal sling. *Urology* 1997; **49**: 41–5.

229 Loveridge K, Malouf A, Kennedy C, Edgington A, Lam A. Laparoscopic colposuspension. Is it cost-effective? *Surg Endosc* 1997; **11**: 762–5.

230 Rhodes P, Jones C, Qureshi H, and Wright K. *Feasibility study of costs, services and quality in continence services*. York: Social Policy Research Unit, University of York, 1996.

231 Clayton J, Smith K, Quershi H, and Ferguson B. *Costs of incontinence to individuals and to services, and users' perceptions of quality and effectiveness of services*. York: Centre for Health Economics, Social Policy Research Unit, University of York, 1996.

232 Williams KS, Assassa RP, Smith NKG, Jagger C, Perry S, Shaw C *et al*. Development, implementation and evaluation of a new nurse-led continence service: a pilot study. *J Clin Nurs* 2000; **9**: 566–73.

233 Shaw C, Williams KS, Assassa RP. Patients' views of a new nurse-led continence service. *J Clin Nurs* 2000; **9**: 574–84.

234 Department of Health. *The new NHS reference costs – 2000*. London: Department of Health, 2000.

235 British Medical Association and the Royal Pharmaceutical Society. *British National Formulary*. London: BMJ Books/Pharmaceutical Press, 2000.

236 Assassa P, Williams KS, Shaw C, Perry SI, Azam U, Dallosso H, Clarke M, McGrother C, Jagger C, Mayne C, the Leicestershire MRC Incontinence Study Team. *Use of health services and treatments for urinary symptoms in the community: a postal survey of 29,268 community residents*. Finland, ICS, 28–31 August, 2000. Unpublished work.

237 Lucas M, Emery S, and Beynon J. *Incontinence*. Oxford: Blackwell Science, 1999.

238 Jackson S, Donovan J, Brookes S, Eckford S, Swithinbank L, Abrams P. The Bristol Female Lower Urinary Tract Symptoms Questionnaire: development and psychometric testing. *Br J Urol* 1996; **77**: 805–12.

239 Lee PS, Reid DW, Saltmarche A, Linton L. Measuring the psychosocial impact of urinary incontinence – the York Incontinence Perceptions Scale (YIPS). *J Am Geriatr Soc* 1995; **43**: 1275–8.

240 Kelleher C. Quality of life and urinary incontinence. *Best Practice & Research in Clinical Obstetrics & Gynaecology* 2000; **14**: 363–79.

241 Abrams P, Khoury S, Wein A. *Incontinence*. WHO – 1st International Consultation on Incontinence, 1998.

242 Yu LC. Incontinence stress index: measuring psychological impact. *Journal of Gerontological Nursing* 1987; **13**: 18–25.

243 Dubeau CE, Kiely DK, Resnick NM. Quality of life impact of urge incontinence in older persons: a new measure and conceptual structure. *J Am Geriatr Soc* 1999; **47**: 989–94.

244 Abrams P, Cardozo L, Khoury S, Wein A. *Incontinence.* Plymouth: WHO – 2nd International Consultation on Incontinence, 2002.

245 Brocklehurst JC. *Promoting continence: clinical audit scheme for the management of urinary and faecal incontinence.* London: Royal College of Physicians, 1998.

246 Cheater F, Lakhani M, Cawood C. *Assessment of patients with urinary incontinence: evidence-based audit protocol for primary health care teams. Clinical governance research and development.* Leicester: University of Leicester, Eli Lilly National Clinical Audit Centre. (Audit protocol; CT15), 1999.

247 Semple DM, Maresh MJA. Effective procedures in gynaecology suitable for audit. London: Royal College of Obstetricians and Gynaecologists, 1999.

248 Blaivas JG, Appell RA, Fantl JA, Leach G, McGuire EJ, Resnick NM *et al.* Definition and classification of urinary incontinence: recommendations of the Urodynamic Society. *Neurourol Urodyn* 1997; **16**: 149–51.

249 Cheater FM, Castleden CM. Epidemiology and classification of urinary incontinence. *Balliere's Clinical Obstetrics and Gynaecology* 2000; **14**: 183–205.

250 The MRC Incontinence Study Team. *Incontinence: a population laboratory approach to the epidemiology and evaluation of care-a progress report.* Leicester, University of Leicester, 2000.

251 Swithinbank LV. The impact of urinary incontinence on the quality of life of women. *World J Urol* 1999; **17**: 225–9.

252 Swithinbank LV, Abrams P. A detailed description, by age, of lower urinary tract symptoms in a group of community-dwelling women. *BJU Int* 2000; **82**: 19–24.

253 Milne JS, Maule MM, Williamson J. Method of sampling in a study of older people with a comparison of respondents and non-respondents. *Brit J Prev Soc Med* 1971; **25**: 37–41.

254 Edwards NI, Jones D. The prevalence of faecal incontinence in older people living at home. *Age and Ageing* 2001; **30**: 503–7.

255 Crome P, Smith AE, Withnall A, Lyons RA. Urinary and faecal incontinence: prevalence and health. *Clinical Gerontology (reviews)* 2001; **11**: 109–13.

256 McGrother CW, Castleden CM, Duffin H, Clarke M. Do the elderly need better incontinence services? *Community Med* 1987; **9**: 62–7.

257 McGrother CW, Castleden CM, Duffin H, Clarke M. A profile of disordered micturition in the elderly at home. *Age and Ageing* 1987; **16**: 105–10.

258 Roe B/Doll H. Prevalence of urinary incontinence and its relationship with health status. *J Clin Nurs* 2000; **9**: 178–87.

259 Feneley RCL, Shepherd AM, Powell PH, Blannin J. Urinary incontinence: prevalence and needs. *Br J Urol* 1979; **51**: 493–6.

260 Akhtar AJ, Brof GA, Crombie A, McLean WMR, Andrews GR, Caird FI. Disability and dependence in the elderly at home. *Age and Ageing* 1973; **2**: 102–11.

261 Akhtar AJ. Refusal to participate in a survey of the elderly. *Gerontol Clin (Basel)* 1972; **14**: 205–11.

262 Maclennan AH, Taylor AW, Wilson DH, Wilson D. The prevalence of pelvic floor disorders and their relationship to gender, age, parity and mode of delivery. *Br J Obstet Gynaecol* 2000; **107**: 1460–70.

263 Lara CNJ. Ethnic differences between Maori, Pacific Island and European New Zealand women in prevalence and attitudes to urinary incontinence. *New Zealand Medical Journal (Obq)* 1994; **107**: 374–6.

264 Hagglund D, Olsson H, Leppert J. Urinary incontinence: an unexpected large problem among young females. Results from a population-based study. *Fam Pract* 1999; **16**: 506–9.

265 Samuelsson EC, Victor FT and Svardsudd KF. Five-year incidence and remission rates of female urinary incontinence in a Swedish population less than 65 years old. *General Obstetrics and Gynecology* 2000; **183**(3): 568–74.

266 Peyrat L, Haillot F, Bruyere F, Boutin JM, Bertrand P, Lanson Y. Prevalence and risk factors of uriinary incontinence in young and middle-aged women. *Br J Urol International* 2002; **89**: 61–6.

267 Vinker S, Kaplan B, Nakar S, Samuels G, Shapira G, Kitai E. Urinary incontinence in women: prevalence, characteristics and effect on quality of life. A primary care clinic study. *Israel Medical Association Journal* 2001; **3**: 663–6.

268 Fultz NH, Herzog AR. Prevalence of urinary incontinence in middle-aged and older women: a survey-based methodological experiment. *Journal of Aging and Health* 2000; **12**: 459–69.

269 Ueda T, Tamaki M, Kageyama S, Yoshimura N, Yoshida O. Urinary incontinence among community-dwelling people aged 40 years or older in Japan: Prevalence, risk factors, knowledge and self-perception. *Int J Urol* 2000; **7**: 95–103.

270 Muscatello DJ, Rissel C, Szonyi G. Urinary symptoms and incontinence in an urban community: prevalence and associated factors in older men and women. *Internal Medicine Journal* 2001; **31**: 151–60.

271 Hording U, Pedersen KH, Sidenius K, Hedegaard L. Urinary incontinence in 45-year-old women – an epidemiologic survey. *Scandinavian Journal of Urology and Nephrology* 1986; **20**: 183–6.

272 Malmsten UGH, Milsom I, Molander U, Norlen LJ. Urinary incontinence and lower urinary tract symptoms: an epidemiological study of men aged 45 to 99 years. *J Urol* 1997; **158**: 1733–7.

273 Milsom I, Ekelund P, Molander U, Arvidsson L, Areskoug B. The influence of age, parity, oral contraception, hysterectomy and menopause on the prevalence of urinary incontinence in women. *J Urol* 1993; **149**: 1459–62.

274 Holtedahl K, Hunskaar S. Prevalence, 1-year incidence and factors associated with urinary incontinence: a population based study of women 50–74 years of age in primary care. *Maturitas* 1998; **28**: 205–11.

275 Kok ALM, Voorhorst FJ, Burger CW, Vanhouten P, Kenemans P, Janssens J. Urinary and fecal incontinence in community-residing elderly women. *Age and Ageing* 1992; **21**: 211–5.

276 Iosif CS and Bekassy Z. Prevalence of genito-urinary symptoms in the late menopause. *Acta Obstet Gynecol Scand* 63, 257–260. 84.

277 Bogren MA, Hvarfwen E, and Fridlund B. Urinary incontinence among a 65-year old Swedish population: medical history and psychosocial consequences. *Vard Nord Utveckl Forsk* 1997; **17**(4): 14–17.

278 Tseng IJ, Chen YT, Chen MT, Kou HY, Tseng SF. Prevalence of urinary incontinence and intention to seek treatment in the elderly. *Journal of the Formosan Medical Association* 2000; **99**: 753–8.

279 Maggi S, Minicuci N, Langlois J, Pavan M, Enzi G, Crepaldi G. Prevalence rate of urinary incontinence in community-dwelling elderly individuals: the Veneto Study. *Journals of Gerontology Series a – Biological Sciences and Medical Sciences* 2001; **56**: M14–M18.

280 Harris T. Aging in the eighties, prevalence and impact of urinary problems in individuals age 65 years and over. *U.S. Department of Health and Human Services* 1986; **121**.

281 Tilvis RS, Hakala SM, Valvanne J, Erkinjuntti T. Urinary incontinence as a predictor of death and institutionalization in a general aged population. *Arch Gerontol Geriatr* 1995; **21**: 307–15.

282 Jolleys JV, Donovan JL, Nanchahal K, Peters TJ, Abrams P. Urinary symptoms in the community: how bothersome are they? *Br J Urol* 74, 551–555. 94.

283 Hannestad YS, Rortveit G, Sandvik H, Hunskaar S. A community-based epidemiological survey of female urinary incontinence: The Norwegian EPINCONT Study. *J Clin Epidemiol* 2000; **53**: 1150–7.

284 Koyama W, Koyanagi A, Mihara S, Kawazu S, Uemura T, Nakano H et al. Prevalence and conditions of urinary incontinence among the elderly. *Methods of Information in Medicine* 1998; **37**: 151–5.

285 Liu C, Andrews GR. Prevalence and incidence of urinary incontinence in the elderly: a longitudinal study in South Australia. *Chinese Medical Journal* 2002; **115**: 119–22.

286 Herzog AR, Fultz N, Brock BM, Brown MB, Diokno AC. Urinary incontinence and psychological distress among older adults. *Psychology and Aging* 1988; **3**: 115–21.

287 Szonyi G, Collas DM, Ding YY, Malonelee JG. Oxybutynin with bladder retraining for detrusor instability in elderly people – a randomized controlled trial. *Age and Ageing* 1995; **24**: 287–91.

288 Ouslander JG, Schnelle JF, Uman G, Fingold S, Nigam JG, Tuico E, Jensen BB. Does oxybutynin add to the effectiveness of prompted voiding for urinary incontinence among nursing-home residents – a placebo controlled trial. *J Am Geriatr Soc* 1995; **43**: 610–7.

289 Jarvis GJ. A controlled trial of bladder drill and drug-therapy in the management of detrusor instability. *Br J Urol* 1981; **53**: 565–6.

290 Madersbacher H, Halaska M, Voigt R, Alloussi S, Hofner K. A placebo controlled, multicentre study comparing the tolerability and efficacy of propiverine and oxybutynin in patients with urgency and urge incontinence. *BJU Int* 1999; **84**: 646–51.

291 Thuroff JW, Bunke B, Ebner A, Faber P, Degeeter P, Hannappel J *et al.* Randomized, double-blind, multicenter trial on treatment of frequency, urgency and incontinence related to detrusor hyperactivity – oxybutynin versus propantheline versus placebo. *J Urol* 1991; **145**: 813–7.

292 Moore KH, Hay DM, Imrie AE, Watson A, Goldstein M. Oxybutynin hydrochloride (3 mg) in the treatment of women with idiopathic detrusor instability. *Br J Urol* 1990; **66**: 479–85.

293 Tapp AJS, Cardozo LD, Versi E, Cooper D. The treatment of detrusor instability in postmenopausal women with oxybutynin chloride – a double-blind placebo-controlled study. *Br J Obstet Gynaecol* 1990; **97**: 521–6.

294 Zorzitto ML, Holliday PJ, Jewett MAS, Herschorn S, Fernie GR. Oxybutynin chloride for geriatric urinary dysfunction – a double-blind placebo-controlled study. *Age and Ageing* 1989; **18**: 195–200.

295 Anderson RU, Mobley D, Blank B, Saltzstein D, Susset J, Brown JS. Once daily controlled versus immediate release oxybutynin chloride for urge urinary incontinence. *J Urol* 1999; **161**: 1809–12.

296 Millard R, Tuttle J, Moore K, Susset J, Clarke B, Dwyer P *et al.* Clinical efficacy and safety of tolterodine compared to placebo in detrusor overactivity. *J Urol* 1999; **161**: 1551–5.

297 Larsson G, Hallen B, Nilvebrant L. Tolterodine in the treatment of overactive bladder: analysis of the pooled phase II efficacy and safety data. *Urology* 1999; **53**: 990–8.

298 Abrams P, Freeman R, Anderstrom C, Mattiasson A. Tolterodine, a new antimuscarinic agent: as effective but better tolerated than oxybutynin in patients with an overactive bladder. *Br J Urol* 1998; **81**: 801–10.

299 Appell RA. Clinical efficacy and safety of tolterodine in the treatment of overactive bladder: A pooled analysis. *Urology* 1997; **50**: 90–6.

300 Van Kerrebroeck P, Kreder K, Jonas U, Zinner N, Wein AN. Tolterodine once-daily: superior efficacy and tolerability in the treatment of the overactive bladder. *Urology* 2001; **57**: 414–21.

Acknowledgements

We would like to acknowledge the contribution of Catherine Cawood and Kathryn West for advice on continence advisory care, Colin Hyde for help with literature reviewing and Lesley Harris for preparation of the manuscript.

3 Dyspepsia

Brendan C Delaney and Paul Moayyedi

1 Summary

Statement of the problem

The term 'dyspepsia' describes a clinical problem referring to a cluster of upper gastrointestinal symptoms that has been defined in many ways. As this chapter is concerned with broad population needs, we have used the 1988 Working Party definition, which includes patients with heartburn. As dyspepsia is a common condition, with costly investigations and treatment, the cost to the NHS has been estimated at £1.1 billion per year (in 1998). Particular concerns in managing dyspepsia are therefore the cost-effective use of resources, the appropriate choice of potentially curative treatments (*Helicobacter pylori* eradication) rather than symptomatic therapies (acid suppression), and the need for prompt diagnosis of upper gastrointestinal malignancy.

Sub-categories

Dyspepsia is a symptom, not a diagnosis. Patients with dyspepsia can be divided into subgroups on the basis of final endoscopic diagnosis, but if we are to accept that endoscopic diagnosis is not cost-effective in all patients, a sub-category 'uninvestigated dyspepsia' is necessary to consider what management is appropriate for patients presenting with a new episode.

- Uninvestigated dyspepsia: patients presenting with a new episode who have not had endoscopic investigation.
- Gastro-oesophageal reflux disease (GORD) refers to patients with symptomatic heartburn and acid regurgitation. Approximately 50% of these patients will also have oesophagitis.
- Peptic ulcer disease can be subdivided into gastric and duodenal ulcers. *Helicobacter pylori* and non-steroidal anti-inflammatory drugs are the predominant causes.
- Oesophageal and gastric cancer.
- Non-ulcer dyspepsia: patients without peptic ulcer, malignancy or oesophagitis on endoscopic investigation.

Prevalence and incidence

Dyspepsia is a chronic, relapsing and remitting symptom. The terms incidence and prevalence are difficult to apply in this context, because of the problem of classifying patients with a history of symptoms, who are currently asymptomatic, but are at high risk of further episodes. In addition, the definition and classification of dyspepsia has changed between ICD-9 and ICD-10. Community surveys vary in their findings according to the definition used. It is estimated that 40% of the population suffer from dyspepsia if reflux symptoms are included, 23% if not. However, the range of the 14 surveys found was wide at 14–48%.

The proportion of patients undergoing endoscopy where a peptic ulcer is detected has fallen dramatically in the past 12 years from 20% in 1989 to 10%. The prevalence of *H. pylori* infection is related to social deprivation in childhood. *H. pylori* infection is declining in the population as successive birth cohorts have a lower risk of childhood acquisition. At present the prevalence of *H. pylori* in 20–30 year olds is 10–20%, rising as a percentage with age to 50–60% in 70 year olds. First generation immigrants from developing countries are very likely to have *H. pylori* infection, as the infection is endemic in these conditions. The fall in peptic ulcer disease may be due to a reduction in recurrent ulcer disease as *H. pylori* is eradicated in patients presenting with peptic ulcer.

Oesophagitis is present in 20% of patients at endoscopy, and may be rising with time, although the condition may be more frequently diagnosed with the availability of effective treatment in the form of proton pump inhibitors.

Gastric cancer is the fifth commonest cancer in the UK. The incidence has been declining steadily, with a concomitant rise in adenocarcinoma of the oesophagus. This may reflect an increasing prevalence of GORD.

Non-ulcer dyspepsia accounts for 60% of cases at endoscopy, and is the commonest sub-category.

Services available and their costs

Consultations for dyspepsia account for between 1.2 and 2.7% of all consultations with general practitioners, rising with age from 355 per 10 000 patient years at age 25–44 to 789 per 10 000 at age 75–84. There is a suggestion from comparisons between the 1990 fourth morbidity survey in general practice and RCGP weekly returns data for 1997 that the consultation rate may have fallen by as much 75%, but comparisons between the two datasets are difficult on account of changing definitions and different population bases.

Qualitative research has shown that between 25 and 50% of patients with dyspepsia will consult their GP. Factors predicting consultation are worry about serious disease, such as cancer or heart disease, and the availability of effective medical therapy.

Prescription Pricing Authority data show a steady rise in the cost of prescribing for dyspepsia since the introduction of proton pump inhibitors (PPIs). In 1999, £471 million was spent, £323 million on PPIs, £124 million on H_2RAs and £24 million on antacids. The costs and numbers of prescriptions for dyspepsia have risen steadily over the past eight years. PPI prescribing has increased steadily, with little substitution of either antacids or H_2 receptor antagonists.

In 2000 there were 539 gastroenterologists working in England and Wales, and it has been estimated that 50% of their workload is accounted for by dyspepsia. Although demand for upper GI endoscopy rose sharply with the availability of 'open access' services to GPs, the rate has stabilised at 1% of the population undergoing the procedure each year. In 2000, £130 million was spent on 451 000 endoscopies. The 2000 NHS reference cost for diagnostic upper GI endoscopy as a day case was £250, but with a very wide range (£52–£1333).

Non-invasive tests for *H. pylori* are also available. Serology is available in most areas, but has poor predictive value where the prevalence of *H. pylori* is low. Near patient tests are also available, but perform less well than serology. Both urea breath tests and stool antigen tests are much more accurate, but either involve the ingestion of a test dose of (non-radioactive) labelled urea and the collection of breath samples for analysis in a mass spectrometer, or collection of stool samples. Both these tests are also more expensive than serology. Several breath test 'kits' are available on NHS prescription, but stool antigen testing is not yet widely available.

The effectiveness of *H. pylori* eradication therapy for peptic ulcer disease and acid-suppression therapy has greatly reduced the role of surgical procedures in dyspepsia. Most gastric surgery is now performed for malignant disease. Most patients are unsuitable for surgery, as the disease is too far advanced at detection, and long-term survival even after surgery is poor at less than 20%.

Effectiveness of services and interventions

Uninvestigated dyspepsia: Symptom patterns are not sufficiently predictive or specific to be of value in managing patients with dyspepsia. Trials comparing acid suppression therapies in uninvestigated patients are either lacking or for short-term outcomes only. PPIs have been the most studied, and have been shown to reduce the proportion of symptomatic patients by 29% compared with antacids and 37% compared with H_2 receptor antagonists. Heartburn responds more than epigastric pain. Management based on an initial endoscopy may be associated with a small reduction in symptoms (12%) compared with empirical acid suppression. Two recent RCTs have shown that *H. pylori* 'test and treat' is as effective as endoscopy, but reduces costs, as only 1/3 of the endoscopies are needed. There is no evidence as to whether 'test and treat' is cost-effective compared to empirical acid suppression as an initial strategy.

Peptic ulcer disease: *H. pylori* eradication is highly effective in both healing and reducing the recurrence rates of both duodenal and gastric ulcers. Ninety-six percent of duodenal ulcers will heal after *H. pylori* eradication, and recurrence rates at one year are reduced to 8%, compared with 83% with 4 weeks of acid-suppression alone (NNT = 1.3).

Oesophagitis: Both H2 receptor antagonists and PPIs are effective in healing oesophagitis (NNTs: H_2 receptor antagonists 6; PPI 2). PPIs are more effective than H2 receptor antagonists (NNT = 3). Both PPIs and H_2 receptor antagonists are also more effective than placebo at reducing heartburn symptoms in patients without oespohagitis (NNTs: H_2 receptor antagonists 8; PPI 5). Eighty percent of patients with successfully treated GORD will suffer relapse within one year without maintenance. Evidence for long-term therapy is less strong, but three RCTs have found a significant reduction in relapse with PPI compared to H2 receptor antagonists.

Non-ulcer dyspepsia: One trial found that antacids were no more effective than placebo, a meta-analysis of trials found no significant reduction in symptoms with H_2 receptor antagonists, although the trials were small and of poor quality. A meta-analysis of trials of PPI against placebo found a significant reduction in symptoms (NNT = 7). *H. pylori* eradication was also associated with a significant reduction in dyspeptic symptoms at one year in a meta-analysis (NNT = 15). Given the uncertainty in trial data, and the potentially important clinical differences between patients, it is important that the response to treatment of all non-ulcer dyspepsia patients is carefully monitored.

Quantified models of care

When the risk of malignancy is low: A discrete event simulation model indicates that endoscopy is not cost-effective in these patients. The choice of strategies should be between empirical acid suppression and *H. pylori* 'test and treat'. The point at which to test for *H. pylori* is sensitive to the underlying likelihood of *H. pylori* infection and the cost of recurrent acid-suppression therapy that could be avoided by successful treatment. However, the additional cost for a month's less symptoms was quite high on switching from empirical acid suppression to 'test and treat', of the order of £50–60 per month. Data from a RCT is awaited to confirm these model findings.

When the risk of malignancy is high: Patients in whom malignancy is suspected should all receive prompt endoscopic investigation. However, patients with overt symptoms such as weight loss or dysphagia are likely to have inoperable cancer. If malignancy is to be detected early, endoscopy needs to be performed in patients without overt symptoms, but at high risk. Previously, an age above 45–55 was used as a crude indicator of risk. Recent data, combined with an economic model, suggests that restricting endoscopy to patients with continuous epigastric pain and/or symptoms of less than one year's duration (in addition to those with alarm symptoms) would improve the cost/life year gained from £50 000/life year to £8400/life year in men. Gastric cancer is less common in women and investigation cannot be justified on economic grounds until age 65.

2 Introduction and statement of the problem

Definitions of dyspepsia

Dyspepsia is derived from the Greek, meaning 'bad digestion'. This vague description is fitting for a constellation of symptoms that has no universally agreed definition. A review of the literature identified 23 different descriptions of dyspepsia[1] and since this review there has been a further international expert meeting to try and reach a consensus.[2] All agree that dyspepsia is a group of symptoms that is thought to arise from the upper gastrointestinal tract and most imply that the term represents a symptom complex and not a diagnosis.

The first influential definition was the 1988 Working Party classification[3] that stated dyspepsia was any symptom considered to be referable to the upper gastrointestinal tract. Symptoms needed to be present for 4 weeks and included upper abdominal pain or discomfort, heartburn, acid reflux, nausea and vomiting. This classification further subdivided patients on the basis of symptom patterns into 'ulcer-like' (epigastric pain), 'reflux-like' (heartburn and acid regurgitation), 'dysmotility-like' (bloating and nausea) and 'unclassifiable'. The Rome I working group[5] suggested that the key symptom needed to define dyspepsia was pain or discomfort centered in the upper abdomen and excluded patients with heartburn or acid reflux as their only symptom.[4] The upper abdominal symptoms needed to be present for more than one month and occur greater than 25% of the time to fulfil the criteria for dyspepsia.

A multinational consensus panel further developed these Rome I criteria.[5] The 'Rome II' criteria state that patients need to have predominant pain or discomfort centred in the upper abdomen for at least 12 weeks in the last 12 months to be classified as having dyspepsia. The British Society of Gastroenterology (BSG), however, took a broader view, stating that dyspepsia was any group of symptoms that alerts doctors to consider disease of the upper gastrointestinal tract.[161] The BSG definition is therefore closer to the 1988 Working Party definition of dyspepsia.

The Rome II criteria were developed to standardise the type of patient enrolled into functional (non-ulcer) dyspepsia trials where organic pathology has been excluded by normal investigations. This important advance will make future non-ulcer dyspepsia trials more comparable but this definition is less relevant for uninvestigated patients. This chapter is concerned with population needs, where the diagnosis is often not established. A broader definition is more appropriate for this purpose and this chapter therefore used the 1988 Working Party and BSG guidelines definition of dyspepsia.[6]

Problems in the management of dyspepsia

Dyspepsia is common, with a primary care consultation rate of 2 per 1000 population per year, and, for many patients, is a lifelong intermittent and relapsing disorder. Dyspepsia drugs have been the single highest cost prescription item in the past two years and 3% of the population may be taking long-term therapy.[7] In any six month period 40% of the population will suffer an episode of dyspepsia, and half of those will consult their general practitioner.[8] The costs of managing dyspepsia outstrip all other conditions in the NHS, £1.1 billion in 1998.[9]

The frequent occurrence of dyspeptic symptoms, the widespread availability of empirical treatments and the high cost of definitive investigation mean that the guiding principle of managing dyspepsia lies in the cost-effective use of both treatments and investigations appropriate to an individual patient. This is in preference to first defining the cause of the symptoms by definitive investigation of all patients. Any assessment of health need relating to dyspepsia must consider both the management of previously uninvestigated cases, and cases where a cause has been established by gastroscopy. This paper attempts to categorise patients according to the potential risk of treatable disease and considers both the treatment of established causes of upper gastrointestinal disease and the evidence relating to the choice of management for uninvestigated cases. In the latter, both direct comparative research evidence and modelling based on case mix and the likely effects of treatments on underlying causes will be used. The two most important factors to consider are the role of testing and eradication of *H. pylori* and the role of endoscopy for the early diagnosis of malignancy.

H. pylori

The gastric pathogen *Helicobacter pylori* is aetiologically implicated in peptic ulcer disease and distal gastric cancer, but is widely present in the population and causes no harm in the majority of patients. A range of invasive and non-invasive tests for *H. pylori* are available. The majority of those investigated by endoscopy do not have significant pathology. Of the conditions that may be detected, most interest has centered on peptic ulcer disease, as this condition may now be cured by the eradication of *H. pylori*. There is also the potential to decrease the incidence of gastric cancer by *H. pylori* eradication. *H. pylori* may also play a role in eradication in functional dyspepsia. A number of strategies for managing dyspeptic patients incorporating non-invasive tests for *H. pylori* followed by either endoscopy or *H. pylori* eradication therapy restricted to those testing positive have been suggested.

The role of endoscopy in detecting early upper gastrointestinal cancer

Some patients with dyspeptic symptoms will prove to have malignancy, principally adenocarcinoma of the stomach or oesophagus. Although most patients with dyspeptic symptoms present at an inoperable stage, some patients may benefit from surgery if investigated promptly by endoscopy.[10] This chapter considers in detail the evidence and potential for early diagnosis of curable malignancy by selective prompt endoscopy in specific subgroups of high risk patients.

3 Sub-categories

Uninvestigated dyspepsia

Uninvestigated dyspepsia describes patients fitting the 1988 Working Party definition of dyspepsia who have not undergone endoscopic investigation. The focus of this chapter is on the cost-effectiveness of initial management strategies for dyspeptic patients in primary care.

The term 'dyspepsia' describes a group of symptoms and is not a diagnosis. However, many patients consulting with dyspepsia are referred for investigation to determine the cause of their symptoms. A diagnosis can then be reached and patients will have one or more of the following diseases.

Gastro-oesophageal reflux disease

Gastro-oesophageal reflux disease (GORD) refers to subjects experiencing reflux of gastric contents into the oesophagus causing symptoms that impair health-related well-being.[11] The distal oesophagus has abnormally prolonged acid and pepsin exposure in the majority of patients with GORD.[12,13] Normal levels of reflux provoke symptoms in a minority of cases, possibly due to increased oesophageal sensitivity.[14,15] Endoscopy may reveal oesophageal mucosal breaks (oesophagitis) in some patients with GORD, but endoscopy results are normal in over 50% of cases.[16]

Peptic ulcer disease

A peptic ulcer is defined as a defect in the gastrointestinal mucosa extending through the muscularis mucosae due to the acid-peptic action of gastric juice. These can be subdivided into gastric and duodenal ulcers, depending on the site of the defect. The traditional view that gastric and duodenal ulcers have distinct symptoms has been shown to be incorrect; indeed, symptoms are inadequate to identify patients with ulcers.[17] H. pylori infection is the main cause of duodenal ulcers, with 95% of cases being associated with this organism. Eighty percent of gastric ulcers are also associated with H. pylori infection, and non-steroidal anti-inflammatory drugs are implicated in most of the remainder.

Non-ulcer dyspepsia

Patients with dyspepsia symptoms with a normal endoscopy are often classified as having non-ulcer dyspepsia. The problem with this definition is that a proportion of these patients will have endoscopy negative reflux disease. It is because of this concern that the Rome II definition excludes patients with predominant heartburn and acid reflux. Patients are then subdivided into 'ulcer-like' and 'dysmotility-like' subgroups. There are several problems with this subclassification of non-ulcer dyspepsia. They all require the patient to have normal investigations whereas the main focus of this chapter will be uninvestigated dyspepsia. Population surveys have shown there is substantial overlap between dyspepsia subgroups[18] and subjects that can be classified often change categories over time.[19] The incomplete separation of the different subgroups and their lack of consistency makes them difficult to apply to populations. The Rome II subgroups have not been prospectively validated and remain speculative. Subgroups do not adequately identify the needs of the population and this paper, therefore, avoids the use of these terms. We use instead a broad definition of dyspepsia, including patients with heartburn and acid regurgitation, and subdivide on the basis of whether the patient has undergone definitive investigation or not.

Barrett's oesophagus

Barrett's oesophagus is a diagnosis made on the basis of both endoscopic and pathologist findings and is defined as columnar-lined oesophageal mucosa.[21] Some suggest that intestinal metaplasia should be seen within the columnar mucosa before a diagnosis of Barrett's oesophagus is made, but as metaplasia is patchy, this requirement is usually thought to be too stringent. Long-segment Barrett's oesophagus is diagnosed when at least 3 cm of the distal oesophagus is lined by columnar epithelium. This has the greatest malignant potential, and surveillance programmes have been recommended for this disorder. Short-segment Barrett's oesophagus is defined as less than 3 cm of columnar-lined oesophageal mucosa and this also has malignant potential.[21] The risk may be less than for long-segment Barrett's oesophagus and the role of surveillance in this disorder is uncertain. There may be no visible columnar-lined oesophagus but intestinal metaplasia may be present in biopsies taken at the gastro-oesophageal junction. The malignant potential of this lesion is uncertain and as 20% of the population have evidence of intestinal metaplasia at the gastro-oesophageal junction,[22] surveillance is not recommended.

Oesophageal neoplasia

Squamous cell carcinoma and adenocarcinoma account for 95% of all oesophageal tumours. Traditionally, squamous carcinoma was the most frequent lesion but in recent years adenocarcinoma has become the predominant disease in Europe and Northern America.[23] Adenocarcinoma of the oesophagus is believed to originate from columnar metaplasia of the oesophagus (Barrett's oesophagus) and endoscopic screening of patients with Barrett's oesophagus has been advocated.

Gastric neoplasia

Adenocarcinoma is responsible for over 95% of all gastric malignancies. Half the patients are inoperable at the time of diagnosis and virtually all of these are dead within five years. The 50% undergoing operative treatment have a 20% five year survival. The overall mortality for this disease in the UK is therefore approximately 90%. Gastric neoplasia is strongly associated with *H. pylori* infection,[24] but as the vast majority of infected individuals do not develop gastric carcinoma, other environmental and genetic factors must be important.

4 Prevalence and incidence

Prevalence and incidence are the two most commonly used measures of disease frequency in epidemiology. Incidence refers to the number of **new cases** of disease per population at risk over a specified time period. Prevalence is the proportion of the population with the disease at a given point in time. Prevalence is concerned with the total number of cases rather than new events and is therefore a function of the incidence and chronicity of the disease. Incidence is the most useful measure for studies evaluating factors associated with disease, whereas prevalence provides information that is useful for health service planning for chronic disorders. Prevalence is relatively simple to calculate for diseases that remain stable until cure or death.

Dyspepsia is a chronic relapsing and remitting disorder, often with an insidious onset, and measuring prevalence in this situation is more problematic. There is no controversy about classifying those subjects with symptoms (either new or ongoing) as having dyspepsia and those that have never had symptoms as not having dyspepsia. The difficult group are those that have had dyspepsia symptoms but are now asymptomatic. These individuals are at high risk of developing recurrent symptoms in the future and therefore may not be 'cured' of their condition. Classifying them as having dyspepsia, however, ignores the fact that a substantial minority will have no further symptoms and could indeed be considered as 'cured'. Including asymptomatic subjects with previous dyspepsia symptoms will therefore overestimate the true prevalence of the disorder whilst excluding them will underestimate the prevalence. This paper will assume asymptomatic subjects with previous symptoms are cured and therefore may be underestimating the true prevalence in the population.

Cross-sectional surveys assessing population dyspepsia rates typically assess the number of subjects with characteristic symptoms over a 3–12 month period. These surveys usually do not usually ascertain whether symptoms are new and are therefore assessing the prevalence of dyspepsia. The commonest causes of dyspepsia are GORD, peptic ulcer disease and non-ulcer dyspepsia. These are all chronic relapsing and remitting disorders and again it is usually the prevalence of the disorder that is measured. The true prevalence of these diseases is hard to establish, however, as endoscopy is needed to obtain the diagnosis. The population at risk is the total adult population and it would be difficult to persuade the general population to undergo endoscopy. Most surveys describe the proportion of patients with upper gastro-intestinal disease in those presenting for endoscopy. This type of study is easier to conduct but the 'population at risk' is those referred for endoscopy and this selected group is not particularly meaningful in public health terms.

A further problem is that there are fundamental differences between the International Classification of Diseases' 9th and 10th revisions in the way that dyspepsia is defined and sub-divided. Under ICD-9 non-ulcer dyspepsia was classed with habitual vomiting and achlorhydria as 'disorders of stomach function' (536). In ICD-10, the term 'functional dyspepsia' is provided (K30), but, following the Rome definition, excludes heartburn symptoms. Similarly, in ICD-9, diseases of the oesophagus (530) do not include symptomatic reflux disease without oesophagitis. ICD-10 uses gastro-oesophageal reflux disease, either with oesophagitis (K21.0) or without (K21.9). Similar problems arise when trying to collect data from primary care. The NHS now stipulates that practice computer systems record data using the Read coding system (currently a 5 digit system). **Table 1** shows the mapping adopted to transfer Read codes, ICD-9 and ICD-10 diagnoses.

Table 1: Read codes and International Classification of Disease codes 9 and 10 used in this chapter.

Main condition	Subgroup	Read (5) Code	ICD-9	ICD-10
GORD		J10..	530	K21.9
	Oesophagitis	J101.	530.1	K21.0
Gastric ulcer		J11..	531	K25
	Perforated gastric ulcer	J1102, J1112, J11y2	531.1, 531.5	K25.1/2/5/6
	Bleeding GU	J1101, J1111, J11y1	531.0, 531.4	K25.0/2/4/6
Duodenal ulcer		J12..	532	K26
	Duodenal scar	J1733, J17y7	537.3, 537.8	–
	Perforated duodenal ulcer	J1202, J1212, J12y2	532.1, 532.5	K26.1/2/5/6
	Bleeding duodenal ulcer	J1201, J1211, J12y1	532.0, 532.4	K26.0/2/4/6
	Peptic ulcer (unspec.)	J13..	533	K27
	Perforated peptic ulcer	J1302, J1312, J13y2	533.1, 533.5	K27.1/2/5/6
	Bleeding peptic ulcer	J1301, J1311, J13y1	533.0, 533.4	K27.0/2/4/6
Functional dyspepsia		J16y.	536.8	K30 (excludes heartburn alone)
	Gastritis and duodenitis	J15..	535	K29

Even if differences in diagnostic criteria, classification and period of data collection are allowed for, there will still be differences between populations and data recorded from community surveys, primary care and secondary care. The data sources available for this chapter are shown in **Figure 1**. Two important sources of data from primary care are the decennial 'Morbidity survey in general practice' conducted by the OPCS (the fourth survey was conducted in 1990–91), and the RCGP 'weekly returns' service. Both these surveys involve general practitioners recording every contact and every diagnosis in their daily work. The RCGP data in particular are valuable for comparing trends, as the same practices collect the data and great effort is put into data monitoring and consistent mapping. Hospital Episode Statistics provide useful information on pathology seen at endoscopy from a secondary care perspective and the Office of National Statistics provides information on upper gastrointestinal malignancy.

Surveys of the proportion of *H. pylori* positive adults are measuring prevalence, as once the organism is acquired it usually becomes a chronic life-long infection. Gastric and oesophageal carcinomas are usually fatal and therefore incidence is the appropriate measure to describe the frequency in the population.

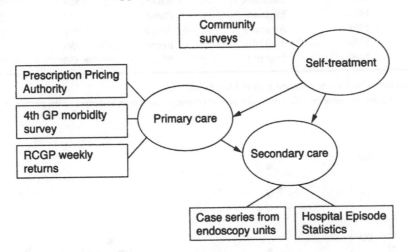

Figure 1: Data sources used in this chapter.

Prevalence of dyspepsia

A review of the literature identified 14 surveys that evaluated the prevalence of dyspepsia in the community in the last 12 years. The pooled estimate of the prevalence of dyspepsia was 34.4% (95% confidence intervals [CI]: 33.9–34.9%) but there was a wide range in the proportion of subjects with dyspepsia ranging from 13% to 48% (*see* **Table 2**). The majority of this variation was due to differences in the definition of dyspepsia. Surveys that included dominant reflux symptoms in the definition gave a prevalence of 39.4% whereas studies that excluded subjects with predominant heartburn and acid regurgitation reported a prevalence of 23.2% (mean difference = 16.2%; 95% CI: 15.3–17.0%; *see* **Figure 2**). A meta-analysis of these trials suggests that dyspepsia is slightly more common in women.

Recent UK trials have tended to use broad definitions of dyspepsia and report a prevalence of 40%.[8,25] The earliest UK study reported a 30% prevalence of dyspepsia in 354 workers in coke oven plants in the 1940s and a 30% prevalence was reported 10 years later in a sample of 5951 English males.[26] A study of Scottish men in 1968 reported a 29% prevalence in 1487 Scottish men.[27] The prevalence of dyspepsia therefore appears to have increased slightly from 30% to 40% in recent years, although the definitions used in the earlier reports may not be comparable to later studies.

Table 2: Population surveys reporting the prevalence of dyspepsia 1988–2000.

Authors	Year of report	Country	Dyspepsia definition	Number studied	% dyspepsia
Jones *et al.*	1989	England	BSG	2,066	38.0
Jones *et al.*	1990	England/Scotland	BSG	7,428	41.8
Bernersen *et al.*	1990	Norway	BSG	1,802	27.5
Talley *et al.*	1992	USA	Rome	835	25.5
Drossman *et al.*	1993	USA	Rome	5,430	25.8
Holtmann *et al.*	1994	Germany	Rome	431	28.8
Talley *et al.*	1994	Australia	Rome	1,528	20.3
Agreus *et al.*	1995	Sweden	BSG	1,156	32.2
Penston *et al.*	1996	Great Britain	BSG	2,112	40.3
Rosenstock *et al.*	1997	Denmark	BSG	3,589	47.8
Kennedy *et al.*	1998	England	Rome	3,169	26.3
Nandurkar *et al.*	1998	Australia	Rome	592	13.2
Talley *et al.*	1998	Australia	Rome	730	12.6
Moayyedi *et al.*	2000	England	BSG	8,350	38.0

BSG: dyspepsia definitions that include epigastric pain and heartburn.

Rome: dyspepsia definitions that only include pain or discomfort centred in the upper abdomen as the predominant symptom.

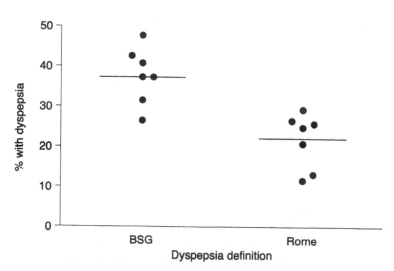

BSG: dyspepsia definitions that include epigastric pain and heartburn
Rome: dyspepsia definitions that only include pain or discomfort centred in the upper abdomen as the predominant symptom

Figure 2: Prevalence of dyspepsia according to dyspepsia definition.

Prevalence of *Helicobacter pylori* infection

The prevalence of *H. pylori* varies widely between countries, with over 80% of Japanese and South American adults infected compared with approximately 40% in the UK and 20% in Scandinavia. Local differences in prevalence will exist where there has been substantial immigration from countries with a higher prevalence of infection. The mode of acquisition of *H. pylori* infection is uncertain, although person to person transmission seems likely. The organism could be transmitted by the faeco-oral or oro-oral route, although *H. pylori* has only rarely been cultured from faeces and saliva.[28] Acute *H. pylori* infection causes a vomiting illness and recent evidence suggests *H. pylori* may be transmitted through vomitus.[29] Whatever the method of transmission, epidemiological data suggests that most individuals acquire the infection in childhood with social deprivation, household crowding[27,30] and number of siblings[31] being important risk factors.

The prevalence of infection is strongly correlated with age. Older individuals are more likely to be infected with *H. pylori* and studies suggest this is an age cohort effect. Socio-economic conditions were poor 70 years ago and so most children were infected with *H. pylori*. The majority of 70-year-olds are therefore *H. pylori* positive, but as childhood socio-economic conditions improved the prevalence fell so that today 10–20% of children are infected.[30] This is consistent with the observation that the incidence of peptic ulcer and distal gastric cancer are falling with time, as these are *H. pylori* related diseases.

H. pylori infection is slightly more common in men,[32] although the difference is small and this is unlikely to explain the gender differences in gastric cancer and peptic ulcer disease.

Prevalence of peptic ulcer disease

Ten percent of patients undergoing endoscopy have a diagnosis of duodenal ulcer (*see* **Figure 3**). This proportion has been falling dramatically over recent years, with 20% of patients having duodenal ulcer in 1989 (*see* **Figure 4**). This observation is confirmed by primary care data. The RCGP figures for the last four years available show a striking 60% decline in the episode rate for duodenal ulcer, from 8.43 to 3.34 consultations per 10 000 patient years (*see* **Figure 5**). Previously, duodenal ulcers were treated with acid suppression, whereas now they are usually permanently cured with a course of *H. pylori* eradication therapy. This striking fall in the prevalence of duodenal ulcer over a short period of time is therefore predictable. There should also be a reduction in the incidence of duodenal ulcer as the prevalence of *H. pylori* falls, but this is unlikely to be as pronounced over short time frames. This is confirmed by the RCGP data that show little change in the rate of newly diagnosed duodenal ulcer disease but a dramatic decline in recurrent episodes (*see* **Figure 5**).

Ten percent of patients endoscoped were diagnosed as having a gastric ulcer (*see* **Figure 3**). This will be an overestimate of the true prevalence as it is recommended that patients with a diagnosis of gastric ulcer have a repeat endoscopy to ensure healing. RCGP data show that the prevalence of gastric ulcer is half to a quarter of duodenal ulcer disease (*see* **Figure 6**). The prevalence of gastric ulcer is also falling dramatically (*see* **Figure 4**).

Duodenal and gastric ulcer differ in their incidence by age and sex. Duodenal ulcer peaks at age 45–64, and is twice as common in males as in females. Gastric ulcer is increasingly common with age and equally as common in females as in males (*see* **Figure 6**). Peptic ulcer disease is more common in patients taking non-steroidal anti-inflammatory drugs (NSAIDs) and bleeding is a particular complication associated with this therapy. Overall there is a 4.7-fold increase in risk of bleeding peptic ulcer in patients taking NSAIDs. This risk increases with age and patients over 60 years of age are 13.2 times as likely to develop bleeding peptic ulcer disease with NSAIDs compared with younger age groups.[33]

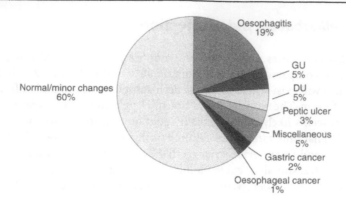

Figure 3: Findings at endoscopy – *Hospital Episode Statistics* 1994.

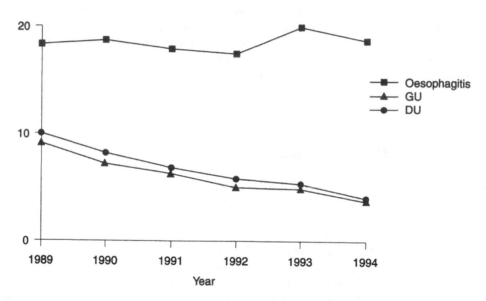

Figure 4: Diagnosis of oesophagitis, duodenal ulcer and gastric ulcer at endoscopy 1989–94 – *Hospital Episode Statistics.*

Prevalence of gastro-oesophageal reflux disease

Gastro-oesophageal reflux disease is more common than peptic ulcer disease, with oesophagitis present in 20% of endoscopy patients (*see* **Figure 3**). This is an underestimate of the prevalence of GORD, as only 25–50% of patients with this disorder have oesophagitis. Hospital Episode Statistics suggest the prevalence of oesophagitis is remaining stable, although this is based on only eight years of follow-up (*see* **Figure 4**). Case series from endoscopy units suggest that the diagnosis of oesophagitis is increasing with time.[30,31,34,35] These studies suggest the prevalence has quadrupled over a 10–20 year period. It is likely

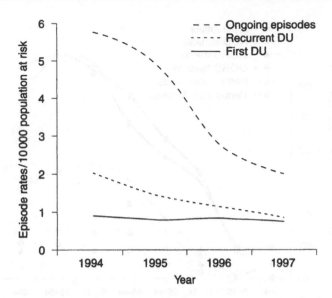

Figure 5: Ongoing, new and first episode rates for duodenal ulcer 1994–97, RCGP.

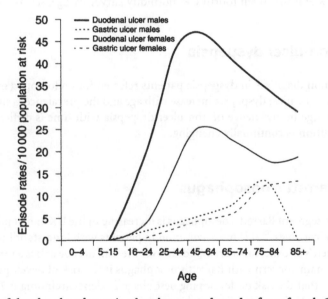

Figure 6: Incidence of duodenal and gastric ulcer by age and gender from fourth GP morbidity survey.

that this reflects a true increase in the prevalence of GORD, but the magnitude of the increase may be overestimated, as the condition is more readily diagnosed with the advent of proton pump inhibitors as effective therapy for the condition. The prevalence of GORD increases with age and is slightly more prevalent in women (*see* **Figure 7**).

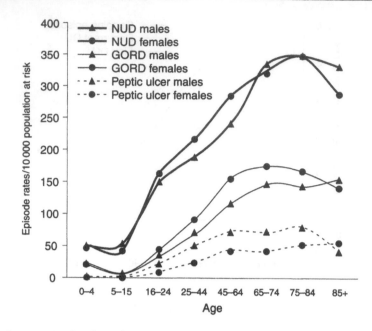

Figure 7: First and new episodes from fourth GP morbidity survey by age, sex and diagnosis.

Prevalence of non-ulcer dyspepsia

This is the most common diagnosis in dyspepsia patients referred for endoscopy (*see* **Figure 3**). Primary care consultations with non-ulcer dyspepsia increase with age and the prevalence is similar in both genders (*see* **Figure 4**). The change in prevalence of non-ulcer dyspepsia with time is difficult to establish as the definition of this condition is continually changing.

Prevalence of Barrett's oesophagus

The prevalence of long-segment Barrett's oesophagus is increasing in the UK and at present the diagnosis is made in 1.4% of all endoscopies.[35] It is more common in patients with long-standing reflux symptoms.[37] The prevalence of Barrett's also increases dramatically over the fifth decade and is a rare diagnosis under the age of 40 years.[38] The main concern with Barrett's oesophagus is the risk of developing adenocarcinoma. Surveys have suggested that the risk of developing oesophageal adenocarcinoma is 1% per year although this may be an overestimate due to publication bias.[39]

Prevalence of gastric and oesophageal cancer

Gastric cancer is the fifth commonest cause of cancer death in the UK. The incidence has declined dramatically in recent years with a concomitant rise in incidence of adenocarcinoma of the oesophagus (*see* **Figure 8**). The overall incidence of upper gastrointestinal malignancy has fallen slightly over recent years. Gastric neoplasia incidence is probably falling because of the decreasing prevalence of *H. pylori* in the UK.

The reasons for the increasing incidence of oesophageal adenocarcinoma are not clear but may relate to the increasing prevalence of GORD in the developed world.[36]

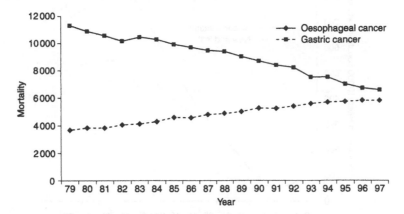

Figure 8: Incidence of gastric and oesophageal cancer in England and Wales 1979 to 1997 from the Office of National Statistics.

5 Services available and their costs

Services for managing dyspepsia are provided in both primary and secondary care. Patients with dyspepsia will consult their general practitioner or present in A&E with dyspeptic symptoms or upper gastrointestinal bleeding. Upper GI endoscopy is primarily provided in secondary care, although some primary care centres and GP-run community hospitals also offer facilities. Most GPs are now able to obtain open access to endoscopy, although waiting times vary widely. Non-invasive tests for *H. pylori* are also available in primary and secondary care.

Primary care services

There are 32 000 general practitioners in England and Wales. Population surveys suggest approximately 25% of subjects with dyspepsia will present with their symptoms to their general practitioner. Data from the fourth GP morbidity survey shows a steady rise in consultation rate for dyspepsia from 355 per 10 000 patient years at age 25–44 to 789 per 10 000 at age 75–84. As age increases, an increasing number of ongoing (chronic) cases add to the burden of disease (*see* **Figure 9**). Total consultations for all conditions were 29 000 per 10 000 person years at risk. Consultations for dyspepsia were thus between 1.2 and 2.7% of total consultations.

Data from the RCGP from 1997 shows a similar pattern, with a rising episode rate with age, but the overall consultation rates are lower, 76 per 10 000 patient years at age 15–44 and 220 at age 65. At age 65, 54% of consultations are for ongoing disease.

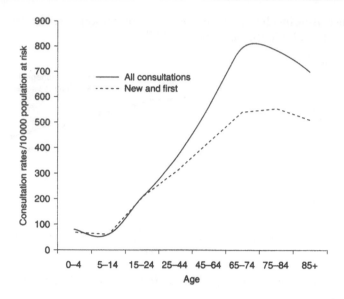

Figure 9: Consultation rates for dyspepsia by age: fourth GP morbidity survey 1991.

Reasons for consultation with dyspepsia

According to the health belief model, the decision to consult the general practitioner is determined by the presence of cues, and the balance between costs and benefits is modified by specific belief in threat from, or vulnerability to, specific conditions.[40,41] A study in the Netherlands examined why patients consult their general practitioner, by means of two questionnaires completed in the waiting rooms of practices by 1000 patients.[42] Multiple logistic regression was used to determine the principal predictors of consultation, and the health belief model showed a 98.9% predictive value for consultation. Perceived efficacy of self-care and perceived need for information also influenced the model, but frequency and duration of complaint did not.

Zola has identified five influences as to whether patients consult a doctor: the availability of medical care; whether the patient can afford it; the availability of non-medical therapies; how the patient perceives the problem; and how the patients' peers perceive the problem. Other triggers are required to force a medicalisation of the symptoms before they are perceived as illness and consultation considered. These triggers are, according to Zola: an interpersonal crisis; perceived interference with personal relationships; sanctioning by another individual, e.g. a relative; interference with work or physical functioning; and setting of external time criteria.[43]

Severity of symptoms

As far as dyspepsia is concerned, several groups have emphasised the poor predictive value of symptoms for upper GI pathology.[44,45] A qualitative study of 46 working class women showed that although complex concepts of multi-factorial causation existed, women were most concerned with finding causal life events with which to invest their symptoms with individual relevance. 'Stomach disease' was most commonly linked to stress and worry.[46] Jones and Lydeard studied a random sample of 69 patients who had consulted their GP in the past six months with dyspepsia and 66 who had not.[47] The patients were interviewed according to a standard schedule, to explore psychological traits, life events and beliefs about dyspeptic symptoms. There was no difference in the frequency, or subjective severity, of symptoms between the two groups. There were significantly more life events in the consulting group. Consulters were significantly more likely to believe that their symptoms were due to serious illness (74% v. 17%) and cancer in particular (29% v. 13%).

Fear of serious illness

Jones and Lydeard's study was essentially positivist in nature, concentrating on facts (in this case the reasons for consulting with dyspepsia), and analysed in a quantitative manner. A qualitative approach to the subject may provide more information about feelings and motives that would be of value in meeting the needs of patients in the consultation. An alternative, interactionist approach to the subject would aim to obtain authentic insight into patients' experiences.[48] In addition, although exploring the issue of vulnerability, Jones and Lydeard's study did not examine the threat component of the health belief model in terms of utility.

A qualitative study of reasons for consultation with dyspepsia was conducted in Birmingham.[49] Consulters and non-consulters with dyspepsia were identified similarly to Jones and Lydeard, but were interviewed in depth and transcribed tapes were subjected to a thematic analysis. Many of the subjects were fatalistic with respect to medical interventions and their ability to significantly alter the prognosis of illness, and the belief in dietary or mechanistic aetiology may reflect patients' expectations of increasing age. Viewed in terms of theories of illness causation, the patients interviewed displayed a predominantly 'personalistic' view. The principal explanations for symptoms lay in the areas of degeneration (age), imbalance (of foods, etc.) and mechanical interpretations of bodily function.

The availability of medical care, the cost to the patient of OTC medication, and the patients' belief in the opportunity for medical intervention to alter the course of serious illness, such as gastric cancer, were all important in this process. The principal predictors of consultation in this analysis were a family or close friend having being diagnosed with a serious condition, and the potential explanation of the patient's own symptoms being due to something similar. The paradoxical feature of some patients expecting the worse but not consulting can be explained within the model by reference to costs and benefits. The medical interventions, for cancer in particular, were perceived as costs, patients either not wishing to be told or not wanting 'to be messed around with'. As in Hackett's study of delay in seeking medical advice at the Massachusetts General Hospital, patients who worried more about cancer tended to delay seeking help more than non-worriers.[50] An element of denial was also evident in the explanation of symptoms as being due to diet or increasing age.

Secondary care services

There are an estimated 539 gastroenterologists working in England and Wales and this figure increases at a rate of approximately 7% per year.[51] There is a wide variation in the number of gastroenterologists working per head of population between Health Authorities (*see* **Figure 10**). Some of this variation may be explained by differences in gastrointestinal disease rates, but this is unlikely to account for the eight-fold differences seen in some regions (*see* **Figure 10**). The number of sessions that each of these gastroenterology consultants undertakes for the NHS each week is uncertain. Cross-sectional studies estimate that dyspepsia accounts for 50% of a gastroenterologist's workload.[52] although national databases do not record this information. General physicians and surgeons are also involved with the secondary care management of dyspepsia, but the proportion of time devoted to this is difficult to quantify.

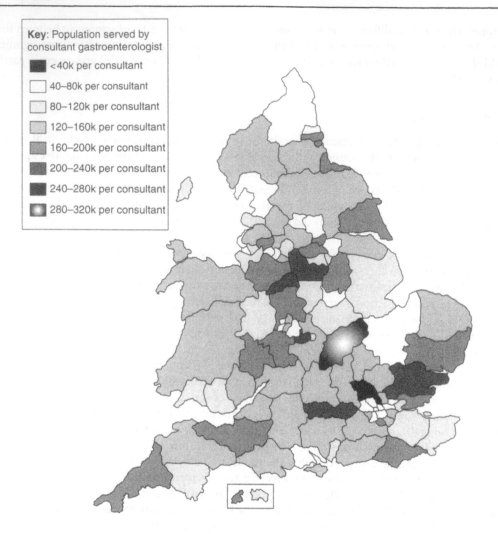

Figure 10: Number of gastroenterologists per head of population in England and Wales by Health Authority.

Investigations available

Dyspepsia is common, and investigation of this symptom complex is therefore likely to be in demand. The investigation of choice until the 1980s was a barium meal but now this has been superseded by endoscopy. This is because upper gastrointestinal endoscopy is perceived to be more accurate, biopsies can be taken of suspicious lesions, and access has improved with development of open access services.[53] The demand for endoscopy doubled in the first five years of the last decade (*see* **Figure 11**). The number of patients having this procedure is now stabilising, with 1% of the population of England having an endoscopy each year (*see* **Figure 11**). There is some variation in endoscopy rates between English regions but it remains a popular procedure throughout the UK (*see* **Table 3**).

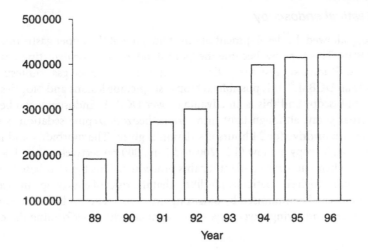

Figure 11: Number of endoscopies performed in England from *Hospital Episode Statistics* 1989–94.

Table 3: Proportion of the population endoscoped by English Health Authority – *Hospital Episode Statistics* 1993.

Region	Total population (thousands)	Number of endoscopies	Endoscopy per 1,000 of population
Northern	3,102	28,563	9.21
Yorkshire	3,708	28,490	7.68
Trent	4,766	35,901	7.53
East Anglia	2,095	13,062	6.24
North West Thames	3,521	23,475	6.67
North East Thames	3,812	23,430	6.15
South East Thames	3,718	22,871	6.15
South West Thames	2,999	20,869	6.96
Wessex	3,154	22,552	7.15
Oxford	2,593	16,863	6.50
South Western	3,331	23,213	6.97
West Midlands	5,290	37,350	7.06
Mersey	2,413	25,383	10.52
Total	48,533	359,243	7.40

Double contrast barium meals

Radiology has been the traditional investigation for upper gastrointestinal disease. Double contrast barium meals (DCBM) provide better gastric mucosal coating and superior images to single contrast methods. DCBM are almost as sensitive as upper gastrointestinal endoscopy in detecting oesophageal cancer, advanced gastric cancer, duodenal and gastric ulceration,[54,56] but are less sensitive at identifying early gastric cancer,[57] oesophagitis and more subtle duodenal inflammation.[58] The other disadvantage of radiology is that biopsies of suspicious lesions cannot be obtained.

Upper gastrointestinal endoscopy

Fibreoptic technology allowed the development of direct imaging of the upper gastrointestinal tract using endoscopy in the 1960s. This has now become the 'gold standard' test for detecting oesophageal, gastric and duodenal lesions. Studies suggest the patient acceptability of upper gastrointestinal endoscopy is similar[59] or greater than DCBM.[60] It is possible to biopsy suspicious lesions and biopsies for *H. pylori* can also be obtained at endoscopy and this is an advantage over DCBM. Endoscopy can be performed with local anaesthetic throat spray, although light intravenous benzodiazepine sedation is often given. The patient is unable to work or drive for 24 hours if sedation is given. The morbidity and mortality rates of upper gastrointestinal endoscopy are low (1 in 200 and 1 in 2000 respectively in the UK),[61] but they still need to be considered when referring a patient for this procedure. This figure is based on secondary-care data and therefore includes high risk patients. It is likely that the risks of endoscopy in healthy patients will be lower. Complications can be minimised by obtaining intravenous access before the procedure, careful monitoring of the patient and giving oxygen via nasal cannulae whilst performing the endoscopy.

Non-invasive tests for Helicobacter pylori

H. pylori causes most peptic ulcer disease, and non-invasive testing for this organism has emerged as an important alternative to imaging the upper gastrointestinal tract in the management of dyspepsia. The three main non-invasive tests for *H. pylori* are serology, faecal antigen tests and the labelled C-urea breath tests.

Serology involves measuring the antibody response to the organism in the patients' serum. This is the cheapest test but also the least accurate, with a 80–90% sensitivity and specificity.[62] This technique can be adapted to provide a near patient test giving a diagnosis within 5 minutes. This is convenient in the primary care setting[63] and some studies have shown sensitivities and specificities approaching 90%.[64] The specificity of near patient *H. pylori* tests have been disappointing in other centres[65] and local validation is important before using these kits in primary care.

- The stool antigen test detects *H. pylori* antigens in the stool and is more accurate with a 92–100% sensitivity and 93–95% specificity.[66,67] The test is more expensive than serology and involves giving a stool sample, which is not acceptable to all patients.
- Urea breath tests use the powerful urease enzyme possessed by *H. pylori* to diagnose the infection.[68] Urea labelled with either ^{13}C or ^{14}C is given orally to the patient and if *H. pylori* infection is present this will be hydrolysed to isotopically labelled CO_2. This is absorbed from the stomach into the blood and excreted by the lungs. The urea breath tests have a sensitivity and specificity >95%[69] and are more accurate than serology.[70] The ^{14}C-urea breath test is simple and cheap[71] but ^{14}C is radioactive and needs to be administered in a medical physics department, which is not ideal for primary care.[68] ^{13}C is not radioactive, so it avoids these problems, but it is difficult to detect, requiring expensive mass spectrometry equipment. There have been a number of technological advances in ^{13}C-urea breath tests, making analysis cheaper[72,73] but the test is still expensive compared with other non-invasive alternatives.

Procedures

The discovery of *H. pylori* and the development of powerful acid suppressive therapy have revolutionised the medical therapy of peptic ulcer and gastro-oesophageal reflux disease. This has made peptic ulcer surgery almost obsolete and anti-reflux surgery is reserved for a selected group of patients with symptoms responsive to medical therapy and documented acid reflux, but who do not wish long-term PPI treatment.

Anti-reflux surgery

The Nissen fundoplication and the Hill posterior gastropexy are the two commonest anti-reflux procedures. The Nissen fundoplication involves mobilisation of the fundus of the stomach that is then wrapped around the lower oesophagus. The gastro-oesophageal junction is sutured to the median arcuate ligament in a Hill posterior gastropexy and the stomach is also held in position by a partial anterior fundic wrap. Surgery is associated with a 1% mortality and a 2–8% morbidity, consisting mainly of gas-bloat syndrome and dysphagia. The short-term success rate of surgery in carefully selected cases is 85% but 10% have a recurrence of symptoms during follow-up.[74] Laparoscopic Nissen fundoplication may make surgery more attractive although one randomised controlled trial suggested it was associated with more morbidity than the open procedure.[75]

Peptic ulcer surgery

The success of *H. pylori* eradication therapy in preventing long-term recurrence of peptic ulcer disease means that ulcer surgery is now rarely performed. Operations that have been recommended include an antrectomy with a gastro-duodenal anastomosis (Billroth I), an antrectomy with gastro-jejunal anastomosis (Billroth II), a vagotomy and pyloroplasty or a highly selective vagotomy.

Surgery for gastric cancer

Surgical resection is the only procedure that provides a potential cure for gastric malignancy. The extent of surgery, however, remains controversial. A total or subtotal gastrectomy with removal of lymph nodes within 3 cm of the stomach (a D1 resection) has been the traditional approach in Europe. This has been shown to have a significantly lower post-operative mortality than more radical surgery removing more distant lymph nodes and performing a splenectomy (a D2 resection) with similar three year survival.[76] The long-term survival from surgery in the UK, however, is disappointing, with only 20% surviving more than five years.[77] The Japanese report less post-operative mortality and better survival with D2 resections.[78] This may be due to the Japanese presenting with gastric cancer at a younger age or more technical expertise at performing radical resections. One report from a UK unit with a high volume of D2 resections reported a 70% five year survival rate[79] and a low post-operative mortality, attributed to preservation of the spleen.[80]

Oesophageal cancer surgery

Oesophageal resection was associated with one of the highest post-operative mortality of any of the routine surgical procedures.[81] The operation now has a <10% post-operative mortality in specialised centres, although five year survival from potentially curative resections is still less than 30%. Randomised controlled trials are currently being conducted to assess whether chemotherapy, radiotherapy or combined adjuvant therapy can improve survival.

Costs of investigations and interventions

The principal costs of investigation are those relating to upper GI endoscopy. The cost of endoscopy varies according to whether it is performed as a day case or inpatient procedure, and whether any therapeutic intervention is performed. However, as with all reference costs, there is a considerable range. The mean cost of day case diagnostic gastroscopy was £250 in 2000, the range £52–£1333, and the interquartile range £203–£380. The mean costs of gastroscopy, with and without intervention, for day case, inpatient and non-elective inpatient are shown in **Table 4**. In 2000, £129.9 million was spent on 451 000 upper GI endoscopies.

Table 4: Cost of upper gastrointestinal endoscopy in England.

	Mean cost diagnostic endoscopy	Mean cost therapeutic endoscopy	Total NHS expenditure 2000 (£ million)
HRG code	F06 & F16	F05 & F15	
Day case	£249, £250	£314, £266	96.8
Elective inpatient	£562, £490	£732, £526	9.8
Non-elective inpatient	£450, £431	£782, £502	23.3

Prescription Pricing Authority data show a steady rise in the cost of prescribing for dyspepsia since the introduction of proton pump inhibitors (PPIs). In 1999, £471 million was spent; £323 million on PPIs, £124 million on H_2RAs and £24 million on antacids. The costs and numbers of prescriptions for dyspepsia have risen steadily over the past eight years (*see* **Figure 12**). Examination of the figures below indicate that PPI prescribing has increased steadily, with little substitution of either antacids or H_2 receptor antagonists (H_2RAs). Costs of H_2RAs have fallen and there was a small levelling off for PPI costs in 1998, presumably as a result of price competition. Omeprazole is due to come off patent in 2002 and this may result in a fall in PPI costs.

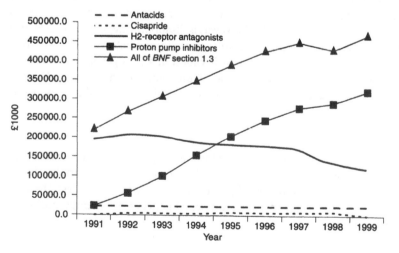

Figure 12: Cost of dyspepsia medication 1991–99.

6 Effectiveness of services and interventions

This evidence-based summary for dyspepsia was largely developed using a recent systematic review funded by the NHS R&D HTA programme,[82] three recently published Cochrane reviews[83–85] and abstracts of recently completed trials.

Management of uninvestigated dyspepsia

Patients presenting with uninvestigated dyspepsia are a common problem in primary care and the appropriate management strategy is uncertain. Symptoms alone are not sensitive and specific enough to make the diagnosis in most cases. One study suggested that 30% of patients with a major pathological lesion would be misclassified, including 50% of ulcer patients.[45] The positive predictive value of 'typical' symptoms for non-ulcer dyspepsia was only slightly better than chance alone.[86] Patients with predominant reflux symptoms (heartburn, acid regurgitation) may have GORD. Although symptoms are not specific for **oesophagitis**, reflux symptoms respond well to acid suppression, particularly with a proton pump inhibitor (PPI), and a 4-week therapeutic trial of PPI may be used to pragmatically define GORD. Epigastric pain in uninvestigated patients and patients with non-ulcer dyspepsia may respond less well.[87]

The choices available to general practitioners are: empirical acid-suppression therapy; early endoscopy (with or without a screening questionnaire); *H. pylori* screening followed by endoscopy of patients who have positive results; and *H. pylori* screening followed by eradication therapy for patients who have positive results.

Empirical anti-secretory therapy/Treat and endoscope

This involves treating dyspeptic patients with antacids, H$_2$ receptor antagonists or proton pump inhibitors and only investigating those that fail to respond. This strategy reserves costly investigation to those patients who are consuming more medication and hence might recover the cost of investigation in decreased prescribing. However, patients with peptic ulcer disease may receive intermittent anti-secretory drugs, responding promptly at each recurrence, whereas *H. pylori* eradication is now the treatment of choice for this group.[88] Nevertheless, empirical anti-secretory therapy or early endoscopy is the usual approach general practitioners take when initially investigating younger patients with dyspepsia.

Antacids

Antacids have been used for centuries to treat dyspepsia and are still the most popular over the counter medication for upper gastrointestinal symptoms. The popularity of antacids in clinical practice has waned since the introduction of H$_2$ receptor antagonists and it is easy to overlook the fact that antacids are safe, cheap and effective drugs. The main disadvantage of antacids is the frequency with which they need to be taken, up to seven times a day. Open use of antacid for symptom relief is common in dyspepsia trials, and no trial has examined antacid v. no treatment.

H$_2$ receptor antagonists

Cimetidine was the first H$_2$ receptor antagonist to be developed and is the cheapest drug in this class. H$_2$ receptor antagonists are also now available over the counter. The main disadvantage with cimetidine is that it competitively displaces dihydrotestosterone from androgen binding sites and gynaecomastia can occasionally occur in men. The newer H_2 receptor antagonists, ranitidine, nizatidine and famotidine, are more potent inhibitors of acid secretion on a weight basis and do not have anti-androgenic side effects. An inconclusive single RCT has compared H_2RA with antacids in primary care. Evidence is lacking as to their relative cost-effectiveness.[89]

Proton pump inhibitors

These drugs irreversibly inhibit the gastric H^+, K^+ ATPase pump and reduce both basal and stimulated gastric acid output more effectively than H_2 receptor antagonists. A systematic review has found that, in the short term, PPIs were more effective at controlling dyspeptic symptoms in unselected patients in primary care than both antacids and H_2RA. Pooled relative risk reductions were −29% (95% CI: −21% to −36%) for PPI:antacids and −37% (95% CI: −15% to −53%) for PPI:H_2RA. The effect on heartburn was highly significant (RRR = 48%; 95% CI: 55% to −40%), but epigastric pain did not respond as well; in fact, for this there was no significant difference between PPI and antacids.[83] Long-term PPI might usefully be limited to patients with either proven oesophagitis[90] or symptoms shown to be responsive to PPIs on careful review.

The National Institute for Clinical Excellence issued guidance on the use of PPIs in July 2000 (NICE Technology Appraisal No. 7). The guidance states that patients with mild symptoms of dyspepsia without a confirmed diagnosis of GORD should not be treated on a long-term basis with PPIs without further investigation. Patients with peptic ulcer should receive testing and treatment of *H. pylori* infection, and patients with non-ulcer dyspepsia should be carefully reviewed for therapeutic response.

Prokinetics

Metoclopramide reduces nausea and vomiting and is more effective than placebo in healing oesophagitis. The drug is cheap and is generally well tolerated but it does cross the blood-brain barrier and occasionally extrapyramidal side effects occur, particularly when large doses are given to elderly subjects. Domperidone has a similar efficacy to metoclopramide, but does not cross the blood-brain barrier and therefore has a much lower propensity to cause extrapyramidal side effects. Cisapride is chemically related to metoclopramide but does not have any anti-dopaminergic activity.[91] The drug has now been withdrawn from the UK as it can prolong the QT interval and could be associated with serious cardiac arrhythmias. There is insufficient evidence to determine the effectiveness of prokinetic agents in unselected dyspeptic patients in primary care.

Combination strategies

In order to limit the prescribing of more expensive and more powerful acid-suppression therapy to patients who seem to need them most to control their symptoms, a number of possible strategies have been proposed. These fall into 'step up' regimens from antacids via H_2RA to PPI, with only patients remaining symptomatic receiving more powerful therapy, or 'step down' from PPI to antacid via H_2RA, aiming to obtain good symptom control at the outset. The role of prokinetics is less clear, being much less commonly used in the UK than in other European countries. Possible strategies include using them first-line in patients with 'dysmotility-like' dyspepsia (predominant nausea, bloating and belching), or trying them after acid suppression had failed.

Initial endoscopy

An alternative strategy is to investigate all dyspeptic patients before initiating a prescription. This strategy takes into account the potential for patients over the age of 50 to have underlying upper gastrointestinal cancer. Approximately one in 300 patients had a potentially curable gastric cancer in a large cohort study of unrestricted early endoscopy in Birmingham.[92] Sufficiently large RCTs are unlikely to be carried out, and cost-effectiveness is likely to be low. At present, patients over the age of 55 with recent onset of symptoms or constant pain and all those patients with symptoms suggestive of malignancy (weight loss, dysphagia, early satiety, jaundice or anaemia) should be investigated by prompt endoscopy under the '2 week rule'.[93]

A meta-analysis of three prospective randomised studies[86,94,95] has indicated that early endoscopy as a strategy may be more effective in terms of cure of dyspeptic symptoms than empirical antacid therapy, particularly in the older age group. Incorporation of a further large trial gives a relative risk of 0.88 (95% CI: 0.77–1.00) for dyspepsia in initial endoscopy compared with usual management.[83]

Initial endoscopy is associated with additional costs. The economic analysis from one of these studies indicates that the incremental cost-effectiveness ratio of initial endoscopy compared with usual management is £1728 per patient additionally free of symptoms at a baseline cost of endoscopy of £246. A sensitivity analysis showed that if the cost of endoscopy could fall to £100 the ICER would fall to only £165.[96]

Non-invasive H. pylori *testing and endoscopy*

H. pylori may be identified by urea breath testing (UBT), serology, stool antigen tests or near patient tests (NPT). UBT and stool antigens are more accurate, but more costly than serology or NPTs. At present there is insufficient evidence as to which test is most cost-effective for initial diagnosis in primary care, but serology or NPT cannot be used as a predictor of cure.

Strategies based on testing for *H. pylori* have been proposed. These include selective endoscopy only in those patients testing positive (test and scope)[97] and *H. pylori* eradication.[98] *H. pylori* is associated with nearly all peptic ulcers in patients not taking non-steroidal anti-inflammatory drugs (NSAIDs). A strategy of screening patients for *H. pylori* with serology or urea breath test and only investigating those infected has been suggested by several groups. This could reduce endoscopies in young dyspeptics by 23–66% whilst detecting almost 100% of peptic ulcers in those not taking NSAIDs.[99] However, a recent primary care-based RCT has shown that test and scope is more costly than usual management in primary care, and does not lead to any difference in dyspeptic symptoms.[100]

Non-invasive H. pylori *testing and eradication*

Two RCTs have found that *H. pylori* eradication therapy is at least as effective in relieving dyspeptic symptoms as endoscopy-guided management. One trial randomised 500 subjects referred by the primary care physician having presented with more than 2 weeks of epigastric pain either to ^{13}C-urea breath test and *H. pylori* eradication if positive or to prompt endoscopy.[101] No difference in symptom-free days was found between the two groups, but the endoscopy rate in the *H. pylori* eradication group was 40% that of the prompt endoscopy group. The other trial randomised 104 *H. pylori* positive subjects under age 45 years to either *H. pylori* eradication or endoscopy.[102] The endoscopy subjects received targeted treatment of *H. pylori* eradication for peptic ulcer alone, PPI for oesophagitis and step-up acid-suppression therapy for non-ulcer dyspepsia. At 12 months follow-up 57% of the 'test and treat' group were symptomatic compared with 70% of the endoscopy group (RR = 0.82; 95% CI: 0.59–1.1).

Both the Lassen and Heaney trials randomised subjects in the secondary care setting. The Lassen trial stipulated that GPs should refer all eligible dyspeptic patients, whereas the Heaney trial entered routine referrals only. It is possible that similar results might not be obtained in primary care, where less severe cases might be treated, eradication rates might be lower, and the potentially reassuring effect of a specialist consultation might not be obtained. Three primary care-based trials are due to report shortly. It is unknown whether *H. pylori* eradication is as effective as empirical acid-suppression therapy as no comparisons have yet been published.

Empirical H. pylori *eradication*

The simplest *H. pylori* management strategy of all would be to prescribe empirical *H. pylori* eradication therapy to all young dyspeptic patients. This avoids the inconvenience and cost of testing for *H. pylori* and a published model[103] has suggested this may be the most cost-effective strategy for managing dyspepsia. Empirical treatment was only slightly cheaper than the screening and treatment strategy and resulted in 50–70% of young dyspeptics who are *H. pylori* negative receiving antibiotics unnecessarily. Whether the increase in antibiotic exposure is worth this small cost saving is debatable, and given current concerns over antibiotic resistance, empirical eradication is not recommended. In addition, 30–40% of patients taking *H. pylori* eradication therapy will suffer temporary side effects (nausea, diarrhoea), although only 1% may need to discontinue treatment.

Management of dyspepsia subgroups after endoscopic investigation

Early endoscopy may not be the appropriate management strategy for young patients presenting with dyspepsia. Nevertheless, in older patients, imaging the upper gastrointestinal tract may be appropriate and endoscopy will be performed in a few young patients with persistent symptoms. These patients will be diagnosed as either having peptic ulcer disease, gastro-oesophageal reflux disease or non-ulcer dyspepsia. We have identified systematic reviews that evaluate pharmacological therapies for these diseases.

Peptic ulcer disease

Peptic ulcer disease is found in less than 10% of patients undergoing endoscopy for dyspepsia. The fourth GP morbidity survey found consultation rates of 0.5% per year and new episode rates of 0.4% per year for peptic ulcer disease. Hospitalisation and surgery rates for uncomplicated ulcers have declined in the US and Europe over the past 30 years; however, the number of admissions for bleeding ulcers is relatively unchanged.[104] Despite advances in treatment, overall mortality has remained at approximately 6–8% for the past 30 years, due in part to increasing patient age and prevalence of concurrent illness.[97]

A systematic review of *H. pylori* eradication therapy for healing duodenal ulcer found seven trials of *H. pylori* triple therapy v. placebo in which *H. pylori* was eradicated in 93% (95% CI: 91–95%) and 96% (95% CI: 94–98%) of duodenal ulcers were healed at 6 weeks.[105] A further systematic review found healing rates in the range 91–97% for *H. pylori* eradication and 20–90% for anti-secretory drugs in 15 RCTs with direct comparison of eradication therapy and 4 weeks of anti-secretory therapy.[106] The same review found that *H. pylori* eradication heals 83% (95% CI: 78–88%) of gastric ulcers and reduces recurrence rates at one year from 49% to 9%. Recurrence of duodenal ulcer was also examined by the systematic reviews. In indirect comparison, both systematic reviews found a highly significant reduction in ulcer recurrence rates. In one, the risk of ulcer recurrence at one year *H. pylori* eradication was 8.8% and 83% with 4–6 weeks histamine H_2 receptor antagonist alone;[105] in the other, duodenal ulcer recurred in 12% of *H. pylori* eradication subjects and 58% anti-secretory subjects.[106]

An RCT of *H. pylori* eradication v. bismuth alone and two small RCTs of *H. pylori* eradication v. PPI in subjects with a bleeding duodenal ulcer have been published. Re-bleeding was reduced from 20% with bismuth alone to 10% with *H. pylori* eradication (RR = 0.5; 95% CI: 0.2–1.2).[107] Pooling the data from the two PPI trials in a meta-analysis gave a RR of 0.07 (95% CI: 0.01–0.52) for recurrent bleeding at 12 months.[108,109]

NSAIDs and NUD are associated with most peptic ulcers not caused by *H. pylori*. Patients with peptic ulcer disease that are taking NSAIDs should discontinue the drug. If this is not possible, proton pump inhibitors have been shown to be more effective than H_2RAs at healing the ulcer and preventing recurrence.[110] Misoprostil also heals NSAID ulcers and prevents relapse, but randomised controlled trials suggest proton pump inhibitors are more effective at preventing relapse and are better tolerated.[111]

The anti-inflammatory properties of NSAIDs are due to the inhibition of cyclooxygenase-2 (COX-2), whereas the protection of the gastro-duodenal mucosa is through COX-1. Highly selective cyclooxygenase-2 (COX-2) inhibitors should therefore have analgesic properties similar to other NSAIDs but with few gastrointestinal adverse events. Two COX-2 selective inhibitors are available, celecoxib and refocoxib, and both are associated with a rate of peptic ulcers similar to placebo and much lower than traditional NSAIDs.[112,113] COX-2 selective inhibitors are worth considering in high risk elderly patients that need to take NSAIDs. These drugs are more expensive than traditional NSAIDs and they are therefore not cost-effective for patients at low risk of bleeding peptic ulcer disease.

Gastro-oesophageal reflux disease

Acute healing of oesophagitis

One systematic review indirectly compared proton pump inhibitors, H2 antagonists and prokinetics in healing oesophagitis.[90] This meta-analysis pooled results across treatment arms to give an overall healing rate for each of the three drugs. This is an inaccurate method of determining the relative effectiveness of therapies. A more appropriate analysis is to compare the relative effects of therapies in each randomised trial and then to pool the data to determine an overall relative effect. We have re-analysed the trial identified in the systematic review by Chiba *et al.* and also updated the articles included using a Medline search.

H_2 receptor antagonists were effective in healing oesophagitis[114–122] (relative risk reduction [RRR] = 21%; 95% CI: 13–28%) (number needed to treat [NNT] = 6; 95% CI: 5–10) (*see* **Figure 13**).

PPIs were also effective[112,113] (RRR = 69%; 95% CI: 25–87%) (NNT = 2; 95% CI: 1–5) (*see* **Figure 14**). PPIs were more effective than H_2RAs in healing oesophagitis in RCTs that compared the two drugs[125–136] (RRR = 50%; 95% CI: 42%–57%) (NNT = 3.3; 95% CI: 2.9–3.9) (*see* **Figure 15**).

One RCT also reported that PPI was superior to a prokinetic in patients with oesophagitis.[137]

Acute healing of endoscopy negative reflux disease

A systematic review reported that proton pump inhibitors were significantly better than placebo, with 60% of the treatment group becoming symptom-free on treatment compared with 33% of the control group (RRR of heartburn on PPI compared with placebo = 32%; 95% CI: 12–47%) in endoscopy negative reflux disease (NNT = 5; 95% CI: 3–12).[138] A further RCT also supports the conclusion that PPI therapy is superior to placebo in endoscopy negative reflux disease.[139] The review also found that H_2 receptor antagonists were more effective than placebo at relieving heartburn (35% v. 22% symptom-free respectively) (RRR = 16%; 95% CI: 5–26%) (NNT = 8; 95% CI: 5–26).

Proton pump inhibitors were superior to H_2 receptor antagonists in two randomised trials that directly compared the two classes of drug, but this did not reach statistical significance (53% symptom free on PPI

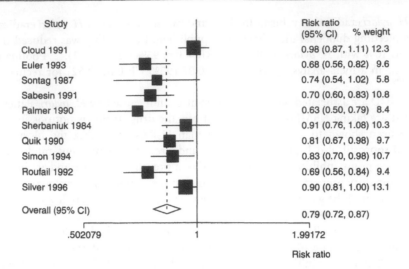

Figure 13: Efficacy of H$_2$ receptor antagonists compared with placebo in oesophagitis.

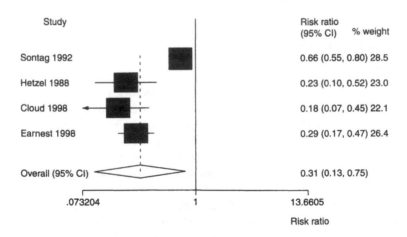

Figure 14: Efficacy of proton pump inhibitors compared with placebo in oesophagitis.

v. 42% on H$_2$ receptor antagonists) (RRR = 31%; 95% CI: 20–61%). We identified a further trial published since this systematic review that reported patients randomised to PPI therapy had significantly lower heartburn scores compared to those allocated to H$_2$ receptor antagonist therapy.[140] The review also found that PPI therapy was superior to prokinetic treatment although the evidence for this came from one trial (40% symptom-free on prokinetic v. 30% on placebo) (RRR = 28%; 95% CI: 8–44%).

Maintenance therapy of oesophagitis and endoscopy negative reflux disease

Eighty percent of patients with successfully treated GORD will have a symptomatic relapse within one year if not given any maintenance therapy. Whilst it is important to give a patient a trial without medication, many will require further courses of treatment. We found no systematic review evaluating the efficacy of medical therapy in preventing relapse in patients with oesophagitis or endoscopy negative reflux disease.

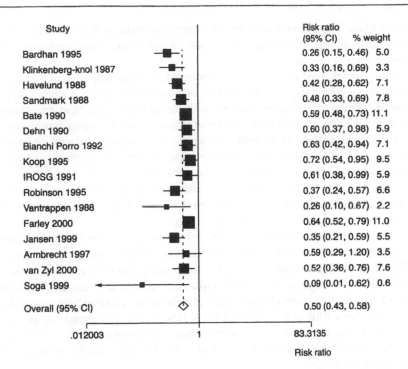

Study	Risk ratio (95% CI)	% weight
Bardhan 1995	0.26 (0.15, 0.46)	5.0
Klinkenberg-knol 1987	0.33 (0.16, 0.69)	3.3
Havelund 1988	0.42 (0.28, 0.62)	7.1
Sandmark 1988	0.48 (0.33, 0.69)	7.8
Bate 1990	0.59 (0.48, 0.73)	11.1
Dehn 1990	0.60 (0.37, 0.98)	5.9
Bianchi Porro 1992	0.63 (0.42, 0.94)	7.1
Koop 1995	0.72 (0.54, 0.95)	9.5
IROSG 1991	0.61 (0.38, 0.99)	5.9
Robinson 1995	0.37 (0.24, 0.57)	6.6
Vantrappen 1988	0.26 (0.10, 0.67)	2.2
Farley 2000	0.64 (0.52, 0.79)	11.0
Jansen 1999	0.35 (0.21, 0.59)	5.5
Armbrecht 1997	0.59 (0.29, 1.20)	3.5
van Zyl 2000	0.52 (0.36, 0.76)	7.6
Soga 1999	0.09 (0.01, 0.62)	0.6
Overall (95% CI)	0.50 (0.43, 0.58)	

.012003   1   83.3135

Risk ratio

Figure 15: Efficacy of omeprazole compared with H_2 receptor antagonists in the treatment of oesophagitis.

Three RCTs compared PPI with an H_2RA (with or without a prokinetic) in people with endoscopically confirmed oesophagitis who had already received a PPI for 4 weeks.[141,142] At 1 year, people treated with daily PPI were significantly less likely to relapse than those on an H_2RA in all three trials. Recent data suggest intermittent PPI therapy may also be effective in controlling long-term GORD symptoms.[143]

An alternative approach to patients who require long-term medication is to offer anti-reflux surgery. Two RCTs have compared medical versus surgical treatment in GORD patients. One reported that surgery was better than maintenance medical therapy that did not include a PPI.[144] A further study has indicated that gastro-oesophageal reflux scores were significantly lower in the surgery arm compared to patients randomised to long-term PPI therapy.[145] There were, however, no statistically significant differences in relapse rates for treatment failures (as defined by the authors) between the two groups after three years.

The National Institute for Clinical Excellence issued guidance on the use of PPIs in July 2000 (NICE Technology Appraisal No. 7). The guidance states that patients with severe GORD symptoms or oesophagitis (or Barrett's) should be treated with a PPI to achieve healing and then stepped down to the lowest possible acid suppression for control of symptoms. Patients with complicated oesophagitis should receive maintenance treatment with a PPI.

Non-ulcer dyspepsia

There has been considerable controversy over the most effective treatments for non-ulcer dyspepsia. Treatments include antacids, H2 receptor antagonists, PPIs, prokinetic agents and *H. pylori* eradication. There have been three reviews of *H. pylori* eradication therapy in non-ulcer dyspepsia, but these have not included recent trials. There have also been no recent systematic reviews of other pharmacological therapies in non-ulcer dyspepsia. We therefore conducted a systematic review with a similar protocol to the uninvestigated dyspepsia review.

Non-ulcer dyspepsia was defined as patients with dyspepsia and with insignificant findings at endoscopy or barium meal and who were not required to have had 24-hour oesophageal pH studies, upper abdominal ultrasounds or computerised tomography. Patients with hiatus hernia, less than five gastric erosions or mild duodenitis were included, as these lesions correlate poorly with dyspepsia symptoms. We included studies evaluating adult patients (age 16–80 years) presenting in secondary care with diagnosis of NUD. All patients must have had either an endoscopic or barium meal examination to exclude peptic ulcer disease. Interventions that were evaluated included antacids, prokinetics, proton pump inhibitors, mucosal protecting agents and *H. pylori* eradication therapy. Trials comparing these therapies with each other or with placebo were included. Global dyspepsia symptoms expressed as a dichotomous outcome (same/worse versus improved) was the principal outcome measure.

One trial has suggested antacids were no more effective than placebo in NUD.[146] A meta-analysis of trials comparing H_2RAs with placebo showed H_2RAs were more effective than placebo (RRR, prokinetics – H_2RA = 29%; 95% CI: 47–4%), but trials were often of poor quality and there was significant heterogeneity between studies.[84] Whilst awaiting further research, H_2RA seem a reasonable choice of treatment for NUD.

Proton pump inhibitors were more effective than placebo in an updated meta-analysis of non-ulcer dyspepsia trials. There was a RRR of 17% (95% CI: 12–21%) in the PPI group compared with placebo (NNT = 7; 95% CI: 6–11) (*see* **Figure 16**). PPI trials were better designed than other classes of drugs and the results are therefore more reliable. Nevertheless, a Markov model suggested that PPIs are unlikely to be a cost-effective treatment for NUD.[82]

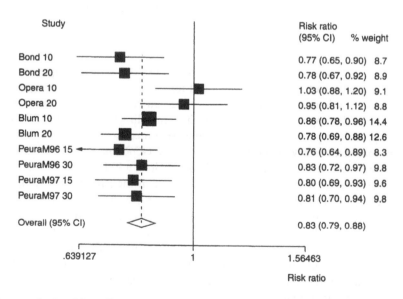

Figure 16: Meta-analysis of the efficacy of PPI therapy compared with placebo in non-ulcer dyspepsia.

Prokinetics were more effective than placebo in a meta-analysis (RRR = 50%; 95% CI: 30–70%), but there was significant heterogeneity between trials.[84] This heterogeneity could be partly explained by year of publication, larger more recent trials being less likely to show an effect. A funnel plot revealed that the results of the prokinetic meta-analysis could be due to publication bias or related quality issues. Most of these trials evaluated cisapride, which has now been withdrawn from the UK market. The relative tolerability and cost-effectiveness of metoclopramide and domperidone in NUD remain to be established.

In a meta-analysis of nine high quality RCTs, *H. pylori* eradication was associated with a 9% (95% CI: 14–4%) relative risk reduction, and an NNT of 15 (95% CI: 10–31) was calculated based on a control event rate of 72% (*see* **Figure 17**).[147] Economic modelling, based on these data, suggests *H. pylori* eradication would be cost-effective with an incremental cost-effectiveness ratio against antacid alone of £56 per month. Sensitivity analysis indicated that *H. pylori* eradication therapy would be cost-effective provided the payer was willing to accept a 20% probability of the policy being incorrect and was willing to pay £75 for each month free of dyspepsia.[147] It is possible that the effect of *H. pylori* eradication in NUD is based on a subgroup of patients with an 'ulcer diathesis' where the treatment prevents the development of future peptic ulcers. This hypothesis is difficult to prove, but provides one explanation as to why an effect is seen, where no association has been observed between chronic *H. pylori* gastritis and dyspeptic symptoms.

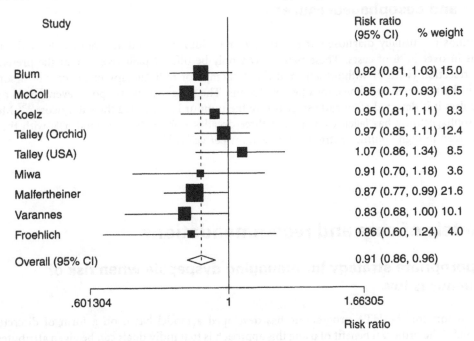

Figure 17: A meta-analysis of *H. pylori* eradication therapy versus placebo antibiotics in non-ulcer dyspepsia.

Given the uncertainty surrounding the definition, aetiology and cost-effectiveness of treatments for NUD, it is essential that patients should be reviewed after treatment changes to determine the most appropriate choice of treatment for each individual patient.

Barrett's oesophagus

Columnar metaplasia in the oesophagus is thought to develop in response to gastro-oesophageal reflux[148] and the management of Barrett's oesophagus aims to relieve reflux symptoms as well as reduce the risk of neoplasia. Reflux symptoms are best treated with proton pump inhibitor therapy. The impact acid suppression has on cancer risk is unclear and needs evaluating in randomised controlled trials. Endoscopic surveillance every two years with quadrantic biopsies every 2 cm has been recommended for patients with no dysplasia that are fit for surgery by the International Society for Diseases of the Esophagus.[149] The consensus was that patients with low-grade dysplasia should have endoscopy annually. Patients with high-grade dysplasia should have a repeat endoscopy with multiple biopsies and a second pathologist should review the histology. If the diagnosis was confirmed, oesophageal resection should be considered.

The risk of oesophageal adenocarcinoma has concerned clinicians, and 70% of a randomly selected group of British Society of Gastroenterology members were offering surveillance[150] The evidence for the efficacy of surveillance has been challenged and economic models have suggested that the cost-effectiveness of this programme may be expensive by UK standards.[151] More evidence is therefore needed before recommendations can be made on the need for surveillance of Barrett's oesophagus.

Gastric and oesophageal cancer

These lesions are usually diagnosed at endoscopy or barium meal and are inoperable at the time of diagnosis in over 50% of cases. These patients can only be offered palliative care at the present time. Surgical resection (with or without adjuvant chemotherapy or radiotherapy in the case of oesophageal cancer) is the treatment of choice for operable lesions. The prognosis is still poor, even for an operable lesion, unless it is detected at an early stage before the tumour has invaded the submucosa.[152] Mortality from oesophagectomy has fallen over the last three decades from 30% to around 5%, with the lowest mortality seen in high volume centres (>50 resections per year).[153]

7 Models of care and recommendations

The appropriate strategy for managing dyspepsia when risk of malignancy is low

A recent report for the HTA programme has developed a model based on a form of discrete event simulation.[82] The principal benefit of using this approach is that individuals can be given attributes: these determine the distribution of time taken in any particular state and the probability of transition to other states. In the dyspepsia model, an individual at any time may or may not be infected with *H. pylori* and may or may not have any combination of duodenal ulcer, gastric ulcer, non-ulcer dyspepsia and reflux dyspepsia.

Five strategies were examined in the model:

1 *H. pylori* eradication for all patients
2 endoscopy for all patients
3 *H. pylori* test, followed by endoscopy if positive
4 *H. pylori* test, followed by eradication therapy if positive
5 initial empirical pharmacological therapy.

Fourteen follow-on prescribing strategies were also specified:

1 prescription antacid only
2 H_2RA only

3 prokinetics only
4 PPI only
5 antacid, H_2RA, PPI, prokinetics and stay
6 antacid, H_2RA/prokinetics, PPI and stay
7 antacid, H_2RA, PPI and stay
8 antacid, H_2RA, PPI, prokinetics and down
9 antacid, H_2RA/prokinetics, PPI and down
10 antacid, H_2RA, PPI and down
11 prokinetics, PPI, H_2RA, antacid and stay
12 PPI, H_2RA/prokinetics, antacid and stay
13 PPI, H_2RA, antacid and stay
14 try PPI or prokinetics until one of them works.

All combinations of strategies were compared. One strategy is said to be simply dominated by another if it is both more costly and less effective. Of the 70 possible combinations of investigation and prescribing strategies, all but nine were eliminated by simple dominance. **Table 5** shows the list of non-dominated options, also shown in **Figure 18**.

Table 5: Non-dominated strategies in the base case.

Point	Investigation strategy	Prescription strategy	Cost over 5 yrs/£	Std. error	Dyspepsia-free months in 5 yrs	Std. error	Extra cost for one month's extra benefit compared to	
							previous	cheapest
A	Medication only	Antacid only	169.05	0.43	35.59	0.056		
B	Test and eradicate	Antacid only	221.60	0.55	36.42	0.058	62.77	62.77
C	Medication only	H_2RA	274.73	0.67	42.25	0.047	9.12	15.86
D	Medication only	Antacid, H_2RA, PPI and down	319.63	0.27	43.12	0.014	51.36	19.98
E	Medication only	PPI, H_2RA, antacid and stay	324.57	0.26	43.17	0.015	105.98	20.51
F	Medication only	Antacid, H_2RA, PPI and stay	328.56	0.88	43.49	0.046	12.57	20.19
G	Medication only	PPI only	357.17	0.89	44.23	0.046	38.41	21.76
H	Test and eradicate	PPI only	395.08	0.93	44.88	0.046	58.73	24.32
I	Test and eradicate	PPI or prokinetic if effective	479.37	1.16	45.13	0.047	329.04	32.50

For points D and E, the number of replications was increased to ensure a statistically significant difference.

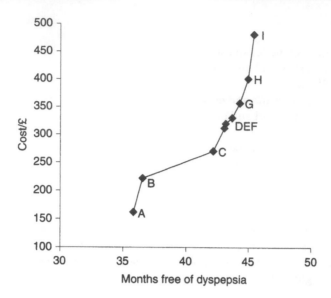

Figure 18: Cost-effectiveness of non-dominated strategies for managing dyspepsia.

All strategies involving endoscopy were dominated. Strategies involving medication only were invariably cheaper, but slightly less effective, than those strategies using an initial *H. pylori* test with the same prescribing strategy. The additional cost of the 'test and eradicate' strategies included the immediate cost of the *H. pylori* test and subsequent eradication therapy in those testing positive. This expense was offset against the cost saving in terms of recurrent ulcers prevented. The additional costs and benefits were both greater in the case where the prescribing strategy is to use antacids, but the ratio between them was lower.

The model was sensitive to the prevalence of *H. pylori*; allowing it to go up to 60% meant that more strategic combinations involving 'test and eradicate', and some involving 'eradicate all', became non-dominated. Varying the effectiveness of medication made more substantial changes to the choice of non-dominated prescribing strategies, as did varying the price. However, the choice of initial strategies remained unchanged.

The appropriate age to promote upper gastrointestinal endoscopy

Endoscopy is not the most cost-effective strategy for managing dyspeptic patients with a low risk of malignancy. The main drive to perform endoscopy is therefore to detect upper gastrointestinal malignancy in a higher risk population, as the prognosis for these cancers is poor unless diagnosed early. Endoscopy is expensive and resources are scarce so it is important to limit this investigation to those that are most likely to benefit.

The traditional method of assessing the cost-effectiveness of life-saving healthcare interventions is in terms of cost/life year saved. We explored the cost-effectiveness of endoscopy at detecting early upper gastrointestinal malignancy, in terms of cost/life year saved, according to age, gender and high risk symptom groups using a Markov model.

Data incorporated into the decision analysis model

The decision analysis model evaluates gastric cancer, as evidence that prompt endoscopy or increased volume of endoscopy increases the proportion of early oesophageal cancer is limited. There is no evidence that investigating patients early will detect a higher proportion of early gastric cancer. There is evidence, however, that more widespread use of endoscopy detects more early gastric cancer (EGC) and this model assumes that reducing waiting times will increase demand for endoscopy. One percent of the population has an endoscopy each year (Finished Consultant Episode data from the Department of Health) and data suggests that doubling the number of endoscopies performed increased the proportion of EGC by 3.75%. The model assumes that if the whole population were endoscoped each year 100% of gastric cancers would be EGC. At present 1% of the population is endoscoped and as demand for endoscopy increases the proportion of EGC detected is given by the following equation giving a heteroscedastic curve (*see* **Figure 19**):

$$EGC = p\_egc \times ied^{\ln(1/p\_egc)/\ln100}$$

Where:

EGC = Total proportion of EGC detected
p_egc = increase in proportion of EGC with each unit increase in endoscopy demand
ied = increase in endoscopy demand

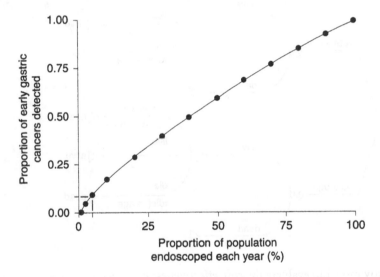

Figure 19: Probability of detecting early gastric cancer with increasing endoscopy demand.

Population surveys indicate only 20% of patients with dyspepsia are currently referred by their general practitioner for endoscopy.[8] There is therefore potential for a five-fold increase in workload assuming all patients would consent to endoscopy. Should this occur, the above equation indicates that there will be approximately a 10 percentage point increase in the proportion of EGCs detected.

The importance of detecting EGC is that 90% of patients survive five years compared with 5% of patients with advanced disease. These figures, together with the cost of endoscopy and gastric surgery, (*see* **Table 6**) were incorporated into a Markov model (*see* **Figure 20**). The model compared a hypothetical early endoscopy strategy allowing everyone with dyspepsia to be investigated with existing services (20% of dyspepsia sufferers presenting to the general practitioner endoscoped, which is equivalent to 1% of the population per year).

Table 6: Data used in the Markov model.

Variable	Baseline	Range for sensitivity analyses
Cost of endoscopy	£246	£186–299
Cost of gastric surgery	£2,405	£1,809–5,015
Survival from EGC	90%	80–99%
Proportion of EGC with each unit increase in endoscopy	3.75%	1%–7.5%

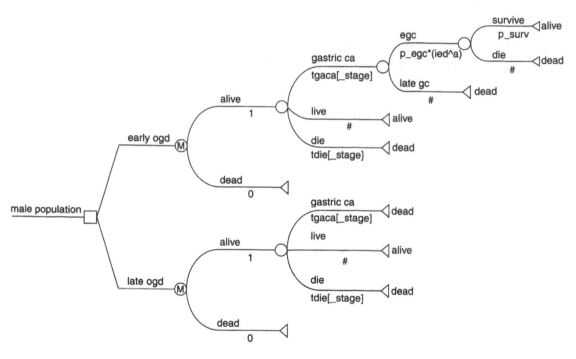

Figure 20: Markov model to evaluate the cost-effectiveness of early endoscopy.

Results

Five hundred and eighty-seven life saving interventions have been evaluated in the United States, and the median cost is approximately £26 000/life year saved.[154] This is expensive by UK standards but could be taken as the upper limit of what would be acceptable to the NHS. The cost-effectiveness analyses were performed with this upper limit in mind.

What is the lowest age limit we can afford to set for endoscoping all men with dyspepsia?

The base case scenario suggests the average cost-effectiveness for endoscoping all men presenting with dyspepsia is £25 241/life year saved. This is superficially attractive, but this figure hides the extra cost of offering endoscopy to younger men. Endoscoping all men over 70 with dyspepsia costs £12 563/life year saved (*see* **Table 7**). Reducing this age limit to 65 costs an extra £15 779/life year saved compared with just offering this service to those over 70. The incremental costs of lowering the age limit further dramatically increases the cost/effectiveness ratio so that endoscoping patients over 40 costs £454 000/life year saved compared with endoscoping patients over 45 (*see* **Table 7**). These data suggest early endoscopy should only be offered to men over 60. This age limit may be unacceptable to many general practitioners and identifying those at higher risk of malignancy may improve the cost-effectiveness ratio, allowing lower age groups to be investigated early.

Table 7: Cost-effectiveness of early endoscopy for all men with dyspepsia.

Age	Cost (£)	Effectiveness (life years saved)	Average c/e*	Incremental cost (£)	Incremental effectiveness	Incremental c/e*
70	91.80	0.00731	12,563	/	/	/
65	123.20	0.00930	13,261	31.40	0.00199	15,779
60	159.80	0.01070	14,995	36.60	0.0014	26,142
55	199.10	0.01170	17,021	39.30	0.001	39,300
50	240.50	0.01250	19,303	41.40	0.0008	51,750
45	283.80	0.01290	21,998	43.30	0.0004	108,250
40	329.20	0.01300	25,242	45.40	0.0001	454,000

* c/e= cost-effectiveness £/life year saved.

Can identifying high risk groups lower the age limit at which early endoscopy is economically feasible?

Data from the group has shown that certain symptoms predict upper gastrointestinal neoplasia. The main concern is that cancer is not missed and therefore the symptom pattern with the lowest negative likelihood ratio should be the most appropriate group to analyse (*see* **Table 8**). Patients with continuous symptoms, anorexia, dysphagia and/or symptoms for less than one year meet this criteria (*see* **Table 8**).

Table 8: Identifying high-risk groups.

Risk group	Sensitivity	Specificity	+ve LR*	−ve LR*
Continuous symptoms and dysphagia	21%	99%	21	0.8
Continuous symptoms and anorexia	23%	98%	12.5	0.79
Continuous symptoms and both of the above	19%	99%	19	0.82
Any of: Continuous symptoms, anorexia, dysphagia, symptoms less than one year**	**92%**	**68%**	**2.875**	**0.11**
Continuous symptoms for less than one year	29%	98%	14.5	0.72
Continuous symptoms for less than one year including either anorexia or dysphagia	22%	99%	22	0.79

* LR=likelihood ratio (from data provided by Peter McCulloch).
** group most appropriate to analyse.

It was assumed that only offering early endoscopy to patients with these symptoms would reduce endoscopy workload by 33% (a range of 10–50% was used in the sensitivity analyses). The Markov model shows selecting this high-risk group is the most cost-effective. The average cost-effectiveness for endoscoping men over 70 with these high-risk symptoms is £8398/life year saved. Offering early endoscopy to all men over 70 costs an extra £45 925/life year saved.

Incremental cost-effectiveness ratios suggest that men over 55 with high-risk symptoms should be offered early endoscopy (*see* **Table 9, Figure 21**).

Table 9: Cost-effectiveness of early endoscopy for men with high risk symptoms.

Age	Cost (£)	Effectiveness (life years saved)	Average c/e*	Incremental cost (£)	Incremental effectiveness	Incremental c/e*
70	54.60	0.00650	8,398	/	/	/
65	73.00	0.0083	8,828	18.40	0.0018	10,222
60	94.30	0.0095	9,950	21.30	0.0012	17,750
55	117.30	0.0104	11,269	23.00	0.0009	25,556
50	141.50	0.0111	12,758	24.20	0.0007	34,571
45	166.70	0.0115	14,521	25.20	0.0004	63,000
40	193.20	0.0116	16,645	26.50	0.0001	265,000

* c/e = cost-effectiveness £/life year saved.

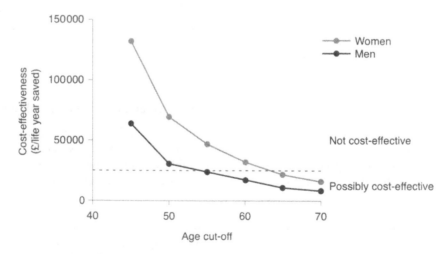

Figure 21: Incremental cost-effectiveness of early endoscopy with age at which endoscopy starts in high risk patients.

The cost-effectiveness of early endoscopy in women

Gastric cancer is less common in women and an early endoscopy strategy will therefore be less cost-effective in women. It is only cost-effective to endoscope women over 65 with the high risk symptoms described above (*see* **Table 10, Figure 21**). Differentiating the age cut-off at which early endoscopy is recommended according to gender may be ethically unacceptable to policy makers. Setting the age cut-off at 55 years for everyone would be more equitable although this is not justified on economic grounds.

Table 10: Cost-effectiveness of early endoscopy for women with high risk symptoms.

Age	Cost (£)	Effectiveness (life years saved)	Average c/e*	Incremental cost (£)	Incremental effectiveness	Incremental c/e*
70	67.80	0.00361	18,799	/	/	/
65	89.20	0.00458	19,460	21.40	0.00097	22,062
60	112.70	0.00529	21,298	23.50	0.00071	33,099
55	137.40	0.00585	23,477	24.70	0.00056	44,107
50	162.60	0.00621	26,174	25.20	0.00036	70,000
45	188.70	0.00641	29,430	26.10	0.00020	130,500
40	215.70	0.00658	32,760	27.00	0.00017	158,823

* c/e = cost-effectiveness £/life year saved.

Sensitivity analyses

The Markov model is based on several assumptions. To evaluate the robustness of the model a maximum and a minimum value was set for each variable (*see* **Table 6**). Worst and best case scenarios were therefore generated for each variable (*see* **Table 11**). The average cost-effectiveness ratios were not affected greatly, indicating that the model is robust (*see* **Table 11**). The model was most affected by the assumptions regarding the proportion of EGC detected for each unit increase in endoscopy.

Table 11: One-way sensitivity analyses for men over 55 with high risk symptoms.

Variable	Range for sensitivity analyses	Worst case (average £/life year saved)	Best case (average £/life year saved)
Cost of endoscopy	£186–299	13,627	8,560
Cost of surgery	£1,809–5,015	11,620	11,189
Survival from EGC	88–99%	12,677	11,331
Proportion of EGC detected with each increase in endoscopy	1–7.5%	27,893	7,067

Assumptions inherent in the model

The decision analysis model was constructed from a health service perspective. A societal perspective would have given higher cost estimates, as travel costs, loss of leisure time and time off work were not considered.

The model did not incorporate any extra medical costs in those surviving longer as a result of early endoscopy. This would make early endoscopy less cost-effective but inclusion of these costs is controversial.

Monetary costs and health benefits were not discounted in the model. Discounting is normal practice, as capital spent on health care now would have been invested and is not worth the same several years later. If a 6% discount rate is used for costs and benefits, the average cost-effectiveness ratio in men over 55 with high risk symptoms increases from £11 269 to £34 808.

The cost-effectiveness calculations were expressed in terms of years of life saved and therefore implicitly all years of life are valued equally. This is a common perspective to take, but it could be argued that many of the life years saved would be in the elderly, some of whom would be frail. This problem could be overcome by incorporating health-related quality of life measures such as Quality Adjusted Life Years (QALYs). Data on QALYs in the normal elderly population is limited and this approach was not taken in this decision analysis model.

The Markov model assumes that gastric cancer cases have no extra comorbidity. Subjects that have early gastric cancers detected therefore have the same age-standardised life expectancy as the general population. If subjects developing gastric cancer are less healthy than the general population, then this model will overestimate the cost-effectiveness of early endoscopy.

The model assumes that all gastric cancers would be detected early if the entire population was endoscoped once a year. This would appear reasonable, as data suggests that time of progression from EGC to advanced cancer is 3 years.[152] The model assumed that all EGC would progress to advanced gastric cancer unless the patient has gastric surgery. Data suggest that some EGC do not progress[155] and this would make an early endoscopy strategy slightly more expensive.

Cost minimisation

Endoscopy is expensive, and although this could be justified in terms of early cancer detected, it would cost billions of pounds to deliver the ideal service. This is clearly not feasible and it is important to minimise costs by reducing the demand for endoscopy in younger age groups. A third of endoscopies are performed in patients under 45.[156] Four randomised controlled trials have shown that screening for *H. pylori* and treating those infected is as effective as endoscopy and less expensive.[102,157–159] A test and treat strategy has also been shown to reduce endoscopy workload in young patients with dyspepsia in clinical practice.[160] Symptomatic treatment or an *H. pylori* screen and treat policy should therefore be encouraged in younger age groups so that existing resources can be used to endoscope those that would most benefit.

Conclusion

Economic analysis suggests that early endoscopy could be advocated for patients over 55 with continuous symptoms, anorexia, dysphagia and/or symptoms less one year. Alternatives to endoscopy should be promoted in younger dyspeptic patients.

8 Outcome measures

Detecting upper gastrointestinal malignancy

Patients seeking health care for dyspepsia are often concerned about the possibility of their symptoms being due to cancer. One of the main aims of the health service should be to detect upper gastrointestinal neoplasia at a treatable stage. Management should focus on detailed investigation of patients at high risk of malignancy and the main determinant of this risk is age. Endoscopy should be encouraged in older age groups and alternative management strategies promoted in younger patients. Assessing whether this has occurred with present forms of data collection is difficult. Hospital Episode Statistics record the number of endoscopies conducted in the UK and the diagnosis. Recording the number of endoscopies in five- or ten-year age bands would make this routine form of data collection more informative.

Routine data collection should be able to evaluate whether a health care intervention is effective as well as whether it has been implemented. Survival from oesophageal and gastric cancer is collected by Cancer Registries and this could be correlated with the number of endoscopies performed within different regions over time. This type of ecological analysis can be difficult to interpret but would act as supportive evidence that increasing endoscopy in older age groups improved survival.

The most important outcome measures to evaluate the efficacy of early diagnostic strategies to detect early upper gastrointestinal malignancy are:

- number of endoscopies in the appropriate age band
- number of gastric and oesophageal cancers detected
- number of early gastric and oesophageal cancers detected
- overall survival from gastric and oesophageal cancer.

Treatment of dyspepsia

Patients also seek health care to relieve symptoms. The health service should therefore aim to improve or cure symptoms. There are a number of validated dyspepsia questionnaires to evaluate response to treatment. This can be measured as a change in dyspepsia score, but a more useful approach is to dichotomise patients into cured (no or minimal symptoms) versus not cured. Cure rates are more meaningful to patients and health care workers than mean change in dyspepsia score. Dyspepsia is a common condition and therefore the cost of the intervention as well as the effect is important.

Routine data collection should be able to assess whether appropriate drugs are prescribed. The most appropriate approach for undiagnosed dyspepsia is less certain. The most effective drugs for gastro-oesophageal reflux disease are PPIs. These drugs are also effective in NUD, as is *H. pylori* eradication therapy. The latter is probably the most cost-effective treatment for NUD and is the treatment of choice for peptic ulcer disease. The most cost-effective therapy to prescribe for undiagnosed dyspepsia on present evidence is PPIs. There is some evidence that reflux symptoms respond well to PPIs, but epigastric pain less well.

At this point, it might be useful to return to the Rome II criteria and label patients with reflux symptoms responding to PPIs as having either endoscopy negative reflux disease or oesophagitis. Some patients with epigastric pain (NUD) will also respond to PPIs. In all patients, a careful review of symptoms' response and either a step-down to H$_2$RA or intermittent PPI therapy should be undertaken. PCOs should be able to obtain audit data from practices as to whether regular reviews of treatment have been undertaken. NICE guidance on PPIs has recommended that PPIs should not be used for more than three months without investigation (either *H. pylori* test and treat or OGD). OGD in young patients without alarm symptoms is not cost-effective; whether *H. pylori* test and treat is more cost-effective than continuing PPI therapy is the subject of an ongoing MRC trial.

The most important outcome measures in evaluating the effects of intervention on dyspepsia symptoms are therefore:

- efficacy of intervention in terms of proportion of patients 'cured'
- cost-effectiveness of the intervention
- appropriateness of drug prescribing
- regular review of patients on long-term treatment.

9 Information and research requirements

Detecting upper gastrointestinal malignancy

Open access endoscopy services have flourished without careful evaluation of the efficacy of this strategy in terms of detection of upper gastrointestinal neoplasia or dyspepsia management. A randomised controlled trial of the efficacy of endoscopy in detecting early neoplastic lesions would be difficult as such, as the sample size needed would be prohibitively expensive. There would also be little equipoise amongst patients and clinicians with the present availability of open access services. Nevertheless, the appropriateness of future expansion of endoscopy services could be evaluated. A cluster randomised trial would be the most appropriate design for this, with certain centres allocated to 'usual care' and others to increased availability of endoscopy.

Treatment of dyspepsia

More information is needed on the appropriate management strategy for dyspepsia. Our model suggests that endoscopy is not a cost-effective option when dyspepsia is the outcome of interest. *H. pylori* test and treat or empirical drug therapy are the most cost-effective options and a randomised controlled trial is needed to evaluate these two options. Whatever the outcome of such a trial, pharmacological therapy will be needed to treat uninvestigated dyspepsia in some patients. Trials suggest PPIs are the most effective therapy but the most cost-effective drug to use is still uncertain.

Many patients will continue to undergo endoscopy where a specific diagnosis can be reached. The evidence that *H. pylori* eradication therapy is the most cost-effective treatment of peptic ulcer disease is conclusive. There is also firm evidence that PPIs are the most effective treatment of GORD. Systematic reviews suggest PPIs and *H. pylori* eradication therapy are also likely to be effective in NUD. Good evidence of cost trials are, however, needed to establish the following:

- the most cost-effective therapy for gastro-oesophageal reflux disease
- the efficacy of H$_2$RA and prokinetic therapy in NUD
- the most cost-effective therapy for NUD.

The main areas of uncertainty relate to cost-effectiveness data. Trials that evaluate this will need to be more pragmatic to reflect what actually occurs in clinical practice. These types of studies usually show that one form of therapy is more effective but also more expensive compared to the alternative. It is useful to know the value of treating dyspepsia in these circumstances, yet we are unaware of any studies that have evaluated this. The value of relief of symptoms either in terms of Quality Adjusted Life Years or in monetary terms would help inform decision makers on the most cost-effective approach to manage dyspepsia.

References

1 Chiba N. Definitions of dyspepsia: time for a reappraisal. *European Journal of Surgery* 1998: **164(suppl 583)**: 14–23.

2 Talley NJ, Stanghellini V, Heading RC, Koch KL, Malagelada JR, Tytgat GN. Functional gastro-duodenal disorders. *Gut* 1999; **45(suppl 2)**: II37–II42.

3 Anonymous. Management of dyspepsia: report of a working party. *The Lancet* 1988; **1**: 576–9.

4 Talley NJ, Colin-Jones D, Koch KL, Koch M, Nyren O, Stanghellini V. Functional dyspepsia: a classification with guidelines for diagnosis and management. *Gastroenterology International* 1991; **4**: 145–60.

5 Talley NJ, Stanghellini V, Heading RC, Koch KL, Malagelada JR, Tytgat GN. Functional gastro-duodenal disorders. *Gut* 1999; **45**: 1137–42.

6 Anonymous. *Dyspepsia management guidelines.* BSG Guidelines in Gastroenterology, 1996.

7 Ryder SD, O'Reilly S, Miller RJ, Ross J, Jacyna MR, Levi AJ. Long-term acid suppressing treatment in general practice. *BMJ* 1994; **308**: 827–30.

8 Jones RH, Lydeard S, Hobbs FDR, Kenkre JE, Williams EI, Jones SJ, Repper JA, Caldow JL, Dunwoodie WMB, Bottomley JM. Dyspepsia in England and Scotland. *Gut* 1990; **31**: 401–5.

9 Asante M, Lord J, Mendall M, Northfield T. Endoscopy for Helicobacter pylori sero-negative young dyspeptic patients: an economic evaluation based on a randomized trial. *Eur J Gastroenterol Hepatol* 1999; **11**: 851–6.

10 Hallissey MT, Allum WH, Jewkes AJ, Ellis DJ, Fielding JW. Early detection of gastric cancer. *BMJ* 1990; **301**: 513–15.

11 Dent J, Brun J, Fendrick AM, Fennerty MB, Janssens J, Kahrilas PJ, Lauritsen K, Reynolds JC, Shaw M, Talley NJ. An evidence-based appraisal of reflux disease management – the Genval Workshop Report. *Gut* 1999; **44**: S1–S16.

12 Robertson DA, Aldersley MA, Shepherd H, Lloyd RS, Smith CL. H2 antagonists in the treatment of reflux oesophagitis: can physiological studies predict the response? *Gut* 1987; **28**: 946–9.

13 Breumelhof R, Smout AJPM. The symptoms sensitivity index: a valuable additional parameter in 24 hour esophageal pH recording. *American Journal of Gastroenterology* 1991; **86**: 160–4.

14 Shi G, Bruley des Varannes S, Scarpignato C, LeRhun M, Galmiche JP. Reflux related symptoms in patients with normal oesophageal exposure to acid. *Gut* 1995; **37**: 457–64.

15 Watson RG, Tham TC, Johnston BT, McDougall NI. Double blind cross-over placebo controlled study of omeprazole in the treatment of patients with reflux symptoms and physiological levels of acid reflux – the 'sensitive oesophagus'. *Gut* 1997; **40**: 587–90.

16 Armstrong D. Endoscopic evaluation of gastro-esophageal reflux disease. *Yale Journal of Biology & Medicine* 1999; **72**: 93–100.

17 Horrocks JC, DeDombal FT. Clinical presentation of pateints with 'dyspepsia'. Detailed symptomatic study of 360 patients. *Gut* 1978; **19**: 19–26.

18 Talley NJ, Zinsmeister AR, Schelck CD, Melton III LJ. Dyspepsia and Dyspepsia Subgroups: A Population-Based Study. *Gastroenterology* 1992; **102**: 1259–68.

19 Agreus L, Svardsudd K, Nyren O, Tibblin G. Irritable bowel syndrome and dyspepsia in the general population. *Gastroenterology* 1995; **109**: 671–80.

20 Spechler SJ, Goyal RK. The columnar lined esophagus, intestinal metaplasia and Norman Barrett. *Gastroenterology* 1996; **110**: 614.

21 Sharma P, Morales TG, Bhattacharyya A, Garewal HS, Sampliner RE. Dysplasia in short-segment Barrett's esophagus: a prospective 3 year follow-up. *Am J Gastroenterol* 1997; **92**: 2012–6.

22 Morales TG, Sampliner RE, Bhattacharyya A. Intestinal metaplasia of the gastric cardia. *Am J Gastroenterol* 1997; **92**: 414–8.

23 Blot WJ, Devesa SS, Kneller RW, Fraumeni JF Jr. Rising incidence of adenocarcinoma of the esophagus and gastric cardia. *Journal of American Medical Association* 1991; **265**: 1287–9.

24 Danesh J. Helicobacter pylori infection and gastric cancer: systematic review of the epidemiological studies. *Alimentary Pharmacology & Therapeutics* 1999; **13**: 851–6.

25 Penston JG, Pounder RE. A survey of dyspepsia in Great Britain. *Alimentary Pharmacology & Therapeutics* 1996; **10**: 83–9.

26 Doll R, Avery Jones F, Buckatzsch MM. *Occupational factors in the aetiology of gastric and duodenal ulcers with estimates of their incidence in the general population*. MRC Special Report Series 276, 7–96. London: HMSO, 1951.

27 Weir RD, Backett EM. Studies of epidemiology of peptic ulcer in a rural community: prevalence and natural history of dyspepsia and peptic ulcer. *Gut* 1968; **9**: 75–83.

28 Kelly SM, Pitcher MC, Farmery SM, Gibson GR. Isolation of Helicobacter pylori from feces of patients with dyspepsia in the United Kingdom. *Gastroenterology* 1994; **107**: 1671–4.

29 Parsonnet J, Shmuely H, Haggerty T. Fecal and oral shedding of Helicobacter pylori from healthy infected adults. *JAMA* 1999; **282**: 2240–5.

30 Mendall MA, Goggin PM, Molineaux N *et al*. Childhood living conditions and Helicobacter pylori seropositivity in adult life. *The Lancet* 1992; **339**: 896–7.

31 Goodman KJ, Correa P. Transmission of Helicobacter pylori among siblings. *The Lancet* 2000; **355**: 358–62.

32 Moayyedi P. H. pylori *screening and eradication in general practice: medical benefits and health economics*. Leeds: University of Leeds, 1999.

33 Garcia Rodriguez LA, Jick H. Risk of upper gastrointestinal bleeding and perforation associated with individual non-steroidal anti-inflammatory drugs. *The Lancet* 1994; **343**: 769–72.

34 Bardhan KD, Royston C, Nayyar AK. Reflux rising! A Disease in Evolution. *Gut* 2000; **46**: A91. (Abstract)

35 Caygill CP, Reed PI, Johnston BJ, Hill MJ, Ali MH, Levi S. A single centre's 20 years' experience of columnar-lined (Barrett's) oesophagus diagnosis. *Eur J Gastroenterol Hepatol* 1999; **11**: 1355–8.

36 Lagergren J, Bergstrom R, Lindgren A, Nyren O. Symptomatic gastroesophageal reflux as a risk factor for esophageal adenocarcinoma. *NEJM* 1999; **340**: 825–31.

37 Lieberman DA, Oehlke M, Helfand M. *Am J Gastroenterol* 1997; **92**: 1293–7.

38 Cameron AJ, Lomboy CT. Barrett's esophagus: age, prevalence and extent of columnar epithelium. *Gastroenterology* 1992; **103**: 1241–5.

39 Shaheen NJ, Crosby MA, Bozymski EM, Sandler RS. Is there publication bias in the reporting of cancer risk in Barrett's esophagus? *Gastroenterology* 2000; **119**: 333–8.

40 Jones RH. Self-care and primary care of dyspepsia: a review. *Fam Pract* 1987; **4**: 68–77.

41 Dean K. Self-care responses to illness: a selected review. *Soc Sci Med* 198; **15**: 673–87.

42 van de Kar A, Knottnerus A, Meertens R, Dubois V, Kok G. Why do patients consult the general practitioner? Determinants of their decision. *British Journal of General Practice* 1992; **42**: 313–16.

43 Zola IK. Studying the decision to see a doctor. Review, critique, corrective. *Advances in Psychosomatic Medicine* 1972; **8**: 216–36.

44 Hansen JM, Bytzer P, deMuckadell OBS. Management of dyspeptic patients in primary care – Value of the unaided clinical diagnosis and of dyspepsia subgrouping. *Scand J Gastroenterol* 1998; **33**: 799–805.

45 Talley NJ, Weaver AL, Tesmer DL, Zinsmeister AR. Lack of discriminant value of dyspepsia subgroups in patients referred for upper endoscopy. *Gastroenterology* 1993; **105**: 1378–86.

46 Blaxter M. The causes of disease. Women talking. *Social Science & Medicine* 1983; **17**: 59–69.

47 Lydeard S, Jones R. Factors affecting the decision to consult with dyspepsia: comparison of consulters and non-consulters. *Journal of the Royal College of General Practitioners* 1989; **39**: 495–8.

48 Oakley A. *Interviewing women, a contradiction in terms*. London: Routledge, 1981.

49 Delaney BC. Why do dyspeptic patients over the age of 50 consult their general practitioner? A qualitative investigation of health beliefs relating to dyspepsia. *British Journal of General Practice* 1998; **48**: 1481–5.

50 Hackett TP, Cassem NH, Raker JW. Patient delay in cancer. *NEJM.* 1973; **289**: 14–20.

51 McIntyre A. Healthy expansion of gastroenterology posts in England and Wales. *BSG News* 2000; **8**: 1.

52 Smith PM, Williams R. A comparison of workloads of physician-gastroenterologists and other consultant physicians. Prepared on behalf of the Clinical Services Committee, British Society of Gastroenterology. *Journal of the Royal College of Physicians of London* 1992; **26**: 167–8.

53 Scott BB. Gastroenterology in the Trent Region in 1992 and a review of changes since 1975. *Gut* 1995; **36**: 468–72.

54 Fraser GM, Earnshaw PM. The double-contrast barium meal: a correlation with endoscopy. *Clinical Radiology* 1983; **34**: 121–31.

55 Hedemand N, Kruse A, Madsen EH, Mathiasen MS. X-ray examination of endoscopy? A blind prospective study including barium meal, double contrast examiniation, and endoscopy of esophagus, stomach, and duodenum. *Gastrointestinal Radiology* 1977; **1**: 331–4.

56 Rogers IM, Sokhi GS, Moule B, Joffe SN, Blumgart LH. Endoscopy and routine and double-contrast barium meal in diagnosis of gastric and duodenal disorders. *The Lancet* 1976; **1**: 901–2.

57 Hamada T, Kaji F, Shirakabe H. Detectability of gastric cancer by radiology as compared to endoscopy. In: Maruyama, M, Kimura K. *Review of clinical research in gastroenterology*, 36–52. Tokyo: Igaku-Shoin, 1984.

58 Dooley CP, Larson AW, Stace NH *et al.* Double-contrast barium meal and upper gastrointestinal endoscopy. A comparative study. *Annals of Internal Medicine* 1984; **101**: 538–45.

59 Dooley CP, Weiner JM, Larson AW. Endoscopy or radiography? – The patient's choice. Prospective comparative survey of patient acceptability of upper gastrointestinal endoscopy and radiography. *American Journal of Medicine* 1986; **80**: 203–7.

60 Stevenson GW, Norman G, Frost R, Somers S. Barium meal or endoscopy? A prospective randomized study of patient preference and physician decision making. *Clinical Radiology* 1991; **44**: 317–21.

61 Quine MA, Bell GD, McCloy RF, Charlton JE, Devlin HB, Hopkins A. Prospective audit of upper gastrointestinal endoscopy in two regions of England: safety, staffing, and sedation methods. *Gut* 1995; **36**: 462–7.

62 Wilcox MH, Dent TH, Hunter JO *et al.* Accuracy of serology for the diagnosis of Helicobacter pylori infection – a comparison of eight kits. *Journal of Clinical Pathology* 1996; **49**: 373–6.

63 Delaney BC and Hobbs FDR. Near patient tests for *Helicobacter pylori* in primary care: how accurate do they need to be? *European Journal of General Practice* 1998; **4**: 149–54.

64 Moayyedi P, Carter AM, Catto A, Heppell RM, Grant PJ, Axon AT. Validation of a rapid whole blood test for diagnosing Helicobacter pylori infection. *BMJ* 1997; **314**: 119.

65 Stone MA, Mayberry JF, Wicks AC *et al.* Near patient testing for Helicobacter pylori: a detailed evaluation of the Cortecs Helisal Rapid Blood test. *Eur J Gastroenterol Hepatol* 1997; **9**: 257–60.

66 Vaira D, Malfertheiner P, Megraud F *et al.* Diagnosis of Helicobacter pylori infection with a new non-invasive antigen-based assay. HpSA European study group. *The Lancet* 1999; **354**: 30–3.

67 Braden B, Teuber G, Dietrich CF, Caspary WF, Lembcke B. Comparison of new faecal antigen test with (13)C-urea breath test for detecting Helicobacter pylori infection and monitoring eradication treatment: prospective clinical evaluation. *BMJ* 2000; **320**: 148.

68 Atherton JC, Spiller RC. The urea breath test for Helicobacter pylori. *Gut* 1994; **35**: 723–5.

69 Moayyedi P, Braunholtz D, Heminbrough E *et al.* Do patients need to fast for a 13C-urea breath test? *Eur J Gastroenterol Hepatol* 1997; **9**: 275–7.

70 Logan RP, Polson RJ, Misiewicz JJ *et al.* Simplified single sample 13Carbon urea breath test for Helicobacter pylori: comparison with histology, culture, and ELISA serology. *Gut* 1991; **32**: 1461–4.

71 Rauws EA. Detecting Campylobacter pylori with the 13C- and 14C-urea breath test. *Scandinavian Journal of Gastroenterology* 1989; **160**: (suppl) 25–6.

72 Murnick DE, Peer BJ. Laser-based analysis of carbon isotope ratios. *Science* 1994; **263**: 945–7.

73 Koletzko S, Haisch M, Seeboth I *et al.* Isotope-selective non-dispersive infrared spectrometry for detection of Helicobacter pylori infection with 13C-urea breath test. *The Lancet* 1995; **345**: 961–2.

74 Lundell L, Dalenback J, Hattlebakk J *et al.* Outcome of Open Antireflux Surgery as Assessed in a Nordic Multicentre Prospective Clinical Trial. *European Journal of Surgery* 1998; **164**: 751–7. (Abstract)

75 Bais JE, Bartelsman JF, Bonjer HJ *et al.* Laparoscopic or conventional Nissen fundoplication for gastro-oesophageal reflux disease: randomised clinical trial. The Netherlands Antireflux Surgery Study Group. *The Lancet* 2000; **355**: 170–4.

76 Cuschieri A, Fayers P, Fielding J *et al.* Postoperative morbidity and mortality after D1 and D2 resections for gastric cancer: preliminary results of the MRC randomised controlled surgical trial. The Surgical Cooperative Group. *The Lancet* 1996; **347**: 995–9.

77 Allum WH, Powell DJ, McConkey CC, Fielding JW. Gastric cancer: a 25-year review. *British Journal of Surgery* 1989; **76**: 535–40.

78 Maruyama K, Okabayashi K, Kinoshita T. Progress in gastric cancer surgery in Japan and its limits of radicality. *World Journal of Surgery* 1987; **11**: 418–25.

79 Sue-Ling HM, Johnston D, Martin IG *et al.* Gastric cancer: a curable disease in Britain. *BMJ* 1993; **307**: 591–6.

80 Griffith JP, Sue-Ling HM, Martin I *et al.* Preservation of the spleen improves survival after radical surgery for gastric cancer. *Gut* 1995; **36**: 684–90.

81 Earlam R, Cunha-Melo JR. Oesophageal squamous cell carcinoma: I. A critical review of surgery. *British Journal of Surgery* 1980; **67**: 381–90.

82 Delaney B, Moayyedi P, Deeks J, Innes MA, Soo S, Barton P *et al.* The management of dyspepsia: a systematic review. *Health Technology Assessment* 2000; **4**: 1–189.

83 Delaney BC, Innes MA, Deeks J *et al.* Initial management strategies for dyspepsia. *Cochrane Database of Systematic Reviews* [computer file] 2000; CD001961.

84 Soo S, Moayyedi P, Deeks J, Delaney B, Innes M, Forman. Pharmacological interventions for non-ulcer dyspepsia. *Cochrane Database of Systematic Reviews* [computer file] 2000; CD001960.

85 Moayyedi P, Soo S, Deeks J *et al.* Eradication of Helicobacter pylori for non-ulcer dyspepsia. *Cochrane Database of Systematic Reviews* [computer file] 2000; CD002096.

86 Bytzer P, Hansen JM, Havelund T, Malchow-Moller A, Schaffalitzky de Muckadell OB. Predicting endoscopic diagnosis in the dyspeptic patient: the value of clinical judgement. *Eur J Gastroenterol Hepatol* 1996; **8**: 359–63.

87 Meineche-Schmidt V, Krag E. Relief of symptoms in patients with reflux-like or ulcer-like dyspepsia after 2 weeks treatment with either omeprazole, cimetidine, or placebo – a Danish multicenter trial in general-practice. *Gastroenterology* 1994; **106**: A539.

88 Agreus L, Talley NJ. Dyspepsia: current understanding and management. *Annu Rev Med* 1998; **49**: 475–93.

89 Paton S. Cost-effective treatment of gastro-oesophageal reflux disease – a comparison of two therapies commonly used in general practice. *Br J Med Econ* 1995; **8**: 85–95.

90 Chiba N, DeGara CJ, Wilkinson JM, Hunt RH. Speed of Healing and Symptom Relief in Grade II to IV Gastroeophageal Reflux Disease: A Meta-analysis. *Gastroenterology* 1997; **112**: 1798–810.

91 Barone JA, Jessen LM, Colaizzi JL, Bierman RH. Cisapride: a gastrointestinal prokinetic drug. *Annals of Pharmacotherapy* 1994; **28**: 488–500.

92 Hallissey MT, Allum WH, Jewkes AJ, Ellis DJ, Fielding JWL. Early detection of gastric cancer. *BMJ* 1990; **301**: 513–15.

93 Axon ATR, Bell GD, Jones RH, Quine MA, McCloy RF. Guidelines on appropriate indications for upper gastrointestinal endoscopy. *BMJ* 1995; **310**: 853–6.

94 Wilson S, Delaney BC, Roalfe A *et al.* Randomised controlled trials in primary care: case study. *BMJ* 2000; **321**: 24–7.

95 Lewin-van den Broek NT. Diagnostic and therapeutic strategies for dyspepsia in primary care. Utrecht: Thesis Universitiet Utrecht, 1999.

96 Delaney BC, Wilson S, Roalfe A *et al.* Cost-Effectiveness of Early Endoscopy for Dyspepsia in Patients of 50 Years of Age and Over: Results of a Primary Care Based Randomised Controlled Trial. *The Lancet* 2000; **356**: 1965–9.

97 Patel P, Khulusi S, Mendall MA *et al.* Prospective screening of dyspeptic patients by Helicobacter pylori serology. *The Lancet* 1995; **346**: 1315–18.

98 Jones RH, Tait CL, Sladen G, Weston-Baker JA. *Helicobacter* test and treat strategy: cost and outcomes in a randomised controlled trial in primary care. *Gastroenterology* 1998; **114**: A20. (Abstract)

99 Sobala GM, Crabtree JE, Pentith JA *et al.* Screening dyspepsia by serology to Helicobacter pylori. *The Lancet* 1991; **338**: 94–6.

100 Delaney B C, Wilson S, Roalfe A, Roberts L, Wearn A, Redman V, Briggs A, Hobbs FDR. A randomised controlled trial of Helicobacter pylori test and endoscopy for dyspepsia in primary care. *BMJ* 2001; **322**: 898–901.

101 Lassen AT, Pedersen FM, Bytzer P, Schaffalitzky dMO. Helicobacter pylori test-and-eradicate versus prompt endoscopy for management of dyspeptic patients: a randomised trial. *The Lancet* 2000; **356**: 455–60.

102 Heaney A, Collins JSA, Watson RGP *et al.* A prospective randomised trial of a 'test and treat' policy versus endoscopy based management in young Helicobacter pylori positive patients with ulcer-like dyspepsia, referred to a hospital clinic. *Gut* 1999; **45**: 186–90.

103 Ebell MH, Warbasse L, Brenner C. Evaluation of the dyspeptic patient: a cost-utility study. *Journal of Family Practice* 1997; **44**: 545–55.

104 Laine L, Hopkins RJ, Girardi LS. Has the impact of Helicobacter pylori therapy on ulcer recurrence in the United States been overstated? A meta-analysis of rigorously designed trials. *Am J Gastroenterol* 1998; **93**: 1409–1415.

105 Moore RA. *Helicobacter pylori and peptic ulcer.* Oxford: Cortecs Diagnostics and The Health Technology Assessment Association, 1995.

106 Penston JG. Review article: clincial aspects of Helicobacter pylori eradication therapy in peptic ulcer disease. *Alimentary Pharmacology & Therapeutics* 1996; **10**: 469–86.

107 Lai K, Hui W, Wong W, Wong BC, Hu WHC, Ching C, Lam S. Treatment of *Helicobacter pylori* in Patients With Duodenal Ulcer Hemorrhage – A Long-Term Randomized, Controlled Study. *The American Journal of Gastroenterology* 2000; **95**: 2225–32.

108 Rokkas T, Karameris A, Mavrogeorgis A, Rallis E, Giannikos N. Eradication of *Helicobacter pylori* reduces the possibility of rebleeding in peptic ulcer disease. *Gastrointestinal Endoscopy* 1995; **41**: 1–4.

109 Jaspersen D, Koerner T, Schorr W, Brennenstuhl M, Raschka C, Hammar CH. *Helicobacter pylori* eradication reduces the rate of rebleeding in ulcer hemorrhage. *Gastrointestinal Endoscopy* 1995; **41**: 5–7.

110 Yeomans ND, Tulassay Z, Juhasz L *et al.* A comparison of omeprazole with ranitidine for ulcers associated with nonsteroidal anti-inflammatory drugs. *N Engl J Med* 1998; **338**: 719–26.

111 Hawkey CJ, Karrasch JA, Szczepanski L *et al.* Omeprazole compared wth misoprostil for ulcers associated with nonsteroidal anti-inflammatory drugs. *N Eng J Med* 1998; **338**: 727–34.

112 Emery P, Zeidler H, Kvien TK *et al.* Celocoxib versus diclofenac in long-term management of rheumatoid arthritis: randomized double blind comparison. *The Lancet* 1994; **354**: 2106–11.

113 Laine L, Harper S, Simon T *et al.* A randomized trial comparing the effect of rofecoxib, a cyclooxygenase 2-specific inhibitor, with that of ibuprofen on the gastroduodenal mucosa of patients with osteoarthritis. *Gastroenterology* 1999; **117**: 776–83.

114 Cloud ML, Offen WW, Robinson M. Nizatidine versus placebo in gastroesophageal reflux disease: A 12 week, multicentre, randomized, double-blind study. *The American Journal of Gastroenterology* 1991; **86**: 1735–42.

115 Euler AR, Murdock RH, Wilson TH, Silver MT, Parker SE, Powers L. Ranitidine is Effective Therapy for Erosive Esophagitis. *The American Journal of Gastroenterology* 1993; **88**: 520–4.

116 Sontag S, Robinson M, McCallum RW, Barwick KW, Nardi R. Ranitidine Therapy for Gastro-esophageal Reflux Disease. *Archives of Internal Medicine* 1987; **147**: 1485–91.

117 Sabesin SM, Berlin RG, Humphries TJ, Bradstreet DC, Walton-Bowen KL, Zaidi S. Famotidine relieves symptoms of gastroesophageal reflux disease and heals erosions and ulcerations. Results of a multicentre, placebo-controlled, dose-ranging study. *Archives of Internal Medicine* 1991; **151**: 2394–400.

118 Palmer RH, Frank WO, Rockhold FW, Wetherington JD, Young MD. Cimetidine 800mg twice daily for healing erosions and ulcers in gastroesophageal reflux disease. *Journal of Gastroenterology* 1990; **12**: S29–S34.

119 Sherbaniuk R, Wensel R, Bailey R *et al.* Ranitidine in the Treatment of Symptomatic Gastro-esophageal Reflux Disease. *Journal of Clinical Gastroenterology* 1984; **6**: 9–15. (Abstract)

120 Roufail W, Belsito A, Robinson M, Barish C, Rubin A. Ranitidine for erosive oesophagitis: A double-blind placebo-controlled study. *Alimentary Pharmacology & Therapeutics* 1992; **6**: 597–607.

121 Simon TJ, Berenson MM, Berlin RG, Snapinn S, Cagliola A. Randomized, placebo-controlled comparison of famotidine 20mg bd or 40mg bd in patients with erosive oesophagitis. *Alimentary Pharmacology & Therapeutics* 1994; **8**: 71–9.

122 Quik RFP, Cooper MJ, Gleeson M, Hentschel E, Schuetze K, Kingston RD, Mitchell M. A comparison of two doses of nizatidine versus placebo in the treatment of reflux oesophagitis. *Alimentary Pharmacology & Therapeutics* 1990; **4**: 201–11.

123 Sontag S, Hirschowitz BI, Holt S, Robinson MG, Behar J, Berenson MM, McCullough A, Ippoliti AF, Richter JE, Ahtaridis G, McCallum RW, Pambianco DJ, Vlahcevic RZ, Johnson DA, Collen MJ, Lyon DT, Humphries TJ, Cagliola A, Berman RS. Two Doses of Omeprazole Versus Placebo in Symptomatic Erosive Esophagitis: The US Multicentre Study. *Gastroenterology* 1992; **102**: 109–18.

124 Hetzel DJ, Dent J, Reed WD, Narielvala FM, Mackinnon M, McCarthy JH, Mitchell B, Beveridge BR, Laurence BH, Gibson GG, Grant AK, Shearman DJC, Whitehead R, Buckle PJ. Healing and Relapse of Severe Peptic Esophagitis After Treatment With Omeprazole. *Gastroenterology* 1988; **95**: 903–912.

125 Bardhan KD, Hawkey CJ, Long RG, Morgan AG, Wormsley KG, Moules IK, Brocklebank D. Lansoprazole versus ranitidine for the treatment of reflux oesophagitis. *Alimentary Pharmacology & Therapeutics* 1995; **9**: 145–51.

126 Klinkenberg-Knol EC, Jansen JB, Festen HPM, Meuwissen SGM, Lamers CBHW. Double-blind multicentre comparison of omeprazole and ranitidine in the treatment of reflux oesophagitis. *The Lancet* 1987; **14**: 349–51.

127 Havelund T, Laursen LS, Skoubo-Kristensen E *et al.* Omerpazole and ranitidine in treatment of reflux oesophagitis: double blind comparitive trial. *BMJ* 1988; **296**: 89–92. (Abstract)

128 Sandmark S, Carlsson R, Fausa O, Lundell L. Omeprazole or Ranitidine in the Treatment of Reflux Esophagitis. Results of a Double-Blind, Randomized, Scandinavian Multicentre Study. *Scandinavian Journal of Gastroenterology* 1988; **23**: 625–32.

129 Bate CM, Keeling PWN, O'Morain C *et al.* Comparison of omeprazole and cimetidine in reflux oesophagitis: symptomatic, endoscopic and histological evaluations. *Gut* 1990; **31**: 968–72. (Abstract)

130 Dehn TCB, Shepherd HA, Colin-Jones D, Kettlewell MGW, Carroll NJH. Double blind comparison of omeprazole (40mg od) versus cimetidine (400mg qd) in the treatment of symptomatic erosive reflux oesophagitis, assessed endoscopically, histologically and by 24 h pH monitoring. *Gut* 1990; **31**: 509–13. (Abstract)

131 Koop H, Schepp W, Dammann HG, Schneider A, Luhmann R, Classen M. Comparative Trial of Pantoprazole and Ranitidine in the Treatment of Reflux Esophagitis. *Journal of Clinical Gastroenterology* 1995; **20**: 192–5.

132 Frame MH. Omeprazole produces significantly greater healing of erosive or ulcerative reflux oesophagitis than ranitidine. *European Journal of Gastroenterology & Hepatology* 1991; **3**: 511–17.

133 Robinson M, Sahba B, Avner D, Jhala N, Greski-Rose PA, Jennings DE. A comparison of lansprazole and ranitidine in the treatment of erosive oesophagitis. *Alimentary Pharmacology & Therapeutics* 1995; **9**: 25–31.

134 Vantrappen G, Rutgeerts L, Schurmans P, Coenegrachts JL. Omeprazole (40 mg) is superior to rantidine in short-term treatment of ulcerative reflux esophagitis. *Digestive Diseases & Sciences* 1988; **33**: 523–9.

135 Soga T, Matsuura M, Kodama Y *et al.* Is a proton pump inhibitor necessary for the treatment of lower-grade reflux esophagitis? *Journal of Gastroenterology* 1999; **34**: 435–40. (Abstract)

136 Bianchi Porro G, Pace F, Peracchia A, Bonavina L, Vigneri S, Scialabba A, Franceschi M. Short-Term Treatment of Refractory Reflux Esophagitis with Different Doses of Omeprazole or Rantidine. *Journal of Clinical Gastroenterology* 1992; **15**: 192–8.

137 Galmiche JP, Barthelemy P, Hamelin B. Treating the symptoms of gastro-oesophageal reflux disease: a double-blind comparison of omeprazole and cisapride. *Alimentary Pharmacology & Therapeutics* 1997; **11**: 765–73.

138 van Pinxteren B, Numans ME, Bonis PA, Lau J. Short-term treatment with proton pump inhibitors, H2-receptor antagonists and prokinetics for gastro-oesophageal reflux disease-like symptoms and endoscopy negative reflux disease. *Cochrane Database of Systematic Reviews* [computer file] 2000; CD002095.

139 Richter JE, Peura D, Benjamin SB, Joelsson B, Whipple J. Efficacy of Omeprazole for the Treatment of Symptomatic Acid Reflux Disease without Esophagitis. *Archives of Internal Medicine* 2000; **160**: 1810–16.

140 Richter JE, Campbell DR, Kahrilas PJ, Huang B, Fludas C. Lansoprazole Compared With Ranitidine for the Treatment of Nonerosive Gastroesophageal Reflux Disease. *Archives of Internal Medicine* 2000; **160**: 1803–9.

141 Dent J, Yeomans ND, Mackinnon M *et al.* Omeprazole v ranitidine for prevention of relapse in reflux oesophagitis. A controlled double blind trial of their efficacy and safety. *Gut* 1994; **35**: 590–8.

142 Vigneri S, Termini R, Leandro G *et al.* A comparison of five maintenance therapies for reflux esophagitis. *NEJM* 1995; **333**: 1106–10.

143 Bardhan KD, Muller-Lissner S, Bigard MA *et al.* Symptomatic gastro-oesophageal reflux disease: double blind controlled study of intermittent treatment with omeprazole or ranitidine. The European Study Group. *BMJ* 1999; **318**: 502–7.

144 Spechler SJ. Comparison of medical and surgical therapy for complicated gastroesophageal reflux disease in veterans. The Department of Veterans Affairs Gastroesophageal Reflux Disease Study Group. *NEJM* 1992; **326**: 786–92.

145 Lundell L, Miettinen P, Myrvold HE, Pedersen SA, Thor K, Lamm M, Blomqvist A, Hattlebakk J, Janatuinen E, Levander K, Nystrom P, Wiklund I. Long-term management of gastro-oesophageal reflux disease with omeprazole or open antireflux surgery: results of a prospective, randomized clincial trial. *European Journal of Gastroenterology & Hepatology* 2000; **12**: 879–87.

146 Nyren O, Adami HO, Bates S *et al.* Absence of therapeutic benefit from antacids or cimetidine in non-ulcer dyspepsia. *NEJM* 1986; **314**: 339–43.

147 Moayyedi P, Soo S, Deeks J, Innes MA, Forman D, Delaney BC. A Systematic Review and Economic Analysis of the Cost-Effectiveness of H Pylori Eradication Therapy in Non-Ulcer Dyspepsia (NUD). *BMJ* 2000; **321**: 659–64.

148 Winters C, Spurling TJ, Chobanian SJ *et al.* Barrett's oesophagus: a prevalent occult complication of gastro-esophageal reflux disease. *Gastroenterology* 1987; **92**: 118–24.

149 Stein HJ. Esophageal cancer: screening and surveillance. Results of a consensus conference held at the VIth world congress of the International Society for Diseases of the Esophagus. *Dis Esoph* 1996; **9(suppl 1)**: S3–S19.

150 Smith AM, Maxwell-Armstrong CA, Welch NT, Scholefield JH. Surveillance of Barrett's oesophagus in the UK. *British J of Surg* 1999; **86**: 276–80.

151 Provenzale D, Schmitt C, Wong JB. Barrett's esophagus: A new look at surveillance based on emerging estimates of cancer risk. *American J Gastroenterol* 1999; **94**: 2043–53.

152 Everett SM, Axon AT. Early gastric cancer: disease or pseudo-disease? *The Lancet* 351, 1350–2. 1998.

153 van Lanschot JJ, Hulscher JB, Buskens CJ, Tilanus HW *et al.* Hospital volume and hospital mortality for esophagectomy. *Cancer* 2001; **91**: 1574–8.

154 Teng TO, Adams ME, Pliskin JS, Safran DG, Siegel JE, Weinstein MC, Graham JD. Five-hundred life-saving interventions and their cost-effectiveness. *Risk Analysis* 1995; **15**: 369–90.

155 Everett SM, Axon AT. Early gastric cancer in Europe. *Gut* 1997; **41**: 142–50.

156 Williams B, Luckas M, Ellingham JMH, Dain A, Wicks ACB. Do young patients with dyspepsia need investigation? *The Lancet* 1988; **ii**: 1349–51.

157 Duggan A, Elliott C, Logan RPH, Hawkey CJ, Logan RFA. Does 'near patient' *H. pylori* testing in primary care reduce referral for endoscopy? Results from a randomised trial. *Gut* 1998; **42**: A82. (Abstract)

158 Lassen AT, Pedersen FM, Bytzer P, Schaffalitzky DMO. *H. pylori* 'test and treat' or prompt endoscopy for dyspeptic patients in primary care. A randomized controlled trial of two management strategies: one year follow-up. *Gastroenterology* 1998; **114**: A196. (Abstract)

159 Jones RH, Tait CL, Sladen G, WestonBaker JA. Helicobacter test and treat strategy: Costs and outcomes in a randomised controlled trial in primary care. *Gastroenterology* 1998; **114**: G0080.

160 Moayyedi P, Zilles A, Clough M, Heminbrough E, Chalmers DM, Axon AT. The effectiveness of screening and treating *Helicobacter pylori* in the management of dyspepsia. *Journal of Gastroenterology & Hepatology* 1999; **11**: 1245–50.

161 Anonymous. *BSG Guidelines in Gastroenterology: Dyspepsia Management Guidelines.* London: British Society of Gastroenterology, September 1996.

4 Black and Minority Ethnic Groups

Paramjit S Gill, Joe Kai, Raj S Bhopal and Sarah Wild

1 Summary

Statement of the problem/introduction

This chapter provides an overview of needs assessment for the Black and Minority Ethnic Groups (BMEGs). These groups are so diverse in terms of migration history, culture, language, religion and disease profiles that in this chapter we emphasise general issues pertinent to commissioning services. This is not a systematic review of literature on all diseases affecting BMEGs – the reader is referred to other chapters in this needs assessment series for details on specific disorders.

A number of general points are first provided as background to the chapter.

(a) As everyone belongs to an ethnic group (including the 'white' population), we have restricted our discussions to the non-white ethnic groups as defined by the 1991 census question. In addition, we do not cover needs of refugees and asylum seekers, whose number is growing within the UK.

(b) Principles of data interpretation are given to highlight important problems such as the interpretation of relative and absolute risk – the relative approach guides research, while the absolute approach guides commissioning.

(c) In the past, data on minority groups has been presented to highlight differences rather than similarities. The ethnocentric approach, where the 'white' group is used as the ideal, and partial analyses are made of a limited number of disorders, has led to misinterpretation of priorities. BMEGs have similar patterns of disease and overall health to the ethnic majority. There are a few conditions for which minority groups have particular health needs, such as the haemoglobinopathies.

(d) The majority of the research on health status and access and utilisation of health services has been skewed towards the South Asian and Afro-Caribbean populations, with little written on the other minority ethnic groups.

(e) There is an assumption that BMEGs' health is worse than the general population, and this is not always the case.

(f) The evidence base on many issues related to minority health is small and needs to be improved.

The historical and current migration patterns are important to local commissioning of services. Migration of communities from minority ethnic groups has been substantial during the latter half of the twentieth century, particularly from British Commonwealth countries such as Jamaica and India.

Problems of defining ethnicity, 'race' and culture are outlined, as they are complex concepts. Ethnicity is multi-dimensional and usually encompasses one or more of the following:

> 'shared origins or social background; shared culture and traditions that are distinctive, and maintained between generations, and lead to a sense of identity in groups; and a common language or religious tradition.'

It is also used as a synonym for 'race' to distinguish people with common ancestral origins. Indeed, 'race' has no scientific value and is a discredited biological term, but it remains an important political and psychological concept. Culture is briefly defined. An individual's cultural background has a profound influence on their health and healthcare, but it is only one of a number of influences on health – social, political, historical and economic, to name but a few.

Ethnic group has been measured by skin colour, country of birth, name analysis, family origin and as self-identified on the census question on ethnic group. All these methods are problematic, but it is accepted that the self-determined census question on ethnic group overcomes a number of conceptual limitations. For local ethnic monitoring, it is good practice to collect a range of information such as religion and languages spoken. There is a marked variation in quality of ethnic minority data collection and caution is advised in interpreting such data. Further training of staff is needed, together with mandatory ethnic coding clauses within the health service contracts.

Sub-categories

As BMEGs are not a homogeneous group, it is not easy to categorise them using standard format as in other chapters. For pragmatic reasons, we have used the following categories in this chapter:

- Indian
- Pakistani
- Bangladeshi
- Afro-Caribbean
- Chinese
- White.

Black and minority ethnic communities comprised, in 1991, 5.5% of the population of England and have a much younger age structure than the white group. It is important to note that almost half of the non-white group was born in the UK, which has important implications for future planning of services. BMEGs are also represented in all districts of Great Britain, with clustering in urban areas.

Prevalence and incidence

This section emphasises the importance of interpreting data on ethnic minority groups with care. One of the major issues is the comparison of health data of minority ethnic groups with those of the ethnic majority (i.e. 'the white population'). This ethnocentric approach can be misleading by concentrating on specific issues and diverting attention from the more common causes of morbidity and mortality. For example, while there may be some differences between ethnic groups in England, cardiovascular, neoplastic and respiratory diseases are the major fatal diseases for all ethnic groups. Even in the absence of specific local data, this principle is likely to hold.

In this section, two approaches are combined to give the absolute and relative disease patterns. Mortality in the UK can only be analysed by country of birth, and analysis has been carried out for people born in the following countries or groups of countries: India, Pakistan, Bangladesh, China/Hong Kong/Taiwan, the Caribbean islands and West/South Africa. In addition, lifestyle and some morbidity data are provided for Indians, Pakistanis, Bangladeshis, Chinese, Afro-Caribbean and white populations.

Due to the diversity and heterogeneous nature of all of the minority ethnic groups, it is not possible to give details of each specific disease by ethnic group. The top five causes of mortality (by ICD chapter) in all BMEGs are:

- diseases of the circulatory system (ICD 390–459)
- neoplasms (ICD 140–239)
- injury and poisoning (ICD 800–999)
- diseases of the respiratory system (ICD 460–519)
- endocrine, nutritional and metabolic diseases, and immunity disorders (ICD 240–279).

Mental health and haemoglobinopathies, which are specific to a number of minority ethnic groups, are also discussed.

Services available

This section provides an overview of services available and their use by minority groups. It focuses upon key generic issues (such as bilingual services) and specific issues (such as the haemoglobinopathies) which are of concern to minority ethnic communities.

On the whole there is no disparity in registration with general practitioner services by ethnic group except that non-registration seems to be higher amongst the African-Caribbean men. Data, from national surveys, show that – in general – minority ethnic groups (except possibly the Chinese) do not underuse either general practitioner or hospital services. After adjusting for socio-economic factors, minority ethnic respondents are equally likely to have been admitted to hospital. However, it appears that use of other community health services is lower than the general population. It is still not clear to what extent institutional racism and language and cultural barriers affect service utilisation.

Even though ethnic monitoring is mandatory within the secondary sector, there still is lack of quality data for adequate interpretation.

Data on cost of services for BMEGs is not available except for language provision and the haemoglobinopathies.

Effectiveness of services and interventions

In general, current evidence on the effectiveness and cost-effectiveness of specific services and interventions tailored to BMEGs is limited. As most studies have excluded individuals from the black and minority ethnic communities, there is a dearth of data on the effectiveness and cost-effectiveness in these groups. The reader is referred to other chapters for details of effectiveness and cost-effectiveness of specific services and interventions aimed at the whole population.

The quality of care provided is considered generally and with reference to cardiovascular disease and the haemoglobinopathies. In addition, specific services, such as communication, health promotion and training interventions, relevant to minority groups are mentioned.

Models of care recommendations

This section provides a generic framework for service development which includes the following points.

(a) Services for BMEGs should be part of 'mainstream' health care provision.
(b) The amended Race Relations Act should be considered in all policies.
(c) Facilitating access to appropriate services by:
   • promoting access – this will entail reviewing barriers to care and provision of appropriate information on services available
   • providing appropriate bilingual services for effective communication
   • education and training for health professionals and other staff
   • appropriate and acceptable service provision
   • provision of religious and dietary choice within meals offered in hospitals
   • ethnic workforce issues, including addressing racial discrimination and harassment within the workplace, and promoting race equality and valuing diversity in the workforce
   • community engagement and participation.
(d) Systematising structures and processes for capture and use of appropriate data.

Details of all services are not covered, as the above framework outlines the principles underpinning them. Service specifications (e.g. cervical screening) that are pertinent to BMEGs are given as examples and can be adapted to other conditions.

Outcome measures, common targets, information and research priorities

The importance of principles guiding further action on priorities are covered in this section, which include:

• national standards of quality of health care to be applied to BMEGs
• emphasis on basic needs, irrespective of similarities or differences between ethnic minority and majority populations
• emphasis on quality of service rather than specific conditions
• focus on a number of priorities rather than a large number
• being guided by priorities identified by, and for, the general population, e.g. *Saving lives: Our Healthier Nation Strategy for England*, as the similarities in the life problems and health patterns of minority ethnic groups exceed the dissimilarities
• considering the impact of policies and strategies in reducing health inequalities amongst BMEGs.

As the development of outcome measures for each disease/condition and ethnic group is in its infancy, existing outcome measures need to be adapted and validated before use.

Further, to improve the quality of care for the BMEGs, the following dimensions of heath services need monitoring: access, relevance, acceptability, effectiveness, efficiency and equity.

National targets for commissioners to achieve have been set and cover:

(a) the development of a diverse workforce
(b) specific diseases and
(c) service delivery issues.

There is a need for further information by ethnic group from primary care, as well as community and cancer screening services. The quality and completeness of ethnic monitoring data from secondary care needs to be improved. There is a need to include ethnic group data on birth/death certificates.

There are many gaps in knowledge and the following are the main priorities for further research:

- the need for incidence data on the major conditions affecting mortality and morbidity
- the evidence base by ethnic group on health status, access to services, health outcomes and cost-effectiveness of interventions is poor and needs to be addressed by all national commissioning bodies
- further evaluation of different models of providing bilingual services, such as physically present interpreters and advocates compared to telephone and telemedicine interpreting
- assessing the effect of racism on health and health care.

2 Introduction and statement of the problem

In this chapter we are not dealing with a specific disease category but a group. Black and Minority Ethnic Groups (BMEGs) are heterogeneous – they are populations grouped together by a concept – that of 'ethnic group'. There are conceptual difficulties with defining the latter and a pragmatic definition has been adopted. We can only provide an **overview** of the issues that commissioners of health services need to consider to meet the needs of these diverse groups. The reader is referred to other sources for details of particular ethnic groups as well as to chapters in this series for specific diseases or services. Some specific areas mentioned in *Saving Lives: Our Healthier Nation* (http://www.archive.official-documents.co.uk/document/cm43/4386/4386.htm) will be discussed, but in addition we want to highlight other priority areas which are also important for these groups.

There are some general points we want to emphasise:

(a) Everyone belongs to an ethnic group (including the 'white' population). We cannot provide a comprehensive review and have restricted our discussions to the non-white ethnic groups as defined by the 1991 census question. In addition, we do not cover needs of refugees and asylum seekers, whose number is growing within the UK. Refugees, again, are a diverse group who have wide-ranging health, social and educational needs, and the reader is referred to Aldous et al.[1] and Jones & Gill.[2]

(b) Principles of data interpretation are given to highlight important problems such as the interpretation of relative and absolute risk – the relative approach guides research, while the absolute approach guides commissioning.[3,4]

(c) In the past, data on minority groups has been presented to highlight differences rather than similarities. The ethnocentric approach, where the 'white' group is used as the ideal, and partial analyses are made of a limited range of disorders, has led to misinterpretation of priorities.[4,5] BMEGs have similar patterns of disease and overall health to the ethnic majority.[6,7] There are a few conditions for which minority groups have particular health needs such as the haemoglobinopathies.

(d) The majority of the research on health status and access and utilisation of health services has been skewed towards the South Asian and Afro-Caribbean populations,[8,9] with little written on the other minority ethnic groups.

(e) There is an assumption that BMEGs' health is worse than the population and this is not always the case.

(f) The evidence base on minority health is now sparse and needs to be improved.

Needs assessment is a relatively new concept and the process is outlined in Chapter One and by Wright et al.[10] This is a complex process for minority ethnic groups due, for example, to cultural diversity, languages spoken, and their genetic susceptibility to specific diseases. These health needs also change with time after migration.[11] This chapter builds upon previous work undertaken on needs assessment and minority ethnic groups which provides further insight into this complex area.[12,13]

Migration

Migration to Britain has been occurring for the past 40 000 years from all over the world so that everyone living in Britain today is either an immigrant or descended from one.[14]

It is important to note that immigrant and ethnic group are not synonymous, and nor should it be assumed that for all minority ethnic groups, immigration is for settlement purposes.[15] 'Immigrant' refers to someone who has arrived in this country for at least a year. **Figure 1** shows the growth of ethnic minority population within the last 30 years with data derived from the Labour Force Survey.[16] Note that this survey underestimates the BMEG population in comparison with the 1991 census.

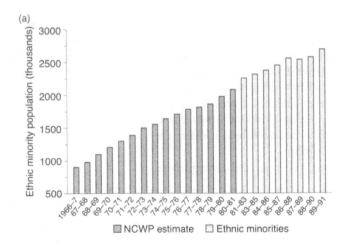

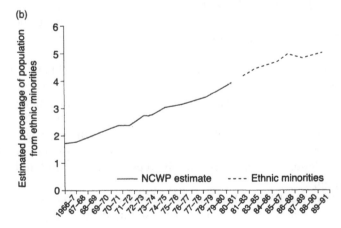

Figure 1: Trend in total ethnic minority population, 1966–67 to 1989–91. NCWP = New Commonwealth and Pakistan ethnic origin.

The reasons for this migration are complex and specific to groups.[17-21] During the late 1940s there was a need for labour, and British Commonwealth citizens were encouraged to come to Great Britain. This migration started with migrants from Jamaica, then the Indians arriving in the 1960s.[22] Under the British Nationality Act of 1948, citizens of the British Commonwealth were allowed to enter Britain freely, to find work, to settle and to bring their families. Many chose this option as a result of employer and government-led recruitment schemes. However, successive immigration policies since the 1960s have significantly reduced this option for persons from the New Commonwealth and Pakistan.[23] Political changes in East Africa ('Africanisation') stimulated a flow of 'Asian' refugees of Indian origin in the late 1960s and early 1970s.[24] The more recent migrants have come from the Sylhet region of Bangladesh, but most migration during the past 30 years or so has consisted of families of the earlier, mainly male, South Asian migrants coming to join their relatives.

Data for international migration for the UK are partial and complex.[25] Most of the data are based on administrative systems – related to control – rather than migrant numbers.[15] However, there is annual variation in net international migration, which contributed a third of the overall population growth.[26] Migration occurs from as well as into the UK.

The majority of people leave the UK due to work, whereas those arriving do so to accompany or join their families. Migrants to the UK are younger than those leaving. Within the UK, Chinese in their twenties are the most mobile group.[26]

Defining ethnicity, 'race' and culture

In this section, an overview of the problems of defining and describing ethnicity is highlighted, together with its measurement. A great deal of confusion surrounds the meaning of 'ethnicity' and it is commonly interchanged with 'race'. The latter is now a discredited biological term but it remains an important political and psychological concept.[27] Social scientists have been debating for some time on what different ethnic groups should be called[28,29] – the so-called 'battle of the name'.[30] This debate has also featured in health services research.[31-35]

What is ethnicity?

Ethnicity is also a multi-dimensional concept that is being used commonly in medical research.[34] It is neither simple nor precise and is not synonymous with 'race'. It embodies one or more of the following: 'shared origins or social background; shared culture and traditions that are distinctive, maintained between generations, and lead to a sense of identity and group; and a common language or religious tradition'.[4] It is also usually a shorthand term for people sharing a distinctive physical appearance (skin colour) with ancestral origins in Asia, Africa, or the Caribbean.[36] This definition also reflects self-identification with cultural traditions and social identity and boundaries between groups. Several authors[4,37] have stressed the dynamic nature and fluidity of ethnicity as a concept.

What is race?

Both race and ethnicity are complex concepts that are appearing in an increasing number of publications.[33] In the United States, the collection of data on race is well established and used extensively for epidemiological, clinical and planning purposes.[38] Buffon in 1749[39] first introduced race into the biological literature. It was explicitly regarded as an arbitrary classification, serving only as a convenient label and not a definable scientific entity. Race, however, carries connotations of genetic determinism and possibly of relative value.[40] It is known that 85% of all identified human genetic variation is accounted for by differences between individuals whereas only 7% is due to differences between what used to be called 'races'.[41] Current consensus is that 'race' has no scientific value[27] as there is more genetic variation within than between groups.[42]

What is culture?

The notion of culture was first defined by Taylor in 1871[43] as:

> 'That complex whole which includes knowledge, belief, art, morals, law, custom and any other capabilities and habits acquired by man as a member of society.'

Anthropologists have further refined this.[44,45] It is seen as a set of guidelines which state 'how to *view* the world, how to experience it *emotionally*, and how to *behave* in it in relation to other people, to supernatural forces or gods, and to the natural environment'.[45] These guidelines are passed on to the next generation to provide cohesion and continuity of a society.

Hence culture is a social construct that is constantly changing and notoriously difficult to measure.[46] 'Culture' is further complicated by societies consisting of *subcultures*[43] in which individuals undergo *acculturation*, adopting some of the attributes of the larger society.[45] Although an individual's cultural background has profound influence on their health and health care, it is only one of number of influences on health – social, political, historical and economic, to name but a few.[33,45,47]

Operationalising ethnicity

Given the importance of ethnicity on health, there are pragmatic grounds for assigning people into ethnicity groups. We would suggest the benefit of collecting data on ethnic group is to help reduce inequalities in health and health care. For the latter, guidelines have been recently produced for studying ethnicity, race and culture.[48]

A number of descriptions have been given to these ethnic groups – i.e. 'ethnic minorities', 'ethnic minority groups' or 'minority ethnic groups'. Note that these groups are not simply minorities in a statistical sense: they are both relatively small in number and in some way discriminated against on account of their ethnic identity.[47] As the title of this chapter states, we have used the term 'minority ethnic groups' to emphasise the question of population size. As stated earlier, we recognise that all individuals in all groups belong to an ethnic group[36] – it is simply that these groups vary in size, and the focus in this chapter is on the non-white group. In addition, the term 'black' has also been used as an inclusive political term to counter the divisive aspects of racism. Debate and controversy continues amongst other minority ethnic groups, as 'black' does not allow them to assert their own individuality in historical, cultural, ethical and linguistic terms.[49]

Several methods used to allocate individuals to ethnic groups are discussed briefly below:

(a) skin colour
(b) country of birth
(c) name analysis
(d) family origin and
(e) 1991 census question on ethnic group.

Skin colour

A classification based on physical traits (phenotype) seems an obvious way to measure ethnicity. Skin colour is subjective, imprecise and unreliable.[4] For example, colour cannot distinguish between the majority 'white' group (i.e. between the Irish and English) and minority ethnic groups (i.e. between Indians, Pakistanis and Bangladeshis).

Country of birth

The country of birth has been commonly used as a proxy for ethnicity,[50,51] as this was readily available – particularly on death certificates. A question on country of birth has been included in each census since 1841. It is an objective but crude method of classification. For example, it does not take account of the diversity of the country of origin of the individual; neither those 'white' people born in countries, such as India, ruled by the British Empire nor the children of immigrants (i.e. 'second-generation immigrants') are identified by this method.[4]

Name analysis

Name analysis has been used in several studies.[52,53,54] South Asian* names are distinctive and relate largely to religion,[55] where endogamy is the norm.[56] The validity of this method has been shown to be good,[55,57] though this will diminish with increasing exogamy.[56]

A software package, developed by Bradford Health Authority and the City of Bradford Metropolitan Council, is available which can identify South Asian names.[58] This program has been shown to have 91.0% sensitivity, 99% specificity and a positive predictive value of 87.5%.[59]

Family origin

This has been used in combination with the census question in a recent study.[60] This approach, based upon country of origin, is relatively straightforward and stable, 'though individuals within particular groups cannot be considered homogeneous in respect of factors related to self-determined ethnicity and health.'[49] Both self-perception and family origin are well related.[60] The difficulty with this approach occurs when an individual responds that they have mixed family origins.[60]

1991 census question on ethnic group

Despite the inclusion in the 1920 Census Act of 'race' as an issue upon which questions might be asked, there has been a long history to the acceptance of an 'ethnic question' in the 1991 census.[61,62] The 1991 census question on ethnic group is a pragmatic, self-determined ethnic group question which was found to be acceptable despite conceptual limitations.[63]

The 1991 census was the first in Great Britain to include a question on ethnic group. Before this, reliable information on ethnic groups was derived from data on country of birth; the Labour Force and General Household Surveys (*see* http://www.data-archive.ac.uk/ for further details).

---

* South Asian refers to individuals who were born in or originate from the Indian subcontinent (India, Pakistan, Bangladesh, Sri Lanka).

The census ethnic question may not meet the needs of all researchers and commissioners, and several authors have suggested that extra information is collected, such as languages spoken and religion, to describe the groups being studied.[4,37,48]

The question also does not deal adequately with people of mixed parentage[64] – most of whom have one minority parent and one white.[60] In addition, the white group conflates a number of groups which have distinct cultural, geographical and religious heritages, i.e. those of Irish, Greek or Turkish origin.

It has been estimated that the census missed 2.2% of the resident population (about 1.2 million people) due to such factors as non-response, one-person households and transient populations, and unpopularity of the community charge.[65] This undercount was not uniform across ethnic groups, age, gender, or geographic areas. To adjust for this, imputed data has been developed (Appendix 1).[66]

Why collect data on ethnic group?

There are two main reasons for this. First, national data was needed to assess the scale of disadvantage and discrimination amongst the Black and Minority Ethnic Groups.[67] Secondly, primary data was required, as it was no longer viable to rely on surrogate measures, i.e. country of birth, for planning.[68]

Coding of ethnic group in the 1991 census

The 1991 census question (**Box 1**) included two categories – 'Black other' and 'Any other ethnic group' – to allow individuals to describe their ethnic group in their words if they felt none of the pre-coded boxes (numbered 0 to 6) was suitable. To deal with these 'written' answers and also with multi-ticking of boxes, the Census Offices developed an extended classification containing 35 categories in all (Appendix 2).

Box 1: The ethnic group question in the 1991 Census of Great Britain

Ethnic group	White	☐	0
	Black-Caribbean	☐	1
Please tick the appropriate box	Black-African	☐	2
	Black-Other	☐	
	please describe ...		
	Indian	☐	3
	Pakistani	☐	4
	Bangladeshi	☐	5
	Chinese	☐	6
If the person is descended from more than one ethnic or racial group, please tick the group to which the person considers he/she belongs, or tick the 'Any other group' box and describe the person's ancestry in the space provided.	Any other ethnic group *please describe ...*	☐	

Due to a number of limitations,[69] including lack of recognition of the significant Irish group resident in this country, the 2001 question as been modified as shown in **Box 2**. A question on religion and country of birth, but not proficiency in English language, has been also added.[69]

Box 2: 2001 Census ethnic group categories

Choose ONE section from a to e, then tick the appropriate box to indicate your cultural background.

a. **White**
- British ☐
- Irish ☐
- Any other White background, *please write in* ☐

b. **Mixed**
- White and Black Caribbean ☐
- White and Black African ☐
- White and Asian ☐
- Any other mixed background, *please write in* ☐

c. **Asian or Asian British**
- Indian ☐
- Pakistani ☐
- Bangladeshi ☐
- Any other Asian background, *please write in* ☐

d. **Black or Black British**
- Caribbean ☐
- African ☐
- Any other Black background, *please write in* ☐

e. **Chinese and other ethnic group**
- Chinese ☐
- Any other, *please write in* ☐

Ethnic monitoring

Ethnic monitoring was introduced in all hospitals in 1995 to enable the NHS to provide services without racial or ethnic discrimination. Currently, the use and the delivery of services vary on these grounds, with or without intent, which hinders the achievement of equity in the NHS.[36] As the census categories may be insufficient to meet the needs of the local population, these categories should be adapted for the particular service and may include items such as religion, language, or dietary requirements.[70]

As there is marked variation in quality of data collection by speciality, particularly mental health services,[71] caution is advised in using this data. Further training of staff is needed together with mandatory coding clauses within contracts.[71]

There is a call for ethnic monitoring to be implemented within the primary care setting,[72] as feasibility has been demonstrated.[73,74]

For local purposes, it is good practice to collect a range of information,[48] such as:

- self-assigned ethnicity (using nationally agreed guidelines enabling comparability with census data)
- country or area of birth (the subject's own, or that of parents and grandparents, if applicable)
- years in country of residence

- religion
- language.

3 Sub-categories

Who are they?

However we define ethnicity (*see* 'What is ethnicity?' above), the 'ethnic label' is a crude indicator of need. For pragmatic reasons we have used the census ethnic question to define ethnic group in this chapter. The more detailed classification is used for the majority of tables in the printed *Country/Region Reports* and the Local *Base Statistics* released in computer-readable form for further analyses by local authorities and researchers. The fourfold classification is used in the Small Area Statistics, a computerised dataset for the 145 000 Enumeration Districts and Output Areas in Great Britain.[75] These are the smallest areas for which census data is released, each containing approximately 200 households.

Pragmatic categorisation

BMEGs are not a homogeneous group, so it is not easy to categorise them using standard format as in other chapters. For pragmatic reasons we have therefore used the following ethnic group (self-assigned/country of birth) categories:

- Indian
- Pakistani
- Bangladeshi
- Afro-Caribbean
- Chinese
- White.

How many are there?

In the 1991 census over 3 million people (5.5% of the population) identified themselves as belonging to one of the non-white ethnic groups (**Table 1**). South Asians (Indians, Pakistanis, Bangladeshis) together formed 2.7% of the British population. 'Black' ethnic groups accounted for 1.6% of the population, with Black-Caribbeans being the largest group. Chinese were 0.3% of the population (**Table 1**).

Age and sex structure

Figure 2 presents age-sex pyramids by ethnic group in which the black shading in each population pyramid represents the percentage of each ethnic group born outside the UK.[16] First note that the minority ethnic groups have a much younger age structure than the white group. The Black-Caribbean population has an hour glass structure, with the bottom half of the structure representing the UK-born children of the first-generation immigrants. Secondly, almost half (46.8%) of the non-white group were born in the United Kingdom.[16]

Also note that Bangladeshi men outnumber the women in the older age groups and the Pakistani pattern is similar, albeit less pronounced. Black-Caribbean women outnumber Black-Caribbean men, though part of this may be due to underenumeration of young Black-Caribbean men (*see* '1991 census question on ethnic group' above). Among other Asians, there is again a preponderance of females.

Table 1: Ethnic group composition of the population in 1991 (percentages).

Ethnic group	Great Britain	England & Wales	England	Wales	Scotland
White	94.5	94.1	93.8	98.5	98.7
Ethnic minorities	**5.5**	**5.9**	**6.2**	**1.5**	**1.3**
Black	*1.6*	*1.8*	*1.9*	*0.3*	*0.1*
Black-Caribbean	0.9	1.0	1.1	0.1	0.0
Black-African	0.4	0.4	0.4	0.1	0.1
South Asian	*2.7*	*2.9*	*3.0*	*0.6*	*0.6*
Indian	1.5	1.7	1.8	0.2	0.2
Pakistani	0.9	0.9	1.0	0.2	0.4
Bangladeshi	0.3	0.3	0.3	0.1	0.0
Chinese & Others	*1.2*	*1.2*	*1.3*	*0.6*	*0.5*
Chinese	0.3	0.3	0.3	0.2	0.2
Total population	54,888.8	49,890.3	47,055.2	2,835.1	4,998.6

Source: Owen 1992[75]

For further details on the major ethnic groups, see Peach 1996.[21]

Estimating future population size of an ethnic group is complicated and has to take into account not only fertility, mortality and net migration, but also ethnic identity.[76] There will, for reasons obvious from **Figure 2**, be more elderly Black-Caribbeans and Indians. This has major implications for health and social care.[77,78]

The assumption that minority elders have supportive extended families is false[79] – the need for health and social care will grow.

Figure 2: Age and sex distribution of persons born within and outside the UK by ethnic group 1991. Note: darker shading represents persons born outside UK.[16]

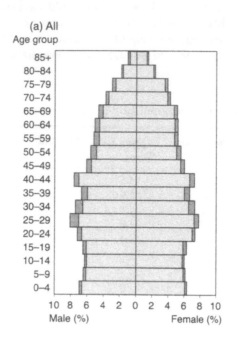

(a) All

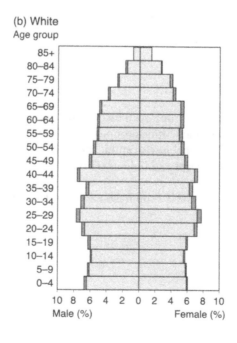

(b) White

(c) Ethnic minorities

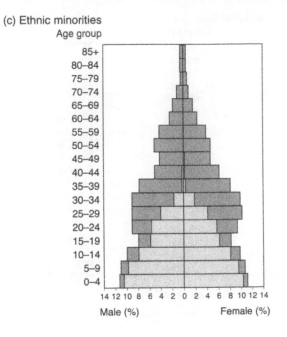

(d) Black

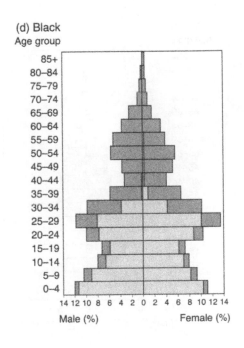

(e) Black Caribbean

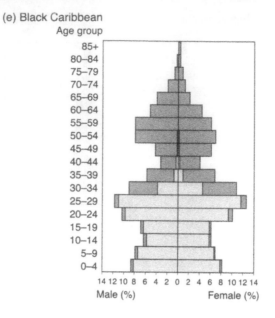

(f) Black African

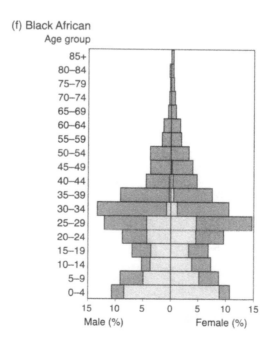

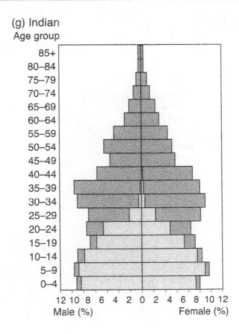

(g) Indian

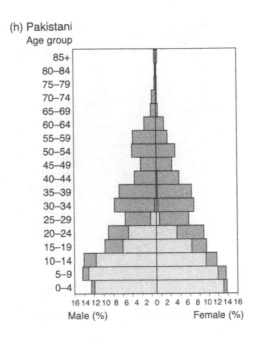

(h) Pakistani

(i) Bangladeshi
Age group

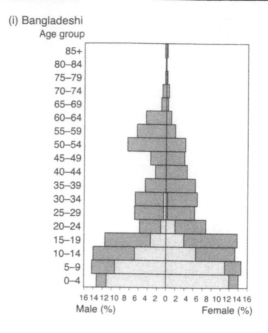

(j) Chinese
Age group

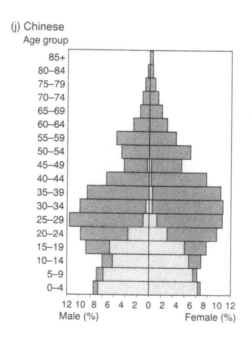

Where are they living?

Black and Minority Ethnic Groups are represented in all districts of Great Britain.[80] The geographical distribution varies across the country, with clustering in urban areas.

Table 2: Regional variations in ethnic composition, within Great Britain 1991.

Region or metropolitan county	Percentage of resident population						
	All ethnic minorities	Black		Indian	Pakistani	Bangla-deshi	Chinese
		Caribbean	African				
South East	9.9	1.9	1.0	2.6	0.8	0.6	0.5
Greater London	20.2	4.4	2.4	5.2	1.3	1.3	0.8
East Anglia	2.1	0.2	0.1	0.3	0.3	0.1	0.2
South West	1.4	0.3	0.1	0.2	0.1	0.1	0.1
West Midlands	8.2	1.5	0.1	3.1	1.9	0.4	0.2
West Midlands MC	14.6	2.8	0.2	5.5	3.5	0.7	0.2
East Midlands	4.8	0.6	0.1	2.5	0.4	0.1	0.2
Yorks & Humberside	4.4	0.4	0.1	0.8	2.0	0.2	0.2
South Yorkshire	2.9	0.5	0.1	0.3	1.0	0.1	0.2
West Yorkshire	8.2	0.7	0.1	1.7	4.0	0.3	0.2
North West	3.9	0.3	0.1	0.9	1.2	0.2	0.3
Greater Manchester	5.9	0.7	0.2	1.2	2.0	0.5	0.3
Merseyside	1.8	0.2	0.2	0.2	0.1	0.1	0.4
North	1.3	0.0	0.0	0.3	0.3	0.1	0.2
Tyne & Wear	1.8	0.0	0.1	0.4	0.3	0.3	0.3
Wales	1.5	0.1	0.1	0.2	0.2	0.1	0.2
Scotland	1.3	0.0	0.1	0.2	0.4	0.0	0.2
Great Britain	5.5	0.9	0.4	1.5	0.9	0.3	0.3

Source: adapted from Owen 1996[16]

Over 70% of the combined ethnic minorities are clustered in two regions of Great Britain, the South East and the West Midlands, which together contain 40% of the total population of Great Britain. These are the only regions of the country where the region's share of minority groups is higher than its share of the total population (**Table 3**). The Black-Caribbean and Black-African groups reside predominantly in the Greater London area. The Indians also reside in Greater London as well as the East and West Midlands. On the other hand, there is a relatively low proportion of Pakistanis in Greater London with their greatest concentration in West Yorkshire and the West Midlands Metropolitan County. The Bangladeshis are found predominantly in Greater London particularly in Tower Hamlets.[81] The Chinese community is much more evenly distributed throughout Great Britain. Detailed geographical spread by district is given in Rees & Philips (1996).[80]

Table 3: Ethnic population by standard regions, Great Britain 1991.

Region	Total	% of Great Britain	Minority	% of minority
North	3,026,732	5.5	38,547	1.3
Yorks and Humberside	4,836,524	8.8	214,021	7.1
East Midlands	3,953,372	7.2	187,983	6.2
East Anglia	2,027,004	3.7	43,395	1.4
South East	17,208,264	31.3	1,695,362	56.2
South West	4,609,424	8.4	62,576	2.1
West Midlands	5,150,187	9.4	424,363	14.1
North West	6,243,697	11.4	244,618	8.1
Wales	2,835,073	5.2	41,551	1.4
Scotland	4,998,567	9.1	62,634	2.1
Great Britain	54,888,844	100.0	3,015,050	100.0

Source: Peach 1996[22]

Social class profile

Table 4 shows that socio-economic position of the minority groups differs significantly. The Chinese, Black-African and Indian males are strongly represented in class I. On the other hand, Black-Caribbean, Pakistani and Bangladeshi are over-represented in classes IV and V.

Table 4: Social class by gender of residents aged 16 and over in Great Britain (%).

	I	II	III (NM)	III (M)	IV	V	Total*
Males							
White	7	29	11	33	15	5	1,226,189
Black-Caribbean	2	17	11	40	22	8	9,803
Black-African	13	25	18	19	17	8	2,839
Indian	13	30	14	23	17	3	18,581
Pakistani	7	23	13	30	22	5	6,547
Bangladeshi	5	11	18	30	31	5	1,970
Chinese	17	21	20	32	8	2	34,334
Females							
White	2	28	39	7	16	8	981,909
Black-Caribbean	1	33	33	7	18	8	10,742
Black-African	4	32	28	7	17	12	2,658
Indian	5	24	35	6	27	3	13,197
Pakistani	4	27	34	7	26	2	2,048
Bangladeshi	5	21	32	9	30	3	393
Chinese	8	30	31	13	13	5	2,797

* Excludes those who were serving in the armed forces and those whose occupation was inadequately described or not stated.

Source: adapted from OPCS/GRO(S) 1993[66]

Females are less well represented in class I than males. The Chinese fare better, with nearly 70% in the higher socio-economic groups (classes I-III (NM)).

Note that this data needs to be interpreted cautiously, as it is recognised that measurement of social class by these groupings is limited. These groupings are not internally homogeneous, so that ethnic minorities could be found in lower occupational grades.[82]

Unemployment

Figure 3 shows the variation in unemployment rates by ethnic group with the Black-Caribbean unemployment rate double the national, Black-African rates three times as high, while Pakistani and Bangladeshi rates being highest of all (29 and 32% respectively).

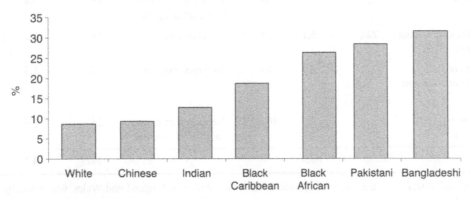

Source: adapted from Owen, 1993[83]

Figure 3: % Unemployment by ethnic group, Great Britain 1991.

4 Prevalence and incidence

Epidemiological approaches

Traditional epidemiological approaches have defined priorities using data on actual and relative mortality, years of life lost, morbidity and loss of social functioning. Ethnicity and race have been used as variables for measurement of such needs by ethnic group. The most popular approach has been to compare the health statistics of ethnic minority groups in relation to those of the population as a whole or the ethnic majority – i.e. in Britain, the 'white' population. Essentially, a disease that is commoner than in the white population is declared a problem and a relatively higher priority than one that is less common than in the white population. This comparative perspective, which is ethnocentric, has some intuitive merit but can also mislead. By concentrating on specific issues, attention may be given to a narrow range of services and drawn away from ensuring that all services are equitable and available to all. This approach has led to some needs of ethnic minorities being ignored, e.g. respiratory diseases and lung cancer.

Table 5: Deaths and SMRs* in male immigrants from the Indian subcontinent (aged 20 and over; total deaths = 4,352).

By rank order of number of deaths				By rank order of SMR			
Cause	Number of deaths	% of total	SMR	Cause	Number of deaths	% of total	SMR
Ischaemic heart disease	1,533	35.2	115	Homicide	21	0.5	341
Cerebrovascular disease	438	10.1	108	Liver and intrahepatic bile duct neoplasm	19	0.4	338
Bronchitis, emphysema and asthma	223	5.1	77	Tuberculosis	64	1.5	315
Neoplasm of the trachea, bronchus and lung	218	5.0	53	Diabetes mellitus	55	1.3	188
Other non-viral pneumonia	214	4.9	100	Neoplasm of buccal cavity and pharynx	28	0.6	178
Total	2,626	60.3	–		187	4.3	–

* Standardised mortality ratios, comparing with the male population of England and Wales, which was by definition 100.
Source: adapted from Senior and Bhopal 1994[4]

This is shown in **Table 5,** which contains data originally presented by Marmot and colleagues.[51] The two columns give radically different perspectives on disease patterns. Generally, when presented using the number of cases, major health problems for minority groups are seen as similar to those of the population as a whole. When presented using the SMR, the differences are emphasised. For example, while there are some differences between ethnic groups in Britain, circulatory diseases, cancer and respiratory diseases are the major fatal diseases for all ethnic groups. Even in the absence of specific local data, this principle is likely to hold: that the important diseases and other health problems of the population generally will also be important to minority ethnic groups. The relative risk approach, which focuses on diseases more or less common in minority ethnic groups, can refine the analysis and interpretation of conclusions reached using simple counts of cases. Interpretation of data has often been misguided by an excessive emphasis on:

- differences rather than similarities
- the uncritical use of 'white populations' as a standard to which minority populations should aspire
- the use of partial analysis and datasets, e.g. looking at a limited number of conditions or particular age groups, leading to misinterpretation of the priorities.

The pattern of disease and interpretation of priorities and needs depends on the mode of presentation of data. The recommendations arising are the following.

- Base the epidemiological component of the needs assessment on ranked causes based on case numbers and disease rates.
- Refine understanding by looking at comparative indices such as the SMR, which will focus attention on inequalities and inequities.
- Draw causal hypotheses based on differences with care, and with due emphasis on social and economic deprivation as explanatory factors.
- Be aware that inferences of biological difference between ethnic/racial groups may be particularly prone to error and misinterpretation, and may harm the standing of minority groups.

In this section we combine the two approaches and give the actual and relative disease patterns. In studying the pattern of disease for health needs assessment, the following are basic items of information:

- the number of cases
- the disease rate, i.e. number of cases per unit of population per unit time, for example 10 cases per 1000 population per year
- the rank position of the disease in question based on the number of cases or rates
- the rate relative to that expected, e.g. the SMR or relative risk
- the rank based on SMRs.

Unfortunately, most existing reports and papers neither present analyses in this format nor provide the information to permit readers to extract it themselves.

Collecting and interpreting epidemiological data for health needs assessment

Questions which are essential to the process of health needs assessment include the following.

- Which ethnic groups are to be studied? Are the ethnic categories used to define population sub-groups acceptable, ethical and accurate?
- What data need to be collected? Have we collected accurate, representative data?
- How do we derive from the data a true picture of the health and health care needs and priorities?

The answer to the first question is usually dictated by the classification used at census. For national studies reliant on census data for denominator information, this is invariably the case. While we may be interested in the pattern of health and disease in Muslims, Punjabis, Hindi-speakers, or those from the Gujarat, such patterns are unlikely to be available, at least from national data. The nearest we can get is the appropriate category at census. Clearly this is a weakness, but the census is the key to building a picture of the ethnic minority communities and analysing and interpreting most epidemiological data, and its limitations are noted (section '1991 census question on ethnic group' above).

Using pragmatic categories can be misleading. For example, one ethnic category that is commonly used is 'South Asian' or 'Asian' as a label for people from India, Pakistan, Bangladesh and Sri Lanka. This label leads to an erroneous view that South Asians are ethnically homogeneous – which may have adverse consequences for health. For example, Bangladeshi men had an extremely high prevalence of current smoking (49%) compared to all South Asian men (26%).[84] Indian men reported a prevalence of 19%, and white men 34%. The same survey showed many important differences by religious affiliation too.

The answer to the second question depends on the underlying purpose. In health needs assessment the challenge is to provide both professionals and members of ethnic minority communities with balanced information to allow them to make informed choices about priority issues and to make rational judgements on the actions to be taken. The value of mortality and morbidity data is self-evident. Despite a national policy for ethnic health monitoring, reliable national statistics on hospital utilisation are not available. Information on the patterns of (non-fatal) ill-health is difficult to obtain. Cancer registrations include country of birth and are published for some areas.

Except in some health authorities with very large ethnic minority populations, local information on causes of death will be hard to make sense of, simply because the numbers of deaths per year will be small. Knowing the make-up of the local ethnic minority community, it is possible to gauge the major health problems by applying the findings from national data to the local populations. Even in the absence of any data on the causes of death in the ethnic group of interest, disease patterns are likely to be similar to the general population, e.g. coronary heart disease, strokes and cancers are major fatal diseases for all ethnic groups in Britain.

Lifestyle is a major determinant of health. All aspects of lifestyle which are important for the general population are important for ethnic minorities, including smoking, alcohol, exercise, diet in relation to chronic disease, and stress. These must not be overlooked when undertaking health promotion with ethnic minorities (there is evidence that this can happen). Other lifestyle issues worth noting in some communities include, e.g. the use of traditional substances such as eye cosmetics that may contain heavy metals, self-treatment with herbal and other remedies, and a strong sense of modesty, especially among women, which may affect the health (vitamin D deficiency) and health care (physical examination).[85] Many such traditional customs have been recorded and much attention has been given to them. However, their overall importance to health is small in comparison with the issues in the above paragraph.

Statistics on self-reported health status and on aspects of lifestyle are in some respects easier to interpret than disease rates, in other respects more difficult. In the two main nationally relevant sources of data – the surveys by the Health Education Authority[86–88] and by the Policy Studies Institute[84] – the main focus is on presenting numbers and percentages, usually giving the figures for the 'white' ethnic majority population. With some simple manipulation of the statistics, ranks can be ascertained and comparisons made. The interpretation of such data in the context of health needs assessment requires the same wary approach outlined for the SMR.

Note that the Health Survey for England for 1999 focused on BMEGs and has produced further useful data. The full anonymised dataset for this survey is available through the Data Archive at Essex University (http://www.data-archive.ac.uk/).

There are some subtle difficulties in comparing ethnic groups in lifestyle and self-reported health. The most important questions to ask are the following.

- Are the populations comparable? It is common practice to draw samples for different ethnic groups using different methods. Differences are inevitable, and may have no relation to ethnicity *per se*, if the samples are different. For example, if some of the ethnic populations are inner city ones, and others are a mix of urban and rural populations, differences will inevitably result.
- Are the data collected equally valid in the different ethnic groups? The concepts underpinning questions (let us say on angina) may be interpreted differently in different ethnic groups. Where questions need translating, the potential pitfalls are magnified.

These limitations need to be remembered in health needs assessment. The validity of health statistics for minority ethnic groups is based on several assumptions: that ethnicity categories and specific ethnic group designations are not only valid but that they are consistently defined and ascertained; also that such categories and designations are completely understood by the populations questioned; that participation and response rates are high and similar for all populations questioned; and that people's responses are consistent over time.

Data

Available data on mortality and lifestyles can be re-analysed or extracted from published documents to provide a foundation in the epidemiological contribution to the health needs assessment process. The demonstration of missing gaps is important to guide future work. National hospital data are not available, and information on disease incidence, as opposed to mortality and prevalence, is unavailable.

Mortality analyses

Limitations of mortality analyses

The accuracy and validity of the numerator (death data) and denominator (population data) and the possibility of numerator-denominator bias should be considered. Death data include information on any person dying in England and Wales and thereby include deaths of visitors, but only include information on residents of England and Wales who die in other countries if these are notified to consulates. Such reporting probably varies across different populations. Recording of country of birth on death certificates, which is reliant on an informant, may be less accurate than on the census, when the person is still alive to provide the information, leading to the possibility of numerator-denominator bias (i.e. where country of birth is recorded differently in census and mortality data). Previous analyses of mortality by country of birth have grouped together countries for which this is a particular issue (e.g. South Asian countries),[51] but this approach obscures potentially important differences between countries of birth. Death certificates do not provide an accurate reflection of prevalence of certain conditions in the general population e.g. diabetes mellitus.[89] Variation in accuracy of cause of death described on death certificates by country of birth has not been studied but may exist. The census excludes people who are not normally residents, but deaths of visitors are included in the numerator. Census data is not complete and no data were obtained for 2.2% of the population in 1991. Underenumeration varied by population and was greatest for Afro-Caribbean men of 20–29 years of age.[90] The effect of underenumeration is to increase apparent mortality rates. As the census occurs only every 10 years, information on population size becomes rapidly inaccurate. Restricting the mortality analyses to the years around the census minimises the effect of population variations. In these analyses we have used four years of mortality data to increase the number of deaths to allow meaningful analysis.

At present, analyses of mortality are limited to the use of country of birth because ethnic group is not available on death certificates. Country of birth is an inexact measure of ethnicity as demonstrated by the cross-tabulation of country of birth by ethnic group given in the 1991 census.[91] For example, of people born in West Africa, 73% described themselves as being of black African origin and 22% described themselves as being of a white ethnic group. Several studies of immigrant populations have suggested that mortality experience tends to approximate to that of the host population with both time and succeeding generations.[51,92] The healthy migrant effect is a term used to describe the fact that migrants as a whole tend to be healthier than the populations they leave and join. There is also, however, the possibility that people migrate as a consequence of ill-health. Country of birth provides no indication of length of stay in that country. Mortality by country of birth is a particularly poor measure of health in children – very few children living in this country were born abroad and mortality statistics are a very incomplete measure of health of children. Socio-economic factors are also likely to influence migration and health.

Some of these limitations can be overcome by analysing data from the Longitudinal Study, a 1% sample of people enumerated by the 1971 census (http://www.statistics.gov.uk/services/longitudinal.asp). Unfortunately, the number of deaths in this dataset is too small for accurate interpretation. We have provided two tables (*see* **Tables 19 and 20**) showing the major causes of death by ethnic group as a means of corroborating the general findings on the major causes of death from the national data.

Methods

The Office for National Statistics provided population and death data for England and Wales. Population data were available from the 1991 census by sex and country of birth in five-year age groups. Death data for the four-year period around the census 1989–92 were available by sex, age, country of birth and underlying cause of death coded using the ninth revision of the International Classification of Diseases (ICD-9).

For this analysis, six countries or groups of countries were studied, as for many countries the numbers of deaths were too small to permit separate tables. West/South Africa denotes data from people born in the Gambia, Ghana, Sierra Leone, Nigeria, Botswana, Lesotho, Swaziland and Zimbabwe. The term Caribbean is used to cover the following countries: Barbados, Jamaica, Trinidad & Tobago, Guyana, Belize, West Indies and other Caribbean islands. Data for people born in Hong Kong, China and Taiwan were combined into a single group that we call Chinese. Data for people born in Bangladesh, India and Pakistan are analysed for individual countries.

Death data are presented in various forms (*see* 'Epidemiological approaches' and 'Collecting and interpreting epidemiological data for health needs assessment' above). The average number of deaths per year over the four-year period is given to provide information on absolute mortality and to permit the reader to assess the reliability of estimates of rates and SMR. Age-standardised death rates per 100 000 population per year were calculated by using the direct method for each sex by five-year age group with 1991 data on population of England and Wales as the standard. Comparisons between standardised rates for men and women are not directly comparable because age distribution differs between men and women. Comparisons between ethnic groups for each sex separately are possible for directly standardised rates within any age group. Population data by country of birth for five age groups are given in Appendix 3.

Standardised mortality ratios (SMRs) were calculated using the indirect method – i.e. reference rates generated from numbers of deaths and population data for England and Wales as a whole by sex and five-year age group applied to populations by country of birth to estimate the expected number of deaths by cause and sex. The SMR is calculated as the ratio of observed to expected deaths for various causes of death, sex and age groups with 95% confidence intervals calculated using the number of deaths over the four-year period. SMRs for individual causes of death were examined for the 20–74 year age group. SMRs cannot be compared either across the sexes or ethnic groups, as age distributions differ by sex and ethnic group, i.e. the SMR can only be compared in relation to the standard for each sex of 100.

The cause-specific mortality tables are presented in rank of the number of deaths by ICD chapter. The main text gives data for the top five causes of death, again at the level of the ICD chapter. In presenting the findings, attention is drawn to the major causes of death, and where the excess is substantial, and the number of deaths is not insignificant, to high SMRs. Readers may also wish to note low SMRs, even though space does not permit the authors to comment in detail.

Mortality patterns

Tables 6–17 summarise the mortality analyses for each country of birth group. The even numbered tables show age-specific death rates for the age groups 0–19 years, 20–44 years, 45–64 years, 65–74 years, 75+ years, and also all age mortality. The odd-numbered tables give the causes of death at ages 20–74 combined. Numbers of deaths in the youngest age group are very small. These tables indicate that SMRs for large age bands can obscure differences that are noted in smaller age bands. SMRs tend to be closer to 100 for older age groups, whereas for younger age groups SMRs tend to exceed 100. As a consequence of smaller numbers of deaths at younger ages, confidence intervals around SMRs tend to be wider. The data confirm that major causes of death are not necessarily associated with high SMRs. Some of the findings of interest are discussed below for each country of birth group.

Indian-born

Table 6(a) shows that while death rates were highest in Indian men aged 75 years and more, most deaths actually occurred in the age group 45–74, reflecting the relatively small size of the population over 75 years. The overall SMR was marginally above the population average (103), with the SMR varying by age – the value of 112 in the 20–44 age group being the most notable finding.

Table 6(b) shows fewer deaths (and lower death rates) in each age group than in **Table 6(a)**, largely reflecting women's better survival compared to men. The overall SMR was 113, indicating that Indian women had higher mortality than the whole population of women. (Men and women cannot, for reasons already discussed, be compared on the SMR or the all age-standardised rate.)

Table 6(a): Age-specific mortality for males born in India (1989–92).

Mortality by age group	Average number of deaths/yr	Directly age-standardised rate/100,000/yr	SMR (95% CI)
Under 20 years of age	4.75	66	93 (56–145)
20–44 years of age	131	137	112 (103–122)
45–64 years of age	1,050	1,355	106 (103–109)
65–74 years of age	653	6,156	102 (98–106)
75+ years of age	478	14,224	95 (91–100)
All ages	2,318	1,156	103 (101–105)

Table 6(b): Age-specific mortality for females born in India (1989–92).

Mortality by age group	Average number of deaths/yr	Directly age-standardised rate/100,000/yr	SMR (95% CI)
Under 20 years of age	4	52	137 (77–227)
20–44 years of age	68	64	93 (82–105)
45–64 years of age	586	852	108 (103–112)
65–74 years of age	568	4,331	122 (117–127)
75+ years of age	657	12,832	113 (109–117)
All ages	1,883	1,281	113 (110–115)

Circulatory diseases, and specifically ischaemic heart disease, were the dominant causes of death in men (**Table 7(a)**) and women (**Table 7(b)**). These SMRs corroborate past analyses showing these diseases as 30–50% more common in Indians compared to the population as a whole.[5,6] The rates/100 000 show that Indian men have much more circulatory disease than women, a point obscured in SMR analyses.

Neoplasms were a dominant cause of death, even though the SMR is lower than in the whole population, and in contrast to the little attention they sometimes receive, the commonest neoplasms in Indians are lung cancer in men and breast cancer in women.

Injury and poisoning was the third ranking cause of death in men, and the fifth in women (**Tables 7(a)** and **7(b)**). The SMR for women was raised.

Table 7(a): Causes of mortality ranked by number: Indian-born men.

Mortality by cause of death (first number is ICD-9 chapter codes) for 20–74 year olds	Average number of deaths per year	Average directly age-standardised death rate per 100,000 per year	SMR (95% CI)
7. DISEASES OF THE CIRCULATORY SYSTEM (390–459)	861	495	134 (130–139)
Chronic rheumatic heart disease (393–398)	5.25	3.1	147 (91–224)
Hypertensive disease (401–405)	12	6.8	145 (107–192)
Ischaemic heart disease (410–414)	668	380	142 (137–147)
Cerebrovascular disease (430–438)	120	73	134 (123–147)
Diseases of arteries, arterioles and capillaries (440–448)	21.25	13	62 (50–77)
2. NEOPLASMS (140–239)	275	160	59 (55–62)
Malignant neoplasm of lip, oral cavity and pharynx (140–149)	8	4.7	89 (61–126)
Malignant neoplasm of nasopharynx (147)	0.5	0.3	64 (8–231)
Malignant neoplasm of oesophagus (150)	14.5	8.6	64 (49–83)
Stomach cancer (151)	13	7.0	42 (31–55)
Colorectal cancer (153/154)	26	15	49 (40–59)
Liver cancer (155)	7.5	4.1	118 (80–169)
Lung cancer (162)	68	40	44 (39–50)
Prostate cancer (185)	38	22	78 (63–96)
Malignant neoplasm of lymphatic and haematopoietic tissue (200–208)	22.5	15	110 (93–129)
17. INJURY AND POISONING (800–999)	94	54	110 (99–122)
Poisoning by drugs, medicinals and biological substances (960–979)	2.25	1.4	177 (81–336)
8. DISEASES OF THE RESPIRATORY SYSTEM (460–519)	87	53	85 (76–95)
Pneumonia and influenza (480–487)	18	11	89 (70–112)
Chronic obstructive pulmonary disease and allied conditions (490–496)	55	35	77 (67–88)
9. DISEASES OF THE DIGESTIVE SYSTEM (520–579)	71	37	158 (140–178)
Diseases of oesophagus, stomach and duodenum (530–537)	11	6.3	103 (74–138)
Cirrhosis (571)	44	21	247 (212–287)
3. ENDOCRINE, NUTRITIONAL AND METABOLIC DISEASES, AND IMMUNITY DISORDERS (240–279)	58	33	230 (201–262)
Diabetes mellitus (250)	51	30	317 (275–364)
Disorders of thyroid gland (240–246)	0	0	0.0 (0–501)
1. INFECTIOUS AND PARASITIC DISEASES (001–139)	21	12	269 (186–375)
Tuberculosis (010–018)	10	6.2	529 (379–717)
6. DISEASES OF THE NERVOUS SYSTEM AND SENSE ORGANS (320–389)	16.5	10	67 (52–85)
Inflammatory diseases of the central nervous system (320–326)	1	0.6	104 (28–267)
Multiple sclerosis (340)	0.75	0.3	24 (5–70)

Table 7(a): Continued.

10. DISEASES OF THE GENITO-URINARY SYSTEM (580–629)	11	6.8	144 (105–192)
Nephritis, nephrotic syndrome and nephrosis (580–589)	7.75	4.8	194 (132–276)
Diseases of male genital organs (600–608)	0.25	0.2	23 (1–128)
5. MENTAL DISORDERS (290–319)	10.5	6.3	109 (78–147)
Senile and presenile organic psychotic conditions (290)	2.5	1.5	61 (29–112)
4. DISEASES OF BLOOD AND BLOOD-FORMING ORGANS (280–289)	5.25	3	137 (85–209)
13. DISEASES OF THE MUSCULO-SKELETAL SYSTEM AND CONNECTIVE TISSUE (710–739)	5.25	3.1	119 (74–182)
14. CONGENITAL ANOMALIES (740–759)	3	2.0	75 (38–130)
16. SYMPTOMS, SIGNS AND ILL-DEFINED CONDITIONS (780–799)	2.5	1.4	88 (42–161)
12. DISEASES OF THE SKIN AND SUBCUTANEOUS TISSUE (680–709)	0.75	0.4	110 (23–321)

Death from diseases of the respiratory system is common and only slightly less common than in the whole population. The importance of digestive disorders as a cause of death is noteworthy, as are the high and relatively high rates of cirrhosis in men (but low in Indian women, *see* **Table 7(b)**).

Diabetes mellitus is substantially commoner in Indians, men and women, than in the population as a whole, and a major killer. For all these diseases the cardiovascular risk factors, including smoking, are of prime importance in either initiating or promoting disease.

The sizeable variations in the SMRs in various conditions are worthy of note, particularly for cirrhosis in men, tuberculosis in men and women and nephritis.

Pakistani-born

Table 8(a) shows, strikingly, that while death rates are highest in the oldest age groups, most deaths occurred in 45–64 year olds (reflecting the population structure). The overall SMR was lower than the population average for men, with an excess only in the under 20 year age group.

Table 8(b) shows that the number of deaths and death rates were lower in women than men. Again, in comparison to the population average for women, there was a raised SMR in the under 20 year age group but overall the SMR was substantially lower than the population average.

In Pakistani men, and to a lesser extent in women, circulatory diseases dominate (**Tables 9(a)** and **9(b)**). In women, the SMR for ischaemic heart disease was only 11% higher than the whole population, with a bigger excess in cerebrovascular disease. As for Indians, neoplasms were the second ranking cause of death. Diabetes mellitus outranked respiratory diseases in men and women. Cirrhosis was, unlike Indians, not especially common in Pakistanis. Injury and poisoning were high in Pakistani men (**Table 9(a)**), but not so in women (**Table 9(b)**).

Table 7(b): Ranked causes of mortality: Indian-born women.

Mortality by cause of death (first number is ICD-9 chapter codes) for 20–74 year olds	Average number of deaths per year	Average directly age-standardised death rate per 100,000 per year	SMR (95%CI)
7. DISEASES OF THE CIRCULATORY SYSTEM (390–459)	413	268	149 (135,164)
Chronic rheumatic heart disease (393–398)	6.75	4.1	97 (64,141)
Hypertensive disease (401–405)	11	7.2	159 (69–313)
Ischaemic heart disease (410–414)	261	178	158 (148–168)
Cerebrovascular disease (430–438)	103	74	146 (119–178)
Diseases of arteries, arterioles and capillaries (440–448)	10	6.7	68 (29–133)
2. NEOPLASMS (140–239)	254	147	70 (61,79)
Malignant neoplasm of lip, oral cavity and pharynx (140–149)	5.75	2	93 (19,272)
Malignant neoplasm of nasopharynx (147)	0.25	0.3	68 (2,381)
Oesophageal cancer (150)	9.25	6.4	88 (35,181)
Stomach cancer (151)	4.25	1	9 (0,50)
Colorectal cancer (153/154)	23	12	58 (35,89)
Liver cancer (155)	5	2.5	132 (36–338)
Malignant neoplasm of trachea, bronchus and lung (162)	22	15	31 (18,48)
Malignant neoplasm of lymphatic and haematopoietic tissue (200–208)	24	15	108 (87,131)
Malignant neoplasm of cervix uteri (180)	13	7.8	65 (30,123)
Malignant neoplasm of female breast (174)	59	32	67 (58,65)
8. DISEASES OF THE RESPIRATORY SYSTEM (460–519)	56	38	91 (68–119)
Pneumonia and influenza (480–487)	15	10	99 (52–169)
Chronic obstructive pulmonary disease and allied conditions (490–496)	30	21	68 (45,99)
3. ENDOCRINE, NUTRITIONAL AND METABOLIC DISEASES, AND IMMUNITY DISORDERS (240–279)	47	30	262 (189–352)
Diabetes mellitus (250)	42	28	333 (238–453)
Disorders of thyroid gland (240–246)	0.5	0.3	0 (0,543)
17. INJURY AND POISONING (800–999)	41	23	142 (121,166)
Poisoning by drugs, medicinals and biological substances (960–979)	0.75	0.4	123 (25,359)
9. DISEASES OF THE DIGESTIVE SYSTEM (520–579)	35	21	99 (67,140)
Diseases of oesophagus, stomach and duodenum (530–537)	6	4	105 (39,228)
Cirrhosis (571)	8.5	4.8	45 (15,105)
1. INFECTIOUS AND PARASITIC DISEASES (001–139)	17	9.7	305 (167–512)
Tuberculosis (010–018)	8.5	5.2	810 (263–1,889)
6. DISEASES OF THE NERVOUS SYSTEM AND SENSE ORGANS (320–389)	13.25	8.5	52 (25–96) (35,328)
Inflammatory diseases of the central nervous system (320–326)	1.0	0.5	43 (18,84)
Multiple sclerosis (340)	2.0	1.1	131 (56–258)

Table 7(b): Continued.

10. DISEASES OF THE GENITO-URINARY SYSTEM (580–629)	12	7.8	155 (42–398)
Nephritis, nephrotic syndrome and nephrosis (580–589)	6.5	4.3	90 (36,185)
13. DISEASES OF THE MUSCULO-SKELETAL SYSTEM AND CONNECTIVE TISSUE (710–739)	10	6.6	44
5. MENTAL DISORDERS (290–319)	3	2.3	(23,77)
Senile and presenile organic psychotic conditions (290)	2.25	1.85	58 (26,110)
4. DISEASES OF BLOOD AND BLOOD-FORMING ORGANS (280–289)	2.75	1.8	100 (50,178)
11. COMPLICATIONS OF PREGNANCY, CHILDBIRTH AND THE PUERPERIUM (630–676)	1.5	1.1	288 (106–627)
14. CONGENITAL ANOMALIES (740–759)	0.75	0.4	22 (4,64)
12. DISEASES OF THE SKIN AND SUBCUTANEOUS TISSUE (680–709)	0.5	0.3	0 (0,549)
16. SYMPTOMS, SIGNS AND ILL-DEFINED CONDITIONS (780–799)	0.5	0.3	45 (5,61)

Table 8(a): Age-specific mortality for males born in Pakistan (1989–92).

Mortality by age group	Average number of deaths/yr	Directly age-standardised rate/100,000/yr	SMR (95% CI)
Under 20 years of age	14	109	124 (94–161)
20–44 years of age	68	111	89 (79–100)
45–64 years of age	365	1,285	101 (96–107)
65–74 years of age	79	4,331	74 (66–83)
75+ years of age	44	8,370	58 (49–67)
All ages	571	887	90 (87–94)

Table 8(b): Age-specific mortality for females born in Pakistan (1989–92).

Mortality by age group	Average number of deaths/yr	Directly age-standardised rate/100,000/yr	SMR (95% CI)
Under 20 years of age	8	55	144 (98–203)
20–44 years of age	43	68	101 (87–118)
45–64 years of age	129	693	91 (83–99)
65–74 years of age	44	2,903	81 (69–93)
75+ years of age	41	6,192	54 (46–63)
All ages	267	772	83 (78–88)

Table 9(a): Ranked causes of mortality: Pakistani-born men.

Mortality by cause of death (first number is ICD-9 chapter codes) for 20–74 year olds	Average number of deaths per year	Average directly age-standardised death rate per 100,000 per year	SMR (95% CI)
7. DISEASES OF THE CIRCULATORY SYSTEM (390–459)	291	489	139 (131–147)
Chronic rheumatic heart disease (393–398)	1.5	1.6	123 (45–268)
Hypertensive disease (401–405)	2.75	3.6	101 (51–181)
Ischaemic heart disease (410–414)	229	372	148 (138–158)
Cerebrovascular disease (430–438)	42	72	149 (127–174)
Diseases of arteries, arterioles and capillaries (440–448)	6.75	13	67 (44–97)
2. NEOPLASMS (140–239)	76	123	48 (43–54)
Malignant neoplasm of lip, oral cavity and pharynx (140–149)	3.5	6.9	108 (59–180)
Malignant neoplasm of nasopharynx (147)	0.25	0.2	81 (2–449)
Malignant neoplasm of oesophagus (150)	1	1.0	13 (4–34)
Stomach cancer (151)	3.5	6.2	35 (19–58)
Colorectal cancer (153/154)	5	7.8	28 (17–44)
Liver cancer (155)	3.5	5.5	158 (86–265)
Lung cancer (162)	17	32	34 (27–43)
Prostate cancer (185)	2.5	20	31 (15–57)
Malignant neoplasm of lymphatic and haematopoietic tissue (200–208)	16	6.2	120 (92–154)
17. INJURY AND POISONING (800–999)	29	36	62 (51–74)
Poisoning by drugs, medicinals and biological substances (960–979)	1	0.8	131 (36–334)
3. ENDOCRINE, NUTRITIONAL AND METABOLIC DISEASES, AND IMMUNITY DISORDERS (240–279)	25	47	258 (210–314)
Diabetes mellitus (250)	23	44	418 (336–514)
Disorders of thyroid gland (240–246)	0	0	0.0 (0–1,559)
8. DISEASES OF THE RESPIRATORY SYSTEM (460–519)	22	40	70 (56–86)
Pneumonia and influenza (480–487)	4.75	8.6	68 (41–106)
Chronic obstructive pulmonary disease and allied conditions (490–496)	14	25	64 (48–84)
9. DISEASES OF THE DIGESTIVE SYSTEM (520–579)	14	19	84 (64–110)
Diseases of oesophagus, stomach and duodenum (530–537)	1.25	1.8	37 (12–85)
Cirrhosis (571)	7.5	10.1	105 (71–150)
1. INFECTIOUS AND PARASITIC DISEASES (001–139)	8.5	13.5	269 (186–375)
Tuberculosis (010–018)	3.25	6	466 (248–796)
6. DISEASES OF THE NERVOUS SYSTEM AND SENSE ORGANS (320–389)	7.25	8	77 (51–110)
Inflammatory diseases of the central nervous system (320–326)	0.25	1	61 (2–341)
Multiple sclerosis (340)	0.5	0.5	40 (5–143)

Table 9(a): Continued.

10. DISEASES OF THE GENITO-URINARY SYSTEM (580–629)	4	6	160 (91–260)
Nephritis, nephrotic syndrome and nephrosis (580–589)	3.25	5	248 (132–424)
Diseases of male genital organs (600–608)	0	0	0 (0–317)
5. MENTAL DISORDERS (290–319)	2.5	5.1	66 (32–122)
Senile and presenile organic psychotic conditions (290)	0.75	2.3	71 (15–209)
13. DISEASES OF THE MUSCULO-SKELETAL SYSTEM AND CONNECTIVE TISSUE (710–739)	1.5	2.4	105 (38–227)
14. CONGENITAL ANOMALIES (740–759)	1.25	1.4	63 (21–148)
16. SYMPTOMS, SIGNS AND ILL-DEFINED CONDITIONS (780–799)	1	0.9	77 (21–197)
4. DISEASES OF BLOOD AND BLOOD-FORMING ORGANS (280–289)	0.5	1.4	38 (5–137)
12. DISEASES OF THE SKIN AND SUBCUTANEOUS TISSUE (680–709)	0.25	0.3	109 (3–608)

Table 9(b): Ranked causes of mortality: Pakistani-born women.

Mortality by cause of death (first number is ICD-9 chapter codes) for 20–74 year olds	Average number of deaths per year	Average directly age-standardised death rate per 100,000 per year	SMR (95% CI)
7. DISEASES OF THE CIRCULATORY SYSTEM (390–459)	73	189	122 (108–137)
Chronic rheumatic heart disease (393–398)	1	1.2	62 (17–158)
Hypertensive disease (401–405)	2.25	5.7	203 (93–385)
Ischaemic heart disease (410–414)	38	107	111 (93–130)
Cerebrovascular disease (430–438)	24	62	159 (129–194)
Diseases of arteries, arterioles and capillaries (440–448)	1.75	1.9	74 (30–152)
2. NEOPLASMS (140–239)	54	106	55 (48–63)
Malignant neoplasm of lip, oral cavity and pharynx (140–149)	1.75	3.8	196 (79–403)
Malignant neoplasm of nasopharynx (147)	0.25	0.6	208 (5–1,157)
Oesophageal cancer (150)	0	0	0 (0–49)
Stomach cancer (151)	2	3.4	75 (32–148)
Colorectal cancer (153/154)	2.75	4.4	32 (16–58)
Liver cancer (155)	0.75	1.0	90 (19–262)
Malignant neoplasm of trachea, bronchus and lung (162)	4.5	10	31 (18–49)
Malignant neoplasm of lymphatic and haematopoietic tissue (200–208)	5	7.8	77 (47–118)
Malignant neoplasm of cervix uteri (180)	1.25	3.5	25 (8–58)
Malignant neoplasm of female breast (174)	13	20	49 (37–64)

Table 9(b): Continued.

Mortality by cause of death (first number is ICD-9 chapter codes) for 20–74 year olds	Average number of deaths per year	Average directly age-standardised death rate per 100,000 per year	SMR (95% CI)
8. DISEASES OF THE RESPIRATORY SYSTEM (460–519)	13.75	46	105 (79–137)
Pneumonia and influenza (480–487)	2.75	9.9	92 (46–165)
Chronic obstructive pulmonary disease and allied conditions (490–496)	7.25	24	82 (55–118)
3. ENDOCRINE, NUTRITIONAL AND METABOLIC DISEASES, AND IMMUNITY DISORDERS (240–279)	13.5	39	316 (237–412)
Diabetes mellitus (250)	12	38	425 (313–563)
Disorders of thyroid gland (240–246)	0.5	0.5	320 (39–1,157)
1. INFECTIOUS AND PARASITIC DISEASES (001–139)	9.5	22	627 (443–860)
Tuberculosis (010–018)	5.75	14	2,219 (1,407–3,329)
·17. INJURY AND POISONING (800–999)	9.5	11	69 (49–95)
Poisoning by drugs, medicinals and biological substances (960–979)	0.5	0.4	92 (11–332)
9. DISEASES OF THE DIGESTIVE SYSTEM (520–579)	6	11	71 (45–105)
Diseases of oesophagus, stomach and duodenum (530–537)	1.25	2.5	96 (31–223)
Cirrhosis (571)	2.25	3.4	63 (29–119)
10. DISEASES OF THE GENITO-URINARY SYSTEM (580–629)	4	5.8	263 (150–427)
Nephritis, nephrotic syndrome and nephrosis (580–589)	3	4.4	480 (248–838)
13. DISEASES OF THE MUSCULO-SKELETAL SYSTEM AND CONNECTIVE TISSUE (710–739)	3	7.0	160 (83–280)
6. DISEASES OF THE NERVOUS SYSTEM AND SENSE ORGANS (320–389)	2.75	4.2	47 (24–84)
Inflammatory diseases of the central nervous system (320–326)	0.25	0.2	90 (2–504)
Multiple sclerosis (340)	0.25	0.5	16 (0–88)
11. COMPLICATIONS OF PREGNANCY, CHILDBIRTH AND THE PUERPERIUM (630–676)	1.5	0.75	408 (150–888)
4. DISEASES OF BLOOD AND BLOOD-FORMING ORGANS (280–289)	1.25	2.3	167 (54–390)
14. CONGENITAL ANOMALIES (740–759)	1.25	2.6	85 (28–198)
5. MENTAL DISORDERS (290–319)	0.5	2.0	30 (4–107)
Senile and presenile organic psychotic conditions (290)	0.5	2.0	77 (9–278)
12. DISEASES OF THE SKIN AND SUBCUTANEOUS TISSUE (680–709)	0.25	0.3	152 (4–844)
16. SYMPTOMS, SIGNS AND ILL-DEFINED CONDITIONS (780–799)	0	0	0 (0–226)

It is noteworthy that infectious and parasitic diseases, though relatively very common (SMR = 335), were the fifth ranking cause of death in Pakistani women.

The data demonstrate the vital importance of controlling cardiovascular risk factors, including smoking, and better control of diabetes in Pakistanis.

Bangladeshi-born

Table 10(a) shows a huge preponderance of deaths in the 45–64 age group, though, as before, death rates rose with age. The SMR was raised, compared to the population average, in this age group, but was substantially lower in the others. For women (**Table 10(b)**), numbers of deaths and death rates were substantially lower than in men. The overall SMR, and SMRs within each age band, were substantially lower than the population average.

Table 11(a) shows that in men, the disease patterns were similar to Indians and Pakistanis (circulatory disease and neoplasms dominating), with an exceptionally high SMR from liver cancer and diabetes. Cirrhosis was a relatively common cause of death in men but not woman.

Table 11(b) shows that the number of deaths in women were small, but neoplasms and circulatory diseases were the commonest cause of death. In women, coronary heart disease rates were relatively low in comparison to the whole population.

Bangladeshi men are in urgent need of interventions to reduce their cardiovascular risk and control diabetes.

Table 10(a): Age-specific mortality for males born in Bangladesh (1989–92).

Mortality by age group	Average number of deaths/yr	Directly age-standardised rate/100,000/yr	SMR (95% CI)
Under 20 years of age	7	47	63 (42–91)
20–44 years of age	11		
	77	50 (36–67)	
45–64 years of age	210	1,725	136 (127–145)
65–74 years of age	22	5,159	88 (71–109)
75+ years of age	4	5,953	40 (23–64)
All ages	255	973	114 (107–121)

Table 10(b): Age-specific mortality for females born in Bangladesh (1989–92).

Mortality by age group	Average number of deaths/yr	Directly age-standardised rate/100,000/yr	SMR (95% CI)
Under 20 years of age	2	16	32 (13–65)
20–44 years of age	12		
	52	81 (59–107)	
45–64 years of age	30	704	82 (68–98)
65–74 years of age	6	2,299	69 (44–103)
75+ years of age	4	4,248	69 (44–103)
All ages	53	620	70 (61–80)

Table 11(a): Ranked causes of mortality: Bangladeshi-born men.

Mortality by cause of death (first number is ICD-9 chapter codes) for 20–74 year olds	Average number of deaths per year	Average directly age-standardised death rate per 100,000 per year	SMR (95% CI)
7. DISEASES OF THE CIRCULATORY SYSTEM (390–459)	128	536	156 (143–170)
Chronic rheumatic heart disease (393–398)	0	0	0 (0–190)
Hypertensive disease (401–405)	0.75	1.8	71 (15–208)
Ischaemic heart disease (410–414)	93	370	151 (136–167)
Cerebrovascular disease (430–438)	29	148	281 (232–337)
Diseases of arteries, arterioles and capillaries (440–448)	1	3.8	27 (7–69)
2. NEOPLASMS (140–239)	52	229	83 (72–95)
Malignant neoplasm of lip, oral cavity and pharynx (140–149)	0.75	19	56 (11–162)
Malignant neoplasm of nasopharynx (147)	0	0	0 (0–693)
Malignant neoplasm of oesophagus (150)	1.25	9	40 (13–94)
Stomach cancer (151)	1.75	9.4	44 (18–90)
Colorectal cancer (153/154)	3.5	19	49 (27–83)
Liver cancer (155)	8.5	27	948 (656–1,324)
Lung cancer (162)	18	91	92 (72–116)
Prostate cancer (185)	0.75	1.4	26 (5–75)
Malignant neoplasm of lymphatic and haematopoietic tissue (200–208)	5.5	25	109 (68–165)
3. ENDOCRINE, NUTRITIONAL AND METABOLIC DISEASES AND IMMUNITY DISORDERS (240–279)	15	52	410 (312–528)
Diabetes mellitus (250)	14	49	670 (506–870)
Disorders of thyroid gland (240–246)	0.25	2.1	1,111 (28–6,191)
9. DISEASES OF THE DIGESTIVE SYSTEM (520–579)	13	41	204 (152–268)
Diseases of oesophagus, stomach and duodenum (530–537)	3.5	17	266 (146–447)
Cirrhosis (571)	6.5	13	235 (153–344)
8. DISEASES OF THE RESPIRATORY SYSTEM (460–519)	11	47	94 (69–127)
Pneumonia and influenza (480–487)	3	14	120 (62–209)
Chronic obstructive pulmonary disease and allied conditions (490–496)	7	31	89 (59–128)
17. INJURY AND POISONING (800–999)	8	29	46 (31–65)
Poisoning by drugs, medicinals and biological substances (960–979)	0.25	7.6	90 (2–503)
1. INFECTIOUS AND PARASITIC DISEASES (001–139)	5.75	16	486 (308–729)
Tuberculosis (010–018)	1	4.3	378 (103–968)
10. DISEASES OF THE GENITO-URINARY SYSTEM (580–629)	2.25	13	242 (110–458)
Nephritis, nephrotic syndrome and nephrosis (580–589)	1	6.8	202 (55–518)
Diseases of male genital organs (600–608)	0	0	0 (0–928)

Table 11(a): Continued.

6. DISEASES OF THE NERVOUS SYSTEM AND SENSE ORGANS (320–389)	1.25	2.2	36 (12–83)
Inflammatory diseases of the central nervous system (320–326)	0.5	0.8	317 (38–1,144)
Multiple sclerosis (340)	0	0	0 (0–190)
4. DISEASES OF BLOOD AND BLOOD–FORMING ORGANS (280–289)	0.25	0.6	51 (1–284)
5. MENTAL DISORDERS (290–319)	0.25	4.1	19 (0–106)
Senile and presenile organic psychotic conditions (290)	0	0	0 (0–265)
12. DISEASES OF THE SKIN AND SUBCUTANEOUS TISSUE (680–709)	0.25	0.5	300 (8–1,670)
14. CONGENITAL ANOMALIES (740–759)	0.25	0.4	33 (1–182)
13. DISEASES OF THE MUSCULO-SKELETAL SYSTEM AND CONNECTIVE TISSUE (710–739)	0	0	0 (0–167)
16. SYMPTOMS, SIGNS AND ILL–DEFINED CONDITIONS (780–799)	0	0	0.0 (0–191)

Table 11(b): Ranked causes of mortality: Bangladeshi-born women.

Mortality by cause of death (first number is ICD-9 chapter codes) for 20–74 year olds	Average number of deaths per year	Average directly age-standardised death rate per 100,000 per year	SMR (95% CI)
2. NEOPLASMS (140–239)	17	173	64 (50–81)
Malignant neoplasm of lip, oral cavity and pharynx (140–149)	1	17.2	404 (110–1,034)
Malignant neoplasm of nasopharynx (147)	0	0	0 (0–2,349)
Malignant neoplasm of oesophagus (150)	0.75	12	163 (34–475)
Stomach cancer (151)	0.5	20	75 (9–272)
Colorectal cancer (153/154)	2	16	92 (40–182)
Liver cancer (155)	0.5	4.1	221 (27–797)
Lung cancer (162)	2	20	56 (24–111)
Malignant neoplasm of lymphatic and haematopoietic tissue (200–208)	1.75	12	95 (38–196)
Malignant neoplasm of cervix uteri (180)	1	5.7	64 (17–164)
Malignant neoplasm of female breast (174)	1.75	17	22 (9–46)
7. DISEASES OF THE CIRCULATORY SYSTEM (390–459)	14.5	154	107 (81–138)
Chronic rheumatic heart disease (393–398)	1	3.2	253 (69–647)
Hypertensive disease (401–405)	0.25	0.9	96 (2–532)
Ischaemic heart disease (410–414)	6.75	73	91 (60–133)
Cerebrovascular disease (430–438)	5.5	57	151 (95–229)
Diseases of arteries, arterioles and capillaries (440–448)	0.5	11	97 (12–349)

Table 11(b): Continued.

Mortality by cause of death (first number is ICD-9 chapter codes) for 20–74 year olds	Average number of deaths per year	Average directly age-standardised death rate per 100,000 per year	SMR (95% CI)
8. DISEASES OF THE RESPIRATORY SYSTEM (460–519)	2.25	26	73 (33–139)
Pneumonia and influenza (480–487)	0.75	12	103 (21–302)
Chronic obstructive pulmonary disease and allied conditions (490–496)	1.25	6.6	61 (20–143)
9. DISEASES OF THE DIGESTIVE SYSTEM (520–579)	2.25	33	97 (44–184)
Diseases of oesophagus, stomach and duodenum (530–537)	0	0	0.0 (0–292)
Cirrhosis	1	5.6	93 (25–237)
17. INJURY AND POISONING (800–999)	2.25	13	49 (22–93)
Poisoning by drugs, medicinals and biological substances (960–979)	0.25	0.5	134 (3–745)
1. INFECTIOUS AND PARASITIC DISEASES (001–139)	1.75	5	385 (155–792)
Tuberculosis (010–018)	0	0	0.0 (0–1,296)
11. COMPLICATIONS OF PREGNANCY, CHILDBIRTH AND THE PUERPERIUM (630–676)	1.25	2.9	1,021 (331–2,382)
3. ENDOCRINE, NUTRITIONAL AND METABOLIC DISEASES, AND IMMUNITY DISORDERS (240–279)	1	17	89 (24–227)
Diabetes mellitus (250)	0.75	16	109 (22–318)
Disorders of thyroid gland (240–246)	0	0	0 (0–2,484)
6. DISEASES OF THE NERVOUS SYSTEM AND SENSE ORGANS (320–389)	0.75	3.0	44 (9–129)
Inflammatory diseases of the central nervous system (320–326)	0	0	0 (0–1,078)
Multiple sclerosis (340)	0	0	0 (0–190)
10. DISEASES OF THE GENITO-URINARY SYSTEM (580–629)	0.75	9.8	191 (39–558)
Nephritis, nephrotic syndrome and nephrosis (580–589)	0	0	0 (0–586)
13. DISEASES OF THE MUSCULO-SKELETAL SYSTEM AND CONNECTIVE TISSUE (710–739)	0.75	2.1	160 (33–468)
14. CONGENITAL ANOMALIES (740–759)	0.5	1.2	103 (12–371)
4. DISEASES OF BLOOD AND BLOOD-FORMING ORGANS (280–289)	0.25	2.9	123 (3–684)
5. MENTAL DISORDERS (290–319)	0.25	2.9	57 (1–315)
Senile and presenile organic psychotic conditions (290)	0	0	0.0 (0–767)
12. DISEASES OF THE SKIN AND SUBCUTANEOUS TISSUE (680–709)	0	0	0.0 (0–2,312)
16. SYMPTOMS, SIGNS AND ILL-DEFINED CONDITIONS (780–799)	0	0	0.0 (0–722)

Chinese/Hong Kong/Taiwan-born

As shown in **Table 12(a)**, deaths were mostly in the 45–74 age group in Chinese men, though death rates were highest in the older age groups. The high number of deaths over 75 years in Chinese women reflects the substantial population in the age group (Appendix 3). The number of deaths (and death rates) were higher in men than women (**Tables 12(a)**, **12(b)**). The SMR was lower in Chinese men and women, compared to the population average, in virtually every age group.

Table 12(a): Age-specific mortality for males born in Hong Kong/China/Taiwan (1989–92).

Mortality by age group	Average number of deaths/yr	Directly age-standardised rate/100,000/yr	SMR (95% CI)
Under 20 years of age	3	65	75 (40–127)
20–44 years of age	20	80	64 (51–79)
45–64 years of age	92	934	75 (68–83)
65–74 years of age	67	5,658	94 (83–106)
75+ years of age	34	11,260	75 (63–89)
All ages	218	919	79 (74–84)

Table 12(b): Age-specific mortality for females born in Hong Kong/China/Taiwan (1989–92).

Mortality by age group	Average number of deaths/yr	Directly age-standardised rate/100,000/yr	SMR (95% CI)
Under 20 years of age	1	10	42 (11–108)
20–44 years of age	18	66	103 (80–129)
45–64 years of age	51	608	77 (67–88)
65–74 years of age	56	3,302	92 (81–105)
75+ years of age	75	10,496	92 (82–103)
All ages	201	1,001	88 (82–94)

In Chinese men and women (**Tables 13(a)** and **(b)**), neoplasms were the top ranking cause of death (lung cancer being in the commonest single cancer in men, and breast cancer in women), with circulatory diseases second. In men, the commonest circulatory disease was ischaemic heart disease, but in women it was cerebrovascular disease. Injury and poisoning was the third ranking cause of death. In both men and women, infections, though an uncommon cause of death, were relatively common, with high SMRs, including for tuberculosis. SMRs for some specific causes were very high, e.g. for liver cancer, naso-pharyngeal cancer and lip/oral/pharynx cancer (**Tables 13(a)** and **(b)**).

Caribbean-born

As shown in **Tables 14(a)** and **(b)**, most deaths occurred in the 45–64 age group, but the death rates were higher in older age groups and in men at each band.

The SMR for men overall shows mortality rates similar to the population average, though the SMR was substantially higher in the age group 20–44 years and substantially lower in those over 75 years. In women, the overall SMR was higher than the population average for women, with a substantial excess in the age groups 20–44 and 45–64.

Table 13(a): Ranked causes of mortality: Chinese born men.

Mortality by cause of death (first number is ICD-9 chapter codes) for 20–74 year olds	Average number of deaths per year	Average directly age-standardised death rate per 100,000 per year	SMR (95% CI)
ALL CANCERS (140–239)	57	252	96 (84–110)
Liver cancer (155)	8	32	1,004 (691–1,410)
Colorectal cancer (153, 154)	7	32	106 (71–154)
Malignant neoplasm of lip, oral cavity and pharynx (140–149)	6	18	493 (312–739)
Malignant neoplasm of nasopharynx (147)	5	15	4,376 (2,674–6,759)
Malignant neoplasm of lymphatic and haematopoietic tissue (200–208)	5	19	102 (63–158)
Lung cancer (162)	15	71	77 (59–100)
Stomach cancer (151)	3	15	79 (41–137)
Oesophageal cancer (150)	1.75	6.8	62 (25–128)
Prostate cancer (185)	1.5	8.9	45 (16–97)
7. DISEASES OF THE CIRCULATORY SYSTEM (390–459)	49	246	61 (53–70)
Ischaemic heart disease (410–414)	27	128	44 (36–54)
Cerebrovascular disease (430–438)	14	71	129 (98–167)
Diseases of arteries, arterioles and capillaries (440–448)	3.5	20	86 (47–144)
Hypertensive disease (401–405)	1.75	7.9	160 (68–347)
Chronic rheumatic heart disease (393–398)	0.5	2.5	110 (13–397)
17. INJURY AND POISONING (800–999)	14	14	74 (56–95)
Poisoning by drugs, medicinals and biological substances (960–979)	0.25	1	94 (2–523)
9. DISEASES OF THE DIGESTIVE SYSTEM (520–579)	8	35	133 (91–188)
Cirrhosis (571)	3.25	13	130 (69–222)
Diseases of oesophagus, stomach and duodenum (530–537)	1.75	8.6	133 (54–275)
8. DISEASES OF THE RESPIRATORY SYSTEM (460–519)	7.5	39	59 (40–84)
Chronic obstructive pulmonary disease and allied conditions (490–496)	5	27	58 (35–89)
Pneumonia and influenza (480–487)	1.25	5.3	45 (15–105)
Infectious/parasitic (001–139)	4.5	17.8	377 (224–596)
TB (010–018)	1	4.3	377 (103–966)
3. ENDOCRINE, NUTRITIONAL AND METABOLIC DISEASES, AND IMMUNITY DISORDERS (240–279)	4.25	15	87 (46–148)
Diabetes (250)	1.75	9	85 (34–175)
Disorders of thyroid gland (240–246)	0	0	(0–3,928)
6. DISEASES OF THE NERVOUS SYSTEM AND SENSE ORGANS (320–389)	1.5	8.4	40 (15–88)

Table 13(a): Continued.

10. DISEASES OF THE GENITO-URINARY SYSTEM (580–629)	1.25	4.8	126 (41–293)
Nephritis, nephrotic syndrome and nephrosis (580–589)	1.25	4.8	244 (79–569)
Diseases of male genital organs (600–608)	0	0	(0–732)
16. SYMPTOMS, SIGNS AND ILL-DEFINED CONDITIONS (780–799)	0.75	1.7	151 (31–440)
4. DISEASES OF BLOOD AND BLOOD-FORMING ORGANS (280–289)	0.5	2.1	94 (11–340)
5. MENTAL DISORDERS (290–319)	0.5	1.8	32 (4–114)
13. DISEASES OF THE MUSCULO-SKELETAL SYSTEM AND CONNECTIVE TISSUE (710–739)	0.25	0.8	45 (1–248)
14. CONGENITAL ANOMALIES (740–759)	0.25	0.6	32 (1–178)
Senile and presenile organic psychotic conditions (290)	0	0	(0–197)
Inflammatory diseases of the central nervous system (320–326)	0	0	(0–584)
Multiple sclerosis (340)	0	0	(0–205)
12. DISEASES OF THE SKIN AND SUBCUTANEOUS TISSUE (680–709)	0	0	(0–1,013)

Table 13(b): Ranked causes of mortality: Chinese-born women Hong Kong/Taiwan.

Mortality by cause of death (First number is ICD-9 chapter codes) for 20–74 year olds	Average number of deaths per year	Average directly age-standardised death rate per 100,000 per year	SMR (95% CI)
ALL CANCERS (140–239)	42	185	88 (75–102)
Malignant neoplasm of lymphatic and haematopoietic tissue (200–208)	3.5	15	110 (60–185)
Lung cancer (162)	3.25	15	41 (22–71)
Stomach cancer (151)	3	13	223 (119–381)
Malignant neoplasm of lip, oral cavity and pharynx (140–149)	2.5	7.7	581 (279–1,068)
Cervical cancer (180)	2.5	9	116 (56–213)
Breast cancer (174)	7	28	60 (40–86)
Colorectal cancer (153, 154)	5	27	113 (69–174)
Malignant neoplasm of nasopharynx (147)	2.25	6	4,300 (1,966–8,162)
Liver cancer (155)	1	3.4	242 (66–620)
Oesophageal cancer (150)	0.75	4.5	74 (15–216)
7. DISEASES OF THE CIRCULATORY SYSTEM (390–459)	25	136	70 (57–85)
Cerebrovascular disease (430–438)	12	62	135 (100–179)
Ischaemic heart disease (410–414)	9	53	43 (30–60)
Hypertensive disease (401–405)	0.75	4.6	116 (24–339)
Diseases of arteries, arterioles and capillaries (440–448)	0.75	3.7	49 (10–144)
Chronic rheumatic heart disease (393–398)	0.5	5.1	124 (45–325)

Table 13(b): Continued.

Mortality by cause of death (First number is ICD-9 chapter codes) for 20–74 year olds	Average number of deaths per year	Average directly age-standardised death rate per 100,000 per year	SMR (95% CI)
17. INJURY AND POISONING (800–999)	11	11	184 (133–247)
Poisoning by drugs, medicinals and biological substances (960–979)	0.75	2.8	428 (88–1,251)
8. DISEASES OF THE RESPIRATORY SYSTEM (460–519)	4	22	53 (30–86)
Chronic obstructive pulmonary disease and allied conditions (490–496)	2.25	12	44 (20–83)
Pneumonia and influenza (480–487)	1.5	8.4	85 (31–184)
3. ENDOCRINE, NUTRITIONAL AND METABOLIC DISEASES, AND IMMUNITY DISORDERS (240–279)	2.5	15	110 (53–202)
Diabetes mellitus (250)	2	11	126 (54–249)
Disorders of thyroid gland (240–246)	0.25	1.7	276 (7–1,537)
1. INFECTIOUS/PARASITIC (001–139)	1.75	7.2	248 (100–511)
TB (010–018)	0.5	2.8	384 (47–1,388)
9. DISEASES OF THE DIGESTIVE SYSTEM (520–579)	1.75	9	41 (17–85)
Diseases of oesophagus, stomach and duodenum (530–537)	1	6.0	133 (36–340)
Cirrhosis (571)	0.5	2.3	32 (4–116)
13. DISEASES OF THE MUSCULO-SKELETAL SYSTEM AND CONNECTIVE TISSUE (710–739)	1.5	6.3	144 (53–312)
10. DISEASES OF THE GENITO-URINARY SYSTEM (580–629)	1	6.3	120 (33–307)
Nephritis, nephrotic syndrome and nephrosis (580–589)	0.25	1.7	71 (2–395)

Table 14(a): Age-specific mortality for males born in Caribbean (1989–92).

Mortality by age group	Average number of deaths/yr	Directly age-standardised rate/100,000/yr	SMR (95% CI)
Under 20 years of age	0.5	39	27 (3–96)
20–44 years of age	63	180	144 (126–162)
45–64 years of age	752	1,273	99 (95–102)
65–74 years of age	296	5,879	97 (91–102)
75+ years of age	86	11,520	79 (71–87)
All ages	1,200	1,062	98 (95–101)

Table 14(b): Age-specific mortality for females born in Caribbean (1989–92).

Mortality by age group	Average number of deaths/yr	Directly age-standardised rate/100,000/yr	SMR (95% CI)
Under 20 years of age	1	32	80 (22–206)
20–44 years of age	54		
	94	148 (129–169)	
45–64 years of age	442	896	116 (110–121)
65–74 years of age	170	3,793	108 (100–116)
75+ years of age	129	10,744	95 (87–103)
All ages	798	1,147	111 (108–115)

Tables 15(a) and (b) show that in both Afro-Caribbean men and women, circulatory disease, neoplasms and endocrine diseases (mainly diabetes) were dominant causes of death. It is worth emphasising that ischaemic heart disease (IHD), which has a low SMR, is the commonest of the circulatory diseases in Caribbean-born men, particularly as this disease may be overlooked in favour of stroke, which has a high SMR. In a similar vein, the low SMR for cancer, including for lung and breast cancer, must not obscure their importance as common causes of death. Endocrine diseases, mainly diabetes, were exceptionally common, with extremely high SMRs in men and women.

The infrequency of deaths from respiratory disease (in absolute and relative terms, especially in women) is notable (**Tables 15(a) and (b)**). High SMRs were particularly notable for hypertensive heart disease and stroke, liver cancer, prostate cancer, tuberculosis, nephritis and deaths from symptoms/ill-defined conditions.

West and South African-born

Tables 16(a) and (b) shows that in men and women most deaths were in the 45–64 age group, but with the usual pattern of rising mortality rates with age. Relative to the whole population of men, the mortality rate was high, especially in the younger age groups.

For women, too, most deaths were in the 45–64 age group, and the number of deaths and death rates was lower than in men. The SMR shows death rates higher than the population as a whole in those aged up to 64 years, and lower thereafter.

The disease pattern in men and women was different, as shown in **Tables 17(a) and 17(b)**. In men, the usual pattern was observed, with circulatory diseases and neoplasms dominant, though IHD had a low SMR. Hypertensive disease and cerebrovascular disease were both common, and had very high SMRs. Injuries and respiratory disease were major killers. Diabetes was relatively common. The high SMRs for liver cancer, infections, symptoms and ill-defined conditions and genito-urinary disorders were noteworthy.

In women, the number of deaths were small but, nonetheless, neoplasms dominated (breast cancer being the commonest) over circulatory diseases. Ischaemic heart disease comprised a small fraction of circulatory deaths and was relatively uncommon, being exceeded by cerebrovascular deaths. Although the SMRs were high for several specific conditions, the number of cases was too low for accurate interpretation (**Tables 17(a) and 17(b)**).

Table 15(a): Ranked causes of mortality: Caribbean-born men.

Mortality by cause of death (first number is ICD-9 chapter codes) for 20–74 year olds	Average number of deaths per year	Average directly age-standardised death rate per 100,000 per year	SMR (95% CI)
7. DISEASES OF THE CIRCULATORY SYSTEM (390–459)	427	358	95 (90–99)
Chronic rheumatic heart disease (393–398)	1.5	1.3	59 (22–129)
Hypertensive disease (401–405)	27	23	471 (386–568)
Ischaemic heart disease (410–414)	210	172	62 (58–67)
Cerebrovascular disease (430–438)	126	108	205 (188–224)
Diseases of arteries, arterioles and capillaries (440–448)	19	15	81 (64–101)
2. NEOPLASMS (140–239)	295	239	89 (84–94)
Malignant neoplasm of lip, oral cavity and pharynx (140–149)	5.25	3.4	83 (51–126)
Malignant neoplasm of nasopharynx (147)	1.25	0.9	236 (77–551)
Malignant neoplasm of oesophagus (150)	11	8.0	66 (48–89)
Stomach cancer (151)	26	20	118 (96–142)
Colorectal cancer (153/154)	21	18	56 (44–69)
Liver cancer (155)	15	13	328 (250–423)
Lung cancer (162)	66	51	59 (52–67)
Prostate cancer (185)	37.5	36	188 (159–221)
Malignant neoplasm of lymphatic and haematopoietic tissue (200–208)	38	30	162 (137–190)
3. ENDOCRINE, NUTRITIONAL AND METABOLIC DISEASES, AND IMMUNITY DISORDERS (240–279)	61	54	375 (329–425)
Diabetes mellitus (250)	50	44	439 (380–504)
Disorders of thyroid gland (240–246)	0.25	0.3	203 (5–1,131)
17. INJURY AND POISONING (800–999)	59	65	128 (112–145)
Poisoning by drugs, medicinals and biological substances (960–979)	3	3.6	471 (243–822)
8. DISEASES OF THE RESPIRATORY SYSTEM (460–519)	43	36	61 (52–70)
Pneumonia and influenza (480–487)	16	13	116 (89–149)
Chronic obstructive pulmonary disease and allied conditions (490–496)	22	19	44 (36–55)
9. DISEASES OF THE DIGESTIVE SYSTEM (520–579)	39	32	128 (109–150)
Diseases of oesophagus, stomach and duodenum (530–537)	7.5	5.9	103 (69–147)
Cirrhosis (571)	14	9	147 (114–186)
6. DISEASES OF THE NERVOUS SYSTEM AND SENSE ORGANS (320–389)	16	14	100 (77–127)
Inflammatory diseases of the central nervous system (320–326)	2.25	2.1	369 (169–700)
Multiple sclerosis (340)	0.25	0.4	12 (0–68)
1. INFECTIOUS AND PARASITIC DISEASES (001–139)	14.75	13	297 (226–383)
Tuberculosis (010–018)	4.5	3.8	387 (237–598)

Table 15(a): Continued.

16. SYMPTOMS, SIGNS AND ILL-DEFINED CONDITIONS (780–799)	9.25	9.9	542 (381–747)
10. DISEASES OF THE GENITO-URINARY SYSTEM (580–629)	9	8.3	170 (119–235)
Nephritis, nephrotic syndrome and nephrosis (580–589)	6	5.9	220 (141–327)
Diseases of male genital organs (600–608)	0.5	0.3	70 (8–251)
5. MENTAL DISORDERS (290–319)	5.75	5.3	99 (63–149)
Senile and presenile organic psychotic conditions (290)	2	2.5	75 (32,147)
4. DISEASES OF BLOOD AND BLOOD-FORMING ORGANS (280–289)	5.25	4.8	207 (128–317)
13. DISEASES OF THE MUSCULO-SKELETAL SYSTEM AND CONNECTIVE TISSUE (710–739)	2.75	2.1	90 (45–162)
14. CONGENITAL ANOMALIES (740–759)	2.25	2.5	93 (42–176)
12. DISEASES OF THE SKIN AND SUBCUTANEOUS TISSUE (680–709)	1	1	221 (60–566)

Table 15(b): Ranked causes of mortality: Caribbean-born women.

Mortality by cause of death (first number is ICD-9 chapter codes) for 20–74 year olds	Average number of deaths per year	Average directly age-standardised death rate per 100,000 per year	SMR (95% CI)
7. DISEASES OF THE CIRCULATORY SYSTEM (390–459)	217	246	137 (128–146)
Chronic rheumatic heart disease (393–398)	2	2.2	47 (20–93)
Hypertensive disease (401–405)	22	23	748 (601–921)
Ischaemic heart disease (410–414)	83	95	86 (77–96)
Cerebrovascular disease (430–438)	76	88	197 (175–220)
Diseases of arteries, arterioles and capillaries (440–448)	7.5	8.1	117 (79–166)
2. NEOPLASMS (140–239)	209	195	91 (85–98)
Malignant neoplasm of lip, oral cavity and pharynx (140–149)	1.25	0.9	59 (19–139)
Malignant neoplasm of nasopharynx (147)	0	0	0 (0–390)
Malignant neoplasm of oesophagus (150)	5	5.4	101 (62–156)
Stomach cancer (151)	10	8	148 (106–202)
Colorectal cancer (153/154)	16	15	73 (56–93)
Liver cancer (155)	4.25	3.5	216 (126–346)
Lung cancer (162)	16	15	41 (32–53)
Malignant neoplasm of lymphatic and haematopoietic tissue (200–208)	28	26	201 (165–242)
Malignant neoplasm of cervix uteri (180)	10	9.4	116 (83–158)
Malignant neoplasm of female breast (174)	61	54	104 (91–117)

Table 15(b): Continued.

Mortality by cause of death (first number is ICD-9 chapter codes) for 20–74 year olds	Average number of deaths per year	Average directly age-standardised death rate per 100,000 per year	SMR (95% CI)
3. ENDOCRINE, NUTRITIONAL AND METABOLIC DISEASES, AND IMMUNITY DISORDERS (240–279)	56	64	569 (496–648)
Diabetes mellitus (250)	50	59	697 (603–801)
Disorders of thyroid gland (240–246)	0.5	0.5	122 (15–442)
9. DISEASES OF THE DIGESTIVE SYSTEM (520–579)	20	19	101 (80–127)
Diseases of oesophagus, stomach and duodenum (530–537)	1	1.2	30 (8–77)
Cirrhosis	6.75	20	103 (81–128)
Poisoning by drugs, medicinals and biological substances (960–979)	1	0.7	193 (53–494)
8. DISEASES OF THE RESPIRATORY SYSTEM (460–519)	19	19	57 (45–71)
Pneumonia and influenza (480–487)	6	6.2	82 (53–123)
Chronic obstructive pulmonary disease and allied conditions (490–496)	11	11	47 (34–63)
6. DISEASES OF THE NERVOUS SYSTEM AND SENSE ORGANS (320–389)	12	12	104 (76–137)
Inflammatory diseases of the central nervous system (320–326)	1	1.2	205 (56–525
Multiple sclerosis (340)	0.5	0.5	16 (2–59)
1. INFECTIOUS AND PARASITIC DISEASES (001–139)	9.5	9	330 (233–453)
Tuberculosis (010–018)	1.5	1.8	269 (55–585)
10. DISEASES OF THE GENITO-URINARY SYSTEM (580–629)	9	9.6	246 (171–342
Nephritis, nephrotic syndrome and nephrosis (580–589)	5.75	5.9	385 (244–577)
13. DISEASES OF THE MUSCULO-SKELETAL SYSTEM AND CONNECTIVE TISSUE (710–739)	5	3.5	110 (67–169)
4. DISEASES OF BLOOD AND BLOOD-FORMING ORGANS (280–289)	4.5	3.4	280 (166,443)
16. SYMPTOMS, SIGNS AND ILL-DEFINED CONDITIONS (780–799)	2.75	1.9	400 (200–716)
5. MENTAL DISORDERS (290–319)	2.5	3.7	70 (34–129)
Senile and presenile organic psychotic conditions (290)	1.25	2	65 (21–152)
14. CONGENITAL ANOMALIES (740–759)	1.75	1.5	84 (34–173)
12. DISEASES OF THE SKIN AND SUBCUTANEOUS TISSUE (680–709)	1	1.1	244 (66–624)
11. COMPLICATIONS OF PREGNANCY, CHILDBIRTH AND THE PUERPERIUM (630–676)	0.5	0.3	205 (25–740)

Table 16(a): Age-specific mortality for males born in West and South Africa (1989–92).

Mortality by age group	Average number of deaths/yr	Directly age-standardised rate/100,000/yr	SMR (95% CI)
Under 20 years of age	7	90	118 (77–172)
20–44 years of age	45	144	112 (96–129)
45–64 years of age	103	1,457	114 (103–125)
65–74 years of age	30	6,324	106 (88–126)
75+ years of age	11	10,507	70 (51–93)
All ages	198	1,116	108 (101–116)

Table 16(b): Age-specific mortality for females born in West and South Africa (1989–92).

Mortality by age group	Average number of deaths/yr	Directly age-standardised rate/100,000/yr	SMR (95% CI)
Under 20 years of age	5	68	151 (94–231)
20–44 years of age	31	93	135 (112–160)
45–64 years of age	44	930	121 (104–140)
65–74 years of age	11	2,976	83 (61–111)
75+ years of age	10	5,909	51 (36–71)
All ages	102	849	107 (97–117)

Table 17(a): Ranked causes of mortality: West and South African men.

Mortality by cause of death (first number is ICD-9 chapter codes) for 20–74 year olds	Average number of deaths per year	Average directly age-standardised death rate per 100,000 per year	SMR (95% CI)
7. DISEASES OF THE CIRCULATORY SYSTEM (390–459)	65	429	113 (100–128)
Chronic rheumatic heart disease (393–398)	0.75	1.2	221 (45–644)
Hypertensive disease (401–405)	5.75	34	764 (484–1,146)
Ischaemic heart disease (410–414)	25	165	58 (47–70)
Cerebrovascular disease (430–438)	20	139	261 (207–325)
Diseases of arteries, arterioles and capillaries (440–448)	2.25	26	88 (40–167)
2. NEOPLASMS (140–239)	46.5	267	106 (92–123)
Malignant neoplasm of lip, oral cavity and pharynx (140–149)	0.75	5.5	78 (16–227)
Malignant neoplasm of nasopharynx (147)	0.25	1.0	241 (6–1,344)
Malignant neoplasm of oesophagus (150)	1.25	8.2	47 (15–110)
Colorectal cancer (153/154)	2.75	18	58 (29–103)
Liver cancer (155)	7	23	1,097 (729–1,586)
Lung cancer (162)	7.75	60	61 (41–86)
Prostate cancer (185)	4.25	37	219 (128–351)
Malignant neoplasm of lymphatic and haematopoietic tissue (200–208)	7.75	31	182 (125–258)

Table 17(a): Continued.

Mortality by cause of death (first number is ICD-9 chapter codes) for 20–74 year olds	Average number of deaths per year	Average directly age-standardised death rate per 100,000 per year	SMR (95% CI)
17. INJURY AND POISONING (800–999)	18	40	82 (65–103)
Poisoning by drugs, medicinals and biological substances (960–979)	1	2.2	256 (70–657)
8. DISEASES OF THE RESPIRATORY SYSTEM (460–519)	10.25	60	118 (85–160)
Pneumonia and influenza (480–487)	5.5	22	240 (150–363)
Chronic obstructive pulmonary disease and allied conditions (490–496)	4	33	73 (42–119)
3. ENDOCRINE, NUTRITIONAL AND METABOLIC DISEASES, AND IMMUNITY DISORDERS (240–279)	6.5	39	185 (121–271)
Diabetes mellitus (250)	4.5	34	297 (176–469)
Disorders of thyroid gland (240–246)	0	0	0.0 (0–5,313)
9. DISEASES OF THE DIGESTIVE SYSTEM (520–579)	5.75	28	111 (70–167)
Diseases of oesophagus, stomach and duodenum (530–537)	1.5	9	159 (58–345)
Cirrhosis (571)	2.5	13	101 (48–185)
1. INFECTIOUS AND PARASITIC DISEASES (001–139)	5.25	20	449 (278–686)
Tuberculosis (010–018)	0.75	5.3	327 (67–956)
6. DISEASES OF THE NERVOUS SYSTEM AND SENSE ORGANS (320–389)	3.25	14	96 (51–165)
Inflammatory diseases of the central nervous system (320–326)	0.5	1.0	319 (39–1,152)
Multiple sclerosis (340)	0	0	0 (0–206)
16. SYMPTOMS, SIGNS AND ILL-DEFINED CONDITIONS (780–799)	3	16	554 (286–967)
10. DISEASES OF THE GENITO-URINARY SYSTEM (580–629)	2.25	10	312 (143–593)
Nephritis, nephrotic syndrome and nephrosis (580–589)	1.5	6.7	393 (144–855)
Diseases of male genital organs (600–608)	0.75	3.2	1,024 (211–2,991)
4. DISEASES OF BLOOD AND BLOOD-FORMING ORGANS (280–289)	1.5	5	354 (130–769)
5. MENTAL DISORDERS (290–319)	1	8.4	67 (18–171)
Senile and presenile organic psychotic conditions (290)	0.25	3.7	97 (2–538)
12. DISEASES OF THE SKIN AND SUBCUTANEOUS TISSUE (680–709)	0	0	0 (0–1,286)
13. DISEASES OF THE MUSCULO-SKELETAL SYSTEM AND CONNECTIVE TISSUE (710–739)	0	0	0 (0–227)
14. CONGENITAL ANOMALIES (740–759)	0	0	0 (0–110)

Table 17(b): Ranked causes of mortality: West and South African women.

Mortality by cause of death (first number is ICD-9 chapter codes) for 20–74 year olds	Average number of deaths per year	Average directly age-standardised death rate per 100,000 per year	SMR (95% CI)
2. NEOPLASMS (140–239)	34	230	111 (93–131)
Malignant neoplasm of lip, oral cavity and pharynx (140–149)	0.25	1.7	61 (41–86)
Malignant neoplasm of nasopharynx (147)	0.25	<1	543 (14–3,026)
Oesophageal cancer (150)	0.5	3.4	61 (20–142)
Stomach cancer (151)	1.25	4.7	164 (53–384)
Colorectal cancer (153/154)	1.75	17	73 (29–151)
Liver cancer (155)	1.75	15	679 (273–1,398)
Malignant neoplasm of trachea, bronchus and lung (162)	1.75	20	46 (18–94)
Malignant neoplasm of lymphatic and haematopoietic tissue (200–208)	3.75	28	163 (71–269)
Malignant neoplasm of cervix uteri (180)	0.75	3.1	35 (7–102)
Malignant neoplasm of female breast (174)	11.75	67	129 (95–171)
7. DISEASES OF THE CIRCULATORY SYSTEM (390–459)	23	220	148 (119–181)
Chronic rheumatic heart disease (393–398)	1.25	4.8	290 (94–676)
Hypertensive disease (401–405)	2.25	12	780 (357–1,481)
Ischaemic heart disease (410–414)	5.25	88	61 (37–94)
Cerebrovascular disease (430–438)	7	50	162 (107–234)
Diseases of arteries, arterioles and capillaries (440–448)	1	11	162 (44–414)
17. INJURY AND POISONING (800–999)	7.5	18	115 (77–64)
Poisoning by drugs, medicinals and biological substances (960–979)	1	1.9	337 (92–864)
3. ENDOCRINE, NUTRITIONAL AND METABOLIC DISEASES, AND IMMUNITY DISORDERS (240–279)	3.5	18	253 (138–424)
Diabetes mellitus (250)	1.25	15	156 (51–364)
Disorders of thyroid gland (240–246)	0.25	0.6	577 (13–3,214)
9. DISEASES OF THE DIGESTIVE SYSTEM (520–579)	2.75	26	98 (49–175)
Diseases of oesophagus, stomach and duodenum (530–537)	0	0	0 (0–253)
Cirrhosis	1.25	6.5	94 (30–218)
4. DISEASES OF BLOOD AND BLOOD-FORMING ORGANS (280–289)	2	4.7	778 (336–1,533)
8. DISEASES OF THE RESPIRATORY SYSTEM (460–519)	1.75	17	49 (20–101)
Pneumonia and influenza (480–487)	0.5	0.8	240 (150–363)
Chronic obstructive pulmonary disease and allied conditions (490–496)	1.25	16	55 (18–128)
1. INFECTIOUS AND PARASITIC DISEASES (001–139)	1.5	5.4	261 (96–567)
Tuberculosis (010–018)	0	0	0 (0–1,011)

Table 17(b): Continued.

Mortality by cause of death (first number is ICD-9 chapter codes) for 20–74 year olds	Average number of deaths per year	Average directly age-standardised death rate per 100,000 per year	SMR (95% CI)
10. DISEASES OF THE GENITO-URINARY SYSTEM (580–629)	1.5	11	310 (114–674)
Nephritis, nephrotic syndrome and nephrosis (580–589)	0.75	7	390 (80–1,139)
6. DISEASES OF THE NERVOUS SYSTEM AND SENSE ORGANS (320–389)	1	1.9	46 (12–117)
Inflammatory diseases of the central nervous system (320–326)	0	0	0.0 (0–830)
Multiple sclerosis (340)	0	0	0.0 (0–206)
16. SYMPTOMS, SIGNS AND ILL-DEFINED CONDITIONS (780–799)	1	8.8	552 (150–1,414)
11. COMPLICATIONS OF PREGNANCY, CHILDBIRTH AND THE PUERPERIUM (630–676)	0.75	0.5	339 (70–991)
13. DISEASES OF THE MUSCULO-SKELETAL SYSTEM AND CONNECTIVE TISSUE (710–739)	0.5	2.1	88 (11–317)
14. CONGENITAL ANOMALIES (740–759)	0.25	0.3	37 (1–205)
5. MENTAL DISORDERS (290–319)	0	0	0.0 (0–153)
Senile and presenile organic psychotic conditions (290)	0	0	0.0 (0–635)
12. DISEASES OF THE SKIN AND SUBCUTANEOUS TISSUE (680–709)	0	0	0.0 (0–1,882)

A note on 'South Asians' and the inclusion of 'East Africans'

A common practice over the last 15 years is the combination of Indians, Pakistanis, Bangladeshis, and sometimes Sri Lankans and East Africans too, into one category, 'South Asians'. As the above tables show, there are similarities and dissimilarities in mortality. Overall, it is probably wise to recognise the substantial heterogeneity in these populations' health needs, even though the study of the separate groups poses additional challenges of smaller population size, and fewer deaths.

We have examined the data for Indians, Pakistanis, Bangladeshis and Sri Lankans as a single group of 'South Asians' together and East Africans separately. The data are not presented here, but we conclude that study of such a South Asian group is reasonable for diabetes, but not for several other causes.

Mortality by ethnic group – the Longitudinal Study

One per cent of the enumerated 1991 census population of England and Wales was identified for the Longitudinal Study (LS) (http://www.statistics.gov.uk/services/longitudinal.asp). Table 18 shows the numbers of Indians, Pakistanis, Bangladeshis, Chinese, Black-Caribbeans, Black-Africans and Whites in the longitudinal study (for this chapter, and analysis, the categories 'black other',' other Asian' and 'other' are excluded). These populations are 'flagged' and traced at the NHS Central Register, from where mortality data are obtained. **Table 18** shows that the population size for the ethnic minority groups is small, especially for Bangladeshi, Chinese and Black African populations. The patterns are likely to be least reliable for them.

Table 18: Population enrolled into the Longitudinal Study by ethnic group from the 1991 census.

	Indian	Pakistani	Bangladeshi	Chinese	Black-Caribbean	Black-African	White
Total	10,450	5,742	2,176	1,521	4,996	1,936	482,189

Source: ONS Longitudinal Study (http://www.statistics.gov.uk/services/longitudinal.asp)

Table 19 ranks the causes, giving numbers of deaths defined by ICD chapter. **Table 19** shows that circulatory diseases were the top ranking cause of death with the exception of Black-Caribbeans, in whom this place was taken by neoplasms.

Table 19: Longitudinal Study: numbers of deaths after 1991 (traced at NHSCR) by ethnic group in approximate rank order* of ICD Chapters.

Underlying cause of death (ICD-9) – broad chapter	Indian	Pakistani	Bangladeshi	Chinese	Black-Caribbean	Black-African	White
Circulatory diseases (ICD-9 = 390–459)	110	42	14	11	56	11	15,953
Neoplasms (ICD-9 = 140–239)	40	22	3	7	65	8	9,931
Respiratory diseases (ICD-9 = 460–519)	39	2	2	7	12	6	5,521
Diseases of digestive system (ICD-9 = 520–579)	21	1	1	1	6	1	1,245
Endocrine, etc. (ICD-9 = 240–279)	19	6	1	–	6	1	502
Infectious and parasitic diseases (ICD-9 = 000–139)	11	1	–	–	4	2	166
Injuries and poisoning (ICD-9 = 800–999)	9	7	1	2	8	–	914
Disease of the nervous system (ICD-9 = 320–389)	4	2	1	2	2	1	639
Genito-urinary diseases (ICD-9 = 580–629)	3	1	–	–	1	1	367
Diseases of the musculo-skeletal system (ICD-9 = 710–739)	1	2	1	–	–	1	247
Ill-defined symptoms (ICD-9 = 780–799)	1	–	–	–	–	–	516
Diseases of blood (ICD-9 = 280–289)	–	–	–	–	1	–	135
Mental disorders (ICD-9 = 290–319)	–	1	–	–	2	–	609
Complications of childbirth (ICD-9 = 630–676)	–	–	1	–	–	–	2
Skin diseases (ICD-9 = 680–709)	–	–	–	–	–	1	66
Congenital anomalies (ICD-9 = 740–759)	–	2	1	–	1	–	65
Conditions originating in perinatal period (760–779)	–	–	–	–	–	–	–

* This ranking is based on rank order in Indians – other groups differ slightly as noted in the text.
Source: ONS Longitudinal Study (http://www.statistics.gov.uk/services/longitudinal.asp)

Table 20 gives the numbers for a small number of specific causes and confirms the burden placed by the specific causes of ischaemic heart disease, stroke, diabetes and the two common cancers. The number of deaths is too low to permit valid sex- and age-specific rates, and hence age-sex adjusted rates, to be calculated. In view of the substantial differences in population structure, rates unadjusted for age and sex would be potentially misleading. The important point is that the ranking of causes of death, as summarised in **Table 20**, is similar to that arising from country of birth analysis. This gives confidence in undertaking health needs assessment for adults based on the data in **Tables 6–17**.

Table 20: Longitudinal Study: some selected causes of death.

Selected cause of death (ICD-9)	Indian	Pakistani	Bangladeshi	Chinese	Black-Caribbean	Black-African	White
Ischaemic heart disease (ICD-9 = 410–414)	70	29	8	6	26	3	8,755
Cerebrovascular disease (ICD-9 = 430–438)	26	9	5	2	15	6	4,085
Diabetes mellitus (ICD-9 = 250)	18	5	1	–	5	–	390
Malignant neoplasm of the trachea, bronchus and lung (ICD = 162)	6	4	2	2	7	–	2,231
Malignant neoplasm of breast (ICD = 174)	5	1	–	–	3	–	829

Source: ONS Longitudinal Study (http://www.statistics.gov.uk/services/longitudinal.asp)

Lifestyle, measures of health and self-reported health

Table 21 summarises the studies from which the data have been extracted. The general findings are summarised below. In comparing different groups, the reader needs to remember that different methods of sampling and questioning in different languages makes precise comparisons between ethnic groups difficult. **Tables 22–27** summarise key data on lifestyles, biochemical measures, anthropometric measures, and self-reported and self-assessed health in six ethnic groups. These data are a sample of the extensive information available. Readers are advised to read the original source to understand the method before utilising the data.

The paucity of research on racism in health is discussed by Bhopal,[7,96] though it is acknowledged as a factor in terms of housing[97] and education.[98] One study from the US found an association between racial discrimination and hypertension,[99] possibly operating via the 'psychosocial pathway'.[100]

Indians

Indians are extremely heterogeneous, so findings are likely to differ in different places, and communities. In particular, religion has an important effect. For example, smoking is much less common in Sikhs than Hindus. The reverse applies to drinking alcohol. That said, the data in **Table 22** show that there are substantial needs in relation to smoking, alcohol and lack of physical activity. In women, the cultural taboo against smoking is holding, for the present.

Lipid profiles in Indians change dramatically after immigration, moving from very low levels towards the high levels of cholesterol in the white population.[101] Vigorous action to alter lipid profiles is warranted.

Table 21: Basic information on sources of data for Tables 22–27.

Study	Date of survey and publication	Age-groups and sample size	Sampling and ethnic classification
Rudat 1994[86]	Survey: 1992 Published: 1994	16–74 3,317 people, mainly in England	Mainly from EDs in England with >10% of population from ethnic minority groups. Population classified on self-report as Indian, Pakistani, Bangladeshi and African-Caribbean.
Nazroo 1997[84]	Survey: 1993/94 Published: 1997	16-plus 8,063 people in England and Wales	Sample from wide range of areas with low ethnicity minority concentrations and high. Ethnic codes based on family origins (groups were White, Caribbean, Indian, African Asian, Pakistani, Bangladeshi, Chinese).
Sproston 1997[87]	Survey: – Published: 1999	16–74 1,022 people in England	Name search using the electoral register. Chinese only.
HEA 2000[88]	Survey: – Published: 2000	16–74 4,452 people in England	EDs where >10% of population was from one of the ethnic groups under study. Personal definition of own ethnicity, categorised into four groups – African-Caribbean, Indian, Pakistani, Bangladeshi.
Bhopal 1999[93]	Survey: 1995–97 Published: 1999	25–74 1,509 people in Newcastle Upon Tyne	Stratified, random samples from Family Health Services Authority Register, categorised as Indian, Pakistani, Bangladeshi and European on basis of name, birthplace of grandparents and self-report.
Harland 1997[94]	Survey: 1991–93 Published: 1997	25–64 1,005 people in Newcastle Upon Tyne	All Chinese resident in the city identified by name search of Family Health Services Register, or recruited via publicity. Europeans identified from FHSA Register as described.
Cappuccio 1998[95]	Survey: 1994–96 Published: 1998	40–59 1,577 people	Name search of lists of 25 general practices, and for Afro-Caribbean, contact with practice staff. Population categorised as White, African origin or South Asian.

Table 22: Selected information on lifestyles, biochemical measures, physical measures and self-reported health status for Indian men and women.

Variable	Measure	Ref.	Number of subjects		Results		Comment
			Male	Female	Male	Female	
Lifestyle factor							
Smoking	current regular smoker (%)	HEA 1994	440	527	20	1	Smoking has decreased in men, but is common, and it has increased slightly in women – most male smokers are over 30, whereas most female are under 30.
		HEA 2000	598	463	15	2	
Alcohol	current drinker (%)	Nazroo	637	66		18	Higher than other South Asian groups but lower than the White population (especially females). Among Indians, Sikhs have higher prevalence than other religious groups.
Physical activity	takes vigorous exercise >20 mins at least 3/week (%)	HEA 2000	290	488	35	17	Fewer older people take such exercise compared with younger people.
Biochemical measure							
Cholesterol	mean (mmol/l)	Bhopal 1999	105	154	5.8	5.4	These values are high, particularly as values in India are very low.
HDL	mean (mmol/l)	Bhopal 1999	105	154	1.3	1.4	A higher level is desirable.
Triglycerides	mean (mmol/l)	Bhopal 1999	105	154	1.7	1.4	Comparatively high, but lower than in Pakistanis and Bangladeshis.
Physical measure							
Waist	mean (cm)	HEA 2000	598	463	88.2	80.5	Waist size is large, though smaller than other South Asian groups.
Height	mean (cm)	HEA 2000	598	463	170.1	156.1	Shorter than the White population, taller than Bangladeshis and Pakistanis.
Weight	mean (kg)	HEA 2000	598	463	71.3	62.6	Weight is high in relation to height.
Waist/hip ratio	mean	HEA 2000	598	463	0.91	0.80	Smallest ratios of the South Asian groups.
BMI	mean	HEA 2000	598	463	24.6	25.6	Mean value is high, particularly in relation to comparable figures from India.
Blood pressure	av. Systolic av. Diastolic (mmHg)	Bhopal 1999	105	154	124 72	123 68	Higher than other South Asian groups, and comparable to the White population.

Table 22: Continued

Self-reported health status

Hypertension	Self-reported (%)	Nazroo 1997	10	6	Hypertension is common. Female values lower than all South Asian groups and the White population.
Diabetes	Self-reported (%)	Nazroo 1997	5.5*	5.5*	Diabetes is extremely common, though lower than other South Asians, but far higher than the White population.
Angina/MI	Self-reported (%)	Nazroo 1997	4.8	2.7	Lower than South Asians and the White population, a surprising finding that needs cautious interpretation.
Mental health	Lacking energy or problem sleeping (%) Anxiety (%) Life not worth living (%)	Nazroo 1997 (a) and (b) (mental health)	28 8 1.9	35 11 2.9	Mental health problems are common. Generally better than Pakistanis and the White population but not as good as Bangladeshis.
Self-assessed general health	Fair/poor health or longstanding illness or registered disabled (%)	Nazroo 1997	27	32	The prevalences are high, though Indians were less likely to report fair/poor health etc. than other South Asian groups and the White population.

* Men and women combined – sex-specific data not given.

Indians are relatively short and obesity (particularly central) is common. Indians born in the UK are growing taller than their parents. Blood pressures vary in different Indian communities, with the best judgement being that levels are similar to the white population – i.e. hypertension is a common disorder.

Diabetes and the associated syndrome of insulin resistance are exceptionally common in men and women. The presence of cardiovascular symptoms is high, and in some studies reflects mortality data.

Mental health problems are present in a substantial proportion of the population.

These data, together with the mortality patterns and other findings in the research literature, show that Indians present health needs that are similar to the population as a whole. Special emphasis is needed to sustain the low prevalence of smoking in women, and vigorous control of all the risk factors for diabetes and cardiovascular diseases.

Pakistanis

Pakistanis are mainly Muslims, whose religion impacts in ways important to health. Although heterogeneity between Pakistani communities should not be overlooked, this is less than in Indians. As with Indians, there are substantial needs in relation to smoking (men) and in promotion of physical activity (**Table 23**). Few people drink alcohol, though the taboo against it may lead to underreporting. Those Pakistanis who do drink may have special difficulties due to social problems arising from admitting to an alcohol problem.

The comments above on lipids and physical measures of health including obesity in Indians, apply with even greater force in Pakistanis, whose rates of heart disease and diabetes are slightly higher than in Indians. The reduction of cardiovascular and diabetes risk factors is the prime health need in Pakistani adults. The indicators of mental health status suggest major needs, as does the high prevalence of self-reporting poor health/longstanding illness.

Overall, these data, combined with the knowledge that Pakistanis are relatively poor, indicate an especial challenge in meeting the health needs of this population.

Bangladeshi

Of the South Asian populations in the UK, the Bangladeshis are the most homogeneous, having in common a single major religion, Islam, and origins from a small country, Bangladesh, and within that many Bangladeshis come from Sylhet. **Table 24** shows that smoking prevalence in Bangladeshi men is exceptionally high, making this the priority public health issue. Although the prevalence of smoking is relatively low in Bangladeshi women, tobacco chewing (with betel nut or paan) is a common practice, and much more so than in Indian or Pakistani women.

The points made on alcohol use in Pakistanis apply to Bangladeshis, too. The exceptionally low rates of physical activity (a major issue) need to be interpreted in the knowledge that most men are in manual occupations.

Lipid patterns in Bangladeshis are problematic, with the apparently low total cholesterol being a result of very low HDL cholesterol. This, together with high triglycerides, signifies a need for dietary advice and change.

Bangladeshis are very short, a reflection of poor nutrition in childhood. In comparison with other ethnic groups, Bangladeshis have less obesity and a lower mean blood pressure. This should not lead to complacency, for their risk of developing cardiovascular disease and diabetes is the highest of all the ethnic groups considered here. It may be that cardiovascular risk is triggered at a lower threshold than in other ethnic groups.

Self-reported health problems are common, though surprisingly, the prevalence of mental health problems is comparatively low. This may simply reflect difficulties of translating questions in comparable ways, or it may arise from social and cultural factors yet to be studied. As Bangladeshis are the poorest of the ethnic minority groups studied here, and the most recent immigrants, one might anticipate their mental health to be worse.

Table 23: Selected information on lifestyles, biochemical measures, physical measures and self-reported health status for Pakistani men and women.

Variable	Measure	Ref.	Number of subjects		Results		Comment
			Male	Female	Male	Female	
Lifestyle factor							
Smoking	current regular smoker (%)	HEA 1994 HEA 2000	456 627	471 517	30 24	2 1	Smoking has decreased in men but is common.
Alcohol	current drinker (%)	Nazroo	582		8	0	Very few Pakistanis drink, mainly for religious reasons. Figures may be underestimates.
Physical activity	takes vigorous exercise >20 mins at least 3/week (%)	HEA 2000	424	426	30	17	Fewer older people take such exercise compared with younger people.
Biochemical measure							
Cholesterol	mean (mmol/l)	Bhopal 1999	156	149	5.6	5.3	These values are high.
HDL	mean (mmol/l)	Bhopal 1999	156	149	1.1	1.3	The levels are undesirably low, and lower than Indians and the White population, though slightly higher than Bangladeshis.
Triglycerides	mean (mmol/l)	Bhopal 1999	156	149	1.8	1.5	Very high, and higher than Indians and the White population, but lower than Bangladeshis.
Physical measure							
Waist	mean (cm)	HEA 2000	627	517	87.6	84.3	The waist size is large, and larger than Indians and Bengalis, and in females, larger than in White females.
Height	mean (cm)	HEA 2000	627	517	170.9	157.9	This population is taller than Indians and Bangladeshis but shorter than the White population.
Weight	mean (kg)	HEA 2000	627	517	72.6	63.8	Weight is undesirably high, and greater than Indians and Bangladeshis, though lighter than the White population.
Waist/hip ratio	mean	HEA 2000	627	517	0.92	0.83	In women, the ratios are higher than Indian and White females.
BMI	mean	HEA 2000	627	517	24.9	26.1	The values are understandably high, and greater than Indians and the White population, though lower than Bangladeshis.
Blood pressure	av. Systolic av. Diastolic (mmHg)	Bhopal 1999	156	149	119 71	116 68	The levels are good, and lower than in Indians and the White population.

Table 23: Continued.

Variable	Measure	Ref.	Number of subjects		Results		Comment
			Male	Female	Male	Female	
Self-reported health status							
Hypertension	Self-reported (%)	Nazroo 1997	1,181		6	12	Male levels lower than Indians and Bangladeshis, though, surprisingly, the rate is double that of Indian women.
Diabetes	Self-reported (%)	Nazroo 1997	1,185		7.6*	7.6*	Extremely high, and the highest of South Asian groups and over three times higher than the White population.
Angina/MI	Self-reported (%)	Nazroo 1997	1,183		6.0	3.8	Common, and higher than in Indians, though lower than Bangladeshis and the White population.
Mental health	Lacking energy or problem sleeping (%) Anxiety (%) Life not worth living (%)	Nazroo 1997 (a) and (b) (mental health)	584		31 10 2.8	41 11 3.1	The prevalences are high, and higher than Indians and Bangladeshis, and for 'life not worth living' higher than in the White population.
Self-assessed general health	Fair/poor health or longstanding illness or registered disabled (%)	Nazroo 1997	1,185		36	39	The prevalences are high, with general health better than Bangladeshis but worse than Indians and the White population.

* Men and women combined – sex-specific data not given.

Table 24: Selected information on lifestyles, biochemical measures, physical measures and self-reported health status for Bangladeshi men and women.

Variable	Measure	Ref.	Number of subjects		Results		Comment
			Male	Female	Male	Female	
Lifestyle factor							
Smoking	current regular smoker (%)	HEA 1994	315	350	42	5	Smoking is extremely common in men. It decreased in men under 30 and increased in those over 30, whereas the opposite was true of women.
		HEA 2000	566	603	46	6	
Alcohol	current drinker (%)	Nazroo	289		4	2	Very few drink, mainly for religious reasons. There may be underreporting.
Physical activity	takes vigorous exercise >20 mins at least 3/week (%)	HEA 2000	357	515	29	12	Fewer older people take such exercise compared to younger people.
Biochemical measure							
Cholesterol	mean (mmol/l)	Bhopal 1999	64	56	5.3	5.3	Lower than other South Asian and White populations, though still higher than desirable.
HDL	mean (mmol/l)	Bhopal 1999	64	56	1.0	1.2	Very low, and lower than other South Asians and the White population. Higher levels are desirable.
Triglycerides	mean (mmol/l)	Bhopal 1999	64	56	2.0	2.0	Very high, and higher than other South Asians and the White population.
Physical measure							
Waist	mean (cm)	HEA 2000	566	603	84.7	80.6	Smallest of all South Asian and White populations, but females have bigger waists than White females.
Height	mean (cm)	HEA 2000	566	603	165.3	152.6	A short population, and smallest among South Asians.
Weight	mean (kg)	HEA 2000	566	603	64.0	55.4	Lightest among South Asians.
Waist/hip ratio	mean	HEA 2000	566	603	0.92	0.85	The ratios are high, and larger than for other South Asians and the White population.
BMI	mean	HEA 2000	566	603	23.4	23.9	Though comparatively low and lowest among South Asian and White populations, a lower BMI is still desirable.
Blood pressure	av. Systolic av. Diastolic (mmHg)	Bhopal 1999	64	56	112 68	109 66	Apparently satisfactory, and lowest of all South Asians and the White population, and yet CHD and stroke mortality rates are still high.

Table 24: Continued.

Variable	Measure	Ref.	Number of subjects		Results		Comment
			Male	Female	Male	Female	
Self-reported health status							
Hypertension	Self-reported (%)	Nazroo 1997		589	10	11	The prevalences are high, bearing in mind mean blood pressure, with males higher than Pakistani males, and females higher than Indian females, but lower than in the White population.
Diabetes	Self-reported (%)	Nazroo 1997		591	7.4*	7.4*	Very high. Higher than Indians and the White population, similar to Pakistanis.
Angina/MI	Self-reported (%)	Nazroo 1997		590	7.6	3.7	Higher than other South Asians but lower than the White population.
Mental health	Lacking energy or problem sleeping (%) Anxiety (%) Life not worth living (%)	Nazroo 1997 (a) and (b) (mental health)		289	28 2 0.3	25 7 1.3	Though mental health problems are common, surprisingly, this population reports better mental health than other South Asian and White populations.
Self-assessed general health	Fair/poor health or longstanding illness or registered disabled (%)	Nazroo 1997		591	36	42	These prevalences are high, and higher than other South Asian and White populations.

* Men and women combined – sex-specific data not given.

Afro-Caribbean

While Afro-Caribbeans come from a diaspora of Caribbean Islands, each with their distinctive characteristics, they have in common a language (English), and are predominantly Christian.

The need for services relating to smoking cessation, alcohol drinking and exercise uptake is clear from the data in **Table 25**. The cholesterol levels are high, but triglycerides are low. The reasons why Afro-Caribbeans have a comparatively low mortality from coronary heart disease despite their unsatisfactory risk profile is unclear. The possibilities of data artefact, or a temporal trend, need to be considered, and the view that African Americans were protected from coronary heart disease (CHD) has not been sustained.[102] An epidemic of CHD may be imminent.

Obesity is common, as in the population as a whole, and weight control is a priority in the light of the high blood pressure and high prevalence of diabetes.

Mental health problems are extremely common, especially in women, and the prevalence of suicidal thoughts is significant. The problem of poor self-assessed health and longstanding illness is an indicator of high levels of health need.

Chinese

China is a vast territory, yet it is surprisingly homogeneous, mainly as a result of its long history as a single political entity and ancient civilisation. Chinese people in Britain are either agnostic, Christian or Buddhist, and most speak Cantonese (87%).

The smoking prevalence is substantial in men, though low in women. There is a need for smoking cessation activity for men, and actions to maintain the low levels in women. The low prevalence of physical exercise is problematic.

The lipid profiles and measures of physique come from a single survey in Newcastle in the early 1990s.[94] In the absence of other data, the cautious interpretation is that the lipid profiles are favourable and Chinese people's physique is slim. This accords with the comparatively low rates of CHD mortality. The challenge for services is to maintain or improve upon this comparatively advantaged position. Mortality data show cardiovascular disease as the second commonest cause of death in Chinese. On self-report (**Table 26**), cardiovascular disease and diabetes are common. There is no room for complacency.

The prevalence of symptoms indicating mental health problems is high in Chinese (excepting suicidal thoughts).

White population

The difficulties in making comparisons have been discussed above. Nonetheless, for interest and reference, some of the comparative data are in **Table 27**. While assessing the health needs of the white population is beyond the remit of this chapter, it would be remiss not to point out that there are multiple and diverse populations captured by the term 'white', and these populations may have distinctive health needs.

A synthesis of current knowledge on the patterns of disease in ethnic minority groups

The following synthesis is based on a reading of the literature, particularly the reports summarised in **Table 27**, and examination of the data tables. Note that preliminary analysis of data collected during the first months of 1999 Health Survey for England broadly substantiate the conclusions presented below and in other sections (for further details, *see* http://www.archive.official-documents.co.uk/document/doh/survey99/hse99-00.htm).

Table 25: Selected information on lifestyles, biochemical measures, physical measures and self-reported health status for Afro-Caribbean men and women.

Variable	Measure	Ref.	Number of subjects		Results		Comment
			Male	Female	Male	Female	
Lifestyle factor							
Smoking	current regular smoker (%)	HEA 1994	527	432	29	17	Smoking is common and has increased in those men under 30 and over 50, but only increased in those women over 30.
		HEA 2000	428	639	29	18	
Alcohol	current drinker (%)	Nazroo	613		87	74	Drinking alcohol is common, and most people drink 'once a week or more'.
Physical activity	takes vigorous exercise >20 mins at least 3/week (%)	HEA 2000	282	483	32	22	Fewer older people take such exercise compared to younger people.
Biochemical measure							
Cholesterol	mean (mmol/l)	Capuccio 1998	197	303	5.5	5.7	The levels are high, though in males they are lower than in the White population, but in females they are higher.
HDL	mean (mmol/l)	Capuccio 1998	197	303	1.3	1.6	The levels are average, with males similar to the White population but females lower than the White population.
Triglycerides	mean (mmol/l)	Capuccio 1998	197	303	0.9	0.8	The levels are desirably low, and lower than the White population.
Physical measure							
Waist	mean (cm)	HEA 2000	174	193	86.6	84.2	Waist size is high in women.
Height	mean (cm)	HEA 2000	174	193	173.8	162.7	The population is tall, with males being slightly shorter than the white population, females taller.
Weight	mean (kg)	HEA 2000	174	193	76.9	73.6	Males lighter than the White population, females heavier.
Waist/hip ratio	mean	HEA 2000	174	193	0.89	0.81	Male ratios less than the White population, female similar to the White population.
BMI	mean	HEA 2000	174	193	25.5	27.5	Male ratios less than the White population, female greater than the White population, and, in the latter at least, too high.
Blood pressure	av. Systolic av. Diastolic (mmHg)	Capuccio 1998	197	303	134 88	134 85	The levels are high, and higher than in any of the other populations described here.

Table 25: Continued.

Self-reported health status						
Hypertension	Self-reported (%)	Nazroo 1997	1,195	15	23	As expected, the prevalences are very high.
Diabetes	Self-reported (%)	Nazroo 1997	1,205	5.9*	5.9*	Very high prevalence, and much higher than the White population.
Angina/MI	Self-reported (%)	Nazroo 1997	1,202	4.3	4.3	As expected, lower than in the White population.
Mental health	Lacking energy or problem sleeping (%)	Nazroo 1997 (a) and (b) (mental health)	614	36	60	Mental health problems are very common, with a particularly high prevalence of affirmative response to the 'life not worth living' question.
	Anxiety (%)			11	14	
	Life not worth living (%)			3.8	3.8	
Self-assessed general health	Fair/poor health or longstanding illness or registered disabled (%)	Nazroo 1997	1,205	34	41	General health reported as poor, and worse than in the White population.

* Men and women combined – sex-specific data not given.

Table 26: Selected information on lifestyles, biochemical measures, physical measures and self-reported health status for Chinese men and women.

Variable	Measure	Ref.	Number of subjects		Results		Comment
			Male	Female	Male	Female	
Lifestyle factor							
Smoking	current regular smoker (%)	HEA Chinese	477	545	21	8	Smoking is common in men, and has increased in those men under 30 and over 50 and increased in women over 30.
Alcohol	current drinker (%)	HEA Chinese	429	491	73	56	Drinking alcohol is common, though the prevalence is lower than in the White population.
Physical activity	takes vigorous exercise >20 mins at least 3/week (%)	HEA Chinese	463	534	17	9	The prevalence is low, and fewer older people take such exercise compared to younger people.
Biochemical measure							
Cholesterol	mean (mmol/l)	Harland 1997	183	197	5.1	4.9	The challenge is to maintain these comparatively low levels.
HDL	mean (mmol/l)	Harland 1997	183	197	1.4	1.6	The challenge is to maintain these satisfactory levels.
Triglycerides	mean (mmol/l)	Harland 1997	183	197	1.0	0.8	The challenge is to maintain these satisfactory levels.
Physical measure							
Waist	mean (cm)	Harland 1997	183	197	83	77	The waist size is satisfactory.
Height	mean (cm)	Harland 1997	183	197	166	155	The population is comparatively short.
Weight	mean (kg)	Harland 1997	183	197	66	56	The weights are satisfactory.
Waist/hip ratio	mean	Harland 1997	183	197	0.89	0.84	Male ratios lower than the White population but females greater than White females, which may reflect small hips, rather than large waists.
BMI	mean	Harland 1997	183	197	23.8	23.5	The level is satisfactory, but increases are to be avoided.
Blood pressure	av. Systolic av. Diastolic (mmHg)	Harland 1997	183	197	123 77	121 75	The levels are average, with males slightly lower than in the White population but females slightly higher.

Table 26: Continued.

Self-reported health status				
Hypertension	Self-reported (%)	Nazroo 1997	4	5	Low, and yet mortality from stroke is comparatively high.
Diabetes	Self-reported (%)	Nazroo 1997	2.2*	2.2*	The prevalence is comparatively low, and similar to the White population.
Angina/MI	Self-reported (%)	Nazroo 1997	4.1	1.7	The prevalence is low, and much lower than in the White population.
Mental health	Lacking energy or problem sleeping (%) Anxiety (%) Life not worth living (%)	Nazroo 1997 (a) and (b) (mental health)	47 5 0	40 10 0	The data, at face value, suggest minor mental health problems are common but serious ones may be less so.
Self-assessed general health	Fair/poor health or longstanding illness or registered disabled (%)	Nazroo 1997	22	30	These figures compare favourably with other ethnic groups.

* Men and women combined – sex-specific data not given.

Table 27: Selected information on lifestyles, biochemical measures, physical measures and self-reported health status for White men and women.

Variable	Measure	Ref.	Number of subjects		Results	
			Male	Female	Male	Female
Lifestyle factor						
Smoking	current regular smoker (%)	Nazroo	2,867		34	37
Alcohol	current drinker (%)	Nazroo	2,866		92	83
Biochemical measure						
Cholesterol	mean (mmol/l)	Bhopal 1999	425	399	5.7	5.6
HDL	mean (mmol/l)	Bhopal 1999	425	399	1.3	1.6
Triglycerides	mean (mmol/l)	Bhopal 1999	425	399	1.4	1.2
Physical measure						
Waist	mean (cm)	HEA 2000			90.3	80.6
Height	mean(cm)	HEA 2000**			175	162
Weight	mean (kg)	HEA 2000			77.2	65.4
Waist/hip ratio	mean	HEA 2000			0.92	0.81
BMI	mean	HEA 2000			25.2	25.1
Blood pressure	av. Systolic	Bhopal 1999			129	121
	av. Diastolic (mmHg)				78	69
Self-reported health status						
Hypertension	Self-reported (%)	Nazroo 1997	2,862		15	17
Diabetes	Self-reported (%)	Nazroo 1997	2,867		2.2*	2.2*
Angina/MI	Self-reported (%)	Nazroo 1997	2,864		8.0	6.2
Mental health	Lacking energy or problem sleeping (%)	Nazroo 1997 (b) (mental health)	2,867		48	62
	Anxiety (%)				12	23
	Life not worth living (%)				1.5	3.3
Self-assessed general health	Fair/poor health or longstanding illness or registered disabled (%)	Nazroo 1997	2,867		31	36

* Men and women combined – sex-specific data not given.

** The physical measures data are from the Allied Dunbar National Fitness Survey, cited in Sproston et al.[87]

Ethnic minority groups are heterogeneous in their health. In terms of both overall health (say, measured by the all-cause SMR or self-reported health) and specific causes (say, coronary heart disease or oral cancers) there is marked heterogeneity. There is also great heterogeneity within ethnic groupings.

There is a common assumption and oft-stated view that the health of Britain's ethnic minorities is worse than expected (judged by the standard of the ethnic majority (white) population). This is at best simplistic, and sometimes wrong. First, such conclusions need to be cautious in the light of the possible weaknesses in the underlying data, particularly those based on mortality statistics. Second, even on the basis of the published statistics, overall measures such as SMRs are often around and sometimes less than 100 in some ethnic minority populations. There is the subtle question of how we judge the level of expected health. Is it right to base the expected level on the white population which, on average, has much higher economic standing? Might it be that, taking into account social and economic factors, the health of ethnic minority groups is about that to be expected? Certainly, overall SMRs in ethnic minority groups tend to be on a par with people in social classes IV and V in the general population. It is worth noting that some of the highest all-cause SMRs are not in the ethnic minority groups but in a sub-group of the white population – Irish and Scots living in England.[103,104]

In many if not most respects, for mortality and morbidity, the ethnic minority groups have similar patterns of disease and overall health to the ethnic majority. This is plain when disease rankings are based on frequency as in **Tables 5**, and **6–17**. In their detailed community-based study of South Asians in Glasgow, Williams *et al.*[105] concluded that 'South Asians were consistently disadvantaged only in terms of anthropometric measures. Otherwise, the many differences were balanced, with disadvantage being concentrated only among South Asian women.' This general conclusion holds in this analysis.

There are some differences in disease pattern that need attention, but not at the expense of potentially more important diseases that show no striking differences (such as respiratory diseases). Conditions which are less common in minority ethnic groups than in the white population tend to be ignored (e.g. lung cancer, the leading cancer in men in most ethnic groups, and among the leaders for women) but may be worth more attention than conditions which are actually less common (though relatively more common than in the white population), e.g. liver cancer.

The differences are complex and vary over time and between ethnic groups. Simplifications may easily mislead. It should be noted that information is most readily available for Afro-Caribbean and South Asian groups, is poor for Chinese origin people, and unavailable for most other groups, e.g. those from the Middle East and many groups of refugees.

With the above provisos, the following generalisations seem to be sound, consistent across studies, and unlikely to be explained by artefacts: the major cause of death, and both the serious and minor health problems, of most ethnic minority communities differ little from those of the population as a whole. For example, coronary heart disease, stroke and cancer are the commonest cause of death, and accidents, poisonings, digestive disorders, respiratory infection and circulatory problems the main reasons for admission to hospital, whichever community you consider. Health professionals caring for ethnic minority patients will usually be confronted with these common problems, and will see the conditions specific to ethnic minorities infrequently. Their problem will be to make the correct diagnosis in the face of communication barriers of one kind or another. However, both health authorities and individual practitioners need to know of the conditions that are rare in the population as a whole and yet sometimes seen in minority ethnic communities. Health authorities may need to modify their service priorities and practitioners may need to consider their approach to diagnosis.

Some of the conditions that are much commoner in one or more minority ethnic groups than the indigenous community include:

- infectious diseases including tuberculosis and malaria
- diabetes mellitus
- perinatal mortality
- hypertension and cerebrovascular disease
- cancer of the oropharynx; cancer of the liver; cancer of the prostate
- haemoglobinopathies
- vitamin D deficiency.

Equally, there are some conditions which are less common in one or more minority ethnic groups relative to the population as a whole, including:

- many cancers, including the common ones of lung and breast

- mental disorders
- diseases of the nervous system and sense organs.

For most specific conditions, the SMR is not consistently high in every ethnic group, for example, ischaemic heart disease is relatively common in Indian, Pakistani, and Bangladeshi populations but relatively uncommon in the Chinese and Afro-Caribbeans.

The above lists are not comprehensive. Health authorities have the difficult task of ensuring that their services cater not only for the common causes of death and disability but also take account of any unusual patterns of disease in their population. Some specific diseases that merit discussion include the following.

- **Diabetes:** This is much commoner in Afro-Caribbean and South Asian minority groups than in the population as a whole. In the Chinese, the prevalence (in Newcastle) is on a par with the white population but on the basis of a higher prevalence of impaired glucose intolerance,[94] there is evidence that a rise is imminent. The causes of the high rates are likely to be a mix of genetic, lifestyle, environmental and economic factors.
- **Coronary heart disease:** This is moderately higher in South Asian groups than in the population as a whole, with increasing evidence that the poorest groups, of Pakistani and Bangladeshi origin, have the highest rates. The causes of the excess are incompletely understood. Recent work[84,93,94] indicates that socio-economic factors are important. The role of the classic risk factors (high blood pressure, lipids, smoking) is clearly important. Central obesity and insulin resistance are two other factors of especial note. Coronary heart disease is one of the foremost killers of other ethnic groups, including Afro-Caribbean and Chinese, even though the rates are lower than in the population as a whole.
- **Stroke:** This is highest in Afro-Caribbean populations, but also the rates are relatively high in the Chinese and South Asian groups. The major known associated risk factor is high blood pressure, which is extremely common in Afro-Caribbeans but not in the others. This tendency to stroke is commonly attributed to genetic factors. Other causes, including racism, are being investigated. Stroke is an extremely important cause of death in all other ethnic minority populations.
- **Respiratory diseases:** These tend to get little attention. The mortality and morbidity from these diseases is usually a little less than in the white comparison populations, which makes them extremely common and important problems which ought not to be neglected.
- **Neoplasms:** Overall, cancers tend to be less common in ethnic minority groups than in the 'white' comparison population (but a dominant problem, nonetheless). Some cancers are strikingly less common, e.g. lung cancer – relating to lower smoking prevalence. Nevertheless, this cancer remains the top ranking cancer in men. For some cancers, the SMRs are strikingly different from the population as a whole. Oropharyngeal cancers are commonest in South Asian groups and prostate cancer in African origin groups. Cancer variations are usually attributed to environmental factors.
- **Infections:** The common respiratory and gastrointestinal infections are dominant and important in all ethnic groups. Diseases that are associated with warm climates, such as malaria, are much more likely in ethnic minority groups. Tuberculosis is dramatically commoner in most ethnic minority groups, particularly South Asian ones. The causes are complex – relating to opportunities for exposure (travel, migration, etc.), immunity and living conditions in the UK. The latter seems to be an important factor maintaining the high level of tuberculosis in South Asians settled in the UK.
- **Haemoglobinopathies:** The haemoglobin disorders – thalassaemias and sickle cell disorders – are important genetic conditions that affect people who originate from Africa, the Caribbean, the Middle East, Asia and the Mediterranean. It is important to distinguish between carriers of haemoglobin disorders, who are very numerous, and people who have a major haemoglobin disorder, who are relatively few.[106] Carriers are healthy but due to recessive inheritance there is risk of having a child with a major disorder. The risk of these disorders in some ethnic groups is shown in **Table 28**.

Table 28: Estimated prevalence of carriers of Hb disorders, affected births and at-risk pregnancies in ethnic minority groups in the UK.

Ethnic group	AS %	AC %	β Thal. %	α^0 Thal. %	Hb E %	Total carriers	Affected births/ 1,000	At-risk pregnancies/ 1,000	Principal risk
White			0.1	+			0.00025	0.001	Thal.
Black-Caribbean	11	4	0.9	+	+	16	5.6	22.4	SCD
Black-African	22	3	1.0			25	15.6	62.4	SCD
Black other	11	4	0.9	+	+	16	5.6	22.4	SCD
Indian	+		4.3		+	4.3	0.46	1.85	β Thal.
Pakistani	+		4.5		+	4.5	1.0	4.0	β Thal.
Bangladeshi			2.8		4.5	7.3	0.826	3.3	Hb E/ β Thal.
Chinese			3.0	5.0	+	8.0	0.85	3.4	α^0 Thal./ β Thal.
Other Asian	+	+	3.0			3.0	0.225	0.9	β Thal.
Other-Other	5		1.0	+		6.0	1.04	4.16	SCD/β Thal.
Cypriot	0.5–1		16.0	1.5		17.5	4.33	17.32	β Thal.
Italian	+		4.0			4.0	0.2	0.8	β Thal.

Source: HEA 1998[107]

AS = sickle cell trait; AC = haemoglobin C trait; β Thal. = beta thalassaemia trait; α^0 Thal. = alpha-zero thalassaemia trait; Hb E = haemoglobin E trait; SCD = sickle cell disorders.

The major haemoglobin disorders are shown in **Box 3** and cover a wide spectrum of clinical severity.

Box 3: The major haemoglobin disorders.

Thalassaemias	Sickle cell disorders
• Beta thalassaemia	• Sickle cell anaemia (Haemoglobin SS)
• Haemoglobin E/beta thalassaemia	• Haemoglobin S/C disease
• Alpha-zero thalassaemia major	• Haemoglobin S/beta thalassaemia
• Haemoglobin H disease	• Haemoglobin S/D disease

Source: HEA 1998[107]

There are estimated to be 600 patients with major beta thalassaemia and 6000 with sickle cell disorder.[107] There is concern about increasing cases of thalassaemia amongst the South Asian communities, probably due to under-utilisation of counselling services.[108,109] The prevalence of these disorders vary by district and the methodology to estimate number within a particular district is given in HEA report[107] and Hickman *et al.* 1999.[110]

- **Childhood mortality:** Perinatal and neonatal mortality rates, and those in the age group 1–14, tend to be higher in most studies. The exception is the comparatively low incidence of sudden infant death syndrome demonstrated in some ethnic minority groups. The causes are complex and poorly understood.

   The high perinatal mortality rate amongst Pakistanis maybe linked to consanguineous marriages,[111] but this remains controversial.[112] Consanguineous marriages are defined as between close relatives, usually between second cousins or closer. These kinship patterns are found throughout the world and not restricted to the Muslim community.[113] These marriages can lead to an increase in rare recessively-inherited disorders, but the effect of this on the disease patterns of the population as a whole has been exaggerated.[113]

- **Mental health:** Numbers of deaths directly attributable to mental illness are small, and mortality data are not helpful to distinguish ethnic differences in prevalence of psychoses and neuroses. Suicide rates among migrants in England and Wales in 1979–93 generally reflect patterns in the country of origin, and migration does not appear to increase the risk of suicide.[114] SMRs for all age groups for suicide in 1988–92 were significantly lower than 100 in men born in Bangladesh, Sri Lanka and Pakistan and for men and women born in the Caribbean commonwealth, although SMRs for suicide among the Caribbean-born were elevated in the 25–34 year age group. SMRs for suicide are significantly higher among women born in India, with marked excess for deaths by burning.[115]

   Migrants to and from a variety of countries have higher rates of admission to psychiatric hospitals than native-born populations and in the United Kingdom African-Caribbeans have higher admission rates and receive a diagnosis of schizophrenia more often than do members of other ethnic groups.[116–8] A prospective study of incident psychosis found that annual incidence of schizophrenia and other non-affective psychoses was higher than the white population in all other minority ethnic groups studied, but the difference was only significant for the black population.[119] Conflicting evidence exists regarding rates of hospital admission for psychosis among people born on the Indian subcontinent, and this may reflect differences between sub-groups of this diverse population. Possible explanations for differences between migrants and native populations include higher incidence of psychiatric disease in the host country, the effect of migration, selection bias of migrants, confounding by socio-economic factors, differences in seeking medical care, prejudice in medical practice, inequitable service utilisation and drug use.

   Descriptive epidemiological studies of use of treatments have suggested that African-Caribbeans have low rates of depression and South Asians have low rates of all mental illnesses.[120] Results of the British Fourth National Survey of Ethnic Minorities provided a different picture, possibly as a consequence of the use of incidence rather than prevalence rates.[121] Rates of mental illness among Asians who had been educated in Britain or who were fluent in English were similar to those of the white population, suggesting the possibility that the instruments used to detect depression were less sensitive among other Asian groups.[122] Similar methodological limitations were suspected in a study of the prevalence of dementia and depression among elderly people in black and ethnic minorities in Liverpool. No differences were found between English speaking ethnic groups and the indigenous populations, but dementia was found to be more prevalent among non-English speaking groups.[123] The prevalence of anxiety and depressive illness was similar in African-Caribbeans and whites in a population-based survey in Manchester.[124] Limitations of this survey include the definitions of the ethnic groups and the low response rates, giving a potentially unrepresentative sample.

- **Sexual health:** Limited information is available concerning the sexual health of ethnic minority populations. South Asian men in Glasgow reported lower use of condoms than non-Asian men.[125] A high prevalence of sexually transmitted disease including gonorrhoea and chlamydia has been reported among Afro-Caribbeans in London, Leeds and Birmingham.[126–9]

   Data from anonymous seroprevalence surveillance suggest that the risk of HIV among pregnant women from sub-Saharan Africa is much higher than that of other populations, such that 76.4% of seropositive newborn babies were delivered to women from this population in 1997–8. Seroprevalence of HIV was highest among women born in East Africa (2.3%) and Central Africa (1.9%), compared with 0.14% overall. There was little evidence of HIV in women born in Southern Asia (0.0081%) and none within UK-born Asian communities.[130]

Data from the General Household Surveys of 1991–5 were used to examine fertility and contraception among ethnic minority women in Great Britain.[131] Fertility in Pakistani/Bangladeshi women was more than double that of white women and was associated with reduced use of contraception. The study highlighted potential unmet family planning needs and the need for cultural sensitivity in provision of family planning services. Married, non-professional Asian women have been found to experience difficulties in using family planning services, largely due to communication problems with health professionals and low levels of personal autonomy.[132] Abortion data are not recorded by ethnic group but there is a rising abortion rate among Bengali women in Tower Hamlets.[133]

- **Nutrition:** Whilst some BMEGs have lower incidence of specific diet-related diseases when resident in their country of origin, this difference gradually reduces as they adopt the more 'western' foods and cooking practices.[134] Further, there are also some diet-related problems that are commoner in BMEGs, such as vitamin D and iron deficiencies amongst South Asian children under 2 years.[135,136] There is an association between low plasma vitamin D and iron deficiency anaemia, particularly in winter.[136,137]

Conclusion

Patterns of health and disease are profoundly influenced by genetic, cultural, socio-economic and environmental factors. Undoubtedly, important differences exist between human populations in such factors. It would be most extraordinary if one of the consequences was not differences in health and disease by ethnicity, which is linked to the factors mentioned. Indeed, such differences between ethnic and racial groups can be shown with ease. The difficulties are not in demonstrating differences but in interpreting their meaning and using them to benefit the population.

Why is a disease more common in one group of people than another? This question lies at the heart of the debate on inequalities in health. Answers to these questions contain essential and unknown truths about the causes of disease. Answers will benefit all populations. Epidemiologists, who attempt to unravel the mystery in the patterns of disease in populations, become intrigued by ethnicity and health research, and particularly the mechanisms by which disease differences occur.

One major explanation, which has had insufficient attention, is the role of socio-economic status. On arrival in Britain most migrants held unskilled jobs. This legacy has been passed to their children (though there are many exceptions) and ethnic minority communities have more than their share of unemployment and low paid work. Much of the health disadvantage associated with ethnic minority groups may not result from their racial and cultural background, but relate to their socio-economic disadvantage. Their health status may be comparable to social classes IV and V in the indigenous population, and the solutions to health problems may also be similar. The problem of inequity and inequality in the health and health care of ethnic minority groups has defied easy solution. The explanation is *not* simply lack of knowledge, interest or even money. Inequalities may widen in the face of both interest and research – the most clear-cut example being the black/white disparity in life expectancy in the USA.[96]

The challenges of gaining, interpreting and utilising information on the pattern of health and disease in ethnic minority groups are great. To avoid traps, health needs assessors should: understand the strengths and limitations of the concepts of race and ethnicity, and the population sub-groupings derived to categorise people; ensure that all the relevant data and modes of presentation are used to produce a balanced analysis; and give due emphasis to both similarities and differences and draw tentative and careful interpretations of the causes of differences. Above all, they should avoid portraying differences as demonstrating the inferiority of some population group – that path has sustained and nourished a racist scientific literature. For health needs assessment, the common diseases and other common health problems deserve the most attention. Health needs assessors must avoid being deflected by the attention given to controversies generated by ethnic differences.

The approach used here has been to focus *first* on the important problems and diseases, then to refine the sense of priority using the relative approach. This approach avoids the piecemeal approach to tackling so-called ethnic health issues. Statistics cannot make coherent policy, without principles that guide their interpretation. This section is therefore as much concerned with the principles of data interpretation as with the data itself.

5 Services available and their costs

Introduction

This section considers services available and their utilisation in so far as data are available. It focuses upon key generic issues of concern to the health care needs of minority ethnic communities. Bilingual services, in particular, are considered. The reader is referred to other chapters for detail upon specific diseases and services, although certain pertinent issues relating to BMEGs are mentioned here.

Access to appropriate services

A central question for health authorities, trusts and Primary Care Organisations (PCOs) is the extent to which minority ethnic populations enjoy equality of access to appropriate health services. Variation in effective access to services may be important sources of inequality in the health experience of different ethnic groups, impacting upon quality and outcomes of care.[84] The variations in health described in section 4 might be partly explained by differences in service use. These may reflect demand for services rather than inequality of access to them. However, differences in demand may also result from a failure of health services to appropriately address the needs of minority ethnic groups.

In addition to levels of ill-health, the demand for, and use of, services will depend upon a wide range of factors including knowledge of services and how to use them, health beliefs and attitudes, the sensitivity of services to differing needs, and the quality of care provided.[138] These raise the key issues for health professionals of effective communication, awareness of attitudes, culture, stereotyping and racism within consultations and broader aspects of service delivery.[139]

Variation in availability and use of services

It must be stated again that even though ethnic monitoring is mandatory for some aspects of secondary care, relevant data remains incomplete and of variable quality for interpretation. However, in some localities, data may be of sufficient quality.[71] There appears to be considerable variation in availability and use of services in different localities. This may reflect several factors including:

- historical lack of performance management of, and variable commitment to, appropriate service development for ethnic minorities
- lack of awareness or relevant training about ethnic health and diversity issues
- professionals' differing attitudes towards people from ethnic minorities

- lack of relevant information (including inadequate ethnic monitoring) and therefore mechanisms to inform clinical audit, service planning and delivery
- nature of the population and variation in demand for services.

It is still not clear to what extent institutional racism and language and cultural barriers affect service utilisation and quality of care. Many services, for example bilingual services, are underdeveloped or may be underused by patients or the professionals facilitating their health care.

Health service utilisation

Primary care services

In general, a high proportion of people from most ethnic groups appear to be registered with a general practitioner – with registration rates of 99–100%,[86,140] but African-Caribbean men have higher non-registration rates (4%). Minority groups are also significantly more likely to attend open GP surgeries than those offering appointments[141] and may wait longer to see their GP.[86,142] With the exception of the Chinese, minority groups have comparable or higher consultation rates with their GP than the general population.[84,86,143,144]

As ethnic monitoring is not yet mandatory within primary care, there is currently little routine data available. However, data (**Tables 29–35**) is available from the National Morbidity Statistics from General Practice study done in 1991.[145] Essentially, 60 practices in England and Wales provided data for one year on face-to-face contact with 502 493 patients. Two percent of these patients were from ethnic minority groups compared to 6% in the 1991 census. The data in the tables are a re-analysis done by ONS and are not identical to those in the published report. This new analysis includes consultations with a nurse (although the study did not record nurse consultations if a doctor was also consulted during the same visit). The standard population for calculating the standardised patient consulting ratios (SPCR) was the entire study population including those for whom there was no ethnicity code (17% of patients). This group's consultation rates were low. As a result the SPCR for the white population is high at 108 for men and 105 for women. The interpreting of the data requires caution as the sample is not representative, the number of people is small, and 95% confidence intervals are not given (for technical reasons). Nonetheless, these are the best data available that provide a national picture. As with the mortality tables, the causes for consultation are ranked by approximate frequency of consultation (based on the numbers for women at all ages).

For each of men and women, in the three age groups and at all ages, the tables show the number of consultations, the consultation rate (crude), the age-standardised consultation rate (both per 10 000 patient-years at risk), and the age-standardised patient consulting ratio, where the entire population in the study provides the standard i.e. 100. The number of people in each age group was small, and this applied particularly to those over 65 years (the exception to this is the white population). The causes of consultation often varied by age and sex, usually in a predictable way. For example, the standardised consultation ratio for infectious and parasitic diseases was higher in children than in adults, diseases of the blood and genito-urinary systems were commoner in women than men, and diseases of the circulatory system were commoner in men than women. The consultation rate for mental disorders in men was half that in women. In all minority ethnic groups, except the Chinese and white groups, boys aged 0–15 years had a higher consultation rate than girls. The interpretation of the patterns is shown in detail for Indians, as an example, and briefly for other groups.

In Indians (**Table 29**), for all diseases, the standardised rates were higher in women than in men – mainly because of substantially higher consultation rates in women 16–64 compared to men. The standardised ratio shows that Indian men had a 12% excess of consultations compared to the whole population, and for women the excess was 2%. The commonest causes of consultation in Indians were factors influencing health status and contact with health services, respiratory problems, musculo-skeletal and connective tissue disorders, problems of the skin, and problems of the nervous system and sense organs. It is noteworthy that at general practice level, diseases of the circulatory system are not one of the dominant problems, and neoplasms are a rare cause of consultation.

Table 29: General practice consultation statistics for Indians. Rates are per 10,000 patient-years at risk.

	Men (no. of people)				Women (no. of people)			
	0–15 (376)	16–64 (905)	65+ (64)	all ages (1,345)	0–15 (344)	16–64 (873)	65+ (86)	all ages (1,303)
All diseases								
Number	1,385	2,932	349	4,666	1,076	4,571	464	6,111
Rate	39,407	34,327	57,546	36,849	33,899	55,057	56,354	49,684
Standardised rate	42,444	34,894	58,403	39,360	34,219	55,943	52,775	51,092
Standardised ratio	108	113	109	112	105	102	89	102
VO1–V82 supplementary classification of factors influencing health status and contact with health services								
Number	171	650	72	893	147	1,091	47	1,285
Rate	4,865	7,610	1,1872	7,052	4,631	13,141	5,708	10,447
Standardised rate	5,215	7,670	10,141	7,434	4,673	13,111	5,326	10,108
Standardised ratio	131	157	139	149	110	98	85	99
460–519 diseases of the respiratory system								
Number	545	451	50	1,046	380	592	67	1,039
Rate	15,507	5,280	8,244	8,261	11,972	7,131	8,137	8,447
Standardised rate	17,040	5,225	10,349	8,407	12,097	7,458	7,009	8,302
Standardised ratio	134	141	121	137	123	112	114	116
710–739 diseases of the musculo-skeletal system and connective tissue								
Number	40	301	42	383	16	580	67	663
Rate	1,138	3,524	6,925	3,025	504	6,986	8,137	5,390
Standardised rate	1,036	3,695	7,182	3,537	498	7,566	8,255	6,281
Standardised ratio	149	118	139	123	79	162	124	151
780–799 symptoms, signs and ill-defined conditions								
Number	146	185	26	357	115	333	40	488
Rate	4,154	2,166	4,287	2,819	3,623	4,011	4,858	3,968
Standardised rate	4,546	2,180	3,723	2,879	3,683	4,030	4,332	4,013
Standardised ratio	177	157	109	161	124	141	130	135
320–389 diseases of the nervous system and sense organs								
Number	126	162	12	300	110	276	37	423
Rate	3,585	1,897	1,979	2,369	3,466	3,324	4,494	3,439
Standardised rate	4,035	1,897	1,809	2,350	3,510	3,348	4,413	3,562
Standardised ratio	101	123	61	109	79	119	122	104
580–629 diseases of the genito-urinary system								
Number	11	41	3	55	24	375	11	410
Rate	313	480	495	434	756	4,517	1,336	3,333
Standardised rate	328	480	456	444	754	4,255	1,091	3,020
Standardised ratio	66	102	70	87	106	88	62	89

Table 29: Continued.

680–709 diseases of the skin and subcutaneous tissue

Number	118	256	15	389	100	288	14	402
Rate	3,357	2,997	2,473	3,072	3,151	3,469	1,700	3,268
Standardised rate	3,429	3,141	2,249	3,097	3,174	3,452	1,432	3,052
Standardised ratio	108	137	134	126	101	125	92	116

001–139 infectious and parasitic diseases

Number	113	110	6	229	92	209	8	309
Rate	3,215	1,288	989	1,809	2,898	2,517	972	2,512
Standardised rate	3,458	1,306	819	1,715	2,907	2,383	842	2,224
Standardised ratio	99	115	118	107	80	98	71	91

800–999 injury and poisoning

Number	65	195	4	264	53	153	32	238
Rate	1,849	2,283	660	2,085	1,670	1,843	3,887	1,935
Standardised rate	1,828	2,239	1,339	2,042	1,686	1,838	4,598	2,279
Standardised ratio	100	105	57	102	113	93	84	97

390–459 diseases of the circulatory system

Number	2	228	91	321	3	146	56	205
Rate	57	2,669	15,005	2,535	95	1,759	6,801	1,667
Standardised rate	44	2,808	16,009	3,795	94	1,951	6,615	2,379
Standardised ratio	118	138	128	135	385	122	98	117

520–579 diseases of the digestive system

Number	22	139	9	170	23	157	20	200
Rate	626	1,627	1,484	1,343	725	1,891	2,429	1,626
Standardised rate	717	1,697	1,408	1,449	740	1,866	2,101	1,683
Standardised ratio	102	133	78	121	134	123	108	123

290–319 mental disorders

Number	12	75	2	89	3	136	26	165
Rate	341	878	330	703	95	1,638	3,158	1,342
Standardised rate	352	893	253	698	93	1,625	2,767	1,516
Standardised ratio	95	76	48	77	48	73	90	73

240–279 endocrine, nutritional and metabolic diseases, and immunity disorders

Number	5	105	14	124	4	106	32	142
Rate	142	1,229	2,308	979	126	1,277	3,887	1,155
Standardised rate	110	1,279	2,156	1,131	120	1,560	3,383	1,586
Standardised ratio	129	178	181	176	60	130	199	139

280–289 diseases of blood and blood-forming organs

Number	4	7	1	12	4	56	7	67
Rate	114	82	165	95	126	675	850	545
Standardised rate	128	84	126	99	128	660	611	546
Standardised ratio	224	170	94	173	213	364	190	320

Table 29: Continued.

	Men (no. of people)				Women (no. of people)			
	0–15 (376)	16–64 (905)	65+ (64)	all ages (1,345)	0–15 (344)	16–64 (873)	65+ (86)	all ages (1,303)
630–679 complications of pregnancy, childbirth and the puerperium								
Number	0	0	0	0	1	48	0	49
Rate	0	0	0	0	32	578	0	398
Standardised rate	0	0	0	0	32	527	0	339
Standardised ratio	0	0	0	0	282	88	0	90
140–239 neoplasms								
Number	0	23	2	25	0	19	0	19
Rate	0	269	330	197	0	229	0	154
Standardised rate	0	251	383	212	0	241	0	152
Standardised ratio	0	81	31	62	0	60	0	48
740–759 congenital anomalies								
Number	5	4	0	9	1	6	0	7
Rate	142	47	0	71	32	72	0	57
Standardised rate	177	48	0	70	30	70	0	50
Standardised ratio	71	154	0	99	37	144	0	91
760–779 certain conditions originating in the perinatal period								
Number	0	0	0	0	0	0	0	0
Rate	0	0	0	0	0	0	0	0
Standardised rate	0	0	0	0	0	0	0	0
Standardised ratio	0	0	0	0	0	0	0	0

The standardised ratio picks out conditions that are relatively common or relatively rare. Surprisingly, the ratio for infectious and parasitic diseases was close to 100. The conditions that were comparatively high were: endocrine disorders; blood; respiratory; circulatory; and symptoms, signs and ill-defined conditions; and those that were comparatively low were: neoplasms; mental disorders; and genito-urinary.

The pattern of consultation for Pakistanis (**Table 30**), shown in **Table 30**, was broadly as described for Indians. Overall, consultation rates for women exceeded those for men. In both men and women, compared to the whole population, there was a 9% excess of consultation in men and 8% in women. For most conditions, the consultation rates were slightly higher than in Indians, but this did not apply to the circulatory system. The substantially raised standardised ratio for endocrine disorders, for digestive system disorders and for symptoms and signs were noteworthy.

Table 31 provides data on Bangladeshis and shows that the general principles described above hold. In men, compared to the population as a whole, there was a 19% excess in the consultation rate, and in women 9%. Among the features that stood out were the high standardised ratios for endocrine diseases and the huge difference in men and women for circulatory disorders. The high standardised ratios for endocrine disorders (particularly in men), for digestive system, for skin, and for symptoms and signs (particularly women) are noteworthy.

Table 30: General practice consultation statistics for Pakistanis. Rates are per 10,000 patient-years at risk.

	Men (No. of people)				Women (No. of people)			
	0–15 (232)	16–64 (399)	65+ (19)	All ages (650)	0–15 (242)	16–64 (320)	65+ (8)	All ages (570)
All diseases								
Number	862	1,431	82	2,375	1,011	1,842	30	2,883
Rate	39,744	37,177	49,370	38,405	44,581	60,815	42,053	53,707
Standardised rate	40,589	37,185	50,218	39,334	45,235	62,502	55,258	57,840
Standardised ratio	109	111	79	109	112	106	81	108
460–519 diseases of the respiratory system								
Number	330	266	15	611	345	264	5	614
Rate	15,215	6,911	9,031	9,880	15,213	8,716	7,009	11,438
Standardised rate	15,594	6,744	10,383	9,085	15,391	8,592	11,926	10,510
Standardised ratio	131	154	84	140	139	133	193	136
VO1–V82 supplementary classification of factors influencing health status and contact with health services								
Number	95	266	7	368	117	402	1	520
Rate	4,380	6,911	4,215	5,951	5,159	13,272	1,402	9,687
Standardised rate	4,478	6,866	3,979	6,030	5,348	12,478	1,244	9,145
Standardised ratio	105	155	96	133	90	101	36	97
780–799 symptoms, signs and ill-defined conditions								
Number	95	88	7	190	123	180	4	307
Rate	4,380	2,286	4,215	3,072	5,424	5,943	5,607	5,719
Standardised rate	4,516	2,286	3,897	2,950	5,456	6,119	4,859	5,772
Standardised ratio	148	172	165	160	180	195	125	187
680–709 diseases of the skin and subcutaneous tissue								
Number	78	102	8	188	108	124	0	232
Rate	3,596	2,650	4,817	3,040	4,762	4,094	0	4,322
Standardised rate	3,697	2,549	4,321	2,992	4,849	4,362	0	3,714
Standardised ratio	124	164	134	145	155	147	0	149
710–739 diseases of the musculo-skeletal system and connective tissue								
Number	10	168	10	188	15	194	6	215
Rate	461	4,365	6,021	3,040	661	6,405	8,411	4,005
Standardised rate	458	4,477	5,759	3,729	672	7,399	7,347	6,055
Standardised ratio	95	146	126	138	105	179	138	167
001–139 infectious and parasitic diseases								
Number	82	62	4	148	128	77	1	206
Rate	3,781	1,611	2,408	2,393	5,644	2,542	1,402	3,838
Standardised rate	3,857	1,585	2,603	2,195	5,699	2,277	1,406	2,807
Standardised ratio	103	129	172	114	141	93	164	119
580–629 diseases of the genito-urinary system								
Number	4	21	0	25	8	189	0	197
Rate	184	546	0	404	353	6,240	0	3,670
Standardised rate	197	468	0	358	367	6,079	0	3,908
Standardised ratio	45	170	0	104	40	121	0	108

Table 30: Continued.

	Men (No. of people)				Women (No. of people)			
	0–15 (232)	16–64 (399)	65+ (19)	All ages (650)	0–15 (242)	16–64 (320)	65+ (8)	All ages (570)
320–389 diseases of the nervous system and sense organs								
Number	83	105	11	199	88	97	4	189
Rate	3,827	2,728	6,623	3,218	3,880	3,203	5,607	3,521
Standardised rate	3,851	2,770	6,708	3,431	3,886	4,112	4,476	4,130
Standardised ratio	91	139	167	113	88	127	125	105
520–579 diseases of the digestive system								
Number	23	89	10	122	37	99	2	138
Rate	1,060	2,312	6,021	1,973	1,632	3,269	2,804	2,571
Standardised rate	1,088	2,405	7,244	2,635	1,647	3,859	14,805	5,290
Standardised ratio	164	162	203	165	228	230	93	226
800–999 injury and poisoning								
Number	44	72	1	117	29	57	2	88
Rate	2,029	1,871	602	1,892	1,279	1,882	2,804	1,639
Standardised rate	2,012	1,776	521	1,694	1,328	2,102	2,489	2,014
Standardised ratio	117	85	52	96	64	118	84	96
290–319 mental disorders								
Number	2	29	0	31	4	43	0	47
Rate	92	753	0	501	176	1,420	0	876
Standardised rate	92	727	0	509	188	1,566	0	1,025
Standardised ratio	43	105	0	90	92	91	0	89
630–679 complications of pregnancy, childbirth and the puerperium								
Number	0	0	0	0	0	33	0	33
Rate	0	0	0	0	0	1,090	0	615
Standardised rate	0	0	0	0	0	851	0	537
Standardised ratio	0	0	0	0	0	180	0	177
280–289 diseases of blood and blood-forming organs								
Number	6	1	0	7	2	29	0	31
Rate	277	26	0	113	88	957	0	578
Standardised rate	289	25	0	81	86	763	0	498
Standardised ratio	436	127	0	269	143	318	0	261
240–279 endocrine, nutritional and metabolic diseases, and immunity disorders								
Number	4	56	6	66	1	27	2	30
Rate	184	1,455	3,612	1,067	44	891	2,804	559
Standardised rate	179	1,598	3,127	1,449	47	905	2,489	1,005
Standardised ratio	411	233	148	237	87	178	161	169
390–459 diseases of the circulatory system								
Number	0	71	3	74	0	22	3	25
Rate	0	1,845	1,806	1,197	0	726	4,205	466
Standardised rate	0	1,955	1,678	1,494	0	858	4,217	1,261
Standardised ratio	0	120	19	99	0	88	43	80

Table 30: Continued.

740–759 congenital anomalies								
Number	4	0	0	4	4	1	0	5
Rate	184	0	0	65	176	33	0	93
Standardised rate	183	0	0	40	179	23	0	50
Standardised ratio	105	0	0	73	158	79	0	125
140–239 neoplasms								
Number	0	35	0	35	0	4	0	4
Rate	0	909	0	566	0	132	0	75
Standardised rate	0	954	0	642	0	158	0	100
Standardised ratio	0	133	0	94	0	47	0	37
760–779 certain conditions originating in the perinatal period								
Number	2	0	0	2	2	0	0	2
Rate	92	0	0	32	88	0	0	37
Standardised rate	96	0	0	21	94	0	0	19
Standardised ratio	175	0	0	174	158	0	0	149

Table 31: General practice consultation statistics for Bangladeshis. Rates are per 10,000 patient-years at risk.

	Men (No. of people)				Women (No. of people)			
	0–15 (232)	16–64 (399)	65+ (19)	All ages (650)	0–15 (242)	16–64 (320)	65+ (8)	All ages (570)
All diseases								
Number	511	663	24	1,198	336	672	17	1,025
Rate	49,323	48,275	34,286	48,318	33,103	56,473	50,421	45,786
Standardised rate	50,862	48,636	26,923	47,335	33,719	58,280	54,109	52,541
Standardised Ratio	115	126	53	119	113	105	103	109
VO1–V82 supplementary classification of factors influencing health status and contact with health services								
Number	69	112	7	188	32	157	1	190
Rate	6,660	8,155	10,000	7,582	3,153	13,194	2,966	8,487
Standardised rate	6,954	8,354	7,853	7,965	3,111	12,487	3,621	9,711
Standardised ratio	127	179	85	152	85	104	78	98
460–519 diseases of the respiratory system								
Number	191	107	4	302	121	63	0	184
Rate	18,436	7,791	5,714	12,180	11,921	5,294	0	8,219
Standardised Rate	19,067	7,462	4,487	10,082	12,351	5,617	0	6,647
Standardised ratio	133	180	53	149	117	106	0	111
780–799 symptoms, signs and ill-defined conditions								
Number	39	45	1	85	36	78	2	116
Rate	3,764	3,277	1,429	3,428	3,547	6,555	5,932	5,182
Standardised rate	3,813	3,124	1,122	3,124	3,649	6,834	6,311	6,091
Standardised ratio	169	234	88	192	160	221	278	193

Table 31: Continued.

	Men (No. of people)				Women (No. of people)			
	0–15 (232)	16–64 (399)	65+ (19)	All ages (650)	0–15 (242)	16–64 (320)	65+ (8)	All ages (570)
680–709 diseases of the skin and subcutaneous tissue								
Number	48	67	1	116	49	42	1	92
Rate	4,633	4,878	1,429	4,679	4,827	3,530	2,966	4,110
Standardised rate	4,953	4,827	1,122	4,542	5,057	3,218	3,621	3,655
Standardised ratio	136	235	108	181	175	150	204	163
001–139 infectious and parasitic diseases								
Number	61	36	0	97	41	39	0	80
Rate	5,888	2,621	0	3,912	4,039	3,277	0	3,574
Standardised rate	5,985	2,562	0	3,191	3,995	3,339	0	3,215
Standardised ratio	162	183	0	166	124	132	0	127
320–389 diseases of the nervous system and sense organs								
Number	33	20	3	56	28	47	3	78
Rate	3,185	1,456	4,286	2,259	2,759	3,950	8,898	3,484
Standardised rate	3,260	1,447	3,365	2,059	2,676	3,658	9,932	3,946
Standardised ratio	91	103	142	97	80	175	271	121
520–579 diseases of the digestive system								
Number	27	68	1	96	5	60	2	67
Rate	2,606	4,951	1,429	3,872	493	5,042	5,932	2,993
Standardised rate	2,670	6,057	1,122	4,798	552	6,129	7,243	4,992
Standardised ratio	390	341	104	342	112	332	207	266
710–739 diseases of the musculo-skeletal system and connective tissue								
Number	4	45	1	50	4	56	3	63
Rate	386	3,277	1,429	2,017	394	4,706	8,898	2,814
Standardised rate	378	3,638	1,122	2,616	360	5,836	9,001	4,886
Standardised ratio	103	150	60	137	72	178	198	160
580–629 diseases of the genito-urinary system								
Number	3	18	0	21	7	49	0	56
Rate	290	1,311	0	847	690	4,118	0	2,501
Standardised rate	271	1,407	0	1,005	704	3,856	0	2,852
Standardised ratio	70	194	0	120	69	104	0	97
800–999 injury and poisoning								
Number	32	43	0	75	11	24	1	36
Rate	3,089	3,131	0	3,025	1,084	2,017	2,966	1,608
Standardised rate	3,112	3,171	0	2,886	1,084	2,313	3,621	2,147
Standardised ratio	127	119	0	120	71	113	185	97
240–279 endocrine, nutritional and metabolic diseases, and immunity disorders								
Number	1	36	2	39	0	28	0	28
Rate	97	2,621	2,857	1,573	0	2,353	0	1,251
Standardised rate	97	2,109	2,244	1,622	0	3,176	0	2,222
Standardised ratio	221	246	170	235	0	183	0	153

Table 31: Continued.

290–319 mental disorders

Number	2	16	2	20	0	9	0	9
Rate	193	1,165	2,857	807	0	756	0	402
Standardised rate	193	1,374	2,244	1,156	0	660	0	461
Standardised ratio	90	109	452	120	0	50	0	41

630–679 complications of pregnancy, childbirth and the puerperium

Number	0	0	0	0	0	9	0	9
Rate	0	0	0	0	0	756	0	402
Standardised rate	0	0	0	0	0	404	0	283
Standardised ratio	0	0	0	0	0	73	0	71

390–459 diseases of the circulatory system

Number	0	47	2	49	1	4	2	7
Rate	0	3,422	2,857	1,976	99	336	5,932	313
Standardised rate	0	2,986	2,244	2,183	91	293	5,379	658
Standardised ratio	0	170	46	144	399	48	99	66

280–289 diseases of blood and blood-forming organs

Number	1	0	0	1	0	5	0	5
Rate	97	0	0	40	0	420	0	223
Standardised rate	107	0	0	26	0	322	0	225
Standardised ratio	177	0	0	103	0	207	0	139

140–239 neoplasms

Number	0	3	0	3	1	1	2	4
Rate	0	218	0	121	99	84	5,932	179
Standardised rate	0	119	0	80	91	105	5,379	526
Standardised ratio	0	90	0	60	118	31	671	70

760–779 certain conditions originating in the perinatal period

Number	0	0	0	0	0	1	0	1
Rate	0	0	0	0	0	84	0	45
Standardised rate	0	0	0	0	0	33	0	23
Standardised ratio	0	0	0	0	0	3,531	0	198

740–759 congenital anomalies

Number	0	0	0	0	0	0	0	0
Rate	0	0	0	0	0	0	0	0
Standardised rate	0	0	0	0	0	0	0	0
Standardised ratio	0	0	0	0	0	0	0	0

Table 32 shows that, for the Chinese, consultation rates were substantially lower than in the population as a whole. Only for symptoms and signs was the standardised ratio distinctly higher in both Chinese men and women compared to the whole population. Chinese men had, overall, lower rates than Chinese women. The consultation rate was markedly higher in men than women for endocrine disorders, but the opposite was true for most other conditions. The male–female disparity was small for circulatory system diseases. The picture portrays an underutilisation of primary care services, possibly in addition to the exceptionally healthy population.

Table 32: General practice consultation statistics for Chinese. Rates are per 10,000 patient-years at risk.

	Men (No. of people)				Women (No. of people)			
	0–15 (232)	16–64 (399)	65+ (19)	All ages (650)	0–15 (242)	16–64 (320)	65+ (8)	All ages (570)
All diseases								
Number	535	602	50	1,187	536	1,445	107	2,088
Rate	32,142	18,004	27,778	22,878	34,048	40,122	40,432	38,379
Standardised rate	31,111	21,280	25,904	23,956	33,926	39,790	38,292	38,371
Standardised ratio	103	84	73	91	97	99	83	98
VO1–V82 supplementary classification of factors influencing health status and contact with health services								
Number	76	98	12	186	88	430	19	537
Rate	4,566	2,931	6,667	3,585	5,590	11,939	7,179	9,871
Standardised rate	4,369	3,262	6,155	3,833	5,628	10,701	6,595	8,993
Standardised ratio	111	100	103	104	121	97	118	102
460–519 diseases of the respiratory system								
Number	174	131	6	311	194	203	14	411
Rate	10,454	3,918	3,333	5,994	12,323	5,636	5,290	7,555
Standardised rate	10,047	4,270	3,392	5,434	12,229	4,841	5,228	6,373
Standardised ratio	102	87	59	94	108	103	65	103
680–709 diseases of the skin and subcutaneous tissue								
Number	47	52	4	103	87	104	6	197
Rate	2,824	1,555	2,222	1,985	5,526	2,888	2,267	3,621
Standardised rate	2,768	1,498	1,966	1,829	5,530	2,790	2,192	3,232
Standardised ratio	91	103	164	100	118	112	77	113
780–799 symptoms, signs and ill-defined conditions								
Number	64	49	6	119	52	121	17	190
Rate	3,845	1,465	3,333	2,294	3,303	3,360	6,424	3,492
Standardised rate	3,727	1,571	2,477	2,146	3,269	3,509	5,947	3,878
Standardised ratio	130	113	124	122	115	126	121	122
580–629 diseases of the genito-urinary system								
Number	16	11	0	27	5	136	4	145
Rate	961	329	0	520	318	3,776	1,511	2,665
Standardised rate	914	355	0	437	324	3,704	1,187	2,603
Standardised ratio	137	83	0	100	57	86	97	84
001–139 infectious and parasitic diseases								
Number	52	24	0	76	51	68	2	121
Rate	3,124	718	0	1,465	3,240	1,888	756	2,224
Standardised rate	3,050	635	0	1,091	3,241	1,773	690	1,879
Standardised ratio	81	71	0	76	88	78	44	81
320–389 diseases of the nervous system and sense organs								
Number	50	33	4	87	23	73	5	101
Rate	3,004	987	2,222	1,677	1,461	2,027	1,889	1,856
Standardised rate	2,890	1,131	1,652	1,575	1,437	2,079	2,003	1,939
Standardised ratio	78	56	52	68	46	74	85	63

Table 32: Continued.

710–739 diseases of the musculo-skeletal system and connective tissue

Number	4	44	3	51	1	85	8	94
Rate	240	1,316	1,667	983	64	2,360	3,023	1,728
Standardised rate	261	1,982	1,239	1,521	70	3,419	2,373	2,576
Standardised ratio	51	52	23	49	17	67	37	59

800–999 injury and poisoning

Number	26	36	0	62	17	64	4	85
Rate	1,562	1,077	0	1,195	1,080	1,777	1,511	1,562
Standardised rate	1,525	1,294	0	1,197	1,081	1,727	1,420	1,547
Standardised ratio	71	52	0	57	72	68	47	68

520–579 diseases of the digestive system

Number	11	25	1	37	12	32	16	60
Rate	661	748	556	713	762	889	6,046	1,103
Standardised rate	644	815	413	732	744	945	6,116	1,788
Standardised ratio	108	72	38	79	134	65	153	84

390–459 diseases of the circulatory system

Number	2	57	3	62	1	43	8	52
Rate	120	1,705	1,667	1,195	64	1,194	3,023	956
Standardised rate	125	2,723	1,867	2,057	63	1,972	3,200	1,803
Standardised ratio	536	86	35	80	268	86	36	74

290–319 mental disorders

Number	7	18	0	25	1	43	1	45
Rate	421	538	0	482	64	1,194	378	827
Standardised rate	442	750	0	598	58	1,068	345	744
Standardised ratio	138	51	0	62	33	51	31	49

630–679 complications of pregnancy, childbirth and the puerperium

Number	0	0	0	0	0	20	0	20
Rate	0	0	0	0	0	555	0	368
Standardised rate	0	0	0	0	0	396	0	250
Standardised ratio	0	0	0	0	0	74	0	73

140–239 neoplasms

Number	1	3	4	8	1	13	0	14
Rate	60	90	2,222	154	64	361	0	257
Standardised rate	68	105	2,909	416	63	505	0	331
Standardised ratio	85	60	105	70	79	86	0	77

240–279 endocrine, nutritional and metabolic diseases, and immunity disorders

Number	1	21	7	29	1	5	1	7
Rate	60	628	3,889	559	64	139	378	129
Standardised rate	56	888	3,833	1,041	63	175	345	182
Standardised ratio	134	99	204	117	125	29	42	35

280–289 diseases of blood and blood-forming organs

Number	0	0	0	0	0	3	2	5
Rate	0	0	0	0	0	83	756	92
Standardised rate	0	0	0	0	0	150	652	206
Standardised ratio	0	0	0	0	0	44	282	64

Table 32: Continued.

	Men (No. of people)				Women (No. of people)			
	0–15 (232)	16–64 (399)	65+ (19)	All ages (650)	0–15 (242)	16–64 (320)	65+ (8)	All ages (570)
740–759 congenital anomalies								
Number	4	0	0	4	2	2	0	4
Rate	240	0	0	77	127	56	0	74
Standardised rate	226	0	0	49	127	36	0	48
Standardised ratio	129	0	0	88	148	136	0	135
760–779 certain conditions originating in the perinatal period								
Number	0	0	0	0	0	0	0	0
Rate	0	0	0	0	0	0	0	0
Standardised rate	0	0	0	0	0	0	0	0
Standardised ratio	0	0	0	0	0	0	0	0

Table 33 shows that the commonest causes of consultation in Caribbeans were similar to other ethnic groups. The most surprising findings were that the rate of consultation for mental disorders was not high, that consultation rates for circulatory diseases were greater in women than men, and that consultations for neoplasms were low.

Table 33: General practice consultation statistics for Caribbeans. Rates are per 10,000 patient-years at risk.

	Men (No. of people)				Women (No. of people)			
	0–15 (232)	16–64 (399)	65+ (19)	All ages (650)	0–15 (242)	16–64 (320)	65+ (8)	All ages (570)
All diseases								
Number	866	1,715	275	2,856	795	3,929	256	4,980
Rate	35,788	31,443	63,836	34,389	32,751	59,443	68,252	52,910
Standardised rate	3,6329	32,203	68,878	36,811	32,318	59,424	63,131	54,680
Standardised ratio	99	111	108	107	102	108	105	106
VO1–V82 supplementary classification of factors influencing health status and contact with health services								
Number	123	244	38	405	112	1,124	31	1,267
Rate	5,083	4,474	8,821	4,877	4,614	17,005	8,265	13,461
Standardised rate	5,220	4,461	7,948	4,980	4,490	15,713	7,080	12,012
Standardised ratio	115	108	133	112	98	116	110	113
460–519 diseases of the respiratory system								
Number	309	277	30	616	268	424	26	718
Rate	12,770	5,079	6,964	7,417	11,041	6,415	6,932	7,628
Standardised rate	12,937	4,985	7,602	7,013	10,938	6,193	6,244	7,143
Standardised ratio	113	135	101	123	110	107	93	108

Table 33: Continued.

580–629 diseases of the genito-urinary system

Number	20	30	9	59	19	362	7	388
Rate	827	550	2,089	710	783	5,477	1,866	4,122
Standardised rate	835	541	2,012	755	776	5,318	1,791	3,815
Standardised ratio	138	151	177	149	95	119	91	117

780–799 symptoms, signs and ill-defined conditions

Number	79	134	19	232	85	248	24	357
Rate	3,265	2,457	4,410	2,794	3,502	3,752	6,399	3,793
Standardised rate	3,313	2,622	4,063	2,920	3,454	3,790	5,924	4,088
Standardised ratio	129	173	153	153	139	146	133	144

710–739 diseases of the musculo-skeletal system and connective tissue

Number	12	166	17	195	11	293	26	330
Rate	496	3,043	3,946	2,348	453	4,433	6,932	3,506
Standardised rate	490	3,058	4,042	2,587	456	5,055	6,341	4,362
Standardised ratio	120	116	117	117	96	121	113	118

680–709 diseases of the skin and subcutaneous tissue

Number	71	122	9	202	92	217	8	317
Rate	2,934	2,237	2,089	2,432	3,790	3,283	2,133	3,368
Standardised rate	2,990	2,218	3,016	2,470	3,732	3,051	1,892	2,988
Standardised ratio	100	110	53	103	115	120	109	118

001–139 infectious and parasitic diseases

Number	86	72	10	168	73	191	2	266
Rate	3,554	1,320	2,321	2,023	3,007	2,890	533	2,826
Standardised rate	3,617	1,257	2,464	1,903	2,984	2,694	522	2,380
Standardised ratio	102	120	135	111	89	119	63	107

390–459 diseases of the circulatory system

Number	0	163	50	213	0	208	55	263
Rate	0	2,988	11,607	2,565	0	3,147	14,663	2,794
Standardised rate	0	3,027	10,493	3,107	0	3,881	13,638	4,777
Standardised ratio	0	143	119	135	0	167	125	155

800–999 injury and poisoning

Number	60	153	8	221	37	203	9	249
Rate	2,480	2,805	1,857	2,661	1,524	3,071	2,399	2,646
Standardised rate	2,453	2,906	1,942	2,708	1,518	2,918	2,367	2,546
Standardised ratio	128	127	152	129	92	122	98	114

320–389 diseases of the nervous system and sense organs

Number	80	98	10	188	73	152	12	237
Rate	3,306	1,797	2,321	2,264	3,007	2,300	3,199	2,518
Standardised rate	3,381	1,834	3,381	2,333	2,973	2,442	2,842	2,616
Standardised ratio	68	93	56	78	72	103	107	92

Table 33: Continued.

	Men (No. of people)				Women (No. of people)			
	0–15 (232)	16–64 (399)	65+ (19)	All ages (650)	0–15 (242)	16–64 (320)	65+ (8)	All ages (570)
240–279 endocrine, nutritional and metabolic diseases, and immunity disorders								
Number	1	67	15	83	5	143	31	179
Rate	41	1,228	3,482	999	206	2,164	8,265	1,902
Standardised rate	43	1,332	3,284	1,242	196	2,800	7,467	3,081
Standardised ratio	93	149	251	164	79	159	242	165
290–319 mental disorders								
Number	5	85	15	105	0	146	14	160
Rate	207	1,558	3,482	1,264	0	2,209	3,733	1,700
Standardised rate	206	1,817	4,230	1,702	0	2,308	4,318	2,193
Standardised ratio	77	81	180	88	0	97	129	93
520–579 diseases of the digestive system								
Number	12	96	26	134	13	101	3	117
Rate	496	1,760	6,035	1,614	536	1,528	800	1,243
Standardised rate	509	1,994	5,523	2,020	516	1,615	706	1,242
Standardised ratio	103	135	199	135	77	99	53	93
630–679 complications of pregnancy, childbirth and the puerperium								
Number	0	0	0	0	0	58	0	58
Rate	0	0	0	0	0	878	0	616
Standardised rate	0	0	0	0	0	729	0	460
Standardised ratio	0	0	0	0	0	109	0	108
140–239 neoplasms								
Number	1	6	6	13	2	28	4	34
Rate	41	110	1,393	157	82	424	1,066	361
Standardised rate	41	115	1,065	194	83	467	1,014	484
Standardised ratio	57	46	95	56	101	78	119	83
280–289 diseases of blood and blood-forming organs								
Number	0	0	13	13	2	29	1	32
Rate	0	0	3,018	157	82	439	267	340
Standardised rate	0	0	7,812	786	83	427	246	328
Standardised ratio	0	0	152	32	139	255	96	224
740–759 congenital anomalies								
Number	4	2	0	6	2	2	3	7
Rate	165	37	0	72	82	30	800	74
Standardised rate	167	37	0	62	80	24	738	157
Standardised ratio	124	120	0	119	94	73	527	99
760–779 certain conditions originating in the perinatal period								
Number	3	0	0	3	1	0	0	1
Rate	124	0	0	36	41	0	0	11
Standardised rate	128	0	0	28	39	0	0	8
Standardised ratio	155	0	0	154	66	0	0	59

Table 34 shows that the overall consultation patterns for Africans were as described for other groups, with an excess, overall, of 11% in men and 8% in women compared to the whole population. The numbers of consultations for each specific cause were too small to sustain a reliable comparison.

Table 34: General practice consultation statistics for Africans. Rates are per 10,000 patient-years at risk.

	Men (No. of people)				Women (No. of people)			
	0–15 (232)	16–64 (399)	65+ (19)	All ages (650)	0–15 (242)	16–64 (320)	65+ (8)	All ages (570)
All diseases								
Number	348	376	14	738	328	1,226	45	1,599
Rate	38,782	23,329	140,000	29,297	32,243	58,584	68,340	50,349
Standardised rate	38,244	23,763	140,000	32,465	31,144	59,633	68,252	54,619
Standardised ratio	112	110	126	111	108	108	105	108
VO1–V82 supplementary classification of factors influencing health status and contact with health services								
Number	62	54	2	118	61	387	2	450
Rate	6,909	3,350	20,000	4,684	5,996	18,493	3,037	14,170
Standardised rate	6,726	4,118	20,000	5,455	5,823	17,848	4,591	13,760
Standardised ratio	141	114	302	127	133	116	81	119
460–519 diseases of the respiratory system								
Number	117	76	2	195	129	154	3	286
Rate	13,039	4,715	20,000	7,741	12,681	7,359	4,556	9,006
Standardised rate	13,157	5,359	20,000	7,862	12,328	6,486	2,908	7,303
Standardised ratio	123	117	379	121	118	98	102	107
780–799 symptoms, signs and ill-defined conditions								
Number	18	25	3	46	22	102	7	131
Rate	2,006	1,551	30,000	1,826	2,163	4,874	10,631	4,125
Standardised rate	1,986	1,426	30,000	2,859	2,116	4,883	10,312	4,932
Standardised ratio	88	123	642	107	97	183	260	155
680–709 diseases of the skin and subcutaneous tissue								
Number	43	25	1	69	30	65	2	97
Rate	4,792	1,551	10,000	2,739	2,949	3,106	3,037	3,054
Standardised rate	4,682	1,301	10,000	2,493	2,731	2,445	2,157	2,472
Standardised ratio	168	97	772	133	70	114	200	100
580–629 diseases of the genito-urinary system								
Number	4	2	1	7	5	87	0	92
Rate	446	124	10,000	278	492	4,157	0	2,897
Standardised rate	419	81	10,000	612	469	3,333	0	2,338
Standardised ratio	105	25	1,647	76	72	103	0	99
710–739 diseases of the musculo-skeletal system and connective tissue								
Number	2	27	0	29	1	83	4	88
Rate	223	1,675	0	1,151	98	3,966	6,075	2,771
Standardised rate	209	1,423	0	1,072	127	5,815	9,181	5,006
Standardised ratio	58	79	0	75	28	148	103	135

Table 34: Continued.

	Men (No. of people)				Women (No. of people)			
	0–15 (232)	16–64 (399)	65+ (19)	All ages (650)	0–15 (242)	16–64 (320)	65+ (8)	All ages (570)
001–139 infectious and parasitic diseases								
Number	34	25	0	59	30	55	2	87
Rate	3,789	1,551	0	2,342	2,949	2,628	3,037	2,739
Standardised rate	3,738	1,289	0	1,807	2,782	2,119	2,157	2,264
Standardised ratio	103	146	0	119	81	103	341	96
320–389 diseases of the nervous system and sense organs								
Number	37	30	0	67	26	56	3	85
Rate	4,123	1,861	0	2,660	2,556	2,676	4,556	2,676
Standardised rate	3,955	1,667	0	2,130	2,631	2,663	6,654	3,122
Standardised ratio	85	124	0	100	76	123	135	101
290–319 mental disorders								
Number	3	25	4	32	3	60	5	68
Rate	334	1,551	40,000	1,270	295	2,867	7,593	2,141
Standardised rate	315	1,913	40,000	3,270	251	3,853	7,034	3,463
Standardised ratio	155	163	1,579	170	105	121	116	120
800–999 injury and poisoning								
Number	14	29	0	43	10	43	6	59
Rate	1,560	1,799	0	1,707	983	2,055	9,112	1,858
Standardised rate	1,564	1,619	0	1,533	879	3,763	7,784	3,623
Standardised ratio	84	85	0	84	64	116	345	107
390–459 diseases of the circulatory system								
Number	0	14	0	14	0	35	11	46
Rate	0	869	0	556	0	1,672	16,705	1,448
Standardised rate	0	1,029	0	739	0	2,344	15,475	3,381
Standardised ratio	0	69	0	64	0	98	98	96
520–579 diseases of the digestive system								
Number	9	38	0	47	3	35	0	38
Rate	1,003	2,358	0	1,866	295	1,672	0	1,197
Standardised rate	943	2,229	0	1,825	265	1,438	0	1,022
Standardised ratio	112	170	0	152	61	138	0	118
140–239 neoplasms								
Number	0	2	0	2	0	10	0	10
Rate	0	124	0	79	0	478	0	315
Standardised rate	0	92	0	66	0	513	0	345
Standardised ratio	0	86	0	66	0	51	0	43
630–679 complications of pregnancy, childbirth and the puerperium								
Number	0	0	0	0	0	28	0	28
Rate	0	0	0	0	0	1,338	0	882
Standardised rate	0	0	0	0	0	917	0	616
Standardised ratio	0	0	0	0	0	98	0	97
280–289 diseases of blood and blood-forming organs								
Number	1	2	0	3	4	6	0	10
Rate	111	124	0	119	393	287	0	315
Standardised rate	105	121	0	112	356	259	0	249
Standardised ratio	210	759	0	398	625	152	0	231

Table 34: Continued.

240–279 endocrine, nutritional and metabolic diseases, and immunity disorders

Number	1	1	1	3	1	18	0	19
Rate	111	62	10,000	119	98	860	0	598
Standardised rate	129	55	10,000	525	127	824	0	581
Standardised ratio	243	27	1,189	71	197	134	0	129

740–759 congenital anomalies

Number	3	1	0	4	3	2	0	5
Rate	334	62	0	159	295	96	0	157
Standardised rate	315	41	0	103	258	132	0	143
Standardised ratio	242	208	0	232	330	236	0	280

760–779 certain conditions originating in the perinatal period

Number	0	0	0	0	0	0	0	0
Rate	0	0	0	0	0	0	0	0
Standardised rate	0	0	0	0	0	0	0	0
Standardised ratio	0	0	0	0	0	0	0	0

Table 35 shows that the white population had, overall, an excess in consultation rates of 8% for men and 5% for women.

Table 35: General practice consultation statistics for Whites. Rates are per 10,000 patient-years at risk.

	Men (No. of people)				Women (No. of people)			
	0–15 (232)	16–64 (399)	65+ (19)	All ages (650)	0–15 (242)	16–64 (320)	65+ (8)	All ages (570)
All diseases								
Number	147,651	339,176	134,810	621,637	146,173	656,481	214,701	101,7355
Rate	34,335	28,909	56,490	33,749	35,540	51,639	60,925	49,993
Standardised rate	34,178	28,536	56,594	33,135	35,455	51,723	60,998	50,080
Standardised ratio	103	111	105	108	103	105	104	105
VO1–V82 supplementary classification of factors influencing health status and contact with health services								
Number	18,432	51,588	14,669	84,689	19,868	16,3997	21,992	20,5857
Rate	4,286	4,397	6,147	4,598	4,831	12,900	6,241	10,116
Standardised rate	4,248	4,341	6,158	4,539	4,807	13,102	6,248	10,286
Standardised ratio	102	112	107	109	103	107	107	106
460–519 diseases of the respiratory system								
Number	47,998	49,592	19,300	116,890	44,471	83,262	24,510	152,243
Rate	11,162	4,227	8,087	6,346	10,813	6,549	6,955	7,481
Standardised rate	11,111	4,207	8,104	6,175	10,787	6,560	6,950	7,465
Standardised ratio	103	113	106	108	103	108	105	106
710–739 diseases of the musculo-skeletal system and connective tissue								
Number	2,114	39,784	13,130	55,028	2,219	51,051	26,997	80,267
Rate	492	3,391	5,502	2,988	540	4,016	7,661	3,944
Standardised rate	495	3,312	5,501	2,963	542	3,953	7,657	3,909
Standardised ratio	105	113	107	111	106	107	106	107

Table 35: Continued.

	Men (No. of people)				Women (No. of people)			
	0–15 (232)	16–64 (399)	65+ (19)	All ages (650)	0–15 (242)	16–64 (320)	65+ (8)	All ages (570)
580–629 diseases of the genito-urinary system								
Number	2,565	6,152	3,851	12,568	3,741	66,142	8,402	78,285
Rate	596	524	1,614	682	910	5,203	2,384	3,847
Standardised rate	594	518	1,619	667	911	5,204	2,389	3,872
Standardised ratio	104	114	108	110	105	108	106	108
320–389 diseases of the nervous system and sense organs								
Number	21,503	24,163	10,637	56,303	21,293	36,583	15,576	73,452
Rate	5,000	2,059	4,457	3,057	5,177	2,878	4,420	3,609
Standardised rate	4,971	2,037	4,465	2,966	5,160	2,866	4,432	3,589
Standardised ratio	105	113	108	109	105	108	107	107
780–799 symptoms, signs and ill-defined conditions								
Number	11,372	18,598	8,482	38,452	11,740	35,965	15,436	63,141
Rate	2,644	1,585	3,554	2,088	2,854	2,829	4,380	3,103
Standardised rate	2,633	1,566	3,572	2,039	2,848	2,829	4,401	3,101
Standardised ratio	102	111	104	107	102	106	104	105
390–459 diseases of the circulatory system								
Number	130	26,299	26,597	53,026	127	25,089	36,642	61,858
Rate	30	2,242	11,145	2,879	31	1,974	10,398	3,040
Standardised rate	30	2,107	11,150	2,743	31	1,914	10,406	2,991
Standardised ratio	99	111	106	108	102	108	105	106
680–709 diseases of the skin and subcutaneous tissue								
Number	12,564	24,574	6,979	44,117	13,077	34,784	10,742	58,603
Rate	2,922	2,095	2,924	2,395	3,180	2,736	3,048	2,880
Standardised rate	2,913	2,093	2,930	2,372	3,174	2,748	3,052	2,884
Standardised ratio	104	113	107	110	103	108	106	106
001–139 infectious and parasitic diseases								
Number	15,833	15,046	2,748	33,627	16,684	31,995	4,875	53,554
Rate	3,682	1,282	1,152	1,826	4,057	2,517	1,383	2,632
Standardised rate	3,665	1,300	1,154	1,796	4,046	2,550	1,385	2,648
Standardised ratio	104	114	107	108	104	109	106	107
290–319 mental disorders								
Number	1,293	20,674	4,295	26,262	1,088	38,510	11,180	50,778
Rate	301	1,762	1,800	1,426	265	3,029	3,173	2,495
Standardised rate	300	1,760	1,809	1,449	265	3,015	3,182	2,498
Standardised ratio	105	112	104	110	104	108	104	107
800–999 injury and poisoning								
Number	8,753	30,286	4,932	43,971	7,055	29,477	11,269	47,801
Rate	2,035	2,581	2,067	2,387	1,715	2,319	3,198	2,349
Standardised rate	2,038	2,599	2,081	2,415	1,717	2,317	3,219	2,352
Standardised ratio	104	114	106	110	104	108	105	106

Table 35: Continued.

520–579 diseases of the digestive system

Number	2,961	17,310	7,646	27,917	2,721	23,431	11,080	37,232
Rate	689	1,475	3,204	1,516	662	1,843	3,144	1,830
Standardised rate	685	1,455	3,211	1,499	660	1,832	3,151	1,825
Standardised ratio	104	113	106	110	105	108	106	107

240–279 endocrine, nutritional and metabolic diseases, and immunity disorders

Number	286	9,611	5,547	15,444	378	16,715	8,583	25,676
Rate	67	819	2,324	838	92	1,315	2,436	1,262
Standardised rate	66	786	2,319	814	92	1,290	2,417	1,245
Standardised ratio	99	112	106	109	104	108	106	107

140–239 neoplasms

Number	436	4,127	4,478	9,041	487	7,503	4,353	12,343
Rate	101	352	1,876	491	118	590	1,235	607
Standardised rate	102	342	1,879	474	119	582	1,235	602
Standardised ratio	105	113	100	107	109	106	102	105

630–679 complications of pregnancy, childbirth and the puerperium

Number	0	0	0	0	46	7,896	13	7,955
Rate	0	0	0	0	11	621	4	391
Standardised rate	0	0	0	0	11	643	4	409
Standardised ratio	0	0	0	0	91	112	116	112

280–289 diseases of blood and blood-forming organs

Number	352	751	1,373	2,476	371	3,225	2,756	6,352
Rate	82	64	575	134	90	254	782	312
Standardised rate	82	61	579	128	90	251	787	311
Standardised ratio	104	112	104	106	104	106	104	105

740–759 congenital anomalies

Number	737	619	144	1,500	458	825	292	1,575
Rate	171	53	60	81	111	65	83	77
Standardised rate	170	53	60	79	111	65	83	77
Standardised ratio	103	115	111	108	100	109	106	105

760–779 certain conditions originating in the perinatal period

Number	322	2	2	326	349	31	3	383
Rate	75	0	1	18	85	2	1	19
Standardised rate	74	0	1	16	84	3	1	18
Standardised ratio	104	135	77	103	103	111	119	104

Other studies have found that consultations with general practitioners are higher amongst Asians (the term 'Asian' has usually not been clearly defined) and increase with age.[143,146,147] It is not possible to determine whether these patterns reflect differences in morbidity and need, varying thresholds and perceptions of illness, differential uptake of services, or a combination of these factors.

Higher GP contact rates may also reflect socio-economic disadvantage, and variation in the quality of care offered to minority ethnic groups, for example, poorer communication within, and outcomes from, consultations from patients' perspectives[86]; the location of many ethnic populations within inner city areas where primary care may be less well developed and under-resourced[16,138]; provision of care insensitive to differing cultural needs; or care based upon stereotypes and negative attitudes about minority groups.[47,148–50]

Ethnic preferences for health professionals

The recent Policy Studies Institute survey[84] found that 40% of Pakistani and Bangladeshi respondents, a third of Chinese and Indian respondents, and under 25% of other ethnic groups including whites surveyed preferred to see a doctor of their own ethnic origin. This preference was much more pronounced for those who spoke limited or no English, and among women who were white, Pakistani, Bangladeshi or Indian. The linguistic and cultural concordance between the patient and GP is more important in the choice of GP than the sex of the GP.[151] Opportunities for Caribbeans to consult a Caribbean GP appear very limited – less than 1% of survey respondents had had access to the latter.[86]

Gender preferences for health professionals

Except for Pakistani men, most men from minority ethnic groups do not appear to express a preference to see a doctor of the same gender.[84] However, women from all minority ethnic groups (except the Chinese) appear more likely than white women to prefer to consult a female doctor.[84] This was the case for Pakistani and Bangladeshi women in particular (75% and 83%, respectively, preferring to see a female doctor) in the recent PSI survey and probably reflects the cultural and religious traditions of Muslim groups.

Although there may be a tendency to overstate the problems of consulting a male GP,[148,152] some Muslim women are reluctant to see a male doctor where physical, and especially gynaecological, examination may be involved.[151,153] The preferences of many minority ethnic women, particularly from South Asian groups, to consult a female doctor of similar ethnicity are currently unlikely to be met.[86] It has been suggested that 'linguistic concordance' again may become more important than gender for some women in this context. Any embarrassment caused through examination by a male doctor may be reluctantly tolerated because of the potential benefit of improved communication with a doctor of similar ethnicity.[151]

Although there is a lack of available information, opportunities to choose health professionals of the same gender and ethnicity appear limited. It is therefore likely that for most women, including those from the BMEGs, the process and quality of current health consultations may be compromised and, for example, result in underreporting of gynaecological, sexual and other women's health issues.

Secondary care services

As routine data of sufficient quality are not available, it is not possible to provide hospital utilisation rates. However Balarajan et al. (1991)[154] note that, after adjusting for socio-economic factors, there appears to be no significant association between ethnic group and hospital utilisation amongst males, though Pakistani females (age 6–44 years) had higher utilisation rates than whites. This overall similarity in hospital utilisation is also supported by Nazroo[84] (**Table 36**) (with the exception of Chinese respondents, who reported lower utilisation). The data also show the expected rise in admission rate, with poorer perceived health amongst all ethnic groups.

Table 36: Hospital inpatient stays in the past year by self-assessed general health.

	White	Caribbean	Indian or African Asian	Pakistani or Bangladeshi	Chinese
Stayed overnight as a hospital inpatient in the last year					
Good/excellent health	7	7	6	7	6
Fair health	16	13	11	14	7*
Poor/very poor health	30	31	31	28	9*
Weighted base	*2,863*	*1,560*	*2,081*	*1,141*	*390*
Unweighted base	*2,856*	*1,197*	*1,992*	*1,769*	*214*

* Small base numbers in the cell make the estimate unreliable.
Cell percentages: age and gender-standardised.
Source: Nazroo 1997[84]

As noted earlier, differences in GP consultation rates between minority ethnic groups and whites are larger than for hospital admission rates, raising the possibility that higher levels of illness among minority groups are not translated into higher admission rates.

GP referrals

GP referral rates vary enormously and are notoriously difficult to disentangle.[155] Some studies have pointed to possible inequities in relation to referral for cardiovascular disease but others have shown no population bias. Differences in referral delay to tertiary cardiovascular services between white and South Asian patients have been suggested.[156] Compared to the white population, South Asians with chronic chest pain may be less likely to be referred for exercise testing and wait longer to see a cardiologist or to have angiography.[157] The barriers do not appear to be a result of patients' interpretations of symptoms or their willingness to seek care. Other factors, related to services and communication with health professionals, might be contributing to inequality of experience.[158] Pending larger scale representative research into these issues, there is a need to ensure equity of services.

Ethnic workforce

There is a dearth of literature and data on the ethnic origin of general practitioners and what is available is from routine statistics and one-off surveys, and has used proxy measures for recording ethnic group, i.e. country of qualification.

Table 37 shows that 16% of GPs have qualified from outside the European Economic Area. The unequal geographical distribution of GPs is well documented,[159] which is particularly marked for overseas qualified GPs. A high proportion of the latter reside within London, West Midlands and the North West. A smaller proportion is found in the South Eastern and Western regions.

Many of these overseas qualified doctors are working in smaller practices, particularly single-handed practices, and are concentrated within conurbations (**Table 37**).[160]

Table 37: Unrestricted principals by country of first qualification (October 1999).

Region	UK	EEA*	Elsewhere	Total
Northern & Yorkshire	3,019	110	463 (13)	3,592
Trent	2,305	75	398 (14)	2,773
Eastern	2,461	118	377 (13)	2,956
London	2,518	167	1,262 (32)	3,947
South Eastern	4,199	141	439 (9)	4,779
South Western	2,912	60	69 (2)	3,041
West Midlands	2,175	79	639 (22)	2,893
North West	2,769	109	727 (20)	3,605
England Total	22,358	859	4,374 (16)	27,591

Source: NHSE Headquarters. Statistics (Workforce) GMS. Leeds, 1999 (http://www.doh.gov.uk/public/gandpmss99.htm)
* European Economic Area.

Table 38 shows the data that is available by ethnic group for hospital medical staff and BMEG doctors form a third of the hospital workforce.

Table 38: All hospital medical staff by ethnic origin (England at 30 September 1999).

All ethnic groups	No.		%	
White	42,777		67.3	
Black	2,412		3.8	
Caribbean		390		0.6
African		1,480		2.3
Other		542		0.9
Asian	11,760		16.8	
Indian		8,781		13.8
Pakistani		1,565		2.5
Bangladeshi		288		0.5
Chinese	1,036		1.6	
Any other ethnic group	5,307		8.4	
Not known	1,382		2.1	
All	63,548		100	

Source: Department of Health (http://www.doh.gov.uk/stats/d_results.htm)

Table 39 shows that 7% of the non-medical workforce are from minority ethnic groups.

Table 39: NHS Hospital and Community Health Services: non-medical staff ethnic origin at 30 September 1999 (England).

	White	Black	Asian	Other	Unknown
All non-medical staff	89.3	3.6	1.6	1.8	3.7
Nursing, midwifery and health visiting (qualified staff)	86.8	4.7	1.6	2.3	4.6
Scientific, therapeutic and technical staff	92.3	2.1	2.4	1.7	1.5
Health care assistants	90.6	4.6	1.5	1.7	1.7
Support staff	90.7	3.9	1.3	1.7	2.4
Ambulance staff	97.8	0.6	0.3	0.5	0.7
Administration and estates staff	92.9	2.5	1.8	1.1	1.7
Other staff	93.9	1.2	2.0	1.4	1.5

Source: Health and Personal Social Services Statistics, England (http://www.doh.gov.uk/public/sb0011.htm)

Figures should be treated with caution as they are based upon organisations reporting 90% or more valid ethnic codes for non-medical staff. Percentages were calculated from numbers of staff expressed as whole-time equivalents.

Bilingual services: interpreter, linkworker and advocate provision

Background

Access to, and use of, appropriate interpreting services is one of the most important health care needs identified by people from ethnic minorities themselves – for effective communication in health encounters.[150,161] Language barriers constitute major obstacles to care for certain ethnic groups, notably South Asian and Chinese populations, especially women and older people from these groups, and for patients from diverse refugee populations. Accurate data upon the proportion of different groups that cannot communicate in English are lacking.

Estimates of functional English literacy among ethnic groups are available.[162] More than a third of non-UK born (and non-UK educated) Bengali and Punjabi speakers were unable to complete a basic test of their name and address on a library card application form in a recent study.[162] In this study, almost three out of four of those born outside the UK were 'below survival level' for functional literacy.

In consultations in primary care, most Caribbean patients appear to share a language with their GP. As many as 80% of South Asian patients may register with a GP of the same or similar ethnicity to themselves[86] which may, at least in part, reflect attempts to reduce communication barriers in consultations. However, available literature is inconsistent on this issue.[138] Such opportunities appear to be much less available for Chinese patients.

However, sharing broad ethnic origin and language with a health professional does not necessarily guarantee a successful consultation. There is evidence that, as with the majority population, issues of gender, status and class, stereotyping and racism may still compromise open communication between patient and professional.[155,163,164] Among those from ethnic minorities who share a language with their GP, a higher proportion report problems with communication than among the English, suggesting wider aspects of communication are important.[86]

The PSI survey[84] found that of those who had difficulty communicating with their GP, less than 10% had had access to a trained interpreter in consultations, and 75% used a friend or relative to translate for them. A third of respondents still felt their GP had not understood them. Similarly, only 30% of Pakistani and Bangladeshi respondents who had been admitted to hospital in the past year had received any form of trained bilingual assistance.

Definitions

Bilingual services can involve workers employed under a number of different titles and roles, which tend to be used interchangeably. They usually fall into a number of broad, **if often overlapping**, categories.

- **Interpreters:** Interpreters translate the meaning and function of messages exchanged between service user and service provider. In practice, many interpreters may play a role in explaining the significance within the patient's cultural context as well as the meanings of words and gestures. The interpreter's role is then to facilitate communication with appropriate cultural sensitivity.
- **Linkworkers or outreach workers:** In addition to interpreting, these workers may provide a more formal link between particular services and the service user, including provision of information about certain services and options. A linkworker may be able to bridge cultural gaps that may arise between patient and professional. This might involve, for example, explaining a patient's concerns in terms understandable to a health professional and relaying health advice in terms consistent with the patient's cultural values, health beliefs and knowledge. They may be employed by a variety of organisations including health authorities, NHS Trusts, local authorities, general practices, community organisations, and charities. However, few schemes are yet established as mainstream services. They have tended to be short-term and their funding opportunistic, so that effective sustained development and evaluation has been lacking.[165]
- **Advocates** – Advocates work from the premise that there is an unequal relationship between patient and health professional. They may fulfil both interpreter and linkworker functions but go beyond, facilitating linguistic and cultural communication to act on behalf of the service user to ensure that service providers know their views of, and preferences for, health care and services. The distinction between interpreter, linkworker and advocacy provision is not clear-cut.

   Many people have problems that overlap or go beyond the responsibilities of different statutory health and social care providers. Linkworkers and advocates can help in interactions with primary care teams, in outpatient clinics, local authority departments and benefits agencies and so on. From a client's perspective, these needs are inter-related and distinguishing between them may be artificial.
- **Language lines** – Telephone interpreter services are beginning to be introduced in some areas.[166] There is growing interest in using telephone language lines, where the interpreter is not physically present during the consultation. They may become useful in response to needs for 24-hour availability, the acute and demand-led nature of some services (particularly in primary care and A&E departments), and the immense diversity of languages in some localities.
- **Translation** – In addition to provision of interpreter and advocacy services, the translation of a wide range of information, for example about health services, health education, hospital menus, etc. is a further key requirement. This includes development and provision of appropriate information, in different media, that are accessible to those who cannot read or speak English.

Factors affecting service use

Provision of interpreting services in the UK is very variable.[167] Even where interpreting services have become established they may be underused by health professionals, who may be unaware of their existence, fail to publicise them appropriately to patients, or lack appropriate skills and training to work effectively with interpreters. Some professionals may be reluctant to engage bilingual services in facilitating communication with patients who cannot speak English.[168]

From patients' perspectives there may be a reluctance to discuss sensitive subjects in the presence of a third party or concerns about confidentiality, particularly in relation to mental ill-health. Such problems are more likely if untrained interpreters or volunteers are used, or in the more common situation of a family member or relative being used as an interpreter. Mistranslation is also more likely in these contexts, adding further difficulty.[151,169]

Using members of the family as interpreters may introduce difficulties due to family relationships, emotional involvement, maturity of the relative concerned if a child, and so on.[170] Unfortunately, many health authorities and professionals have tended to rely upon such informal mechanisms for communication. It is increasingly regarded as unprofessional and unethical for family members, and particularly children, to be asked to interpret in health encounters.[168,171]

Current models for interpreting service provision

There are a wide variety of existing service models in the NHS for interpreter/advocacy provision. They are based upon different collaborations between HAs and Trusts and local authority or voluntary sector. Some services are centrally co-ordinated at HA level, others are organised at NHS Trust level or have been stimulated by specific service developments. Most appear to provide interpreter rather than dedicated advocacy services, or a mixture where staff sometimes fulfil advocacy roles.

Some HAs have attempted to establish minimum standards of comprehensive provision, while others provide neither co-ordinated nor apparently adequate provision.[167] Some continue to rely upon untrained volunteers or family members translating for patients. The range of elements variously include:

- full-time or sessional trained interpreters
- volunteer and ad hoc interpreters (e.g. minority ethnic health staff)
- patient advocates
- telephone interpreter services
- translation services for health service/education information
- bilingual health care staff.

Table 40 summarises the main characteristics of differing interpreting/advocacy/translation services provided in four selected health authorities.

Table 40: Summary of the main characteristics of interpreting, advocacy and translation services in four health authorities' studies.

Health authority	Key language groups catered for by the health authority	Health authority backed interpreter/advocacy provision in primary care?	Interpreter/advocacy provision within acute hospitals?	Interpreter/advocacy provision within mental health? In community care?	Interpreter/advocacy provision within obstetrics?	Translation provision
Birmingham	*Birmingham Health Authority:* Urdu, Mirpuri, Pahari, Punjabi, Sindhi, Pushto, Hindi, Gujarati, Kutchi, Bengali, Creole, Patois, Bangla, Sylheti, Arabic, Vietnamese, Cantonese, Hakka, Mandarin, Swahili, Hausa.	*Birmingham Health Authority:* Some general practices do not provide interpreting service provision; others, however, do. A pilot scheme is currently in operation whereby ethnic monitoring is undertaken in return for free authority funded provision.	*City Hospital NHS Trust:* Have paid professional interpreters. *The Royal Orthopaedic NHS Trust:* Use bilingual staff volunteers to provide service. *Birmingham Heartlands:* Have paid professional interpreters. *University Hospital Birmingham:* A professional service is provided. *Birmingham Children's Hospital:* £8,000 interpreting costs.	*Northern Birmingham Community Health NHS Trust:* The Trust uses paid professional interpreters. *Northern Birmingham Mental Health NHS Trust:* The Trust uses Express Interpreting and Translating Services. *South Birmingham Mental Health NHS Trust:* A professional service is provided. *South Birmingham Community:* A professional service is provided.	*South Birmingham Community NHS Trust:* Has provision as a result of the Asian mother and baby campaign. *Birmingham Women's Hospital:* A professional service is provided using linkworkers and interpreters.	There is a general lack of information about such provision.
Ealing, Hammersmith and Hounslow	*Ealing, Hammersmith and Hounslow Health Authority:* Urdu, Punjabi, Gujarati, Farsi, Somali, Turkish, Armenian, Albanian, Serbo-Croat, Arabic, Far Eastern, Eastern European languages, Kurdish, and Afghani. Some of those requiring provision are refugees.	*Ealing, Hammersmith and Hounslow Health Authority:* General practitioners are provided with a telephone interpreting service sponsored by the health authority, as well as some face to face interpreter provision.	*Ealing Hospitals NHS Trust:* The Trust employs an interpreter and employs other interpreters via an agency. *The Hammersmith Hospitals NHS Trust:* Provision is provided by Language Line and Hammersmith and Fulham Commission for Racial Equality.	*Hounslow and Spelthorne Community and Mental Health NHS Trust:* Have a bilingual support worker supporting five child health clinics a week, and provide interpreting support to the Department of Child and Adolescent Psychiatry, Health Visiting Services, Mental Health Services, and others. Language Line is also used a little.		*Ealing, Hammersmith and Hounslow Health Authority:* When translation is required, it tends to be needed for four major languages. However, the health authority infrequently provides leaflets and when it does these are not usually translated.

Table 40: Continued.

West London Health Care Trust: Some agency and freelance interpreting is provided. *West Middlesex University Hospital:* A limited professional interpreting service is provided. *Language Line:* Provides services to the health authority.	*Riverside Mental Health Trust:* The Trust buys in interpreting services. *Riverside Community:* A professional service is used.	*Hounslow and Spelthorne Community and Mental Health NHS Trust:* Patient information, and mental health audio cassettes are translated into five Asian languages including Bengali, Somali, Arabic and Farsi, whilst health visiting leaflets are translated into Somali, Punjabi, Urdu. *West London Health Care NHS Trust* Obtain a limited amount of translation. *West Middlesex University:* Not clear. *The Riverside Mental Health Trust:* Not clear. *The Hammersmith Hospitals NHS Trust:* Three leaflets have been translated into Bengali, Urdu, Farsi, Arabic, Turkish, Polish, Greek, Spanish, Somali.

Table 40: Continued.

Health authority	Key language groups catered for by the health authority	Health authority backed interpreter/ advocacy provision in primary care?	Interpreter/advocacy provision within acute hospitals?	Interpreter/advocacy provision within mental health? In community care?	Interpreter/ advocacy provision within obstetrics?	Translation provision
Leicestershire	*Leicester Health Authority:* Urdu, Gujarati, Hindi, Punjabi, Bengali, Chinese, Polish, and other languages.	*Leicester Health Authority:* Primary care providers are encouraged to establish their own arrangements for the provision of interpreter services based upon health authority guidelines. Currently some provision is from the Fosse Trust.	*Leicester General:* The Trust use a combination of hospital volunteer interpreters, professional agency interpreters, Language Line and hospital employed linkworkers in maternity. *Leicester Royal Infirmary:* The trust has its own interpreters. It also has the use of professional trained interpreters. It has access to Language Line via the Fosse NHS Trust. *Glenfield NHS Trust:* Provision is concentrated in cardiology. Some secondary provision is provided by provider units, and Language Line is sometimes used. Generally, though, professional provision is lacking as expenditure in this area is low.	*Leicester Mental Health Service NHS Trust:* Has two interpreters with a command of seven different languages. *Fosse Community NHS Trust:* The Trust obtains interpreting provision from the Ujala Resource Centre.	*Leicester General Hospital:* Identified obstetrics as a major speciality user. *Leicester General NHS Trust:* There are linkworkers earmarked for maternity.	*Health authority:* There is a general lack of translation provision at health authority level. Health authority projections suggest that £500,000 would be required to provide what is regarded as 'adequate' provision. *Leicester General Hospital:* Not clear. *Leicester Royal Infirmary:* Not clear.
Newcastle and North Tyneside	*Newcastle and North Tyneside Health Authority:* Bengali, Sylheti, India, Pakistani, Punjabi, Urdu, Hindi, Chinese, Hakka, Mandarin, Serbo-Croat, Arabic, Farsi, French, Italian, and others.	*Newcastle Interpreting Service:* Provision to primary care sector is the largest sector now that the health authority sponsors provision.	*Newcastle Interpreting Service:* Trusts obtain trained interpreters via the 'Newcastle Interpreting Service for Health and Social Services'. All Trusts within the health authority encourage the use of professional interpreting provision from this service.	*Newcastle Interpreting Service:* Interpreters are trained to operate in a Mental Health context as required.	*Newcastle Interpreting Service:* Provision to obstetrics is not discernibly different.	*Newcastle and North Tyneside Health Authority:* There is a patchy provision of leaflets. It was considered that more use of audio material is required due to a lack of written skills. *Newcastle City Health NHS Trust:* Not clear.

Important note: The sources of the information are indicated in *italics*.
Source adapted from Clark 1998[167]

Preventive care

Childhood immunisation

Uptake of childhood immunisation appears similar to or higher among most ethnic minority groups, particularly South Asian groups, than the majority population.[172–5] Socio-economic or communication difficulties might, paradoxically, contribute to higher levels of immunisation amongst some ethnic minorities when fears about safety may have dissuaded parents from other white groups from having their children immunised.[174]

Cervical and breast screening

Again, there is no routine ethnic monitoring within the cancer screening services, and data are available only from a number of local studies. Further, as not all studies have taken account of socio-economic factors, interpretation of such information must be guarded.

Existing evidence about uptake of cervical screening amongst ethnic minority groups is equivocal. Although uptake has generally been found to be low (and knowledge about cervical smears to be poor),[176–8] more recent studies have found similar rates to the majority population.[148,179] However, uptake amongst South Asian women appears consistently lower and this has been attributed to poorer knowledge and greater population mobility.[148,176,180]

Lack of basic accessible information about cervical smears, and cultural attitudes and beliefs have been suggested as dominant reasons for low uptake.[86,176,178,181] Such research has been criticised for promulgating unhelpful generalisations and stereotypes of minority ethnic women in failing to acknowledge the dynamic nature of minority ethnic groups, and their experiences of racism and inequalities within health services. This work has also been questioned for advancing too simplistic a focus upon improving information to increase uptake of screening.[182]

Available evidence about uptake of breast screening is again equivocal but suggests lower uptake amongst minority ethnic populations compared to white women.[183,184] At the practice level, no significant difference between screening rates and ethnicity exist.[180,185] This is supported by studies using individual level data.[186,187]

Health promotion and education

Provision of health promotion services is usually encompassed as part of health promotion units' general role, working from district or locality bases resourced by health and/or local authorities. Some have designated workers with an ethnic minority brief. Some NHS Trusts have their own dedicated units or a service may be part of a local linkworker scheme that may support particular clinical service areas (for example CHD, diabetes or sexual health). These services may typically provide some of the following:

- sources of translated written and audio-visual material
- development/dissemination of accessible and appropriate information in suitable media
- raising of community awareness of health issues
- health promotion initiatives and events in community settings.

There is a lack of information about utilisation of such services but, anecdotally, uptake of such services is in general perceived to be low.

Other community health services

There are few available data concerning the use of community health services outside general practice. Studies limited to some minority ethnic groups have found generally lower use of, or receipt of care from, community nursing[188,189] and dental and chiropody services.[190] A more recent study found white respondents were more likely to have made use of most other services (**Table 41**), although there was generally little variation among ethnic groups.[84]

Table 41: Other health and social services used in the past year (cell percentages).

	White	Caribbean	Indian	African Asian	Pakistani	Bangladeshi	Chinese
% who have used the service							
Dentist	62	53	45	46	50	25	47
Physiotherapist	9.0	6.5	5.8	4.1	3.9	0.6	7.9
Psychotherapist	1.1	0.7	0.5	0.8	0.8	0.6	1.3
Alternative practitioner	5.7	2.9	1.7	3.0	1.3	0.6	3.8
Health visitor or District Nurse	7.4	8.7	4.2	4.1	4.8	6.9	6.8
Social worker	3.8	5.2	2.2	1.1	1.7	1.7	2.5
Home help	2.1	1.0	0.3	0.1	1.8	0.8	0
Age- and gender-standardised	0.7	0.9	0.2		1.7		0
Meals on wheels (age 65+)	3.2	1.8	0	*	3.1*	*	*
Age- and gender-standardised	2.2	1.7	0		2.0		*
Other	6.9	4.4	1.2	2.9	1.3	2.7	2.3
Weighted base	*2,863*	*777*	*646*	*390*	*417*	*138*	*195*
Unweighted base	*2,862*	*609*	*638*	*348*	*578*	*289*	*104*

* Small base numbers in the cell make the estimate unreliable.
Source: Nazroo 1997[84]

However, use of dentists by minority ethnic groups appears considerably lower than the white majority population, particularly amongst Bangladeshis.[84] There is growing concern about oral health in minority communities, particularly among children, and early evidence that different approaches for preventive dentistry may be required among Asian populations.[191,192]

The limited evidence available suggests that use of complementary or alternative therapies (including, for example, use of hakims, Ayurvedic remedies) in minority ethnic communities tends to be additional to rather than alternative to NHS service use – as with the majority population.[85,193] It is also important to note the increasing trend to consult practitioners of alternative medicine within the general population.[194] There appears to be no identifiable good evidence that some minority ethnic communities may be particularly likely to seek treatment when overseas (e.g. visiting relatives).

Local authority, community and voluntary services

Local authorities (LAs) provide a range of services important to the health of minority ethnic communities. Recent initiatives have often developed from Community Care legislation creating certain statutory responsibilities for some groups. In addition, some LAs have mobilised joint finance initiatives or used Single Regeneration Budget projects to stimulate both service provision and community development for ethnic minorities. There is considerable variation between localities, but provision may include services for: people with mental ill-health; older people (including day and respite care, and residential services); adults and children with disabilities; carers; refugees; and people with HIV and AIDS. A wide range of examples of service strategies, initiatives and provision are detailed in a variety of LA reports available centrally from LARRIE, Layden House, 76–86 Turnmill St, London EC1M 5QU.

Many local authorities have been considerably more proactive than statutory health agencies in developing and implementing standards for good practice in service provision for minority ethnic communities, including appropriate training for social workers, teachers and other staff. However, in general, there appears to be underutilisation of services such as home care support and meals on wheels by minority ethnic communities.[84]

LAs often play a key role in supporting provision for ethnic minorities in the voluntary and community group sector, sometimes including delivery of specific social care services (see, for example, Wandsworth Social Care Provider Project, 1996 – available from LARRIE).

Voluntary sector provision is, in general, provided by people from ethnic minorities, with less secure funding, and there is evidence that currently the more mainstream voluntary sector has yet to cater for black people.[195] Although there are many active and thriving voluntary and community organisations, it has been argued that some minority ethnic communities may not be able to provide the degree of support some of their members may require: few people from ethnic minorities report attending community groups and associations other than religious ones, and these did not prevent feelings of isolation.[196,197]

Specific services

Details for all diseases and conditions are not provided, except for the haemoglobinopathies, due in part to lack of data. Pertinent issues for specific conditions are mentioned to highlight the provision and uptake of services amongst these groups.

In general, amongst South Asians and Afro-Caribbeans, current provision of renal replacement therapy for end stage renal failure is inadequate given the higher prevalence in these groups.[198] This is of concern, as the transplantation services cannot meet the growing need for organs with over 6556 waiting for a suitable organ, of which 9.7% are from the BMEGs.[199] This problem is compounded by tissue typing incompatibility between the Asian and other ethnic groups, so that Asians have to wait longer for suitable organs.[200]

It is also noted that there is low uptake of cardiac rehabilitation services by minority ethnic communities.[201]

Amongst the palliative care community, there is a belief that minority ethnic communities do not use their services.[202,203] This cannot be substantiated as there is lack of reliable data on usage of palliative services by BMEGs.

Haemoglobinopathies

Beta-thalassaemia is characterised by severe anaemia and usually diagnosed in early childhood.[204,205] Patients require regular blood transfusion and iron chelation therapy to minimise iron overload – the sequelae of which lead to death. The goals of transfusion include correction of anaemia, suppression of erythropoesis, and inhibition of gastrointestinal absorption of iron. Transfusion regimens which achieve these goals in addition to relatively lower rates of iron accumulation are now advocated.[206]

Prognosis is improving and most with severe disorder live to their mid-thirties. Indeed, those who find a suitable bone marrow donor and do not show pathological changes related to the disease or its treatment can be considered to be 'cured'.[207]

Symptoms for sickle cell disease can start between 3–6 months of age and result in anaemia and painful thrombotic episodes – some producing permanent disability.[208] Life-threatening complications include acute chest syndrome, stroke, and splenic or hepatic sequestration.[209] They also have increased risk of sudden death secondary to infection, so that prophylactic penicillin is required, especially during the first five years of life. Life expectancy for sickle cell anaemia has increased, with median survival of 42 years in men and 48 years in women.[210]

Although services for these patients are available, they are delivered inadequately and inequitably, particularly the screening and counselling services.[211]

Racism in service delivery

In consulting minority ethnic patients about their health needs, the experience of negative or prejudiced attitudes of professionals and services is commonly highlighted.[139] This demands broad social and institutional change, but it underlines the need to sensitise professionals to issues of prejudice, stereotyping and racism, and to address their attitudes to others through appropriate training.[168,212] Different forms of racism may occur.[138]

- **Direct racism:** Where a health worker treats a person less favourably simply by virtue of the latter's ethnicity.
- **Indirect or institutional racism:** Where, although ostensibly services are provided equally to all people, the form in which they are provided inevitably favours particular groups at the expense of others. For example, lack of provision of information in languages other than English or facilities to pray that are limited to those of Christian faith.
- **Ethnocentrism:** Where inappropriate assumptions are made about the needs of people from minority ethnic groups on the basis of the majority experience. For example, that the gender of the health professional is not important to the patient.

From the perspectives of patients, these forms often overlap, and result in discriminatory treatment. Racism has usefully been defined as 'prejudice plus power'.[197] Many minority ethnic patients' relative lack of power to contest assumptions and prejudices lends racism its force in their experience of health care. Interactions between health professionals and minority ethnic service users are as much shaped by broader social assumptions and stereotyping as by the existence of direct prejudice.[138]

Racism in health service delivery has been clearly described.[148,213–5] It remains a pervasive feature of wider society and public institutions, including the NHS.[216,217] Evidence about how racism affects interactions between NHS staff and minority ethnic users and patterns of service use or outcome is growing.[47,153,218,219] Ethnocentrism among health professionals, for example, has been shown to affect the experience of mental health services by minority ethnic users.[220] Illustrative examples are given below.

The interpretation of this research is difficult and varied.[138] Explanations offered for professionals' attitudes have included the social distance between the GPs and their patients,[217] the gap of culture and communication between GPs and patients,[153] and the inner city context of many patients' problems.[219] Although direct racism is certainly present in the delivery of health care to minority ethnic populations, more complex problems also arise through difficulties of communication and ethnocentrism, which may also result in less satisfactory service provision.

The nature of institutional racism is more elusive, partly because of a lack of conceptual clarity about its meaning.[221] The recent McPherson inquiry highlighting this issue in the police service may add momentum for discussion and change within the NHS.[222] Common examples include lack of provision of interpreting services in NHS Trusts or primary care, and the failure of health authorities and others to provide information about services in appropriate media, so that minority ethnic populations are disadvantaged in terms of their ability to make use of them.

Costs of services for minority ethnic communities

General health services

We have been unable to locate any cost-effectiveness studies involving minority ethnic groups in the UK although there is an English Languages Difficulties Adjustment weighting in the recent resource allocation formula.[223]

Bilingual services: interpreter, linkworker and advocate provision

Available information from the published and 'grey literature' (including health authority and Trust reports) provides a range of crude cost estimates for some services.[167] Methods for modelling costs have been suggested, though their current limitations are acknowledged.[167] The necessary quality of data is lacking. In particular, there is a lack of data describing precise costs associated with procedures and conditions, or in linking consistent categories of ethnic group with epidemiological and operational service provision.

Accurate information on the utilisation and cost of such services is currently limited. The average hourly cost of providing trained interpreters in health contacts is estimated to be between £26 and £30 including training, management and infrastructure.[167] This work attempted to identify total costs for interpreting/advocacy and translation in the 13 HAs that were studied. Costs are outlined in **Table 42** (for year 1997/98) by primary care, acute hospital sector, mental health/community trust sector, and total for acute sector. Key broad cost issues to consider are:

- the need for and use of bilingual, advocacy and translation services to facilitate access and effectiveness of generic services
- ethnic variation in the prevalence and cost of managing 'common' conditions
- incidence of conditions specific to minority ethnic groups
- the need for local community consultation and research to enable appropriate local services.

There is considerable variation in approaches adopted by different health authorities. Key points are the following.

- Certain activity requires funding to *initiate* service development and provision, and may not be directly related to population size.
- A recent review for the NHSE concluded that some additional costs can be identified and appear to be unavoidable.[224]

Table 42: Costs arising due to the provision of interpreter and translation services.

Health authority	Interpreter/ advocacy costs in primary care	Interpreter/ advocacy costs in acute hospitals	Interpreter/advocacy costs in mental health and community	Other interpreter/ advocacy costs	Total interpreter/ advocacy costs to the acute sector (i.e. excluding primary care)	Translation and other media (costs)
Birmingham	Not identified	*City Hospital NHS Trust:* The total cost of interpreting within the Trust was £131,126. *The Royal Orthopaedic Hospital NHS Trust:* Total cost for interpreting services was £674 (staff and volunteers are re-deployed from other departments). *Birmingham Heartlands NHS Trust:* Costs for employed interpreters/advocates are £32,017. *University Hospital Birmingham:* Provision costs £16,000.	*Northern Birmingham Community Health NHS Trust:* The total cost of interpreters was £67,725 (excluding advocacy costs). *North Birmingham Mental Health NHS Trust:* A professional service is provided via a contractual arrangement. *South Birmingham Mental Health NHS Trust:* A professional interpreting service is provided at a cost of £15,545. *South Birmingham Community:* £15,545.	*Birmingham Women's Hospital:* £49,835. *Birmingham Children's Hospital:* £37,000.	*City Hospital NHS Trust:* £131,126. *The Royal Orthopaedic Hospital:* £674. *Birmingham Heartlands NHS Trust:* £32,017. *University Hospital Birmingham:* £16,000. *Northern Birmingham Community Health NHS Trust:* The cost of three full-time interpreters was £42,725 + £25,000, which was the cost of the bank of interpreters = £67,725. *Northern Birmingham Mental Health NHS Trust:* £7,763. *South Birmingham Mental Health NHS Trust:* £15,545. *Birmingham Women's Hospital:* £49,835. *Birmingham Children's Hospital:* £37,000. *Total identifiable acute costs:* £357,685.	*City Hospital NHS Trust:* Data not provided. *The Royal Orthopaedic Hospital:* Data not provided. *Birmingham Heartlands NHS Trust:* Data not provided. *University Hospital Birmingham:* Data not provided. *Northern Birmingham Community Health NHS Trust:* Data not provided. *Northern Birmingham Mental Health NHS Trust:* Data not provided. *South Birmingham Mental Health NHS Trust:* Data not provided. *Birmingham Women's Hospital:* Data not provided. *Birmingham Children's Hospital:* Data not provided. *Total identifiable costs:* £0.

Table 42: Continued.

Bradford	A small proportion of the budget for Airedale NHS Trust is used to provide interpreting, but largely for one GP practice. (Likely to be around £30,000 – i.e. this is approximate allocation funded by GMS.)	*Bradford Hospitals NHS Trust:* £100,000 for a service based in paediatrics, maternity, antenatal and out-patients. *Airedale NHS Trust:* £29,600 for a service co-ordinator plus provision to the Women and Children's Directorate.	*Airedale NHS Trust:* Community provision costs £17,162 whilst mental health provision costs £49,000 + £2,000 = £68,162.	*Bradford Community Health Council Advocacy Service:* Ethnic minority advocacy service is employed at a cost of £25,000 per annum. *Bradford Community NHS Trust:* £132,000 is spent including family planning clinics, infant welfare clinics, dental clinics speech and language therapy, ante-natal clinics, and immex clinics. Allowing for £30,000 allocation costs to trusts are c.£102,000.	*Bradford Hospitals NHS Trust:* £100,000. *Airedale NHS Trust:* £95,792. *Bradford Community NHS Trust:* £102,000. *Bradford Community Health Council Advocacy Service:* £25,000. *Total identifiable acute costs:* £322,792.	*Bradford Health Authority:* Translation of the annual report, a radio advertising campaign to inform access to physicians, a radio campaign to encourage the take-up of dental provision, and translation of two letters at a total cost of £4,660. *Bradford Hospitals NHS Trust:* Very little outside translation. Therefore not costed. *Airedale NHS Trust:* Not identified. *Bradford Community NHS Trust:* Not separately identifiable. *Total identifiable costs:* £4,660.
Coventry	*Language Line:* Very limited service to GPs, breakdown of costs not available.	*Language Line:* Provide a very limited service to the Walsgrave Hospital Trust and Coventry and Warwickshire Hospital Trust + to GPs.	*Lamb St interpreting centre:* £47,180; 30 hours for co-ordinator (25% spent interpreting) + sessional interpretation (150–160 hrs per month average). Figure includes travel, office and communication costs.	N/A	*Lamb St interpreting centre:* £47,180. *Language Line:* £944.70. *Total identifiable acute costs:* £48,124.70.	*Total identifiable costs:* £2,342 at the Lamb St Centre.

Table 42: Continued.

Health authority	Interpreter/advocacy costs in primary care	Interpreter/advocacy costs in acute hospitals	Interpreter/advocacy costs in mental health and community	Other interpreter/advocacy costs	Total interpreter/advocacy costs to the acute sector (i.e. excluding primary care)	Translation and other media (costs)
Doncaster	No health authority backed provision. Cost of GP use of outside interpreters is not identifiable.	*Doncaster Health Care NHS Trust:* Interpreting costs cannot be identified. *Doncaster Royal Infirmary:* Hospital largely relies on voluntary provision from bilingual staff, so the costs in 1997/98 were said to be less than or equal to £200 for emergency use of outside interpreters.	No specialist service in mental health or community health.	Figures not broken down.	*Doncaster Health Care NHS Trust:* Interpreting costs cannot be identified. *Doncaster Royal Infirmary:* Identifiable costs less than or equal to £200. *Total identifiable acute costs: £200.*	*Doncaster Health Care NHS Trust:* Translating costs were £647. *Doncaster Royal Infirmary:* Translation costs cannot be identified. *Total identifiable costs: £647.*
Ealing, Hammersmith, and Hounslow	Beginning to sponsor interpreting at a primary care this year at a projected cost of £25,000 p.a. for Language Line and some face-to-face interpreting.	*West London Health Care Trust:* Some provided but costings not broken down by speciality. *Ealing Hospitals NHS Trust:* Some provided but costings not broken down by speciality. *Hammersmith Hospitals NHS Trust:* Projected full year costs of £52,720 (including £775 for Language Line). *West Middlesex University NHS Trust:* £5,500.	*West London health Care Trust:* Some provided but costings not broken down by speciality. *Hounslow and Spelthorne Community and Mental Health NHS Trust:* Total interpreting costs were £17,548 (including Language Line). *Riverside Mental Health NHS Trust:* £14,702.07. *Riverside Community Trust:* Costs in 1997/98 are £27,000–28,000.	Figures not broken down.	*West London Health Care Trust:* Total costs £21,058 (including Mental Health and Community provision). *Ealing Hospitals NHS Trust:* A Trust interpreter costs £14,000 whilst agency interpretation costs are £15,000 = £29,000. *Hammersmith Hospitals NHS Trust:* Projected full year costs of £52,720 (including £775 for Language Line). *West Middlesex Hospitals NHS Trust:* Costs are thought to be around £5,500.	

Table 42: Continued.

				Riverside Mental Health NHS Trust: Costs in 1997/98 are £14,702. Hounslow and Spelthorne Community Mental Health: £17,548. Riverside Community Trust: Costs in 1997/98 were around £27,000–28,000. Total identifiable acute costs: £167,528–168,528.	*West London Health Care Trust: 27 translations carried out by freelance interpreters at £385. Ealing Hospitals NHS Trust: Not clear. Hammersmith Hospitals NHS Trust: Not clear. Hounslow and Spelthorne Community and Mental Health NHS Trust: c.£3,000 translation budget. Riverside Mental Health NHS Trust: Not clear. Riverside Community NHS Trust: Not clear. Total identifiable costs: £10,385–13,385.*
East London and City	*East London and City Health Authority: £22,680 for primary care Advocacy.*	*East London and City Health Authority: Figures not broken down.*	*East London and City Health Authority: Figures not broken down.*	*East London and City Health Authority: Complaints department spent £135.50 on interpreting.*	*East London and City Health Authority: Overall spending for 1997/98 is £2,335,975 (including complaints). Total identifiable acute costs: £2,335,975.*	*East London and City Health Authority: £1,203 was spent on translation of a conciliation leaflet + £6,700 on other translations (via an agency) + £20,000 on the production of videos in community languages. Total identifiable costs: £27,903.*
Kensington & Chelsea, and Westminster	c.£60,000.	c.£145,000.	c.£95,000.	Figures not broken down.	c.£240,000 for mainstream interpreting service + £68,000 for the interpreting dimension of health authority funded projects. Overall total is around £308,000. *Total identifiable acute costs: £308,000.*	Excluding print runs: £18,000–24,000. *Total identifiable costs: £18,000–24,000.*

Table 42: Continued.

Health authority	Interpreter/ advocacy costs in primary care	Interpreter/ advocacy costs in acute hospitals	Interpreter/advocacy costs in mental health and community	Other interpreter/ advocacy costs	Total interpreter/ advocacy costs to the acute sector (i.e. excluding primary care)	Translation and other media (costs)
Leicestershire	*Actual:* At present the budget is £5,000.	*Leicester General Hospital:* Costs cannot be identified. *Leicester Royal Infirmary:* £6,981. *Glenfield Hospital NHS Trust:* Currently use volunteers so costing is not available.	*Leicestershire Mental Health Service Trust:* £41,550 to cover two full-time staff and office costs. *Fosse Community Health Trust:* The total cost is £12,473.	Figures not broken down.	*Leicester General Hospital:* Costs not identifiable. *Leicester Royal Infirmary:* £6,981. *Glenfield Hospital NHS Trust:* No identifiable costs. *Leicester Mental Health:* £41,550. *Fosse Community Health Trust:* Spent £35,835 on interpreters. *Language Line:* Total health authority-wide spending of £1,914. *Total identifiable acute costs:* £86,280.	*Leicester General Hospital:* Costs not identifiable. *Leicester Royal Infirmary:* Costs not identifiable. *Glenfield Hospital NHS Trust:* Costs not identifiable. *Leicester Mental Health:* Costs not identifiable. *Fosse Community Health Trust:* £8,500. *Total identifiable costs:* £8,500.
Newcastle and North Tyneside	£19,400.	Figures not broken down.	Figures not broken down.	Figures not broken down.	*Total identifiable acute costs:* £40,600.	Reported translation costs at Newcastle Interpreting Service for Health and Social Services: £1,645 + translation cost of maternity information into Arabic, Bengali, Cantonese, Hindi, Punjabi, and Urdu was £391.50. *Total identifiable costs:* £2,037.

Table 42: Continued.

North West Anglia	Figures not broken down.	Figures not broken down.	Figures not broken down.	*Peterborough District Hospital NHS Trust:* Costs of CINTRA interpretation are £10,980. *North West Anglia Health Care Trust:* Costs of CINTRA interpreting are £4,846. *Language Line:* Costs of telephone interpreting for the health authority are £4,681. *Total identifiable acute costs: £20,507.*	*Peterborough District Hospital NHS Trust:* Costs of CINTRA provided interpretation are £60. *North West Anglia Health Care Trust:* Costs of CINTRA provided translation £48. *Total identifiable costs: £108.*
Salford and Trafford	Figures not broken down.	Figures not broken down.	Figures not broken down.	*Salford and Trafford Health Authority:* Report total district interpreting costs to be £31,500. *Total identifiable acute costs: £31,500.*	*Salford and Trafford Health Authority:* Report total district translating costs to be £10,500. *Total identifiable costs: £10,500.*
Sandwell	Figures not broken down.	Figures not broken down.	*Black Country Mental Health Trust:* Costs not identifiable, and much voluntary provision anyway.	*Sandwell Health Care Trust:* £68,595. *Black Country Mental Health Trust:* Not identifiable. *Total identifiable acute costs: £68,595.*	*Health Authority Translation Unit:* Costs to Sandwell £10,090. *Total identifiable costs: £10,090.*

Table 42: Continued.

Health authority	Interpreter/advocacy costs in primary care	Interpreter/advocacy costs in acute hospitals	Interpreter/advocacy costs in mental health and community	Other interpreter/advocacy costs	Total interpreter/advocacy costs to the acute sector (i.e. excluding primary care)	Translation and other media (costs)
Warwickshire		*North Warwickshire NHS Trust:* Estimated costs of £7,000 during 1997/98 + Language Line at £1,836 for North Warwickshire and the former Rugby NHS Trust = £8,836 + £13,000 = £22,836. *Warwick Hospital:* Figures not broken down to this level. *George Eliot Hospital NHS Trust:* Figures not broken down to this level. *Language Line (not included in above figures):* £1,838.	Figures in main totals.	*North Warwickshire NHS Trust:* A bilingual co-worker providing advocacy and interpreting provision works part-time at a cost of £8,000. A proportion of the Race Equality Officer's time is spent working as an advocate at a cost of £5,000 = £13,000.	*North Warwickshire NHS Trust:* £7,000 + £13,000 = £20,000. *Warwick Hospital NHS Trust:* £757 for provision from November 1997–Mar 1998. Therefore for whole year projection = £752 × 2 = £1,514. *South Warwickshire Combined Care:* £431. *George Eliot NHS Trust:* £6,300. *Language Line:* £1,836. *Total identifiable acute costs:* £31,081.	*North Warwickshire NHS Trust:* Spends an estimated £3,000 per annum on written translation. *Warwick Hospital NHS Trust:* Translation is not provided. *South Warwickshire Combined Care:* Not identifiable. *George Eliot NHS Trust:* Not identifiable. *Total identifiable costs:* £3,000.

Source: Clark *et al.* 1998[167]

- However, there are other areas of need where minority ethnic populations may have diminished health care costs, or where provision of services specific to these communities may be desirable or alternative to (but not necessarily more costly than) existing provision (for example, provision of vegetarian meals or employment of female health professionals).
- The process of drawing attention to minority ethnic needs may lead to service developments that are relevant and desirable to people from the majority population, for example provision of options for vegetarian meals or facility to consult a health professional of the same gender.

Haemoglobinopathies

Zeuner et al.[225] have estimated that total lifetime treatment costs over 60 years for patients with thalassaemia major and sickle cell anaemia are £490 000 and £173 000, respectively.

6 Effectiveness of services and interventions

Evidence on the effectiveness and cost-effectiveness of specific services and interventions tailored to BMEGs is limited. The reader is referred to other chapters for details of effectiveness and cost-effectiveness of specific services and interventions aimed at the whole population or specific ethnic minority groups. Indeed, the information base to support policies are only partially available as mortality statistics (*see* 'Mortality analyses'), hospital episode and general practitioner data – all problematic.[226] The haemoglobinopathies are mentioned in this section as the evidence base is growing. It is also important to note that as most studies have excluded individuals from the black and minority ethnic communities, there is a dearth of data on effectiveness and cost-effectiveness in these groups.[227,228]

Assessment of the quality of clinical care may become more readily available as:

- ethnic monitoring becomes more systematised in secondary care, and if it becomes statutory and more widely adopted in primary care
- clinical governance strategies are implemented and evaluated, including greater measurement of clinical outcomes.

Note that the level of evidence is based on criteria given in Appendix 4, where the emphasis is on study design only.

Quality of care

Primary care

- Level of evidence – III to II-3.

The national BMEG survey showed ethnic minority respondents, particularly Bangladeshis, were less likely than the general population to feel that time their GP spent with them was adequate.[86] The PSI survey[84] found that the preferences of some ethnic minority patients for doctors of similar ethnicity and gender to themselves were unlikely to be met. Patients' accounts of their unsatisfactory experiences of consultations consistently raise concerns about effective communication, use and availability of interpreters and other bilingual workers, and the communication skills and attitudes of health professionals.[150,161]

A dominant issue for all services, from patients' perspectives, is quality of effective communication (*see* below). There is limited evidence suggesting the quality of primary care of minority groups might be poorer than the majority population in terms of achieving effective communication.[86]

Secondary care

- Level of evidence – III to II-3.

Failure to communicate the availability of female GPs appears to act as a barrier to uptake of maternity and gynaecology services for some women.[229] Research concerning the quality of secondary services offered to minority ethnic groups is sparse, but suggests lower quality of care, in terms of inequalities of access and poorer treatment, compared to the majority population. For example, lower quality of obstetric[230] and diabetic care.[231]

Overall, levels of 'satisfaction' with some NHS services are not that dissimilar (though usually slightly less) than those of the majority population,[84,86,138] even when specific questions are asked about recently utilised services.[232,233] It has been suggested that the challenge of meeting the needs of minority ethnic groups – at least to their own 'satisfaction' – should not be regarded as insurmountable.[13]

Cardiovascular disease

- Level of evidence – I.

There is a dearth of literature comparing efficacy of interventions on CVD risk factors among minority ethnic communities. However, the risk factors are essentially the same but their distribution is different so that preventive strategies have to be tailored to account for this.

Pharmacological treatment of hypertension is effective[234] and in general black patients have lower levels of renin than whites, and are more salt-sensitive than whites.[235] Hence beta-blockers, ACE inhibitors and AII antagonists are less likely to be as effective as diuretics and calcium channel blockers among black patients.

Haemoglobinopathies

- Level of evidence – II-3 to I.

There are two main components of treatment of sickle cell disease – preventative and supportive. These patients are susceptible to infections (particularly pneumococcus, salmonella species, meningococcus and haemophilus). Preventative treatments include prophylactic penicillin from four months of age, which reduces pneumoccocal infections by 84%,[236] but there is debate on the appropriate age to stop; immunisation against pneumococcus and haemophilus; and education on avoiding precipitating conditions and support of parents.[237] Supportive therapies include treatment of acute crises with fluid therapy, pain relief, and blood transfusion. Hydroxurea is also effective in some patients in decreasing incidence of acute chest syndrome and the need for blood transfusion.[238] Bone marrow transplantation is also available for selected children.[239]

The clinical course of β-Thalassaemia is more predictable and morbidity and mortality reduced by regular blood transfusions[240] and subcutaneous desferrioxamine to reduce iron overload.[241] The latter itself leads to complications[242] and problems with compliance.[243] Oral iron chelators are available but have not been fully evaluated.[244] Bone marrow transplantation is curative and indicated in children who have not had any complications.[245]

Screening programmes including pre-natal diagnosis have resulted in a marked reduction in the birth rate of affected children in Greece, Cyprus, Italy and Sardinia[246] but no UK studies have been reported.

Effective communication

- Level of evidence – III to I.

There is an extensive literature demonstrating that good communication is important and valuable in terms of health care, clinical outcomes and efficiency.[247–9] However, there is a paucity of research concerning the effectiveness of strategies to improve communication with 'non-English speaking' and culturally diverse patients.

Language and cultural differences can create barriers, misunderstandings and misconceptions in health professional–patient relationships and therefore the outcomes of health contacts.[169,250] This may clearly compromise active participation in management plans, which can facilitate better outcomes.[251] Patients themselves repeatedly highlight ineffective communication as causes of unsatisfactory experiences of health services.[150,161] Three key factors are:

- **Generic issues in common with the majority population:** for example, the importance of being given time, taken seriously, listened to, being examined and given appropriate explanation are emphasised (*see* below).
- **Absence of, or limited shared language with professionals:** for example, the PSI survey[84] found opportunities to consult a bilingual primary care professional were often limited. Of those who had difficulty communicating with their GP, less than 10% had had access to a trained interpreter in consultations, and 75% used a friend or relative to translate for them. A third of respondents still felt their GP had not understood them. Similarly, only 30% of Pakistani and Bangladeshi respondents who had been admitted to hospital in the past year had received any form of trained bilingual assistance.
- Patients from minority ethnic communities may also experience **negative stereotyping or racist attitudes** from professionals or find them insensitive to cultural issues.[150,161,217,218] Communication difficulties may clearly serve to reinforce these pre-existing inequalities of experience.[252]

A review focusing upon communication issues specifically between people from minority ethnic communities and health professionals[253] identified examples of good practice that appeared to be related to effectiveness, but there is a lack of sound evaluation to date. Research concerning the effectiveness of translated written and audio-visual materials is also lacking.[253]

Evidence relating to use of interpreters remains limited but is beginning to accumulate.

A report of services across London suggested that medical consultations across languages without the use of a trained interpreter were three to four times longer in duration, and appeared to compromise effective diagnosis and management.[254] The use of full-time or experienced sessional interpreters who have undergone training appears to result in high quality of interpreting, diminishing problems associated with inadequate communication.[253] Moreover, such provision may improve the health and wellbeing of minority ethnic patients.[255]

There is no firm evidence available concerning the effectiveness of telephone interpreter services, though North American research suggests this can be very effective and popular.[256] While offering the advantage of ready and potentially 24-hour availability, adequacy of interpreting may be compromised by not being physically present to interpret non-verbal cues and signs. However, with further experience, this provision may prove more cost-effective in some contexts than face to face interpreting, for example for rare languages and out of hours provision.

There is limited published research about the effectiveness of bilingual linkworker or advocacy programmes.[257] Such work tends to be problematic to evaluate and difficult to generalise beyond specific schemes. This research base needs to be strengthened. However, the literature suggests linkworkers may make a valuable contribution in many services, such as new patient health checks in primary care, women's health and mental health.[258] Linkworkers have been employed to encourage uptake of breast and cervical screening,[181,259] but evidence for their effectiveness in health promotion is mixed.[260] They have been successfully trained in managing patients with diabetes and asthma, though resolution of medicolegal issues is needed before these clinical roles can develop.[261]

Some linkworker initiatives have helped challenge individual and institutional racism in the NHS.[262] There is some evidence suggesting bilingual advocates may affect the quality of service obtained by minority ethnic patients. Women from minority ethnic groups in East London who had contact with a bilingual advocate experienced significantly better obstetric outcomes in terms of length of antenatal stay, onset of spontaneous labour and normal vaginal delivery than women who had no such contact.[263] Although this research had limitations, these differences may have arisen from better quality of contact between health professionals and women supported by advocates.

Effectiveness of health promotion interventions

- Level of evidence – I.

A review by White et al.[264] has revealed a dearth of relevant research on nutritional interventions promoting healthy eating among BMEGs. Most interventions were based in the USA, thus limiting generalisability and interpretation from these studies.

Health education campaigns to reduce vitamin deficiency have had little success in changing dietary practice.[134] An alternative effective policy to recommending supplements to prevent vitamin D deficiency in South Asians is still awaited.

Only two randomised trials have evaluted interventions specifically targeted at the BMEGs, both aimed at increasing uptake of breast[259] and cervical[265] screening. The former showed no effect, possibly due to contamination and lack of statistical power, and the latter showed that visits and home visits were effective. Caution is needed in interpreting study by McAvoy,[265] as results may not be generalisable as the sample was drawn from a previous study on use of health services and there was over-representation of Muslims.

Training for service delivery in an ethnically diverse society

- Level of evidence – III.

The development of relevant training of health professionals to respond appropriately to the needs of diverse groups is slowly beginning to gain momentum.[212] However, sound evaluation of its effectiveness is not yet available and is unlikely to accrue until such training itself is perceived as necessary.[212] For interpreters to be used well and cost-effectively, staff training in how to identify language needs and work with the interpreter is necessary.[266,267]

7 Models of care and recommendations

Introduction

This section suggests a *generic* framework comprising key recommendations and desirable components for services. These are based upon available experience of good practice and limited extant research. The information provided should usually be regarded as *starting points* for inclusion in local Health Improvement Programmes and service development. Other chapters in this series offer specific recommendations in relation to specific disease areas, and relevant models are also provided elsewhere,[12] though selected issues for certain conditions are briefly highlighted here.

Services for black and ethnic minority groups should be part of 'mainstream' health care provision and all policies should include needs of this group.[227] This ensures that race and equality issues are integrated into corporate and departmental policy development, day-to-day management processes and evaluation mechanisms so that all personnel are competent not just a few specialists.

As the majority of the BMEGs reside in deprived urban areas, the effects of wider social circumstances[268] have to be considered and strategies developed which also tackle these.[269]

Framework for care

Current policy contexts of clinical governance and PCO-led locality-oriented service development[270] may offer particular opportunities to enhance care for minority ethnic communities in the UK.[139] The following key elements for a service framework are recommended across primary, community and secondary health services (**Box 4**). They might appropriately form part of clinical governance strategies developed by PCGs and Trusts, and area Health Improvement Plans, to reflect local health needs. Note that following the MacPherson report[216] all public services, including the NHS, now have to comply with the amended Race Relations Act (2000). This legislation should be considered in all policies for health care. Further, the principles of equity of health care, stated as ensuring equal access and use of available health care for equal need, with equal equality for all need to be incorporated.[156,271]

Box 4: Framework for developing services

---

1 Facilitating access to appropriate services

- Promoting access
- Providing appropriate bilingual services for effective communication
- Education and training for health professionals and other staff:
  - to enable effective working with bilingual services
  - for cultural awareness and competence (including gender preferences)
  - for sensitivity to attitudes: stereotyping, prejudice, racism
- Appropriate and acceptable service provision
- Ethnic workforce issues
- Community engagement and participation

2 Systematising structures and processes for capture and use of appropriate data

- Ethnic monitoring and audit of quality of care

Delivering suggested framework

Practical examples of good practice where elements of this framework have been addressed or developed in the NHS are available[272] (Appendices 5–8). These should be drawn upon in considering local development and implementation. Robust evaluation of effectiveness is limited at present. However, this evidence base should develop with further experience and greater commitment to appropriate data collection and use, including ethnic monitoring.

Firm performance management at central, regional and local levels of the NHS, including the delivery of clinical governance, will be crucial to the successful further development and delivery of effective and appropriate services (and their evaluation) suggested here. This implies political commitment.

In developing Health Improvement Plans and service specifications and monitoring provision, it is important that specific responsibility for minority ethnic communities is held by a designated team that includes a manager, or managers, with sufficient power and status to execute tasks effectively.

Facilitating access to appropriate services

Promoting access: reviewing barriers

Similar principles apply to all services. Primary care teams, community services and Trusts can make themselves more accessible to people from minority ethnic communities by **reviewing barriers to access**, including:

(a) **Patient information on available services:** Are leaflets, audio-visual displays/resources and surgery/clinic/hospital signs readily available, accurate and appropriate to local communities in relevant languages?

(b) **Physical accessibility and appointment systems:** Is there appropriate flexibility of provision in terms of the need for longer appointments where interpreting is required, timing of surgeries and clinics? Are facilities secure and well lit? For example, in the recent PSI survey 58% of people from minority ethnic groups avoid going out at night and 35% visit shops at certain times only because of concerns about racial harassment.[49]

(c) **Empowering reception staff:** Receptionists and other administrative or clerical staff often provide the first important point of contact with, and can play an important role in facilitating access to, services. Are they enabled through service organisation and training (*see* below) to, for example:
- facilitate telephone access for appointments
- promote access to relevant information about services
- liaise with bilingual services as appropriate
- be sensitive to possible gender preferences for health professional
- appropriately seek and record ethnic monitoring data?

(d) **Primary care:** Given consistently high levels of minority ethnic registration and use of primary care and General Practitioner services in comparison with other health services, the GP and primary care colleagues are a particularly crucial point of contact and access with health services than is already the case for the majority population.

(e) **Providing appropriate bilingual services for effective communication:** The vital importance of negotiating language and other barriers by providing interpreting, linkworker and advocacy services to work with health services has been highlighted. The need for more comprehensive, appropriate and flexible provision of these services is crucial. In many areas such services are underdeveloped and availability poor.[167,253]

Key issues for successful development and implementation are:

- **Explicitly budgeting for, and mainstreaming, provision as integral to health services:** This implies unequivocal and effective performance management at all levels (*see* above). This should be aligned to continuing and appropriate resource allocation. It is recommended that a statutory responsibility should be assigned (for example to HAs) to provide adequate services for its local population.

  A cost formula has recently been suggested by a team at the University of Warwick as offering, albeit with limitations, an estimate of funding required to provide 'adequate' interpreting and advocacy provision per person with language needs.[167]

- **Management:** Dedicated management of services, including senior managerial commitment and usually a designated service manager, is suggested for needs assessment, effective planning, co-ordination, quality assurance and end delivery. Clear objectives should be derived and related to service level agreements with appropriate community involvement.

- **Predicting need:** Few schemes are based upon formally assessed needs, preventing establishment of clear objectives for service delivery. Effective needs assessment should be developed in tandem with development of better ethnic monitoring data (for example, establishing linguistic needs, literacy, and the number of health contacts in which an interpreter would have been indicated in those services used by non-English speaking patients).

  A range of estimates of functional literacy in five minority linguistic groups (Bengali, Chinese, Gujarati, Punjabi, Urdu) and some refugee groups (Bosnian, Kurdish, Tamil and Somali) has been derived.[162] The same report also provides a mechanism for predicting need for interpreter provision against local census data. This should be complemented by local community consultation in configuring services (*see* below).

- **Health professional and other staff training:** This should be regarded as a priority for both pre-and post-registration training.

  Health professionals need to learn skills to identify interpreting needs and to be able to work effectively with interpreters and linkworkers/advocates if these services are to be used well and cost-effectively in health services. This includes recognising that allowing friends or family to interpret for patients is usually unsatisfactory. Consideration of these training issues and suggestions and resources for practical training are becoming available.[212]

- **Effectively publicising availability of services among communities and how to access them.**

- **Mechanisms for quality assurance and evaluation:** This should include monitoring and categorisation of service uptake, and the setting of minimum standards for recruitment, training and supervision of staff. The use of trained bilingual workers (including language lines) whenever possible is advocated, with the use of volunteers acceptable only in emergencies.

- **Mechanisms for patient feedback and complaints.**

- **Tensions that need to be anticipated in developing services include:**
  - bilingual workers such as linkworkers and advocates being employed on low A&C grades, which lowers their perceived status by other professionals
  - developing ways of integrating linkworkers into established primary care and other health teams to improve effectiveness and mutual support, and avoid suspicion from health care professionals
  - quality assurance and co-ordination of recognised and accredited training for bilingual workers, in particular to facilitate access into traditional health care professions where minority ethnic communities are under-represented.

Examples of linkworker and advocacy service models in primary care are discussed in a recent review.[258] This also offers a checklist for HAs and PCOs seeking to establish or develop local services (Appendix 6) that considers strategic frameworks, assessing needs, defining roles, management and supervision, monitoring and evaluation, recruitment and training, administration.

The role of effective communication in relation to addressing the mental health needs of people from minority ethnic communities warrants special note. Detection, assessment and management of mental ill health are peculiarly and critically dependent upon effective communication (both linguistically and in terms of cultural sensitivity to conceptual models). Hence appropriate training for professionals to work with bilingual services here are crucial, including recognition of the limitations and challenges involved within the context of mental health.

Training for health professionals and other staff

The importance of addressing the training of health professionals to work effectively with bilingual services is highlighted earlier. But achieving effective communication means more than negotiating language barriers. Health professionals' attitudes and their awareness of them are equally important. Although further experience in health professional education is needed, **learning to value ethnic diversity** as an integral part of consultation skills has recently been advocated.[139,212] The importance of instigating this has been highlighted by the MacPherson Report (1999),[216] which defined institutional racism as:

> *The collective failure of an organisation to provide an appropriate and professional service to people because of their colour, culture or ethnic origin. It can be seen or detected in processes, attitudes and behaviour which amount to discrimination through unwitting prejudice, ignorance, thoughtlessness and racist stereotyping which disadvantages ethnic minority people. . .*
>
> *[Racism] persists because of the failure of the organisation openly and adequately to recognise and address its existence and causes by policy, example and leadership. Without recognition and action to eliminate such racism it can prevail as part of the ethos or culture of the organisation. It is a corrosive disease.*

While a general recognition of the differing needs of ethnic groups is important, this means learning generic skills to respond flexibly to encounters where diversity has an impact, and in particular to assess and respond to each patient as an *individual*, and to variations in patients' culture in its broadest sense.[212] As with the majority population, professionals must acknowledge the cultural context in which health and illness is expressed. Any patient, black or white, will have a particular ethnicity, education, socio-economic background, set of health beliefs and experiences, for example. In particular, there is a need for professionals to recognise and be sensitive to the socio-economic disadvantage and inequalities of opportunity that many from minority ethnic communities experience. Responding to this diversity demands development of a heightened awareness of, and sensitivity to, stereotyping, prejudice and racism – and how this can be challenged.[139,212]

Given that no training can prepare professionals for all issues, training should primarily adopt these generic principles.[212] However, more specific training should, where feasible and appropriate, enable professionals to work competently with local communities. This should include acquiring relevant cultural knowledge, for example, about patterns of disease and presentation, beliefs, diet, religion and caring for dying patients of different faiths. Health staff should be able to show cultural sensitivity but must avoid relying upon stereotyped notions of culture or language ability in communicating with and caring for clients.

Training in valuing diversity requires care. It may challenge attitudes and suggest fundamental change within professionals themselves. It is important not to underestimate the strong discomfort that may be generated. This field is relatively new to health professional education in the UK and further experience is required.[86,168] One resource offers practical suggestions and guidance for promoting small group interactive learning about culture, communication, racism, working with interpreters, and placing the needs of ethnic minorities in context. Although intended primarily for those training undergraduate medical students and GP registrars, it should be useful for other health professionals in pre- and post-registration training.[168]

For success, such training must start to become embedded in the education and accreditation of all health professionals: from pre-registration to post-registration, including induction courses at the commencement of posts.[212,273] These are crucial first steps. Overlooking them, and thus failing to address professionals' awareness and attitudes, may explain why important initiatives such as ethnic monitoring have faltered.

Training professionals: mental health of minority ethnic communities

This is a fundamental requirement for appropriate mental health service provision. There may be considerable unmet need for psychological support among minority ethnic groups in primary care[274] who are much less likely to be referred for psychological therapies. There is a strong case for appropriate training of primary care professionals in awareness and detection of psychological problems in minority ethnic groups, particularly where assessments are likely to be compromised by language difficulties.[121,275]

Need for mental health services (based upon observed diagnosis) among South Asian populations is probably underestimated.[276] Major concerns with psychiatric practices in relation to minority ethnic groups[46,277] and their theoretical and ideological basis[138,278] have been recognised for some time, particularly in relation to African and Caribbean communities. The experience of psychiatric services is different and often less satisfactory for many people from ethnic minorities compared to the white majority.[279]

Training should include:

- the central importance of effective communication between patient and professional, including working with bilingual services
- ethnic variations in mental ill-health
- the importance of social inequalities and racism in contributing to experience of mental ill-health
- cultural influences and variation in the expression and communication of distress
- issues of detection and management
- awareness of racism and stereotyping in terms of impact upon patients and professionals' attitudes and behaviour
- recognition that psychiatric diagnoses and categories developed in Western cultures may not be applicable to others and may contribute to racism and ethnocentrism.[46]

Appropriate and acceptable service provision

While services should be acceptable to all patients, they should be sensitive to the cultural values and beliefs of people from minority ethnic communities. As indicated earlier, staff training is vital, in addition to the provision of the following.

Appropriate and acceptable choices across services

Do meals meet religious and dietary requirements? This would imply, for example:

- local policy detailing responsibilities for meeting dietary needs
- awareness and information about these requirements for catering managers, suppliers and health staff

- recording these requirements on patient and nursing records
- training programmes for dieticians, health visitors and catering staff
- menus available in relevant languages, including information for patients indicating food content and preparation
- food choices in canteens, etc.
- monitoring of the quality and appropriateness of food choices.

Is there appropriate religious support? For example:

- is there a place of worship for those admitted to hospital?
- are there quiet rooms, mortuary or prayer space not dominated by symbols of the majority religion and suited to religious observance and preparation of the dead by other faiths?

Are female doctors and other female health professionals available in relevant contexts such as obstetrics and gynaecology?

Are health promotion and education information and programmes adapted to cultural and religious backgrounds and provided in appropriate media and languages?

Separate or mainstream provision

Debate about the advantages and disadvantages of providing 'dedicated' ethnically separate services for different clinical areas or enhancing existing provision integral to mainstream services arise frequently, in particular in relation to mental health care.

Elements of some services may be appropriately specific to certain groups, for example linkworkers focusing upon improving care of heart disease and diabetes within some services.

In mental health, a register of psychiatrists with particular interest or expertise in transcultural psychiatry has been developed that indicates ethnicity, languages spoken, special experience and readiness to be contacted (Royal College of Psychiatrists, 17 Belgrave Square, London SW1X 8PG; Tel: 020 7235 2351).

However, the large number of differing ethnic groups usually precludes development of several separate comprehensive services. Moreover, doing so may lead to undesirable marginalisation of minority ethnic needs and short-term interventions at the expense of improving more appropriate mainstream service delivery. Requirements particular to different localities should be based upon needs assessment including local community consultation and service user involvement.

Ethnic workforce

The NHS is the largest employer in England, with over 7% of staff non-medical staff from the BMEGs. (http://www.doh.gov.uk/public/stats1.htm) It should recruit and develop workers reflecting the local community and provide equality of opportunities and outcome. It should have policies to tackle and monitor racial harassment within its workforce (see http://www.doh.gov.uk/race_equality/index.htm and www.cre.gov.uk/publs/dl_phccp.html for further information).

Health authorities, Primary Care Organisations (PCOs) and Trusts should implement equal opportunities and proactive recruitment policies that as far as possible enable their workforces to reflect the ethnic diversity of local communities. The employment of bilingual health workers/professionals is clearly desirable but there is a relative lack of people from minorities entering health professions, in particular in nursing.[267] It should be noted that the Race Relations Act (1976) specifically allows employers to appoint using ethnic or linguistic criteria on the basis of, for example, a genuine occupational qualification such as appropriate linguistic skills.

In supporting its workforce, organisational culture and recruitment, services must have clearly defined procedures in place for dealing with racism and racial harassment towards or from staff and patients. These policies need to be publicised to both staff and patients.

In general practice, a particular issue for services is the imminent retirement of a cohort of doctors from minority ethnic backgrounds who have sustained general practice in many inner city and other largely disadvantaged areas.[280] Some patients have countered their linguistic disadvantage by consulting such doctors who are fluent in their own language.[151] This gap in service experience and provision needs to be anticipated and opportunities from new flexibilities and developments in primary care might be used, for example salaried general practitioner schemes and nurse practitioner-led services.

Recruitment, in particular to nursing and professions allied to medicine, presents challenges. Cultural or material constraints, lack of educational opportunities, and discrimination must be explored and addressed appropriately. Proactive and creative outreach approaches may help, for example by awareness raising and discussion in schools and colleges to encourage young people to apply for and enter health-related and health professional courses at local institutions.

Approaches need to be allied to engaging local communities in partnerships. Strategies that empower and develop community members through training and accredited qualifications may facilitate routes to health-related higher education and health professions. Examples of such practice are emerging. They include community parents as 'paraprofessionals' in health and social care roles,[281] and health researcher and health development worker projects.[164,282]

Community engagement and participation

Local communities – organisations, voluntary groups, individuals – should be engaged and their participation secured, wherever possible, in the framework for services suggested in this section. Many issues for appropriate service provision (for example, health education and promotion or effective access to services) – and therefore approaches to community participation – are likely to be shared with other communities of interest, in particular those from disadvantaged white populations.

A range of approaches can be used,[283,284] including community development and participatory research strategies.[164,285] These approaches need to evolve within new health service contexts, in particular of Primary Care Organisations (PCO). PCO-led decision-making now offers important opportunities to advance service development that is responsive to local communities' needs. Local communities should be enabled to have active roles in shaping and supporting all aspects of services outlined. These include roles in:

- community consultation and research about needs, appropriateness and quality of service
- service design, acceptability and delivery
- health professional training
- health promotion interventions
- minority ethnic recruitment to the NHS workforce
- approaches to ethnic monitoring and audit of quality of care.

Systematising the capture and use of appropriate data: ethnic monitoring

HAs, PCOs and Trusts need to know the size, geographical distribution and socio-economic character-istics of their local ethnic minority populations. This information should include languages spoken, religions and lifestyles. Such information needs to be collected consistently and appropriately. These requirements appear axiomatic but the continuing failure of the NHS to realise and monitor them systematically must be addressed. They are crucial to the effective development and evaluation of services for minority ethnic populations.

Ethnic monitoring data is clearly a pre-requisite for defining populations, successful needs assessment, planning and audit of services. The statutory requirement to compile basic ethnic monitoring data within the acute hospital sector needs to be further developed. It must be extended elsewhere in the NHS to the community care sector and, crucially, to the primary care sector. Again, for success, performance management is a critical starting point. In tandem, the introduction of such initiatives need to be carefully researched and evaluated.

Issues of variation in quality, and good practice for local ethnic monitoring are outlined in section 3. Particular concerns are ensuring data goes beyond ethnic origin (usually by census group) to relate to language and other needs. Functional literacy is related to non-UK birth, underlining the importance of recording birthplace. Staff need to be aware of the purpose of data collection and supported by training to seek information sensitively and accurately.

Effective models that can help primary care teams collect essential data about patients' ethnicity, language and culture are now available.[74,286] This information must then be used to plan and improve quality of care through audit and evaluation.

Integration with wider policy initiatives

In reviewing, developing or providing services for minority ethnic communities, opportunities should be sought that may be, or are being, presented by local initiatives seeking to address the exclusion and inequalities experienced by marginalised and disadvantaged communities.

These may provide momentum for service innovations, or the development of existing services and their evaluation. They may entail creative and holistic approaches that move beyond traditional models of health service provision and integration with more socially oriented approaches to health improvement. These include urban regeneration programmes (Single Regeneration Budget), Health Action Zones, New Deal for Communities, SureStart and new flexibilities likely to arise from modernising and integrating health and social services.[270]

Specific services

The following are examples of services which highlight pertinent issues relating to BMEGs and can be adapted to other conditions.

Mental health

A comprehensive review of the psychiatric care received by people with severe mental illness from different ethnic groups in Birmingham, made recommendations for service development provided in Appendix 5.[279] This identifies the need for consultation with local ethnic minority communities, staff training, greater accessibility of social and psychological therapies, models of community-based care and home treatment alternatives to hospital admission.

The new National Service Framework for Mental Health (http://www.dh.gov.uk/assetRoot/04/07/72/09/04077209.pdf) rehearses similar recommendations in relation to minority ethnic communities, in particular highlighting training for health professionals.

Cervical screening

Recommendations for equitable and quality cervical screening services in primary care have been developed and are summarised in Appendix 7.[182]

Health education and promotion

Overall, black people may not be aware, or made aware, of the range of services available. When they are made aware, many express a wish to use them but may be inhibited in using them – or find that these services do not cater for their needs. Such provision often ignores the needs of people from ethnic minorities or marginalises them by focusing upon the difference in their cultural practices from the white 'norm'.[287]

It is clear that health promotion activities for minority ethnic communities can be improved. For example, the smaller proportion of people from ethnic minorities who have given up smoking (e.g. Bangladeshi men) compared to the white majority[84] would suggest health promotion messages have been less successful or strategies have not led to motivation to behaviour change.

In forming strategies, HAs, PCOs and Trusts should note that the health education needs of minority ethnic groups may be very similar to the majority population, but that appropriate methods for targeting and delivery may require a different, flexible approach.[288] Examples include:

- improving uptake of preventive services/screening – for example by proactive household by household invitation to Bangladeshi families[289]
- cervical screening uptake – targeted home visiting and information video can be superior to translated written material[265]
- information about primary care services and preventive advice – using videos and interactive computer and video packages.[149]

In order to determine appropriate health promotion interventions, health professionals need to establish the community's views and aspirations; their reactions to proposed methods and settings; and the effects of interventions upon not only target behaviour/knowledge/ill-health but also the wider social and cultural aspects of the community's life.[288,290]

Interventions need to be sensitive to both similarities and differences in health beliefs and illness.[291] Moreover, they must go beyond understanding cultural issues and recognise the material constraints faced by many people from minority ethnic communities. The relatively disadvantaged socio-economic status of many ethnic minority populations and its impact upon their health cannot be ignored.[84]

Haemoglobinopathies

Haemoglobinopathy counselling centres are sited mostly in areas of high prevalence, but services are not yet comprehensive.[106] Awareness of these disorders amongst health professionals has been suggested for low uptake of screening services.

For both thalassaemia and sickle cell anaemia, survival is expected to rise.[225] Provision for health information, screening, pre-natal and antenatal counselling services and professional development is patchy and poorly co-ordinated.[106] Utilisation of prenatal diagnosis for haemoglobin disorders is low and varies by region.[109] Initial provision was provided by enthusiastic individuals and voluntary groups in areas of high prevalence.[292]

There is also a need for appropriate interpreting services, as only 4 out of 34 haemoglobinopathy counsellors in England spoke one or more Asian languages.[293]

A model service specification for these disorders is given in Appendix 8.

8 Outcome measures

As there is still a need for further work on delivering services to BMEGs, there are a number of principles[3,294] to guide further action on priorities based on equity:

- national standards of quality of health care to be applied to BMEGs
- emphasis on basic needs, irrespective of similarities or differences between ethnic minority and majority populations
- emphasis on quality of service rather than specific conditions
- focus on a number of priorities rather than a large number
- be guided by priorities identified by, and for, the general population, e.g. *Saving lives: Our Healthier Nation Strategy for England*, as the similarities in the life problems and health patterns of minority ethnic groups exceed the dissimilarities
- consider impact of policies and strategies in reducing health inequalities amongst BMEGs.

Outcome measures

As the development of outcome measures for each disease/condition and ethnic group is in its infancy, general (i.e. SF-36) and disease specific (i.e. Rose Angina questionnaire) measures can be used as in the majority ethnic group. But there are a number of problems to overcome before translation and use of these measures in routine clinical practice.[295] It is vital to get as accurate a restatement of meaning as possible rather than linguistic precision[296] before validated instruments can be applied to specific minority ethnic populations.

To maximise the quality of care for the BMEGs, the following dimensions are still applicable for the development and monitoring of care provided by the health service: access, relevance, acceptability, effectiveness, efficiency and equity.[297]

Targets

Using national guidance, targets have or need to be set in the following areas:

Developing a diverse workforce

Each health authority is to implement *The Vital Connection: An equalities framework for the NHS strategy* (http://www.dh.gov.uk/assetRoot/04/03/50/54/04035054.pdf). This document provides a framework for action and targets in implementing this framework. The key elements are an equality statement and agreed national equality standards and indicators (details will be available from the above website in due course). The framework is underpinned by three strategic aims.

- To recruit, develop and retain a workforce that is able to deliver high quality services that are accessible, responsive and appropriate to meet the needs of different groups and individuals.
- To ensure that the NHS is a fair employer, achieving equality of opportunity and outcomes in the workplace.
- To ensure that the NHS uses its influence and resources as an employer to make a difference to the life opportunities and the health of its local community, especially those shut out or disadvantaged.

Building on the *Working Together*[298] document, which set targets for achieving a representative workforce and tackling racial harassment, specific targets from April 2000 for NHS organisations have been set.

- Each local employer should be able to demonstrate a year on year increase in the level of confidence that staff have in their ability to tackle racial harassment at work, as measured through the annual survey.
- Each local employer should agree a target percentage reduction in the level of harassment at work and have arrangements in place to be able to demonstrate this progress year on year.
- Each local employer should meet the criteria to use the Employment Service disability symbol ('Two Ticks') by April 2001.
- All NHS boards should undertake training on managing equality and diversity by April 2001.
- A national target should be in place to increase ethnic minority representation in executive posts at board level to 7% by end of March 2004 across all sectors of the NHS.
- A national target should be in place to increase women's representation in executive posts at board to 40% by end of March 2004 across all sectors of the NHS.

Specific diseases

As outlined in *Saving lives: Our Healthier Nation Strategy for England* (http://www.webarchive.org.uk/pan/11052/20050218), targets to achieve by the year 2010 have been set for specific priority areas. These are not provided for specific minority ethnic groups and we advocate the following:

- **cancer:** to reduce the death rate in people under 75 by at least a fifth
- **coronary heart disease** and **stroke:** to reduce the death rate in people under 75 by at least two fifths
- **accidents:** to reduce the death rate by at least a fifth and serious injury by at least a tenth
- **mental illness:** to reduce the death rate from suicide and undetermined injury by at least a fifth.

The National Service Frameworks detail implementation plans to achieve the above targets and the following four are due to be published by spring of 2001: coronary heart disease, mental health, older people and diabetes (http://www.webarchive.org.uk/pan/11052/20050218).

Service delivery

(a) Provide an explicit statement by commissioning groups on embedding equality and diversity within Health Improvement Programmes. This includes racial prejudice and harassment.
(b) Develop a strategy to address 'culturally competent' services that emphasises not only clinically effective services but also the linguistic, cultural and religious preferences of individuals receiving the care. Ensure that these are reflected in their local Health Improvement Plans.
(c) Develop a local policy on screening/counselling for haemoglobinopathies (*see* Appendix 8).
(d) Set local target to ensure quality data on ethnic group status within secondary care.

9 Information and research requirements

Information needs

(a) Ethnic monitoring in primary care should be mandatory as in secondary care. Indeed, this should be extended to community and cancer screening services as well. The quality and completeness of this data needs to be improved to utilise routine datasets currently available.

(b) There is a need to include ethnic group data on birth/death certificates.

Further research

Research on BMEGs to date has concentrated on a number of minority groups, and the research that has been funded has been on short-term project funding so that full evaluation by rigorous methodologies has tended to be neglected. Further, most studies have neglected to recruit individuals from minority ethnic communities so that generalisability is limited. Research involving minority groups is also relevant to the needs of the majority 'white' population. This includes increased awareness of diversity within the population and its implications for practice; improved access to specific communities; and appreciation of the holistic approach to managing conditions within the health service. This chapter has highlighted many gaps in knowledge, and the following are the main priorities for further research amongst the BMEGs.

- There is a need for incidence data on the major conditions affecting mortality and morbidity.
- The evidence base by ethnic group on health status, access to services, health outcomes and cost-effectiveness of interventions is poor and needs to be addressed by all national commissioning bodies.
- Further evaluation is needed of different models of providing bilingual services, such as physically present interpreters and advocates compared to telephone and telemedicine interpreting.
- Assessment the effect of racism on health and health care is needed.

Conclusions

Needs assessment for black and minority groups is a complex task and the evidence base to guide decision-making is growing. Nevertheless, commissioners should assess the size of their local population; begin to address priorities for their population within their Health Improvement Plans; develop services to meet these; and monitor outcomes of care. This depends on having an effective, systematic ethnic monitoring within their provider services. We have highlighted issues and the dearth of data and hope that the ideas and frameworks will help. Some further resources are listed in Appendix 9.

Note that since completion of this chapter, an initial update on two surveys has been undertaken as shown in Appendix 10.

Appendix 1: Adjustment factors for estimated undercoverage by age, sex and ethnic group in the 1991 census, Great Britain

| Age | Ethnic group | | | | | | | | | Other groups | |
	Total	White	Black-Caribbean	Black-African	Black-Other	Indian	Pakistani	Bangla-deshi	Chinese	Asian	Other
Persons, all ages	1.02	1.02	1.03	1.05	1.04	1.03	1.03	1.03	1.03	1.03	1.03
0–4	1.03	1.03	1.04	1.04	1.04	10.3	10.3	10.4	1.03	1.04	1.04
5–9	1.03	1.03	1.03	1.03	1.03	1.03	1.03	1.03	1.03	1.03	1.03
10–14	1.02	1.02	1.02	1.02	1.02	1.02	1.02	1.02	1.02	1.02	1.02
15–19	1.02	1.02	1.02	1.02	1.02	1.02	1.02	1.02	1.02	1.02	1.02
20–24	1.06	1.06	1.09	1.09	1.08	1.07	1.08	1.09	1.09	1.08	1.08
25–29	1.07	1.07	1.10	1.11	1.09	1.08	1.09	1.10	1.09	1.08	1.09
30–34	1.03	1.03	1.04	1.05	1.04	1.04	1.04	1.05	1.04	1.04	1.04
35–39	1.01	1.01	1.01	1.01	1.01	1.01	1.01	1.01	1.01	1.01	1.01
40–44	1.01	1.01	1.01	1.01	1.01	1.01	1.01	1.01	1.01	1.01	1.01
45–79	1.00	1.00	1.00	1.00	1.00	1.00	1.00	1.00	1.00	1.00	1.00
80–84	1.02	1.02	1.02	1.02	1.02	1.02	1.02	1.02	1.02	1.02	1.02
85+	1.04	1.04	1.04	1.04	1.04	1.04	1.04	1.04	1.04	1.04	1.04
Males, all ages	1.03	1.03	1.05	1.07	1.06	1.04	1.04	1.04	1.05	1.05	1.05
0–4	1.04	1.04	1.04	1.04	1.04	1.04	1.04	1.04	1.04	1.04	1.04
5–9	1.03	1.03	1.03	1.03	1.03	1.03	1.03	1.03	1.03	1.03	1.03
10–14	1.02	1.02	1.02	1.02	1.02	1.02	1.02	1.02	1.02	1.02	1.02
15–19	1.03	1.03	1.03	1.03	1.03	1.03	1.03	1.03	1.03	1.03	1.03
20–24	1.10	1.10	1.14	1.15	1.14	1.12	1.14	1.14	1.14	1.13	1.13
25–29	1.10	1.10	1.16	1.17	1.15	1.13	1.15	1.16	1.14	1.14	1.14
30–34	1.05	1.05	1.07	1.08	1.07	1.06	1.07	1.08	1.06	1.06	1.07
35–39	1.02	1.02	1.02	1.02	1.02	1.02	1.02	1.02	1.02	1.02	1.02
40–44	1.02	1.02	1.02	1.02	1.02	1.02	1.02	1.02	1.02	1.02	1.02
45–79	1.00	1.00	1.00	1.00	1.00	1.00	1.00	1.00	1.00	1.00	1.00
80–84	1.01	1.01	1.01	1.01	1.01	1.01	1.01	1.01	1.01	1.01	1.01
85+	1.01	1.01	1.01	1.01	1.01	1.01	1.01	1.01	1.01	1.01	1.01
Females, all ages	1.01	1.01	1.02	1.02	1.03	1.02	1.02	1.02	1.02	1.02	1.02
0–4	1.03	1.03	1.03	1.04	1.03.	1.03	1.03	1.03	1.03	1.03	1.03
5–9	1.02	1.02	1.02	1.02	1.02	1.02	1.02	1.02	1.02	1.02	1.02
10–14	1.01	1.01	1.01	1.01	1.01	1.01	1.01	1.01	1.01	1.01	1.01
15–19	1.01	1.01	1.01	1.01	1.01	1.02	1.02	1.01	1.01	1.01	1.01
20–24	1.03	1.03	1.04	1.04	1.04	1.03	1.04	1.04	1.04	1.04	1.04
25–29	1.03	1.03	1.05	1.05	1.05	1.04	1.05	1.05	1.04	1.04	1.04
30–34	1.01	1.01	1.02	1.02	1.02	1.02	1.02	1.02	1.02	1.02	1.02
35–39	1.00	1.00	1.00	1.00	1.00	1.00	1.00	1.00	1.00	1.00	1.00
40–44	1.01	1.01	1.01	1.00	1.01	1.01	1.01	1.01	1.01	1.01	1.01
45–79	1.00	1.00	1.00	1.00	1.00	1.00	1.00	1.00	1.01	1.01	1.00
80–84	1.02	1.02	1.03	1.03	1.02	1.03	1.03	1.03	1.02	1.03	1.03
85+	1.06	1.06	1.06	1.06	1.06	1.06	1.06	1.06	1.05	1.06	1.06

Note: Derived entirely from factors by age, sex, and area of residence.
Source: OPCS/GRO(S) 1993, p.7[66]

Appendix 2: Full ethnic group classification

Code*	Category
0	White
1	Black-Caribbean
2	Black-African
3	Indian
4	Pakistani
5	Bangladeshi
6	Chinese
	Black-Other: non-mixed origin
7	British
8	Caribbean Island, West Indies or Guyana
9	North African, Arab or Iranian
10	Other African countries
11	East African, Asian or Indo-Caribbean
12	Indian subcontinent
13	Other Asian
14	Other answers
	Black-Other: mixed origin
15	Black/White
16	Asian/White
17	Other mixed
	Other ethnic group: non-mixed origin
18	British – ethnic minority indicated
19	British – no ethnic minority indicated
20	Caribbean Island, West Indies or Guyana
21	North African, Arab or Iranian
22	Other African countries
23	East African, Asian or Indo-Caribbean
24	Indian subcontinent
25	Other Asian
26	Irish
27	Greek (including Greek Cypriot)
28	Turkish (including Turkish Cypriot)
29	Other European
30	Other answers
	Other ethnic group: mixed origin
31	Black/White
32	Asian/White
33	Mixed White
34	Other mixed

* Codes 0 to 6 are the pre-coded boxes in the question (*see* **Box 1**).

Appendix 3: Population sizes according to 1991 census by sex and age group for selected countries of birth

Males Age-group Country of birth	0–19	20–44	45–64	65–74	75+	Total
East Africa	9,410	81,545	18,700	1,527	368	111,550
West/South Africa	8,256	33,679	9,593	992	265	52,785
Caribbean	3,161	32,844	53,755	11,487	2,406	103,653
Bangladesh	20,132	19,588	14,208	1,146	201	55,275
India	8,177	86,544	74,803	17,498	7,364	194,386
Pakistan	19,291	61,386	29,624	4,396	1,109	115,806
Hong Kong/China	6,622	26,698	9,529	1,996	789	45,634

Females Age-group (years) Country of birth	0–19	20–44	45–64	65–74	75+	Total
East Africa	9,346	76,236	16,920	1,571	477	104,550
West/South Africa	8,618	37,740	7,878	577	321	55,134
Caribbean	3,360	46,797	53,590	8,728	2,945	115,420
Bangladesh	17,356	23,424	7,557	408	188	48,933
India	7,786	99,331	68,823	18,658	11,032	205,630
Pakistan	16,301	65,777	22,742	2,761	1,309	108,890
Hong Kong/China	6,116	27,337	8,060	2,327	1,503	45,343

Appendix 4: Quality of Evidence

I: Evidence obtained from at least one properly designed randomised controlled trial.

II-1:   Evidence obtained from well-designed controlled trials without randomisation.

II-2:   Evidence obtained from well-designed cohort or case-control analytic studies, preferably from more than one centre or research group.

II-3:   Evidence obtained from multiple time series with or without the intervention. Dramatic results in uncontrolled experiments (such as the results of the introduction of penicillin treatment in the 1940s) could also be regarded as this type of evidence.

III: Opinions of respected authorities, based on clinical experience, descriptive studies, or reports of expert committees.

IV: Evidence inadequate and conflicting.

Appendix 5: Findings and recommendations for mental service development[279]

Recommendations

Service development

All patients admitted to an in-patient facility should be give oral and written information about the reason for their admission, details of the staff who are to care for them, including their availability, and, where appropriate, their status under the Mental Health Act. The latter should include the type of section under which the patient is detained, the maximum length of detention and the right of appeal. A dated copy of this written information should be lodged in the patient's file. Medical Records staff should verify that this has been done.

The ethnic dimension in the Health of the Nation targets must be emphasised and, in particular, there should be an explicit acknowledgement that the social outcome for black people with mental health problems need to be improved. This should form part of contract negotiations between health purchasers and provider Trusts.

In areas with substantial minority ethnic groups, service providers should set up a regular process of consultation with service users from black and Asian backgrounds and also, local black communities. We recommend setting up an ethnic minority consultation forum to include representatives of local black communities, black service users, service providers, general practitioners, health purchasers and black voluntary groups.

There should be a system of monitoring the use of the Mental Health Act according to ethnicity. Regular data on this should be available and standards should be set up in each provider Trust with the aim of achieving uniform detention rates for all ethnic groups. Service purchasers should insist on targets that can be set on admission rates and detention rates for each provider unit with the aim of equalising the service usage of people from different minority ethnic groups.

There is an urgent need to review the availability, accessibility and appropriateness of social and psychological therapies for black and Asian patients. Referral rates and acceptance rates within such services must be monitored according to ethnicity.

Trusts providing psychiatric care in inner city areas in particular should be encouraged to develop alternative informal services for black service users with the emphasis on social care and culturally based interventions. Such services should form part of a network of social care available locally, including supporting housing schemes, cultural therapy centres and other informal systems of non-medical care. These alternative services should be evaluated and monitored on a regular basis. There is an urgent need to develop alternatives to hospital admission. Given the intrinsic problems associated with in-patient care – their reliance on coercion and control, which are made more explicit in the case of ethnic minority clients – alternative interventions such as community-based crisis residential facilities, and home treatment services ought to be developed as in integral part of the spectrum of care available to all patients.

Training

All staff who are likely to have contact with black patients (both inside and outside the health service) must be given special training on culture and mental health, the impact of racism on the perceptions of staff, the common stereotypes and discriminatory attitudes and behaviour of the staff.

Furthermore, staff must have specific training in strategies of engagement with people experiencing serious mental illness. All provider Trusts serving populations containing ethnic minority groups should identify someone in senior management trained to take specific responsibility for ethnic minority issues. This should include the nature and adequacy of service provision for ethnic minorities, training on ethnicity and mental health for the staff, monitoring service usage by ethnicity, consultation with local ethnic minority groups and achieving targets set in advance on a year to year basis.

All staff should receive basic training in the principles of community-based care and the alternative service models which are available where traditional hospital based care is no longer appropriate or is not acceptable to the community being served.

Staff should have basic training in the place and techniques of service evaluation in the development of higher service standards and evidence-based intervention.

Appendix 6: Linkworkers in primary care: checklist for HAs and PCOs[258]

This checklist is designed to remind commissioners and providers of primary care of questions that may be relevant to them in establishing and supporting linkworkers in primary care. There will be further points that need to be added in the light of local experience as primary care develops. Few schemes have, or are likely to have, addressed all questions in a wholly satisfactory way. However, working towards comprehensive answers to the questions raised in the checklist should enable schemes to be more effective and sustainable and should provide a framework for increasing quality in linkworker schemes as well as better training and support for linkworkers themselves.

Strategic framework

- Is there an agreed strategy for improving ethnic minority health and access to health services?
- How does the linkworker scheme contribute to the development of a local strategy for improving ethnic minority health and access to health services?
- Who is involved in developing a local health strategy for improving ethnic minority health and access to health services?
- Are there robust links between the NHS, local authorities, voluntary organisations and the wider community in developing a local strategy?

Assessing need

Has there been an assessment of the local need for linkworkers that:

- Uses demographic information about the local population?
- Uses projections on future population changes?
- Uses morbidity and mortality data?
- Uses current information on language needs?
- Reflects discussions with local communities on need?
- Involves all types of primary health care staff (not only GPs)?
- Reaches out to engage small minority communities, and those who may be less well represented by effective community organisations?
- Includes discussions with the appropriate local authorities?
- Includes an audit of existing relevant, local services?
- Is there a mechanism for recording unmet need that falls outside the scope of existing services for ethnic minorities?

Defining the linkworker's tasks

- Has there been explicit discussion to clarify the role(s) of linkworkers, and to define the nature and scope of what they will do, and what they will not do?
- Have professional and lay interests been taken into account in defining tasks and priorities?

Management and supervision of linkworkers

- How will linkworkers be line managed and to whom will they be accountable?

- If joint funded, are there clear management arrangements that are acceptable to all funders?
- Has the line manager sufficient time in which to manage postholders, bearing in mind the likelihood of front-loading of management time at the outset of new schemes?
- What means of appraisal will be used to assess linkworkers' performance, and how will the appraiser develop competencies to carry out this appraisal?
- Are there clear Service Level Agreements in place between commissioners and providers?
- Is there a means by which linkworkers can access professional advice from someone other than a line manager, if required?
- Has there been discussion/decisions on whether/how to involve local communities in management arrangements?

Funding

- Has there been a clear estimate of the overall costs of starting up and maintaining linkworking?
- Is the cost of linkworkers (including management and administration) to be met through mainstream funding?
- What is the duration of the funding commitment?
- Has full use been made of available external funding sources?
- If funding is time-limited, what arrangements are in place to secure future funding?
- If long-term funds are unlikely to be available, has a full assessment been made of the case for and against establishing short-term schemes?

Monitoring and evaluation

- What performance measures and indicators of outcome have been agreed?
- Is there agreement on what would constitute a successful outcome of linkworker involvement?
- Does the process of agreeing and reviewing performance measures and outcomes include professional and lay interests?
- What monitoring arrangements are in place to ensure an appropriate level and quality of service?
- How can the community be involved in monitoring and evaluating services?

Recruitment and selection of postholders

- Is there a clear job description for the post(s)?
- Is there a clear person specification that relates to the job description?
- Does the person specification pay proper regard to valuing applicants' life experiences, voluntary and community activity, and show evidence of understanding of the needs of the communities to be served?
- Has there been consultation with local communities on the relevance of the job description and person specification?
- Who will be involved in the selection of postholders? Will there be community/lay involvement in selection, and if so, how?
- Where will posts be advertised and publicised in order to maximise access by relevant communities?

Training

- What arrangements have been made for induction training?
- What arrangements are in place for in-service training?

- Are there effective links with local colleges, etc. to ensure their input to curriculum development and delivery of training programmes?
- Have there been discussions with professionals, community workers, community organisations and patients on content of training courses?
- Does the training programme for linkworkers include:
  - communication and language skills?
  - understanding how the NHS works?
  - input on local policies?
  - understanding of other relevant services (e.g. social services)?
  - cultural and religious issues?
  - assertiveness and confidence-building?
  - input on relevant health/medical issues?
  - needs assessment?
  - community development?
  - negotiating skills?
  - information on anti-discrimination legislation?
- How will training be financed?
- Have local communities been invited to contribute to training courses?
- Have arrangements been made to ensure that all colleagues (including doctors of all levels of seniority) have access to training to enable them to understand the roles of linkworkers and to work effectively with them?
- Is anti-discrimination training and equal opportunities training mandatory and available for all staff?

Administration and support

Have arrangements been made for:

- desks and office space?
- health and safety provision?
- access to telephones, bleeps, etc?
- clerical/secretarial assistance?
- name badges?
- advising switchboard and local information services of start date, availability of workers?
- out-of-hours cover?
- cover for sickness, holidays and study leave?

Appendix 7: Recommendations for cervical screening services for women from ethnic minority communities in primary care[182]

The following are suggestions for health authorities, and the new Primary Care Commissioning Groups in particular, to consider as an integral part of their commissioning strategy in the development of an equitable and quality screening service in primary care.

There is a responsibility upon the screening services to ensure that ethnic minority women, particularly those whose first language is not English, are informed of the purpose and the procedure of the cervical screening programme.

The screening service should uphold the principle of informed choice. Opportunistic screening of ethnic minority women without information should be actively discouraged.

In order to address the issue of inequality of access to the cervical screening service, ethnic monitoring, and auditing of uptake among ethnic minority women should form part of the health improvement programme in primary care.

Health professionals who have the responsibility for smear-taking should undergo a programme of intercultural communication.

Where a district has a sizeable ethnic minority population, a "Community Health Educator Model" should be adopted to facilitate access to the service by ethnic minority women as an integral part of primary care with due regard to language support. The spirit of partnership between health promotion departments, ethnic minority communities and primary care in developing this model should be stressed.

Inter-district collaboration, and pooling and sharing resources are essential strategies in addressing the issue of small and scattered ethnic minority populations, such as typify the Chinese, Vietnamese and Yemeni communities in the UK.

A Cervical Screening Training Pack for Minority Women should be distributed to all Public Health and Health Promotion Departments in England and Wales.

As a principle of good practice, smear-taking medical professionals in primary care should make use of photo-audio pack tools for informing ethnic minority women who may have language needs before they proceed with a smear test.

Further research is needed to test the robustness of Community Health Educator models in the context of women from areas of low uptake who do not experience language differences.

Appendix 8: Model service specification for haemoglobinopathy services[107]

Health promotion should be included in all relevant contracts. These specifications are relevant for commissioners and providers of services including voluntary organisations.

The level of service that is appropriate in each area will depend on the number of people at risk, but all purchasers should ensure that staff understand about the management of patients with haemoglobin disorders in emergencies and that services are purchased from centres that meet these specifications.

1   A senior manager has responsibility for co-ordinating and developing services for haemoglobin disorders.

Health promotion

2   There is a strategy for haemoglobin disorders developed with health and local authorities, providers, GP's voluntary agencies, trade unions and business, covering:
   • the general population
   • at-risk groups
   • people affected and their carers
   • police, prison and probation services
   • employers and businesses.
3   The health promotion programme includes:
   • working on needs identified with community groups
   • supporting local self-help groups
   • developing appropriate health information
   • professional development.
4   There is a programme for raising awareness about haemoglobin disorders, including:
   • schools and further education colleges
   • primary care
   • employers
   • religious and community groups
   • local authority services
   • the media.
5   There is a range of materials available in appropriate languages including:
   • leaflets
   • posters
   • audio and video cassettes
   • drama and teaching packs for schools.
6   These materials have been selected and developed with local users and the district health promotion service.
7   Health promotion materials are available free to GPs, antenatal clinics, health centres and within the community.

Primary care

8 All GPs with significant numbers of people from relevant ethnic groups on their lists are encouraged to take part in haemoglobinopathy screening, including:
  - preconception advice for women of child-bearing age, including family planning
  - opportunistic screening
  - testing partners and family members of carriers
  - screening new patients joining the practice.
9 There is information and guidelines on patient care for GPs including:
  - appropriate care for acute illness
  - routine screening for signs of long-term consequences
  - appropriate strategies for maintaining good health and avoiding situations which can precipitate ill health.
10 All staff involved with haemoglobin disorders are trained in giving accurate information.
11 Appropriate information is distributed to practices to be given to patients about screening and self-management.
12 All GPs are informed of the results of tests on their patients and neonates born to patients.

Screening

General and opportunistic screening

13 All screening services should be associated with an adequate educational and counselling service.
14 There are protocols for screening programmes including:
  - informed consent
  - confidentiality
  - report back of test results
  - communication of test results to GPs.
15 There is a quality control programme to check the accuracy of results of screening tests.
16 Those tested are issued with a certificate of testing, showing the result of their blood test, their carrier status and the centre responsible for the test.
17 Preconception advice is included in all family planning and fertility clinics.
18 Opportunistic screening is offered at 'well woman' and 'well men' clinics.
19 The coverage and take-up of screening is monitored.

Antenatal screening

20 Antenatal screening is offered early enough to allow at-risk couples be identified by ten weeks of pregnancy.

Neonatal screening

21 There is a protocol for determining which neonates are screened.
22 Neonatal screening is carried out in association with phenylketouria and hypothyroidism screening at one to two weeks of life.
23 Parents and GPs are informed of the results of neonatal screening and the implications of these results.
24 Results are included in the child health record.

Counselling

25 There are counselling services available:
  - Before screening
  - After screening
  - For families of carriers and patients
  - Associated with long-term management of patients with major disorders.
26 Information is offered to all people with positive results in the language if their choice.
27 Counsellors work as part of a multidisciplinary team dealing with all aspects of care in hospitals and the community.
28 Counsellors have training in:
  - counselling
  - genetic counselling and haemoglobin disorders.
29 There sufficient specialist haemoglobinopathy counsellors to meet the needs of both primary health care and hospitals.
30 Counselling services are:
  - available in appropriate languages
  - sensitive to cultural and religious needs of users
  - appropriate to the needs of young people.
31 Counselling services are widely advertised and accessible, including drop-in sessions for people worried about the condition or those who think they may need a test.
32 Counsellors have links with local groups for those affected and their families, and offer them support.

Professional development

33 A training programme about the haemoglobin disorders and appropriate management is provided for key staff, specifying the objectives, volume, methods and evaluation of training.
34 Training is provided to key workers including:
  - haematology staff
  - accident and emergency staff
  - maternity services staff
  - child health services
  - the primary care team
  - school health services.
35 Training in genetics and genetic counselling is multidisciplinary to encourage co-operation between the profession and agencies.

Joint working

36 Haemoglobin disorders are identified in the community care plan.
37 There are guidelines for schools, youth workers, child and family services, housing and environmental health on haemoglobin disorders.

Monitoring and evaluation

38 Services are regularly monitored to assess their appropriateness and effectiveness, including:
  - regular reports from providers
  - monitoring services by user groups

- clinical audit (including medical audit in primary care)
- user surveys to get feedback on whether health promotion messages are received and how effective they are
- community liaison to get feedback from the community on its needs, the appropriateness of materials and the effectiveness of campaigns
- complaints received.

Appendix 9

In addition to the resources listed in the main text and the references, listed below are website addresses resources that may help in assessing health care needs locally. This is not an exhaustive list, but provides 'gateways' to other sites.

The King's Fund is an independent health care charity working for better health in London. They also work nationally and internationally and carry out research and development work to bring about better health policies and services.

- http://www.kingsfund.org.uk/health_topics/black_and.html

The Centre for Research in Ethnic Relations is an national academic centre for research and teaching in the field of ethnic relations and houses unique collections of primarily British non-book materials covering a wide range of issues in ethnic relations. The 'Ethnic Health File' of the Clinical Sciences Library, University of Leicester, is included in the main database.

- http://www.warwick.ac.uk/fac/soc/CRER_RC/

The Health Development Agency (HDA) is a special health authority that aims to improve the health of people in England. There are many links to other sites through its database (HealthPromis, http://healthpromis.hda-online.org.uk/).

- http://www.nice.org.uk/page.aspx?0=295458

The Department of Health (England) site provides information on many topics relevant to ethnic minority communities.

- http://www.doh.gov.uk/

The Office of National Statistics contains the latest comprehensive range of official UK statistics and information about statistics. In addition, information on all the major national surveys on health and health care can be accessed.

- http://www.statistics.gov.uk/

The **Accessible Publishing of Genetic Information** (ApoGI) site provides genetic information both to health workers and to affected individuals.

- http://www.chime.ucl.ac.uk/APoGI/

The Health Care Needs Assessment site has a number of epidemiologically based needs assessment reviews relevant to the health of ethnic minority communities.

- http://hcna.radcliffe-oxford.com/bemgframe.htm

The **General Medical Council** has issued guidance that highlights best practice and current legislation in diversity and equality issues:

- http://www.gmc-uk.org/guidance/library/valuing_diversity.asp

Appendix 10: Update on surveys

In this appendix we update the health needs assessment using two surveys: the 2001 Census and the Health Survey for England (HSE) 1999 that focused on the health of minority ethnic groups. PG updated the Census 2001 and RB the Health Survey for England data.

Census 2001

As shown in **Box 2**, the Census 2001 question was significant as it asked questions on people of Irish descent and mixed parentage. Also, for the first time, the Northern Ireland 2001 Census included an ethnic group question thereby providing a comprehensive picture of the UK population ethnic group.

However, both the Scotland and Northern Ireland Census Offices adopted a modified version of the ethnic group question to that used in England and Wales (**Table A10.1**). In both England and Wales and Scotland, a 'two-tier' question was used: people were first invited to choose whether they were 'white', 'mixed', 'Asian', 'Black' or 'Other' and then directed to choose a more specific category within these broad groups. In Northern Ireland, a single-tier question was used. The relationship of the three questions and the way in which they relate to the 1991 Census categories is detailed in **Table A10.1**.

Census data is available by country at: http://www.statistics.gov.uk/statbase/explorer.asp?CTG=3&SL= &D=4712&DCT=32&DT=32#4712 (for England & Wales), http://www.scrol.gov.uk/scrol/common/ home.jsp (for Scotland) and http://www.nisra.gov.uk/Census/Census2001Output/standard_tables1.html (for Northern Ireland).

Ethnic composition of the UK

In the 2001 Census over 4.6 million people (7.9%) identified themselves as belonging to one of the non-white ethnic groups. South Asians formed 3.5%, with the Black group accounting for 2.0% and the Chinese 0.4%. Note that in the UK there are 677 117 (1.2%) people belonging to the mixed ethnic group category (**Table A10.2**).

Geographical distribution across the UK

Although the BMEG population is distributed throughout the UK, there are large clusters particularly in the London region (45%), followed by the West Midlands (12.8%) and the North West (8.1%) regions. Not surprisingly, the largest proportion of the mixed ethnic group reside in the London region (33.4%), which also has the largest proportion of the Black ethnic group (**Table A10.3**).

Unemployment rates

There is large variation in unemployment rate by ethnic group (**Figure A10.1**) with the highest rate amongst males except for the Pakistani and Bangladeshi groups where it is higher in females (**Figure A10.1**). Overall, the highest rates are found in Men – Other Black followed by the mixed group (White/ Black-Caribbean).

Table A10.1: Census ethnic group classification in 1991 and 2001.

1991 Great Britain Equivalent	England and Wales	Scotland	Northern Ireland
White	White: British	White Scottish Other White British	White
	White: Irish	White Irish	
	White: Other White	Other White	Irish Traveller
Black – Other	Mixed: White and Black Caribbean Mixed: White and Black African	Any Mixed Background	Mixed
Other – Other	Mixed: White and Asian Mixed: Other Mixed		
Indian	Asian or Asian British: Indian	Asian, Asian Scottish or Asian British: Indian	Indian
Pakistani	Asian or Asian British: Pakistani	Asian, Asian Scottish or Asian British: Pakistani	Pakistani
Bangladeshi	Asian or Asian British: Bangladeshi	Asian, Asian Scottish or Asian British: Bangladeshi	Bangladeshi
Other – Asian	Asian or Asian British: Other Asian	Asian, Asian Scottish or Asian British: Any other Asian background	Other Asian
Caribbean	Black or Black British: Caribbean	Black, Black Scottish or Black British: Caribbean	Black Caribbean
African	Black or Black British: African	Black, Black Scottish or Black British: African	Black African
Other	Black or Black British: Other Black	Black, Black Scottish or Black British: Other Black	Other Black
Chinese	Chinese or other ethnic group: Chinese	Asian, Asian Scottish or Asian British: Chinese	Chinese
Other – Other	Chinese or other ethnic group: Other Ethnic Group	Other ethnic Background	Other ethnic group

Table A10.2: Ethnic group composition of the population in 2003 (%).

	Great Britain	England & Wales	England	Wales	Scotland	Northern Ireland	United Kingdom
White	91.9	91.3	90.9	97.9	98.0	99.3	92.1
Ethnic minorities	**8.1**	**8.7**	**9.1**	**2.1**	**2.0**	**0.7**	**7.9**
Mixed	1.2	1.3	1.3	0.6	0.3	0.2	1.2
Black	2.0	2.2	2.3	0.2	0.2	0.1	2.0
Black-Caribbean	1.0	1.1	1.1	0.1	0.0	0.0	1.0
Black-African	0.8	0.9	1.0	0.1	0.1	0.0	0.8
South Asian	3.6	3.9	4.1	0.8	1.0	0.1	3.5
Indian	1.8	2.0	2.1	0.3	0.3	0.1	1.8
Pakistani	1.3	1.4	1.4	0.3	0.6	0.0	1.3
Bangladeshi	0.5	0.5	0.6	0.2	0.0	0.0	0.5
Chinese & Other	1.3	1.3	1.4	0.5	0.6	0.3	1.2
Chinese	0.4	0.4	0.4	0.2	0.3	0.2	0.4
Total population	57,103,927	52,041,916	49,138,831	2,903,085	5,062,011	1,685,267	58,789,194

Table A10.3: Regional distribution of ethnic groups.

	Share of UK population by ethnic group					
	White	Mixed	South Asian	Black	Chinese & Other	Minority ethnic groups
ENGLAND	82.5	95.0	96.5	98.6	92.8	96.2
North east	4.5	1.8	1.5	0.3	1.9	1.3
North west	11.7	9.2	10.3	3.6	7.6	8.1
Greater Manchester (Met County)	4.2	4.9	6.3	2.6	3.9	4.8
Yorkshire and Humber	8.6	6.6	10.1	3.0	4.7	7.0
West Yorkshire (Met County)	3.4	3.7	8.3	1.8	2.4	5.1
East Midlands	7.2	6.4	7.5	3.4	4.4	5.9
West Midlands	8.6	10.8	17.5	9.1	7.0	12.8
West Midlands (Met County)	3.8	8.1	15.6	8.3	5.3	11.1
East	9.5	8.6	5.2	4.2	6.7	5.7
London	9.4	33.4	35.2	68.1	45.0	44.6
Inner London	3.4	15.9	12.3	39.6	17.9	20.5
Outer London	6.1	17.5	22.9	28.6	27.0	24.1
South east	14.1	12.7	7.8	5.0	11.8	8.4
South west	8.9	5.5	1.3	1.8	3.7	2.4
WALES	5.2	2.6	1.1	0.6	2.0	1.3
SCOTLAND	9.2	1.9	2.3	0.7	4.4	2.2
NORTHERN IRELAND	3.1	0.5	0.1	0.1	0.8	0.3
GREAT BRITAIN	96.9	99.5	99.9	99.9	99.2	99.7

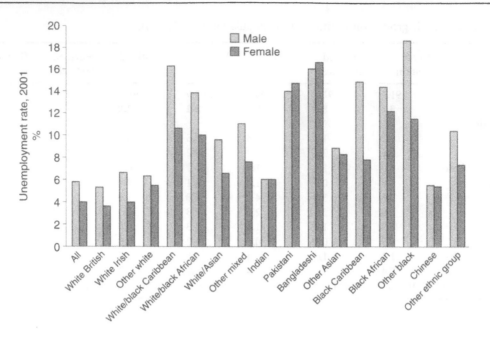

Figure A10.1: Unemployment rates by ethnic group and gender, England and Wales, 2001.

Age and sex structure

Figures A10.2–A10.12 show the age–sex pyramids for each ethnic group in Great Britain. The relative younger age profile of the minority ethnic groups is noted particularly in the mixed ethnic group.

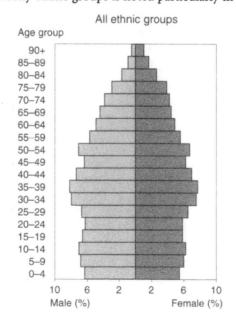

Figure A10.2: Population pyramid for all ethnic groups in Great Britain, 2001.

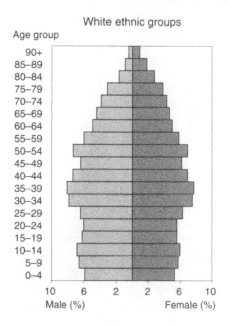

Figure A10.3: Population pyramid for white ethnic groups in Great Britain, 2001.

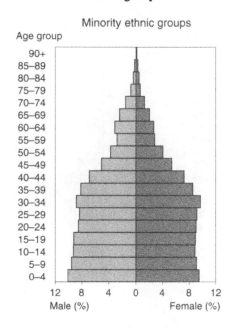

Figure A10.4: Population pyramid for minority ethnic groups in Great Britain, 2001.

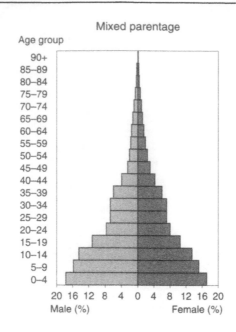

Figure A10.5: Population pyramid for mixed parentage groups in Great Britain, 2001.

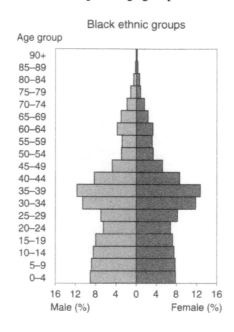

Figure A10.6: Population pyramid for black ethnic groups in Great Britain, 2001.

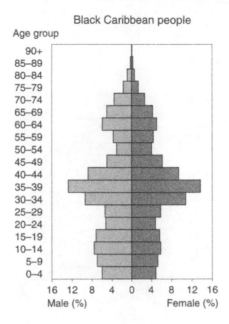

Figure A10.7: Population pyramid for black Caribbean people in Great Britain, 2001.

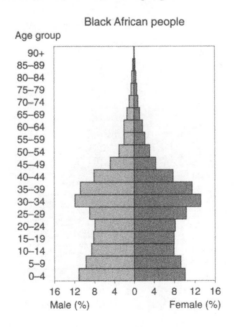

Figure A10.8: Population pyramid for black African ethnic people in Great Britain, 2001.

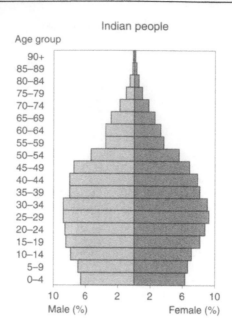

Figure A10.9: Population pyramid for Indian people in Great Britain, 2001.

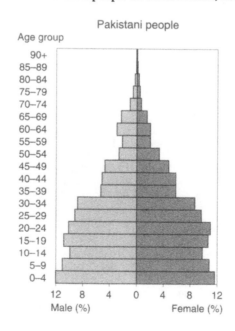

Figure A10.10: Population pyramid for Pakistani people in Great Britain, 2001.

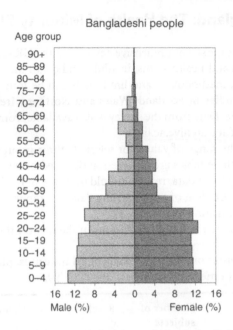

Figure A10.11: Population pyramid for Bangladeshi people in Great Britain, 2001.

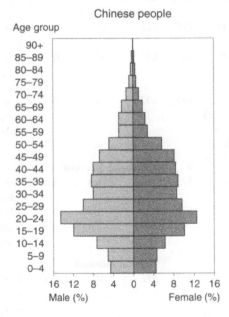

Figure A10.12: Population pyramid for Chinese people in Great Britain, 2001.

Health Survey for England: The Health of Minority Ethnic Groups 1999

This survey comprises the single most comprehensive database in the UK on ethnicity and health lifestyles, socio-economic circumstances and health status, in adults and children.

Further details of the scope, methodology and limitations can be found on www.doh.gov.uk/public/ hse99.htm. Pending similar studies in Scotland, Wales and Northern Ireland, results from this survey should be extrapolated with care. Data from the survey is also available from the UK Data Archive based at the University of Essex (www.data-archive.ac.uk/).

Tables A10.4–A10.9 show the range of values for selected ethnic groups (see also Tables 22–27). For simplicity, results reported in these tables are not age-standardised or weighted for sample size.

Note also that in interpreting these data, readers should be aware of the low response rate for a number of variables/ethnic groups; the problem of self-reporting data in a range of languages and the cautionary remarks made in the main text around Tables 21–27.

By and large, these data support the main conclusions in the text on the health needs of BMEGs.

Table A10.4: Selected information on lifestyles, biochemical measures, physical measures, and self-reported health status for Indian men and women in the HSE '99.

Variable	Measure	Number of subjects		Results		Comment
		Male	Female	Male	Female	
Lifestyle factor						
Smoking	Current smoker (%)	620	651	23	6	The gradual rise in prevalence expected is shown in these data (**Table 22**).
Alcohol	Current drinker (%)	612	645	67	37	The prevalence is much higher in Indian women than in Nazroo's study.[84]
Physical activity in last month	No vigorous activity (%) for 30 minutes or more in last 4 weeks	626	657	30	35	A wide range of activities, including occupational, were included. The scale of the task is great.
Biochemical measure						
Cholesterol	Mean (mmol/l)	379	376	5.4	5.0	These values are high, particularly as values in India are very low.
HDL	Mean (mmol/l)	379	376	1.3	1.4	A higher level is desirable.
Triglycerides	Mean (mmol/l)	187	179	2.3	1.5	Values are higher than reported by Bhopal *et al.* in all groups.[93]
Physical measure						
Height	Mean (cm)	557	612	170.2	156.1	The HSE '99 shows that younger people are taller than older ones in every ethnic group.
Weight	Mean (kg)	548	573	73.2	62.7	
Waist/hip ratio	Mean	467	461	0.92	0.81	
BMI	Mean	527	572	25.2	25.9	The mean value is high, particularly in relation to comparable figures from India and noting that the cut-off for overweight ought to be much lower for South Asians.

Table A10.4: Continued.

Blood pressure	av. Systolic	401	418	134	126	Higher than other South Asian
	av. Diastolic			78	72	groups, and comparable to the White
	(mmHg)					population. The HSE '99 method gives
						a higher reading than standard methods.
	Self-reported health status					
Hypertension	Self-reported (%)	401	408	35.7	16.1	Hypertension is common. However,
	and self-measured					we need to remember the method of
						measurement reads high.
Diabetes	Self-reported (%)	626	657	7.7	4.7	Diabetes is extremely common.
						Remember that self-reporting only
						picks up about 50% of those with
						diabetes.
Angina	Self-reported (%)	626	657	5.4	1.7	These figures show the burden of
						CHD in South Asian population.
Mental health	GHQ-12 score of	565	546	16	23	Mental health problems are common.
	4 or more (%)					A score of 4 or more of the GHQ-12
						is equivalent to needing review for
						possible psychiatric problems.
Self-assessed general health	Very good (%)	626	655	28	19	

Table A10.5: Selected information on lifestyles, biochemical measures, physical measures and self-reported health status for Pakistani men and women.

Variable	Measure	Number of subjects		Results		Comment
		Male	Female	Male	Female	
		Lifestyle factor				
Smoking	Current regular smoker (%)	605	634	26	5	Smoking showing some rise in women in other surveys.
Alcohol	Current drinker (%)	601	631	10	3	Modest rise in comparison to other surveys.
Physical activity	No vigorous activity (%) for 30 minutes or more in last 4 weeks	620	643	32	39	A wide range of activities, including occupational, were included. The scale of the task is great.
		Biochemical measure				
Cholesterol	Mean (mmol/l)	301	281	5.0	4.8	
HDL	Mean (mmol/l)	301	281	1.1	1.4	The levels are undesirably low in men.
Triglycerides	Mean (mmol/l)	108	77	2.1	1.6	
		Physical measure				
Height	Mean (cm)	575	599	171.9	158.2	
Weight	Mean (kg)	557	551	75.1	66.1	Weight is undesirably high.
Waist/hip ratio	Mean	387	403	0.90	0.82	
BMI	Mean	556	550	25.4	26.5	The mean value is high, particularly in relation to comparable figures from India and noting that the cut-off for overweight ought to be much lower for South Asians. The values are high.

Table A10.5: Continued.

Variable	Measure	Number of subjects		Results		Comment
		Male	Female	Male	Female	
Blood pressure	av. Systolic av. Diastolic (mmHg)	319	361	130 73	123 69	The levels are lower than in Indians and the White population but the risk of stroke and CHD is high so needs to be lowered.
			Self-reported health status			
Hyper-tension	Self-reported and measured (%)	319	361	25.5	12.3	
Diabetes	Self-reported (%)	620	643	8.7	5.3	Extremely high and yet less than half the true value.
Angina/MI	Self-reported (%)	620	643	2.9	1.5	
Mental health	GHQ-12 score of 4 or more (%)	488	464	18	22	
Self-assessed general health	Very good (%)	620	643	32	25	

* See notes on Table A10.4, which are generally relevant to this table.

Table A10.6: Selected information on lifestyles, biochemical measures, physical measures and self-reported health status for Bangladeshi men and women.

Variable	Measure	Number of subjects		Results		Comment
		Male	Female	Male	Female	
			Lifestyle factor			
Smoking	Current regular smoker (%)	520	549	44	1	Smoking is extremely common in men. The low value in women is likely to be an underestimate.
Alcohol	Current drinker (%)	512	540	4	1	There may be underreporting.
Physical activity	No vigorous activity (%) for 30 minutes or more in last 4 weeks	533	563	49	54	The Bangladeshi population is the most inactive of the groups studied.
			Biochemical measure			
Cholesterol	Mean (mmol/l)	198	176	5.0	4.7	Higher than desirable.
HDL	Mean (mmol/l)	198	176	1.1	1.3	Very low, and lower than other South Asians and the general population. Higher levels are desirable.
Triglycerides	Mean (mmol/l)	60	35	2.5	2.0	Very high.

Table A10.6: Continued.

				Physical measure		
Height	Mean (cm)	475	517	165.9	153.3	A short population, though younger people substantially taller than older ones.
Weight	Mean (kg)	414	411	65.5	56.6	Lightest among South Asians.
Waist/hip ratio	Mean	273	288	0.90	0.84	The ratios are high, indicating that there is central obesity even though Bangladeshis tend to be light.
BMI	Mean	409	408	23.8	24.1	Though comparatively low and lowest among South Asian and White populations, a lower BMI is still desirable.
Blood pressure	av. Systolic av. Diastolic (mmHg)	214	258	127 73	120 70	Lowest of all South Asians and the general population, and yet CHD and stroke mortality rates are still high.
				Self-reported health status		
Hypertension	Self-reported and measured (%)	214	258	23.6	12.3	On this measure BP prevalence is high.
Diabetes	Self-reported (%)	533	563	10.6	5.9	Very high.
Angina	Self-reported (%)	533	563	3.9	1.3	
Mental health	GHQ-12 score of 4 or more (%)	402	424	26	23	This population reports better mental health than other South Asian and general populations and that despite worse economic circumstances.
Self-assessed general health	Very good (%)	533	563	18	17	Self-assessed health is power.

* See notes on Table A10.4, which are generally relevant to this table.

Table A10.7: Selected information on lifestyles, biochemical measures, physical measures and self-reported health status for Black Caribbean men and women.

Variable	Measure	Number of subjects		Results		Comment
		Male	Female	Male	Female	
				Lifestyle factor		
Smoking	Current smoker (%)	540	741	35	25	Smoking is common.
Alcohol	Current drinker (%)	525	726	87	82	Drinking alcohol is common.
Physical activity	No vigorous exercise (%) for 30 minutes or more in last 4 weeks	547	748	24	25	A wide range of activities, including occupational, were included. The scale of the task is great.

Table A10.7: Continued.

Variable	Measure	Number of subjects		Results		Comment
		Male	Female	Male	Female	
Biochemical measure						
Cholesterol	Mean (mmol/l)	285	368	5.0	4.9	
HDL	Mean (mmol/l)	285	368	1.5	1.6	The levels are satisfactory.
Triglycerides	Mean (mmol/l)	124	174	1.5	1.1	The value for males is higher than expected, Caribbeans usually have low TGs.
Physical measure						
Height	Mean (cm)	483	671	174.2	162.8	
Weight	Mean (kg)	475	639	79.6	74	
Waist/hip ratio	Mean	363	513	0.88	0.82	
BMI	Mean	466	618	26.2	28.0	BMI levels are high and in men tend to reflect muscle mass, but in women obesity.
Blood pressure	av. Systolic av. Diastolic (mmHg)	287	432	136 75	129 72	Unusually, these levels are not particularly high compared to other ethnic groups possibly reflecting effective treatment. Nonetheless stoke is very common in this population, and average blood pressure too high.
Self-reported health status						
Hypertension	Self-reported and measured (%)	287	432	41.9	28.8	As expected, the prevalences are high.
Diabetes	Self-reported (%)	547	748	7.8	7.9	Very high prevalence.
Angina	Self-reported (%)	547	748	1.9	2.2	
Mental health	GHQ-12 score of 4 or more (%)	492	686	16	23	
Self-assessed general health	Very good (%)	545	746	32	27	

* See notes on Table A10.4, which are generally relevant to this table.

Table A10.8: Selected information on lifestyles, biochemical measures, physical measures and self-reported health status for Chinese men and women.

Variable	Measure	Number of subjects		Results		Comment
		Male	Female	Male	Female	
Lifestyle factor						
Smoking	Current smoker (%)	297	359	17	9	
Alcohol	Current drinker (%)	293	358	70	59	
Physical activity	No vigorous activity (%) for 30 minutes or more in last 4 weeks	301	361	31	31	The prevalence is low.

Table A10.8: Continued.

Biochemical measure						
Cholesterol	Mean (mmol/l)	149	175	5.1	5.1	Surprising not lower than other minority groups.
HDL	Mean (mmol/l)	149	175	1.3	1.6	The challenge is to maintain these satisfactory levels.
Triglycerides	Mean (mmol/l)	77	101	1.6	1.5	Compared with Harland *et al.*'s data[94] these levels are high.
Physical measure						
Height	Mean (cm)	285	346	168	156.2	The population is comparatively short.
Weight	Mean (kg)	287	343	68.2	57.4	The weights are satisfactory.
Waist/hip ratio	Mean	196	249	0.88	0.81	
BMI	Mean	409	408	24.1	23.6	Increases are to be avoided as it is likely that the threshold of BMI for overweight in Chinese is low, e.g. about 23 or less.
Blood pressure	av. Systolic	173	219	131	125	
	av. Diastolic (mmHg)			76	71	
Self-reported health status						
Hypertension	Self-reported and measured (%)	173	219	27.9	22.5	Mortality from stroke is comparatively high.
Diabetes	Self-reported (%)	301	361	4.2	2.6	The prevalence is comparatively high, e.g. compared to Harland *et al.*, and maybe heralding an epidemic of diabetes in Chinese.
Angina	Self-reported (%)	301	361	1.8	0.4	The prevalence is low.
Mental health	GHQ-12 score of 4 or more (%)	264	328	3	8	The data, at face value, suggest fewer psychological/psychiatric difficulties, but cross-cultural measurement of this type is difficult.
Self-assessed general health	Very good (%)	301	361	29	26	

* See notes on Table A10.4, which are generally relevant to this table.

Table A10.9: Selected information on lifestyles, biochemical measures, physical measures and self-reported health status for general population men and women.

Variable	Measure	Number of subjects		Results	
		Male	Female	Male	Female
		Lifestyle factor			
Smoking	Current regular smoker (%)	3,543	4,224	27	1
Alcohol	Current drinker (%)	3,516	4,201	93	87
Physical activity	No vigorous activity (%) for 30 minutes or more in last 4 weeks	3,558	4,240	23	28
		Biochemical measure			
Cholesterol	Mean (mmol/l)	4,874	5,458	5.5	5.6
HDL	Mean (mmol/l)	4,874	5,458	1.3	1.6
Triglycerides	Mean (mmol/l)	181	237	1.7	1.4
		Physical measure			
Height	Mean (cm)	3,282	3,908	174.6	161.2
Weight	Mean (kg)	3,274	3,792	81.2	68.4
Waist/hip ratio	Mean	6,095	7,135	0.91	0.81
BMI	Mean	3,204	3,699	26.6	26.4
Blood pressure	av. Systolic	5,409	6,483	137	133
	av. Diastolic (mmHg)			76	72
		Self-reported health status			
Hypertension	Self-reported (%)	5,401	6,483	40.8	32.9
Diabetes	Self-reported (%)	7,193	8,715	3.3	2.5
Angina	Self-reported (%)	7,193	8,715	5.3	3.9
Mental health	GHQ-12 score of 4 or more (%)	3,389	4,052	15	19
Self-assessed general health	Very good (%)	3,558	4,239	35	31

* See notes on Table A10.4, which are generally relevant to this table.

References

1 Aldous J, Bardsley M, Daniel R, Gair R, Jacobson B, Lowdell C, Morgan D, Storkey M, Taylor G. *Refugee Health in London. Key issues for public health.* The Health of Londoners Project, 1999.

2 Jones D, Gill P. Refugees and primary care: tackling the inequalities. *BMJ* 1998; **317**: 1444–6.

3 Bhopal R. Setting priorities for health care. In: Rawaf S, Bahl V (eds). *Assessing health needs of people from minority ethnic groups.* London: Royal College of Physicians, 1998.

4 Senior PA, Bhopal R. Ethnicity as a variable in epidemiological research. *BMJ* 1994; **309**: 327–30.

5 Bhopal RS. Health Care for Asians: Conflict in need, demand and provision. In: *Equity. A prerequisite for health.* The proceedings of the 1987 Summer Scientific Conference of the Faculty of Community Medicine. Faculty of Community Medicine and the World Health Organisation 1988; 52–5.

6 Bhopal RS, Donaldson LJ. Health education for ethnic minorities: current provision and future directions. *Health Educ J* 1988; **47**: 137–40.

7 Bhopal R. Is research into ethnicity and health racist, unsound, or important science? *BMJ* 1997; **314**: 1751–5.

8 Donovan J. Black People's Health: A different approach. In: Rathwell T, Phillips D (eds). *Health Race & Ethnicity.* London: Croom Helm, 1986.

9 Gillam S. Ethnicity and the use of health services. *Postgrad Med J* 1990; **66**: 989–93.

10 Wright J, Williams R, Wilkinson JR. Health needs assessment: Development and importance of health needs assessment. *BMJ* 1998; **316**: 1310–3.

11 Elford J, Ben-Schlomo Y. Geography and migration. In: Kuh D & Ben-Schlomo Y (eds). *A Life Course Approach to Chronic Disease Epidemiology.* Oxford: OUP, 1997.

12 Rawaf S, Bahl V. *Assessing health needs of people from minority ethnic groups.* London: Royal College of Physicians, 1998.

13 Mackintosh J, Bhopal R, Unwin N, Ahmad N. *Step by Step Guide to Epidemiological Health Needs Assessment for Ethnic Minority Groups.* Newcastle: University of Newcastle, 1998.

14 Commission for Racial Equality. *Roots of the future. Ethnic diversity in the making of Britain.* London: Commission for Racial Equality, 1996.

15 Salt J. Immigration and ethnic group. In: Coleman D, Salt J (eds). *Ethnicity in the 1991 Census Volume One. Demographic characteristics of the ethnic minority populations.* London: HMSO, 1996.

16 Owen D. Size, structure and growth of the ethnic minority populations. In: Coleman D, Salt J (eds). *Ethnicity in the 1991 Census Volume One. Demographic characteristics of the ethnic minority populations.* London: HMSO, 1996.

17 Ballard R, Ballard C. The Sikhs – The Development of South Asian Settlement in Britain. In: Watson JL (ed). *Between Two Cultures. Migrants and minorities in Britain.* Oxford: Blackwell, 1977.

18 Robinson V. The Development of South Asian Settlement in Britain and the Myth of Return. In: Peach C, Robinson V, Smith S (eds). *Ethnic Segregation in Cities.* London: Croom Helm, 1981.

19 Visram R. *Ayahs, Lascars and Princes: Indians in Britain 1700–1947.* London: Pluto Press, 1986.

20 Henley A. The Asian Community in Britain. In: Coombe V & Little A (eds). *Race & Social Work: A Guide to Training.* London: Routledge, 1986.

21 Peach C. *Ethnicity in the 1991 Census Volume Two. The ethnic minority populations of Great Britain.* London: HMSO, 1996.

22 Peach C. Introduction. In: Peach C (ed). *Ethnicity in the 1991 Census Volume Two. The ethnic minority populations of Great Britain.* London: HMSO, 1996.

23 Martin I. The Development of UK Immigration Control. In: Coombe V, Little A (eds). *Race & Social Work: A Guide to Training.* London: Routledge, 1986.

24 Taylor C. Asians in Britain – origins and lifestyles. In: McAvoy B, Donaldson L (eds). *Health Care for Asians*. Oxford: OUP, 1990.

25 Coleman DA. United Kingdom statistics on immigration: development and limitations. *International Migration Review* 1987/8; **21**: 1138–69.

26 Champion T. Population Review: (3) Migration to, from and within the United Kingdom. *Pop Trends* 1996; **83**: 5–16.

27 LaVeist TA. Beyond dummy variables and sample selection: what health services researchers ought to know about race as a variable. *Hlth Services Res* 1994; **29**: 1–16.

28 Banton M. *The Idea of Race*. London: Tavistock, 1977.

29 Cole M. 'Black and ethnic minority' or 'Asian, black and other minority ethnic': A further note on nomenclature. *Sociology* 1993; **27**: 671–3.

30 Banton M. The battle of the name. *New Community* 1987; **14**: 170–5.

31 Bhopal RS, Phillimore P, Kholi HS. Inappropriate use of the term 'Asian': an obstacle to ethnicity and health research. *J Public Health Med* 1991; **13(4)**: 244–6.

32 Bhopal R. Ethnicity and race as epidemiological variables: centrality of purpose and context. In: Macbeth H, Shetty P (eds). *Health and Ethnicity*. London: Taylor and Francis, 2001.

33 Sheldon TA, Parker H. Race and ethnicity in health research. *J Public Health Med* 1992; **14(2)**: 104–10.

34 Mckenzie KJ, Crowcroft NS. Race, ethnicity, culture and science. *BMJ* 1994; **309**: 286–7.

35 Williams DR. The concept of race in health services research: 1966 to 1990. *Hlth Services Res* 1994; **29(3)**: 261–73.

36 Gill PS, Johnson M. Ethnic monitoring and ethnicity. *BMJ* 1995; **310**: 890.

37 Mckenzie KJ, Crowcroft NS. Describing race, ethnicity, and culture in medical research. *BMJ* 1996a; **312**: 1050.

38 Hahn RA. The state of federal health statistics on racial and ethnic groups. *JAMA* 1992; **267**: 268–71.

39 Montague A. *The Concept of Race*. Toronto: Collier-Macmillan, 1964.

40 Cooper R. Race, Disease and Health. In: Rathwell T, Phillips D (eds). *Health Race & Ethnicity*. London: Croom Helm, 1986.

41 Lewontin RC. *The Doctrine of DNA: Biology as Ideology*. London: Penguin, 1992.

42 Hill AVS. Molecular markers of ethnic groups. In: Cruickshank JK and Beevers DG (eds). *Ethnic Factors in Health and Disease*. Sevenoaks: Wright, 1989.

43 Leach E. *Social Anthropology*. Glasgow: Fontana, 1982.

44 Keesing RM. *Cultural Anthropology: A Contemporary Perspective*. New York: Holt, Rinehart and Winston, 1981.

45 Helman CG. *Culture, Health and Illness*. London: Butterworth and Co Ltd, 1990.

46 Fernando S. *Mental health, race and culture*. London: Macmillan, 1991.

47 Ahmad WIU. *'Race' and health in contemporary Britain*. Buckingham: OUP, 1993.

48 British Medical Journal. Guidelines on describing race, ethnicity, and culture in medical research. *BMJ* 1996; **312**: 1094.

49 Modood T. Culture and Identity. In: Modood T, Berthoud R, Lakey J, Nazroo J, Smith P, Virdee S, Beishon S (eds). *Ethnic Minorities in Britain. Diversity and Disadvantage*. London: Policy Studies Institute, 1997.

50 Cruickshank JK, Beevers DG, Osbourne VL, Haynes RA, Corlett JCR, Selby S. Heart attack, stroke, diabetes, and hypertension in West Indians, Asians and whites in Birmingham, England. *BMJ* 1980; **281**: 1108.

51 Marmot MG, Adelstein AM, Bulusu L, Shukla V. *Immigrant mortality in England and Wales 1970–78*. (OPCS Studies on Population and Medical Subjects: No. 47). London: HMSO, 1984.

52 Balarajan R, Bulusu L, Adelstein AM, Shukla V. Patterns of mortality among migrants to England and Wales from the Indian sub-continent. *BMJ* 1984; **289**: 1185–7.

53 McKeigue PM, Marmot MG, Adelstein AM, Hunt SP, Shipley MJ, Butler SM *et al.* Diet and risk factors for coronary heart disease in Asians in NW London. *The Lancet* 1985; **ii**: 1086–9.

54 Barker RM and Baker MR. Incidence of cancer in Bradford Asians. *J Epid & Comm Hlth* 1990; **44**: 125–9.

55 Nicoll A, Bassett K, Ulijaszek SJ. What's in a name? Accuracy of using surnames and forenames in ascribing Asian ethnic identity in English populations. *J Epidemiol Community Health* 1986, 40: 364–8.

56 Coleman D. Ethnic intermarriage in Great Britain. *Population Trends* 1985; **40**: 4–10.

57 Ecob R, Williams R. Sampling Asian minorities to assess health and welfare. *J Epid Comm Hlth* 1991; **45**: 93–101.

58 Bradford Health Authority. Nam Pehchan computer software (version 1.1). New Mill, Victoria Road, Saltaire, Shipley, West Yorkshire BD18 3LD.

59 Cummins C, Winter H, Cheng KK, Maric R, Silcocks P, Varghese C. An assessment of the Nam Pehchan computer program for the identification of names of south Asian origin. *J Public Health Med* 1999; **21**: 401–6.

60 Berthoud R, Modood T, Smith P. Introduction. In: Modood T, Berthoud R, Lakey J, Nazroo J, Smith P, Virdee S, Beishon S (eds). *Ethnic Minorities in Britain. Diversity and Disadvantage.* London: Policy Studies Institute, 1997.

61 Bulmer M. On the Feasibility of Identifying 'Race' and 'Ethnicity' in Censuses and Surveys. *New Community* 1980; **8**: 3–16.

62 Bulmer M. A Controversial Census Topic: Race and Ethnicity in the British Census. *J Official Statistics* 1986; **2(4)**: 471–80.

63 Teague A. Ethnic group: first results from the 1991 Census. *Population Trends* 1993; **72**: 12–7.

64 Berrington A. Marriage patterns and inter-ethnic unions. In: Coleman D, Salt J (eds). *Ethnicity in the 1991 Census: Volume 1: Demographic characteristics of the ethnic minority populations.* London: HMSO, 1996.

65 Raleigh VS, Balarajan R. Public Health and the 1991 census. *BMJ* 1994; **309**: 287–8.

66 OPCS/GRO(S). *1991 Census ethnic group and country of birth, Great Britain.* London: HMSO. Table (i) (Adjustment factors for estimated undercoverage) (Topic Report) (CEN91 EGCB), 1993.

67 Anwar M. Ethnic classifications, ethnic monitoring and the 1991 census. *New Community* 1990; **16(4)**: 607–15.

68 Ratcliffe P. Social geography and ethnicity: a theoretical, conceptual and substantive overview. In: Ratcliffe P (ed). *Ethnicity in the 1991 Census Volume Three. Social geography and ethnicity in Britain: geographical spread, spatial concentration and internal migration.* London: HMSO, 1996.

69 Moss C. Selection of topics and questions for the 2001 Census. *Population Trends* 1999; **97**: 28–36.

70 Jones A. *Making Monitoring Work. A guide to the successful implementation of ethnic record keeping and monitoring systems for service delivery.* University of Warwick: Centre for Research in Ethnic Relations, 1996.

71 Lay-Yee R, Gilthorpe MS, Wilson RC. *An Audit of Ethnic Monitoring.* University of Birmingham: Department of Public Health and Epidemiology, 1998.

72 Heath I. The role of ethnic monitoring in general practice. *Br J Gen Pract* 1991; **41**: 310–1.

73 Pringle M, Rothera I. Practicality of recording patient ethnicity in general practice: descriptive intervention study and attitude survey. *BMJ* 1996; **312**: 1080–2.

74 Sangowawa O, Bhopal R. Can we implement ethnic monitoring in primary health care and use the data? A feasibility study and staff attitudes in North East England. *Public Hlth Med* 2001; in press.

75 Owen D. 1991 Census Statistical Paper No 1. *Ethnic Minorities in Great Britain: Settlement Patterns.* Centre for Research in Ethnic Relations: University of Warwick, 1992.

76 Warnes T. The age structure and ageing of the ethnic groups. In: Coleman D, Salt J (eds). *Ethnicity in the 1991 Census Volume One. Demographic characteristics of the ethnic minority populations.* London: HMSO, 1996.

77 Butt J, Mirza K. *Social Care and Black Communities.* London: HMSO, 1996.

78 Lowy AGJ, Woods KL, Botha JL. The effects of demographic shift on coronary heart disease mortality in a large migrant population at high risk. *J Public Health Med* 1991; **13**: 276–80.

79 Department of Health/Social Services inspectorate. *They look after their own, don't they?: The report of community care services for black and ethnic minority older people.* London: Department of Health, 1998.

80 Rees P, Phillips D. Geographical spread: the national picture. In: Ratcliffe P (ed). *Ethnicity in the 1991 Census Volume Three. Social geography and ethnicity in Britain: geographical spread, spatial concentration and internal migration.* London: HMSO, 1996.

81 Eade J, Vamplew T, Peach C. The Bangladeshis: the encapsulated community. In: Peach C (ed). *Ethnicity in the 1991 Census Volume Two. The ethnic minority populations of Great Britain.* London: HMSO, 1996.

82 Davey Smith G, Shipley MJ, Rose G. Magnitude and causes of socioeconomic differentials in mortality: further evidence from the Whitehall Study. *J Epid Comm Health* 1990; **44**: 265–70.

83 Owen D. *1991 Census Statistical Paper No 3. Ethnic Minorities in Great Britain: Economic Characteristics.* Centre for Research in Ethnic Relations: University of Warwick, 1993.

84 Nazroo JY. *The Health of Britain's Ethnic Minorities.* London: Policy Studies Institute, 1997.

85 Bhopal RS. The interrelationship of folk, traditional and western medicine within an Asian community in Britain. *Soc Sc Med* 1986; **22**: 99–105.

86 Rudat K. *Black and Minority ethnic groups in England.* London: HEA, 1994.

87 Sprotson K, Pitson L, Whitfield G, Walker E. *Health and lifestyles of the Chinese population in England.* London: Health Education Authority. 1–337, 1999.

88 Health Education Authority. *Black and minority ethnic groups in England: the second health and lifestyles survey.* London: HEA, 2000.

89 Goldacre MJ. Cause-specific mortality: understanding uncertain tips of the disease iceberg. *J Epidemiol Comm Health* 1993; **47**: 491–6.

90 Bulmer M. The ethnic group question in the 1991 Census of population. In: Coleman D, Salt J (eds). *Ethnicity in the 1991 Census Volume One. Demographic characteristics of the ethnic minority populations.* London: HMSO, 1996.

91 OPCS/GRO(S). *1991 Census ethnic group and country of birth, Great Britain.* London: HMSO. Table A (Ethnic group full and summary classifications) (Topic Report)(CEN91 EGCE), 1993.

92 Winter H, Cheng KK, Cummins C, Maric R, Silcocks P, Varghese C. Cancer incidence in the south Asian population of England (1990–92). *Br J Cancer* 1999; **79**: 645–54.

93 Bhopal R, Unwin N, White M, Yallop J, Walker L, Alberti KGMM, Harland J, Patel S, Ahmad N, Turner C, Watson B, Kaur D, Kulkarni A, Laker M, Tavridou A. Heterogeneity of coronary heart disease risk factors in Indian, Pakistani, Bangladeshi, and European origin populations: cross sectional study. *BMJ* 1999; **319**: 215–20.

94 Harland JO, Unwin N, Bhopal RS, White M, Watson B, Laker M, Alberti KG. Low levels of cardiovascular risk factors and coronary heart disease in a UK Chinese population. *J Epidemiol Community Health* 1997; **51**: 636–42.

95 Cappuccio FP, Cook DG, Atkinson RW, Wicks PD. The Wandsworth Heart and Stroke Study. A population-based survey of cardiovascular risk factors in different ethnic groups. Methods and baseline findings. *Nutr Metab Cardiovasc Dis* 1998; **8**: 371–85.

96 Bhopal RS. The spectre of racism in health and health care: lessons from history and the USA. *BMJ* 1998; **316**: 1970–3.

97 Lakey J. Neighbourhoods and housing. In: Modood T, Berthoud R, Lakey J, Nazroo J, Smith P, Virdee S, Beishon S (eds). *Ethnic Minorities in Britain. Diversity and Disadvantage*. London: Policy Studies Institute, 1997.

98 Modood T, Acland A. *Race and Higher Education*. London: Policy Studies Institute, 1998.

99 Krieger N, Sidney S. Racial discrimination and blood pressure: the CARDIA study of young black and white adults. *Am J Public Health* 1996; **86**: 1370–8.

100 Marmot MG, Bosma H, Hemingway H, Brunner E, Stansfeld S. Contribution of job control and other risk factors to social variations in coronary heart disease incidence. *The Lancet* 1997; **350**: 235–9.

101 Bhatnagar D, Anand IS, Durrington PN, Patel DJ, Wandr GS, Mackness MI, *et al.*. Coronary risk factors in people from the Indian subcontinent living in west London and their siblings in India. *The Lancet* 1995; **345**: 405–9.

102 Gillum RF. The epidemiology of cardiovascular disease in black Americans. *N Engl J Med* 1996; **335**: 1597–9.

103 Wild S, McKeigue P. Cross sectional analysis of mortality by country of birth in England and Wales, 1970–92. *BMJ* 1997; **314**: 705–10.

104 Harding S, Maxwell R. Differences in mortality of migrants. In: Drever FWM (ed). *Health Inequalities*. London: Office for National Statistics, 1997, 108–21

105 Williams R, Bhopal R, Hunt K. Health of a Punjabi ethnic minority in Glasgow: a comparison with the general population. *J Epidemiol Community Health* 1993; **47**: 96–102.

106 Modell B, Anionwu A. In: *Ethnicity and health: reviews of literature and guidance for purchasers in the areas of cardiovascular, mental health and haemoglobinopathies*. NHS Centre for Reviews and Dissemination/Social Policy Research Unit. CRD: York University, 1996. Report No 5.

107 Health Education Authority. *Sickle cell and thalassaemia: achieving health gain. Guidance for commissioners and providers*. London: HEA, 1998.

108 Gill PS, Modell B. Thalassaemia in Britain: a tale of two communities. *BMJ* 1998; **317**: 761–2.

109 Modell B, Petrou M, Layton M, Varnavides L, Slater C, *et al.*. Audit of prenatal diagnosis for haemoglobin disorders in the United Kingdom: the first 20 years. *BMJ* 1997; **115**: 779–83.

110 Hickman M, Modell B, Greengross P, Chapman C, Layton M, Falconer S, Davies SC. Mapping the prevalence of sickle cell and beta thalassaemia in England: estimating and validating ethnic-specific rates. *Br J Haematol* 1999; **104(4)**: 860–7.

111 Bundey S, Alam H, Kaur A, Mir S, Lancahire RJ. Why do UK-born Pakistani babies have high perinatal and neonatal mortality rates? *Paediat Perinat Ep* 1991; **5**: 101–14.

112 Ahmad WIU. Reflections on the consanguinity and birth outcome debate. *J Public Health Med* 1994; **16**: 423–8.

113 Alwan A, Modell B, Bittles, Czeizel A, Hamamy H. *Community control of genetic and congenital disorders*. Alexandria: World Health Organization, 1997.

114 Raleigh VS, Balarajan R. Suicide levels and trends among immigrants in England and Wales. *Health Trends* 1992; **24**: 91–4.

115 Raleigh VS. Suicide patterns and trends in people of Indian subcontinent and Caribbean origin in England and Wales. *Ethn Health* 1996; **1(1)**: 55–63.

116 Dean G, Walsh D, Downing H, Shelley E. First admissions of native-born and immigrants to psychiatric hospitals in south-east England 1976. *Brit J Psychiatry* 1981; **139**: 506–12.

117 McGovern D, Cope RV. First admission rates for first and second generation Afro-Caribbeans. *Social Psychiatry* 1987; **22**: 139–49.

118 Littlewood R, Lipsedge M. Some social and phenomenological characteristics of psychotic immigrants. *Psychol Med* 1981; **11**: 289–302.

119 King M, Coker E, Leavey G, Hoare A, Johnson-Sabine E. Incidence of psychotic illness in London: comparison of ethnic groups *BMJ* 1994; **309**: 1115–9.

120 Cochrane R, Bal SS. Mental hospital admission rates of immigrants to England: a comparison of 1971 and 1981. *Soc Psychiatry Psychiatr Epidemiol* 1989; **24**: 2–11.

121 Nazroo JY. *Ethnicity and Mental Health. Fourth National Survey of Ethnic Minorities.* London: Policy Studies Institute, 1997.

122 Nazroo JY. Rethinking the relationship between ethnicity and mental health. *Soc Psychiatry Psychiatr Epidemiol* 1998; **33**: 145–8.

123 McCracken CG, Boneham MA, Copeland JR, Williams KE, Wilson K, Scott A, McKibbin P, Cleave N. Prevalence of dementia and depression among elderly people in black and ethnic minorities. *Br J Psychiatry* 1997; **171**: 269–73.

124 Shaw CM, Creed F, Tomenson B, Riste L, Cruickshank JK. Prevalence of anxiety and depressive illness and help seeking behaviour in African Caribbeans and white Europeans: two phase general population survey. *BMJ* 1999; **318**: 302–6.

125 Bradby H, Williams R. Behaviours and expectations in relation to sexual intercourse among 18–20 year old Asians and non-Asians. *Sex Transm Infect* 1999; **75**: 162–7.

126 Low N, Daker-White G, Barlow D, Pozniak AL. Gonorrhoea in inner London: results of a cross sectional study. *BMJ* 1997; **314**: 1719.

127 Lacey CJN, Merrick DW, Bensley DC, Fairley I. Analysis of the sociodemography of gonorrhoea in Leeds, 1989–93 *BMJ* 1997; **314**: 1715–8.

128 De Cock KM, Low N. HIV and AIDS, other sexually transmitted diseases, and tuberculosis in ethnic minorities in United Kingdom: Is surveillance serving its purpose? *BMJ* 1997; **314**: 1747.

129 Shahmanesh M, Gayed S, Ashcroft M, Smith R, Roopnarainsingh R, Dunn J, Ross J. Geomapping of chlamydia and gonorrhoea in Birmingham. *Sex Transm Infect* 2000: 76: 268–72.

130 Ades AE, Walker J, Botting B, Parker S, Cubitt D, Jones R. Effect of the worldwide epidemic on HIV prevalence in the Untied Kingdom: record linkage in anonymous neonatal seroprevalence surveys. *AIDS* 1999; **13**: 2437–43.

131 Raleigh VS, Almond C, Kiri V. Fertility and contraception among ethnic minority women in Great Britain. *Health Trends* 1997; **29**: 109–13.

132 Hennink M, Cooper P, Diamond I. Asian women's use of family planning services. *Br J Fam Plann* 1998; **24**: 43–52.

133 Burton R, Savage W. Knowledge and use of postcoital contraception: a survey among health professionals in Tower Hamlets. *Br J Gen Pract* 1990; **40**: 326–30.

134 Bush H, Williams R, Sharma S, Cruickshank K. *Opportunities for and barriers to good nutritional health.* London: HEA, 1997.

135 Lawson M, Thomas M, Hardiman A. Iron status of children aged two years living in England. *Arch Dis Child* 1998; **78**: 420–6.

136 Lawson M, Thomas M. Vitamin D concentrations in Asian children aged 2 years living in England: population survey *BMJ* 1999; **318**: 28.

137 Grindulis H, Scott PH, Belton NR, Wharton BA. Combined deficiency of iron and vitamin D in Asian toddlers. *Arch Dis Child* 1986; **61**: 843–8.

138 Smaje C. *Health, 'Race' and Ethnicity. Making sense of the evidence.* London: King's Fund Institute, 1995.

139 Kai J. Valuing ethnic diversity in primary care. *Br J Gen Pract* 1999; **49**: 171–3.

140 Benzeval M, Judge K. Access to health care in England: continuing inequalities in the distribution of general Practitioners. *J Public Health Med* 1996; **18**: 33–40.

141 Nzegwu F. *Black people and health care in contemporary Britain.* Reading: International Institute for Black Research, 1993.

142 Hopkins A, Bahl V. *Access to health care for people from black & ethnic minorities.* London: Royal College of Physicians, 1993.

143 Balarajan R, Yuen P, Soni Raleigh V. Ethnic differences in general practice consultations. *BMJ* 1989; **299**: 958–60.

144 Carr-Hill RA, Rice N, Roland M. Socioeconomic determinants of rates of consultation in general practice based on fourth national morbidity survey of general practices. *BMJ* 1996; **312**: 1008–13.

145 McCormick A, Fleming D, Charlton J. *Morbidity Statistics from General Practice.* Fourth national study 1991–1992. London: HMSO, 1995.

146 Johnson M. Inner city residents, Ethnic minorities and Primary Health Care in the West Midlands. In: Rathwell T, Phillips D (eds). *Health Race & Ethnicity.* London: Croom Helm, 1986.

147 Gillam SJ, Jarman B, White P, Law R. Ethnic differences in consultation rates in urban general practice. *BMJ* 1989; **299**: 953–7.

148 Pilgrim S, Fenton S, Hughes T, Hine C, Tibbs N. *The Bristol Black and Ethnic Minorities Health Survey Report.* Bristol: University of Bristol, 1993.

149 NHS Ethnic Health Unit. *Good Practice Quality Indicators in Primary Health Care.* Leeds: NHS Ethnic Health Unit, 1996.

150 Yee L. *Breaking barriers: towards culturally competent general practice. A consultation project for the Royal College of General Practitioners Inner City Task Force.* London: Royal College of General Practitioners, 1997.

151 Ahmad WIU, Kernohan EEM, Baker MR. Patients' choice of general practitioner: influence of patients' fluency in English and the ethnicity and sex of the doctor. *J Roy Coll Gen Pract* 1989; **39**: 153–5.

152 Rashid A, Jagger C. Attitudes to and perceived use of health care services among Asian and non-Asian patients in Leicester. *Br J Gen Pract* 1992; **42**: 197–201.

153 Wright C. Language and communication problems in an Asian community. *J Roy Coll Gen Pract* 1983; **33**: 101–4.

154 Balarajan R, Raleigh VS, Yuen P. Hospital care among ethnic minorities in Britain. *Health Trends.* 1991; **23**(3): 90–3.

155 Roland MO, Bartholomew J, Morrell DC, McDermot A, Paul E. Understanding Hospital Referral rates: a user's guide. *BMJ* 1990; **301**: 98–102.

156 Goddard M, Smith P. *Equity of Access to Health Care.* York: Centre for Health Economics, University of York, 1998.

157 Lear JT, Lawrence IG, Burden AC, Pohl JEF. A comparison of stress test referral rates and outcome between Asians and Europeans. *J Roy Soc Med* 1994; **87**: 661–2.

158 Chaturvedi N, Rai H, Ben-Schlomo Y. Lay diagnosis and health care seeking behaviour for chest pain in South Asians and Europeans. *The Lancet* 1997; **350**: 1578–83.

159 Gravelle H, Sutton M. *inequality in the geographical distribution of GPs in England and Wales 1974– 1995.* National Primary Care Research and Development Centre, July 1999.

160 Smith DJ. *Overseas Doctors in the National Health Service.* London: Policy Studies Institute, 1980.

161 Fassil J. *Primary health care for black and minority ethnic people: a consumer perspective.* Leeds: NHS Ethnic Health Unit, 1996.

162 Carr-Hill R, Passingham S, Wolf A, Kent N. *Lost Opportunities: The language skills of linguistic minorities in England and Wales.* The Basic Skills Agency, 1996.

163 Bowes AM, Domokos TM. South Asian women and health services: a study in Glasgow. *New Community* 1993; **19**: 611–26.

164 Kai J, Hedges C. Minority ethnic community participation in needs assessment and service development in primary care: perceptions of Pakistani and Bangladeshi people about psychological distress. *Health Expectations* 1999; **2**: 7–20.

165 Gillam S, Levenson R. Linkworkers in primary care. *BMJ* 1999; **319**: 1215.

166 Leman P. Interpreter use in an inner city accident and emergency department. *J Accid Emerg Med* 1997; **14**(2): 98–100.

167 Clark M, Owen D, Szczepura A, Johnson MRD. *Assessment of the costs to the NHS arising from the need for interpreter and translation services.* CRER and CHESS: University of Warwick, 1998.

168 Kai J, Spencer J, Wilkes M, Gill P. Learning to value ethnic diversity – what, why and how? *Medical Education* 1999; **33**: 616–23.

169 Ebden P, Carey O, Bhatt A, Harrison B. The bilingual consultation. *The Lancet* 1988; **i**: 347.

170 Poss JE, Rangel R. Working effectively with interpreters in the primary care setting. *Nurse Pract* 1995; **20**: 43–7.

171 Jones D, Gill P. Breaking down language barriers. *BMJ* 1998; **316**: 1476.

172 Johnson M, CrossM, Cardew S. Inner-city residents, ethnic minorities and primary health care. *Postgraduate Med J* 1983; **59**: 664–7.

173 Baker M, Bandaranayake R, Schweiger M. Difference sin rate of uptake of immunisation among ethnic groups. *BMJ* 1984; **288**:1075–8.

174 Bhopal R, Samim A. Immunization uptake of Glasgow Asian children: paradoxical benefit of communication barriers. *Community Med* 1988; **10**: 215–20.

175 Martineau A, White M, Bhopal R. No sex difference in immunisation rates of British South Asian Children: the effect of migration? *BMJ* 1997; **314**: 642–3.

176 Doyle Y. A survey of the cervical screening service in a London district, including reasons for non-attendance, ethnic responses and views on the quality of the service. *Soc Sci & Med* 1991; **32**: 953–7.

177 Firdous R, Bhopal R Reproductive health of Asian women: a comparative study with hospital and community perspectives. *J Pub Hlth* 1989: 103: 307–15.

178 McAvoy B, Raza R. Asian women: (i) contraceptive knowledge, attitudes and usage (ii) contraceptive services and cervical cytology. *Health Trends* 1988; **20**: 11–4.

179 Bradley S, Friedman E. Cervical cytology screening: a comparison of uptake among 'Asian' and 'non-Asian' women in Oldham. *J Public Health Med* 1993; **15**: 46–51.

180 Hoare T. Breast screeining and ethnic minorities. *Br J Cancer* 1996; **74**(supp): 38–54.

181 Naish J, Brown J, Denton B. Intercultural consultations: investigation of factors that deter non-English speaking women from attending their general practitioners for cervical screening. *BMJ* 1994; **308**: 1126–8.

182 Chiu LF. *Woman to Woman – promoting cervical screening among minority ethnic women in primary care.* Department of Health Promotion, Rotherham Health Authority, 1998.

183 Atri J, Falshaw M, Gregg R, Robson J, Omar RZ, Dixon S. Improving uptake of breast screening in multiethnic populations: a randomised controlled trial using practice reception staff to contact non-attenders. *BMJ* 1997; **315**: 1356–9.

184 Liao X, McIlwaine G. The health status and health needs of Chinese population in Glasgow. *Scot Med J* 1995; **40**: 77–80.

185 Majeed FA, Cook DG, Given-Wilson R, Vecchi P, Polienicki J. Do general practitioners influence the uptake of breast cancer screening? *J Med Screening* 1995; **2**: 119–24.

186 Botha JL, Manku-Scott TK, Moledina F, Williams A. Indirect discrimination and breast screening. *Ethnicity and Disease* 1993; **3**: 189–95.

187 Sutton, Bickler G, Sancho-Aldridge J, Saidi G. Prospective study of predictors of attendance for breast cancer screening in inner London. *J Epid & Comm Hlth* 1994; **48**: 65–73.

188 Hek G. Contact with Asian elders. *J of District Nursing* 1991; 13–15.

189 Norman A. *Triple Jeopardy: Growing Old in a Second Homeland.* London: Centre for Policy on Ageing, 1985.

190 Ebrahim S, Patel N, Coats M, Grieg C, Gilley J, Bangham C, Stacey S. Prevalence and severity of morbidity among Gugarati Asian elders: a controlled comparison. *Fam Pract* 1991; **8**: 57–62.

191 Holt RD. Caries in the pre-school child: British Trends. *J of Dentistry* 1990; **18**: 296–9.

192 Bedi R. Ethnic indicators of dental health for young Asian schoolchildren resident in areas of multiple deprivation. *Brit Dent J* 1989; **166**: 331–4.

193 Ahmad WIU. The maligned healer: the 'hakim' and western medicine. *New Community* 1992; **18**: 521–36.

194 Emslie M, Campbell M, Walker K. Complementary therapies in a local health care setting. *Complementary Therapy and Medicine* 1996; **4**: 39–42.

195 Bowling B. *Elderley people from ethnic minorities: a report on four projects.* London: Age Concern Institute of Gerontology, 1990.

196 Fenton S. *Race, Health and Welfare.* University of Bristol (Department of Sociology): Bristol, 1985.

197 Atkin K, Rollings J. *Community Care in a Multi-Racial Britain: A Critical Review of the Literature.* HMSO: London, 1993.

198 Roderick PJ, Ferris G, Feest TG. The provision of renal replacement therapy for adults in England and Wales: recent trends and future directions. *QJM* 1998; **91**: 581–7.

199 United Kingdom Transplant Support Service Authority. *Statistics prepared by the United Kingdom Transplant Support Service Authority from the National Transplant Database maintained on behalf of the UK Transplant Community, February 2000.*

200 Randhawa G. The impending kidney transplant crisis for the Asian population in the UK. *Public Health* 1998; **112**: 265–8.

201 Effective Health Care Bulletin. *Cardiac Rehabilitation.* University of York, 1998 (No 4).

202 Smaje C, Field D. Absent minorities? Ethnicity and the use of palliative care services. In: Hockey J, Small N (eds). *Death, Gender and Ethnicity.* London: Routledge.

203 Gaffin J, Hill D, Penso D. Opening doors: improving access to hospice and specialist palliative care services by members of the black and minority ethnic communities. Commentary on palliative care. *Br J Cancer Suppl* 1996; **29**: S51–3.

204 Higgs D. Alpha-thalassaemia. *Ballieres Clin Haematol* 1993; **6**: 117–50.

205 Thein SL. Beta-thalassaemia. *Ballieres Clin Haematol* 1993; **6**: 151–75.

206 Cazzola M, Bornga-Pignatti C, Locatelli F, Ponchio L, Beguin Y, De Stefano P. A moderate transfusion regimen may reduce iron overloading in β-thalassaemia major without producing excessive expansion of erythropoesis. *Transfusion* 1997; **37**: 135–40.

207 Weatherell D. Bone marrow transplantation for thalassaemia and other inherited disorders of haemoglobin. *Blood* 1992; **80**: 1379–81.

208 Serjeant GR. The clinical features of sickle cell disease. *Ballieres Clin Haematol* 1993; **6**: 93–115.

209 Roberts-Harwood M, Davies SC. Current management in sickle cell disease. *Haematology* 1998; **3**: 419–27.

210 Platt OS, Brambilla DJ, Rosse WF, Milner PF, Castro O, Steinberg MH, Klug PP. Mortality in Sickle Cell Disease. Life Expectancy and Risk Factors for Early Death. *N Engl J Med* 1994; **330**: 1639–44.

211 Modell B, Harris R, Lane B, Khan M, Darlison M, Petrou M, Old J, Layton M, Varnavides L. Informed choice in genetic screening for thalassaemia during pregnancy: audit from a national confidential inquiry. *BMJ.* 2000; **320**: 337–41.

212 Kai J (ed). *Valuing Diversity – a resource for effective health care of ethnically diverse communities.* London: Royal College of General Practitioners, 1999.

213 Kushnick L. Racism, the National Health Service, and the health of black people. *Int J Hlth Services* 1988; **18**: 457–70.

214 Larbie J. *Black women and the maternity services.* London: Health Education Council/National Extension College, 1985.

215 Wilson A. *Finding a voice: Asian women in Britain.* London: Virago, 1978.

216 MacPherson W. *Report for the Stephen Lawrence Inquiry.* London: The Stationery Office, 1999.

217 Ahmad W, Baker M, Kernohan E. General practitioners' perceptions of Asian and non-Asian patients. *Fam Practice* 1991; **8**: 52–6.

218 Bowler I. 'They're not the same as us': midwives' stereotypes of South Asian descent maternity patients. *Sociology of Hlth & Illness* 1993; **15**: 157–78.

219 Fenton S. Racism is harmful to your health. In: Cox J, Bostock S (eds). *Racial discrimination in the health service.* Newcastle under Lyme: Penrhos, 1989.

220 Littlewood R, Lipsedge M. *Aliens and Alienists.* London: Unwin Hyman, 1989.

221 Knowles C. Afro-Caribbeans and schizophrenia: how does psychiatry deal with issues of race, culture and ethnicity? *J Social Policy* 1991; **20**: 173–90.

222 McKenzie K. Something borrowed from the blues? *BMJ* 1999; **318**: 616–7.

223 NHS Executive. *Resource Allocation: Weighted Capitation Formulas.* NHSE July 1999; catalogue no.15995.

224 Johnson MRD, Clark M, Owen D, Szczepura A. *The Unavoidable Costs of Ethnicity: A Review for the NHSE. CRER and CHESS.* University of Warwick, 1998.

225 Zeuner D, Ades AE, Karnon J, Brown J, Dezateux C, Anionwu EN. *Antenatal and neonatal haemoglobinopathy screening in the UK: review and economic analysis.* Leeds: The Health Technology Assessment Panel, NHS Executive, 1999.

226 Aspinall PJ. Ethnic groups and our healthier nation: whither the information base? *J Public Health Med* 199; **21**: 125–32.

227 Alexander Z. *Study of Black, Asian and Ethnic Minority Issues.* London: Department of Health, 2000.

228 Johnson M. *Involvement of Black and Ethnic Minority Consumers in Health Research.* De Montfort University: Mary Seacole Centre, 1998.

229 Baxter C. The case for bilingual workers within maternity services. *BJ Midwifery* 1997; **5**: 568–72.

230 Clarke M, Clayton D. Quality of obstetric care provided for Asian immigrants in Leicestershire. *BMJ* 1983; **286**: 621–3.

231 Hawthorne K. Asian diabetics attending a British hospital clinic: a pilot study to evaluate their care. *Br J Gen Pract* 1990; **40**: 243–47.

232 Madhok R, Bhopal R, Ramaiah S. Quality of hospital service: a study comparing 'Asian' and 'non'Asian' patients in Middlesborough. *J Public Health Med* 1992; **14**: 217–79.

233 Madhok R, Hameed A, Bhopal R. Satisfaction with health services among Pakistani population in Middlesborough, England. *J Public Health Med* 1998; **20**: 295–301.

234 Ebrahim S. Detection, adherence and control of hypertension for the prevention of stroke: a systematic review. *Health Technol Assessment* 1998; **2(11)**.

235 Materson BJ, Reda DJ, Cushman WC, Massie BM, Freis ED, Kochar MS, Hamburger RJ, Fye C, Lakshman R, Gottdiener J, Ramirez EA, Henderson WG, for the Department of Veterans Affairs Cooperative Study Group on Antihypertensive Agents. Single-Drug Therapy for Hypertension in Men – A Comparison of Six Antihypertensive Agents with Placebo. *N Engl J Med* 1993; **328**: 914–21.

236 Gaston M, Verter JI, Joel I, Woods G, Pegolow C, Kelleher J *et al.*. Prophylaxis with oral penicillin in children with sickle cell anaemia: a randomized trail. *N Engl J Med* 1986; **314**: 1594–9.

237 Lee A, Thomas P, Cupidore L, Serjeant B, Serjeant G. Improved survival in homozygous sickle cell disease: lessons from a cohort study. *BMJ* 1995; **311**: 1600–2.

238 Charache S, Terrin ML, Moore RD, Dover GJ, Barton FB, Eckert SV, McMahon RP, Bonds DR. Effect of Hydroxyurea on the Frequency of Painful Crises in Sickle Cell Anemia. *N Engl J Med* 1995; **332**: 1317–22.

239 Walters MC, Patience M, Leisenring W, Eckman JR, Scott JP, Mentzer WC, Davies SC, Ohene-Frempong K, Bernaudin F, Matthews DC, Storb R, Sullivan KM. Bone marrow transplantation for sickle cell disease. *N Engl J Med* 1996; **335(6)**: 369–76.

240 Cao A, Galanello R, Rosatelli MC, Argiolu F, DeVirgilis S. Clinical experience of management of thalassaemia: the Sardinian experience. *Semin Hematol* 1996; **33**: 66–75.

241 Brittenham GM, Griffith PM, Nienhuis AW, McLaren CE, Young NS, Tucker EE, Allen CJ, Farrell DE, Harris JW. Efficacy of desferoxamine in preventing complications of iron overload in patients with thalassaemia major. *N Engl J Med* 1994; **331**: 567–73.

242 Giardian PJ, Grady RW. Chelation therapy in beta-thalassaemia: the benefits and limitations of desferoxamine. *Semin Hematol* 1995; **32**: 304–12.

243 Ratip S, Modell B. Psychological and sociological aspects of the thalassaemias. *Semin Hematol* 1996; **33**: 53–65.

244 Barman Balfour JA, Foster RH. Deferipone: a review of its clinical potential in iron overload in beta-thalassaemia major and other transfusion-dependent diseases. *Drugs* 1999; **58**: 553–78.

245 Giardini C, Galimberti M, Lucarelli G. Bone marrow transplantation in thalassaemia. *Ann Rev Med* 1995; **46**: 319–30.

246 Cao A, Galanello R, Rosatelli MC. Prenatal diagnosis and screening of the haemoglobinopathies. *Ballieres Clin Haematol* 1998; **11**: 215–38.

247 Serrano AC. Language barriers in pediatric care. *Clin Pediatrics* 1989; 193–4.

248 Street RL. Physicians' communication and patients' evaluations of paediatric consultations. *Med Care* 1991; **29**: 1146.

249 Audit Commission. *What seems to be the matter: Communication between hospitals and patients.* Audit Commission report. London: HMSO, 1994.

250 Jain C, Naryan N, Naryan K, Pike L, Clarkson M, Cox I, Chatterjee J. Attitudes of Asian patients in Birmingham to general practitioner services. *J Roy Coll of Gen Pract* 1985; **35**: 416–18.

251 Kaplan SH, Greenfield S, Ware JE. Assessing the effects of physician-patient interactions on the outcomes of chronic disease. *Med Care* 1989; **27**(3): S110.

252 Balarajan R, Soni Raleigh V. *The Health of the Nation: Ethnicity and Health.* London: Department of Health, 1993.

253 Johnson MRD. *Ethnic Minorities, Health and Communication: A research review for the NHS Executive and West Midlands Regional Health Authority.* Research paper in ethnic relations. No 24. ESRC, 1996.

254 Stewart P, Bartram M. *Now we're talking.* London: Consumer Congress Trust, 1996.

255 Ntshona MS. Are professional interpreters needed in the South African health care services. *S Afr Med J* 1997; **87**(9): 1143.

256 Hornberger JC, Gibson CD, Wood W et al.. Eliminating language barriers for non-English speaking patients. *Med Care* 1996; **34**(8): 845–56.

257 Bahl V. *Asian Mother and Baby Campaign: A report by the Director.* London: Department of Health and Social Security, 1987.

258 Levenson R, Gillam S. *Linkworkers in primary care.* London: King's Fund, 1998.

259 Hoare T, Thomas C, Biggs A, Booth M, Bradley S, Friedman E. Can the uptake of breast screening by Asian women be increased? A randomized controlled trial of a linkworker intervention. *J Public Health Med* 1994; **16**: 179–85.

260 Mason D. A rose by any other name . . .?: categorisation, identity and social science. *New Community* 1990; **17**: 123–33.

261 Khanchandani R, Gillam S. The ethnic minority linkworker: a key member of the primary health care team? *Brit J Gen Pract* 1999; **49**: 993–4.

262 Cornwell J, Gordon P. *An Experiment in Advocacy: The Hackney Multi-Ethnic Women Health Project.* King's Fund Centre: London, 1984.

263 Parsons L, Day S. Improving obstetric outcomes in ethnic minorities: an evaluation of health advocacy in Hackney. *J Public Health Med* 1992; **14**: 183–91.

264 White M, Carlin L, Adamson A, Rankin J. *Effectiveness of interventions to promote healthy eating in people from ethnic minority groups: a review.* London: Health Education Authority, 1998.

265 McAvoy B, Raza R. Can health education increase the uptake of cervical smear testing among Asian women? *BMJ* 1991; **302**: 833–6.

266 Giacomelli J. A review of health interpreter services in a rural community: a total quality management approach. *Aust J Rural Health* 1997; **5(3)**: 158–64.

267 Phelan M. Parkman S. Work with an interpreter. *BMJ* 1995; **311**: 555–7.

268 Acheson D. *Independent Inquiry into Inequalities in Health.* London: The Stationery Office, 1998.

269 Arblaster L, Entwistle V, Lambert M, Forster M, Sheldon T, Watt I. *Review of the research on the effectiveness of health service interventions to reduce variations in health.* York: CRD: York University, 1996. Report No 3.

270 Secretary of State for Health. *The New NHS: Modern, Dependable.* London: HMSO, 1997.

271 Whitehead M. *The concepts and principles of equity in health.* Copenhagen: WHO: Regional Office for Europe, 1990.

272 Bhopal RS, Parsons L. A draft policy for adoption by health authorities, purchasers and providers of health care. In: A Hopkins, V Bahl (eds). *Access to Health Care for People from Black and Ethnic Minorities.* London: Royal College of Physicians, 1993; 199–200.

273 British Medical Association. *Multicultural health care: current practice and future policy in medical education.* London: BMA, 1995.

274 Lloyd K. Ethnicity, Primary Care and Non-psychotic disorders. *Int Rev of Psychiatry* 1992; **4**: 257–66.

275 Cochrane R, Sashidharan SP. Mental health and ethnic minorities: a review of the literature and implications for services. In: *Ethnicity and Health.* York: Centre for Reviews and Dissemination, University of York, 1996: 105–26.

276 Williams R, Eley S, Hunt K, Bhatt S. Has pyschological distress among UK South Asians been under-estimated? A comparison of three measures in the West of Scotland population. *Ethnicity and Health* 1997; **2**: 21–9.

277 Fernando S. *Race and Culture in Psychiatry.* London: Tavistock, 1988.

278 Sashidharan SP, Francis E. Epidemiology, ethnicity and schizophrenia. In: Ahmad WIU (ed). *'Race' and health in contemporary Britain.* Buckingham: OUP, 1993.

279 Commander M, Sashidharan S, Odell S, Surtees P. Access to mental health care in an inner city health district. Pathways into and within specialist psychiatric services. *Br J Psychiatry* 1997; **170**: 312–6.

280 Taylor DH Jr, Esmail A. retrospective analysis of census data on general practitioners who qualified in South Asia: who will replace them as they retire? *BMJ* 1999; **318**: 306–10.

281 Kai J, Foreman B, Solanki B, Khan S. Facilitating work, social support and health in an ethnically diverse community: The Sparkbrook community parents experience. In: Kai J, Drinkwater C (eds). *Primary Care in Urban Disadvantaged Communities.* Oxford: Radcliffe Medical Press; 2004.

282 Allen L, Kai J. *Newcastle Minority Ethnic Health Development Project: Report of an Evaluation 1998–2000.* Newcastle City NHS Health Trust; in press.

283 Jordan J, Dowswell T, Harrison S, Lilford R, Mort M. Whose priorities? Listening to users and the public. *BMJ* 1998; **316**: 1668–70.

284 NHS Executive. *In the Public Interest, Developing a Strategy for Public Participation in the NHS.* London: HMSO, 1998.

285 Dockery G. Rhetoric or reality? Participatory research in health: setting the context. In: Koning de K, Martun M (eds). *Participatory Research in Health.* London: Zed Books, 1996.

286 Silvera M, Kapasi R. *Implementation strategy for the collection and use of ethnicity information in general practice.* London: Primary Care Ethnicity Project. Brent and Harrow Health Authority, 1998.

287 Pearson M. The Politics of Ethnic Minority Health Studies. In: Rathwell T, Phillips D (eds). *Health Race & Ethnicity.* London: Croom Helm, 1986.

288 Bhopal R, White M. Health promotion for ethnic minorities: past present and future. In: Ahmad WIU (ed). *'Race' and Health in Contemporary Britain*. Buckingham: Open University Press, 1993.

289 Lee E. General Practice screening clinic for Bangladeshi families. *Br J Gen Pract* 1994; **44**: 268–70.

290 Rankin J, Bhopal R. Understanding of heart disease and diabetes in a South Asian community: cross-sectional study testing the 'snowball' sample method. *Public Health* 2001; **115**: 253–60.

291 Greenhalgh T, Helman C, Chowdhury AM. Health beliefs and folk models of diabetes in British Bangladeshis: a qualitative study. *BMJ* 1998; **316**: 978–83.

292 Prashar U, Anionwu EN, Brozovic M. *Sickle cell anaemia: who cares?* London: Runnymede Trust, 1985.

293 Anionwu EN. Ethnic origin of sickle and thalassaemia counsellors: does it matter: In: Kelleher D, Hillier S (eds). *Researching cultural differences*. London: Routledge, 1996.

294 Bhopal RS. *The public health agenda and ethnic minority ethnic health. Proceedings of the US/UK symposium on minority ethnic health 2000*. London: Department of Health, 2001.

295 Gill PS, Jones D. Cross-cultural adaptation of outcome measures. *Eur J Gen Pract* 2000; **6**: 120–1.

296 Brislin RW. Comparative research methodology: crosscultural studies. *Int J Psychol* 1976; **11**: 215–29.

297 Maxwell R. Quality assessment in health. *BMJ* 1984; **288**: 1470–1.

298 *Working Together Securing a Quality Workforce for the NHS* published under cover of HSC 1998/162 and 1999/169 (NHS Human Resources Framework Document).

Acknowledgements

This chapter would not have been possible without the help of many individuals, too numerous to list in full, and include the following: Naseer Ahmad; Sheila Bailey; Michael Chan; John Charlton; Sue Clifford; Sharon Denley; Carol Fraser; Seeromanie Harding; John Haskey; Lorna Hutchison, Mark Kroese; Janet Logan; Mark Johnson; David Owen; Hamid Rehman; Jeremy Shuman; and Annaliese Werkhoven. Many thanks also to Velda Osborne and her colleagues for allowing use of the ONS Longitudinal Study and members of the LS User Support Programme at the Centre for Longitudinal Studies (CLS), Institute of Education. Note that the views expressed in this publication are those of the authors only.

Tables 2 and 3, and Figures 1 and 2 are reproduced with permission of ONS Publications.

Box 3, Table 28 and Appendix 8 are reproduced with permission of Health Promotion England.

Contributions

- PG, JK and RB were involved in the complete process from conception, detailed planning, writing, revising and editing of all sections. PG edited the whole chapter and led on sections 1, 2, 3 and 8; RB took the lead for section 4 with help from SW, who helped with analysis, interpretation and editing of data; and JK led on sections 5, 6 and 7.

5 Hypertension

Richard J McManus and Jonathan Mant

1 Summary

Introduction

Hypertension – that is, raised blood pressure – affects up to a third of adults in England. It is asymptomatic in the majority of cases but predisposes to significant morbidity and mortality, particularly due to stroke and coronary heart disease (CHD). It is also a risk factor in some renal disease and may accelerate cognitive decline. Both the treatment of hypertension and its sequelae are associated with significant costs to the NHS: stroke and CHD alone consume almost 9% of the total budget.

Treatment can significantly reduce risk of stroke and CHD. However, achieving these gains depends on identification of cases and community surveys suggest that only a third of those with raised blood pressure receive treatment and only a third of these are controlled below commonly accepted targets.

The definition of thresholds for hypertension is problematic due to evidence of a log-linear relationship between blood pressure and risk at all levels of blood pressure. This had led to variations in definition between various national and international guidelines. Furthermore, evidence is emerging in stroke at least that lowering blood pressure is worthwhile whatever the baseline level.

Sub-categories

Due to the problems with definition of blood pressure we have taken a pragmatic approach to the sub-categories used and have broadly kept to those definitions recommended by the Joint British Societies Statement. The sub-categories used are as follows:

- **Group 1:** *Raised blood pressure – level sufficient to merit treatment regardless of cardiovascular risk.* Definition: For people without diabetes, blood pressure ≥160/100 mmHg (either diastolic alone, systolic alone or both) *or* evidence of target organ damage with blood pressure below 160/100 mmHg. The level of blood pressure along with the overall cardiovascular risk dictates the degree of urgency.
- **Group 2:** *Raised blood pressure – treat on basis of underlying cardiovascular risk.* Definition: sustained systolic blood pressure in the range 140–159 *or* sustained diastolic blood pressure 90–99 mmHg with no evidence of target organ damage. In this group, overall cardiovascular risk dictates the need for treatment.
- **Group 3:** *Raised blood pressure and diabetes.* Definition: blood pressure ≥140/90 mmHg with co-existing diabetes mellitus. In this group the presence of diabetes lowers the treatment threshold whatever other cardiovascular risk factors are present.

- **Group 4:** *Malignant or accelerated hypertension.* Definition: hypertensive emergency with bilateral retinal haemorrhages and exudates.
- **Group 5:** *Secondary hypertension.* Definition: hypertension with clear underlying cause, often reno-vascular or endocrine.
- **Group 6:** *White coat hypertension.* Definition: blood pressure raised in the presence of medical personnel but not otherwise and with no evidence of target organ damage.

Literature on the epidemiology of hypertension tends to combine groups 1, 2 and 3 under the umbrella term of essential hypertension, i.e. hypertension with no discernible cause. This pragmatic grouping will also be used where applicable in this chapter.

Prevalence and incidence

The prevalence and incidence is summarised in **Table 1**.

Table 1: Prevalence and incidence of hypertension.

Category	Prevalence	Incidence	Comment
Essential hypertension (sub-categories 1–3)	36.5% >16 years raised or on treatment 9.6% >16 years on treatment (both figures from community survey)	<1% per year in under 30s 4–8% in those aged 60–79	Prevalence and incidence both rise with age. Community surveys tend to overestimate prevalence of hypertension.*
Diabetes and hypertension (sub-category 3)	Prevalence in newly presenting diabetics 40%	No data	Current prevalence probably higher as study quoted used conservative cut-off figure (>160/90).
Malignant or accelerated hypertension (sub-category 4)	1–2/100 000 population	No data	
Secondary hypertension (sub-category 5)	10%	No data	Primary hyperaldosteronism comprises half of all cases.
White coat hypertension (sub-category 6)	7–35%	No data	Wide variation between studies depending on definition and method of measurement.

*Blood pressure measured on one occasion will overestimate presence of hypertension compared to the recommended three occasions.

Services available and their costs

Diagnosis

The diagnosis of hypertension depends on clinical evaluation usually in primary care, including blood pressure measurement with further investigations indicated if pressures remain consistently raised. More specialised investigations may be required if there is suspicion of secondary or white coat hypertension.

Screening

No national community screening programme exists for hypertension and blood pressure is commonly measured opportunistically in primary care. The prevalence of untreated hypertension suggests that current methods may be inadequate.

Treatment

Treatment for hypertension may be divided into three categories: non-pharmacological aimed at lowering blood pressure (diet, exercise and stop smoking), pharmacological aimed at lowering blood pressure (i.e. antihypertensive medication) and pharmacological aimed at reducing other cardiovascular risk factors (i.e. cholesterol lowering and anti-platelet agents).

Setting

The majority of care for hypertension (>90%) occurs in primary care on an outpatient basis. Smaller numbers are seen in hospital outpatients (mostly for assessment of possible secondary causes) with very few inpatient episodes per year.

Costs

The main direct costs of hypertension are due to medication which varies widely in costs depending on class of drug from £20/patient/year to over £300/patient/year. A typical PCT would expect to spend well over £1 million on antihypertensive medication per year.

Effectiveness of services and interventions

Diagnostic tests

Measurement of blood pressure using a sphygmomanometer is the standard method of diagnosis. More than one measurement on at least three occasions is required due to the natural variability of blood pressure. Measurement may be performed using a mercury, aneroid or electronic sphygmomanometer. All of these methods may be inaccurate, principally due to operator or device errors.

Screening for hypertension

Little evidence for systematic screening for hypertension over and above opportunistic case finding exists. The prevalence of untreated hypertension in the community suggests that current practice is not effective.

Opportunistic screening has the potential to reach the vast majority of patients registered with a GP within a five year time period.

Non-pharmacological treatment

Evidence from small RCTs has shown that small but significant reductions of blood pressure (1–3 mmHg) are possible following non-pharmacological treatment including exercise, weight loss, reduced salt intake, and reduced alcohol intake. Stopping smoking does not reduce blood pressure but reduces overall cardiovascular risk.

Pharmacological treatment

Unequivocal evidence from numerous large RCTs and meta-analyses now exists that reduction of blood pressure using antihypertensive medication is effective at reducing stroke and CHD. This strong evidence applies to both men and women when analysed separately. The latest meta-analyses including data from the ALLHAT trial as well as other recent RCTs suggests that the major benefits from lowering blood pressure are proportional to the reduction in blood pressure achieved and are independent of the agent used, at least for diuretics, beta-blockers, ACE inhibitors and calcium antagonists.

Absolute benefit from lowering blood pressure in terms of absolute risk reductions is dependent on baseline risk and so most advantage comes from treating the elderly and those with co-morbidities such as diabetes. Evidence for current treatment targets is flawed but suggests that a target of <140/85 mmHg as suggested by the Joint British Societies is reasonable for those without diabetes.

Population treatment

Population approaches to lowering blood pressure are attractive in that relatively small reductions in pressure across a whole population can theoretically result in large gains for that population. Interventions such as supermarkets lowering salt content in food have the potential to realise such gains.

Cost-effectiveness

Most of the evidence for the cost-effectiveness of antihypertensive treatment comes from modelling exercises and suggests that treatment is most cost-effective for those who are older or at higher risk for some other reason.

Models of care and recommendations

Guidelines for hypertension treatment

The British Hypertension Society (BHS) recommends that treatment is required for all patients with a sustained blood pressure greater than 160/100 mmHg and not required for those with a blood pressure below 140/90 mmHg. Between these limits, treatment will depend on evidence of end organ damage, coronary heart disease risk ≥15% over 10 years or the presence of diabetes. For those receiving treatment then target blood pressures should be 140/85 mmHg for those without diabetes and 140/80 mmHg for those with diabetes. Choice of antihypertensive agent may be influenced by co-morbidities but in general the evidence suggests that cheaper alternatives are as effective as more expensive classes. In combining drugs, the BHS 'ABCD' rule (ACE inhibitor or beta-blocker first line for under-55s combined with a calcium antagonist or diuretic (which are first line for over-55s)) is a reasonable one.

A quantified model for hypertension care

An opportunistic but systematically carried out method for screening in primary care is suggested. Treatment costs of those diagnosed with this method will vary dependent on the choice of medication. Assuming a five year cycle of screening, a PCT of 100 000 population will require 14 300 screening blood pressure checks per year and will treat an additional 2100 individuals per year over and above those currently receiving treatment. Total yearly additional costs will vary between £440 000 and £1.35 million depending on the choice of antihypertensives used. Overall, a five year screening programme will cost approximately £2.4 million – £8.9 million per 100 000 population over and above current costs, depending on the drugs used (i.e. more than doubled from current levels).

Approaches to audit and outcome measures

Most audit for hypertension on a national basis will now be geared towards the new General Medical Services contract for primary care which came into force in April 2004. This includes the following criteria for people with hypertension:

- **BP 1:** The practice can produce a register of patients with established hypertension (Yes/No).
- **BP 2:** The percentage of patients with hypertension, whose notes record smoking status at least once (standard max 90%).
- **BP 3:** The percentage of patients with hypertension who smoke, whose notes contain a record that smoking cessation advice has been offered at least once (standard max 90%).
- **BP 4:** The percentage of patients with hypertension in which there is a record of the blood pressure in the past 9 months (standard max 90%).
- **BP 5:** The percentage of patients with hypertension in whom the last blood pressure (measured in last 9 months) is 150/90 or less (standard max 70%).

Research priorities

Key areas for research in hypertension include:

- robustly powered studies with appropriate clinically relevant end points (i.e. mortality and major morbidity) to determine the efficacy of non-pharmacological measures in the treatment of hypertension
- further studies examining the effect of increased user involvement in the treatment and control of hypertension
- community-based studies evaluating the benefit of generic antihypertensive medication post stroke
- long-term community-based studies with clinically relevant end points evaluating the implementation of treatment for hypertension on the basis of risk rather than blood pressure thresholds.

2 Introduction and statement of the problem

Hypertension as a major health issue

Over a third of adults in England can be categorised as having hypertension.[1] Hypertension is asymptomatic, but is associated with significant morbidity and premature mortality, primarily from stroke and coronary heart disease.[2] It is also an important cause of renal disease,[3] and may have a role in accelerating cognitive decline.[4] Both the treatment of hypertension and its sequelae are associated with significant costs to the NHS – coronary heart disease has been estimated to account for 2.5% and stroke 6% of total NHS expenditure.[5]

Treatment of hypertension is associated with important reductions in risk of stroke and coronary heart disease. A 10–12 mmHg reduction in systolic and a 5–6 mmHg reduction in diastolic blood pressure has been shown to lead to a highly significant reduction in relative risk of stroke (38%, 95% CI 31–45%) and coronary heart disease (16%, 95% CI 8–23%) – see section 6.[6] Therefore in theory, substantial reductions in the burden of coronary heart disease and stroke could be achieved by optimal treatment of blood pressure. However, to translate this trial-demonstrated efficacy into community-based effectiveness, people with hypertension need to be identified, treated, and their blood pressure controlled. The 'Rule of Halves' as stated in 1972 was that: '50% of hypertensives are unknown; 50% of the known hypertensives are untreated and that 50% of those treated are not controlled'.[7] Ebrahim estimated that if the rule of halves still applied, the effect on stroke risk reduction of treating hypertension in the community will have been reduced to 5%.[8] Similarly, the risk reduction for coronary heart disease will have been lessened from 16% to 2%. While there is some evidence that a greater proportion of hypertensive people have been identified and treated in recent years, there is still substantial under-treatment of hypertension in the community as described in section 5.

Definitions of hypertension

As outlined in section 3, the definition of hypertension is problematic. Blood pressure is a continuous variable, and any cut-off between normal and abnormal is to some extent arbitrary. Indeed, in the last decade, emphasis in treating hypertension has changed from consideration of the blood pressure alone, to consideration of blood pressure in the context of the underlying risk of cardiovascular disease in a given individual. The higher the risk of cardiovascular disease, the greater the potential benefit in terms of absolute risk reduction for an individual in lowering their blood pressure. Thus, guidelines recommend lower treatment thresholds for initiating antihypertensive therapy in people with other risk factors for cardiovascular disease (see section 7), such as diabetes, hyperlipidaemia and smoking. Indeed, the implications of the PROGRESS trial are that in people who have had a stroke, treatment should be considered in people who are traditionally thought to be normotensive.[9] Thus, the terminology is switching from 'treating hypertension' to 'lowering blood pressure'.

Purpose and scope of this chapter

The aim of this chapter is to provide the background information for commissioners of health care – a responsibility being taken over by primary care trusts in England – to inform their decision making on policy with regard to hypertension services. The chapter does not address the sequelae of hypertension, which are dealt with in separate chapters in this series. The chapter does comment on treatment of hypertension in the context of some specific diseases, such as diabetes, but readers should cross-refer to the other chapters that address these diseases (including diabetes, coronary heart disease and stroke).

Key questions for commissioners of health care include:

- choice of antihypertensive agents, which has significant cost implications, given the ten-fold difference in costs of different drugs (*see* section 5)
- how to improve population coverage, given the evidence from the Health Survey for England of significant under-diagnosis and under-treatment of hypertension (*see* section 5)
- how to ensure optimal blood pressure lowering in people at high risk of cardiovascular disease.

A particular issue in relation to the latter point is blood pressure lowering in the elderly. There is good evidence from systematic reviews of randomised controlled trials that treatment of elderly people with hypertension is an effective way to reduce risk of stroke and coronary heart disease (*see* section 6).[10,11] Despite this, surveys have consistently demonstrated, as shown in section 5, that general practitioners have a higher threshold for treating hypertension in older patients.[12]

There are two complementary strategies to reducing morbidity from hypertension. One is to identify and treat individuals with high blood pressure. This is sometimes referred to as the 'high risk' approach.[13] An alternative strategy is to aim to lower blood pressure in the population as a whole, the so-called 'population strategy'. The attraction of the population strategy is that it will lower risk in the whole population, and not just in high risk individuals, and therefore has the potential to lead to greater reductions in stroke and coronary heart disease than strategies focusing on those individuals with higher blood pressure. While the focus of much preventive health care is on identifying and treating at-risk individuals, commissioners of health care have important public health responsibilities, which include taking this broader population-based perspective on preventive strategy. Therefore, population-based strategies to lower blood pressure in the population are included within the scope of this chapter, although the responsibility for implementation is wider than health care commissioners alone.

3 Sub-categories

The categorisation of blood pressure is of necessity an arbitrary exercise, as there is a continuum of cardiovascular risk associated with the level of blood pressure: the higher the blood pressure, the higher the risk of both stroke and coronary events.[2,14] Within this continuum, all but the highest blood pressures produce little in the way of symptoms for the patient and so these cannot form the basis of a categorisation. Qualitative terms such as mild, moderate and severe have been used to label increasing levels of blood pressure but without universal acceptance of the definition of these terms.[15]

In the majority of patients with asymptomatic hypertension, it has become commonplace to use level of cardiovascular risk to guide the level at which intervention to lower blood pressure is required.[16-18] In determining cardiovascular risk, two broad categories of risk factor must be taken into account: fixed and modifiable. Age, sex and family history are the most important fixed risk factors, whilst modifiable factors include smoking, serum cholesterol, diabetes (in terms of control), blood pressure, left ventricular hypertrophy, diet and exercise status.[19] Many of these risk factors have been combined in a set of risk equations derived from multifactorial analysis of the results from 12 years of follow-up of the subjects in the Framingham Heart Study.[20] Estimations of the risk of a number of cardiovascular end points can then be made for patients without current cardiovascular disease and may be used to inform thresholds for intervention at various levels of blood pressure.

Evidence of end organ damage is another factor which affects the intervention threshold for blood pressure control. High blood pressure affects the heart, kidneys, brain and eye – so-called 'end organs' – via vascular damage to both the small (resistance) arteries and arterioles and large (conduit) arteries. Whilst there is universal agreement that end organ damage is important, there is no agreed definition of what constitutes damage. One scheme adapted from that proposed in Canadian guidelines is shown in **Table 2.**[21]

Table 2: Definitions of hypertensive end organ damage (adapted from Myers *et al.* 1989[21]).

Target organ	Evidence of damage
Heart and peripheral vasculature	a) Left ventricular hypertrophy with strain demonstrated by electrocardiography or echocardiography. b) A history or symptoms of angina pectoris. c) A history or electrocardiographic evidence of myocardial infarction. d) A history or symptoms of intermittent claudication.
Brain	Previous history of transient ischaemic attack or cerebrovascular accident.
Kidney	Serum creatinine >150mmol/l.
Eye	Evidence of hypertensive retinopathy.

This difficulty in categorisation is reflected in the differences in recommendations from various national and international bodies for the diagnosis and treatment of hypertension. Of these recommendations, those of the World Health Organization,[22] and the national guidelines of New Zealand,[17] Canada,[21] US[16] and UK[18] are the best known and most cited. Whilst there are many similarities between these guidelines there are also important differences. These differences include the definitions of both treatment thresholds and target blood pressure.

The key differences between the guidelines in terms of definition of hypertension that warrants treatment are summarised in **Table 3.**

Table 3: Blood pressure thresholds for treatment (adapted and updated version of Swales, 1994 to include current versions of guidelines[14]).

Guideline	Absolute treatment threshold: Diastolic blood pressure (mmHg)	Absolute treatment threshold: Systolic blood pressure (mmHg)	Period of observation (months)	Treatment threshold in presence of other risk factors (mmHg)
Canada[23]	90 if aged under 60 105 if over 60	160	3–6	90
Britain[18]	100	160	4–6	140/90
USA[24]	90	140	1 week–2 months	120/80
New Zealand[17]	100	170	6	150/90–170/100 depending on overall cardiovascular risk
WHO/ISH[22]	95	150	3–6	140/90

All of the guidelines recognise that overall cardiovascular risk affects treatment threshold. Both the New Zealand and British guidelines advocate formally estimating risk, using a series of tables or a computer program, before considering treatment for patients lying within their definition of mild hypertension. All of the authorities agree on the need for treatment of sustained hypertension above the threshold of 170/100 and none recommend treatment below 130/85. Between these two values there is considerable variation in the level and associated cardiovascular risks at which treatment is advocated.

The importance of blood pressure control in diabetes is now well established. People with diabetes derive more benefit from blood pressure reduction than those without diabetes.[18,25] Moreover, there is good evidence that lowering blood pressure in those with type 2 diabetes reduces both micro and macrovascular changes.[26] In view of this we have separated outpatients in this group as a separate sub-category.

A special sub-category of hypertension is malignant hypertension, which is defined by WHO as the presence of bilateral retinal haemorrhages and exudates in the presence of severe hypertension – typically with a diastolic blood pressure greater than 130 mmHg.[27] Malignant hypertension is accompanied by a number of clinical features, the most common of which are left ventricular hypertrophy, headache, visual impairment and renal failure.[28] The relevance of this sub-category is that urgent treatment is required to limit the risk of serious complications, most notably the onset of renal failure.

As already discussed, most patients with hypertension are asymptomatic and have no discernible cause for their raised blood pressure. However, around 10% have a clearly defined cause for their hypertension.[29,30] These form another important sub-group. In most cases, the underlying cause is endocrine (principally normokalaemic hyperaldosteronism), renal or vascular.[29,30] These will be discussed as a separate sub-group as they are important not only in their own right, but in view of the implications for the investigation of the majority of patients with hypertension.

White Coat Hypertension is a description of the phenomenon whereby the blood pressure rises simply in association with the procedure of having it measured. This can be effectively identified using ambulatory blood pressure measurement and although patients do not generally need treatment, it is appropriate to consider this as a separate sub-category, since patients with this condition are at higher risk of subsequently developing true hypertension.[31]

In view of a lack of a universally accepted sub-categorisation of hypertension, this document has used the following sub-categories. The first three groups correspond to the blood pressure thresholds suggested in 1998 by the Recommendations of the Joint British Societies:[32]

- **Group 1:** *Raised blood pressure – level sufficient to merit treatment regardless of cardiovascular risk.* Definition: For people without diabetes, blood pressure $\geq$160/100 mmHg (either diastolic alone, systolic alone or both) *or* evidence of target organ damage with blood pressure below 160/100 mmHg. The level of blood pressure along with the overall cardiovascular risk dictates the degree of urgency.
- **Group 2:** *Raised blood pressure – treat on basis of underlying cardiovascular risk.* Definition: sustained systolic blood pressure between 140–159 *or* sustained diastolic blood pressure 90–99 mmHg with no evidence of target organ damage. In this group, overall cardiovascular risk dictates the need for treatment.
- **Group 3:** *Raised blood pressure and diabetes.* Definition: blood pressure $\geq$140/90 mmHg with co-existing diabetes mellitus. In this group the presence of diabetes lowers the treatment threshold whatever other cardiovascular risk factors are present.
- **Group 4:** *Malignant or accelerated hypertension.* Definition: hypertensive emergency with bilateral retinal haemorrhages and exudates.
- **Group 5:** *Secondary hypertension.* Definition: hypertension with clear underlying cause, often reno-vascular or endocrine.
- **Group 6:** *White coat hypertension.* Definition: blood pressure raised in the presence of medical personnel but not otherwise and with no evidence of target organ damage.

Literature on the epidemiology of hypertension tends to combine groups 1, 2 and 3 under the umbrella term of essential hypertension, i.e. hypertension with no discernible cause. This pragmatic grouping will also be used where applicable in this chapter.

4 Prevalence and incidence

Essential hypertension (sub-categories 1–3)

Most community surveys measuring the prevalence of hypertension do not differentiate patients on the basis of cause of hypertension, but rather by other criteria such as age, sex and ethnicity. Essential hypertension (sub-categories 1–3) makes up around 95% of all cases and so the overall figures are presented here as broadly representative of the population burden of essential hypertension. The major sources of data are the Health Survey for England (HSE) 1998[1] and the General Practice Research Database (GPRD).[33] The Health Survey for England sampled a population of almost 16 000 drawn from 720 postcode districts stratified for health authority and social class of head of household. Hypertension was defined as a mean resting blood pressure ≥140/90 mmHg or receiving treatment for hypertension. Blood pressure readings were taken on one occasion and although multiple measurements were made, this does not correspond to the definition of true hypertension, which requires that the elevation of blood pressure is sustained.[18] Furthermore, the threshold adopted by the Joint British Societies and in the sub-categories of this chapter for hypertension was 160/100 or 140/90 in the presence of significant coronary heart disease risk due to presence of other risk factors. For both of these reasons, the estimates from the HSE are likely to overestimate the true prevalence of hypertension. The GPRD comprises electronic data from the computer records of over 350 general practices throughout the UK.[33] It provides an alternative estimate of the prevalence of treated hypertension, defined as an ever-recorded diagnosis of hypertension in combination with treatment with an antihypertensive agent.

Prevalence by age and sex

Overall hypertension is more common in men than women and rises in prevalence with age. The rise with age is more pronounced in women who have a higher prevalence in the over-65 age group. Using the HSE definition of hypertension, over a third of the adult population have raised blood pressure, and the majority of people over the age of 55. Figures are presented in **Table 4** for men, women and overall derived from the Health Survey for England 1998.[1]

Despite the higher prevalence of hypertension in men than women, the prevalence of treated hypertension is higher in women than men. This finding is echoed in the GPRD data (*see* **Table 5**), which shows a similar pattern of age specific prevalence of treated hypertension to that of the HSE. The overall standardised rate is lower in the GPRD as this is a prevalence for all ages, whereas the HSE gives an overall prevalence for adults (aged 16 or over).

Prevalence by region

Table 6 shows age and sex standardised prevalence by region. Prevalence varies in men from 35% in the North West Region, to 43% in Northern and Yorkshire Region.

Prevalence by socioeconomic group

There is an association between social class and hypertension, with higher rates in the lower social classes – see **Table 7**.

Table 4: Prevalence (%) of hypertension by age and sex.[1]

	Age							Total
	16–24	25–34	35–44	45–54	55–64	65–74	>75	
Males								
Overall	16.0	20.5	26.1	42.3	59.8	69.9	72.8	40.8
On treatment	0	0.3	2.3	7.2	17.4	20.6	22.6	8.5
>140/90, untreated	16.0	20.2	23.8	35.4	42.4	49.3	50.2	32.3
Females								
Overall	4.2	6.9	13.2	30.8	51.6	72.8	77.6	32.9
On treatment	0.1	0.5	2.4	6.2	15.5	30.0	31.8	10.5
>140/90, untreated	4.0	6.4	10.8	24.6	36.0	42.9	45.8	22.5
Overall	9.7	13.2	19.0	36.1	55.4	71.4	75.7	36.5
On treatment	0.1	0.4	2.4	6.7	16.4	25.6	28.1	9.6
>140/90, untreated	9.5	12.8	16.7	29.5	38.9	45.9	47.6	27.0

Table 5: Prevalence (%) of treated hypertension by age and sex: GPRD data for 1998.[33]

	Age							Overall (standardised)
	0–34	35–44	45–54	55–64	65–74	75–84	>85	
Males	0.2	2.0	7.3	16.4	25.9	28.1	20.1	6.0
Females	0.2	2.1	7.9	18.8	30.2	37.5	29.1	7.1

Table 6: Standardised prevalence (%) of hypertension by region.[1]

	Northern & Yorks	North West	Trent	West Midlands	Anglia & Oxford	North Thames	South Thames	South & West
Males	43.0	35.1	38.4	39.2	38.3	36.5	38.5	42.2
Females	36.0	30.6	32.9	32.4	33.8	31.2	32.4	34.2

Table 7: Standardised prevalence (%) of hypertension[a] by social class.[1]

	I	II	IIINM	IIIM	IV	V
Men	34.3	38.0	37.2	41.8	35.2	40.2
Women	31.4	31.3	34.4	34.2	34.4	35.9

[a] Defined as BP >140/90 mmHg or on treatment for hypertension.

Prevalence by ethnic group

The data presented in **Table 8** are taken from the HSE minority ethnic group report 1999.[34] Some of these figures are likely to be imprecise due to the small numbers of representatives in a number of ethnic groups surveyed, most notably the Chinese. In general, the prevalence of hypertension is lower in minority ethnic groups than it is in the general population. The exception to this is the high prevalence of hypertension in the Black Caribbean group associated with cardiovascular disease. It is difficult to judge whether the prevalence of hypertension is genuinely lower in minority ethnic groups, or whether this reflects treatment patterns.

Table 8: Observed prevalence (%) of hypertension[a] by ethnic group amongst those with and without CVD conditions.[b][34]

	Black Caribbean	Indian	Pakistani	Bangladeshi	Chinese	Irish	All
Males							
with CVD	78	59	61	45	64[c]	61	71
without CVD	36	32	20	19	24	37	38
Females							
with CVD	67	62	51	43	35[c]	53	65
without CVD	23	20	12	9	22	24	30

[a] Defined as: on treatment for hypertension or with recorded blood pressure >140/90.

[b] Defined as self-reported presence of angina, heart attack, stroke, heart murmur, irregular heart rhythm, 'other heart trouble' or diabetes.

[c] Very small numbers of Chinese individuals with CVD were included in the survey.

Incidence of hypertension

In terms of a health care needs assessment for hypertension, prevalence is a much more useful concept than incidence. What is relevant in this context is ascertaining the number of people who, on the basis of their blood pressure and other risk factors for cardiovascular disease, would benefit from treatment to lower their blood pressure. Since treatment will usually be long-term, prevalence will be the major determinant of this need rather than incidence. However, incidence does give an indication of the numbers of new patients that warrant treatment over a given period of time.

The incidence of hypertension increases with age from <1–2% in people aged 20–29 to 4–8% aged 60–79.[35] Incidence is higher in younger men than women, but higher in older women than men. Factors associated with higher incidence of hypertension include obesity, excessive use of alcohol, salt consumption, and lack of exercise.[35]

Trends in mean blood pressure in the population

As well as looking at number of 'cases', which is how prevalence and incidence data deal with hypertension, it is also useful to look at the mean level of blood pressure in the population. Firstly, as already emphasised, blood pressure is a continuous variable, and any cut-off between cases and non-cases is to some extent arbitrary. Secondly, in terms of population strategies to lower blood pressure (*see* 'Non-pharmacological' in section 5), the mean blood pressure is a more useful indicator.

Trends in age-specific systolic and diastolic blood pressure from 1994–98 in men and women are shown in **Figures 1–4**, drawing on data from the HSE.[1]

Between 1994 and 1998, there is some evidence of small falls in the age-specific mean blood pressures of the English population. Over the five year period, the age-specific mean blood pressures for men went down on average by 1.7/0.9 mmHg, and for women by 2.7/1.2 mmHg. If real, these small declines in blood pressure would be clinically important in terms of leading to corresponding falls in the incidence of stroke and coronary heart disease (*see* section 6). The decline in blood pressure appeared to be slightly more pronounced in older people: in men, the blood pressure of people aged 75 and over went down by 2/2 mmHg, and in women by 4.5/2.8 mmHg. US data over a longer time scale (1960–1980) also offer evidence of a decline in blood pressure over time.[35] The age-adjusted mean systolic blood pressure went down by 4–8 mmHg in men and 6–8 mmHg in women. Again, the decline was greater in the older age groups.

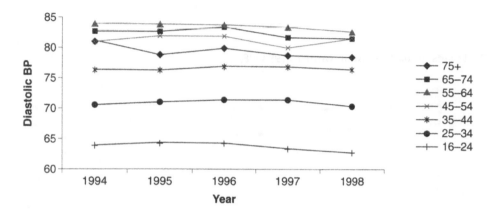

Figure 1: Trends in diastolic BP in men: 1994–98.

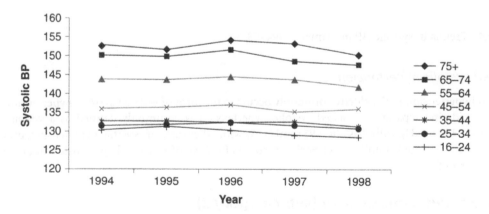

Figure 2: Trends in systolic BP in men: 1994–98.

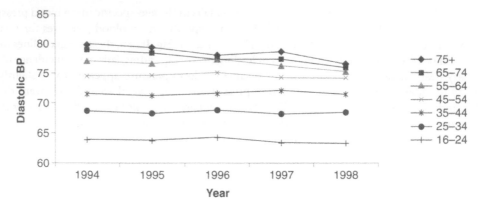

Figure 3: Trends in diastolic BP in women: 1994–98.

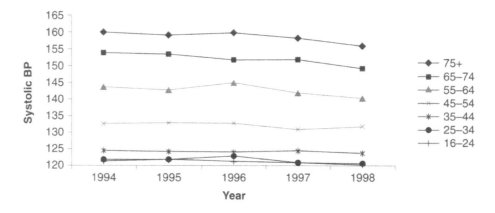

Figure 4: Trends in systolic BP in women: 1994–98.

Isolated systolic hypertension

Essential hypertension in the elderly commonly occurs in the form of isolated systolic hypertension and is worth considering separately. Isolated systolic hypertension is commonly defined as a systolic blood pressure of >160 mmHg with diastolic <95 mmHg. As with other cases of essential hypertension, prevalence rises with age – isolated systolic hypertension accounts for 25% of essential hypertension in people aged over the age of 80.[36]

Diabetes and hypertension (sub-category 3)

Although diabetics with raised blood pressure commonly have essential hypertension, their overall increase in cardiovascular risk and the effect of hypertension on microvascular disease mean that it is helpful to consider this group separately. In the Hypertension in Diabetes Study, the prevalence in newly presenting adult diabetics was found to be 34.7% in men, and 46.5% in women.[37] In this study, hypertension was defined as a blood pressure >160/90, or on antihypertensive therapy. Therefore, the prevalence of hypertension appears higher in people with diabetes than those without, given the overall prevalence is similar to that obtained by the HSE which used the lower definition of >140/90 (see above).

Malignant or accelerated hypertension (sub-category 4)

Precise figures on the prevalence of malignant hypertension are rare. A series from one large hypertension unit in the West Midlands approximated a prevalence of 1–2/100 000 population.[38]

Secondary hypertension (sub-category 5)

The prevalence of secondary hypertension was until recently thought to be around 5%. This was based on a number of 'classical series' but more recent work suggests that this is probably higher, at least 10%, with primary hyperaldosteronism an important cause. Secondary hypertension is important as treatment of the underlying cause may be life-saving and lead to normotension.

Two older studies provide data on the prevalence of secondary hypertension. Data from a Swedish population sample are available from a primary prevention trial in Goteborg.[29] 7455 men were initially screened, of whom 1159 were found to be hypertensive or already on treatment for hypertension (15.5%). Subsequent investigation of 689 of these patients revealed 40 to have secondary hypertension (5.8% of hypertensives). Secondary hypertension was further broken down into renal parenchymal disease (63%), renovascular disease (10%) and other forms of secondary hypertension (27%). The cut-off for hypertension was very high by modern standards (175/115 mmHg) and the series included four patients with renal tuberculosis so the numbers are not directly comparable with a current population.

A further Swedish series, this time in secondary care, (a retrospective analysis of 1000 consecutive patients attending another hypertension unit) found 47 (4.7%) to have an identifiable secondary cause of hypertension: renal parenchymal disease in 21, renal artery stenosis in 10, endocrine hypertension in 13 and hydronephrosis in 3.[30]

More recent investigations into the prevalence of primary hyperaldosteronism have suggested that the prevalence of this abnormality amongst hypertensives may itself be as high as 3–18%.[39] The reason for this difference is that previous studies used hypokalaemia as a screening tool before looking for hyperaldosteronism, whereas more modern studies screen using direct measurement of serum aldosterone and the ratio of serum aldosterone to plasma renin activity. The upper limits of the prevalence range are disputed as there is concern as to selection bias in the populations concerned.[39] Overall it is probably reasonable to assume that around 5% of those thought previously to have essential hypertension have primary hyperaldosteronism.

A summary of the results of studies that investigated the epidemiology of secondary hypertension is shown in **Table 9**.

Table 9: Proportion of patients with secondary hypertension – summary of studies.

	Proportion in each category (range %)
Essential hypertension	72.6–95.3
Renal hypertension	2.4–17.2
Renovascular hypertension	0.6–6.1
Primary hypokalaemic aldosteronism	0.1–0.4
Primary normokalaemic aldosteronism	3–18
Phaeochromocytoma	0.2–0.7
Cushing's syndrome	0.1–0.3
Endocrine, other	0.1–0.4
Oral contraceptives	1.5–5.0
Coarctation of the aorta	0.2–0.6
Other	1.0–3.7

Adapted from Danielson and Dammstrom (1981).[30]

White coat hypertension (sub-category 6)

Estimates of the prevalence of white coat hypertension vary between series from around 7–35%. A widely quoted secondary care series found a 21% (61/292 subjects) prevalence of normal daytime ambulatory blood pressure in patients with untreated borderline hypertension (persistently raised diastolic clinic measurements 90–104 mmHg).[40] A more recent Canadian series, again in secondary care, investigated patients with blood pressure above 140/90 mmHg despite taking at least two antihypertensive agents. They found 37/103 of these patients to have a white coat response.[41] A primary care study using home blood pressure measurement rather than ambulatory monitoring found a 27% prevalence of white coat hypertension in an untreated population of 236 patients.[42] This study also reported that 17% (45 of 258) of poorly-controlled hypertensives had white coat hypertension. The phenomenon of higher blood pressure in the presence of medical staff has also been reported in people with established hypertension.[22]

Hypertension as a risk factor for disease

Observational studies have found a continuous relationship between level of blood pressure and risk of stroke and CHD. In a study combining the results of nine major prospective observational studies, a difference in blood pressure of 9/5 mmHg was associated with a difference in stroke risk of 34% and CHD risk of 21%.[2] An individual participant data meta-analysis including 61 prospective studies and 1 million adults found that between ages 40–69, each difference in usual systolic blood pressure of 20 mmHg was associated with a more than doubling of mortality rates from ischaemic heart disease and other vascular causes.[43]

Similar results have been found when the risk reduction obtained by antihypertensive treatment is examined. A systematic review of antihypertensive treatment trials found a mean reduction in stroke of 38% (95% CI 31–45) for mean Diastolic Blood Pressure (DBP) reduction of 5–6 mmHg over 2–3 years. The equivalent mean reduction in CHD was 16% (8–23%). Given that CHD is more common than stroke, the absolute reduction in CHD events through treating hypertension is closer to the absolute reduction in stroke events, though the overall effect of treatment is still to prevent more strokes than coronary events (treatment vs control: 934 vs 1104 CHD events compared with 525 vs 835 strokes).[6]

The latest publication from the Blood Pressure Trialists Collaboration reports no significant difference in the relative risk reductions for total major cardiovascular events between Angiotensin Converting Enzyme Inhibitors (ACE inhibitors), calcium antagonists, diuretics and beta-blockers, so choice of agent within these classes does not appear to be a particular issue.[44]

Benefit from blood pressure lowering also occurs in isolated systolic hypertension (ISH): a meta-analysis of trials of treatment of ISH found relative hazard ratios for 10 mmHg higher initial Systolic Blood Pressures (SBP) were 1.26 (p=0.0001) total mortality; 1.22 (p=0.02) stroke but only 1.07 (p=0.37) coronary events.[45]

Summary of epidemiology at primary care trust level

Table 10 shows a breakdown of the number of people expected to suffer from hypertension by sub-category in a population of 100 000.

Table 10: Prevalence of hypertension and sub-categories in primary care trust (PCT) of 100,000 population.[1,29,30,38,41]

	Prevalence
All hypertension	29,100
Treated hypertension	7,500
Elderly isolated systolic hypertension (age >70)	900
Malignant hypertension	1
Secondary hypertension	375
White coat hypertension	750
Assuming 21% of the population are under the age of 16.	

5 Services available and their costs

This section describes the services that are available to diagnose and treat hypertension, and the different settings within which that care is provided. It also provides some data on current use of services and costs. It does not comment on whether these services are effective (covered in section 6) or whether they should be available (covered in section 7).

Diagnosis

Clinical evaluation

Patients with hypertension will have a process of evaluation consisting of history (including any symptoms, lifestyle factors, cardiovascular risk factors, past medical history, possible precipitants and family history), examination (of cardiovascular system) and repeated blood pressure measurements. In primary care this will typically be carried out by the general practitioner in conjunction with the practice nurse. The patient themselves may undertake self-monitoring of blood pressure as part of this process.[42]

Routine diagnostic investigation

Routine investigations performed in primary care on patients with hypertension typically include urine testing, blood tests and electrocardiography (ECG). These aim to screen for end organ damage as well as test for other risk factors for cardiovascular disease. The precise tests used will depend on the suspicion of a secondary cause of hypertension and this will largely depend on the age of the patient. The evidence for routine investigation and recommendations for appropriate investigation are covered in subsequent sections. A summary of the tests which may be carried out in the investigation of hypertension is provided in **Table 11**.

Table 11: Baseline investigations for hypertension (adapted from BHS Guidelines 1999 and The Sixth Report of the Joint National Committee on Prevention, Detection, Evaluation, and Treatment of High Blood Pressure (JNC VI) 1997).[16,18]

Investigation	Rationale
Performed on most patients	
Urinalysis: protein and blood	Evidence of end organ damage and investigation of possible secondary cause for hypertension (Renal)
Serum creatinine and electrolytes	Investigation of possible secondary cause for hypertension: Hypokalaemia/increased plasma sodium (Endocrine – Conn's syndrome) Elevated serum creatinine (Renal)
Blood glucose	Risk assessment (diabetes)
Serum total: HDL cholesterol	Risk assessment (Framingham Risk score for primary prevention)
ECG	Evidence of end organ damage and risk assessment (investigation of possible left ventricular hypertrophy)
Performed on selected patients	
Note: it is unlikely that all of these investigations would be performed on a single patient but rather that a clinician would be guided by the clinical picture	
Creatinine clearance	Further investigation of renal dysfunction (end organ damage and/or secondary cause of hypertension)
Microalbuminuria	Screening for evidence of early renal; dysfunction (end organ damage principally)
24-hour urinary protein	Further investigation of renal dysfunction (end organ damage and/or secondary cause of hypertension)
Urine microscopy and culture	Investigation of haematuria and/or proteinuria (possible urinary tract infection)
Urinary catecholamines	Investigation of possible secondary cause for hypertension: Phaeochromocytoma
Aldosterone/renin ratio	Investigation of possible secondary cause for hypertension: Diagnosis of hyperaldosteronism
Uric acid	Investigation of possible secondary cause for hypertension: Gout
Thyroid stimulating hormone	Investigation of possible secondary cause for hypertension: Hyperthyroidism
Serum calcium	Investigation of possible secondary cause for hypertension: Hyperparathyroidism
Chest X-ray	Investigation of possible cardiomegaly (left ventricular hypertrophy)
Echocardiogram	Further investigation of possible left ventricular hypertrophy or other structural abnormality or dysfunction of heart

Special investigations for secondary hypertension

Patients referred to secondary care for consideration of possible secondary hypertension will typically have a more intensive and/or invasive set of investigations. These will again involve blood, urine and ECG but may also include chest X-ray, ultrasonography, echocardiography and other more complex screening tests. Key conditions that these screening tests will aim to test for are: renal artery stenosis, endocrine causes of hypertension (including phaeochromocytoma, Conn's disease) and renal parenchymal disease (including glomerulonephritis, renal cystic disease). These tests and their rationale are summarised in **Table 11**.

Special investigations for white coat hypertension

Patients with suspected white coat hypertension will receive further evaluation of their blood pressure in a non-health care setting. Typically this might involve either home blood pressure monitoring or ambulatory blood pressure measurement. Both will usually involve automated electronic measurement. Ambulatory measurement consists of a portable device which measures blood pressure at regular intervals (half-hourly–hourly) over a 24 hour period. Results are usually expressed in terms of mean blood pressure (overall, day and night). Home measurement involves an individual recording their own BP over a period of days or weeks.

Cost of equipment is likely to be a barrier to the widespread adaptation of both these types of measurement. Ambulatory measurement is most often available in specialised settings and home measurement generally requires an individual to purchase equipment. Alternatives to this include short-term loaning until blood pressure is controlled or self-measurement at the practice.

Screening for hypertension

Routine health checks

Blood pressure is routinely checked in UK primary care in many different circumstances. These include health checks when a patient registers with a new general practice; contraceptive and obstetric encounters for women; Accident and Emergency encounters for non-minor injury; and private medical checks performed for insurance or other reasons.

Community screening programmes

No national community screening programme exists in the UK but various models have been studied both in the UK and US. These include schemes for blood pressure screening in pharmacies, work places and even door to door screening.[8]

Treatment

Non-pharmacological

Patients presenting with new hypertension are routinely offered advice on aspects of lifestyle to both lower blood pressure and affect other risk factors. This includes diet (increase fruit and vegetables, less salt, less alcohol, weight loss), exercise (increase) and smoking (stop). A summary of the effect of these treatments is presented in 'Non-pharmacological treatment of hypertension' in section 6 and **Table 21**.

Pharmacological: blood pressure lowering

Pharmacological treatment of blood pressure can be subdivided on the basis of class of drug. In the UK, the recent British Hypertension Society guidelines recommend the 'ABCD rule' for uncomplicated hypertension.[46] This is the use of ACE inhibitors or beta-blockers as first line in the under-55s and calcium antagonists or diuretics in the over-55s. Other choices may be relevant in the case of co-existing disease or lack of efficacy of first line drugs. The utilisation of various classes of antihypertensive is presented in **Table 12**. Figures from both the general practice research database 1998[33] and Health Survey for England 1996[1] are included. The former includes all patients receiving each class of drug and gives absolute numbers whereas the later is by proportion of patients with hypertension. Thus, the most commonly used class of agent are diuretics – 48% of treated hypertensives are on this class of drug. The GPRD data are not hypertension-specific, so are more difficult to interpret since each of these therapies have other indications (such as ischaemic heart disease).

Data from the HOT study suggest that less than one third of hypertensive patients will be adequately controlled on monotherapy and that a similar proportion will require three or more agents for control.[25] Overall the mean use of antihypertensive drugs was just under 2 per patient and depending on choice of drugs, costs can be expected to vary from £20 to £455.[47]

Table 12: Choices of antihypertensive drugs by class.

Drug class	GPRD 1998 All persons prescribed drugs per 1000 patients[33]		Drug class	HSE 1996[48] % of persons on hypertensive medication		
	Male	Female		Males	Females	All adults
Diuretics	37.8	61.2	Diuretics	39	54	48
Beta-blockers	38.0	44.5	Beta-blockers	38	35	36
Drugs affecting the renin-angiotensin system	34.9	28.0	ACE inhibitors	25	19	22
Nitrates, calcium antagonists and potassium channel activators	45.0	36.6	Calcium antagonists	36	28	31
			Other drugs affecting blood pressure	4	3	1

Inevitably trends in drug prescription have changed over time both in terms of new classes of drugs (principally ACE inhibitors) gaining in popularity and also in the proportion of patients receiving combination therapy. **Table 13** shows the change in prescription over time for the classes of drug both by absolute number (rate of prescription per 1000 patients) and by net ingredient cost (NIC).

Pharmacological: other interventions to lower cardiovascular risk

Patients with hypertension, particularly those at highest overall risk, may benefit from other pharmacological measures to lower their cardiovascular risk, namely aspirin and cholesterol-lowering drugs.[18]

Setting of treatment

Hypertension is largely managed in primary care with only complicated or difficult-to-control cases being referred to hospital. A number of distinct models of care exist within either setting as described below.

Table 13: Change over time in prescription of antihypertensive drugs by rate[33] and cost (NIC data from Prescription Pricing Authority; Personal Communication Dr John J Ferguson).

Year		Diuretics	Beta-blocker	ACE inhibitor[c]	Calcium channel blocker[d]
1994	Rate[a]	35.7	35.7	24.1	42.5
	NIC[b]	60,954	88,428	147,023	160,161
1995	Rate	35.7	36.0	26.9	43.3
	NIC	55,590	81,511	170,364	178,918
1996	Rate	36.3	36.2	30.1	44.2
	NIC	51,641	79,283	193,297	197,796
1997	Rate	37.0	36.8	32.4	44.7
	NIC	48,349	77,361	200,003	212,031
1998	Rate	37.8	38.0	34.9	45.0
	NIC				

[a] Rate of prescription per 1,000 patients.
[b] Net ingredient cost (£000s). The NIC refers to the cost of the drug before discounts and does not include any dispensing costs or fees.
[c] The rate data for ACE inhibitors includes all drugs in chapter 2.5 of the BNF including all renin-angiotensin system drugs, alpha-blockers.
[d] Rate data includes nitrates and potassium channel activators.

Episodic treatment

Traditionally the standard method of care in primary care, this model depends on the patient attending periodically for blood pressure measurement as well as screening for end organ damage, consideration of management changes and other risk factor modification.

Structured care

This involves primary care teams following a structured care programme, typically using protocols and recording data on blood pressure, management changes and risk factors in a systematic fashion, perhaps using a computer template. A further key feature of structured care is systematic recall of patients. Structured care can be provided by both medical and/or nursing staff either within normal 'open' surgeries or at set times of the week in a special clinic.

Shared clinics

Shared clinics involve GPs and hospital specialists sharing the management of patients either with alternate visits, 'virtually' via IT links, or sometimes by sharing a clinic on the same site on a periodic basis.[49] This model allows specialist advice for complex cases while retaining the majority of patients within primary care.

Hospital clinics

Hospital clinics receive referrals from general practitioners and typically see either newly diagnosed patients where a secondary cause is suspected or patients with established hypertension where blood pressure control has proved hard to achieve. Length of follow-up of patients will depend on local workload and whether a secondary cause is established.

In-patient hospital care

Hypertension *per se* is an uncommon cause of hospital admission. Patients with malignant or accelerated hypertension are admitted to hospital, and uncontrolled hypertension may be a presenting feature of underlying disease such as renal or endocrine which may precipitate hospital admission. Hypertension is a co-morbidity in many other conditions that lead to hospital admission. This is illustrated by **Table 16** (*see* 'In-patient data' below) which shows Hospital Episode Statistics for England for 1996/7.

Data on service use

The overall consultation rate for all people with essential hypertension is 420 persons per 10 000 person years at risk. As expected this varies considerably with age and sex as can be seen in **Table 14**.

Table 14: Patient consulting rates for hypertension per 10,000 person years at risk.[50]

	Total	0–4	5–15	16–24	25–44	45–64	65–74	75–84	85+
All essential hypertension	420	1	0	9	98	813	1,656	1,430	663
Male essential hypertension		1	1	9	100	760	1,488	1,118	511
Female essential hypertension		1	0	10	96	869	1,791	1,615	713

Uptake of treatment

Another way of looking at service use is to consider what proportion of people with hypertension have been diagnosed, and what proportion of people with hypertension are on antihypertensive therapy. The Health Survey for England provides some data on this, as shown in **Table 15**. In this survey, blood pressure was measured three times on one occasion and so the proportions of people found with untreated hypertension are likely to be overestimates if compared with the number with sustained raised blood pressure over a period of weeks or months. Nevertheless, only the minority of people with hypertension appear to be currently receiving treatment.

Table 15: Blood pressure status by age and sex.

	16–24	25–34	35–44	45–54	55–64	65–74	>75	Total
	%	%	%	%	%	%	%	%
Men								
Normotensive[1] (untreated)	84	79.5	73.9	57.7	40.2	30.1	27.2	59.2
Treated hypertension[2]	0	0.3	2.3	7	17.4	20.6	22.6	8.5
Untreated hypertension[3]	16	20.2	23.8	35.4	42.4	49.3	50.2	32.3
Women								
Normotensive[1] (untreated)	95.8	93.1	86.8	69.2	48.4	27.2	22.4	67.1
Treated hypertension[2]	0.1	0.5	2.4	6.2	15.5	30	31.8	10.5
Untreated hypertension[3]	4	6.4	10.8	24.6	36	42.9	45.8	22.5

[1] Normotensive: untreated and with mean BP <140/90.

[2] Treated hypertension: on treatment for hypertension.

[3] Untreated hypertension: BP>140/90 and not receiving treatment for hypertension.

In-patient data

Table 16 shows Hospital Episode Statistics (HES) data relating to hospital admissions in England & Wales in 1996/97. Over this period, there were 20 times as many hospital episodes with hypertension coded as a secondary diagnosis as opposed to a primary diagnosis (i.e. the major reason for the admission). For the vast majority of cases where hypertension was a secondary diagnosis, this was coded as essential hypertension (96%). Where hypertension was the primary cause of the episode, essential hypertension remained the commonest cause (58%), but often in association with renal disease (35%).

Table 16: Hospital episodes associated with a primary or secondary diagnosis of hypertension. Hospital Episode Statistics Data for England & Wales 1996/7.

ICD-10 Diagnosis	Primary cause of episode		Secondary diagnosis	
	No. of admissions (% of total hypertensive admissions)		No. of admissions (% of total hypertensive admissions)	
Essential hypertension (I10x)	8,716	(58.2)	283,016	(96.3)
Hypertension with heart disease (I11.0, I11.9)	771	(5.2)	1,574	(0.5)
Hypertension with renal disease (I12.0, I12.9, I15.0, I15.1)	5,249	(35.1)	8,632	(2.9)
Hypertension with heart & renal disease (I13.0, I13.1, I13.2, I13.9)	191	(1.3)	233	(0.1)
Hypertension with endocrine cause (I15.2)	4	(0)	22	(0)
Other secondary hypertension (I15.8, I15.9)	35	(0.2)	291	(0.1)
Totals	14,966	(100)	293,768	(100)

Source: National Casemix Office[51]

Estimated costs for hypertension detection and management

Drugs

A primary care trust (PCT) serving 100 000 patients would expect to spend over £1 million annually on drugs from the main classes used in hypertension. A more detailed breakdown is shown in **Table 17**.

Table 17: Estimated drug costs by antihypertensive drug class.

	Actual National NIC (£000s) 1997 data	Estimated PCT NIC (£000s) 1997 data[a]	Urban West Midlands PCT (£000s) 2000 data[a]
Diuretics	48,349	93	139
Beta-blockers	77,361	149	191
Drugs affecting the renin-angiotensin system	200,003	385	436
Nitrates, calcium antagonists and potassium channel activators	212,031	389	580
Total	537,744	1,016	1,346

Sources: Dr JJ Ferguson as above and Personal Communication Mr J Horgan, SW Birmingham PCT

[a] Scaled for population of 100,000.

The costs of the individual drugs for a 28 day course are shown in **Table 18**.

Table 18: Costs of commonly used antihypertensive agents.[47]

	Example used for price (generic where relevant)	**Cost of 28 days treatment (£)**
Diuretics	Bendrofluazide 2.5mg	0.74
Beta-blockers	Atenolol 50mg	0.85
ACE inhibitors	Enalapril 10mg	5.20
AT II	Losartan 50mg	17.23
Calcium antagonists	Amlodipine 5mg	11.85
Alpha-blocker	Doxazosin 4mg	14.08

Source: BNF 44
ACE inhibitor: angiotensin converting enzyme inhibitor; AT II: angiotensin II receptor blocker.

GP time

A stable hypertensive patient will require approximately two consultations per year regarding hypertension plus blood and urine monitoring as a minimum. A consultation for hypertension with a GP or nurse practitioner has been estimated to cost in the order of £20.[52,53]

Hospital time

Data for this are available from the National Reference Costs 2002.[54] The average cost of a first outpatient appointment for General Medicine (a typical route for referral) is £104 (range £66–143) with follow-up appointments considerably cheaper at £66 (£47–69).

Patient time

It is difficult to estimate this cost, due to the methodological problems such as what assumptions should be made with regard to loss of earnings. One study has suggested that the average costs incurred by patients attending a GP surgery are around £5, compared to £15 for attending medical outpatients.[55] These costs are made up from a survey of patients attending each type of clinic in terms of time and transport costs (both measured from origin of journey back to origin). Time was costed at 1996 average earnings. The greater costs incurred at outpatients reflects both longer time taken and greater transport costs.

6 Effectiveness of services and interventions

The grading of the quality of evidence in this section takes into account both the nature of the evidence (grade 1–4) and the size of the effect (A–E). The definitions are given in the introductory chapter to this series.

Diagnostic tests

Measurement of blood pressure

Natural variation in blood pressure

Blood pressure varies throughout the day and with the performance of various activities.[56] There is also often a variation between arms and with the technique used for measurement (*see* **Table 19**). In view of these variations, recommendations for blood pressure measurement include taking two or three readings of blood pressure at each office visit and only making a diagnosis on the basis of a sustained rise in blood pressure on three separate occasions.[18]

Table 19: Effect of routine activities on blood pressure.[57]

Activity	Effect on blood pressure (mmHg)	
	Systolic Blood Pressure	**Diastolic Blood Pressure**
Attending a meeting	+20	+15
Commuting to work	+16	+13
Dressing	+12	+10
Walking	+12	+6
Talking on the telephone	+10	+7
Eating	+9	+10
Doing desk work	+6	+5
Reading	+2	+2
Watching television	+0.3	+1
Sleep	−10	−8

Mercury sphygmomanometers versus automated sphygmomanometers

Blood pressure has been measured indirectly using a mercury sphygmomanometer with little change for almost 100 years.[58] Measurements are taken using the appearance and disappearance of the Korotkoff sounds I and V.[59] The vast majority of treatment trials for hypertension have used this method of measurement as the basis for their end points.[6] The use of mercury sphygmomanometers is however open to inaccuracy and bias.[56,60,61]

Areas of potential bias include patient factors, operator error and machine error (*see* **Table 20**). Patient factors such as talking, ambient temperature variation or drinking alcohol can make significant differences to blood pressure. Avoidable operator errors include terminal digit preference (rounding of BP to nearest 0 or 5), threshold bias (avoidance of recording readings around a treatment or diagnostic threshold) and inability to accurately distinguish Korotkoff sounds. The position of a person's arm when performing a measurement as well as the size of cuff used can also make a significant difference. Considerable evidence exists regarding poor maintenance and lack of calibration of equipment.[62] The effect of these on recorded blood pressure is harder to estimate but could certainly be significant.

Furthermore, mercury is an environmental pollutant that is due to be phased out.[63] A number of automated electronic sphygmomanometers now exist which are accurate enough to be recommended for routine use.[63] Transferring to electronic blood pressure measurement appears to be associated with a reduction in bias due to rounding but no consistent change in recorded blood pressure.[64]

Table 20: Potential sources of bias in blood pressure measurement (adapted from McAlister *et al.* 2001[56]).

Source of bias	Mean variation of measured blood pressure from actual blood pressure	
	Systolic Blood Pressure	Diastolic Blood Pressure
Operator factors		
Terminal digit preference	Rounding to nearest 10 or 5 mmHg	Rounding to nearest 10 or 5 mmHg
Threshold bias	Increased frequency of recorded BP just below threshold	Increased frequency of recorded BP just below threshold
Inability to distinguish Korotkoff sounds	Wide variation	Wide variation
Position of patient's arm	↓ or ↑ 8 mmHg for every 10 cm above or below heart level	↓ or ↑ 8 mmHg for every 10 cm above or below heart level
Failure to support arm	↑ 2 mmHg	↑ 2 mmHg
Cuff too small	↓ 8 mmHg	↑ 8 mmHg
Patient factors		
Talking	↑ 17 mmHg	↑ 13 mmHg
Acute exposure to cold	↑ 11 mmHg	↑ 8 mmHg
Acute ingestion of alcohol	↑ 8 mmHg for ≤3 hours	↑ 7 mmHg for ≤3 hours
Supine rather than sitting	No effect; ↑ 3 mmHg in supine position	↓ 2–5 mmHg in supine position
Equipment factors		
Poorly calibrated machine	Unquantifiable but potentially clinically significant	Unquantifiable but potentially clinically significant

Setting of measurement: home versus office readings

The standard method of measuring blood pressure is in an 'office' setting (hospital outpatient or primary care surgery).[18] Blood pressure measured in these circumstances may be affected by the 'white coat effect'.[65] The recent availability of relatively affordable accurate automated electronic sphygmomanometers has made self-measurement of blood pressure in the home a realistic alternative for some people.[66] Absolute values of home measurement tend to be lower than office measurements and so a different normal range needs to be adopted. A meta-analysis of home blood pressure measurement studies concluded that a threshold for normotension of ≤135/85 mmHg was appropriate for home measurement.[67] However, many machines currently on the market have not been adequately evaluated for accuracy.[63]

One UK primary care study has evaluated the use of home blood pressure measurement by patients borrowing equipment from a practice and found this method to be feasible.[42] A recent small study in Hampshire found self-measurement in the surgery to be broadly comparable with measurement by a nurse and acceptable to patients.[68] Key issues in self-measurement are the training of individuals to use the equipment satisfactorily and ongoing calibration of that equipment.[61] Few long-term large scale randomised studies (>100 patients per group for >6 months) exist providing evidence with respect to the effectiveness of self-measurement compared to office.

Ambulatory versus one-off readings

The results of ambulatory blood pressure monitoring correlate more closely with target organ damage than those from office measurements.[69] Some consensus on reference ranges for ambulatory blood pressure monitoring has been achieved with 24-hour readings of ≤135/85 mmHg considered normal.[70] The major issues with ambulatory measurement are the lack of availability due to cost even in very developed countries such as the USA and the paucity of evidence of effectiveness in treating individuals on the basis of ambulatory measurements as opposed to one-off readings.[71]

The accuracy of one-off readings can be improved by multiple readings on the same occasion although it may take several readings on more than one occasion to reach a steady state.[72] The reasons for this include regression to the mean and cuff response. In the former, the natural variation in an individuals' blood pressure means that a single measurement will not be a good representation of an individuals' true mean blood pressure. In cuff response, the defence reaction of an individual to cuff inflation is attenuated over time as blood pressure measurement becomes more familiar. As a result, most consensus guidelines (see above, guidelines) recommend multiple readings over time before a diagnosis of hypertension is made, the number and time period recommended being dependent on the level of blood pressure recorded.

Tests for end organ damage and/or underlying cause

Tests performed are either to exclude a possible secondary cause for hypertension (for instance renal disease tested for using serum creatinine and urinalysis) or to look for end organ damage secondary to prolonged raised blood pressure (for instance the use of ECG or echocardiography to test for left ventricular hypertrophy). A list of standard and possible tests along with the rationale for doing them appears in section 5.

Screening for hypertension

Systematic versus opportunistic

Systematic screening aims to cover a population by systematically calling up a population to be screened in a clinic or by visiting them at home. Opportunistic screening is performed when a person presents themselves for some other reason (for instance attends the general practitioner for contraceptive advice). The latter may lead to similar rates of coverage provided that opportunistic attendance is high enough: in the UK around 90% of patients will visit their general practitioner over three years, and the consultation rate is rising.[73,74] Trials that have examined the yield of unknown hypertensive patients from systematic compared to opportunistic methods have shown little difference in detection rates for hypertension.[8]

Different settings for systematic and opportunistic screening

Practice-based

An RCT of practice-based systematic screening (two invitations to attend for screening two years apart) compared to control (i.e. opportunistic detection) in two UK practices resulted in a 73% population coverage for the first round of screening and 66% for the repeat screening round. No difference was found compared to control in prevalence of diastolic blood pressure >95 mmHg five years after initial screening (10.8% vs 10.9%).[75] A Canadian RCT compared nurse-led case finding with usual care. After 5 years the nurses had measured blood pressure on 91% of the target population compared with 80% by usual care.[76] Case finding by Norwegian general practitioners was compared to systematic screening using a before and after design. Almost 90% of cases identified by screening had already been detected by case finding.[77] One study in Bristol examined the effect of calculating cardiovascular risk in patients with hypertension and found no effect in terms of a reduction of patients' cardiovascular risk (measured in terms of reducing risk below a prespecified threshold of a 10% 5 year cardiovascular risk).[78] However, a reduction in systolic blood pressure compared to usual care was seen in the group where risk had been calculated using a chart but not in those whose risk was calculated using a computer program.

Community-based

A number of studies attempting case finding by 'health fairs' in shopping malls or housing blocks have been unsuccessful in achieving even modest rates of participation.[8] A US RCT based on the population of three apartment blocks achieved 43% coverage with door to door screening compared with invitation to a central site of 8%.[79]

Possible adverse consequences of screening

Labelling

There are conflicting results from studies studying the effect of labelling in hypertension suggesting that although labelling may have detrimental effects in terms of absenteeism following diagnosis, these effects can be mitigated by an intervention programme.[8]

Non-pharmacological treatment of hypertension (quality of evidence B I-2)

Evidence for the effectiveness of non-pharmacological intervention in hypertension comes from observational studies or small trials with end points in terms of blood pressure reduction rather than cardiovascular morbidity or mortality. The evidence for the effectiveness of exercise, weight loss, salt restriction and a low fat, high fruit and vegetable diet is presented in **Table 21**. Many of the trials of non-pharmacological interventions are relatively short in duration and individuals often find that exercise and weight loss in particular are difficult to maintain in the longer term.

Table 21: Effectiveness of lifestyle interventions for lowering blood pressure in people with primary hypertension.[80]

Intervention	Mean decrease in BP (mmHg)	Number of RCTs (people)	Participants	Duration (weeks)	Mean change in targeted factor	Reference and evidence rank
Exercise	4/3	54 (2,419)	Sedentary adults >18	>2	At least 15 min aerobic 3x per week	[81] BI-1
Salt restriction	4/2. 2/0.5	58 (2,161) 28 (1,131)	Mean age 49 Mean age 47	1–52 4	118 mmol/day 60 mmol/day	[82] BI-1 [82]
Weight loss	3/3	18 (2,611)	55% male, mean age 50	2–52	3–9% of body weight (mean weight 85 kg)	[83] BI-1
Low fat high fruit and vegetable diet	5.5/3	1 (459)	50% male, mean age 44	8		[84] BI-1

Exercise (quality of evidence B I-1)

The evidence from randomised studies for exercise reducing blood pressure shows small but significant reductions in the short term (regimes lasting at least 2 weeks) when compared to no exercise but trial evidence from longer studies (6 months or more) is equivocal with smaller non-significant reductions.[81,85] One large observational study suggests that those performing regular exercise several times per week have lower all cause and cardiovascular mortality (all cause mortality RR 0.43, 95% CI 0.22 to 0.82; cardiovascular mortality RR 0.33, 95% CI 0.11 to 0.94).[86]

Salt restriction (quality of evidence B I-1)

Randomised studies have shown that dietary salt restriction leads to small but significant reductions in blood pressure. The effect appears to be related to the extent of salt restriction with greater reductions in BP resulting from greater reductions in salt intake. A recent systematic review found that a mean reduction of 118 mmol/l (= 6700 mg; 2000 mg = one level teaspoon of salt) for 1 month led to a reduction of 3.9 mmHg (95% CI 3.0 mmHg to 4.8 mmHg) in systolic blood pressure and 1.9 mmHg (95% CI 1.3 mmHg to 2.5 mmHg) in diastolic blood pressure.[82] Hooper *et al.* have looked at the longer term effects of salt restriction advice and found smaller but still significant reductions in systolic blood pressure but not diastolic blood pressure at follow-ups between 13 and 60 months.[87] Despite these robust findings of benefit in terms of blood pressure reduction, there is no satisfactory evidence of the effects of salt restriction on mortality and morbidity and subsequently there has been much debate in the literature regarding the 'real life' benefits.[88] Whilst there is debate on the efficacy of salt restriction on 'hard' end points, the evidence of any harm from salt restriction is weak due to methodological problems.[89]

Weight loss (quality of evidence B I-1)

Relatively small reductions of weight (of the order of around 5 kg) over short periods of time have been shown to be associated with small reductions of blood pressure (around 3 mmHg) in hypertensive patients. A systematic review found that in 6 RCTs where antihypertensive regimens were not varied during the intervention period, losing weight (mean weight 85kg; mean reduction 3–9%) reduced blood pressure by 3.0/2.9 mmHg, compared to no weight loss.[83]

Diet (quality of evidence B I-2)

One study has found that a diet low in fat and high in fruit and vegetables taken for 8 weeks lowered blood pressure by 5.5/3 mmHg compared to a 'control diet' low in magnesium and calcium. The results from this should be interpreted with caution due to the short duration and the fact that all food eaten by subjects in the study was prepared in a central kitchen, a setting unlikely to be reflected in usual daily life.[84] A systematic review on the effects of potassium supplementation on blood pressure found that supplementation (60–100 mmol per day) led to a mean reduction of blood pressure of 3/2 mmHg.[90] Fish oils taken in large quantities (3g daily) led to a reduction in blood pressure of 3/2 mmHg.[91] There is insufficient evidence on the efficacy of other forms of dietary intervention including calcium and magnesium supplementation to judge effectiveness of blood pressure lowering in hypertensives.[92]

Pharmacological treatment

Treatment of raised blood pressure leads to benefit in terms of total death rate, cardiovascular death rate, stroke, major coronary events and congestive heart failure. Absolute benefit is dependent on absolute risk, which depends on age and level of blood pressure.

Effects of lowering blood pressure

Various reviews and meta-analyses have been performed on the effects of treatment of hypertension. The data presented here are from Collins and Peto's 1994 update of their 1990 *The Lancet* meta-analysis and from a subsequent individual patient data analysis by Gueyffier.[6,93] The Collins meta-analysis used data derived from four large and 13 small unconfounded randomised trials of pharmacological treatment reported between 1965 and 1992. Gueyffier used individual patient data from seven of the larger trials with considerable overlap between the two reviews. The sample sizes in the trials ranged from under 100 to over 17 000 with totals of 47 653 and 40 777 patients used by Collins and Gueyffier respectively. Most of the trials used a stepped approach to therapy with a diuretic being the main first line treatment used. Mean follow-up was for 4–5 years. Treatment was compared to either placebo or usual care. Treatment resulted in approximately a 5–6 mmHg reduction in diastolic blood pressure (reductions in systolic BP not available for all studies but likely to have been about double the diastolic reduction). Collins provides overall data for men and women whereas Gueyffier breaks down by gender.

Total death rate (quality of evidence C I-1)

Total mortality was significantly reduced but the absolute figures have not been quoted by Collins and Peto.[6] They equate to approximately a 12% relative risk reduction. Gueyffier quotes OR for total mortality in favour of treatment for women of 0.91 (95% CI 0.81–1.01, p=0.094) and for men of 0.88 (0.8–0.97, p=0.013).[93]

Cardiovascular death rate (quality of evidence A I-1)

Cardiovascular death rate was reduced by 21% in the treatment group compared to control in Collins and Peto's review.[6] Gueyffier quotes ORs of 0.86 (0.74–1.01, p=0.068) for women and 0.80 (0.70–0.91, p=<0.001) for mean, again in favour of treatment.[93]

Stroke (quality of evidence A I-1)

A highly significant reduction in relative risk of stroke was seen of 38% (95% CI 31–45%). Results for fatal and non-fatal stroke were similar.[6] Gueyffier's review also found highly significant reductions in stroke for both men and women (OR in favour of treatment 0.63 (0.52–0.73) women and 0.66 (0.56–0.78) for men, both p<0.001).[93]

Major coronary events (quality of evidence A I-1)

A highly significant reduction in relative risk of major coronary events was seen of 16% (95% CI 8–23%).[6] Gueyffier's review also found reductions in coronary events in favour of treatment (OR 0.85 (0.72–1.01, p=0.059) women and 0.82 (0.73–0.92, p=<0.001)).[93]

Congestive heart failure (quality of evidence A I-1)

No results for congestive heart failure are given by either Collins' or Gueyffier's reviews. A third meta-analysis also by Gueyffier (and using very similar trials to the Collins review) found an OR for congestive heart failure of 0.54 (0.43–0.68) in favour of treatment in trials on older people.[94] The result for younger people was non-significantly in favour of treatment but this is likely to be due to lack of power in view of very few events.

Adverse effects compared to placebo

Gueyffier's 1996 meta-analysis showed no increase in non-cardiovascular mortality or major morbidity in those receiving antihypertensive treatment as compared to placebo.[93] Treatment of hypertension *per se* does not appear to influence quality of life adversely: for patients in the HOT study, the lower the achieved blood pressure, the better the quality of life.

What drugs have been shown to be effective?

Placebo controlled trials, or new drugs compared to old drugs of proven efficacy

Most placebo controlled trials with major morbidity/mortality as end points have used diuretics and/or beta-blockers and it is this evidence that is presented above. Newer agents have typically been evaluated against secondary end points such as blood pressure reduction achieved or compared to older drugs of proven efficacy. The results of randomised comparisons and systematic reviews for the individual classes of antihypertensive are presented below. It is likely that the bulk of benefit from these drugs comes from their effect on blood pressure which lowers risk of cardiovascular disease and in particular stroke to levels approaching those expected from observational studies of the effect of blood pressure in populations.[95]

Diuretics and beta-blockers (quality of evidence A I-1)

See above for results from meta-analysis of trials of diuretics (typically thiazide diuretics ± amiloride) and/or beta-blockers compared with placebo in the treatment of hypertension. Of note is the fact that the doses of thiazides used in many of these trials was typically much higher than in common use today (e.g. bendrofluazide 10mg vs 2.5mg in current practice). Lower doses have a lower incidence of side effects albeit at marginally lower effects on blood pressure.[96] Two systematic reviews have compared diuretics with beta-blockers.[97,98] No significant difference was found in terms of blood pressure reduction but although diuretics were found to reduce coronary events, no evidence was found that beta-blockers reduce coronary events. However, beta-blockers are known to reduce coronary events in other circumstances, e.g. post-myocardial infarction.[99]

Angiotensin converting enzyme inhibitors (quality of evidence A I-1)

A systematic review of ACE inhibitors for lowering blood pressure found similar effects in terms of outcome to older drugs.[100] Recent RCTs have given conflicting results over whether ACE inhibitors confer benefit in addition to the direct effect on lowering blood pressure.[101,102] The HOPE study compared an ACE inhibitor with placebo in people at high cardiovascular risk (history of ischaemic heart disease or diabetes plus a risk factor) but not necessarily with hypertension.[101] This found significant benefit for the intervention group in terms of a composite primary end point of myocardial infarction, stroke, or death from cardiovascular causes despite only modest blood pressure reduction (136/76 in the ramipril group vs 139/77 in the placebo group at the end of the trial). Similarly, the PROGRESS post stroke trial found significant benefit in terms of the intervention comprising a diuretic and ACE inhibitor with a reduction in blood pressure of 9/4 mmHg.[102] The benefits were seen in patients with high and 'normal' blood pressure at base line. Wing *et al.* from Australia performed an open label study in healthy older people comparing ACE inhibitors and diuretics as first line treatment with no limit on other classes of treatment used as 'add on' if required. Patients were included with blood pressures of over 140/90 without recent cardiovascular events, contraindications to ACE inhibitor or diuretics and without significant renal impairment. They found a hazard ratio for a cardiovascular event or death with ACE inhibitor treatment of 0.89 (95% CI 0.79–1.00; p=0.05) despite similar blood pressure reductions (26/12 mmHg), suggesting that ACE inhibitors might have additional beneficial effects apart from their impact on blood pressure.[103]

However, the recently reported results from the ALLHAT study comparing a diuretic, ACE inhibitor and calcium antagonist have cast doubt on a special effect from ACE inhibitors, with no difference found in all cause mortality between the groups with over 33 000 people randomised.[104] Any differences between classes were in terms of secondary outcomes, in favour of the diuretic, and likely to be due to small differences in achieved blood pressure. Similarly, the prospective meta-analysis conducted by the Blood Pressure Lowering Treatment Trialists Collaboration, which included both ALLHAT and Wing *et al.*'s results, found no difference between ACE inhibitors and calcium antagonists, or diuretics or beta-blockers in terms of total major cardiovascular events.[44]

Calcium antagonists (quality of evidence A I-1)

Calcium antagonists reduced blood pressure to equivalent levels compared with diuretics but considerable controversy has surrounded possible adverse effects in comparison with other classes of antihypertensive treatment. Evidence from previous observational studies, small RCTs and meta-analyses has suggested that calcium antagonists are inferior at protecting against heart failure and cardiovascular events, particularly MI, in comparison to other classes of drugs.[105–107] However, data from the ALLHAT study suggests that the differences between calcium antagonists and other classes of drugs with respect to CHD, all cause mortality and cardiovascular disease are negligible and may have been due to either differences in achieved blood pressure or chance findings in previous smaller studies.[104] The one secondary outcome where the calcium channel blocker performed poorly in comparison to the diuretic was in terms of a 38% higher risk of heart failure. This secondary outcome included deaths, hospitalisations and treated non-hospitalised patients and may be in part explained by the fact that the use of diuretics may mask a clinical diagnosis of heart failure by reducing oedema. The latest publication by the Blood Pressure Trialists Prospective Meta-analysis Collaboration found no significant difference between calcium antagonists, ACE inhibitors, beta-blockers and diuretics in terms of cardiovascular events, death or total mortality but found that ACE inhibitors, beta-blockers and diuretics were all superior to calcium antagonists for heart failure that caused death or admission to hospital.[44]

Alpha-blockers (quality of evidence B I-1)

The best evidence for the use of alpha-blockers in hypertension again comes from the ALLHAT trial, in which the alpha-blocker – diuretic arm was terminated and reported early.[108] This found that although no difference was seen in the main end point of fatal CHD or non-fatal MI, the alpha-blocker (doxazosin) performed significantly worse with respect to both the combined CVD end point (25% increase) and congestive heart failure (doubling of risk). These results need to be interpreted cautiously because the diuretic arm achieved a small but significantly greater reduction in systolic blood pressure (2 mmHg) which may be enough to explain some or all of the increased risk (especially in non-CHF CVD), and again the clinical diagnosis of CHF is likely to have been reduced in the diuretic group. Nevertheless, the degree of increased risk is probably significant enough to avoid the first line use of alpha-blockers unless there is good reason in terms of drug intolerance or co-morbidity, particularly benign prostatic hypertrophy.

Angiotensin II receptor antagonists (quality of evidence A I-I)

Angiotensin II antagonists (AT II blockers) are a more recent development in hypertension and work by blocking a different part of the renin-angiotensin pathway than ACE inhibitors. A systematic review has examined the evidence for efficacy in terms of blood pressure reduction and found the various compounds in this group to be broadly similar.[109] One large RCT has compared cardiovascular end points for an AT II blocker with that of a beta-blocker in patients with hypertension and left ventricular hypertrophy and found a reduction in the primary end point of combined cardiovascular mortality and morbidity.[110] These results need to be interpreted with caution in view of the fact that the AT II group attained slightly lower blood pressure and the major effect seen was on stroke which is most affected by blood pressure reduction. In addition, patients in the AT II group were more likely to have received other drugs including a thiazide diuretic (see above for comments regarding the efficacy of diuretics in the ALLHAT study).

Nitrates and potassium channel activators (quality of evidence B III)

Both these classes of drugs tend to reduce blood pressure but are not routinely used or licensed for the treatment of hypertension. Both medications have their main role in the treatment of ischaemic heart disease which is a common co-morbidity in people with hypertension. No RCTs exist of these therapies in terms of effects on morbidity and mortality but it would be expected that any blood pressure reduction achieved from their use would lead to similar effects as seen in other classes of medication.

Other antihypertensive classes (quality of evidence A III)

Three other classes of antihypertensive medication are in use in the UK but usually as third line therapy or on a historical basis. These are vasodilator antihypertensive drugs (e.g. hydralazine), centrally acting antihypertensives (e.g. clonadine, moxonadine) and adrenergic neurone blocking drugs (e.g. guanethidine). These older classes of drugs have not in general been used in any of the modern randomised comparisons although hydralazine, clonidine and reserpine were part of the titration scheme used in the ALLHAT study.[104] Again, on the basis of blood pressure lowering, the effects of these medications on cardiovascular effects would be expected to be similar to diuretics and beta-blockers.

Other pharmacological interventions to lower cardiovascular risk

Evidence exists for the use of both aspirin and cholesterol-lowering drugs in patients with hypertension. The following section refers to the use of these interventions in the primary prevention of cardiovascular disease, i.e. in patients without other indications such as previous stroke or myocardial infarction.

Anti-platelet therapy (quality of evidence A I-1)

The evidence for the use of anti-platelet therapy (in most cases low dose aspirin) in patients at increased cardiovascular risk (hypertension or other risk factor) has been summarised in a systematic review.[80] This gives an estimate of approximately 1.2 events avoided per 1000 person years in a total pool of over 50 000 patients. Treatment is associated with a risk of haemorrhage (major extracranial and intracranial) of similar magnitude. The choice to treat asymptomatic patients with aspirin must therefore depend both on absolute risk of cardiovascular event and likelihood of haemorrhage. The BHS guidelines recommend treatment with aspirin only in individuals over the age of 50, with blood pressure controlled below 150/90 and a 10 year cardiovascular risk of $\geq$15%.[18]

Cholesterol lowering (quality of evidence A I-1)

Several systematic reviews and subsequent RCTs have shown that although cholesterol lowering therapy reduces CHD risk when used for primary prevention, it does not have an effect on overall mortality.[111] This is likely to be due to the fact that the absolute risk of cardiovascular disease in patients with hypertension (or other risk factors) but not frank cardiovascular disease is too low for benefit to be clearcut. The ALLHAT study, which in addition to antihypertensives studied the use of pravastatin 40 mg against 'usual care', found no benefit in terms of either all cause mortality or CHD.[112] Prior to the landmark '4S' study, concerns had been raised regarding a possible excess of violent death due to cholesterol lowering.[113,114] The '4S' study randomised 4444 people with coronary heart disease and moderately raised cholesterol to simvastatin or placebo and was the first cholesterol lowering study to find a reduction in all cause mortality (30%). Subsequent meta-analysis of statin cholesterol lowering trials has found no evidence of increased risk of accidental death, suicide or trauma.[115] Jackson *et al.* have attempted to quantify the level of risk at which the potential harm from cholesterol lowering might out weigh potential benefits.[116] The conclusions reached were that for those at low CHD risk (<13% 10 year CHD risk) the evidence for an overall benefit in terms of mortality was poor and that absolute safety had not been demonstrated for this group. Above this level, however, benefits outweighed risk. However, the results of the recent ASCOT trial cholesterol lowering arm showed benefit from lipid lowering (atorvastatin 10 mg) compared to placebo in terms of non-fatal MI and fatal CHD for patients with a 10 year CHD risk of approximately 10% (although off antihypertensive treatment this risk would have been approximately doubled).[117] These results, along with those from the Heart Protection Study (simvastatin 40 mg vs placebo for 20 536 UK adults (aged 40–80 years) with coronary disease, other occlusive arterial disease, or diabetes), suggest that benefit from statins is still present at lower risks, with little evidence of significant adverse effects.[118]

Adverse effects of drug therapy

Trial data on adverse effects suggests that with modern therapies, around 2% of patients will suffer adverse effects from treatment.[25] These are mostly dose-related and clearly linked to the individual drug classes, for instance ankle swelling with calcium channel blockers, cough with ACE inhibitors or cold extremities with beta-blockers. Most trial designs are not appropriate for identifying rare events which may only occur after years of treatment. Case control or cohort designs are most appropriate in these circumstances.

A systematic review of individual patient data from RCTs found no evidence of increased non-cardiovascular mortality in patients treated with diuretics or beta-blockers compared to placebo.[94]

A systematic review investigated the association between diuretic use and renal cell carcinoma.[119] 12 studies were reviewed, 9 case control and 3 cohort. A small but significant increase in renal cell carcinoma was found (OR in case control studies 1.55 (95% CI 1.42 1.71, p<0.00001)). The significance of these results is unclear: renal cell carcinoma is rare, many millions of people worldwide take diuretics, and there is a possibility that the results are confounded by an effect of hypertension on renal cell carcinoma or vice versa.

A secondary analysis of the treatment of mild hypertension study examined the differences in rate of sexual dysfunction between acebutolol, amlodipine, chlorthalidone, doxazosin, enalapril or placebo.[120] After 2 years chlorthalidone was associated with a higher rate of erectile problems than the other groups or placebo. Baseline levels of erectile dysfunction (ED) were 14% and related to age. Although the chlorthalidone group had higher rates of ED, the absolute numbers were small due to small sample sizes.

Numerous other side effects have been reported from the various classes of antihypertensive and are summarised in **Table 22**.

Table 22: Side effects of commonly used classes of antihypertensive.[47]

Drug class and example	Side effects
Thiazide diuretics *Bendrofluazide*	Postural hypotension and mild gastrointestinal effects; impotence (reversible on withdrawal of treatment); hypokalaemia (see also notes above), hypomagnesaemia, hyponatraemia, hypercalcaemia, hypochloraemic alkalosis, hyperuricaemia, gout, hyperglycaemia and altered plasma lipid concentration; less commonly rashes, photosensitivity; blood disorders (including neutropenia and thrombocytopenia – when given in late pregnancy neonatal thrombocytopenia has been reported); pancreatitis, intrahepatic cholestasis and hypersensitivity reactions (including pneumonitis, pulmonary oedema, severe skin reactions) also reported.
Beta-blockers *Propranolol*	Bradycardia, heart failure, hypotension, conduction disorders, bronchospasm, peripheral vasoconstriction (including exacerbation of intermittent claudication and Raynaud's phenomenon), gastrointestinal disturbances, fatigue, sleep disturbances; rare reports of rashes and dry eyes (reversible on withdrawal), exacerbation of psoriasis; see also notes above.
Alpha-blockers *Doxazosin*	Postural hypotension; dizziness, vertigo, headache, fatigue, asthenia, oedema, somnolence, nausea, rhinitis; less frequently abdominal discomfort, diarrhoea, vomiting, agitation, tremor, rash, pruritus; rarely blurred vision, epistaxis, haematuria, thrombocytopenia, purpura, leucopenia, hepatitis, jaundice, cholestasis and urinary incontinence; isolated cases of priapism and impotence reported.
ACE inhibitors *Captopril*	ACE inhibitors can cause profound hypotension and renal impairment (in patients with severe bilateral renal artery stenosis), and a persistent dry cough. They may also cause angioedema (onset may be delayed), rash (which may be associated with pruritus and urticaria), pancreatitis and upper respiratory-tract symptoms such as sinusitis, rhinitis and sore throat. Gastrointestinal effects reported with ACE inhibitors include nausea, vomiting, dyspepsia, diarrhoea and constipation. Altered liver function tests, cholestatic jaundice and hepatitis have been reported. Blood disorders including thrombocytopenia, leucopenia, neutropenia and haemolytic anaemia have also been reported. Other reported side-effects include headache, dizziness, fatigue, malaise, taste disturbance, paraesthesia, bronchospasm, fever, serositis, vasculitis, myalgia, arthralgia, positive antinuclear antibody, raised erythrocyte sedimentation rate, eosinophilia, leucocytosis and photosensitivity, tachycardia, serum sickness, weight loss, stomatitis, maculopapular rash, photosensitivity, flushing and acidosis.
AT II blockers *Candesartan*	Side-effects are usually mild. Symptomatic hypotension may occur, particularly in patients with intravascular volume depletion (e.g. those taking high-dose diuretics). Hyperkalaemia occurs occasionally; angioedema has also been reported with some angiotensin-II receptor antagonists. See notes above; also upper respiratory-tract and influenza-like symptoms including rhinitis and pharyngitis; abdominal pain, back pain, arthralgia, myalgia, nausea, headache, dizziness, peripheral oedema, rash also reported; rarely urticaria, pruritus, blood disorders reported.
Calcium antagonists *Amlodipine*	Headache, oedema, fatigue, nausea, flushing, dizziness, gum hyperplasia, rashes (including rarely pruritus and very rarely erythema multiforme); rarely gastrointestinal disturbances, dry mouth, sweating, palpitations, dyspnoea, drowsiness, mood changes, myalgia, arthralgia, asthenia, peripheral neuropathy, impotence, increased urinary frequency, visual disturbances; also reported, jaundice, pancreatitis, hyperglycaemia, thrombocytopenia, vasculitis, angioedema, alopecia, gynaecomastia.

Comparisons between different drug classes (quality of evidence A I-1)

As discussed above in the individual drug class sections, there is little convincing evidence of a differential effect in terms of cardiovascular morbidity and mortality or all cause mortality between the various classes of antihypertensives, at least with regard to diuretics, beta-blockers, ACE inhibitors and calcium channel blockers. For an individual person with hypertension the choice may well be influenced by co-morbidities such as heart failure, diabetes or benign prostatic hypertrophy. Blood pressure lowering in patients with hypertension and co-existing heart failure in particular is more effectively treated with diuretics, ACE inhibitors or beta-blockers rather than calcium antagonists. Furthermore, individuals may achieve better results in terms of blood pressure lowering with different drugs: in one small trial, 56 hypertensive patients were randomised between and then rotated in turn through four drug classes comprising a diuretic, beta-blocker, ACE inhibitor and calcium antagonist.[121] Rotation around the four classes doubled the chance of controlled blood pressure on monotherapy as compared to the first drug randomised to.

Class effects vs specific drugs (quality of evidence A I-1)

The effect of antihypertensive drugs in reducing stroke and coronary heart disease risk appears to be largely due to the blood pressure lowering properties of these drugs and so would be expected to be a class effect rather than specific to a given drug.[104] This is in keeping with epidemiological studies showing the association of lower blood pressure with lower cardiovascular risk. The recent HOPE trial using the ACE inhibitor ramipril found a significant reduction in its combined outcome of myocardial infarction, stroke or cardiovascular death despite apparently very modest blood pressure effects (2.4 mmHg/1 mmHg).[122] However, a sub-study of HOPE involving 24-hour blood pressure monitoring of a sample of the subjects found that the mean blood pressure lowering achieved by ramipril was sufficiently lower than that of the control group to explain the reduction in risk seen.[123] Thus, the 'additional' benefits of ramipril can probably be explained by blood pressure lowering alone.

Older drugs vs newer drugs

The best evidence for benefit from the treatment of hypertension comes from studies of the older classes of drugs, namely diuretics and beta-blockers. See above for further details. The evidence from the ALLHAT study and meta-analyses suggests that little if any important differences exist between old and new drugs given equivalence of blood pressure lowering.[104]

Treatment in specific circumstances

Isolated systolic hypertension (quality of evidence A I-1)

A meta-analysis has investigated the effects of treating isolated systolic hypertension (systolic >160 mmHg and diastolic <95 mmHg) in patients aged 60 years or more.[45] Eight trials containing 15 963 patients were examined with a median follow-up of 3.8 years. The relative hazard associated with a 10 mmHg higher initial systolic blood pressure was 1.26 (p=0.0001) for total mortality and 1.22 (p=0.02) for stroke but not significantly raised for coronary events. Treating systolic hypertension reduced total mortality by 13% (95% CI 2–22, p=0.02), cardiovascular mortality by 18%, all cardiovascular complications by 26%, stroke by 30% and coronary events by 23%. Absolute benefits of treatment were increased for men vs women (NNT 18 vs 38), at or above age 70 (NNT 19 vs 39) and in patients with previous cardiovascular complications (NNT 16 vs 37).

Older people (quality of evidence A I-1)

Older people are at higher absolute risk for all types of cardiovascular disease and so will tend to receive greater benefit in terms of absolute risk reduction for any given reduction in blood pressure. Gueyffier's meta-analysis which included seven trials in older patients (mean age >65) found significant risk reductions in terms of congestive heart failure (46% risk reduction), stroke (34% risk reduction), cardiovascular mortality (23% risk reduction), major coronary events (21% risk reduction) and all cause mortality (10% risk reduction).[93] The absolute risk reduction was of the order of 10 events avoided for 1000 patients treated for one year (all end points combined, NNT 100). This is in contrast to the results in the same review for younger patients where the only significant reduction was seen in terms of stroke risk (down 49% vs placebo), but even this was a small reduction in absolute terms (NNT 1000 for one year to prevent one event). Messerli examined ten trials involving over 16 000 patients aged ≥60 and compared results from those using diuretics with those using beta-blockers.[98] The diuretics were found to be superior in terms of preventing all outcomes studied (cerebrovascular events, fatal stroke, coronary heart disease, cardiovascular mortality, and all cause mortality) and beta-blockers were found only to have a significant effect in stroke prevention, not CHD. This study was not a formal meta-analysis but rather a comparison of the results from the individual trials.

Insufficient evidence currently exists with respect to patients aged over 80 of the efficacy of blood pressure lowering, particularly in terms of mortality. A meta-analysis using data from 1670 elderly people included in trials of blood pressure lowering found that treatment prevented 34% (95% CI 8–52) of strokes. There was a significant decrease in the rate of major cardiovascular events and heart failure, by 22% and 39%, respectively. No treatment benefit was seen for cardiovascular death, and a non-significant 6% (−5 to 18) relative excess of death from all causes.[124]

Minority ethnic groups (quality of evidence A I-1)

Many of the large randomised trials in hypertension have previously included few patients from minority ethnic groups. Responses to the standard classes of antihypertensive will be different depending on ethnicity: African and African-Caribbean people respond better to diuretics and calcium antagonists than to beta-blockers, ACE inhibitors or AT II blockers.[125–128] This applies only to monotherapy and these differences in efficacy are eliminated when used in combination. The recent consensus statement on the management of high blood pressure in African Americans differs in two key ways from guidelines for other ethnic groups: lower blood pressure targets are recommended for diabetes or non-diabetic renal disease (namely <130/80) and combination therapy is recommended first line for patients presenting with blood pressure ≥150/100 mmHg.[129] The ALLHAT study included 35% black and 19% Hispanic patients. Results for chlorthalidone vs amlodipine showed no difference in outcomes for black vs non-black but lisinopril showed poorer blood pressure response, which presumably explains the observed increased risk of stroke and combined CVD for blacks receiving lisinopril compared to those receiving chlorthalidone.[104]

Secondary prevention of stroke (A I-1)

The effect of blood pressure reduction post stroke is covered in detail in the stroke chapter, but briefly, the PROGRESS study has recently confirmed the benefit of blood pressure reduction in this group of people.[130]

Diabetes

See under 'Treatment by sub-category' below.

Treatment targets (quality of evidence A I-1)

The Hypertension Optimal Treatment Trial (HOT) investigated the effect of treating blood pressure in over 18 000 hypertensives to three predetermined treatment targets, namely 90, 85 and 80 mmHg.[25] No significant difference was found between the groups in terms of major cardiovascular events, stroke or total mortality, but a small difference in terms of myocardial infarction was achieved when comparing the 80 and 90 mmHg target groups. This apparent paucity of effect was probably due to a combination of small differences in achieved blood pressure between the three groups (85.5, 83.2 and 81.2 mmHg) and fewer than expected cardiovascular events, which lowered the power of the study. A secondary analysis of events in relation to achieved blood pressure found the lowest incidence of major cardiovascular events at a mean achieved BP of 130–140/80–85 mmHg. Reduction of blood pressure below these values was not associated with further reduction in event incidence.

Achieving currently recommended levels of blood pressure reduction will require combination therapy in the majority of patients. For example, in the HOT study, the mean number of drugs per patient at final follow-up was 1.8, with almost 60% needing two or more medications (*see* **Table 23**).

Table 23: The proportion of patients taking antihypertensive drugs at the final visit of the HOT Study.

Number of medications	Proportion taking
0 drug	1.9%
1 drug	37.9%
2 drugs	43.8%
3 drugs	13.6%

Source: data on file, Astra Zeneca. Personal communication from Paul Sellwood

Treatment by sub-category

This section refers back to the sub-categories defined in section 3.

Groups 1 & 2 (essential hypertension) (A I-1)

The absolute effect of treatment is directly proportional to absolute level of baseline risk. Older (>65 years) patients are in general at higher risk. On average, treating 1000 older adults for 1 year can be expected to prevent five strokes (95% CI 2–8), three coronary events (95% CI 1–4) and four cardiovascular deaths (1–8). Similar blood pressure reductions in middle aged (<65) hypertensives prevent only one stroke (0–2) per thousand person years of treatment, with no significant effect on coronary events or mortality.[93]

Group 3 (hypertension and diabetes) (A I-1)

Treatment of blood pressure in patients with diabetes is at least as effective as in those without, due to increased absolute risk of cardiovascular disease.[131] Elderly hypertensive diabetics have double the risk of stroke, cardiovascular events and all cause mortality compared to non-diabetics.

With regard to target blood pressure, the BHS guidelines recommend 140/80 as goal BP for diabetics, based on a sub-group analysis of the HOT trial.[18,25] This same data has been interpreted by others as suggesting lower targets (130/80 or lower).[132]

Tighter blood pressure control in patients with diabetes has been associated with reduction in risk of deaths and complications related to diabetes (progression of diabetic retinopathy and reduction in visual acuity).[26] Sub-group analysis of the 1501 patients with diabetes in the Hypertension Optimal Treatment Trial found a reduction in major cardiovascular events (RR 2.06 (95% CI 1.24–3.4)), and cardiovascular mortality (RR 3.0 (1.28–7.08), p=0.016) in the group randomised to a target diastolic blood pressure of 80 mmHg compared to a target of 90 mmHg. These reductions were not seen in the study population as a whole but this is likely to be due to the much higher event rate in the diabetic population.[133] The benefit of intensive treatment appears to be independent of whether low-dose diuretics, beta-blockers, angiotensin-converting enzyme inhibitors or calcium antagonists are used as first line treatment.[134] Diabetics with proteinuria or impaired renal function benefit from even lower BP (systolic <125 mmHg).[135]

Group 4 (malignant hypertension) (A I-1)

Patients with malignant hypertension need emergency treatment of their blood pressure. Early trials of lowering very high blood pressure leave no doubt as to the efficacy of treatment.[136]

Group 5 (secondary hypertension) (A II-1)

Treatment of the underlying cause of secondary hypertension may lead to improvements in blood pressure. In a retrospective study of 1000 secondary care hypertensive patients, 47 were found to have some form of secondary hypertension, of whom 18 had blood pressure improved or normalised after operative treatment of the underlying cause or cessation of oral contraception.[120]

Group 6 (white coat hypertension) (C III)

Treatment of white coat hypertension is generally considered unnecessary and there is evidence that although clinic BP may be lowered by treatment, little effect is seen on ambulatory BP.[137]

Population approaches to lower blood pressure (C I-I)

Population level interventions to reduce blood pressure are attractive in theory. Evidence from both observational studies and treatment trials shows that lower blood pressure is associated with better prognosis from a wide range of cardiovascular outcomes. Initiatives might include programmes aimed at smoking cessation, increasing exercise, reducing salt in processed foods (for example bread) or healthier eating (the 'five fruit a day' campaign). Higher cigarette prices (e.g. by higher taxes) have been shown to reduce cigarette consumption.[138] The evidence from the effect of instituting smoke-free workplaces shows a reduction in overall tobacco consumption.[139] A modelling exercise published this year suggested that salt reduction on a population basis (possibly by legislation for processed food) was one of the most cost-effective methods of reducing blood pressure.[140] A number of supermarket chains have now agreed to reduce the salt content in processed food in response to concerns raised by amongst others the Department of Health.[141] A systematic review of physical activity promotion (11 studies) found that interventions that encouraged walking and did not require attendance at a central facility were most likely to lead to sustainable increases in overall physical activity.[142] Initial evaluations of the 'five-a-day' programme suggest that it is possible to increase fruit and vegetable intake.[143]

Cost-effectiveness studies

When considering the cost-effectiveness of blood pressure lowering treatment a number of factors need to be taken into account. Many of these have already been considered earlier in this section, and include:

- treatment threshold
- treatment target
- perspective of costs
- blood pressure lowering vs effect on cardiovascular risk
- antihypertensive vs other interventions to lower cardiovascular risk.

Pearce *et al.* performed a cost minimisation analysis based on the number needed to treat (NNT) to prevent one stroke, MI or death from a meta-analysis of 15 major trials of antihypertensive treatment.[10] This US study found an NNT of 86 for middle aged patients with uncomplicated mild hypertension and 29 for elderly patients. The results are presented in **Table 24**. The drugs used and costs are based on US prices, but the price differentials are similar in the UK. Diuretic therapy remained most cost-effective, even under the unlikely assumption that newer drugs were 50% more effective at preventing these events than diuretics.

Table 24: Wholesale drug acquisition costs to prevent one MI, stroke or death among patients with uncomplicated mild-to-moderate hypertension.[a]

Drug class	Most common treatment			Least expensive treatment		
	Treatment	Middle aged	Elderly	Treatment	Middle aged	Elderly
Diuretic	HCTZ	£3,400	£1,100	HCTZ	£3,400	£1,100
β-blocker	Atenolol	£75,000	£25,300	Propranolol	£39,100	£13,200
ACE inhibitor	Enalopril	£111,500	£37,700	Trandolapril	£67,300	£22,700
α-blocker	Terazosin	£138,800	£46,800	Doxazosin	£108,000	£36,400
Calcium blocker	Nifedipine GITS	£247,300	£83,400	Nisoldipine	£91,800	£31,000

[a] Costs converted from dollars at rate of $1.4=£1.

The cost-effectiveness of antihypertensive treatment in the UK has recently been evaluated in a modelling exercise by Montgomery and colleagues.[144] They produced a Markov model comparing the effects of treatment for hypertension versus non-treatment and taking into account age, sex, cardiovascular risk, costs and patient preferences. The range of cardiovascular risk considered was from <0.1% per year to almost 30%. The costs of antihypertensive treatment used were fairly conservative, being less than £80 per year for all groups. Antihypertensive treatment resulted in gains in life expectancy for all groups considered but these were small in those at low risk of cardiovascular disease. In all but the oldest age groups, treatment was effective but cost more. In the oldest high risk group, treatment resulted in cost savings. Incremental cost-effectiveness for those at low risk ranged from £1000 to £3300 per quality adjusted life year (QALY) gained and from £30 to £250 per QALY in those at higher risk.

Because the cost-effectiveness of antihypertensive medication varies with absolute risk of stroke and CHD, the costs involved in the intensive treatment of non-insulin dependent diabetics, a high risk group, has been examined. The study was part of the long running UKPDS trial and found that the cost-effectiveness ratio of intensive treatment compared favourably to many accepted health care programmes. The incremental costs are shown in **Table 25**.[145]

Table 25: Incremental costs associated with tight blood pressure control compared to less tight control.[145]

	Costs and effects discounted at 6% per year	Costs discounted at 6% per year, effects not discounted
Incremental cost per extra year free from end points	£1,049	£434
Incremental cost per life year gained	£720	£291

7 Models of care and recommendations

Summary of guidelines for hypertension treatment

Diagnostic thresholds

There is variation in national and international recommendations with respect to diagnostic thresholds in hypertension. The following strategy represents a degree of consensus between the international guidelines and importantly reflects the BHS guideline.[18] Patients with sustained blood pressure over 160/100 need treatment, but the decision for those in the range 140–159/90–99 will depend on the presence of other factors, namely evidence of end organ damage, diabetes or a raised 10 year CHD risk.

No data exist on the proportions of patients requiring treatment in a UK population and the effect of treatment in terms of events prevented, but a group from New Zealand have performed a modelling exercise by extrapolating data from a risk factor survey to the population of Auckland residents.[146] This study showed that a change to treatment on the basis of cardiovascular risk would result in a greater number of cardiovascular events being averted with fewer patients treated, compared to current treatment (largely on the basis of absolute level of blood pressure), even if a conservative threshold of 20% 5 year cardiovascular (CVS) risk were used.

A Swedish review has considered treatment thresholds in the light of cost-effectiveness.[147] For patients aged over 45 cost savings result at a threshold above 100 mmHg, whereas in younger patients, even blood pressure above 105 mmHg was associated with costs per life year gained as high as £28 300–42 200 (1992 prices).

Treatment targets

The various guidelines give similar recommendations on treatment targets as indicated in **Table 26**. One study of 876 patients from 18 UK general practices found that the proportion of patients with controlled hypertension varied between 17.5% and 84.6%, depending on which guidelines were used.[148]

Choice of antihypertensive drug

The latest guideline from the British Hypertension Society regarding treatment choice is the 'ABCD algorithm'.[46] The recommendations for choice of first line antihypertensive drug are as follows:

1   In younger non-black patients either angiotensin-converting enzyme inhibitors or angiotensin receptor blockers (A) or in some circumstances beta-blockers (B) should be used as an initial therapy.

Table 26: Target blood pressure and first line treatment for uncomplicated hypertension (adapted and updated from Swales, 1994[14]).

Guideline	Target diastolic blood pressure (mmHg)	Target systolic blood pressure (mmHg)	First line treatment
Canada[23]	<90	<140	In uncomplicated cases, low dose thiazide diuretics, β-blockers, or ACE inhibitors in under 60s; low dose thiazide or long acting hydropyridine calcium antagonists in over-60s
Britain[18]	<85	<140	ABCD algorithm (*see* section 5)
USA[24]	<90	<140	Thiazide diuretics alone or in combination
DM/Renal Dis	<80	<130	with ACE inhibitors, or beta-blockers (uncomplicated hypertension)
New Zealand[17]	70–80	120–140	Low dose thiazide diuretics or β-blockers
WHO/ISH[22]			Patient factors determine choice from:
(older)	<90	<140	diuretics, β-blockers, ACE inhibitors,
(younger)	<85	<130	calcium antagonists, α adrenoceptor blockers or angiotensin II antagonists

In older or black (i.e. African-Caribbean) patients calcium channel blockers (C) or diuretics (D) should be used initially.

2   The majority of patients need a combination of drugs in order to achieve a blood pressure target of 140/85 mmHg (140/80 mmHg in diabetics).

3   When two drugs are needed, A (or B) should be combined with C or D, and for triple therapy A+C+D should be used.

The guideline goes on to recommend the use of fixed dose combinations, provided appropriate cost-effective choices are available.

Additional treatments to lower cardiovascular risk

The BHS guideline recommends the addition of aspirin and/or a statin to people with hypertension at higher risk of cardiovascular disease:[18]

- **aspirin:** over 50 years of age, CHD risk >15% over 10 years and BP controlled below audit threshold of 150/90
- **statin:** cholesterol >5mmol/l if current cardiovascular disease, otherwise in the presence of CHD risk >30% over 10 years.

Table 27: Compelling and possible indications, contraindications and cautions for major classes of antihypertensive drug (taken from Guidelines for management of hypertension, BHS).[18]

Class of drug	Compelling indications	Possible indications	Possible contraindications	Compelling contraindications
α-blockers	Prostatism	Dyslipidaemia	Postural hypotension	Urinary incontinence
ACE inhibitors	Heart failure LV dysfunction Type 1 diabetic Nephropathy	Chronic renal disease Type 2 diabetes Nephropathy	Renal impairment[a] Peripheral vascular disease[b]	Pregnancy Renovascular disease
AT II blockers	ACE inhibitor-induced cough	Heart failure Intolerance of other antihypertensive drugs	PVD[b] Pregnancy Renovascular disease	
β-blockers	Myocardial infarction Angina	Heart failure[c]	Heart failure Dyslipidaemia PVD	Asthma/COPD Heart block
Calcium antagonists (dihydropyridine)	Elderly ISH	Elderly Angina		
Calcium antagonists (rate limiting)	Angina	Myocardial infarction	Combination with β-blockade	Heart block Heart failure
Thiazides	Elderly		Dyslipidaemia	Gout

[a] ACE inhibitors may be beneficial in chronic renal failure but should only be used with caution, close supervision and specialist advice when there is established and significant renal failure.
[b] Caution with ACE inhibitors and AT II blockers in peripheral vascular disease because of the association with renovascular disease.
[c] Beta-blockers may worsen heart failure but may also be used to treat heart failure.
COPD: chronic obstructive pulmonary disease; ISH: isolated systolic hypertension; PVD: peripheral vascular disease.

Follow-up

Site of follow-up

The vast majority of hypertensive patients will be followed up in the community under the care of a general practitioner. Follow-up clinics may often be run by a practice nurse. Patients requiring continued follow-up in a secondary care setting may include those with poorly controlled hypertension, those with secondary hypertension and those requiring special monitoring.

Frequency of follow-up

The BHS guideline recommends follow-up of people receiving treatment for hypertension at between 3–6 month intervals once stable but points out that the frequency of follow-up for an individual will depend on multiple factors including severity of hypertension, variability of blood pressure and compliance with treatment.[18]

Those not currently receiving treatment who have previously been hypertensive or who have borderline blood pressures should be reviewed yearly.

Follow-up regime

The BHS guideline recommends the following routine for follow-up visits:

- measure BP and weight
- enquire about general health, side effects and treatment problems
- reinforce non-pharmacological measures
- test urine for proteinuria (annually)
- systematic follow-up including computerised recall for patients not otherwise attending.

Special groups

Diabetes mellitus

Treatment targets for those people suffering from diabetes are lower following evidence for this from the HOT study.[25] The BHS recommends a treatment target of <140/80 and commencement of treatment with a sustained blood pressure of ≥140/90 in diabetics.[18]

Elderly

Treatment targets and thresholds for the elderly are no different than for other groups.[18] However, as increasing age is a key risk factor for CHD, people will be eligible for risk-based care at lower levels of blood pressure. Furthermore, many older people will have isolated systolic hypertension. The evidence for treating this group of people is good, particularly with respect to stroke protection (*see* 'Hypertension as a risk factor for disease' in section 4, p.416).

Pregnancy

The BHS guideline recommends that careful distinction be made between those with new onset (or newly recognised) chronic hypertension (i.e. BP ≥140/90 mmHg before 20 weeks gestation) and pre-eclampsia.[18] Raised BP prior to 20 weeks usually means that hypertension preceded pregnancy. If chronic hypertension is diagnosed then secondary causes should be sought. Exclusion of phaeochromocytoma using urinary catecholamines is particularly important as it can cause sudden death in pregnancy.

Sub-categories

Guideline recommendations for people falling in sub-categories 1–3 have been covered above. The BHS guideline recommends admission for immediate treatment for people in group 4 (malignant or accelerated hypertension).[18] Recommendations for diagnosis and treatment of group 5 (secondary hypertension) will depend on the underlying cause (for example surgery for those with phaeochromocytoma). The BHS guideline recommends referral to secondary care of those where such a secondary cause is suspected. The BHS guideline does not give specific recommendations for people in group 6 (white coat hypertension). JNC VI states that in people in whom a raised clinic blood pressure is the only abnormality, ambulatory blood pressure monitoring may identify a group at relatively low risk of morbidity.[16]

Towards a quantified model

Figure 5 (page 448) represents a simple model for the detection and treatment of hypertension encompassing community and secondary care facilities. Figures from the Health Survey for England suggest that around 36.5% of the adult population screen positive for hypertension (or are already receiving treatment) using a threshold of 140/90 for mean blood pressure taken three times on one occasion (*see* section 4, **Table 4**).[1] Only 26% of those screening positive for hypertension were currently being treated, which suggests that around a quarter (27%) of the adult population require further follow-up to determine whether or not their blood pressure requires treatment.

Detecting hypertension

Detecting of previously unrecognised hypertension could be done opportunistically, using a systematic untargeted screening system or by using targeting to prioritise systematic screening. A recent modelling exercise compared non-targeted and targeted systematic screening and concluded that targeting people for primary prevention in order of estimated coronary heart disease risk (calculated using known patient data or population estimates where this was not available) was more efficient.[149] However, as discussed in section 6, over 90% of a primary care population will consult their GP in a three-year period. The initial screening of blood pressure could feasibly be done opportunistically in a consultation without the need for systematic screening, apart from chasing up low attenders as required. The BHS guidelines suggest a five-yearly opportunistic screen.[18]

Guidelines recommend making a diagnosis of hypertension over a period of time (3–6 months) unless the BP on presentation is particularly high. This is because many people's blood pressure will reduce over time due to a combination of accommodation to the measurement procedure and regression to the mean. For example, one study found that in a group with mild to moderate untreated hypertension, mean blood pressure dropped by 8.5/4.5 mmHg between two readings taken one week apart. In this study around 20% of patients were misclassified as hypertensive or not after four readings at weekly intervals.[72]

For example, a population of 100 000, of which 21% are below the age of 16 will contain 71 500 adults not currently taking antihypertensives (**Figure 5**). Screening this population on a five year cycle would require 14 300 additional blood pressure readings per year. Data from the Health Survey for England suggest that 4260 (27%) would screen positive (i.e. BP >140/90 and not currently on treatment). Each person screening positive will need at least two additional screening visits to confirm or refute the diagnosis of hypertension requiring an additional 8500 nurse appointments per year. Assuming that each visit takes 10 minutes (to take account of lifestyle advice and appropriate rest periods prior to measurement) then at £10 per consultation, this will cost £85k per year or £0.43m over five years (**Table 28**).[53]

It is not clear what proportion of hypertension screen positive adults will be categorised as hypertensive after such a period of monitoring. Using current BTS guidelines then those with sustained blood pressure of $\geq 160/100$ mmHg would be treated automatically with those falling between 140–159/90–99 being treated on the basis of their coronary heart disease risk or other risk factors (pre-existing cardiovascular disease or diabetes).[18] However, blood pressure tends to drop on repeated measurement and only a proportion of those screening positive will be high risk and so this will reduce the number requiring treatment.[72] The HSE found that a third of those screening positive at a threshold of 140/90 had a blood pressure $\geq 160/95$. For the purposes of this example, it will be assumed that half of those screening positive to a BP >140/90 will require treatment after further evaluation (i.e. 2100 per year or 10 500 over five years) (**Figure 5**).

Each newly diagnosed person with hypertension will need baseline investigations at the very least. Costs for investigation are likely to be low for the majority of patients comprising urinalysis, simple blood tests and ECG. The actual costs of these in primary care are difficult to quantify but using the NHS reference costs then a figure of £100 (£90 for the ECG and £10 for the blood and urine tests) is appropriate.[54] If 2100 additional patients require investigating then this will equate to £210,000 of additional baseline investigations costs per year (**Table 28**).

Between 5–10% are likely to require referral for additional investigation and/or treatment. Assuming 200 are referred per year then each will require a consultation and further costs for investigation. These will include the baseline consultation (£79), and ECG (£100 as above), and may include an echocardiogram (£72–103), further pathology tests such as 24-hour urinary protein collection (£5–20 depending on number and type of test ordered) or 24-hour blood pressure monitoring (cost not available but likely to be of the order of £100 based on ECG/echo costs). It would seem realistic to assume that an average secondary care consultation with associated investigation will cost of the order of £200 (i.e. £80,000–160,000). Ongoing costs will depend on frequency of follow-up.

The additional treatment costs incurred by detecting new cases will depend to a great extent on the classes of drug used. Assuming each patient requires two medications to adequately control blood pressure (1.8 was the mean in the HOT study) then the mean additional yearly cost could range from (BNF 44: BDZ 2.5 mg £9.67 + atenolol 50mg £11.08) £20 per patient per year to (losartan 50mg £224.61 + amlodipine 10 mg 230.73) £455 per patient per year. Aspirin and cholesterol lowering medication will inflate this further (**Table 28**).

Ongoing costs in terms of follow-up and follow-up investigation once blood pressure has been controlled will comprise two consultations per year (one GP (£15) and one practice nurse (£10)), urea and electrolytes (£5) for those on a diuretic or drug affecting the renin angiotensin system (likely to be the majority) and urinalysis (<£1 so ignored). This gives a total of £30 per year non-drug ongoing costs.

Table 28 and **Table 29** show a breakdown of likely costs of such a screening programme. Overall, a five year screening programme will cost approximately £2.4 million–£8.9 million per 100 000 population over and above current costs, depending on the drugs used (i.e. more than doubled).

Table 28: Additional yearly costs of screening and treating for hypertension over and above current costs using 5-year rolling programme.

Activity	Number of people[a]	Unit cost	Cost per year
Adult population not currently taking antihypertensives	71,500		
Initial screening for hypertension	14,300 per year		Assume zero additional cost as opportunistic
Follow-up screening (2 visits @ £10 each)	4,260 per year	£20	£85,000
Baseline investigations	2,100 per year	£100	£210,000
Secondary ref/investigations	200 per year	£200	£40,000
Low cost combination drug treatment	2,100 per year	£20	£42,000
High cost combination drug treatment	2,100 per year	£455	£956,000
Ongoing monitoring	2,100 per year	£30	£63,000
Yearly additional non-drug costs			£398,000
Yearly additional drug costs			£42,000–£956,000
Yearly total additional costs			£440,000–£1,350,000

[a] Assumes population of 100,000 of which 79,000 are adults of which 7,500 are currently receiving antihypertensive treatment.

Table 29: Estimated additional cost of 5 year programme to screen and treat hypertension.

	Non-drug costs (screening, investigation & monitoring)[a]	Drug costs[b]
Year one	£398,000	£42,000–£956,000
Year two	£461,000	£84,000–£1,910,000
Year three	£524,000	£126,000–£2,870,000
Year four	£587,000	£168,000–£3,820,000
Year five	£650,000	£210,000–£4,780,000
Total five year costs[c]	£2,620,000	£630,000–£13,380,000

[a] Ongoing monitoring costs are cumulative as more people require monitoring each year (£63,000 extra per year).
[b] Ongoing drug costs are cumulative as more people are treated each year of the cycle.
[c] An assumption has been made that both the population and cost remain static throughout. (*See* Figure 5 overleaf.)

Treating hypertension

The Health Survey for England showed that only between a quarter and a third of treated hypertensives are currently being treated adequately (to below 140/90 mmHg in this case).[1] Data from the HOT study (*see* 'Treatment targets' in section 6) found that for non-diabetics the optimum blood pressure in terms of morbidity and mortality was 138/83.[25] For those with diabetes, benefit was gained from still lower pressures. Subsequently the British Hypertension Society has recommended a target of below 140/85 for people without diabetes and below 140/80 for those with diabetes. Data from the HOT study suggest that most people will require two or more medications to achieve this target.

So, returning to the population of 100 000 used in the example above, 7500 patients from the adult population already receiving treatment will require monitoring at a yearly cost of £30 and £20–£455 depending on treatment chosen. This equates to £1.13 million monitoring and £750 000–£17.06 million treatment over 5 years.

Conclusions for the model

The two main priorities for purchasers in the management of hypertension are therefore to extend the current reach of detection using a largely opportunistic model and then to ensure that those being treated are receiving adequate medication to control blood pressure below recommended limits. This should be done in the context of an individual's overall cardiovascular risk unless blood pressure is above 160/100. Given that current provision is limited, treatment of people at the highest risk, namely those with current cardiovascular disease (coronary heart disease, vascular disease or stroke) should be the first priority. This exercise is likely to require significant funding of the order of several million pounds per PCT. The largest influence on cost over and above this level is the choice of drug. The BHS recommendations of 'ABCD' can be achieved with both low cost or high cost combinations and choice will depend at least in part on individual patient characteristics. However, given the evidence of equivalence of benefit from the four major classes, low cost combinations will be more cost-effective.[46,104] For those patients with side effects or poor control, new more expensive medications will be appropriate.

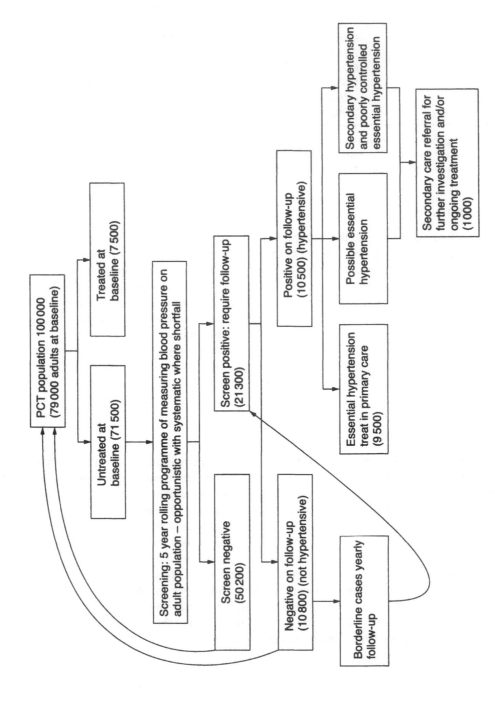

Figure 5: Model for the detection and treatment of hypertension (numbers indicate population screened in a 5 year cycle).

8 Outcome measures

A number of national audit and outcome indicators are currently in use by various primary care organisations.

British Hypertension Society Guideline

The British Hypertension Society Guideline recommends the following audit criteria for primary care:[18]

- the proportion of all adults in the practice who have had a blood pressure measurement in the last 5 years
- the proportion of all hypertensives given non-pharmacological advice
- the proportion of all hypertensives given antihypertensive therapy
- the proportion of hypertensives receiving antihypertensive therapy who have suboptimal control, i.e., blood pressure levels >150 mmHg systolic and >90 mmHg diastolic BP
- the proportion of patients lost from follow-up; or of treated patients who have not been reviewed within the last 6 months
- the use of aspirin and statins by those who require secondary prevention; or their use when indicated for primary prevention, i.e. when the estimated 10 year CHD risk is >15% (aspirin) or >30% per year (statins).

New General Medical Services Contract

The new General Medical Services Contract for General Practitioners has, since April 2004, awarded quality points and therefore resources to practices performing the following criteria for people with hypertension:

- **BP 1:** The practice can produce a register of patients with established hypertension (Yes/No).
- **BP 2:** The percentage of patients with hypertension, whose notes record smoking status at least once (standard max 90%).
- **BP 3:** The percentage of patients with hypertension who smoke, whose notes contain a record that smoking cessation advice has been offered at least once (standard max 90%).
- **BP 4:** The percentage of patients with hypertension in which there is a record of the blood pressure in the past 9 months (standard max 90%).
- **BP 5:** The percentage of patients with hypertension in whom the last blood pressure (measured in last 9 months) is 150/90 or less (standard max 70%).

The performances of practices in respect of these criteria are likely to become the major data from audit available on a national scale in England due to the fact that every practice with a GMS contract will be paid according to them.

National Service Framework for Coronary Heart Disease

Standard four of the National Service Framework for Coronary Heart Disease states:[150]

> General practitioners and primary health care teams should identify all people at significant risk of cardiovascular disease but who have not yet developed symptoms and offer them appropriate advice and treatment to reduce their risks.

The relevant NSF milestones with respect to hypertension are contained in the second step, which concerns those at high risk for CHD (>30% 10 year CHD risk) but without evidence of frank disease at present:

- **Milestone 2:** Every practice should have:
  - a systematically developed and maintained practice-based register of people with clinical evidence of CHD, occlusive vascular disease *and* of people whose risk of CHD events is >30% over ten years in place and actively used to provide structured care to those at high risk of CHD.
- **Milestone 3:** Every practice should have:
  - a protocol describing the systematic assessment, treatment and follow-up of people at high risk of CHD, including those without evidence of existing arterial disease but whose risk of CHD events is >30% over 10 years, agreed locally and being used to provide structured care to people with CHD.
- **Milestone 4:** Every practice should have:
  - clinical audit data no more than 12 months old available that describes all the items listed below
  - clinical audit data recording the following interventions and risk factors:
    - advice about how to stop smoking including advice on the use of nicotine replacement therapy
    - information about other modifiable risk factors and personalised advice about how they can be reduced (including advice about physical activity, diet, alcohol consumption, weight and diabetes)
    - advice and treatment to maintain blood pressure below 140/85 mmHg
    - add statins to lower serum cholesterol concentrations *either* to less than 5 mmol/l (LDL-C to below 3 mmol) *or* by 30% (whichever is greater)
    - meticulous control of blood pressure and glucose in people who also have diabetes.

Overview of audit criteria and National Standards

At the time of writing, none of these audit criteria have been in widespread use, nor have there been nationally available figures for the performance of practices with respect to the various criteria. The new GP contract is the most likely to change this state of affairs in that as GP income will be directly related to performance against these criteria, it is likely that at least summary figures will be available.

9 Information and research requirements

Key areas for research in hypertension include:

- robustly powered studies with appropriate clinically relevant end points (i.e. mortality and major morbidity) to determine the efficacy of non-pharmacological measures in the treatment of hypertension
- further studies examining the effect of increased user involvement in the treatment and control of hypertension
- community-based studies evaluating the benefit of generic antihypertensive medication post stroke
- long-term community-based studies with clinically relevant end points evaluating the implementation of treatment for hypertension on the basis of risk rather than blood pressure thresholds.

Update

The bulk of this chapter was written in 2003/4 prior to both the implementation of the new General Medical Services (nGMS) Contract for General Practitioners and the publication of the most recent guidelines from the National Institute for Clinical Excellence (NICE) and the British Hypertension Society (BHS). Furthermore, these guidelines are now in the process of being updated again following publication of several new studies, particularly relating to the use of beta-blockers in hypertension.

Key recent changes relevant to the chapter include:

- National prevalence of recognised hypertension has increased to around 11% (Quality and Outcomes Framework of nGMS; slightly lower in the 2003 version of Health Survey for England due to different definitions).
- Two systematic reviews and the Anglo-Scandinavian Cardiac Outcomes Trial (ASCOT) results have cast doubt on the efficacy of beta-blockers in the treatment of hypertension as compared to other classes of antihypertensive.
- The forthcoming update of the NICE hypertension guideline will use a cost-effectiveness model to dictate choice of antihypertensive therapy taking into account both benefits (in terms of reduction of cardiovascular events) and significant side effects (principally in terms of risk of diabetes). It is expected to relegate beta-blockers to fourth line treatment behind calcium channel blockers, thiazide diuretics and ACE inhibitors to bring NICE and BHS guidance together.

References

1 Erens R, Primatesta P (eds). *Health Survey for England '98.* No. 6. Joint Health Surveys Unit. London: HMSO, 1999, pp. 1–368.
2 MacMahon S, Peto R, Cutler J, Collins R, Sorlie P, Neaton J, Abbott R, Godwin J, Dyer A, Stamler J. Blood pressure, stroke, and coronary heart disease. Part 1, Prolonged differences in blood pressure: prospective observational studies corrected for the regression dilution bias. *The Lancet* 1990; **335**: 765–74.
3 Klag MJ, Whelton PK, Randall BL, Neaton JD, Brancati FL, Ford CE, Shulman NB, Stamler J. Blood pressure and end-stage renal disease in men. *New England Journal of Medicine* 1996; **334**: 13–18.
4 Glynn RJ, Beckett LA, Hebert LE, Morris MC, Scherr PA, Evans DA. Current and remote blood pressure and cognitive decline. *JAMA* 1999; **281**: 438–45.
5 Department of Health. *The Health of the Nation.* London: HMSO, 1992, pp. 1–126.
6 Collins R, Peto R. Antihypertensive Drug Therapy: Effects on Stroke and Coronary Heart Disease. In: Swales JD (ed.). *Textbook of Hypertension.* Oxford: Blackwell Scientific Publications, 1994, pp. 1156–64.
7 Wilber JA, Barrow JG. Hypertension – a community problem. *American Journal of Medicine* 1972; **52**: 653–63.
8 Ebrahim S. Detection, adherence and control of hypertension for the prevention of strokes: a systematic review. *Health Technology Assessment* 1998; **2**: i–iv.
9 Effects of ramipril on cardiovascular and microvascular outcomes in people with diabetes mellitus: results of the HOPE study and MICRO-HOPE substudy. Heart Outcomes Prevention Evaluation Study Investigators. *The Lancet* 2000; **355**: 253–9.
10 Pearce KA, Furberg CD, Psaty BM, Kirk J. Cost-minimization and the number needed to treat in uncomplicated hypertension. *American Journal of Hypertension* 1998; **11**: 618–29.

11 Mulrow C, Lau J, Cornell J, Brand M. Pharmacotherapy for hypertension in the elderly. *Cochrane Database Syst Rev* 1998, Issue 2. Art. No.: CD000028. DOI: 10.1002/14651858. CD00028.

12 Marques-Vidal P, Tuomilehto J. Hypertension awareness, treatment and control in the community: is the 'rule of halves' still valid? *J Hum Hypertens* 1997; **11**: 213–20.

13 Rose G. *The strategy of preventive medicine.* Oxford: Oxford University Press, 1992, pp. 1–135.

14 Swales JD. Guidelines for treating hypertension. In: Swales JD (ed.). *Textbook of Hypertension.* Oxford: Blackwell Scientific Publications, 1994, pp. 1195–221.

15 WHO Expert Committee. *Hypertension Control.* WHO Technical Reports. Serial Number 662. Geneva: World Health Organisation, 1996.

16 The sixth report of the Joint National Committee on prevention, detection, evaluation, and treatment of high blood pressure. *Arch Intern Med* 1997; **157**: 2413–46.

17 Jackson R, Barham P, Bills J, Birch T, McLennan L, MacMahon S, Maling T. Management of raised blood pressure in New Zealand: a discussion document. *BMJ* 1993; **307**: 107–10.

18 Ramsay L, Williams B, Johnston G, MacGregor G, Poston L, Potter J, Poulter N, Russell G. Guidelines for management of hypertension: report of the third working party of the British Hypertension Society. *J Hum Hypertens* 1999; **13**: 569–92.

19 Robson J. Information needed to decide about cardiovascular treatment in primary care. *BMJ* 1997; **314**: 277–80.

20 Anderson KM, Odell PM, Wilson PW, Kannel WB. Cardiovascular disease risk profiles. *American Heart Journal* 1991; **121**: 293–8.

21 Myers MG, Carruthers SG, Leenen FH, Haynes RB. Recommendations from the Canadian Hypertension Society Consensus Conference on the Pharmacologic Treatment of Hypertension. *CMAJ* 1989; **140**: 1141–6.

22 1999 World Health Organization – International Society of Hypertension Guidelines for the Management of Hypertension. Guidelines Subcommittee. *J Hypertens* 1999; **17**: 151–83.

23 Feldman RD, Campbell N, Larochelle P *et al.* 1999 Canadian recommendations for the management of hypertension. Task Force for the Development of the 1999 Canadian Recommendations for the Management of Hypertension. *CMAJ* 1999; **161**: S1–17.

24 Chobanian AV, Bakris GL, Black HR, Cushman WC, Green LA, Izzo JL, Jr., Jones DW, Materson BJ, Oparil S, Wright JT, Jr., Roccella EJ. The Seventh Report of the Joint National Committee on Prevention, Detection, Evaluation, and Treatment of High Blood Pressure: the JNC 7 report. *JAMA* 2003; **289**: 2560–72.

25 Hansson L, Zanchetti A, Carruthers SG, Dahlof B, Elmfeldt D, Julius S, Menard J, Rahn KH, Wedel H, Westerling S. Effects of intensive blood-pressure lowering and low-dose aspirin in patients with hypertension: principal results of the Hypertension Optimal Treatment (HOT) randomised trial. HOT Study Group. *The Lancet* 1998; **351**: 1755–62.

26 Tight blood pressure control and risk of macrovascular and microvascular complications in type 2 diabetes: UKPDS 38. UK Prospective Diabetes Study Group. *BMJ* 1998; **317**: 703–13.

27 Isles C. Hypertensive Emergencies, A: Malignant Hypertension and Hypertensive Encephalopathy. In: Swales JD (ed.). *Textbook of Hypertension.* Oxford: Blackwell Scientific Publications, 1994, pp. 1233–48.

28 Vaughan CJ, Delanty N. Hypertensive emergencies. *The Lancet* 2000; **356**: 411–17.

29 Berglund G, Andersson O, Wilhelmsen L. Prevalence of primary and secondary hypertension: studies in a random population sample. *BMJ* 1976; **2**: 554–6.

30 Danielson M, Dammstrom B. The prevalence of secondary and curable hypertension. *Acta Med Scand* 1981; **209**: 451–5.

31 O'Brien E, Beevers G, Lip GY. ABC of hypertension. Blood pressure measurement. Part III – automated sphygmomanometry: ambulatory blood pressure measurement. *BMJ* 2001; **322**: 1110–14.

32 Anonymous. Joint recommendations of the British Cardiac Society, British Hyperlipidaemia Society, British Hypertension Society, British Diabetic Association on the Prevention of coronary heart disease in clinical practice. *Heart* 1998; **80**: 1–28.

33 *Key Health Statistics from General Practice.* Series MB6 No.2. London: Office for National Statistics, 2000, pp. 1–175.

34 Department of Health. *Health Survey for England 1999.* www.doh.gov.uk/public/hs99ethnic.htm. London: Department of Health, 2000.

35 Whelton PK, Jiang He, Klag MJ. Blood Pressure in Westernised Populations. In: Swales JD (ed.). *Textbook of Hypertension.* Oxford: Blackwell Scientific Publications, 1994, pp. 11–21.

36 Staessen J, Amery A, Fagard R. Isolated systolic hypertension in the elderly. *J Hypertens* 1990; **8**: 393–405.

37 Hypertension in Diabetes Study (HDS): I. Prevalence of hypertension in newly presenting type 2 diabetic patients and the association with risk factors for cardiovascular and diabetic complications *J Hypertens.* 1993; **11**: 309–17.

38 Lip GY, Beevers M, Beevers G. The failure of malignant hypertension to decline: a survey of 24 years' experience in a multiracial population in England. *J Hypertens* 1994; **12**: 1297–305.

39 Quinkler M, Lepenies J, Diederich S. Primary hyperaldosteronism. *Exp Clin Endocrinol Diabetes* 2002; **110**: 263–71.

40 Pickering TG, James GD, Boddie C, Harshfield GA, Blank S, Laragh JH. How common is white coat hypertension? *JAMA* 1988; **259**: 225–8.

41 MacDonald MB, Laing GP, Wilson MP, Wilson TW. Prevalence and predictors of white-coat response in patients with treated hypertension. *CMAJ* 1999; **161**: 265–9.

42 Aylett M, Marples G, Jones K. Home blood pressure monitoring: its effect on the management of hypertension in general practice. *Br J Gen Pract* 1999; **49**: 725–8.

43 Lewington S, Clarke R, Qizilbash N, Peto R, Collins R. Age-specific relevance of usual blood pressure to vascular mortality: a meta-analysis of individual data for one million adults in 61 prospective studies. *The Lancet* 2002; **360**: 1903–13.

44 He FJ, MacGregor GA. Effect of modest salt reduction on blood pressure: a meta-analysis of randomized trials. Implications for public health. *J Hum Hypertens* 2002; **16**: 761–70.

45 Staessen JA, Gasowski J, Wang JG, Thijs L, Den Hond E, Boissel JP, Coope J, Ekbom T, Gueyffier F, Liu L, Kerlikowske K, Pocock S, Fagard RH. Risks of untreated and treated isolated systolic hypertension in the elderly: meta-analysis of outcome trials. *The Lancet* 2000; **355**: 865–72.

46 Brown MJ, Cruickshank JK, Dominiczak AF, MacGregor GA, Poulter NR, Russell GI, Thom S, Williams B. Better blood pressure control: how to combine drugs. *J Hum Hypertens* 2003; **17**: 81–6.

47 Anonymous. *British National Formulary No 44.* London: British Medical Association and Royal Pharmaceutical Association of Great Britain, 2003.

48 Prescott-Clarke P, Primatesta P (eds). *Health Survey for England '96.* Joint Health Surveys Unit. No. 6. London: HMSO, 1998, pp. 1–368.

49 McGhee SM, McInnes GT, Hedley AJ, Murray TS, Reid JL. Coordinating and standardizing long-term care: evaluation of the west of Scotland shared-care scheme for hypertension. *Br J Gen Pract* 1994; **44**: 441–5.

50 Office of Population Censuses & Surveys. *Morbidity statistics from general practice 1991/2* (MSGP4). London: HMSO, 1994.

51 Department of Health. *Hospital Episode Statistics Data.* London: Department of Health, 2003.

52 Venning P, Durie A, Roland M, Roberts C, Leese B. Randomised controlled trial comparing cost effectiveness of general practitioners and nurse practitioners in primary care. *BMJ* 2000; **320**: 1048–53.

53 Netten A, Curtis L. *Unit Costs of Health and Social Care 2002.* Personal Social Services Research Unit, 2003.

54 *National Reference Costs 2002.* www.doh.gov.uk/nhsexec/refcosts.htm. London: Department of Health, 2003.

55 Kernick DP, Reinhold DM, Netten A. What does it cost the patient to see the doctor? *Br J Gen Pract* 2000; **50**: 401–3.

56 McAlister FA, Straus SE. Evidence based treatment of hypertension: Measurement of blood presssure: an evidence based review. *BMJ* 2001; **322**: 908–11.

57 Padwal R, Straus SE, McAlister FA. Evidence based management of hypertension. Cardiovascular risk factors and their effects on the decision to treat hypertension: evidence based review. *BMJ* 2001; **322**: 977–80.

58 O'Brien E. Ave atque vale: the centenary of clinical sphygmomanometry. *The Lancet* 1996; **348**: 1569–70.

59 O'Brien ET, Petrie JC, Littler WA *et al. Blood Pressure Measurement: Recommendations of the British Hypertension Society.* London: BMJ, 1997, pp. 1–27.

60 Rose G, Holland WW, Crowley EA. A sphygmomanometer for epidemiologists. *The Lancet* 1964; **i**: 296–300.

61 Neufeld PD, Johnson DL. Observer error in blood pressure measurement. *CMAJ* 1986; **135**: 633–7.

62 Markandu ND, Whitcher F, Arnold A, Carney C. The mercury sphygmomanometer should be abandoned before it is proscribed. *J Hum Hypertens* 2000; **14**: 31–6.

63 O'Brien E, Waeber B, Parati G, Staessen J, Myers MG. Blood pressure measuring devices: recommendations of the European Society of Hypertension. *BMJ* 2001; **322**: 531–6.

64 McManus RJ, Mant J, Hull MRP, Hobbs FDR. Does changing from mercury to electronic blood pressure measurement influence recorded blood pressure? An observational study. *Br J Gen Pract* 2003; **53**: 953–6.

65 Lerman CE, Brody DS, Hui T, Lazaro C, Smith DG, Blum MJ. The white-coat hypertension response: prevalence and predictors. *J Gen Intern Med* 1989; **4**: 226–31.

66 O'Brien E, Mee F, Atkins N, Thomas M. Evaluation of three devices for self-measurement of blood pressure according to the revised British Hypertension Society Protocol: the Omron HEM-705CP, Philips HP5332, and Nissei DS-175. *Blood Press Monit* 1996; **1**: 55–61.

67 Thijs L, Staessen JA, Celis H, de Gaudemaris R, Imai Y, Julius S, Fagard R. Reference values for self-recorded blood pressure: a meta-analysis of summary data. *Arch Intern Med* 1998; **158**: 481–8.

68 Little P, Barnett J, Barnsley L, Marjoram J, Fitzgerald-Barron A, Mant D. Comparison of acceptability of and preferences for different methods of measuring blood pressure in primary care. *BMJ* 2002; **325**: 258–9.

69 Perloff D, Sokolow M, Cowan R. The prognostic value of ambulatory blood pressures. *JAMA* 1983; **249**: 2792–8.

70 O'Brien E, Staessen JA. What is 'hypertension'? *The Lancet* 1999; **353**: 1541–3.

71 Prasad N, Isles C. Ambulatory blood pressure monitoring: a guide for general practitioners. *BMJ* 1996; **313**: 1535–41.

72 Brueren MM, Petri H, van Weel C, van Ree JW. How many measurements are necessary in diagnosing mild to moderate hypertension? *Fam Pract* 1997; **14**: 130–35.

73 Rowlands S, Moser K. Consultation rates from the general practice research database. *Br J Gen Pract* 2002; **52**: 658–60.

74 Cook DG, Morris JK, Walker M, Shaper AG. Consultation rates among middle aged men in general practice over three years. *BMJ* 1990; **301**: 647–50.

75 D'Souza MF, Swan AV, Shannon DJ. A long-term controlled trial of screening for hypertension in general practice. *The Lancet* 1976; **1**: 1228–31.

76 Bass MJ, McWhinney IR, Donner A. Do family physicians need medical assistants to detect and manage hypertension? *CMAJ* 1986; **134**: 1247–55.

77 Holmen J, Forsen L, Hjort PF, Midthjell K, Waaler HT, Bjorndal A. Detecting hypertension: screening versus case finding in Norway. *BMJ* 1991; **302**: 219–22.

78 Montgomery AA, Fahey T, MacKintosh C, Sharp DJ, Peters TJ. Estimation of cardiovascular risk in hypertensive patients in primary care [In Process Citation]. *Br J Gen Pract* 2000; **50**: 127–8.

79 Cooke CJ, Meyers A. The role of community volunteers in health interventions: a hypertension screening and follow-up program. *Am J Public Health* 1983; **73**: 193–4.

80 Murphy M, Foster C, Sudlow C, Nicholas J, Mulrow C, Ness A, Pignone M. Primary prevention. *Clin Evid* 2002; 91–123.

81 Whelton SP, Chin A, Xin X, He J. Effect of aerobic exercise on blood pressure: a meta-analysis of randomized, controlled trials. *Ann Intern Med* 2002; **136**: 493–503.

82 Graudal NA, Galloe AM, Garred P. Effects of sodium restriction on blood pressure, renin, aldosterone, catecholamines, cholesterols, and triglyceride: a meta-analysis. *JAMA* 1998; **279**: 1383–91.

83 Mulrow CD, Chiquette E, Angel L, Cornell J, Summerbell C, Anagnostelis B, Grimm R, Jr., Brand MB. Dieting to reduce body weight for controlling hypertension in adults. *Cochrane Database Syst Rev* 1998, Issue 4. Art. No.: CD000484. DOI: 10.1002/14651858. CD000484.

84 Appel LJ, Moore TJ, Obarzanek E, Vollmer WM, Svetkey LP, Sacks FM, Bray GA, Vogt TM, Cutler JA, Windhauser MM, Lin PH, Karanja. A clinical trial of the effects of dietary patterns on blood pressure. DASH Collaborative Research Group. *N Engl J Med* 1997; **336**: 1117–24.

85 Ebrahim S, Smith GD. Lowering blood pressure: a systematic review of sustained effects of non-pharmacological interventions. *J Public Health Med* 1998; **20**: 441–8.

86 Engstrom G, Hedblad B, Janzon L. Hypertensive men who exercise regularly have lower rate of cardiovascular mortality. *J Hypertens* 1999; **17**: 737–42.

87 Hooper L, Bartlett C, Davey SG, Ebrahim S. Systematic review of long term effects of advice to reduce dietary salt in adults. *BMJ* 2002; **325**: 628.

88 Alderman MH. Salt, blood pressure and health: a cautionary tale. *Int J Epidemiol* 2002; **31**: 311–15.

89 Alderman MH, Madhavan S, Cohen H, Sealey JE, Laragh JH. Low urinary sodium is associated with greater risk of myocardial infarction among treated hypertensive men. *Hypertension* 1995; **25**: 1144–52.

90 Whelton PK, He J, Cutler JA, Brancati FL, Appel LJ, Follmann D, Klag, MJ. Effects of oral potassium on blood pressure. Meta-analysis of randomized controlled clinical trials. *JAMA* 1997; **277**: 1624–32.

91 Morris MC, Sacks F, Rosner B. Does fish oil lower blood pressure? A meta-analysis of controlled trials. *Circulation* 1993; **88**: 523–33.

92 Hale WA, Chambliss ML. Should primary care patients be screened for orthostatic hypotension? *J Fam Pract* 1999; **48**: 547–52.

93 Gueyffier F, Froment A, Gouton M. New meta-analysis of treatment trials of hypertension: improving the estimate of therapeutic benefit. *J Hum Hypertens* 1996; **10**: 1–8.

94 Gueyffier F, Boutitie F, Boissel JP, Pocock S, Coope J, Cutler J, Ekbom, Fagard R, Friedman L, Perry M, Prineas R, Schron E. Effect of antihypertensive drug treatment on cardiovascular outcomes in women and men. A meta-analysis of individual patient data from randomized, controlled trials. The INDANA Investigators. *Ann Intern Med* 1997; **126**: 761–7.

95 Turnbull F. Effects of different blood-pressure-lowering regimens on major cardiovascular events: results of prospectively-designed overviews of randomised trials. *The Lancet* 2003; **362**: 1527–35.

96 Law MR, Wald NJ, Morris JK, Jordan RE. Value of low dose combination treatment with blood pressure lowering drugs: analysis of 354 randomised trials. *BMJ* 2003; **326**: 1427.

97 Psaty BM, Smith NL, Siscovick DS, Koepsell TD, Weiss NS, Heckbert SR, Lemaitre RN, Wagner EH, Furberg CD. Health outcomes associated with antihypertensive therapies used as first-line agents. A systematic review and meta-analysis. *JAMA* 1997; **277**: 739–45.

98 Messerli FH, Grossman E, Goldbourt U. Are beta-blockers efficacious as first-line therapy for hypertension in the elderly? A systematic review. *JAMA* 1998; **279**: 1903–7.

99 Freemantle N, Cleland J, Young P, Mason J, Harrison J. Beta blockade after myocardial infarction: systematic review and meta regression analysis. *BMJ* 1999; **318**: 1730–7.

100 Neal B, MacMahon S, Chapman N. Effects of ACE inhibitors, calcium antagonists, and other blood-pressure-lowering drugs: results of prospectively designed overviews of randomised trials. Blood Pressure Lowering Treatment Trialists' Collaboration. *The Lancet* 2000; **356**: 1955–64.

101 The Heart Outcomes Prevention Evaluation Study Investigators. Effects of an Angiotensin-Converting-Enzyme Inhibitor, Ramipril, on Cardiovascular Events in High-Risk Patients. *N Engl J Med* 2000; **342**: 145–53.

102 Randomised trial of a perindopril-based blood-pressure-lowering regimen among 6,105 individuals with previous stroke or transient ischaemic attack. *The Lancet* 2001; **358**: 1033–41.

103 Wing LM, Reid CM, Ryan P, Beilin LJ, Brown MA, Jennings GL, Johnston CI, McNeil JJ, Macdonald GJ, Marley JE, Morgan TO, West MJ. A comparison of outcomes with angiotensin-converting–enzyme inhibitors and diuretics for hypertension in the elderly. *N Engl J Med* 2003; **348**: 583–92.

104 ALLHAT Research Group. Major outcomes in high-risk hypertensive patients randomized to angiotensin-converting enzyme inhibitor or calcium channel blocker vs diuretic: The Antihypertensive and Lipid-Lowering Treatment to Prevent Heart Attack Trial. *JAMA* 2002; **288**: 2981–97.

105 Psaty BM, Heckbert SR, Koepsell TD, Siscovick DS, Raghunathan TE, Weiss NS, Rosendaal FR, Lemaitre RN, Smith NL, Wahl *et al*. The risk of myocardial infarction associated with antihypertensive drug therapies. *JAMA* 1995; **274**: 620–5.

106 Tatti P, Pahor M, Byington RP, Di Mauro P, Guarisco R, Strollo G, Strollo F. Outcome results of the Fosinopril Versus Amlodipine Cardiovascular Events Randomized Trial (FACET) in patients with hypertension and NIDDM. *Diabetes Care* 1998; **21**: 597–603.

107 Pahor M, Psaty BM, Alderman MH, Applegate WB, Williamson JD, Cavazzini C, Furberg CD. Health outcomes associated with calcium antagonists compared with other first-line antihypertensive therapies: a meta-analysis of randomised controlled trials. *The Lancet* 2000; **356**: 1949–54.

108 Major cardiovascular events in hypertensive patients randomized to doxazosin vs chlorthalidone: the antihypertensive and lipid-lowering treatment to prevent heart attack trial (ALLHAT). ALLHAT Collaborative Research Group. *JAMA* 2000; **283**: 1967–75.

109 Conlin PR, Spence JD, Williams B, Ribeiro AB, Saito I, Benedict C, Bunt AM. Angiotensin II antagonists for hypertension: are there differences in efficacy? *Am J Hypertens* 2000; **13**: 418–26.

110 Dahlof B, Devereux RB, Kjeldsen SE *et al.* Cardiovascular morbidity and mortality in the Losartan Intervention For Endpoint reduction in hypertension study (LIFE): a randomised trial against atenolol. *The Lancet* 2002; **359**: 995–1003.

111 Pignone M, Phillips C, Mulrow C. Use of lipid lowering drugs for primary prevention of coronary heart disease: meta-analysis of randomised trials. *BMJ* 2000; **321**: 983–6.

112 ALLHAT Research Group. Major outcomes in moderately hypercholesterolemic, hypertensive patients randomized to pravastatin vs usual care: The Antihypertensive and Lipid-Lowering Treatment to Prevent Heart Attack Trial. *JAMA* 2002; **288**: 2998–3007.

113 Muldoon MF, Manuck SB, Matthews KA. Lowering cholesterol concentrations and mortality: a quantitative review of primary prevention trials. *BMJ* 1990; **301**: 309–14.

114 Scandinavian Simvastatin Survival Study Group. Randomised trial of cholesterol lowering in 4444 patients with coronary heart disease: the Scandinavian Simvastatin Survival Study (4S). *The Lancet* 1994; **344**: 1383–9.

115 Muldoon MF, Manuck SB, Mendelsohn AB, Kaplan JR, Belle SH. Cholesterol reduction and non-illness mortality: meta-analysis of randomised clinical trials. *BMJ* 2001; **322**: 11–15.

116 Jackson PR, Wallis EJ, Haq IU, Ramsay LE. Statins for primary prevention: at what coronary risk is safety assured? *Br J Clin Pharmacol* 2001; **52**: 439–46.

117 Sever PS, Dahlof B, Poulter NR, Wedel H, Beevers G, Caulfield M, Collins R, Kjeldsen SE, Kristinsson A, McInnes GT, Mehlsen J, Nieminen M, O'Brien E, Ostergren J. Prevention of coronary and stroke events with atorvastatin in hypertensive patients who have average or lower-than-average cholesterol concentrations, in the Anglo-Scandinavian Cardiac Outcomes Trial–Lipid Lowering Arm (ASCOT-LLA): a multicentre randomised controlled trial. *The Lancet* 2003; **361**: 1149–58.

118 MRC/BHF Heart Protection Study of cholesterol lowering with simvastatin in 20,536 high-risk individuals: a randomised placebo-controlled trial. *The Lancet* 2002; **360**: 7–22.

119 Grossman E, Messerli FH, Goldbourt U. Does diuretic therapy increase the risk of renal cell carcinoma? *Am J Cardiol* 1999; **83**: 1090–3.

120 Grimm RHJ, Grandits GA, Prineas RJ, McDonald RH, Lewis CE, Flack JM, Yunis C, Svendsen K, Liebson PR, Elmer PJ. Long-term effects on sexual function of five antihypertensive drugs and nutritional hygienic treatment in hypertensive men and women. Treatment of Mild Hypertension Study (TOMHS). *Hypertension* 1997; **29**: 8–14.

121 Dickerson JE, Hingorani AD, Ashby MJ, Palmer CR, Brown, MJ. Optimisation of antihypertensive treatment by crossover rotation of four major classes. *The Lancet* 1999; **353**: 2008–13.

122 Yusuf S, Sleight P, Pogue J, Bosch J, Davies R, Dagenais G. Effects of an angiotensin-converting-enzyme inhibitor, ramipril, on cardiovascular events in high-risk patients. The Heart Outcomes Prevention Evaluation Study Investigators. *N Engl J Med* 2000; **342**: 145–53.

123 Svensson P, de Faire U, Sleight P, Yusuf S, Ostergren J. Comparative effects of ramipril on ambulatory and office blood pressures: a HOPE Substudy. *Hypertension* 2001; **38**: E28–E32.

124 Gueyffier F, Bulpitt C, Boissel JP, Schron E, Ekbom T, Fagard R, Casiglia E, Kerlikowske K, Coope J. Antihypertensive drugs in very old people: a subgroup meta-analysis of randomised controlled trials. INDANA Group. *The Lancet* 1999; **353**: 793–6.

125 Saunders E, Weir MR, Kong BW, Hollifield J, Gray J, Vertes V, Sowers JR, Zemel MB, Curry C, Schoenberger J. A comparison of the efficacy and safety of a beta-blocker, a calcium channel blocker, and a converting enzyme inhibitor in hypertensive blacks. *Arch Intern Med* 1990; **150**: 1707–13.

126 Rahman M, Douglas JG, Wright JT, Jr. Pathophysiology and treatment implications of hypertension in the African-American population. [Review] [177 refs]. *Endocrinology & Metabolism Clinics of North America* 1997; **26**: 125–44.

127 Cushman WC, Reda DJ, Perry HM, Williams D, Abdellatif M, Materson BJ. Regional and racial differences in response to antihypertensive medication use in a randomized controlled trial of men with hypertension in the United States. Department of Veterans Affairs Cooperative Study Group on Antihypertensive Agents. *Arch Intern Med* 2000; **160**: 825–31.

128 Materson BJ, Reda DJ, Cushman WC, Massie BM, Freis ED, Kochar MS, Hamburger RJ, Fye C, Lakshman R, Gottdiener J, Ramirez EA, Henderson WG, The Department of Veterans Affairs Cooperative Study Group on Antihypertensive Agents. Single-Drug Therapy for Hypertension in Men – A Comparison of Six Antihypertensive Agents with Placebo. *N Engl J Med* 1993; **328**: 914–21.

129 Douglas JG, Bakris GL, Epstein M *et al.* Management of high blood pressure in African Americans: consensus statement of the Hypertension in African Americans Working Group of the International Society on Hypertension in Blacks. *Arch Intern Med* 2003; **163**: 525–41.

130 Bales A. Hypertensive crisis. How to tell if it's an emergency or an urgency. *Postgrad Med* 1999; **105**: 119–26, 130.

131 Messerli FH, Grossman E, Goldbourt U. Antihypertensive therapy in diabetic hypertensive patients. *Am J Hypertens* 2001; **14**: 12S–16S.

132 McAlister FA, Zarnke KB, Campbell NR *et al*. The 2001 Canadian recommendations for the management of hypertension: Part two – Therapy. *Can J Cardiol* 2002; **18**: 625–41.

133 Kjeldsen SE, Hedner T, Jamerson K, Julius S, Haley WE, Zabalgoitia M, Butt AR, Rahman SN, Hansson L. Hypertension optimal treatment (HOT) study: home blood pressure in treated hypertensive subjects. *Hypertension* 1998; **31**: 1014–20.

134 Grossman E, Messerli FH, Goldbourt U. High blood pressure and diabetes mellitus: are all antihypertensive drugs created equal? *Arch Intern Med* 2000; **160**: 2447–52.

135 Weir MR. Diabetes and hypertension: how low should you go and with which drugs? *Am J Hypertens* 2001; **14**: 17S–26S.

136 Effects of treatment on morbidity in hypertension. Results in patients with diastolic blood pressures averaging 115 through 129 mmHg. *JAMA* 1967; **202**: 1028–34.

137 Pickering TG. White coat hypertension: time for action. *Circulation* 1998; **98**: 1834–6.

138 Chaloupka FJ, Wechsler H. Price, tobacco control policies and smoking among young adults. *J Health Econ* 1997; **16**: 359–73.

139 Chapman S, Borland R, Scollo M, Brownson RC, Dominello A, Woodward S. The impact of smoke-free workplaces on declining cigarette consumption in Australia and the United States. *Am J Public Health* 1999; **89**: 1018–23.

140 Murray CJ, Lauer JA, Hutubessy RC, Niessen L, Tomijima N, Rodgers A, Lawes CM, Evans DB. Effectiveness and costs of interventions to lower systolic blood pressure and cholesterol: a global and regional analysis on reduction of cardiovascular-disease risk. *The Lancet* 2003; **361**: 717–25.

141 *Supermarket war on salt*. BBC Online. 5 January 2004.

142 Hillsdon M, Thorogood M. A systematic review of physical activity promotion strategies. *Br J Sports Med* 1996; **30**: 84–9.

143 Department of Health. *Executive Summary Of The Pilot Initiatives Evaluation Study*. London: Department of Health, 2003.

144 Montgomery AA, Fahey T, Ben Shlomo Y, Harding J. The influence of absolute cardiovascular risk, patient utilities, and costs on the decision to treat hypertension: a Markov decision analysis. *J Hypertens* 2003; **21**: 1753–9.

145 Gray A, Clarke P, Farmer A, Holman R. Implementing intensive control of blood glucose concentration and blood pressure in type 2 diabetes in England: cost analysis (UKPDS 63). *BMJ* 2002; **325**: 860.

146 Baker S, Priest P, Jackson R. Using thresholds based on risk of cardiovascular disease to target treatment for hypertension: modelling events averted and number treated. *BMJ* 2000; **320**: 680–85.

147 Lindholm LH, Werko L. Cost effectiveness analyses have been carried out in Sweden. *BMJ* 1996; **313**: 1203b–1204.

148 Fahey TP, Peters TJ. What constitutes controlled hypertension? Patient based comparison of hypertension guidelines. *BMJ* 1996; **313**: 93–6.

149 Marshall T, Rouse A. Resource implications and health benefits of primary prevention strategies for cardiovascular disease in people aged 30 to 74: mathematical modelling study. *BMJ* 2002; **325**: 197.

150 Department of Health. *National Service Framework for Coronary Heart Disease*, Chapter 2: Preventing coronary heart disease in high risk patients. London: DoH, 2000.

Acknowledgements

The authors would like to thank Dr JJ Ferguson and Mr J Horgan for access to prescribing data.

6 Obesity

John Garrow and Carolyn Summerbell

1 Summary

Statement of the problem

In 1976, a study group in the UK reported to the DHSS/Medical Research Council: 'We are unanimous in our belief that obesity is a hazard to health and a detriment to well-being. It is common enough to constitute one of the most important medical and public health problems of our time... '[1] In 1979, the US Department of Health published a similar report.[2] In the past twenty five years, many expert committees have issued the same warning, but the problem of obesity is rapidly becoming more serious in both developed and third world countries. The World Health Organization (WHO)[3] now calls it a 'global epidemic', and has concluded that the changing nature of the environment towards greater inducement of obesity (or the 'Obesogenic Environment') is mainly to blame.[4]

Obesity in adults is defined for epidemiological purposes as body mass index (BMI) > 30 kg/m.[2] The crude relationship of BMI (a convenient index of fatness) to all-causes mortality risk is shown in Figure 2: minimum risk is observed between BMI 20 and 25, and mortality increases both below and above this range. It is now known that the increased mortality among thinner subjects is largely related to cigarette smoking and pre-existing disease, and that in weight-stable non-smokers an increased risk of heart disease, diabetes and musculoskeletal disorders becomes evident even below BMI = 25 kg/m.[2] Obesity causes insulin insensitivity, which is an important causal factor in diabetes, heart disease, hypertension and stroke. Adipose tissue converts androgens to oestrogens, which probably explains the reproductive disorders and sex-hormone-sensitive cancers to which obese people are predisposed, and the increased cholesterol flux associated with obesity increases the risk of gallstones and associated diseases. The increased mechanical load increases liability to osteoarthritis and sleep apnoea. Obesity also carries psychosocial penalties. Thus there are many routes by which obesity is a detriment to well-being. All these penalties (except the risk of gallstones) decrease with weight loss.

The health consequences of obesity in children are less well defined, but the risks of diabetes, hypertension, heart disease and perceived poor health are greater among adults who were obese at age 18 years than in those who were of normal weight at age 18 years. Obesity also carries psychosocial penalties for fat children, who are likely to be teased, so there is good reason to try to prevent obesity in childhood.

It is difficult to explain why, when there have been repeated warnings from clinical scientists that obesity is a serious health hazard, there has been no effective control of the problem. We offer four possible explanations.

First, the academic view that obesity per se is not the problem. This arose because studies on cardiovascular risk factors in 50-year-old men showed that if age, cigarette smoking, blood pressure and serum cholesterol were already entered into a multiple regression equation, then adding weight status did not improve prediction of which men would have a heart attack. This was interpreted to mean that if blood pressure and cholesterol were controlled, then obesity could be ignored. The reasoning was false, since (as indicated above) obesity itself predisposes to hypertension and dyslipidaemia, and also to many other important diseases as well as heart attacks.

The second argument is that obesity is determined by our genes, and therefore untreatable. Certainly there have been recent advances in our understanding of the genetics of obesity, but it is obvious that the rapid increase in prevalence in the past two decades does not reflect a change in the gene pool of the population, since genetic change can only occur between successive generations. A large part of the cause of the global epidemic must therefore be environmental (the 'Obesogenic Environment'), and hence (in principle) treatable.

A third factor is that obesity is a feminist issue. Social psychologists have rightly pointed out that many normal-weight young women try to lose weight to achieve an unrealistic female stereotype of excessive thinness. This is true, and regrettable, especially as some resort to cigarette smoking as a method for weight control. However, it is not an argument for neglecting the real health problem of true obesity.

The fourth problem is related to the third. There is frantic media interest in magic weight loss cures, so the public is bombarded with conflicting misinformation about the causes, consequences and cures for overweight.

For whatever reason, the National Health Service (NHS) and the Health Development Agency (HDA) have been very muted in their response to the obesity challenge, and have hoped that with general advice about healthy lifestyles, some help from the private sector, or perhaps the ever-hoped-for 'superdrug', the problem would go away. This policy has been a spectacular failure, as highlighted by a House of Commons Health Committee Report on Obesity published in May 2004.[5]

Sub-categories

Obesity is a condition that (like hypertension) begins at some arbitrary threshold and becomes increasingly severe. For a given level of obesity in adults the health hazards are greatest among those who are young with existing co-morbidities, or have family histories of obesity-related diseases (diabetes, heart disease, hypertension). For a given amount of fat, a central (intra-abdominal) distribution is more metabolically harmful than a peripheral distribution. The objective of treatment is to manage existing co-morbidities, and in all cases is to reduce fat mass to normal limits, maintain that loss and (if necessary) support the self-esteem of the patient. Healthcare needs are determined by an iterative process, which is described in section 7.

Among children, the objective is to prevent the development of obesity, rather than to achieve fat loss in children who have become obese. Children with obese parents, or who are showing excessively rapid weight gain during primary school years, are most in need of help.

Prevalence and incidence

The prevalence of obesity in adults in the UK has been rising steadily since the programme of national monitoring was started in 1980 (Table 5). The most recent figures available (2002) show that the prevalence of obesity in men was 23%, and in women 25%. In 2002 the prevalence of obesity in boys was 6%, and in girls 7%. The trend data shows how obesity has risen dramatically in the last 25 years, but it is not possible to estimate incidence with confidence since a large number of people are oscillating above and below the thresholds which define obesity and overweight.

Services available and their cost

In 2000 the National Audit Office (NAO) found that it was unusual for GPs and other health professionals to use a protocol for the management of obesity, although the majority of those asked reported that they would find a protocol useful.[6] It can be assumed that this situation has improved a little with time. The NAO survey also found that the primary care team wanted improved access to onward referral options for their overweight and obese patients, and training on obesity management. The variety and quantity of referral options remains limited and patchy across the UK.

The best available estimate of the direct and indirect costs of obesity were calculated for 1998 as part of the NAO report.[6] The NAO estimated that it cost at least £½ billion a year in treatment costs to the NHS, and possibly in excess of £2 billion to the wider community, in 1998. The direct cost is driven primarily by the cost of treating of the secondary disease attributable to obesity, and particularly coronary heart disease (CHD), hypertension and type 2 diabetes. A recent Health Technology Assessment (HTA) report on obesity published in 2004 concluded that the cost of diet and exercise together appear comparable to the cost of drug treatments in obese individuals with risk factors.[7]

Effectiveness of services and interventions

A convenient, but imperfect, measure of the effectiveness of obesity treatment is the weight loss achieved during treatment, and the extent to which it is maintained after active treatment ceases. Ideally, such measurements should be made over a period of several years. It is difficult to achieve high follow-up rates over long periods, so most trials of obesity treatment are characterised by a rather high drop-out rate, and a large variability in weight loss within a group of patients on the same treatment. This makes design of good randomised control trials (RCTs) very difficult. For example, in trials comparing orlistat with placebo, the standard deviation of weight loss within groups was of similar magnitude to the mean weight loss of the group, so it was necessary to recruit several hundred subjects to show statistically significant differences between the orlistat and placebo groups. The interventions which have been shown to be effective are analysed in section 6. It is evident that dietary treatments which are aimed at reducing total energy intake are most effective in causing weight loss in obese people. Decreasing dietary fat, or increasing fibre, are effective only to the extent that they reduce energy intake, which is a rather small effect when such diets are designed to be eaten ad libitum. Very-low-calorie diets cause greater weight loss than low calorie diets in the short term, but in the longer term this advantage disappears. Exercise alone does not cause significant weight loss, but causes a modest improvement in weight loss (and has other health advantages) when combined with a low-energy diet. Drugs licensed for the treatment of obesity cause a modest increased weight loss (effect size B) when added to a low-energy diet. Gastric surgery produces massive weight loss by enforcing a low-energy intake by the patient. The results of studies to manage obesity in children have yielded results that are too variable to summarise with confidence, but targeting a decrease in sedentary behaviour appears to be a useful strategy in both the prevention and treatment of obesity in children.

Quantified models of care

In section 7, a quantified model of care is proposed: the numbers of patients requiring care in a population of 100 000 is estimated in Table 10. For overweight and obese adults there are three levels of service provision: Level 1 is a slimming club in the community led by a non-medical healthcare worker. For those requiring further assessment, Level 2 is based on the primary care team, and Level 3, on a specialist in a referral hospital. The process is iterative, so estimates of the workload at each level depend on the efficacy of management offered at the other levels, and that offered in the private sector.

The prevention of obesity in children is a different problem. Reasons are given for choosing the primary school years as an optimum stage at which to manage children who are in the highest tenth of BMI at age 5. The objective is not to cause weight loss, but to limit weight gain between the ages of 5 and 12 years.

Outcome measures and audit methods

A crude but robust audit measure is the BMI of the population served, and the weight loss achieved, and maintained, by those adults treated for overweight or obesity. The success of the programme for preventing obesity in children can be assessed by measuring the prevalence of overweight in schoolchildren at age 12 years. This does not address the other objective of improving the psychological status of weight-reduced adults, for which there is no simple audit method.

Information and research requirements

There are many questions to which we need answers. For example:

- the influence of dietary fat intake on obesity prevalence and treatment
- the efficacy of different preventative programmes, especially those involving exercise
- the relative influence of genetics and environment to the familial aggregation of obesity
- the efficacy of strategies for maintenance of weight loss
- the cost of preventing and treating obesity
- the relationship between the amount and rate of weight loss, and the reduction of co-morbidities such as hypertension, heart disease, diabetes, gallstones, osteoarthritis and sleep apnoea.

Introduction and statement of the problem

Introduction

The main purpose of this chapter is to help healthcare commissioners in England to develop purchasing plans for the prevention and treatment of obesity in both the primary and secondary care setting. In theory, this needs assessment activity should be easy. We have good data on the prevalence (but not incidence) of obesity in England (section 4) and the effect this has on health (sections 2 and 3), a number of systematic reviews on the efficacy of interventions for obesity (section 6), and information on costs (section 5). The main difficulty for healthcare commissioners is assessing the optimum field for service provision, i.e. where need, supply (section 5) and demand (section 2) are congruent. For obesity, there is poor overlap between need, supply and demand; we suggest that some of this difficulty is a result of the lack of training on weight management (and nutrition in general) given to medical students, and poor provision for catch-up courses for doctors once qualified (section 5). At the end of this chapter (section 7) we make recommendations of what we believe obesity health services should look like.

What is obesity?

Adults

Obesity is a condition in which body fat stores are enlarged to an extent that impairs health. Obese people tend to die young, and hence are not profitable subjects for life insurance. To guide doctors doing insurance examinations, life insurance companies have for many years published tables of 'desirable weight', based on the mortality experience of people they have insured. As more data become available for analysis it emerges that this desirable range corresponds closely to the range of BMI from 18.5 to 25. The index is calculated by dividing the individual's weight (kg) by the square of his or her height (m). Thus a person who weighed 65 kg and who was 1.73 m tall would have a BMI of $65/(1.73 \times 1.73) = 21.7$, which is in the desirable range. In practice, it is usually more convenient to use a chart such as that shown in Figure 1, which shows the boundaries of BMI 18.5, 25, 30, 35 and 40.

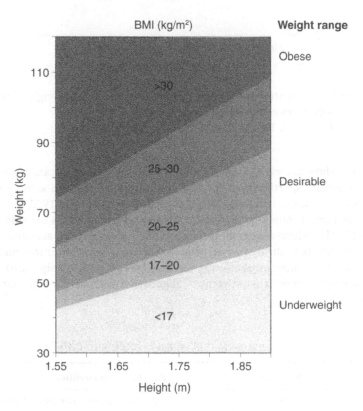

Figure 1: Weights and heights determining the boundaries between individuals who are underweight, normal weight, pre-obese or obese in grade I, grade II or grade III. A person on these boundaries would have a BMI of 18.5, 25.0, 30.0, 35.0 or 40.0 kg/m^2 respectively.[3]

It is arbitrary to choose a value for BMI above which a person is deemed obese: mortality starts to increase significantly somewhere between 25 and 30, and increases rapidly at values of BMI above 30, as shown in Figure 2.

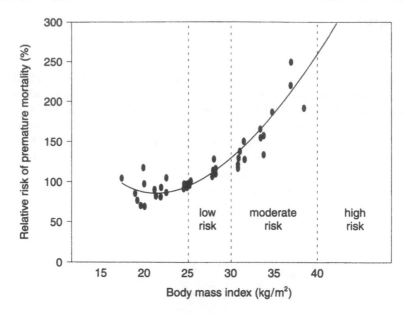

Figure 2: Relative risk of premature mortality with increasing BMI. The weight and height determining the grades of overweight and obesity are shown in Figure 1.
Source: Bray. *Ann Int Med* 1985; **104**: 1052–62.

Very thin people also show decreased longevity (but they usually die from cancer and chronic infectious diseases such as tuberculosis, rather than the non-communicable diseases associated with obesity), so below 18.5 there is increased mortality. At a WHO consultation meeting in 1997, it was proposed that the thresholds shown in Table 1 should be used to classify overweight in adults according to BMI.[8]

The weakness of BMI as a basis for defining obesity is that it does not take account of the distribution of body fat, which also affects health risks (see below). The most popular simple measure of abdominal adiposity is the ratio of circumferences of waist and hips (WHR, or waist/hip ratio). However, there are arguments for using simply waist circumference.[9] Suggested thresholds for waist circumference classification are shown in Table 2.

Table 1: Classification and risk of overweight in adults according to BMI.[3]

Classification	BMI (kg/m²)	Risk of co-morbidities
Underweight	< 18.5	Low (but risk of other clinical problems increased)
Normal range	18.5–24.9	Average
Overweight	> 25	
Pre-obese	25–29.9	Increased
Obese class I	30.0–34.9	Moderate
Obese class II	35.0–39.9	Severe
Obese class III	> 40.0	Very severe

Table 2: Sex-specific waist circumferences that denote increased risk of metabolic complications of obesity in adult Caucasians.

	Risk of complications	
	Increased	Substantially increased
Men	> 94 cm (~37 in)	> 102 cm (~40 in)
Women	> 80 cm (~32 in)	> 88 cm (~35 in)

Children

The simple classification shown in Table 1 for obesity in adults is not applicable to children, since the ratio of velocity of weight gain to height gain changes during normal growth, especially around puberty. Many different methods are currently in use to estimate body fatness or relative weight, and for each method, various cut-off levels are used to describe overweight or obesity. These problems have been discussed in more detail elsewhere.[10] To encourage consistency in defining fatness, the International Task Force on Obesity has developed an international reference population and BMI standards to classify overweight and obesity, using age- and sex-specific curves.[11] BMI charts for boys and girls, based on these standards, should be used (published by the Child Growth Foundation, London). The BMI of a boy or girl on the 50th centile at age 1 year is 17.5 kg/m^2, falls to 15.5 kg/m^2 at age 6 years, and climbs to 21 kg/m^2 at age 18 years.

In the case of adults, the bands of BMI can be related to health risk as indicated in Figure 2. However, it is difficult to base a definition of obesity in children related to the health risks in adult life because there are too few longitudinal studies on which these judgements can be made. Even if these data were available, this task would be a tricky one since children often cross many centiles of weight-for-height, especially children under the age of 5 years. However, obesity in childhood is recognised as a significant health risk, as explained in more detail below, since obese adolescents are at increased risk of obesity in adult life[12] and at increased risk of mortality, independent of adult weight.[13]

Summary

The classification of obesity in both adults and children simply requires the accurate measurement of height, weight and waist circumference. However, as with most measurements there are potential errors involved. The most common error, particularly common in primary care, is a result of self-reported height and/or weight.[14] Tall, thin individuals are more likely to under-report their height, and shorter, fatter individuals to overestimate their height and underestimate their weight. It is important that weight and height are measured, and measured correctly; weight in light clothing and height without shoes. Weighing scales should be calibrated regularly, and height sticks should be checked to make sure that they are correctly placed. The good news for health commissioners is that the assessment of obesity is remarkably cheap!

Why is obesity important?

There is increasing recognition that obesity is important in causing many of the major non-communicable diseases with which it was previously classified merely as an associated condition. On 1st June 1998 the American Heart Association announced that it was upgrading obesity from a 'contributing risk factor' to a 'major risk factor for coronary heart disease'.[15] Obesity is a lifelong disease, not just a cosmetic issue nor a matter for moral judgement.

Adults

Obesity and total mortality

The main cause of the premature death rate among obese people is heart disease: hypertension, coronary thrombosis and congestive heart failure are all significantly more common among obese people than among normal-weight controls. Of course age and cigarette smoking are important contributors to the risk of heart disease in both obese and non-obese people, but obesity increases the risk (Figure 3). High blood pressure, raised concentration of plasma low-density cholesterol and a low concentration of high-density cholesterol fractions are all important risk factors, but weight gain makes these factors worse, and weight loss makes them better.

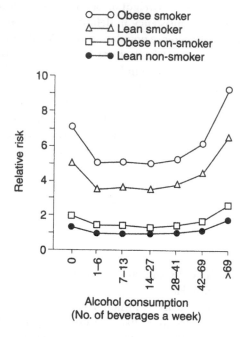

Figure 3: Relative risks (RR) of mortality in relation to alcohol intake at specified levels of smoking and BMI. (RR set at 1.00 for lean, non-smoker with alcohol intake of one to six beverages a week.) *Source*: Gronbaek *et al. BMJ* 1994; **308**: 302–6.

The way in which cigarette smoking and adult weight gain confuse the relationship between obesity and mortality is well illustrated in Table 3, which summarises results from a large study of nursing personnel by Manson *et al.* in 1995.[16]

On inspection of the relative risk of death during the 14-year follow-up of these women it appears that those in the whole group with a BMI between 19 and 27 kg/m^2 have the least mortality risk (0.8 relative to 1.0 for those with a BMI < 19). Only in the range 27.0–28.9 does the risk rise to the level of those < 19 kg/m^2, and above 29 the risk is definitely increased. However, when those women who had never smoked are analysed separately, a different story emerges. Among non-smokers the mortality risk starts to increase at

Table 3: Influence of BMI, history of cigarette smoking, and adult weight gain, on relative mortality risk in 30–55-year-old women followed for 14 years.

BMI	< 19	19.0–21.9	22.0–24.9	25.0–26.9	27.0–28.9	29.0–31.9	> 32.0
All women							
Adj. RR[a]	1.0	0.8	0.8	0.8	1.0	1.2	1.5
95% CI[b]		0.7–0.9	0.7–0.9	0.7–0.9	0.9–1.1	1.0–1.3	1.3–17
Women who never smoked							
Adj. RR	1.0	1.0	1.1	1.1	1.4	1.7	1.9
95% CI		0.8–1.3	0.9–1.3	0.8–1.3	1.1–1.8	1.4–2.2	1.5–2.5
Women who never smoked and had stable weight[c]							
Adj.RR	1.0	1.2	1.2	1.3	1.6	2.1	2.2
95% CI		0.8–1.6	0.9–1.7	0.9–1.9	1.1–2.5	1.4–3.2	1.4–3.4

[a] Relative risk of death from all causes adjusted for age, smoking, menopausal status, use of oral contraceptives and post-menopausal hormones, and parental history of myocardial infarction before age 60 years.
[b] 95% confidence interval for relative risk.
[c] Excluding first four years of follow-up and women with > 4 kg weight change during those four years.

22 kg/m^2 and is significantly increased at 27 kg/m^2, so the increased mortality among the women < 19 kg/m^2 disappears when the smokers are removed from the analysis. An even greater change occurs if the analysis is restricted to those women who had never smoked, and who had not either died or gained > 4 kg in the first four years of follow-up. Now the J-shaped curve has disappeared, the minimum mortality is with the thinnest women, and a significant increase in mortality risk occurs above 27 kg/m^2. Some of the women who died within four years of enrolment in the survey probably had a disease at that time, which may explain why they were thin and also why they died. This example has been considered in some detail because crude data on mortality do not provide reliable information on the health risks of obesity if the confounding effects of cigarette smoking, adult weight gain and previous disease are not allowed for. If these factors are removed, a woman aged 30–55 years is more than twice as likely to die in the next 14 years if her BMI is > 29 kg/m^2 than if it was < 19 kg/m^2.

The effect of age on excess mortality from all causes associated with obesity is controversial. In a large cohort of obese persons (n=6193), obesity-related excess mortality declined with age at all levels of obesity.[17] This is not because obesity causes less ill health in older people, but because in older people death from causes unrelated to obesity becomes more common.

It is important to note that the obesity-related health risks cited above do not necessarily apply to populations of different ethnic origins. However, a systematic review[18] concluded that differences in absolute risk by ethnicity are not relevant to individuals in a clinical setting.

It is also important to note that there is evidence which suggests that being fit may reduce the hazards of obesity.[19]

Obesity: socioeconomic consequences

From the viewpoints of human suffering and healthcare expenditure, morbidity is as important as mortality. Obesity causes disability as well as death. Rissanen et al.[20] analysed data from the Finnish Social Security system and found that the risk of drawing a disability pension increased significantly with BMI, even within the 'desirable' range of 20–25 kg/m^2; one quarter of all disability pensions in women and half as many in men were due to obesity. These disabilities arose mainly from cardiovascular and musculo-skeletal disease.

The impact of obesity on a number of specific diseases is outlined below (e.g. Figure 4).

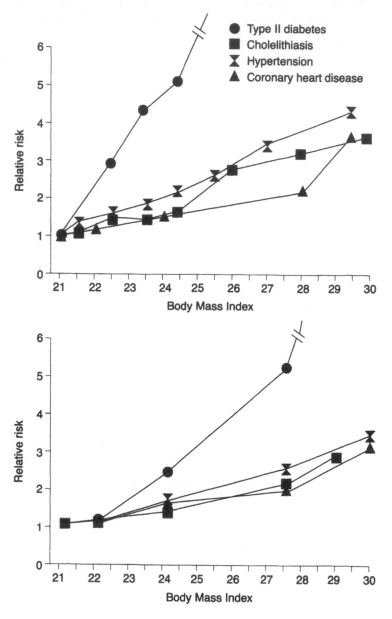

Figure 4: Relationship between BMI up to 30 and relative risk of type II diabetes, hypertension, CHD, and cholelithiasis. (a) Relations with women, initially 40–65 years old who were followed up for 18 years; (b) Relations with men, initially 40-65 years old, who were followed up for ten years. *Source*: Willett *et al. NEJM* 1995; **273**: 461–5.

Obesity, insulin sensitivity and diabetes

Type II diabetes is not as impressive a cause of mortality among obese people as heart disease, but it is itself a risk factor for heart disease, and also a very important cause of morbidity from neuropathy, nephropathy and eye disease.

The relationship between obesity and type II diabetes is very tight, and the risk of type II diabetes increases sharply with increasing BMI, particularly in men (Figures 4 and 5). A man more than 140% of average weight is 5.2 times more likely to die of type II diabetes than a normal-weight man, and for women the mortality ratio is 7.9 times for a similar degree of overweight.[21] A classic study of experimental obesity in Vermont has shown that the association between obesity and reduced insulin sensitivity (which is the primary problem in type II diabetes mellitus) is a causal one. Young male volunteers, with no family history of type II diabetes or obesity, overate for six months so they increased their weight by 21%, of which 73% was fat, and they then showed significant changes in biochemistry in the direction of type II diabetes. After weight loss to normal values these changes reverted to normal.[22] Even among pre-pubertal children obesity is associated with peripheral and hepatic insulin resistance.[23]

Although type II diabetes is not directly the cause of most of the excess mortality among obese people, the metabolic defect underlying type II diabetes is clearly the result of obesity,[24] which itself predisposes to hypertension and heart disease. These defects are reversible with weight loss, with corresponding improvement in mortality. A deliberate weight loss of 0.5–9.0 kg is associated with a 30–40% reduction in type II diabetes-related mortality.[25]

Coronary heart disease

The main cause of the excess mortality among obese people is coronary heart disease (CHD). Obesity is itself strongly related to hypertension and stroke (Figure 4), particularly in young people.[26] However, these risk factors improve when obese people lose weight.[27] After adjustment for age and smoking, the risk of a fatal or non-fatal myocardial infarction (MI) among women > 29 kg/m^2 is three times that among lean women.[16,28] High blood pressure, high triacylglycerol and high low-density lipoproteins favour the formation of atheromatous lesions, but obese people have the added hazard of abnormalities of blood clotting factors, which further increase the risk of thrombosis and MI.[29] These abnormalities improve with therapeutic weight reduction.[30]

Cancer

A very large survey by the American Cancer Society found that the mortality ratio for cancer among men who were 40% overweight was 1.33, and for women 1.55. The most important increase is for breast cancer in post-menopausal women, but there is also an increased risk of cancer of the endometrium, uterus, cervix, ovary and gall bladder in women, and of the colon, rectum and prostate in men.[31] Intentional weight loss of 0.5–9.0 kg is associated with a decrease of 40–50% in mortality from obesity-related cancers.

Osteoarthritis

Degenerative disease of weight-bearing joints is a very common complication of obesity, particularly in the knees of middle-aged women, and causes significant disability.[20] Unlike the risk of heart disease or diabetes, the risk of osteoarthritis is related to the total amount of fat, and not in particular to the amount of intra-abdominal fat.[32]

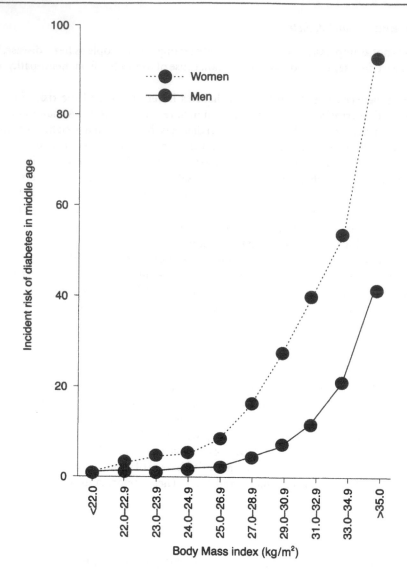

Figure 5: Relative risk of Type II diabetes with increasing weight.
Source: Colditz *et al. Ann Int Med* 1995; **122**: 481–6.

Gallstones

Obese people have a higher output of cholesterol in bile, with a lower concentration of bile salts, so their bile is constantly in danger of forming gallstones (Figure 4). Rapid weight loss increases the release of cholesterol from adipose tissue, and hence increases the load to be excreted in bile.[33] Bile stasis contributes to biliary infections, and also to the risk of gall-bladder cancer, mentioned above.

Reproductive disorders

Obesity is associated with disorders of menstrual function, fertility and childbirth. Examination of obese pregnant women is particularly difficult, whether by abdominal palpation, ultrasound or laparoscopy. The difficulty in monitoring fetal well-being in severely obese mothers partly explains their increased rate of caesarian section. However, even moderate degrees of obesity are associated with an increased incidence of hypertension, toxaemia, gestational diabetes, urinary tract infections and fetal macrosomia.[34] There is also an increased risk of neural tube defects in the children of obese mothers: among women over 70 kg in weight, dietary intake of folic acid does not have the same protective effect as it has in leaner women.[35,36]

Sleep apnoea

Obesity causes inefficiency of respiratory function by several mechanisms. The mechanical load of fat on the chest wall increases the mechanical work of inspiration, especially when the subject is recumbent, and a large mass of intra-abdominal fat tends to push the liver upwards, thus decreasing the intrathoracic space. There is also a mismatch of pulmonary ventilation and perfusion, so much of the blood flowing through the lung capillaries is at the base of the lung, where ventilation is poor. These problems may cause the Pickwickian syndrome of chronic hypoxia and carbon dioxide retention, which may manifest itself as inappropriate somnolence, vividly described by Dickens in the fat boy in *The Pickwick Papers*, and obstructive sleep apnoea (OSA). This is a serious condition, which is associated with pulmonary hypertension and right-sided heart failure. Data from the Swedish Obese Subjects (SOS) study show that OSA was an important contributor to morbidity in severe obesity, and contributed to cardiovascular mortality.[37] Respiratory function improves when obese people lose weight.[38]

Psychological and social disorders

The health hazards of the obese person, which have been listed above, become increasingly evident as the person becomes older: heart disease, hypertension, stroke, osteoarthritis, cancer and gallstones are all conditions which occur mainly in older people, so the obese young person does not experience these as a threat. However, the psychological and social penalties of obesity fall mainly on the child and young adult. Indeed, there is a view, often promoted in the media, that the penalties of obesity are mainly due to social discrimination, so if society treated obese people with respect and tolerance it would cease to be a problem.[39] This is wrong: the health hazards of obesity listed above would remain, however respectfully obese people were treated, but there is compelling evidence that our society discriminates against fat people.[40]

Social discrimination continues through adult life. Sonne-Holm and Sorensen[41] showed that, for a given parental social class, intelligence and education, severely obese people achieved less favourable social status than non-obese people. In the US, Gortmaker *et al.*[42] studied a nationally representative sample of 10 039 men and women who were 16 to 24 years old in 1981, and obtained follow-up data on 65–79% of the cohort seven years later. Women who were initially above the 95th centile for BMI had completed fewer years in school, were less likely to be married and had higher rates of household poverty than the women who had not been overweight, independent of their baseline socioeconomic status and aptitude-test scores. However, people with chronic conditions such as asthma and musculo-skeletal abnormalities did not differ from non-overweight people in these ways.

In the general population, those who are overweight or obese are not significantly more depressed than lean people.[40] Among those who are depressed, it is difficult to establish if this is caused by obesity or caused by dieting in an unsuccessful attempt to reverse the obesity. Among the severely obese, there have been numerous reports of psychopathology: for example volunteers for the SOS study, both men and women, showed very poor ratings for mental well-being, and more symptoms of anxiety and depression than the reference population. The score on psychometric scales were as bad as, or worse than, those of patients with chronic pain, generalised malignant melanoma or tetraplegia after neck injury.[43] It is particularly important for doctors or dietitians who are treating obese patients to remember that their duty is to help to restore the self-esteem of obese patients, as well as to help them to lose their excess weight. This point is considered again when discussing treatment of obesity.

It is useful to note that there is some evidence that weight concerns vary with ethnic group.[44,45]

All of these penalties of obesity decrease with weight loss, with the exception of the risk of gallstone formation. During weight loss in an obese person, the cholesterol in adipose tissue is mobilised and the bile may become even more liable to form cholesterol stones.

Fat distribution and health risk

A study in Gothenburg, Sweden, showed that people with a high WHR (indicating that fat was largely in the abdominal cavity, rather than subcutaneously on the limbs) had a greater risk of heart disease and diabetes than people with a similar amount of fat distributed peripherally.[46] This probably relates to the insulin insensitivity which is caused by a high flux of free fatty acids in the portal circulation, because intra-abdominal fat cells can release fatty acids very rapidly. However, further studies have shown that the increased mortality among men was not significantly related to WHR when the follow-up period was extended to 20 years,[47] and the central distribution of fat is associated with both cigarette smoking and a high alcohol intake, which may have contributed to some of the observed excess mortality risk.

Children

Effect on adult morbidity and mortality

There is limited evidence for an association between adolescent obesity and increased risk of adult morbidity[10] and mortality.[13] Must et al.[13] showed that obesity in adolescence predicts a broad range of adverse health effects that are independent of adult weight after 55 years of follow-up: the risks of morbidity from CHD and atherosclerosis are increased among men and women who were overweight as adolescents.

There is better evidence that the childhood period is important for adult obesity (and all the associated health risks, as described above) because tracking of overweight, albeit moderate, is observed between childhood and adulthood. This topic has been reviewed.[10,48] The figures vary according to the definition of obesity and length of follow-up, but fat children have a high risk of going on to become fat adults. For example, in the 1958 British birth cohort, 38% of boys and 44% of girls above the 95th BMI centile at age 7, were obese at age 33.[49] Even so, only a small proportion of fat adults were fat in childhood. It is likely that there are factors operating in early adulthood that promote obesity, but there may also be factors operating in childhood that promote adult obesity. It is still a matter of debate whether there are particular stages in childhood, during which physiological alterations increase the risk of later obesity. These stages are termed critical periods, and may include the prenatal period, the adiposity rebound (second rise in adiposity occurring at about 6 years), and puberty.[50]

Parental fatness has also been identified by a systematic review as the most important predictor in childhood of adult obesity,[12] although the contribution of genes and inherited lifestyle factors to the parent–child fatness association remains largely unknown. Other important risk factors in childhood of adult obesity included social factors, birth weight, timing or rate of maturation, physical activity, dietary factors and other behavioural or psychological factors. The relationship between low socioeconomic status

(SES) in childhood and increased fatness in adulthood is remarkably consistent, but when fatness is measured in childhood, the association with SES is less consistent. Studies investigating SES were generally large, but very few considered confounding by parental fatness. Women who change social class (social mobility) show the prevalence of obesity of the class they join, an association which is not present in men, and the influence of other social factors such as family size, number of parents at home and childcare have been little researched. Parsons et al.[12] found good evidence from large and reasonably long-term studies, for an apparently clear relationship for increased fatness with higher birth weight, but in studies which attempted to address potential confounding by gestational age, parental fatness or social group, the relationship was less consistent. The relationship between earlier maturation and greater subsequent fatness was investigated in predominantly smaller, but also a few large studies. Again, this relationship appeared to be consistent, but in general, the studies had not investigated whether there was confounding by other factors, including parental fatness, SES, earlier fatness in childhood, or dietary or activity behaviours. Studies investigating the role of diet or activity were generally small, and included diverse methods of risk factor measurement. There was almost no evidence for an influence of activity in infancy on later fatness, and inconsistent but suggestive evidence for a protective effect of activity in childhood on later fatness. No clear evidence for an effect of infant feeding on later fatness emerged, but follow-up to adulthood was rare, with only one study measuring fatness after the age of 7 years. Again, confounding variables were seldom accounted for. A few, diverse studies investigated associations between behaviour or psychological factors and fatness, but mechanisms through which energy balance might be influenced were rarely addressed.

Effects during childhood

Obese children are more prone to physical ailments, and are also liable to underperform at school relative to their potential.[11] The health consequences of obesity in youth have been reviewed;[51,52] increased blood lipids, glucose intolerance, hypertension and increases in liver enzymes associated with fatty liver, have all been observed to be more common in obese children or adolescents. The diseases to which obese children are more liable are tabulated in Table 4.[8]

Table 4: Health consequences of childhood obesity.

High prevalence	Intermediate prevalence	Low prevalence
Faster growth	Hepatic steatosis	Orthopaedic complications
Psychosocial	Abnormal glucose metabolism	Sleep apnoea
Persistence into adulthood	Persistence into adulthood	Polycystic ovary syndrome
(for late onset and severe	(depending on age of onset	Pseudotumour cerebri
obesity)	and severity)	Cholelithiasis
Dyslipidaemia		Hypertension
Elevated blood pressure		

The main penalties of obesity experienced by children are social isolation and peer problems.[53] Although there is little evidence to suggest that self-esteem is significantly affected in obese young children, on reaching the teenage years the effect is striking. Obese children are believed by their peers at school to be lazy, dirty, stupid, ugly, cheats and liars, and these perceptions have been reported by children as young as 9 years old.[54]

Overweight adolescent women have a lower educational attainment, lower incomes and are less likely to marry than those not overweight.[42] If these relationships are indeed causal, then they imply far-reaching consequences for costs to health services, and the total healthcare.

Why does the NHS think that obesity is not important?

The dramatic effect which obesity has on quality of life, morbidity and mortality (and equally how these can be reversed with weight loss) has resulted in repeated and strongly worded reports by national and international expert committees that 'obesity is one of the most important public health hazards of our time'.[8,18,55–57] There is a stark contrast between these authoritative warnings, and the absence in any country of any effective preventative or treatment programme to reverse the increasing prevalence of obesity. In the UK, a target for obesity was omitted from all current UK Government health policy documentation, including *Our Healthier Nation: Saving Lives*.[58] However, the Health Development Agency (HDA) produced an Evidence Briefing on 'The management of obesity and overweight'[59] which lists useful strategies, and NICE has produced guidance on the use of orlistat,[60] sibutramine[61] and surgery[62] for the management of obesity reviews and guidance on drugs and surgery. The difficulty for health care providers is how best to use these separate guidance strategies in the management of obesity. This was one of the many concerns highlighted by the House of Commons Health Committee.[5] An obesity strategy, and guidance on the management of obesity, are required to help tackle the problem of obesity in the UK. The good news is that NICE, in collaboration with the HDA, has started to work on these documents, and outputs were expected by summer 2006. In the interim, the guidance produced by the Scottish Inter-collegiate Guidelines Network (SIGN) should be used.[63] So why has the health service refused to treat obesity seriously? We do not have hard evidence on which to base an answer to this crucial question, but believe there are several factors that, in varying proportion, inhibit health services from controlling obesity. Some of these obstacles have a factual basis, others are based in misapprehension of the facts. If progress is to be made these obstacles need to be removed. Their nature and basis is briefly reviewed below.

'Obesity per se is not a health hazard'

In the 1950s, international epidemiology was in its infancy. Keys and colleagues set up a prospective study of the factors which predisposed to CHD. They recruited healthy men aged 40–59 years in seven countries (USA, Japan and five European countries), and found after 15 years of follow-up that adiposity did not significantly predict mortality if age, cigarette smoking, blood pressure and cholesterol were already entered into a multiple regression equation.[64] This finding led public health policy makers to the view that obesity per se was benign, and that the real villains were smoking, blood pressure and cholesterol. The flaw in the argument, as described above, is that obesity itself predisposes to hypertension and hypercholester-olaemia, but even when these factors are allowed for, obesity remains an independent risk factor for heart disease and total mortality both in men[65] and women.[25]

'Obesity is genetically determined, and hence untreatable'

The genetics of obesity in some laboratory rodents has been extensively explored, and it has been shown that the genetically determined absence of 'leptin' entirely accounts for the obesity of some strains of mouse. The role of leptin in the aetiology of obesity in human subjects is not clear: obese people have high, not low, leptin concentrations. There is also good evidence from twin studies that the susceptibility to weight gain in a given environment is affected by hereditary factors, probably by the interaction of many genes. However, it is obvious that the recent dramatic increase in the prevalence of obesity in the UK cannot be ascribed to a change in the genetic make-up of the population because genetic make-up can change over generations, not during the lifetime of an individual. Obesity is determined by the interaction between genes and environment, and is greatly influenced by psychosocial factors and cognitive actions. Environmental and lifestyle factors can certainly be changed, and it is by this route that obesity can be prevented or treated in the individual and in the community.

'Fat is a feminist issue'

Orbach[66] made the valid point that many young women struggled vainly to achieve unphysiological thinness in order to meet a feminine stereotype which was thought to be attractive, and they would be better if they gave up this futile endeavour. This is true, and it should remind healthcarers that it is important not to damage the self-esteem of obese people when trying to help them to lose weight. However, it is not a valid argument against providing help for those who are obese, so they can avoid the health hazards listed above.

Orbach's original thesis has been taken further by pressure groups who claim that health education campaigns designed to control obesity are a form of unfair discrimination, analogous to racism, and should be made illegal. Health educators who say (truthfully) that obesity is unhealthy, and can be avoided or reversed by lifestyle changes, may be accused of 'victim blaming'. No doubt this in part explains the very muted response of government organisations to the obesity problem.

Media misinformation

There is huge public demand (described below) for an easy solution to the problem of weight loss, so it is not surprising that an unlimited amount of bizarre advice, magic potions and pseudo-science is on offer to the bemused consumer. This is part of the price we pay for freedom of expression, but it is an obstacle to those who try to offer reliable guidance about the health hazards of obesity, and what can and should be done to avoid them.

Public demand and putting the NHS services for obesity into context

Demand may be defined as what the public would be willing to pay for, or might wish to use, in a system of free healthcare. The public demand for help to acquire the perfect body is immense; it is a national obsession, particularly among women. This is one of the key differences in the planning of obesity health services as compared with those for other diseases. The public demand is catered for by the many sources of help from outside the health service. Help in the form of specialist magazines and books, slimming clubs and slimming foods has soared in the past 20 years. The fact that so many people within England seek advice on obesity from outside the health service highlights two important issues for health services commissioners.

- Most individuals who would benefit from losing weight probably use non-NHS services, but only a minority also demand help from, or are offered help by, the NHS. Unfortunately the constant background information on dieting from other sources is usually more compelling. The patient may request advice from the health professional regarding a specific diet or food which they have heard will enhance their weight loss (or even cause weight loss without the tedium of dieting). Regardless of the credibility of reported claims for such diets or foods, it is important that the health professional addresses them seriously and does not dismiss them as simply ridiculous; if the patient thought that these claims were ridiculous he or she would not have asked for advice on them in the first place. We suggest that effective care in this field requires provision of services by both the NHS and others working in close collaboration.

* Demand for obesity services is greater than the need for them since many individuals who seek advice on weight management are not overweight or obese. However, it is also important to recognise that these individuals might benefit from sound advice on lifestyle issues through the health promotion services.

Children are quite different from adults in terms of non-NHS sources of help on weight management. The sources mentioned above are targeted only at adults, and this provides the NHS with a niche on this childhood obesity 'market'. Earlier in this section we highlighted the risks of childhood obesity, and in section 7 we suggest ways in which the NHS may deliver services to this vulnerable group.

Prospect for new effective treatments

Readers of this chapter will be aware that the media are constantly heralding a 'breakthrough' in the treatment or prevention of obesity, since such items are effective in selling newspapers. The two developments that have received most attention recently are the discovery of the hormone leptin and the licensing of two anti-obesity drugs: orlistat and sibutramine. The evidence relating to these compounds is reviewed later in the chapter. The purpose of this short note is to consider the possibility that they will revolutionise the management of obesity and thus render the contents of this chapter obsolete.

Leptin is a hormone, released from adipose tissue, which has the effect of reducing food intake in genetically obese mice, and curing their obesity and infertility. Initially, therefore, there was great optimism that it would have similar effects in obese human subjects. It was found, however, that obese human subjects did not (like obese mice) have abnormally low levels of leptin, but abnormally high levels. So far (except in a single case of a rare genetic disorder) leptin has not been shown to be therapeutically effective in human obesity.

Orlistat is a drug that inactivates the enzymes that digest fat in the human small intestine, and thus reduces fat absorption by about 30%. The results of RCTs are reviewed in section 6. In very large, multicentre, international trials orlistat has been shown to cause greater weight loss in obese subjects on a low-fat diet than that observed in control subjects; this difference is statistically significant (since the trials involved about 1000 subjects) but clinically not very impressive.

Sibutramine promotes a sense of satiety through its action as a serotonin and noradrenaline re-uptake inhibitor. In addition, it may have an enhancing effect on thermogenesis through stimulation of peripheral noradrenergic receptors.

In a French trial,[67] patients with BMI > 30 were screened using a four-week treatment on a very-low-calorie diet; only those who lost > 6 kg in this phase entered the trial. An intention to treat analysis showed the mean weight change after one year among 81 patients on sibutramine (10 mg) was –5.2 kg, and among 78 patients on placebo was +0.5 kg. In an American trial,[68] 1463 patients were screened, 1047 were randomised and 683 completed the 24-week study. The weight loss at completion ranged from 1.2% in the placebo group to 9.4% among those on a dose of 30 mg/day. These results show that sibutramine causes weight loss which is statistically greater than placebo, but not impressive compared with the initial overweight of the volunteers, and with a large variation in response between individuals.

We are confident that, at least for the next decade, the health problems associated with obesity, and the methods available for effective treatment, will be little changed from the present situation. We do not expect that a new therapeutic 'breakthrough' will greatly affect the assumptions on which this chapter is based.

3 Sub-categories

Sub-categories of obesity related to risk of associated diseases

Health risk, in terms of mortality, increases progressively from normality to very severe obesity (section 2, Figure 2). At each weight, this health risk is greatest in young people, people with diabetes or hypertension, and people with a relatively high WHR. The costs of obesity, both to the individual and to the community, arise mainly from the co-morbidities rather than from obesity itself (*see* section 5).

From the viewpoint of healthcare planners there is a dilemma. One strategy (which has been widely adopted in the past) is to plan to treat the co-morbidities – heart disease, stroke, hypertension, diabetes, osteoarthritis, gallstones, certain cancers, reproductive disorders, sleep apnoea, psychological and social disorders – and ignore the underlying obesity. This strategy is superficially plausible, since patients with these co-morbidites clearly need treatment. However, experience shows that the strategy is expensive and ineffective if the underlying obesity is allowed to increase.

An alternative strategy is to seek to prevent the development of obesity by health education campaigns that promote physical activity and healthy diets of low energy density. This also fails for several reasons. First, people will not adopt healthier lifestyles unless the facilities are available to modify their diet and exercise more in conditions that are affordable and safe, and unless they have a clear understanding of the relationship between overweight and health risk. These requirements are not met at present. Second, a campaign to prevent overweight and obesity is inadequate to meet the needs of a population in which over half of all adults are already overweight, and one quarter of all adults are already obese. Third, campaigns that exhort adults to 'fight the flab' do not address the problem of increasing obesity among children. Government and health authorities potentially have some control over the diet and physical activity of schoolchildren, but this opportunity is not being effectively used to prevent obesity at its earliest stage.

The solution to the dilemma lies in the ability of healthcare planners to take a broader view of the problem of obesity, and integrate its three sub-categories. These are:

- **Obese patients with existing co-morbidities**. These are the most visible component of the problem, to which the most attention is at present paid. With better management of the other two components there will be fewer patients in this category, and so costs in this sector will decrease, and the level of public health will improve.
- **Obese individuals who do not yet have co-morbidities**. These are the people who are at present least well served by the NHS.
- **Adults and children who are not obese, but particularly at risk to become obese** (see below).

The evidence for categorising the health risk in children by degree of obesity is not available. Section 7 describes the evidence which suggests that primary school children, compared with younger or older children, are more effectively managed.

Sub-categories of the non-obese population who are most likely to become obese (predictors of obesity)

It is important to state at the outset that anybody is at risk of becoming obese, so long as they consume more energy than they use. Adults who are most likely to become obese are:

- those who were previously obese and who have lost weight
- smokers who have stopped smoking

- those who change from an active to an inactive lifestyle
- those with poor educational achievement.

Children at high risk of becoming obese adults (as detailed in section 2) are:

- children who have high weight-for-height
- children who have obese parents.

4 Prevalence and incidence

Adults

The prevalence of obesity, particularly in the developed world, has increased particularly rapidly over the past two decades. The WHO calls it a 'global epidemic'.[3] The prevalence of obesity in UK adults and children, compared with those living in other European countries, is shown in Figures 6, 7, and 8.

There are good data for England showing the prevalence of obesity in the UK (Table 5). The prevalence of overweight and obesity in the UK population was first determined in 1980, in a survey of a representative sample of 5000 men and 5000 women aged 16–64 years. At that time, the proportion of men in the 'pre-obese' stage was 34%, and 6% were obese; for women there were 24% in the 'pre-obese' stage and 8% were obese.

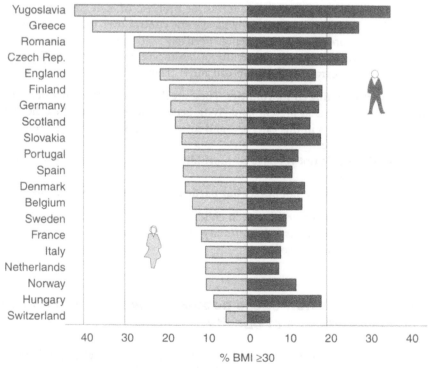

Collated by the IOTF from recent surveys

Figure 6: Prevalence of obesity (%) in adults in selected European countries in 2002 (IOTF data). *Source*: With kind permission of IOTF.

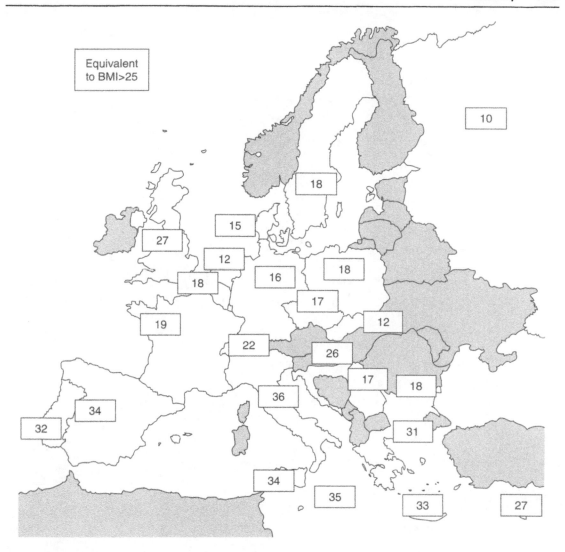

Figure 7: Prevalence of overweight (%) in children aged 7–11 years in selected European countries in 2002 (IOTF data).
Source: With kind permission of IOTF.

The prevalence was higher among the older subjects. Another survey carried out in 1987 using the same methodology showed an alarming increase in the prevalence of obesity (BMI > 30), which overall had increased from 6 to 8% in men and from 8 to 12% in women. The increase occurred in all age groups, but particularly among women aged 25–34 years, in whom the prevalence appears to have doubled over the seven-year interval. From 1990 there has been a regular cycle of surveys (Health Surveys for England) which continue to show an increasing prevalence of obesity: the trend up to 2002 (which is the latest year for which data are available at the time of writing is shown in Table 5. The data on prevalence become available about two years after the fieldwork is done, and the prevalence among adult men and women in the UK has increased by approximately one percentage point annually over the past decade. It is therefore

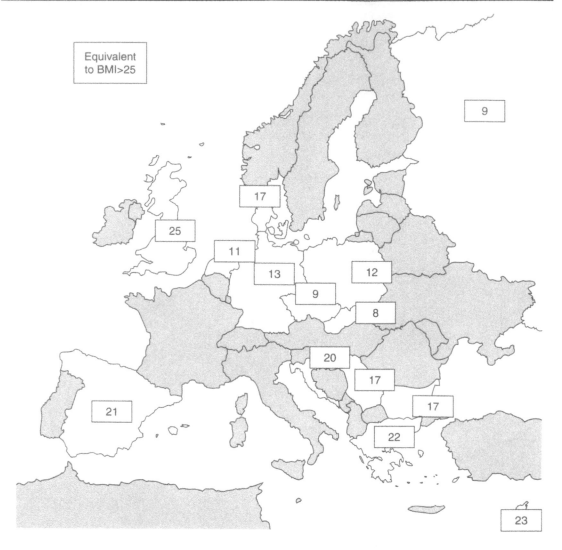

Figure 8: Prevalence of overweight (%) in children aged 14–17 years in selected European countries in 2002 (IOTF data).
Source: With kind permission of IOTF.

reasonable to estimate that the prevalence will be more than 25% among both men and women by the year 2005. Serial surveys in other countries show a similar trend.

It is evident that, since the first survey in 1980, the prevalence of obesity in the UK has more than tripled among both men and women. The general level of obesity in affluent countries ranges from the strikingly low values in Japan, through moderate levels in Netherlands and Sweden, to the high levels in USA and Australia. Among less affluent countries there is also a huge range from low levels in Brazil to astonishingly high levels in Samoa. Despite these differences the trend towards increasing obesity is evident everywhere, whatever the baseline level.

Table 5: Prevalence of obesity (%) in England 1980–2002.

BMI	1980	1993[a]	2000[a]	2002[a]
Men				
Healthy weight: 20–25	Not available	37.8	29.9	29.6
Overweight: 25–30	Not available	44.4	44.5	43.4
Obese: > 30	6	13.2	21.0	22.1
Morbidly obese: > 40	Not available	0.2	0.6	0.8
Women				
Healthy weight: 20–25	Not available	44.3	39.0	37.4
Overweight: 25–30	Not available	32.2	33.8	33.7
Obese: > 30	8	16.4	21.4	22.8
Morbidly obese: > 40	Not available	1.4	2.3	2.6
	1984[b]	1994[b]	2000[c]	2001/2[e]
Boys				
Healthy weight: 20–25	94.0[d]	89.3[d]	74.9[d]	72.0[d]
Overweight: 25–30	5.4	9.0	20.3	22.0
Obese: > 30	0.6	1.7	4.8	6.0
Morbidly obese: > 40	Not available	Not available	Not available	Not available
Girls				
Healthy weight: 20–25	89.4[d]	83.9[d]	66.6[d]	63.0[d]
Overweight: 25–30	9.3	13.5	26.6	29.0
Obese: > 30	1.3	2.6	6.8	8.0
Morbidly obese: > 40	Not available	Not available	Not available	Not available

Sources:
[a] Health Survey for England, various years.
[b] Data for children aged 4–12 in England only. Data extracted from POST report 199, September 2003, Improving children's diet – trends pp. 23–4.
[c] Data for children aged 2–19 in England only. Data extracted from the national office for statistics website: (www.statistics.gov.uk/cci/nugget.asp?id=718), diet and nutrition section.
[d] Healthy weights are calculated as 100 – (%obese + %overweight), and thus include those with BMI < 20.
[e] Data provided by IOTF (personal communication).

Relation to age, social class and region

Adults

Sex

In those aged 16–24 years, mean BMI in men is 23.8 in men, and 24.2 in women. Among those aged 16–64 years, mean BMI is 26.2 kg/m^2 in men and 25.8 kg/m^2 in women. In all adults, 65.5% of men and 56.5% of women are overweight or obese. A greater proportion of men (43.4%) than women (33.7%) are overweight, but slightly lower proportions of men (22.1%) than women (22.8%) are obese. Among those aged 16–64 years, 21.4% of men and 21.9% of women are obese.

Age

Men and women tend to reach a maximum prevalence of obesity between 55–64 years, after which BMI starts to decline.

Social class

The prevalence of obesity is inversely related to social class, but there is no satisfactory explanation for this observed association.

Region

There are no marked regional differences in the prevalence of obesity in the UK when the effects of age, social class and smoking habit are allowed for. In men aged 16–24 years, the prevalence of being overweight is lowest in the South East (19.8%) and highest in Yorkshire and Humber (28.4%), while in women it is lowest in London (18.5%) and highest in East England (24.3%). The prevalence of obesity in men is lowest in the South West (5.9%) and highest in the North East (14.5%). In women, obesity is lowest in London (9.3%) and highest in the West Midlands (17.3%).

Smoking and ethnicity

Data on obesity by smoking or ethnicity in 2002 is not published in the *Health Survey for England*.

Incidence

Incidence of obesity is impossible to measure, since there is so much variability in weight with time in any individual. At any moment there will be quite a lot of people oscillating above and below any given threshold of severity.[69]

Children

Sex and age

Using BMI charts (published by the Child Growth Foundation, London), 5.5% of boys and 7.2% of girls aged 2–15 were obese in 2002. Mean BMI falls between age 2 and age 5 or 6. It then increases fairly rapidly to adulthood. Compared with males, females have a slightly higher BMI during adolescence.

Social class, region and ethnicity

Data on childhood obesity by social class, region, and ethnicity in 2002 are not published in the *Health Survey for England*.

Incidence

Incidence of obesity is even more difficult to measure in children since variability in weight and height is greater during growth.

5 Services available and their costs

What happens at present and why?

Obesity has features that do not apply to the other major causes of ill health and disability (e.g. hypertension, cancer or diabetes) with which the health service should cope. A patient with such an illness has probably been diagnosed by a doctor, and looks to medical aid (NHS or private or alternative) for treatment. The problem is one that is known only to those whom the patient chooses to inform, and it carries no social stigma.

In contrast, obesity is usually a condition the patient has self-diagnosed, it is obvious to the public and it does carry a social stigma in many cases. It is unusual for the obese person to seek medical aid in the first instance. The media is full of advice on what to do, so typically the obese person who eventually has a medical consultation gives a history of a series of self-help measures, which did not have a satisfactory outcome. This gives doctors the impression that the self-help measures are invariably ineffective, but this is not so: medical referrals are always self-help failures, but self-help successes do not register in the medical statistics. Field studies of unselected populations show that those who are now overweight were often previously normal weight, and those now of normal weight were often previously overweight.[69]

So, from the viewpoint of the primary care physician seeing an obese patient in surgery, the patient has typically 'tried everything' without satisfaction, and hopes that the GP will have a pill which will solve the problem. The patient already carries a large amount of misinformation about obesity: especially about the rate of weight loss which is to be expected, since this is routinely exaggerated by some commercial weight-loss organisations and magazines. The patient is a self-help failure who may well have been told by the previous therapist that his or her failure indicates a rare metabolic abnormality with which he or she expects the GP to deal. This is not a basis on which a successful consultation can be expected.

This unsatisfactory situation is made much worse by the fact that the GP has had little or no training on how to manage obesity unless, in exceptional circumstances, they attended a postgraduate course,[70] and has no clinical guidelines on which to anchor the consultation and help with decision making.

The next part of this section outlines, for doctors (GPs and consultants), practice nurses (PNs) and dietitians, information about treatments offered and delivery of this service. As there are no significant services that specifically tackle the prevention of obesity or childhood obesity in the UK, the information below is restricted to the treatment of adult obesity. The final part of this section deals with the cost of obesity.

How is obesity managed in primary care?

The first NHS port of call for the obese patient is the GP who can manage the patient him or herself, or refer them to a PN or a dietitian. Information is available on how GPs and PNs manage obesity from a survey conducted by the National Audit Office in 1999.[6] A sample of 1200 GPs and 1200 PNs were surveyed by post, and 20 GPs and 16 PNs took part in face-to-face interviews. The responses showed that management of obesity within general practice consists broadly of three types, depending on the degree of obesity and the extent of clinical complications:

- general lifestyle advice
- general lifestyle advice plus drug therapy
- onward referral to specialist.

Of note, only 4% of GPs used a protocol for managing overweight or obese patients, and many of those in use had been developed independently by the practice. Figure 9 shows the most frequent responses to the question 'What factors might help you in developing further your approach to managing your overweight and obese patients'. 63% of GPs and 85% of PNs believed that national clinical guidelines or a protocol would be 'useful' or 'very useful'. Since this NAO survey was carried out, many PCTs have now developed their own obesity strategy. However, these are variable in quality, and rarely evidence based. There is no formal system for logging local and regional obesity strategies, but the Association for the Study of Obesity website (www.aso.org.uk) provides a list of those made available to them, and links to the documents if possible. The good news is that the National Institute for Clinical Excellence (NICE) is committed to produce guidance for the prevention and treatment of obesity by the end of 2007.

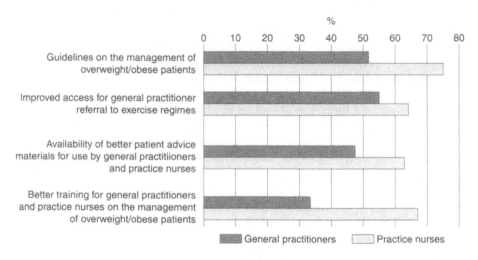

Figure 9: Factors which general practitioners and practice nurses said would assist them in advising and treating patients.[6]

66% of GPs felt that treating patients for overweight or obesity was the responsibility of the primary care team, and 75% thought they had a role to play in referring obese patients to appropriate specialists. [2% neither treated obese patients personally nor referred them to specialists.] Figure 10 shows the referral options most commonly used by GPs. Since this NAO survey was carried out, many PCTs have developed possible referral options to alleviate pressure on the primary care team. Some PCTs now have arrangements with commercial weight loss companies, some have helped develop community based programmes/ self-help groups, and many have developed their exercise on prescription service. Indeed, improved access for referral to exercise regimes was a factor which GPs and PNs said would assist them in managing their overweight and obese patients (Figure 9). It is worth noting that access to the referral options mentioned above is variable by region.

68% of PNs and 33% of GPs stated that better training would assist them in managing their overweight and obese patients (Figure 9). This important point is picked up later in this section.

Referral to a hospital consultant who runs a specialist obesity clinic is unusual, simply because there are so few specialist obesity clinics. In the UK in 2004 there were 10 clinics for adults and 4 for children. Kopelman has argued that there should be more obesity clinics in the NHS.[71] Specialist obesity clinics are usually multidisciplinary, and often have a (limited) facility to refer patients on to a clinical psychologist or surgeon. An audit of one such specialist clinic (run by Prof. Kopelman at the Royal London Hospital)

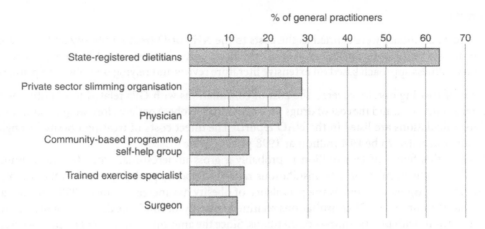

Figure 10: Referral options most commonly used by general practitioners.[6]

showed that 69% of patients were treated by diet alone, 23% by diet and anti-obesity drugs, and 7% by psychological interventions.[72,73] Surgical treatment for obesity in the UK is rare, and procedures are carried out at variable rates across the country.[74]

What do dietitians do?

From a survey conducted in 1998, only one out of 99 NHS dietetic services questioned did not accept overweight or obese client referrals for management.[73] The majority (87%) of respondents allocated up to 30 minutes for a new client appointment. Although 27% had no specific policy about the number of follow-up appointments during a 'course' of treatment, 20% offered one or two follow-up appointments; 35% offered three or four; 16% offered five or more, and only 2% offered no follow-up. Most follow-up appointments were every four weeks (8% were three weeks or more frequently; 50% were every four weeks; 35% were five weeks or less frequently, and data for 7% were missing). The duration of follow-up appointments was as follows: 24% were allocated less than 11 minutes; 73% 11–20 minutes; 2% 21–30 minutes).

The majority of dietetic services did not prioritise (or match) patients for different dietary treatments. Of those who did, criteria such as existing disease, other risk factors, diagnosed eating disorder, degree of fatness, weight history and mental health or learning difficulties were used to identify different approaches for management. However, no common strategies for matching patients to treatments could be identified. Most dietetic services (78%) saw overweight or obese clients only on an individual basis; 20% offered treatment on a combination of individual and group styles. Very few (only 23%) had a protocol, although some others (20%) stated that they currently had protocols under development.

The economic cost of obesity

The National Audit Office[6] conducted a survey to estimate the cost (direct and indirect) of obesity in England in 1998.

Direct costs

The direct costs of obesity were defined as the costs to the NHS of 1) treating obesity and 2) treating the associated disease that can be attributed to it. These direct costs were estimated by taking a prevalence-based, cost-of-illness approach based on extensive literature review and relying on published primary data.

1) The cost of treating obesity covered the cost of consultations with GPs related to obesity, the cost of hospital attendances, and the cost of drugs prescribed to help obese patients lose weight. Sources of data used for calculations are listed in the NAO report.[6] The direct costs of treating obesity in England in 1998 were estimated to be £9.4 million at 1998 prices (Table 6).

   Of note, this figure of £9.4 million is probably a gross underestimate for 2005 for a number of reasons. First, the number of GP consultations related to obesity probably matches the prevalence of obesity in the population, and as the prevalence of obesity has increased since 1998, one can assume that so has the number of GP consultations relating to obesity. Second, the data do not include the cost of consultations with practice nurses or dietitians. Since the amount of time spent by practice nurses on monitoring and advising patients exceeds that spent by most GPs, the cost of primary care interventions for obesity is likely to be significantly greater than that indicated by GP consultations alone. Third, at the time of the NAO survey (1998), orlistat had just been licensed in the UK (in Autumn of 1998), and sibutramine was yet to be licensed. Therefore, the annual cost of prescriptions for these anti-obesity medications in 1999 and beyond is likely to be considerably higher than £0.8 million.

Table 6: Total cost of obesity in England in 1998.[6]

Cost component	Cost (£m)
Cost of treating obesity	
General Practitioner consultations	6.8
Ordinary admission	1.3
Day cases	0.1
Outpatient attendances	0.5
Prescription	0.8
Total costs of treating obesity	9.5
Cost of treating the consequences of obesity	
General Practitioner consultations	44.9
Ordinary admissions	120.7
Day cases	5.2
Outpatient attendances	51.9
Prescription	247.2
Total costs of treating the consequences of obesity	**469.9**
Total direct costs	**479.4**
Indirect costs	
Lost earnings due to attributable mortality	827.8
Lost earnings due to attributable sickness	1,321.7
Total indirect costs	**2,149.5**
GRAND TOTAL	**2,628.9**

2) The cost of treating the consequences of obesity covered the cost of treating diseases such as CHD. The cost of treating these diseases was estimated by calculating the relevant population attributable risk proportion. The proportion of these diseases in the population that was attributable to obesity was then establised using systematic review. [Of note, there were a number of potentially important disease areas that were excluded from this analysis because of a lack of data, e.g. depression and back pain.] Further details of methodology used are provided in the NAO report.[6] The direct costs of treating the consequences of obesity in England in 1998 were estimated to be £469.9 million at 1998 prices (Table 7).

Table 7: The cost of treating the consequences of obesity in England in 1998.[6]

	Attributable cases (% of total cases)	Cost of general practitioners (£m)	Cost of hospital contacts (£m)	Cost of prescriptions (£m)	Total cost (£m)	Proportion of total costs (%)
Hypertension	794,276 (36)	25.5	7.7	101.6	134.8	29
Type II diabetes	270,504 (47)	7.9	36.7	78.9	123.5	26
Angina pectoris	90,776 (15)	2.8	35.3	46.6	84.7	18
Myocardial infarction	28,027 (18)	0.6	41.6	0.0	42.2	9
Osteoarthritis	194,683 (12)	4.7	14.5	15.6	34.8	7
Stroke	20,260 (6)	0.5	15.7	0.5	16.7	4
Gallstones	8,384 (15)	0.2	10.2	0.4	10.8	2
Colon cancer	7,483 (29)	0.4	10.0	0.0	10.4	2
Ovarian cancer	1,543 (13)	0.1	3.8	0.1	4.0	1
Gout	96,549 (47)	2.2	0.0	1.7	3.9	1
Prostate cancer	809 (3)	0.0	0.9	1.7	2.6	1
Endometrial cancer	834 (14)	0.0	1.1	0.1	1.2	0
Rectal cancer	126 (1)	0.0	0.2	0.1	0.3	0
Total		44.9	177.7	247.3	469.9	100

Indirect costs

Earnings lost due to premature mortality

The NAO estimated that over 31 000 deaths in England in 1998 were attributed to obesity; approximately 6% of all deaths. This represents over 275 000 life years lost due to obesity. Some 9000 of these deaths occurred before the age of 65, resulting in a loss of over 40 000 years of working life up to state retirement age alone. The associated lost earnings in England due to obesity in 1998 was estimated to be £827 million at 1998 prices.

Earnings lost due to sickness absence

The NAO estimated that there were over 18 million days of sickness attributable to obesity in 1998. Further details of methodology used are provided in the NAO report.[6] Of note, this is almost certainly an underestimate since the days of absence recorded were only based on medically certified days of incapacity where a claim to benefit was made (no data on self-certified days of sickness were available). On this basis, estimated lost earnings due to sickness absence attributable to obesity in England in 1998 was £1322 million at 1998 prices.

In summary, the direct cost of obesity to the NHS in England in 1998 was at least £480 million, equivalent to about 1.5% of NHS expenditure in that year (Table 6). The direct cost is driven primarily by the cost of treating the secondary diseases attributable to obesity, which accounted for 98% of the total. The most significant cost drivers by far are CHD, hypertension, and type II diabetes, followed by osteoarthritis and stroke. The indirect cost of obesity in England in 1998 represented by lost earnings was estimated to be £2149 million. Combining the direct and indirect costs, the total cost of obesity in England in 1998 was £2.6 billion, or 0.3% of UK Gross Domestic Product.

Cost of individual treatments

More detailed information on the costs of individual treatments for obesity are provided in a recently published report.[7] This report reviewed systematically health economic evaluations of obesity treatments and assessed the cost to the NHS of these treatments. The report concluded that:

Targeting high-risk individuals with drugs or surgery was likely to result in a cost per additional life-year or quality-adjusted life-year (QALY) of no more than £13 000. There was also suggestive evidence of cost-savings from treatment of people with type II diabetes with metformin. Targeting surgery at people with severe obesity and impaired glucose tolerance was likely to be more cost effective, at £2329 per additional life-year.

Economic modelling of diet and exercise over 6 years for people with impaired glucose tolerance was associated with a high initial cost per QALY, but by the sixth year the cost per QALY was £13 389. Results were sensitive to the quality of life weights, for which there were very limited data. Results did not include cost savings from disease other than diabetes, and therefore may be conservative.

The cost of diet and exercise together appear comparable to treatments, for example drugs, in obese individuals with risk factors, such as impaired glucose tolerance.

6 Effectiveness of services and interventions

Assessment of effectiveness

To assess the effectiveness of interventions for the treatment of obesity we have relied primarily on systematic reviews of RCTs. Randomised controlled trials are (almost) the best source of evidence for assessing the efficacy of healthcare interventions, including lifestyle interventions. Results from systematic reviews (and meta-analysis) of several RCTs which address the same question are even better.[75] A conclusion based on several RCTs, selected by previously defined criteria, is likely to be nearer the truth than one based on a group of RCTs which happen to support the reviewer's own prejudices.

There have been a wealth of good systematic reviews (and reviews of reviews) on the treatment of obesity published in the past few years, and a number of others were published in 2004/5 (Table 8a). [NICE is committed to produce guidance for the prevention and treatment of obesity by the end of 2007.] For the purpose of this chapter, we have chosen to use information and data from the most recent of the good systematic reviews listed in Table 8b. Thus, we have used the information and data from the Health Technology Assessment (HTA) review on obesity[7] for evidence of the efficacy of treatments for obesity in adults. We have used the information and data from two Cochrane reviews for evidence of the efficacy of interventions for the prevention[76] and treatment[77] of obesity in children. We have used the information and data from the Health Development Agency review of reviews on obesity[59] for evidence of the efficacy of interventions for the prevention of obesity in adults.

The findings from these four reviews are all based on sound methodology, but vary a little in their inclusion criteria; these differences are highlighted in Table 8b. Full reports of these four reviews contain details of the methodologies they employed and findings. All four reports are available free at the relevant websites (Table 8a).

Table 8a: Systematic reviews on the management of obesity published from 2002.

Source (country)	Referenced as	Population	Year published	Search date	URL
Systematic reviews					
Calgary (Canada)	Calgary	Children	2004	2004	www.calgaryhealthregion.ca
HTA (UK)	HTA	Adults	2004	Spring 2001	www.ncchta.org
NHMRC (Australia)	NHMRC	All	2003	May 2001	www.obesityguidelines.gov.au
US PSTF (US)	USPSTF	Children	2004	Feb 2003	www.ahrq.gov/clinic/uspstfix.htm
US PSTF (US)	USPSTF	Adults	2003	Feb 2003	www.ahrq.gov/clinic/uspstfix.htm
SBU (Sweden)	SBU	All	2002	2002	www.sbu.se
Cochrane (International)	Summerbell *et al.*	Children	2003	July 2002	www.nelh.nhs.uk
SIGN (Scotland)	SIGN	Children	2003	Dec 2001	www.sign.ac.uk
NHS CRD (UK)	NHS CRD	Children	2002	July 2002	www.york.ac.uk/inst/crd
Cochrane (International)	Campbell *et al.*	Children	2002	July 2002	www.nelh.nhs.uk
HTA-surgery (UK)	HTA-surgery	Adults	2002	Summer 2001	www.ncchta.org
HTA-sibutramine (UK)	HTA-sibutramine	Adults	2002	June 2000	www.ncchta.org
HTA-orlistat (UK)	HTA-orlistat	Adults	2001	June 2000	www.ncchta.org
Reviews of reviews					
CIHR (Canada)	CIHR	All	2003	May 2003	www.caphc.org/partnerships_obesity.html
HDA (UK)	HDA	All	2003	Oct 2002	www.hda.nhs.uk/evidence

The outcome presented in this chapter is weight loss. This is not, of course, the only measure of efficacy in a treatment for obesity, but it is one measure of outcome that is normally reported, and this enables us to make comparisons between treatments.

Estimates of the effectiveness, where known, are graded by the size of the effect where:

Mean weight loss attributable to intervention
A* = large weight loss   >10 kg
A = strong beneficial effect   5–10 kg
B = moderate beneficial effect   2–5 kg
C = measurable beneficial effect   Significant difference
D = no measurable effect   No significant difference
E = harms of the treatment outweigh its benefits

Table 8b: Inclusion criteria for systematic reviews from which information was used for this chapter.

Reference	Population and intervention	Study design	Minimum follow-up
HTA (2004)[7]	Treatment of obesity in adults	RCTs	At least 1 year
Campbell *et al.* (2004)[76]	Prevention of obesity in children	RCTs and CCTs	At least 3 months
Summerbell *et al.* (2004)[77]	Treatment of obesity in children	RCTs	At least 6 months
HDA (2003)[59]	Treatment and prevention of obesity in adults & children	various	various

and quality of the supporting evidence where:

I-1 = Evidence from several consistent or one large RCT(s)

I-2 = Evidence obtained from at least one properly designed RCT

II-1 = Evidence obtained from well-designed controlled trials without randomisation, or from well-designed cohort or case-control analytic studies

II-2 = Evidence obtained from multiple time series with or without the intervention

III = Opinions of respected authorities, based on clinical experience, descriptive studies, or reports of expert committees

IV = Evidence inadequate and conflicting

Effectiveness of treatments

Obesity inevitably follows a prolonged period during which energy intake (in food and drink) exceeds energy output (in resting metabolism, exercise, metabolic response to various thermogenic stimuli, and energy losses in excreta). Therefore effective treatment inevitably requires a reversal of energy balance, so output exceeds input, and body fat is burned off to meet the deficit. However it has recently been recognised that a large part of the cause of the 'global epidemic' of obesity is environmental. The availability and commercial promotion of cheap palatable snack foods tends to increase energy intake. The labour-saving devices that reduce the need for manual work, and the increasing tendency to watch, rather than participate in, vigorous leisure activities tends to decrease energy output. Together these tendencies create an 'obesogenic' environment.

For estimates of effectiveness of treatments for obesity in this chapter we have relied primarily on a systematic review of RCTs in HTA 2004.[7] The authors of this review adopted the entry criteria that NICE suggest for drug trials, and therefore included only randomised controlled trials of people with BMI > 28 kg/m^2 at entry and a follow-up for at least 1 year. It is very difficult to conduct trials of dietary or lifestyle treatments that meet these criteria, since the control group are required to make no effort to control their obesity for a year, which is an unrealistic requirement. Having set these selection criteria the authors comment: 'Limitations in the evidence available for the reviews, particularly inadequate sample size and reporting, lack of long-term follow-up and few quality of life data, mean that most results should be interpreted with caution.' We have therefore used data from other sources that HTA 2004 excluded. For each type of treatment the effectiveness, and the quality of the supporting evidence, is graded as described in the above section.

Since dietary treatments are economical, widely used and suitable for the great majority of obese people, they will be discussed first, then exercise, drug treatment, behaviour therapy, surgery and various combinations of these treatments.

Effectiveness of patient-centred interventions

Dietary treatments

The largest intentional weight loss in an obese patient ever reported in a peer-reviewed medical journal was achieved on a diet supplying 800 kcal/day for 2 years.[78] The patient's weight fell from 310 kg to 90 kg as an inpatient in a metabolic unit. Such treatment today is economically and socially impractical, but this exceptional case shows that there is no limit to the amount of weight that can be lost by dieting, if the patient can actually keep to the diet.

Effects of 600 kcal/day deficit or low-fat diet versus control

This 'slightly hypocaloric' diet[79] was extensively used as a 'control' diet in RCTs of drug treatments (see below). Theoretically, if a person consumes a diet supplying 600 kcal/day less than expenditure their weight should decrease by 600 g/week, or 31 kg at 12 months, since the excess weight in obese people has an energy value of 7000 kcal/kg.[80] The observed weight losses in the trials below are much less than this theoretical value, indicating that the treatment subjects did not strictly observe the diet, or that the control group were not strictly non-dieting.

Listed below are meta-analyses of RCTs reviewed in HTA 2004,[7] in which can be found references for the individual trials. This review analyses the change in body weight (kg), total cholesterol, LDL cholesterol, HDL cholesterol, triglyceride, HbA_{1c}%, fasting plasma glucose and blood pressure. Only weight changes will be quoted here, since the beneficial changes in risk factors (where available) are closely proportionate to the weight change.

A meta-analysis of 12 RCTs found that, compared with non-dieting controls, the 600 kcal/day deficit or low-fat diets were associated with an overall weighted mean difference (WMD) weight change at 12 months of −5.31 kg (95% CI −5.86 to −4.77 kg). There was evidence of statistical heterogeneity, although the direction of effect was consistent across all studies. When 12-month weight changes from studies with imputed values were compared with studies with no assumed values, the weight changes were −4.52 kg (95% CI −5.67 to −3.36 kg) compared with −5.55 kg (95% CI −6.17 to −4.94 kg). When 12-month weight loss from RCTs with participants with cardiovascular risk factors was compared with RCTs with participants with no reported risk factors, a clearer difference between studies emerged (−4.19 kg, 95% CI −4.90 to −3.48 kg; compared with −6.98 kg, 95% CI −7.83 to −6.12 kg, respectively).

At 18 months weight change was −1.15 kg (95% CI −2.76 to 0.45 kg), 24 months −2.35 kg (95% CI −3.56 to −1.15 kg), 30 months 0.70 kg (95% CI −1.78 to 3.18 kg), 36 months −3.55 kg (95% CI −4.54 to −2.55 kg) and at 60 months −0.20 kg (95% CI −2.03 to 1.63 kg). After 12 months only a maximum of three studies provided data towards any one comparison.

Quality of supporting evidence = I-1   Size of effect = A

In the cluster RCT the weight change at 12 months was −0.88 kg (SD 4.0 kg) for the diet group and 1.3 kg (SD 3.0 kg) for the control group, which was not found to be a statistically significant difference.

The two studies that were associated with the least mean difference in weight change also had populations with the largest mean BMI of 34.0 kg/m.[2]

One death occurred in the control arm of the Hypertension Prevention Trial (HPT) study and two deaths in the intervention arm of the TAIM Phase I study. Two deaths in the intervention group and one in the control group occurred in the study by Hankey and colleagues, three deaths in the Hypertension Optimal Treatment (HOT) study and four deaths in the first year of the study by Swinburn and colleagues (group allocation not known). One diagnosis of cancer occurred in year 2 of the study by Wood and colleagues, and two cancers and one cardiac event in the Oslo Diet and Exercise Study (ODES) (allocation unknown).

Swinburn and colleagues found that 47% of the participants developed diabetes or impaired glucose tolerance, compared with 67% in the control group. After 1 year the investigators for the Dietary Intervention Study of Hypertension (DISH) reported that 59.5% of participants allocated to diet remained off medications, compared with 35.3% of controls (reported p=0.0015). The investigators for the HOT study also reported that people in the diet intervention arm required fewer medications between 1 year and 30 months, a difference that was consistently statistically significant. In the HPT 9% of intervention and control groups required drug treatment for hypertension during the 3 years of study.

One study reported no effect of diet counselling by doctor and dietitian or dietitian alone on subsequent use of medication. The same study reported that the cost of an extra kilogram weight loss was Aus$9.76 for the doctor/dietitian group and Aus$7.30 for the dietitian group.

Effects of low-calorie diet (LCD) versus control

An RCT on cancer patients showed that, compared with the control group, the LCD was associated with a WMD weight change at 12 months of –6.25 kg (95% CI –9.05 to –3.45 kg), at 24 months of –7.00 kg (95% CI –10.99 to –3.01 kg) and at 36 months of –6.10 kg (95% CI –10.71 to –1.49 kg).

Quality of supporting evidence I-2   Size of effect = B

Three breast cancers occurred in the intervention group and one in the control group. Three people died from breast cancer in the intervention group and five people in the control group. There were two deaths from other causes in each of the two groups.

Effects of very low-calorie diet (VLCD) versus control in an obese population with asthma

At 12 months VLCD compared with control was associated with a WMD weight change of –13.40 kg (95% CI –18.43 to –8.37 kg). After 1 year the difference in forced expiratory volume in 1 second between VLCD and control groups was 7.6% (95% CI 1.5 to 13.8%), forced vital capacity 7.6% (95% CI3.5 to 11.8%) and peak expiratory flow 6.2% (95% CI –1.4 to 13.7%).

Quality of supporting evidence = I-2   Size of effect = A*

During the year of follow-up 18 out of 19 participants in the control group and 16 out of 19 participants in the VLCD group had at least one exacerbation of asthma. The median number of exacerbations was 1 (range 0–7) in the control group and 1 (range 0–4) in the VLCD group (reported p=0.001). Overall reduction in rescue medication was 0.5 doses in the VLCD group and zero doses in the control group. Thirteen out of 19 participants in the control group needed a course of oral steroids during the year and ten out of 19 participants in the VLCD group.

Effects of low-calorie diet versus 600 kcal/day deficit or low-fat diet

At 12 months an LCD compared with a low-fat diet was associated with a WMD weight change of 1.63 kg (95% CI –1.26 to 4.52 kg).

Effects of very low-calorie diet versus low-calorie diet

Compared with LCD, VLCD was associated with an overall WMD weight change at 12 months of –0.15 kg (95% CI –2.73 to 2.43 kg) and at 18 months of –1.13 kg (95% CI –5.32 to 3.06 kg). Thus, there was no evidence to suggest that VLCD was associated with a significantly greater weight loss than LCD at any of the time-points.

Effects of protein-sparing modified fast (PSMF) versus low-calorie diet

At 12 months the PSMF compared with LCD was associated with an overall WMD weight change of –3.57 kg (95% CI –7.36 to 0.22 kg), at 18 months 0.69 kg (95% CI –1.58 to 2.96 kg), at 24 months of –2.17 kg (95% CI –4.88 to 0.54 kg), at 36 months of –1.51 kg (95% CI –5.43 to 2.41 kg) and at 60 months of 0.20 kg (95% CI –5.68 to 6.08 kg). There were no statistically significant changes in lipids at 18 months in one study in diabetics, although the same study found an association between the PSMF diet and reduced HbA_{1c} of –2.60% (95% CI –4.36 to –0.84%) and fasting plasma glucose of –4.5 mmol/l (95% CI –7.07 to –1.93 mmol/l) at 18 months.

Quality of evidence = I-2   Size of effect = B

Effects of 220 kcal vs 800 kcal diet for 24 weeks[81]

In the 20-week outpatient phase of this trial obese women on a diet supplying 220 kcal/day lost 19.9 kg, and those on 800 kcal/day lost 14.2 kg. However lean tissue contributed a larger proportion of the weight lost in the former group.

Quality of evidence II-1   Size of effect A*

Effectiveness of exercise

Effects of diet and exercise versus control

In these studies initial BMI was 27.9 to 31.3 kg/m², and the diet was either low fat, or one designed to cause a 600 kcal/day energy deficit. The exercise was up to three supervised sessions of 45–60 minutes weekly. Diet plus exercise versus no treatment was associated with an overall WMD weight change at 12 months of –4.78 kg (95% CI –5.41 to –4.16 kg). Weight loss at 24 months was still evident, with diet plus exercise associated with a WMD weight change of –2.70 kg (95% CI –3.60 to –1.80 kg).

Diet plus exercise compared with controls demonstrated a statistically significant effect on lipids, blood pressure and fasting plasma glucose at 12 months, and fasting plasma glucose at 24 months.

Quality of evidence = I-1   Size of effect = B

Effectiveness of drug treatments

The intervention which is most readily investigated by RCT is a drug trial, since either active drug or placebo can be administered in randomised double-blind conditions. Furthermore drug trials are usually very well managed, since the licensing of a new drug depends on the quality of evidence of efficacy presented to the licensing authority. In the UK at present (2004) only two drugs are licensed for the treatment of obesity.

Orlistat

This drug is from Roche Laboratories – trade name Xenical. It inhibits the activity of intestinal lipase, and thus reduces by about 30% the digestion and absorption of dietary fat from the gut.

Effects of orlistat 360 mg/day and diet versus placebo and diet

The added effect of orlistat 360 mg/day on weight reduction produced an overall WMD weight change at 12 months of –3.01 kg (95% CI –3.48 to –2.54 kg).

Quality of evidence = I-1   Size of effect = B

The added effect of orlistat 360 mg/day on weight maintenance produced an overall weight change after 12 months of –0.85 kg (95% CI –1.50 to –0.19 kg) with evidence of heterogeneity in these four studies.

All the risk factors for the 1-year weight reduction phase showed beneficial changes, except for HDL cholesterol, which showed a small decrease, and triglycerides (TGs). There was evidence of heterogeneity for HbA_{1c}, fasting plasma glucose and TGs for this 12-month weight reduction phase. This may have related to the inclusion of people with diabetes in two studies. After 12 months of orlistat in people with diabetes a change in HbA_{1c} of –0.27% (95% CI –0.38 to –0.15%) compared with the control group was observed, and –0.11% (95% CI –0.20 to 0.02%) for non-diabetics compared with controls. Similarly, for fasting glucose the observed change was –0.58 mmol/l (95% CI –0.80 to –0.36 mmol/l) for diabetics compared with controls and –0.16 mmol/l (95% CI –0.27 to –0.05 mmol/l) for non-diabetics. However, for TGs observed changes were less marked between diabetics compared with controls (–0.05 mmol/l, 95% CI –0.19 to 0.09 mmol/l) and non-diabetics (0.05 mmol/l, 95% CI –0.03 to 0.14 mmol/l). For the 12-month weight maintenance phase there were no added benefits on risk factors.

Two weight reduction studies produced an overall WMD weight change at 24 months of –3.26 kg (95% CI –4.15 to –2.37 kg). By 24 months the beneficial effects of orlistat on risk factors were still seen, with the exception of triglycerides and systolic blood pressure (SBP).

One death occurred in the orlistat arm of the study by Broom and colleagues from cancer and one death in the orlistat arm of the study by Hauptman and colleagues from acute myocardial infarction (MI). One death from brainstem infarction occurred in the orlistat arm of the study by Lindgarde and colleagues.

Davidson and colleagues reported four cases of breast cancer in year 1, three of these cases in participants treated with orlistat and one case in a participant treated with placebo (one in each group had evidence of breast cancer on mammograms before study entry). Rossner and colleagues reported one participant with cholelithiasis. Rossner also reported one participants with breast cancer in the placebo group and three participants with breast cancer in the 120-mg orlistat group (of whom two had mammogram evidence of cancer before recruitment). Sjostrom and colleagues reported one participant with gastrointestinal cancer in the placebo/placebo group during the 2 years of the study.

All the orlistat studies reported gastrointestinal adverse events, such as oily stools and faecal incontinence, to be more common in the orlistat groups than in the placebo groups.

In two studies vitamin supplementation was routinely given to all participants. Where reported, vitamin supplementation *per protocol* was always required more commonly in the orlistat groups than in the placebo groups.

Hollander and colleagues reported that the average dose of oral sulfonylureas decreased more in the orlistat than in the placebo group (–23% versus –9%, respectively, p=0.0019).

Effects of orlistat 360 mg/day for 52 weeks and diet versus placebo for 24 weeks and diet then orlistat 360 mg/day for 28 weeks and diet

At 12 months 52 weeks of orlistat 360 mg/day was associated with a WMD weight change of –0.69 kg (95% CI –2.85 to 1.47 kg) compared with the placebo/orlistat group. The orlistat group had changes at 12 months in total cholesterol of –0.29 mmol/l (95% CI –0.65 to 0.07 mmol/l), LDL cholesterol of –0.51 mmol/l (95% CI –0.76 to –0.26 mmol/l) and fasting plasma glucose –0.30 mmol/l (95% CI –0.75 to 0.15 mmol/l). However, all these results are from only one study.

During the double-blind phase of 24 weeks 86.6% of participants on orlistat and 42.3% of participants on placebo experienced gastrointestinal side-effects. One participant required a cholecystectomy in the placebo/orlistat group and one participant developed a stroke in the 52-weeks orlistat 360 mg/day group.

Sibutramine

This drug from Abbott Laboratories (trade name Reductil) is a serotoninergic and adrenergic re-uptake inhibitor that enhances satiation.

Effects of sibutramine (10 mg/day) and diet versus placebo and diet

Sibutramine and diet compared with diet in the three weight reduction studies was associated with an overall WMD weight change at 12 months of –4.12 kg (95% CI –4.97 to –3.26 kg). The weight reduction study by Apfelbaum and colleagues was associated with a weight change at 15 months of –3.70 kg (95% CI –5.71 to –1.69 kg). The STORM weight maintenance study was associated with a weight change at 18 months of –3.40 kg (95% CI –4.45 to –2.35 kg).

Quality of evidence I-1   Size of effect = B

At 12 months sibutramine in the weight reduction studies showed beneficial effects on HDL cholesterol and triglycerides, as did the sibutramine group in the STORM weight maintenance study. At 18 months in the STORM study HDL and triglycerides were still significantly improved.

At 12 months, SBP showed a WMD change of 1.16 mmHg (95% CI –0.60 to 2.93 mmHg) in two weight reduction studies. Diastolic blood pressure showed a WMD change of 2.04 mmHg (95% CI 0.89 to 3.20 mmHg).

One person required a cholecystectomy in the sibutramine group of the study by Apfelbaum and colleagues. One person was also withdrawn from the placebo group in this study because of the development of hypertension. Adverse events did not appear to differ between the treatment arms for this study, with the exception of constipation, which was more common with sibutramine (OR 4.14, 95% CI 1.31 to 13.10), although the confidence interval was wide.

In the study by Smith and colleagues one participant withdrew from the 10-mg sibutramine group owing to four drop attacks within 2 weeks of the start (history of epilepsy) and one participant withdrew from the 15-mg sibutramine group owing to palpitations due to frequent ventricular ectopic beats. Dry mouth was also significantly more frequent in both sibutramine groups than in participants on placebo (OR 11.42, 95% CI 2.72 to 47.87).

In the study by McMahon dry mouth and constipation were also the adverse events reported as being significantly more frequent in the group on sibutramine ($p < 0.05$). Eight out of 150 participants discontinued sibutramine as a result of hypertension, compared with one out of 74 participants on placebo (OR 4.11, 95% CI 0.50 to 33.52).

The STORM study found dry mouth, constipation, increased blood pressure, insomnia and nausea to be more than twice as frequent in the sibutramine participants. One participant in each of the sibutramine and placebo groups was withdrawn as a result of hypertension. Of the participants with hypertension taking sibutramine, two needed an increase in therapy and two a decrease.

Effects of SSRIs and diet versus placebo and diet

Other SSRIs (e.g. fluoxetine, femoxetine or sertraline) had no apparent added effect on weight loss or maintenance or any of the reported risk factors. At 12 months the added effect of SSRIs on weight reduction was associated with an overall WMD weight change of −0.33 kg (95% CI −1.49 to 0.82 kg).

The study by Bitsch and Skrumsager assessed weight at 12 months in 37 participants and reported a median change in weight of −6.6 kg for the femoxetine group and −8.8 kg for the placebo group.

O'Kane and colleagues reported one serious adverse event of colonic malignancy in the placebo group of a fluoxetine trial. Wadden and colleagues reported no difference in depression scores between participants on sertraline and placebo; other studies did not report on mood. Goldstein and colleagues, Wadden and colleagues and Bitsch and Skrumsager reported significantly more adverse events in the SSRI groups, which were expected side-effects of the drugs.

Metformin

Metformin is a biguanide that decreases glugoneogenesis and increases peripheral utilisation of glucose. It is mainly prescribed for the treatment of diabetes mellitus.

Effects of metformin (up to 1700 mg daily) and diet versus placebo and diet

Metformin for weight reduction was associated with a WMD effect on weight at 12 months of −1.09 kg (95% CI −2.29 to 0.11 kg) and at 24 months of −0.50 kg (95% CI −4.02 to 3.02 kg). At a median of 5 years metformin was associated with a WMD weight change of −0.12 kg (95% CI −1.13 to 0.89 kg), at 10 years of −0.37 kg (95% CI −1.67 to 0.93 kg) and at 15 years of −2.71 kg (95% CI −6.98 to 1.56 kg). The longer term data were only available for the UKPDS study.

Metformin had a beneficial effect on total cholesterol at 12 and 24 months and on fasting plasma glucose at 12 months. At a median of 5 years metformin was associated with a WMD in fasting plasma glucose of −1.30 mmol/l (95% CI −1.91 to −0.69 mmol/l), 10 years of −0.34 mmol/l (95% CI −1.10 to 0.42 mmol/l) and 15 years of −1.51 mmol/l (95% CI −3.76 to 0.74 mmol/l). The UKPDS was associated with a WMD in HbA_{1c} at a median of 5 years of −0.46% (95% CI −0.98 to 0.06%) and 15 years of −2.31% (95% CI −3.85 to −0.77%).

At 12 months the control arms were associated with a greater reduction in SBP and diastolic blood pressure (DBP) than the metformin arms and at 24 months this was statistically significant. The WMD effect on SBP at 24 months was 10.00 mmHg (95% CI 3.21 to 16.79 mmHg) and on DBP at 24 months was 5.00 mmHg (95% CI 0.56 to 9.44 mmHg). It should be noted these data at 24 months were derived from one study with small numbers of participants and that the confidence intervals are wide.

One death and no new cases of diabetes were reported in the metformin group of the BIGPRO 1 study and five new cases of diabetes occurred in the placebo group (OR for developing diabetes 0.09, 95% CI 0.00 to 1.64). Teupe and Bergis reported one MI in the treatment group at 1 year. Diarrhoea was more commonly reported for patients on metformin in BIGPRO 1 and the study by Teupe and Bergis.

The UKPDS reported outcomes of total mortality, and deaths for MI, stroke and all-cause cancers at a median period of 10 years. For all-cause mortality the OR was 0.62 (95% CI 0.42 to 0.91) in favour of metformin, for MI mortality the OR was 0.51 (95% CI 0.28 to 0.94). For cerebrovascular mortality the OR was 0.80 (95% CI 0.28 to 2.26) and for all-cause cancer mortality it was 0.73 (95% CI 0.36 to 1.49).

Acarbose

Acarbose inhibits the action of pancreatic amylase, and hence delays the digestion and absorption of carbohydrates from the gut. It is mainly prescribed for the treatment of diabetes mellitus.

Effects of acarbose (up to 600 mg/day) and diet versus placebo and diet in an obese population with type II diabetes

Over 12 months acarbose was associated with a WMD weight change of –0.79 kg (95% CI –1.53 to – 0.05 kg). Over 12 months acarbose was associated with a WMD change in HbA_{1c} of –0.76% (95% CI –1.05 to –0.47%) and in fasting plasma glucose of –1.36 mmol/l (95% CI –1.96 to –0.75 mmol/l). The authors reported that lipids did not change in participants who received acarbose, but the data were not provided. Acarbose led to significant decreases in the doses of metformin, sulfonylurea and insulin prescribed. Acarbose was more frequently associated with gastrointestinal adverse effects, classified as mild. Four participants on insulin (one receiving acarbose and three receiving insulin) required correction of severe hypoglycaemia.

Effectiveness of behaviour therapy

Behaviour therapy is a treatment for obesity that was introduced by Stuart[81] who reported excellent results in 8 patients who lost 17.1 kg in 12 months (see below). Behaviour therapy does not in itself cause weight loss, but enables patients to adhere more strictly to the prescribed diet. The therapy is based on the assumption that behaviour is acquired and maintained by environmental events, so it can be relearned if the environment is altered to promote this change. Stuart's patients were therefore required to eat only in a special room in their house, at specified times, and with a specified place setting. Everything related to food and eating was recorded in a diary. They weighed themselves 4 times daily. They were taught how to cope with self-defeating thoughts about dieting.

Many attempts have been made to make this therapy less onerous, while retaining its efficacy, so now the term 'behaviour therapy' is used to describe many different combinations of psychological strategies to enable the patient to achieve greater control over their eating behaviour. Behaviour is placed after drug therapy in this chapter because, like sibutramine, behaviour therapy does not in itself cause weight loss, but makes it easier for patients to follow a prescribed diet, and thus lose weight.

Effects of diet and behaviour therapy versus control

In these studies the mean BMI at baseline was 34 kg/m^2. The control group received 'minimal' treatment, and the diet and behaviour therapy group were contacted 13 to 40 times in the initial year.

The meta-analysis of diet and behaviour therapy compared with no treatment showed a WMD weight change at 12 months of –7.21 kg (95% CI –8.68 to –5.75 kg) and at 24 months of –1.80 kg (95% CI –4.77 to 1.17 kg).

Quality of evidence = I-1 Size of effect = A*

At 12 months diet and behaviour therapy demonstrated beneficial effects on HDL cholesterol, with a weighted mean difference of 0.11 mmol/l (95% CI 0.06 to 0.17 mmol/l), triglycerides –0.58 mmol/l (95% CI –0.98 to –0.17 mmol/l), SBP –3.39 mmHg (95% CI –5.91 to –0.86 mmHg) and DBP –3.37 mmHg (95% CI –5.16 to –1.58 mmHg). At 24 months the study by Wing and colleagues showed significant beneficial effects on total cholesterol only, WMD –0.30 mmol/l (95% CI –0.58 to –0.02 mmol/l), but the number of participants in this study was small.

In the cluster RCT by Kaplan and colleagues, mean body weight in the groups ranged from 89.9 to 92.2 kg. All participants received an equal number of contacts and an active initial treatment period of 10 weeks. LCD plus behaviour therapy was associated with a mean weight change at 18 months of –1.68 kg, but weight change was not reported for the control group. At 18 months the diet and behaviour group was associated with a mean change in HbA_{1c} of –0.46% compared with 0.36% in the control group. Quality of well-being was also assessed, and was increased by 0.03 units in the diet and behaviour group and decreased by 0.04 units in the control group at 18 months.

No deaths or serious adverse events were reported in any of the studies. Wing and colleagues reported that the risk of developing diabetes was 7% in the control group and 30.3% in the diet and behaviour therapy group.

Effects of diet and behaviour therapy and exercise versus control

Diet, behaviour therapy and exercise compared with control from 11 studies was associated with an overall WMD weight change at 12 months of –4.00 kg (95% CI –4.47 to –3.54 kg).

Quality of evidence = I-1   Size of effect = B

Diet, behaviour therapy and exercise was associated with a WMD weight change at 30 months of –4.68 kg (95% CI –6.08 to –3.28 kg, two trials) and at 36 months of –2.00 kg (95% CI –2.66 to –1.34 kg, one trial).

In the cluster RCT by Kaplan and colleagues, the authors reported that at 18 months participants' weight was 'essentially constant' in the LCD, behaviour therapy and exercise group. Change in weight was not reported for the control group at 18 months. At 18 months the diet, behaviour therapy and exercise group was associated with a mean change in HbA_{1c} of –1.48% compared with 0.36% in the control group. The authors reported that for 100 participants receiving the diet, exercise and behaviour therapy programme 4.7 well-years would be produced, compared with the control (0.047 well-years for each participants, where 0 = death and 1 = optimal function).

In the study by Wing and colleagues, two out of 40 control participants and five out of 40 participants assigned diet, exercise and behaviour therapy developed type II diabetes mellitus at 2 years.

Two participants with MI were reported in the active treatment group and four in the control group (which includes non-obese participants) of the Trial of Non-pharmacological Interventions in the Elderly (TONE) study. Two participants with cerebrovascular accident were also reported in the control group (which includes non-obese participants), and none in the intervention group. In the TONE study the hazard ratio for the primary end-point (recurrence of hypertension and cardiovascular events) was 0.65 (95% CI 0.50 to 0.85) for those randomised to weight loss alone compared with controls. One participant with breast cancer and one with pancreatic cancer were reported, but it was unclear which groups these people came from.

One death was reported in the intervention group and one in the control group of Trials of Hypertension Prevention (TOHP) I. The relative risk for developing hypertension for the intervention group was 0.66 (95% CI 0.46 to 0.94). In TOHP II five people randomised to weight loss died (three cardiovascular disease deaths) and two people in the usual care group died. The relative risk of developing hypertension for the weight loss group was 0.87 (p=0.06) at 48 months.

Effects of family versus individual treatment

The family-based intervention from four studies was associated with an overall WMD weight change at 12 months of –2.96 kg (95% CI –5.31 to –0.60 kg).

Quality of evidence = I-1   Size of effect = B

At 18 months two family-based intervention studies were associated with an overall WMD weight change of –1.08 kg (95% CI –3.04 to 0.87 kg). At 24 months one family-based study was associated with an overall WMD weight change of –5.61 kg (95% CI –10.98 to –0.24 kg). At 43 months one family-based study was associated with an overall WMD weight change of –0.75 kg (95% CI –6.95 to 5.45 kg) and at 48 months

−1.55kg (95% CI −7.88 to 4.78 kg); however after 18 months the number of participants contributing to this comparison was very small.

At 18 months Wing and colleagues were unable to demonstrate any difference between family and individual approaches for weight change, HbA_{1c} or fasting plasma glucose, in a study with a small number of participants.

There were no reported deaths or serious adverse events in any of the included studies.

Effects of group versus individual treatment

Compared with individual treatment the group administered intervention for three studies was associated with an overall WMD weight change at 12 months of 1.59 kg (95% CI −1.81 to 5.00 kg).

Effects of diet and behaviour therapy versus diet

The additional effect of behaviour therapy on diet was associated with an overall WMD weight change at 12 months of −7.67 kg (95% CI −11.97 to −3.36 kg), at 18 months of −4.18 kg (95% CI −8.32 to −0.04 kg), at 36 months of −2.91 kg (95% CI −8.60 to 2.78 kg) and at 60 months of 1.90 kg (95% CI −3.75 to 7.55 kg).

Quality of evidence = I-2 Size of effect = A

Thus, there was a significant added effect of behaviour therapy on weight change at 12 and 18 months, but not at 36 or 60 months. The number of participants contributing to the comparisons decreased over time so the sustained effect of behaviour therapy cannot readily be assessed. In the cluster RCT by Phenix, where meeting time was the unit of randomisation, mean body weight in the groups ranged from 79 to 86 kg. Phenix evaluated the added effects to diet of two forms of behaviour therapy, which were overt behaviour therapy and cognitive behaviour therapy. The added effect of overt behaviour therapy to an LCD was associated with a weight change at 12 months of −3.26 kg compared with −4.82 kg in the diet-only group. The added effect of cognitive behaviour therapy to an LCD was associated with a weight change at 12 months of −6.68 kg compared with −4.82 kg in the diet-only group.

No deaths or serious adverse events were reported in any of the included studies.

Added effect of any intervention over diet

Comparing all treatments assessed as an adjunct to diet at 12 months, behaviour therapy was associated with the greatest WMD weight change of −7.67 kg (95% CI −11.97 to −3.36 kg).

Sibutramine was associated with a WMD weight change of −4.12 kg (95% CI −4.97 to −3.26 kg), orlistat −3.01 kg (95% CI −3.48 to −2.54 kg), exercise −1.95 kg (95% CI −3.22 to −0.68 kg) and metformin −1.09 kg (95% CI −2.29 to 0.11 kg), acarbose −0.79 kg (95% CI −1.53 to −0.05 kg) and behaviour therapy plus exercise −0.67 kg (95% CI −4.22 to 2.88 kg).

At 18 months, exercise was associated with improved weight loss when added to diet, and the additional behaviour therapy was just significant. At 24 months, orlistat was associated with enhanced weight loss when added to diet, and exercise enhanced weight loss when added to diet and behaviour therapy.

The effect of exercise was similar at 36 months. At 60 months behaviour therapy as an adjunct to diet could not be shown to prevent weight gain.

At 12 months orlistat added to diet was associated with lowered DBP and SBP, HbA_{1c}, total cholesterol and glucose, whereas sibutramine increased DBP. At 12 months acarbose added to diet was associated with lowered HbA_{1c} and glucose.

Only one study assessed the added effect of behaviour therapy and exercise to diet and was unable to demonstrate any significant effect on weight or any risk factor at 12 months and 24 months.

The addition of exercise to diet and behaviour therapy was associated with significantly increased weight loss at 12 and 24 months.

Comparisons of treatments versus controls

Few studies compared LCD or VLCD with control, but there was a trend for these diets to produce more weight loss at 1 year than the 600 kcal/day deficit or low-fat diet. One VLCD study was associated with the greatest WMD weight change at 12 months of -13.40 kg (95% CI –18.43 to –8.37 kg). At 24 and 36 months there was some suggestion that LCDs were more effective than 600 kcal/day deficit diets.

Diet and exercise, diet and behaviour therapy, and diet, behaviour therapy and exercise were all associated with significantly greater weight loss than control at 12 months.

In terms of mode of delivery, participants appeared to lose less weight in a group setting than when receiving treatment on an individual basis at all time-points, and this reached statistical significance at 24 months. Participants also appeared to lose more weight when accompanied by their spouse or a friend than when unaccompanied, and this was statistically significant at 12 and 24 months.

Surgery

The HTA 2004 review makes little mention of the efficacy of surgery in the treatment of obesity. In this case also there are problems about entry criteria. By far the largest trial of the effectiveness of surgical treatment is the Swedish Obese Subjects (SOS) trial, that started in 1987.[83] It is intended to recruit 2000 matched patient pairs, and to follow them for 10 years. It is not a randomised trial (the patient having surgery is matched (on 18 variables) with a similar patient who is having non-surgical treatment) therefore it is not included in any Cochrane review. So far 1879 patient pairs have been recruited. After 8 years the weight loss in the surgical group was 28±15 kg, and 0.5±8.9 kg among controls. The weight loss in the surgical patients (as percent body weight) was 33±10% after gastric bypass, 23±10% after vertical banded gastroplasty, and 21±12% after gastric banding. The two-year incidence of diabetes in the surgical patients is 32 times less than in the matched controls, and with hypertension it is 2.6 times less than in controls.

Effects of surgery and diet and behaviour therapy versus surgery

One RCT reported weight change in patients after bariatric surgery. The mean BMI at baseline was 48.9 kg/m^2 for the diet and behaviour group, and 47.6 kg/m^2 for the minimal intervention group. At 12 months diet and behaviour therapy compared with the minimal intervention was associated with a WMD weight change of –10.03 kg (95% CI –22.29 to 2.23 kg) and at 24 months of –10.56 kg (95% CI –23.17 to 2.05 kg). The number of participants in the study was small. The dropout rate was 47% in 2 years, and it was unclear if intention-to-treat (ITT) analysis had been used.

Critical evaluation of the HTA review[7]

The HTA 2004 systematic review presents the weight loss and change in risk factors, compared with control groups, of obese patients who were initially BMI > 28 kg/m^2, and who consented to be randomised to active or control groups, and were followed for at least 12 months. These entry criteria are reasonable for comparing drug trials of orlistat or sibutramine (with which the review is mainly concerned) but not for assessing the effectiveness of diet, exercise or surgery as treatments for obesity. There have been some RCTs comparing diet with 'control', but it is very difficult to recruit obese people who are randomised to the non-diet control group who will remain for 12 months making no effort to obtain some help elsewhere to lose weight. RCTs of exercise very rarely are able to recruit individuals with BMI > 28 kg/m^2, because such people are incapable of prolonged vigorous exercise.[82]

Run-in periods, drop-outs, and ITT analysis

Ideally, patients in an RCT should be typical of all patients with the condition under study, and they should all complete the protocol as planned. In real life these ideal conditions are rarely achieved, so the trial protocols are designed to cope with patients who enrol in the study, but do not comply with the protocol, or who drop out before the trial is designed to end. For example, in a trial of orlistat,[81] all 743 entrants had a run-in period of 4 weeks on placebo and diet, and the 688 patients who took > 75% of the capsules prescribed were then randomised to orlistat or placebo. Therefore the patients who entered the trial were not typical of all the patients screened – they were those selected for being more compliant.

In all long-term drug trials some patients drop out, and these are usually those who are making poor progress. If the analysis is confined to those who complete the trial the results are falsely favourable to the treatment, especially if more patients drop out from the active than from the control group. To avoid this error ITT (intention to treat) analysis is used, but in the case of weight loss trials this also involves bias, since when a patient drops out the last recorded weight is assumed to be the weight at termination of the trial. We know that this is unduly favourable, because when patients drop out of trials their weight does not usually remain constant, but they tend to regain the weight they have lost.

For these reasons, when comparing trials of different interventions for weight loss, we must consider factors such as the starting weight of participants, the selection of compliant responders, and the analysis of drop-outs. Unfortunately this important information is often not provided in the HTA 2004 review.

Prevention of obesity in adults

Three reviews have investigated the prevention of obesity and overweight in adults.[84,85,86] Two of these reviews[84,85] looked at the same three community-based studies, but there was a subtle difference in their conclusions. One review[84] stated that *'community-based education programmes linked with financial incentives may be effective (based on one study) but more research is required'*, whereas the other review[85] concluded that, based on the very limited evidence to date, *'community-based obesity prevention methods have not been proven effective. There is insufficient evidence to recommend in favour of, or against, community-based obesity prevention programmes.'* In all the studies, the mean weight of the intervention and control communities did not differ significantly during a three to seven year follow-up period. However, one review[85] also concluded that, given the health risks and financial costs associated with obesity, *'priority should be given to the prevention of obesity over weight loss interventions'*.

A systematic review of interventions to prevent weight gain in both children and adults[86] identified 11 papers describing five distinct interventions in schools and four in the wider community. Five of the studies were RCTs and half targeted individuals with a low income or a socially disadvantaged background. All the studies had a follow-up of at least one year, except one which followed up after six weeks. Due to the variability of study designs, samples and outcome variables, the authors found it difficult to identify effective types of interventions. The review reported positive changes in half of the interventions that measured diet and physical activity by self-report. Effects on observed weight were mixed, with two studies finding no significant differences, two studies reporting less weight gain in the intervention group and one study finding less weight gain only in sub-groups; the other four studies did not report on the effect on weight. Only one of the five RCTs reported a significant effect on weight. This intervention involved a correspondence programme and a mix of behaviour change methods including goal setting, self-monitoring and contingencies. Overall, the authors concluded that *'future interventions might be more effective if they were explicitly based on methods of behaviour change that have been shown to work in other contexts. Effective interventions would be more easily replicated if they were explicitly described. Effectiveness might be more precisely demonstrated if more objective measures of physical activity and diet were used, and if the follow-up was over a longer period.'*

In summary, the evidence from the three identified reviews[84,85,86] was found to be mixed and inconclusive in terms of effectiveness. Considering the potential scale of obesity and overweight and the associated health, economic and social consequences, the development of effective strategies to prevent obesity is a priority. Therefore, there is an urgent need for further research.

There is inconclusive evidence regarding the effectiveness of community-based interventions (for example, seminars, mailed educational packages and mass media participation) for the prevention of obesity and overweight in adults.

Quality of supporting evidence = I-2   Size of effect = too variable to summarise (due to the different types and combinations of interventions used)

Obesity in children

Treatment of obesity in children[77]

Eighteen randomised controlled trials, with 975 participants, were included in this review. Five studies (n=245 participants) investigated changes in physical activity and sedentary behaviour. Two studies (n=107 participants) compared problem-solving with usual care or behavioural therapy. Nine studies (n=399 participants) compared behavioural therapy with varying degrees of family involvement, with no treatment or usual care or mastery criteria and contingent reinforcement. Two studies (n=224 participants) compared cognitive behavioural therapy with relaxation.

These 18 studies shared similar goals and objectives. However, there were multiple differences in terms of study design (particularly comparisons) and quality (particularly sample size and thus power), and outcome measures. Most of the studies included in this review were too small to have the power to detect the effects of the treatment. A meta-analysis wasn't conducted since so few of the trials included the same comparisons and outcomes. Therefore, results are synthesised in a narrative format.

The results suggest that there may be some additional benefit to behaviour therapy where parents, rather than the child, are given the primary responsibility for behaviour change. In addition, relaxation may be as effective as behavioural therapy. Although there were many trials which focused on changing levels of physical activity and/or sedentary behaviour, these trials were too small to draw any conclusions from with confidence. However, there are some data from these trials in favour of a reduction in sedentary behaviour. Compliance to lifestyle advice was assessed in a minority of the included studies.

Physical activity is recommended for everybody regardless of their weight because of the proven health benefits, although these are not as clear in childhood. Therefore, children should be encouraged to increase their levels of physical activity, even if there is no great benefit in terms of weight reduction.

Most studies were generated in the United States of America among children aged between 7 and 12 years. Interventions to reduce obesity may vary in effect depending on the age of the child since children are metabolically, developmentally, emotionally and nutritionally different in each of the three childhood phases (i.e. infancy, childhood and adolescence). Most studies were underpowered (15/18 randomised fewer than 23 children to at least one group). Seven of the included studies were carried out by the same research team in the US, which has implications for generalising the results of this review to other contexts. Many of the 18 included trials were run from a specialist obesity clinic within a hospital setting.

The proposed relationship between treating obesity and eating disorders, particularly in young populations, may limit the enthusiasm of healthcare workers to treat obesity in children. However, while eating disorders are clearly important public health issues and while dieting may be a risk factor for eating disorders in some people, the literature about this relationship remains equivocal. It is important to acknowledge that the proportion of the population who are obese far exceeds the proportion of the population who have eating disorders.

In summary, the limited evidence makes it difficult to conclude that one strategy or combination of strategies is more important than others in the treatment of childhood obesity. However, the existing literature provides some useful insights regarding 1) the potential of a reduction in children's sedentary behaviours, 2) the delivery of behaviour therapy, and 3) the use of relaxation as effective treatments for childhood obesity. The practicalities of delivering effective advice on lifestyle changes to overweight children will vary with the wide span of social, ethnic and economic circumstances. However, obesity is known to cluster in families, and interventions should be targeted to children whose parents are overweight as a priority.

Quality of supporting evidence = I-1   Size of effect = too variable to summarise (due to the many different types and combinations of interventions used)

NOTE: The SIGN guideline (2003)[63] on childhood obesity provides practical guidance for healthcare workers who treat overweight and obese children.

Prevention of obesity in children[76]

Ten studies were included in this review, seven of which were long-term (follow-up at least 1 year from baseline) and three of which were shorter term (follow-up at least 3 months from baseline). These ten studies shared similar goals and objectives, but multiple differences in terms of study design and quality, target population, theoretical underpinning of intervention approach, and comparable outcome measures, precludes the opportunity to combine results. However, it seems reasonable to suggest that a concentration on strategies that encourage a reduction in sedentary behaviours and an increase in physical activity may be fruitful.

Most studies were generated in the United States of America among children aged between 7 and 12 years. The diversity of the studies limits the generalisability and reproducibility of the findings. Documentation of the characteristics of non-participants and those who are lost to follow-up, whilst difficult to achieve, would be extremely useful in broadening our understanding of the implications of these study findings. Clearly, generalisability would be improved by designing interventions that target a range of communities.

The small number and diverse nature of studies in this area is likely to reflect a number of conceptual, methodological and possibly ethical challenges facing researchers. The environment in many countries, in which driving physiological goals to be sedentary and well fed are overwhelmingly supported by an increasingly complex socio-political environment, may make any attempt to change the status quo seem unrealistic. Therefore, interventions in this area may be considered to be too difficult to pursue. A further conceptual challenge is posed by our limited understanding of the interface between individuals' behaviours and the environment.

This review highlights a paradoxical situation. At a time in which we see obesity prevention nominated as a public health priority, we find a research environment that currently lacks the power to set clear directions for obesity prevention activity across a range of groups at risk.

In summary, there is limited quality data on the effectiveness of obesity prevention programmes and as such no generalisable conclusions can be drawn. Concentration on strategies that encourage reduction of sedentary behaviours and an increase in physical activity may be fruitful.

Quality of supporting evidence = I-2   Size of effect = D

NOTE: The SIGN guideline (2003)[63] on childhood obesity provides practical guidance for healthcare workers who are involved in preventing children from becoming overweight and obese.

Effectiveness of healthcare professional-centred interventions[87]

Eighteen studies were included involving 446 providers and 4158 patients. Five were professional-oriented interventions (the use of reminders and training) and the sixth was a study of professional and organisational interventions of shared care. Twelve studies compared either the deliverer of weight loss interventions or the setting of interventions. The studies identified for this review are heterogeneous in terms of participants, interventions, outcomes, and settings. In addition, only a small number of different interventions have been evaluated rigorously. Along with small sample-sizes and reasonably high drop-out rates among patients, it is difficult to draw firm conclusions on how the management of obesity might be improved from the available evidence.

The two reminder studies indicate that this may be a promising approach to changing doctors' practice. More information is necessary to be able to indicate whether this finding is generalisable across other settings and health professionals. It is not possible to say whether the change in practice may result in a reliable change in patient outcomes.

It is not possible to tell from the evidence whether training might be a useful approach to changing the behaviour of practice nurses. Two studies assessed the effect of a brief educational intervention on obesity management to GPs and both showed that a cheap and quick intervention of this type may be promising in terms of changing practice, at least in the short term. However, a recent study that involved the entire primary care team found no change in patient outcomes at one year.[88]

One study indicated some positive effects in the short term from encouraging shared care between GPs and a hospital service, but these were not sustained over the long term. It seems that additional strategies might be necessary to attempt to ensure the maintenance of improvements among patients.

The findings from studies evaluating different settings and deliverers are inconclusive. Most are small and of limited quality, and do not appear to demonstrate any consistent setting or deliverer effects. However, one study comparing inpatient and outpatient treatments is interesting in that it offers a novel approach to obesity management. In this study, benefits were seen in the inpatient group, including in the longer term. It would be useful to know whether these findings can be replicated on a larger scale across different settings. However, the cost of such an approach to obesity management may prove prohibitive. Without good quality studies including reliable cost effectiveness analyses, it is not possible to say whether the health benefits are worth the additional financial outlay.

Given the large number of commercially run weight loss programmes in some countries, it would be interesting to know whether interventions delivered by health professionals are more effective than those delivered by lay people. We identified one such study. This study found that mean weight loss at one year in weight loss clinics run by a professional therapist was greater than that in weight loss clinics run by a self-help weight clinic leader who had previously been trained by the professional therapist in behavioural therapy.

It would also be interesting to know if less resource-intensive interventions (such as programmes delivered in the home) are cost effective relative to more intensive face to face treatments, but based on the available evidence we cannot say whether this might be so.

There were no studies assessing whether negative attitudes amongst providers were impinging on good practice and whether interventions to change attitudes might result in improved clinical decisions. Given that much commentary has been passed on the possible implications of negative views toward this group of patients, it is surprising there have been no rigorous evaluations of strategies to improve negative attitudes and related practices.

There were no studies comparing whether organisational interventions designed to change the structure of services for overweight and obese people are more effective than educational or behavioural interventions for health professionals. The rationale behind this comparison was that changes in the provision of weight loss services may be more effective than attempting to change health professionals' practice on an individual basis. That is, health professionals could utilise a service rather than think about what to do with overweight and obese patients themselves, thereby overcoming negative perceptions of patients and treatment efficacy, as well as knowledge and time barriers. Along with more general evaluations of interventions to implement obesity services, such comparisons would be of interest.

In summary, health professionals, and in particular primary care providers, have the potential to access large numbers of patients. We currently have little information about how practice or the organisation of care in this area might be improved, although reminder systems, brief training interventions, shared care, inpatient care and dietitian-led treatments may all be worth further investigation.

Effectiveness and cost

In section 7 we suggest how the NHS could most effectively spend the resources allocated for obesity.

7 Models of care and recommendations

Objectives of treatment

In the treatment of patients with established obesity there are three objectives:

- to assist the patient to achieve a weight at which the health risks of obesity are reduced to the lowest possible level for this patient
- to help the patient to maintain this weight loss indefinitely
- to maintain, or restore if necessary, the patient's self-esteem.

Target weight and rate of weight loss

Some guidelines emphasise that 'priority in obesity management should be on weight maintenance and modest weight loss, rather than a return to ideal or normal weight'.[56] The reasoning behind this advice is that there can be a substantial reduction in mortality and risk factors in overweight people who lose 5–10 kg in one year, and that repeated failures to achieve normal weight amplify a patient's depression and lack of self-esteem. These are valid arguments, but there is no evidence that a patient who is, say, 40 kg overweight does better if advised to lose 5–10 kg than if advised to lose 30–40 kg. If the patient who is 40 kg overweight is aged 65 years, short in stature and crippled with osteoarthritis of hips or knees, it is quite likely that a loss of 5–10 kg is as much as can reasonably be achieved. In this situation, the modest weight loss may reduce the health risks to the lowest possible level for this patient, and thus achieve the first objective above.

On the other hand, if the 40 kg-overweight patient is aged 25 years and otherwise fit, but has a family history of diabetes or heart disease, a loss of only 5–10 kg is unlikely to be the optimum for reduction of health risk. Thus the appropriate target weight loss should be assessed in the light of the individual circumstances, rather than by the application of any fixed rule.

Concerning the optimum rate of weight loss there is consensus that a rate greater than 1 kg/week is undesirable, since it is likely to cause excessive loss of lean tissue.

Priority for treatment: obesity or co-morbidity?

In section 3, three sub-categories of obesity were identified: obese patients with existing co-morbidities, obese patients without co-morbidities and non-obese individuals with special risk factors for the development of obesity. At present the usual policy is to treat the co-morbidities of the first group, and to ignore the remainder.

This policy may not be appropriate. French *et al.*[89] studied the effect of weight change between the ages of 18 and 50 years on disease prevalence later in life. They obtained by postal questionnaire reported weight change between the ages of 18 and 50 years in 41 837 women, and were able to classify the weight change pattern of 17 252 of these women into one of five classes. The pattern of the remaining 23 710 women (mostly weight gainers) would not fit into these patterns, and they were excluded from the series. Between age 18 and 30 years those in whom weight changed by less than 5% were classified 'weight stable'. Those in whom weight increased, or decreased, by 5 kg or more were classified as 'weight gainers' or 'weight losers'. A similar designation was used for weight change between the age of 30 and 50 years. The number of women who showed each of the five patterns of weight gain, and their subsequent odds ratio of developing diabetes, high blood pressure, heart attack, other heart disease, cancer or perceived poor health, is shown in Table 9. The data are also analysed separately for those who were, or were not, overweight at age 18 years. Three important messages emerge from this table.

1   Weight loss of 5 kg or more between the age of 18 and 30 years is uncommon: it was observed in only 8% of the population, half of whom regained this lost weight during the period between 30 and 50 years of age. The largest group (47%) are those who gain at least 5 kg between 18 and 30, and again between 30 and 50 years.
2   The odds ratio for diabetes, hypertension, heart attack, other heart disease and perceived poor health (but not cancer) is significantly increased in those women who gained weight compared with those whose weight was stable. The diseases most strongly associated with weight increase are diabetes and hypertension.
3   Eight percent (712 of 9153) of the women were overweight at age 18. In virtually every instance, the odds ratio of the diseases analysed (except cancer) is markedly higher among those who were overweight at 18 compared with those who were not.

This indicates that a policy of laissez faire is not justified. Individuals who are overweight at age 18 years, or who gain more than 5 kg during adult life, have a significantly increased risk of developing the co-morbidities of obesity. Both medically and economically it may be better to prevent this weight gain than to treat the co-morbidity when it arises.

Table 9: Pattern of reported weight change in 17 252 women between age 18 and 50 years, and subsequent health. 95% confidence interval for odds ratio includes 1.0; values are shown in parentheses.[89]

Proportion of women		28%	4%	4%	17%	47%
Weight change*						
Age 18–30 years		stable	loss	loss	gain	gain
Age 30–50 years		stable	stable	gain	stable	gain
Odds ratio of reporting disease at age 62 years						
Diabetes	(a)	1.0	(0.6)	2.3	3.8	6.6
	(b)	5.5	(1.4)	7.5	8.9	19.1
Hypertension	(a)	1.0	(0.8)	1.8	1.8	3.2
	(b)	2.0	(1.2)	3.1	6.3	7.6
Heart attack	(a)	1.0	(1.3)	1.9	1.6	2.0
	(b)	(1.5)	(1.6)	2.0	5.4	3.5
Other heart disease	(a)	1.0	(1.3)	1.8	1.7	1.8
	(b)	(1.3)	2.0	(1.1)	2.6	2.9
Cancer	(a)	1.0	(1.2)	(1.6)	(0.8)	(0.9)
	(b)	(1.0)	(0.8)	(0.6)	(1.0)	(1.1)
Perceived poor health	(a)	1.0	(1.1)	1.7	1.3	2.1
	(b)	(1.4)	1.5	2.4	2.1	4.5

*Stable = < 5 kg change, loss = 5 kg+ loss, gain = 5 kg+ gain.
(a) not overweight at age 18 years, (b) overweight at age 18 years.

Health gain from weight loss

The data presented above show that weight gain in adult life is a common event, and is associated with greater risks of ill health. In adults, there is conflicting evidence about the health effects of weight loss, or fat loss. This evidence is reviewed at length in a systematic review.[18] Most of the evidence comes from prospective cohort studies. In particular, there are strong epidemiological data, which show that weight loss is associated with *increased* total mortality. This has led some commentators to conclude that, although weight gain is bad for health, losing the excess weight does not confer any benefit.

This paradox has been resolved by a secondary analysis of data from the Tecumseh and the Framingham studies.[90] In these two studies, change in body weight, and also in fat mass (by skinfolds) was recorded. They found that each standard deviation in weight loss *increased* the mortality hazard by 29% and 39% respectively in the two studies. Contrarily, each standard deviation of fat loss *reduced* the hazard rate by 15% and 17% respectively. This supports the interpretation that unintentional weight loss in the general population is a sign of ill health, but that intentional fat loss in obese people is beneficial.

The reason why evidence relating intentional weight loss to health outcomes comes from cohort studies is obvious; although one can randomise individuals to different types of treatments for obesity, one cannot randomise them to weight-loss or no weight-loss groups. Indeed, this problem was the topic of a workshop convened in 1997 by the National Institutes of Health and Centres for Disease Control and Prevention.[91] The workshop participants agreed that a well-designed RCT should be undertaken to estimate the magnitude and direction of the long-term health benefits of intentional weight loss. The results of this study, and those from the SOS study will provide much better evidence. Data on sick leave and disability pension from the SOS study at four years have been published.[92] Severely obese patients who underwent surgical treatment for obesity lost more weight and experienced a reduction in sick leave and disability pension compared with controls, particularly patients aged 47–60 years.

Matching patients to resources

It is obvious that the number of people involved, and type of care needed, varies greatly between the sub-groups identified in section 3. The relatively small number of obese people with established co-morbidities urgently need medical care, whereas the large number of non-obese people at high risk to develop obesity do not. This suggests that the appropriate model of care should have different levels ranging from low-cost advice centres, which are easily accessible to concerned members of the public and capable of coping with large numbers, to tertiary referral centres capable of providing medical care for the most complex problems.

- Level 1 is essentially a self-help group, which may be guided by a health professional – either a state registered dietitian[93] or a specially trained public health nurse.[94] It is aimed at management of overweight people for whom the SIGN[56] target of weight maintenance or modest weight loss is entirely suitable. It is also suitable for the long-term follow-up of patients who have been assessed and/or treated at Level 2 or 3. The GP of the individual attending a Level 1 centre should be so informed, to ensure that there is no medical contraindication to the proposed weight management plan.
- Level 2. For those individuals who do not achieve satisfactory results at Level 1, or whose obesity or co-morbidity is sufficiently severe to justify it, the next step is to Level 2. This is based on a primary care doctor who may, having assessed the patient, refer back to Level 1. The assessment of current disease and risk factors at Level 2, which is suggested by the SIGN[56] guidelines includes the following:
  - measurement of weight, height and waist: BMI calculated
  - risk factors assessed (e.g. smoking)
  - blood pressure measured
  - urine tested for glucose
  - plasma γ-glutamyl transferase
  - total plasma cholesterol
  - thyroid-stimulating hormone.

  Advice on risk factor management and dietary advice may be offered at level 2, or the patient may be sent back with a referring letter to level 1 for this advice and further follow-up.
- Level 3. The last step, which is appropriate for a small minority of difficult cases, is Level 3, based on a specialist in a tertiary referral centre. Any attempt to quantify the workload at each of these levels involves assumptions about the efficacy of each level (especially Level 1) and the criteria that are used to make the judgement that a change to another level is indicated. Furthermore, if the system works well the prevalence of obesity will decrease, and hence the load at every level will decrease also (see below).

Integration within the NHS and relationship with private facilities

The components of the above model, which involve NHS resources (Levels 2 and 3), should be integrated with NHS activities elsewhere. Clearly the existing facilities for managing diabetes, heart disease, osteoarthritis, etc., should be available to obese patients entering through the Level 1 route, and conversely patients who enter treatment for a co-morbidity, and who are also overweight, should have access to the Level 1 facilities.

Any model of obesity management based on the NHS will run in parallel with other non-NHS facilities, such as commercial clinics, slimming clubs, health farms and leisure centres. At present there is justifiable suspicion and even hostility between NHS and non-NHS healthcare providers in the field of obesity, since there are many charlatans who are untrained and unregulated in the private sector. Another problem is that under rule 51.3 of the Advertising Standards Agency, slimming clubs are not allowed to advertise themselves as treating obesity (BMI > 30 kg/m^2) because this is a medical condition which should be treated 'under the supervision of a suitably qualified health professional'. This is a commendable attempt to protect the public from exploitation by charlatans, but it also limits the ability of well-run private facilities to provide much-needed Level 1 facilities.

Logistics of the proposed model

Since a very large proportion of the population need help from this model it is logistically necessary to prioritise services to those who would derive most benefit from weight control. The only health *benefit* associated with obesity is a protection against osteoporosis: probably this is partly because adipose tissue contains aromatase, which converts androgens to oestrogens, and hence tends to preserve skeletal mass in post-menopausal women. The health hazards of obesity are greater in young people than in older ones, and weight loss is easier to achieve in younger people, so there are grounds for offering help primarily to younger adults.[95] Management of obesity in children requires a different approach. The implications of this policy related to demographic patterns are discussed below.

Age structure of a model population of 100 000, and of those requiring obesity management services

The age structure of the population of England and Wales is shown in Table 10, divided into five categories. For three of these (pre-school children, secondary school children and retired adults) the case for providing obesity management services is much weaker than for the remaining two – primary school children and pre-retirement adults. The reasons for these priorities are indicated above.

Table 10: Age structure of a model population of 100 000 people in the UK, and the numbers requiring obesity management services.

Category	Age (years)	Number	Annual recruits intake	Requiring management	
				Annual number	Total
Pre-school	0–4	6,400	1,280	nil	nil
Primary school	5–11	8,900	1,270	120	840
Secondary school	12–15	5,000	1,270	nil	nil
Pre-retirement	16–64	63,600	1,270	NK	38,000
Retired	> 65	16,100	NK	nil	nil
Total		100,000			840 primary school 38,000 adults

NK = not known.

For purposes of the following calculation, the population is assumed to be of a constant size, and numbers have been rounded to give no more than three significant figures. In the model population of 100 000 with a typical age structure there will be 8900 primary school children aged 5–11 years, with an annual intake of 1270. Among each year's entry 9% will be above the 91st centile, giving an annual intake of 120 children, who are in this category for seven years, giving a total of 840 primary school children requiring management of their overweight. Facilities for children are discussed later in this section.

The other sector requiring help are the pre-retirement adults of which there are 63 600. With the 2002 prevalence of overweight and obesity in the UK population there will (at any given time) be about 38% or 24 000 who are overweight (BMI 25–30), and about 23% or 14 000 who are obese (BMI >30). To achieve the second objective of treatment given at the start of this section, help should be available to 38 000 young adults (aged 16–64 years) who are overweight or obese.

Weight management clinics required to help 38 000 overweight adults

Although typically a population of 100 000 people will at any given moment have about 38 000 who need help with weight management, it will not be the same 38 000 from one year to the next. In Table 10, the annual intake of overweight adults is shown as 'not known'. Within a population individuals are constantly passing above and below whatever threshold is used to define an 'overweight' category[96] so it is not possible to identify a subsection of the population who are particularly at risk for obesity. The facility must therefore be some form of clinic capable of dealing with those individuals who are overweight, and who perceive themselves to be in need of help at this time.

For reasons given above, it is not possible to estimate how many people in a population of 100 000 would wish to use a Level 1 facility. Some indication can be gained from the experience of Bush et al.[93] in Harrow, and of Karvetti and Hakala[94] in Finland. The Harrow Slimming Club operated in a northern suburb of London, and registered 1090 members in 50 courses over a period of ten years. On average, therefore, each year there were five 10-week courses, which were attended by 109 people. Karvetti and Hakala recruited 243 overweight people in six weeks in the city of Turku, which has a population of about 160 000 and 'several' health centres. If a district with a population of 100 000 had five clinics, and each clinic ran ten courses per year for 20 people per course, this would provide facilities for 1000 members per year. This would probably be an adequate facility, because a family member (usually a mother of children) who attended the course would often be able to transmit what she had learned to other members of the family.

Level 2 help should be available by referral of Level 1 members who have additional problems. If this is estimated to be 10% of those attending at Level 1, then there would be 100 referrals per year to GPs of overweight people with additional problems. This would not be a great burden, since it would be fewer than ten patients per year to individual GPs.

If there were ten specialist centres in the UK, then each Level 3 facility would serve about 600 districts. If practitioners at Level 2 referred 98% of the patients back to Level 1 for management, and 2% on to Level 3, then each specialist unit would receive about 1200 referrals per year. Assessment at Level 3 would initially involve an outpatient consultation with a specialist (and preferably also a dietitian), for which about 30 minutes would be required, so a clinic session of 2.5 hours would provide slots for five new patients. At this input, the Level 3 facility would have to run about five clinics per week. At present there is no experience of a national Level 3 facility such as that suggested, so the estimate of workload is a guess which would have to be modified in the light of experience, and in the light of the confounding factors mentioned at the start of this section.

Facilities required to manage 38 000 overweight adults

The facilities needed at Level 1 are easily provided by local authority school health clinics, which are not used in the evenings. The most important requirement is a good leader – preferably a state registered dietitian or specially trained health nurse. A room in which it is possible to conduct seminar-type teaching with a group of up to 25 members, and facilities for weighing the members of the group and for showing audiovisual teaching aids is also required.

The facilities required at Level 2 are normally found in the surgery premises of GPs. These are for a clinical consultation, physical examination and assessment according to the SIGN[56] guidelines. These are weight, height and waist measurement, blood pressure, urine glucose, plasma γ glutamyl transferase, plasma cholesterol and thyroid-stimulating hormone.

The facilities for Level 3 care will normally be in a teaching hospital. Apart from the advantage of the facilities mentioned below, it is important that the management of obesity at this level should be part of the education of healthcare students. In addition to the normal clinical and diagnostic facilities, there should be a physician with a special interest in obesity, full dietetic support, and preferably facilities for measuring resting metabolic rate by indirect calorimetry and for measuring body composition by dual emission x-ray absorptiometry (DEXA) or bioimpedance. The consultant physician needs to have the option of referral for advice to a surgeon or clinical psychologist, and to be familiar with the indications for drug treatment. It is very helpful to have the option to use up to three hospital beds, so that patients who have been referred from a distance can be admitted for investigation if necessary.

Hospital admission 'to get the patient started on a diet' is a waste of resources. Of course it is possible to initiate weight loss in a metabolic ward, but that has no long-term benefit because if the patient is totally unable to diet outside hospital the prognosis is hopeless. However a brief admission (up to three weeks) may be justified in some cases to establish the type of diet and exercise programme which a given patient can reasonably be expected to maintain in the long term. Even the most highly motivated patients do not adhere to dietary restrictions as rigidly at home as they do in a well-run metabolic ward.[97]

Management of obesity in children

There is good evidence that childhood obesity is a risk for ill health in adulthood (*see* section 2), but data on the effects of intentional weight control in childhood on health outcomes are lacking. Table 9 shows that the subsequent health problems of women who are already overweight at the age of 18 years are significantly greater than of those who are not overweight at age 18 years, so it is evidently necessary to prevent excessive weight gain in childhood.

The change in BMI from birth to age 20 years is shown in Figure 11. At birth the average baby is approximately 50 cm long and weighs 3.4 kg, giving a BMI of 13.6. In the first year of life, the normal child trebles its birth weight and grows to 75 cm, giving a BMI of 17.5. Over the next four years height increases more rapidly than weight, so BMI decreases, and the nadir of the 50th centile line is below 16 kg/m^2 at age 5 years. During this period of rapid height growth there are potential dangers of causing permanent stunting if energy intake is restricted. In fact, fat babies often do not stay fat,[98] so it seems prudent to delay weight control measures until after the age of 5 years. By age 12, the 50th centile line has risen to 18 $kg/m.^2$ The broken arrow in Figure 11 shows that if a child who was on the 91st centile at age 5 years *did not increase BMI* over the next seven years, he or she would then be on the 50th centile of weight-for-height. A strategy by which this might be achieved is discussed below. The rationale for ceasing weight control measures at age 12 years is that children during and after puberty become much more economically and emotionally independent, and some rebellion against adult authority is a normal phenomenon. If the proposed

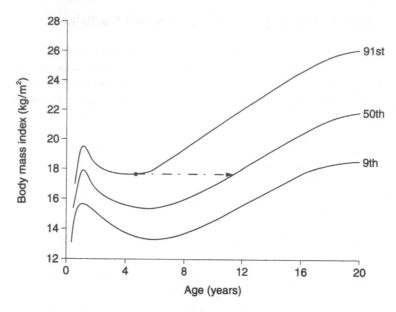

Figure 11: The relationship of BMI to age in a child on the 9th, 50th or 91st centile between birth and age 20 years. The broken horizontal arrow shows that if a child aged 5 years, who is then on the 91st centile, maintains a constant BMI over the next seven years, then by age 12 years he or she would be on the 50th centile of weight-for-height. The years of primary schooling offer an opportunity to prevent obesity in adolescents.[11]

programme has achieved its objective by age 12 years there will be little need for weight control in the secondary school years.

Indeed, a primary school-based intervention study in two towns in northern France is currently assessing the impact of an educational programme in all 6–12-year-olds. The study began in 1992, and body weight evolution will be reported after the ten-year follow-up.[99]

Facilities required to manage overweight among 840 primary school children

A child on the 50th centile for BMI at age 5 years has a weight of 19 kg, height 1.15 m, BMI = 14.4 kg/m.^{2} By age 12 years the corresponding values are weight 40 kg, height 1.5 m, BMI = 17.8 kg/m.^{2} A child with the same height but who is travelling along the 91st centile for BMI will weigh 23 kg, BMI = 17.4 kg/m^2 at 5 years, and by 12 years will weigh 50 kg, BMI = 22.2 kg/m.^{2} Therefore the 50th-centile child will gain 21 kg over the seven years in primary school, while the 91st centile child will gain 27 kg. However, if the 91st-centile child gained only 17 kg (instead of 27 kg) and continued to achieve the same height growth, the result would be that the two children would converge to the same value of BMI, as shown by the broken arrow in Figure 11. In terms of energy balance, an increase of weight by 21 kg indicates a storage of 147 Mcal (600 MJ), and an increase of 17 kg indicates a storage of 119 Mcal (500 MJ). The difference in rate of energy storage between the two over a period of seven years is approximately 11 kcal (46 kJ)/day.

The purpose of this calculation is to show that the degree of average daily energy restriction that is required to convert an overweight 5-year-old into a normal-weight 12-year-old is very small. It can be achieved by substituting fruit and low-energy drinks for sweets and high-energy drinks, and by encouraging extra exercise. It should be noted that weight *loss* is not part of the objective: what is required is a slowing of weight gain.

The problem with this lies not in the thermodynamics, but in the social implications of weight control of young children. Great care is required that well-intentioned schemes do not make matters worse by causing social stigmatisation of the overweight child. It is for this reason that Figure 11 has the 9th centile line also, in order that underweight children are also selected as having special healthcare needs, as would children with problems of hearing or vision. It seems likely that the ideal model would be for children at entry to primary school entry to have their BMI determined. Those who fell below the 9th, or above the 91st, centile line in Figure 11 would be referred to a special needs nurse, who would undertake monitoring of weight and height growth of these children during the next seven years. This should be done with the minimum of fuss, and with the help of the child's parents, teachers and school physical education and catering staff, with referral to a paediatrician if necessary.

8 Outcome measures

The simplest criterion of the prevalence of obesity among adults is measured height and weight so that BMI can be calculated. BMI can be audited at any level, and a cross-sectional sample is measured annually by the Health Surveys for England. The success of a programme to manage obesity will also be indicated by the decrease in co-morbidities such as heart disease, diabetes, gallstones, osteoarthritis, sleep apnoea, some sex-hormone-sensitive cancers and the psychopathologies associated with severe obesity. These criteria, though important, are difficult to interpret, since changes in the prevalence of these diseases may be confounded by changes not associated with obesity status, such as cigarette smoking.

The success of a programme for preventing obesity in children can be assessed by measuring the prevalence of overweight in children at age 12 years.

9 Information and research requirements

There are many questions to which we need answers. For example:

* the influence of dietary fat intake on obesity prevalence and treatment
* the efficacy of different preventative programmes, especially those involving exercise
* the relative influence of genetics and environment to the familial aggregation of obesity
* the efficacy of strategies for maintenance of weight loss
* the cost of preventing and treating obesity.

A more extensive list of topics that require further research is set out in recent reports.[7,11,59]

References

1 Waterlow JC (chairman). *Research on obesity: report of a DHSS/MRC group.* London: HMSO, 1976.

2 Bray GA (ed.). *Obesity in America.* NIH Publication No 79–358. Washington: US Dept of Health Education and Welfare, 1979.

3 World Health Organization. *Obesity: Preventing and Managing the Global Epidemic.* Report of a WHO Consultation. WHO Technical Report Series no. 894. WHO: Geneva, 2000.

4 World Health Organization. *Report of a Joint WHO/FAO Expert Consultation. Diet, Nutrition and the Prevention of Chronic Diseases.* WHO Technical Report Series no. 916. WHO: Geneva, 2002.

5 House of Commons Health Committee. *Obesity.* Third Report of Session 2003–2004. Volume 1. House of Commons. The Stationery Office, London, 2004.

6 National Audit Office. *Tackling obesity in England.* London: The Stationery Office, 2001.

7 Avenell A, Broom J, Brown TJ, Poobalan A, Aucott L, Stearns C *et al.* Systematic review of the long-term effects and economic consequences of treatments for obesity and implications for health improvement. *Health Technol Assess* 2004; **8**/21. Available at www.ncchta.org

8 World Health Organization (WHO), International Obesity Task Force (IOTF). *Obesity: preventing and managing the global epidemic.* Report of a WHO consultation on obesity, Geneva, June 3–5 1997. Geneva: WHO, 1998.

9 Seidell JC, Flegal KM. Assessing obesity: classification and epidemiology. *Br Med Bull* 1997; **53**: 238–52.

10 Power C, Lake JK, Cole TJ. Measurement and long-term health risks of child and adolescent fatness. *Int J Ob* 1997; **21**: 507–26.

11 IOTF. Obesity in children and young people: a crisis in public health. *Obesity Reviews* 2004; **5** (suppl 1): 1–104.

12 Parsons T, Power C, Logan S, Summerbell CD. Childhood predictors of adult obesity: a systematic review. *Int J Ob* 1999; **23** (suppl 8): S1–107.

13 Must A, Jacques PF, Dallai GE, Bajema CJ, Dietz WH. Long term morbidity and mortality of overweight adolescents. *N Engl J Med* 1992; **327**: 1350–5.

14 Crawley HF, Portides G. Self-reported versus measured height, weight and body mass index amongst 16–17 year old British teenagers. *Int J Ob* 1995; **19**: 579–84.

15 Eckel RH, Krauss RM, for the AHA Nutrition Committee. American Heart Association call to action: obesity as a major risk factor for coronary heart disease. *Circulation* 1998; **97**: 2099–100.

16 Manson JE, Willett WC, Stamfer MJ, Colditz GA, Hunter DJ, Hankinson SE, Hennekins CH, Speizer FE. Body weight and mortality among women. *N Engl J Med* 1995; **333**: 677–85.

17 Bender R, Jockel K-H, Trautner C, Spraul M, Berger M. Effect of age on excess mortality in obesity *JAMA* 1999; **281**: 1498–504.

18 The National Heart, Lung, and Blood Institute (NIH). *Clinical guidelines on the identification, evaluation, and treatment of overweight and obesity in adults.* Bethesda, Maryland: National Institutes of Health, 1998. Available at website: www.nhlbi.nih.gov/guidelines/obesity/ob_gdlns.pdf

19 Lee CD, Blair BN, Jackson AS. Cardiorespiratory fitness, body composition, and all-cause and cardiovascular disease mortality in men. *Am J Clin Nutr* 1998; **69**: 373–80.

20 Rissanen A, Heliovaara M, Knekt P, Reunanen A, Aromaa A, Maatela J. Risk of disability and mortality due to overweight in a Finnish population. *BMJ* 1990; **301**: 835–6.

21 Lew EA, Garfinkel L. Variations in mortality by weight among 750,000 men and women. *J Chronic Dis* 1979; **32**: 563–76.

22 Sims EAH, Danforth E Jr, Horton ES, Bray GA, Glennon JA, Salans LB. Endocrine and metabolic effects of experimental obesity in man. *Recent Progress Hormone Res* 1973; **29**: 457–96.

23 Hoffman RP, Armstrong PT. Glucose effectiveness, peripheral and hepatic insulin sensitivity in obese and lean prepubertal children. *Int J Ob* 1996; **20**: 521–5.

24 Scheen AJ, Paquot N, Letiexhe MR, Paolisso G, Castillo MJ, Lefebvre PJ. Glucose metabolism in obese subjects: lessons from OGTT, IVGTT and clamp studies. *Int J Obes* 1995; **19** (suppl 3): S14–S20.

25 Williamson DF, Pamuk E, Thun M, Flanders D, Byers T, Heath C. Prospective study of intentional weight loss and mortality in never-smoking overweight US white women aged 40–64 years. *Am J Epid* 1995; **141**: 1128–41.

26 Chen Y, Rennie DC, Reeder BA. Age-related association between body mass index and blood pressure: the Humbolt study. *Int J Obes* 1995; **19**: 825–31.

27 Dattilo AM, Kris-Etherton PM. Effects of weight reduction on blood lipids and lipoproteins: a meta-analysis. *Am J Clin Nutr* 1992; **56**: 320–8.

28 Manson JE, Colditz GA, Stamfer MJ, Wuillett WC, Rosner B, Monson RR, Speizer FE, Hennekens CH. A prospective study of obesity and risk of coronary heart disease in women. *N Engl J Med* 1990; **322**: 822–9.

29 Meade TW, Ruddock V, Stirling Y, Chakrabati R, Miller GJ. Fibrinolytic activity, clotting factors and long-term incidence of ischaemic heart disease in the Northwick Park study. *The Lancet* 1993; **342**: 1076–9.

30 Ernst E, Matrai A. Normalisation of hemorheological abnormalities during weight reduction in obese patients. *Nutrition* 1987; **3**: 337–9.

31 Garfinkel L. Overweight and cancer. *Ann Intern Med* 1985; **103**: 1034–6.

32 Davis MA, Neuhaus JM, Ettingrer WH, Mueller WH. Body fat distribution and osteoarthritis. *Am J Epid* 1990; **132**: 701–7.

33 Spirt BA, Graves LW, Weinstock R, Bartlett SJ, Wadden TA. Gallstone formation in obese women treated by a low-calorie diet. *Int J Ob* 1995; **19**: 593–5.

34 Galtier-Dereure F, Montpeyroux F, Boulot P, Bringer J, Jaffiol. Weight excess before pregnancy: complications and cost. *Int J Ob* 1995; **19**: 443–8.

35 Shaw GM, Velie EM, Schaffer D. Risk of neural tube defect-affected pregnancies among obese women. *JAMA* 1996; **275**: 1093–6.

36 Werler MM, Louik C, Shapiro S, Mitchell AA. Pre-pregnant weight in relation to risk of neural tube defects. *JAMA* 1996; **275**: 1089–92.

37 Grunstein RR, Stenlof K, Hedner J, Sjostrom L. Impact of obstructive apnoea and sleepiness on metabolic and cardiovascular risk factors in the Swedish Obese Subjects (SOS) study. *Int J Ob* 1995; **19**: 410–18.

38 Harman EM, Block AJ. Why does weight loss improve the respiratory insufficiency of obesity? *Chest* 1986; **90**: 153–4.

39 Chernin K. *The Tyranny of Slenderness.* London: The Women's Press, 1981.

40 Wadden TA, Stunkard AJ. Social and psychological consequences of obesity. *Ann Intern Med* 1985; **103**: 1062–7.

41 Sonne-Holm S, Sorensen TI. Prospective study of attainment of social class of severely obese subjects in relation to parents social class, intelligence and education. *BMJ* 1986; **292**: 586–9.

42 Gortmaker SL, Must A, Perrin JM, Sobol AM, Dietz WH. Social and economic consequences of overweight in adolescence and young adulthood. *N Engl J Med* 1993; **329**: 1008–12.

43 Sullivan M, Karlsson J, Sjostrom L, Backman L, Bengtson C, Bouchard C, Dahlgren S, Jonsson E, Larsson B, Lindstedt S, Naslund I, Olbe L, Wedel H. Swedish obese subjects (SOS) – an intervention study of obesity. Baseline evaluation of health and psychosocial functioning in the first 1743 subjects examined. *Int J Ob* 1993; **17**: 503–12.

44 Ogden J, Chanana A. Explaining the effect of ethnic group on weight concern: finding a role for family values. *Int J Ob* 1998; **22**: 641–7.

45 Striegel-Moore RH, Wilfley DE, Caldwell MB, Needham ML, Brownell KD. Weight-related attitudes and behaviors of women who diet to lose weight: a comparison of black dieters and white dieters. *Ob Res* 1996; **4**: 109–16.

46 Lapidus L, Bengtsson C, Larsson B, Pennert K, Rybo E. Sjostrom L. Distribution of adipose tissue and risk of cardiovascular disease and death: a 12 year follow-up of participants in the population study of women in Gothenburg, Sweden. *BMJ* 1984; **289**: 1257–61.

47 Larsson B. Regional obesity as a health hazard in men – prospective studies. *Acta Med Scand Suppl* 1988; **723**: 45–51.

48 Serdula MK, Ivery D, Coates RJ, Freedman DS, Williamson DF, Byers T. Do obese children become obese adults? A review of the literature. *Prev Med* 1993; **22**: 167–77.

49 Power C, Lake JK, Cole TJ. Body mass index and height from childhood to adulthood in the 1958 British born cohort. *Am J Clin Nutr* 1997; **66**: 1094–101.

50 Dietz WH. Critical periods in childhood for the development of obesity. *Am J Clin Nutr* 1994; **59**: 955–9.

51 Dietz WH. Health consequences of obesity in youth: childhood predictors of adult disease. *Pediatrics* 1998; **101** (suppl): 518–25.

52 Weiss R, Dziura J, Burgert TS, Tamborlane WV, Taksali SE, Yeckel CW, Allen K, Lopes M, Savoye M, Morison J, Sherwin RS, Caprio S. Obesity and the metabolic syndrome in children and adolescents. *N Engl J Med* 2004; **350**: 2362–74.

53 Stunkard A, Burt V. Obesity and the body image. II. Age at onset of disturbances in the body image. *Am J Psychiatry* 1967; **123**: 1443–7.

54 Hill AJ, Silver EK. Fat, friendless and unhealthy: 9-year-old children's perception of body shape stereotypes. *Int J Ob* 1995; **19**: 423–30.

55 Royal College of Physicians (RCP). *Clinical Management of Overweight and Obese Patients with Particular Reference to the Use of Drugs.* London: RCP, 1998.

56 Scottish Intercollegiate Guidelines Network (SIGN). *Obesity in Scotland: integrating prevention with weight management.* Edingburgh: SIGN, 1996. Also available (updated version) at website: http://show.cee.hw.ac.uk/sign/home.htm

57 British Nutrition Foundation (BNF). *Obesity.* Report of the British Nutrition Foundation Task Force (J Garrow, chairman). Oxford: Blackwell Science, 1999.

58 Department of Health. *Our Healthier Nation: saving lives.* London: HMSO, 1999.

59 Health Development Agency. The management of obesity and overweight: An analysis of reviews of diet, physical activity and behavioural approaches. Evidence Briefing. October 2003.

60 NICE, National Institute for Clinical Excellence (2001) Orlistat for the treatment of obesity in adults. Guidance No 22. Available at: www.nice.org.uk

61 NICE, National Institute for Clinical Excellence (2001) Guidance on the use of Sibutramine for the treatment of obesity in adults. Guidance No 31. Available at: www.nice.org.uk

62 NICE, National Institute for Clinical Excellence (2002) Guidance on the use of surgery to aid weight reduction for people with morbid obesity. Guidance No 46. Available at: www.nice.org.uk

63 Scottish Intercollegiate Guidelines Network Obesity in Scotland. Management of obesity in children and young people. Guideline No 69, Published by Scottish Intercollegiate Guidelines Network, Edinburgh, 2003. Also available at website: www.sign.ac.uk/

64 Keys A, Menotti A, Aravanis C, Blackburn H, Djordevic BS, Buzina R, Dontas AS, Fidanza F, Karvonen MJ, Kimura N, Mohacek I, Nedeljkovic S, Puddu V, Punsar S, Taylor HL, Conti S, Kromhout D, Toshima H. The seven countries study: 2289 deaths in 15 years. *Prev Med* 1984; **13**: 141–54.

65 Hubert HB. The nature of the relationship between obesity and cardiovascular disease. *Int J Cardiol* 1984; **6**: 268–74.

66 Orbach S. *Fat is a Feminist Issue.* London: Hamlyn, 1978.

67 Apfelbaum M, Vague P, Ziegler O, Hanotin C, Thomas F, Leutenegger E. Long-term maintenance of weight loss after a very-low-calorie diet: a randomized blinded trial of the efficacy and tolerability of sibutramine. *Am J Med* 1999; **106**: 179–84.

68 Bray GA, Blackburn GL, Ferguson JM, Greenway FL, Jain AK, Mendel CM, Mendels J, Ryan DH, Schwartz SL, Scheinbaum ML, Seaton TB. Sibutramine produces dose-related weight loss. *Ob Res* 1999; **7**(2): 189–98.

69 Jeffery RW, Folsom AR, Leupker RV, Jacobs DR, Gillum RF, Taylor HL, Blackburn H. Prevalence of overweight and weight loss behaviour in a metropolitan adult population: the Minnesota heart survey experience. *Am J Public Health* 1984; **74**: 349–52.

70 Summerbell CD. Teaching nutrition to medical doctors: the potential role of the State Registered Dietitian. *J Hum Nutr Diet* 1996; **9**: 349–56.

71 Kopelman, P. Place of obesity clinics in the NHS. *Brit J Hosp Med* 1993; **49** (8); 533–5.

72 Grace C, Summerbell C, Kopelman P. An audit of dietary treatment modalities and weight loss outcomes in a specialist obesity clinic. *J Hum Nutr Diet* 1998; **11**(3): 197–202.

73 Cowburn G, Summerbell C. A survey of dietetic practice in obesity management. *J Hum Nutr Diet* 1998; **11**: 191–6.

74 Wilkinson J, Summerbell C, Macknight N, Bailey K, Chappel D. Use of surgery to aid weight reduction – experience of two regions of Northern England – a database study. *Int J Ob* 2005; **29**: 204–7.

75 Summerbell CD, Higgins JPT. Systematic reviews and meta-analysis. *BNF Bulletin* 1997; **22**: 111–8.

76 Campbell K, Waters E, O'Meara S, Kelly S, Summerbell C. Interventions for preventing obesity in children (Cochrane Review). In: The Cochrane Library, Issue 2, 2004. Chichester, UK: John Wiley & Sons, Ltd.

77 Summerbell CD, Ashton V, Campbell KJ, Edmunds L, Kelly S, Waters E. Interventions for treating obesity in children (Cochrane Review). In: The Cochrane Library, Issue 2, 2004. Chichester, UK: John Wiley & Sons, Ltd.

78 Bortz WM. A 500 pound weight loss. *Amer J Med* 1969; **47**: 325–31.

79 Sjostrom L, Rissanen A, Andersen T, Boldrin M, Golay A, Koppeschaar HP *et al.* Randomised placebo-controlled trial of orlistat for weight loss and prevention of weight regain in obese patients. European Multicentre Orlistat Study Group. *The Lancet* 1998; **352**: 167–72.

80 Webster JD, Hesp R, Garrow JS. The composition of excess weight in obese women estimated by body density, total body water and total body potassium. *Hum Nutr Clin Nutr* 1984; **38C**: 299–306.

81 Stuart RB. Behavioural control of overeating. *Behav Res Ther* 1967; **5**: 357–65.

82 Garrow JS, Summerbell CD. Meta-analysis: effect of exercise, with or without dieting, on the body composition of overweight subjects. *Eur J Clin Nutr* 1995; **49**: 1–10.

83 Torgerson JS, Sjostrom L. The Swedish Obese Subjects (SOS) study – rationale and results. *Int J Obes* 2001; **25**: 52–4.

84 NHS CRD (Centre for Reviews and Dissemination). A systematic review of the interventions for the prevention and treatment of obesity, and the maintenance of weight loss. CRD Report 10, 1997, University of York. Also available at website: http://www.york.ac.uk/inst/crd/obesity.htm

85 Douketis JD, Feightner JW, Attia J, Feldman WF, with the Canadian Task Force on Preventative Health Care. Periodic health examination, 1999 update: 1. Detection, prevention and treatment of obesity. *J Can Med Ass* 1999; **160**: 513–25.

86 Hardeman W, Griffin S, Johnston M, Kinmonth AL, Wareham NJ. Interventions to prevent weight gain: a systematic review of psychological models and behaviour change methods. *Int J Ob* 2000; **24**: 131–43.

87 Harvey EL, Glenny A-M, Kirk SFL, Summerbell CD. Effective Professional Practice: a systematic review of health professionals' management of obesity. *Int J Ob* 1999; **23**(12): 1213–22.

88 Moore H, Summerbell CD, Greenwood D, Tovey P, Griffiths J, Henderson M, Hesketh K, Woolgar S, Adamson AJ. Improving the management of obesity in primary care: a cluster randomised trial. *BMJ* 2003; **327**: 1085–9.

89 French SA, Jeffery RW, Folsom AR, McGovern P, Williamson DF. Weight loss maintenance in young adulthood: prevalence and correlations with health behaviour and disease in population-based sample of women aged 55-69 years. *Int J Ob* 1996; **20**: 303–10.

90 Allison DB, Zannolli R, Faith MS, Heo M, Pietrobelli A, Van Itallie TB, Pi-Sunyer FX, Heymsfield SB. Weight loss increases and fat loss decreases all-cause mortality rate: results from two independent cohort studies. *Int J Ob* 1999; **23**: 603–11.

91 Yanovski SZ, Bain RP, Williamson DF. Report of a National Institute of Health – Centers for Disease Control and Prevention Workshop on the feasibility of conducting a randomised clinical trial to estimate the long-term health effects of intentional weight loss in obese persons. *Am J Clin Nutr* 1999; **69**: 366–72.

92 Narbro K, Agren G, Jonsson E, Larsson B, Naslund I, Wedel H, Sjostrom L. Sick leave and disability pension before and after treatment for obesity: a report from the Swedish Obese Subjects (SOS) study. *Int J Ob* 1999; **23**: 619–24.

93 Bush A, Webster J, Chalmers G, Pearson M, Penfold P, Brereton P, Garrow JS. The Harrow slimming club: Report on 1090 enrolments in 50 courses, 1977–1986. *J Hum Nutr Diet* 1988; **1**: 429-36.

94 Karvetti RL, Hakala P. A 7-year follow-up of a weight reduction programme in Finnish primary health care. *Eur J Clin Nutr* 1992; **46**: 743–52.

95 Andres R, Elahi D, Tobin JD, Muller DC, Brant L. Impact of age on weight goals. *Ann Int Med* 1985; **103**: 1030–3.

96 French SA, Jeffery RW, Folsom AR, Williamson DF, Byers T. Weight variability in a population-based sample of older women: reliability and intercorrelation of measures. *Int J Ob* 1995; **19**: 22–9.

97 Garrow JS, Webster JD, Pearson M, Pacy PJ, Harpin G. Inpatient-outpatient randomised comparison of Cambridge diet versus milk diet in 17 obese women over 24 weeks. *Int J Obes* 1989; **13**: 521–9.

98 Poskitt EME, Cole TJ. Do fat babies stay fat? *BMJ* 1977; **1**: 7–9.

99 Basedevant A, Boute D, Borys JM. Who should be educated? Education strategies: could children educate their parents? *Int J Ob* 1999; **23** (suppl 4): S10–S13.

7 Chronic Pain

Henry J McQuay, Lesley A Smith and R Andrew Moore

1 Summary

Introduction and statement of the problem

Chronic pain is conveniently defined as any pain that persists for at least three months despite sensible treatment. It ultimately affects almost half of all adults and is most likely to occur in older people. Chronic pain is known to have significant effects on health and well-being and is a major cause of lost work days. Prevalence data alone does not capture the burden of pain, or the disability which goes with the pain. For many conditions there is no certain remedy, so that health care needs have to consider prevalence, the burden of the pain (and disability), and just how treatable the pain is. In addition, health care needs for chronic pain extend from community through to hospital care. Patients with some chronic pain conditions, such as migraine, may manage with over the counter medications; others will require prescription medication and some will need other interventions. One organisational dilemma is the overlap of pain management between community and hospital care and the overlap between pain services and other hospital services. Between primary care and the pain service there are several groups of patients who may need referral. Between the pain clinic and other hospital services the reality is that patients who fail to respond to the best endeavours of the other services find their way to the pain clinic.

Sub-categories

The sub-categories used in this chapter are based on demand in a clinic which rarely refuses referrals and which has mature relationships with other services. The main categories of pain are musculoskeletal, cancer, face/head, neuropathic, vascular, chronic postoperative and medically unexplained painful syndromes. The most problematic growth in demand is for medically unexplained painful syndromes.

Prevalence and incidence

Chronic pain is common. One in two people report chronic pain lasting for three months or more, rising to two in three over 67 years. In a Primary Care Trust population of 100 000 people there would be about 5000 to 10 000 people with severe chronic pain. Roughly half the problems will be musculoskeletal, with back pain and arthritis predominant. Pain due to nerve damage and chronic postoperative pain are two of the other big categories. Musculoskeletal conditions have the most severe impact on quality of life.

Services available

Possible interventions include drugs, the conventional analgesics from paracetamol up to morphine, the unconventional analgesics for nerve pain, antidepressants and anticonvulsants, injections including continuous infusion devices, psychological behavioural management, and operations. Patients with chronic pain who fail to respond to the best endeavours of other services find their way to the pain clinic. The pain clinic may offer injection treatments, more expert handling of neuropathic pain medication and psychological expertise unavailable in the other services.

A total of 85% of Trusts provide a chronic pain service, which can vary from the 'spoke' provision with a single-handed consultant in a district hospital to the 'hub' in the university hospital with a multi-disciplinary clinic offering a wider range of interventions. Limited cost data suggests a Primary Care Trust covering 100 000 patients should be budgeting between £100 000 and £200 000 per year for chronic pain services, allowing ten consultant sessions per 100 000 patients. Canadian data shows that users of speciality pain clinic services incur less direct health care expenditure than non users with similar conditions, about £1000 per patient per year. Without adequate provision for chronic pain management these people will bounce ineffectively and expensively around the health care system.

Effectiveness

There is a strong evidence base for pain management, for both efficacy and safety. Of the many interventions, pharmacological, non-pharmacological, invasive and non-invasive, from which to choose there is good evidence of effectiveness for many of the drug treatments, for behavioural management and for some of the invasive options. There is evidence that some of the alternative therapies do not improve pain, but may help patients cope better.

Models of care

The provision of chronic pain services should not be taken in isolation. Many treatments, drugs or procedures, are common to the different service providers; the additional expertise found in the pain service is prescribing expertise and the ability to do particular invasive procedures. The ideal promoted widely in the developed world is chronic pain services which are multidisciplinary. The medical components of such multidisciplinary services include rehabilitation, neurology, orthopaedic and psychiatric, together with clinical psychology, physiotherapy and pharmacy inputs as integral to the chronic pain service. The fact that 85% of Trusts surveyed had a chronic pain clinic is evidence that there is a perceived need for the service. There is little evidence as to what constitutes the optimal form of the service, and very little evidence on resource use and benefit gained. The current satellite and hub model of DGH and regional centre works to an extent, but there has been a dearth of organisational research into service provision. The need for good liaison with other specialities favours decentralised rather than centralised arrangements.

For the future, chronic pain, like other specialities, needs studies of complex interventions to show how to make the best of the interventions we have.

2 Introduction and statement of the problem

Chronic pain is conveniently defined as any pain that persists for at least three months despite sensible treatment, sweeping aside subtle distinctions between conditions which are always painful and conditions which are sometimes painful. Surveys that have examined the extent and significance of 'generic' chronic pain in the community have come to remarkably similar conclusions. Chronic pain ultimately affects almost half of all adults[1-6] and is most likely to occur in older people.

Chronic pain is known to have significant effects on health and well-being[7] and is a major cause of lost work days, from back pain[8] to migraine,[9] so it is important to define the extent of the problem systematically to specify health care needs. In 1999, The International Association for the Study of Pain published a book on the epidemiology of pain.[10] This should be referred to for greater detail on some of the conditions mentioned throughout the chapter.

Other publications have focused on the prevalence of chronic pain due to specific disease states, such as back pain,[8,11] fibromyalgia,[12] arthritis[13] and terminal and palliative care.[14] The aim of this chapter is to consider the prevalence and treatment options and thus the need for services for the pain conditions likely to be seen in chronic pain clinics.

Organisation and perception

One common organisational dilemma is the overlap of pain management between community and hospital care, and a common source of confusion is the overlap between the pain service and other hospital services. Between primary care and the pain service there are several groups of patients who may need referral:

- patients who fail to respond to conventional analgesics and need active management of neuropathic pain, which may involve use of 'off-label' medication
- patients requiring injection procedures not available in the community
- patients who need large doses of opioids
- patients without clear diagnosis and who are difficult to manage
- patients needing services not available in the community, e.g. devices or specialist psychological input.

Between the pain clinic and other hospital services the reality is that patients who fail to respond to the best endeavours of the other services find their way to the pain clinic. The pain clinic may offer injection treatments, more expert handling of neuropathic pain medication and psychological expertise unavailable in the other services. Apparent overlaps are often minimised by local understandings. Out of back pain triage, for instance, orthopaedics may retain younger less disabled patients and refer the older and more disabled to the pain clinic. The argument that the pain clinic service could be subsumed by another service, for instance by an orthopaedic clinic, ignores the fact that the special skills of the pain clinic are of value across a variety of pain conditions which the orthopaedic clinic would not want to see. The learning, maintenance and governance of those special skills require critical mass and demand, both of which would be lost or diluted if the pain clinic was subsumed by other services.

There is a striking contrast between the standing of palliative care and that of chronic pain. Both began at roughly the same time, but palliative care, unlike chronic pain, has formal recognition and is seemingly better presented to health commissioners. A coherence has emerged about the clinical framework for palliative care which is less obvious for chronic pain. Both services are necessary, but presenting a more coherent case for chronic pain would be a great deal easier with better data. In this context it is fair to say that absence of data does not mean absence of benefit. The data needed is more management and audit rather than research.

3 Sub-categories

The pain classification in **Table 1** is the basis for the sub-categories of chronic pain used in this chapter. This was developed from the simple manoeuvre of auditing clinics for one month. This is a classification by demand in a clinic which rarely refuses referrals and which has mature relationships with other services, and joint clinics with psychiatry, neurosurgery and neurology. Cancer has been included because pain clinics commonly provide invasive options for cancer pain at the behest of the palliative care team. The classification does not use mechanism of pain, apart from the generic grouping of neuropathic pain, and is a static snapshot. The most problematic growth in demand is for medically unexplained painful syndromes.

Table 1: Pain classification.

Musculoskeletal	Back*	degenerative disc disease
		osteoporotic collapse
		stenosis
		facet joint
		post-trauma/surgery
		ankylosing spondylitis*
		no clear pathology
	Neck*	degenerative disc disease
		whiplash*
	Fibromyalgia*/myofascial	polymyalgia rheumatica*
	Arthritis	osteoarthritis, rheumatoid
Cancer	Breakthrough cancer pain*	neuropathic, movement related, poor control with oral morphine
MUPS (medically unexplained painful syndromes)		non-cardiac chest pain
		abdominal
		pelvic
		chest pain
Face/head pain	Migraine*	
	Headache*	
	Trigeminal neuralgia*	
	Dental	atypical facial*
Neuropathic		diabetic neuropathy*
		postherpetic neuralgia*
		multiple sclerosis*
		post stroke*
		repetitive strain injury
		reflex sympathetic dystrophy (CRPS1)
		traumatic
Vascular	Peripheral	claudication*/Raynaud's*
	Central	angina*
Chronic postoperative pain		pain after amputation (phantom* and stump)
		chronic postoperative breast pain*
		chronic postoperative thoracotomy pain*
		chronic postoperative cholecystectomy pain*

* Asterisk means prevalence and incidence discussed below.

4 Prevalence and incidence

Chronic pain overall

Chronic pain affects almost half of all adults (**Table 2**).[1-6] Not all of this chronic pain is severe, or the conditions disabling, but chronic pain is likely to occur in older people, and in the largest UK survey[6] half of those with chronic pain had severe pain or were moderately disabled.

This recent data[6] shows that the prevalence of chronic pain in the community is high. Particular population groups can differ significantly in the prevalence of chronic pain and severe chronic pain, though the importance for practice of such significant differences is not easy to perceive.[15] The causes of any variations include differences in sampling methods, diversity in disease definitions used and differences in populations studied. The main thrust of all the findings, though, is for the bulk of chronic pain to have musculoskeletal causes (**Table 2**), and to occur more frequently in older people.[6] Chronic pain may be particularly common in older people in nursing homes or long-term care institutions.[16] In a Primary Care Trust population of 100 000 people there would be about 5000 to 10 000 people with severe chronic pain.

Sub-categories of chronic pain

Information was sought on the prevalence and incidence of the pain conditions marked with an asterisk in **Table 1**, using the methods detailed in Appendix 1. The prevalence and incidence of the sub-categories of pain that have not been covered in depth elsewhere are presented.

Musculoskeletal pain

Musculoskeletal disorders are the commonest cause of chronic incapacity, and half are due to back pain.

Back pain

A health care needs assessment on low back pain is published in the Health Care Needs Assessment second series[13] but it is also considered here as it is an important cause of chronic pain.

Back pain is one of the commonest causes of disability and absence from work, particularly during the productive middle years of adult life.[8] Seven percent of UK adults consult their GP each year, and back pain costs the NHS more than £500 million a year.[8] While 90% or more of patients with back pain recover within three months, those that do not may recover slowly and their demand for care is high.

Most recent reports estimating the burden of low back pain have focused mainly on acute back pain. There is less reliable data for chronic pain. One of the reasons for this is the lack of agreement about definitions of chronic back pain, the different time periods used and the intermittent nature of back pain.

Table 3 summarises the relevant reports. In addition, for self-reported low back pain in the community 6% of the population reported pain persisting for at least a year and 3% were still unable to work a year later.[11] In a primary care trust population of 100 000 people there might be as many as several thousand with back pain that is disabling and limiting.

Table 2: Prevalence of chronic pain.

Reference	Type of study	Sample source	Disease definition	Sample size	Age range	Overall prevalence
Andersson 1994[1]	Prospective questionnaire	Random sample of 15% of the 25–74 population of two Swedish primary care districts	Chronic pain duration longer than 3 months	1,806 questionnaires sent, 1,609 responded (89%)	25–74	High prevalence, 50,000/100,000 in men and women, with high intensity pain about 30% of this. Greater in older population. Musculoskeletal had highest prevalence.
Brattberg et al. 1989[2]	Postal survey	Randomly chosen individuals in a single Swedish county	Obvious pain, longer than 6 months' duration	1,009 questionnaires sent, 672 responded (67%)	18–84	38 000/100,000 in men and 42,000/100 000 in women. Peak age 45–64. Musculoskeletal had the highest prevalence.
Birse & Lander 1998[3]	Cross-sectional telephone survey	Random sample of households, and of individuals within households, in Edmonton, Canada	Chronic pain was recurrent or persistent pain of at least 6 months' duration	592 individuals, 410 responded (69%)	Over 18	35,000/100,000 in men and 66,000/100,000 in women. Peak age younger and older women and older men. Musculoskeletal had the highest prevalence. Accidents and medical or surgical procedures were most common antecedants of chronic pain.
Bowsher et al. 1991[4]	Cross-sectional telephone survey	Random selection of households in Great Britain	Chronic pain defined as lasting on or off for more than the last 3 months	2,942, 1,037 respondents (35%)	Over 15	11,500/100,000 had chronic pain. This was higher in women than men (1.5 to 1). Prevalence higher in older age groups.
Chrubasik et al. 1998[5]	Cross-sectional postal survey	Every 71st person in a county in Baden-Würtenberg, Germany	Prolonged pain in preceding 6 months	2,127 questionnaires sent, 1,420 responded (67%)	18–80	47,000/100,000 reported prolonged pain, and in 87% it had lasted over a year, and in about half the pain was severe. In about 29% of respondents pain was severe or intolerable and had lasted more than a year. Musculoskeletal pain predominated.
Elliott et al. 1999[6]	Cross-sectional postal survey	Random sample of adults in Grampian region of Scotland	Pain or discomfort that persisted continuously or intermittently for longer than 3 months	5,036 questionnaires sent, 3,605 returned (72%)	Over 25	50,000/100,000 reported chronic pain (47,000/100,000 of general population). About half had severe pain or disability. Prevalence higher in older people. Musculoskeletal pain predominated.

Table 3: Chronic back pain.

Reference	Type of study	Sample source	Disease definition	Sample size	Age range (years)	Overall prevalence (per 100,000)	Occurrence
Cassidy et al. 1998[17]	Retrospective survey, PSAQ	General population, random selection residents of Saskatchewan province, Canada	Point prevalence data obtained by question 'do you have LBP at the present time?' Lifetime prevalence data by question 'have you ever had LBP in your lifetime?' Mannequin diagram for location of LBP Chronic pain questionnaire for 6 month period prevalence graded in severity PI (range 0–100) disability (range 0–6)	n=2,184 recruited, 55% (n=1,133) response rate	20 to 69	*Age-adjusted point prevalence: 28,400/ 100,000 (25,600 to 31,100) *Age-adjusted lifetime prevalence: 84,100/ 100,000 (81,900 to 86,300) *Age-adjusted 6 month period prevalence: Grade 1: Low intensity/ low disability = 48,900/ 100,000 Grade 2: High intensity/ low disability = 12,300/ 100,000 Grade 3 & 4: high disability/moderately to severely limiting = 10,700/100,000	
Davies et al. 1995[18]	Prospective 3 year survey, questionnaire and examination by physician at clinic consultation	Patients attending 10 pain clinics with back pain, North Britain	Consultant diagnosis of back pain	n=2,007, all reported on	median age 48.5 (IQR 40–60)		Occurrence: 35,000/ 100,000 complaining of pain in low back only Duration of pain: 73% > 2 years 27% > 10 years Pain intensity: 54% moderate, 18% severe, 40% unable to work (as stated by patient) Putative cause of pain: Degenerative: 56% Trauma: 21% Failed surgery: 16% No definite cause: 15%

Table 3: Continued.

Reference	Type of study	Sample source	Disease definition	Sample size	Age range (years)	Overall prevalence (per 100,000)	Occurrence
Thomas *et al.* 1999[19]	Prospective 1 year survey, questionnaire + clinical exam	Patients with low back pain, registered with two GPs, Manchester, UK	Persistent disabling low back pain defined as presence of both low back pain and disability Pain rated by VASPI 0–10% scale, disability rated by Hanover back pain activity schedule 0 to 100% scale	n=442, 67% (n=246) response rate, n=180 analysed	18–75		Occurrence: at 1 week after consultation: 73% at 3 months: 48% at 12 months: 42% Period prevalence persistent disabling low back pain at each follow-up visit: 34%

Abbreviations: PSAQ – postal self-assessed questionnaire; * age-adjusted to 1995 Saskatchewan mid-year population; LBP = low back pain; PI = pain intensity; IQR = inter quartile range; VASPI = visual analogue pain intensity; DHSS = Department of Health and Social Security.

Ankylosing spondylitis

Disease prevalence

The prevalence of ankylosing spondylitis (AS) correlates with the prevalence of HLA-B27 antigen, and for the UK is estimated to be 1 to 2% of the population.[20] There are surveys using strict diagnostic criteria from Europe and North America (**Table 4**). The largest population-based survey was in Norway, based on 21 329 randomly selected subjects.[21] The prevalence of AS was 1100 to 1400/100 000, and was between four and six times higher in men than in women. In a prospective study of 273 blood donors in Berlin, the prevalence of AS was 900/100 000.[22] A large American population-based survey using retrospective record review of Minnesota residents between 1935 and 1989 found an age- and sex-adjusted incidence of 7.3 per 100 000 person-years (95% CI 6.1–8.4). The age-adjusted incidence was four times higher in men at 11.7 per 100 000 person-years (95% CI 9.6–13.8) than in women at 2.9 per 100 000 person-years (95% CI 2.0–3.9).[23]

Pain prevalence

Of 14 539 AS patients who completed a back pain questionnaire, 2907 complained of pain.[21] In a retrospective survey of 121 AS patients in Norway, 71 of the 100 responders reported daily pain and 60 used analgesics every day.[26] In the Minnesota study back pain was reported by 96% and neck pain by 27% at presentation.[23] Pain will therefore be a chronic feature for between 25% and 50% of AS patients. In a primary care trust population of 100 000 people there would be about 30 new cases of AS with pain a year.

Neck pain

Seven population-based surveys have examined the prevalence of self-reported neck pain in random samples of the general population (**Table 5**). With the exception of one Canadian and one British study, all were Scandinavian. There were no studies reporting the incidence of chronic neck pain.

The prevalence of chronic neck pain in adults was of the order of 5000 to 20 000/100 000, with most estimates about 10 000/100 000 (**Table 5**). There was some evidence that prevalence was higher in women than in men. Significantly disabling chronic neck pain affected 5000/100 000 in Canada.[28] In a primary care trust population of 100 000 people there would be about 5000 cases.

Whiplash

One nine-year prospective study of patients admitted to an accident and emergency department was conducted in the UK, to determine the prevalence and incidence of neck sprain following a road traffic accident (RTA).[32] Of 6149 patients admitted following injuries sustained in an RTA, 46% (2801) were diagnosed with neck sprain.

A 25 year retrospective medical record review in Holland determined the prevalence of neck sprain in all patients admitted to an accident and emergency department either due to an RTA[33] or due to injury from another cause.[34] Of 1374 neck sprain patients 51% (694) were sustained in a car accident and 49% (680) were not (NCA). For NCA, the five year period prevalence rates increased over time from 6.5 per 100 000 (1970 to 1974) to 28.5 per 100 000 (1990 to 1994). The age group at highest risk was 15 to 19 year olds with a prevalence of 39.2 per 100 000; accidental falls caused 25% and sports 24%. For neck sprain due to RTA, five year period prevalence rates increased over time from 34 per 100 000 (1970 to 1974) to 402 per 100 000 (1990 to 1994). The age groups at highest risk were 25 to 29 year olds with prevalence of 28.3 per 100 000, and 40 to 44 year olds with prevalence of 27.9 per 100 000.

There appears to have been a ten-fold increase over 25 years in the prevalence of neck sprain, particularly following RTA.

Table 4: Chronic pain due to ankylosing spondylitis.

Reference	Type of study	Sample source	Disease definition	Sample size	Age range	Incidence	Overall prevalence	Male prevalence	Female prevalence
Braun et al. 1998[22]	Survey and prospective screening with questionnaire and physical examination	Blood donors resident in Berlin, HLAB27-positive age- and sex-matched with HLAB27 negative blood donors	AS diagnosis using modified New York criteria: radiographs showing bilateral changes in SI joints > grade II	n=320 recruited, n=273 (85.3%) responded to initial questionnaire	18–65 years		AS diagnosed in 9/140 B27-positive donors calculated prevalence in population Berlin = 860/100,000		
Carbone et al. 1992[23]	Retrospective review of medical records, 1935–1989	General population, residents Rochester county, Minnesota, USA	Modified New York criteria for AS: Radiographic evidence of sacroiliitis with 1/3 clinical criteria (inflammatory back pain 3 month duration, limitation of movement of lumbar spine in sagittal and frontal planes, reduced chest expansion)	Population for Rochester 1930 = 18,931; 1990 = 69,995	All ages	Incidence rates calculated assuming the entire population is at risk: age- and sex-adjusted rate = 7.3/100,000 (6.1–8.4) Men: age-adjusted 11.7/100,000 (9.6–13.8) Women: age-adjusted 2.9/100,000 (2.0–3.9)			

Table 4: Continued.

Study	Method	Population	Diagnostic criteria	n	Age	Prevalence
Gran et al. 1985[21]	Prospective survey 1979–80, postal SAQ, clinical exam	General population, residents of Tromsø, Norway random selection (n=449, 56%) further selected for clinical examination	New York diagnostic criteria, definite AS defined as X-ray changes of sacroiliac joints	n=21,329 recruited, n=14,539 responded, (68.2%)	Adults aged 20–54	1,100 to 1,400/100,000; 1,900 to 2,200/100,000; 300 to 600/100,000
Julkunen and Korpi 1984[24]	Health examination surveys, part of mini-Finland health survey, clinical exam and X-ray	General population, three population samples in Finland Study 1 and 2 were random samples, study 3 includes 196 patients with back pain	study 1: diagnosis by X-ray 10 × 10 of chest study 2: normal-sized chest X-ray study 3: lumbar spine X-ray	study 1: n=6,176 study 2: n=750 study 3: n=580	study 1 = 30+ yrs study 2 = 30+ yrs. Study 3 = 30 to 64 yrs	study 1: 400/100,000 study 2: 1,600/100,000 study 3: 1,000/100,000
Underwood and Dawes 1995[25]	Prospective study of patients presenting with back pain over 1 year	Suburban general practice in England	Short screening questionnaire, plus detailed diagnosis by one observer	6,600 patients	All ages	30/100,000 in 1 year (2 of 313 patients presenting with back pain)

Table 5: Chronic neck pain.

Reference	Type of study	Sample source	Disease definition	Sample size	Age range (years)	Prevalence (per 100 000)		
						Overall	**Male**	**Female**
Anderson et al. 1993[1]	Prospective survey, PSAQ with a drawing of neck	General population, random selection of patients registered with two primary health care districts, Sweden	Persistent or regular recurrent pain more than 3 months in the neck	n=1,806, 90% (n=1,624) response rate	25–74		14,500/100,000	19,100/100,000
Bovim et al. 1994[27]	Retrospective survey, PSAQ	General population, random selection of residents Norway	Questionnaire asked about troublesome neck pain within the last year, and duration Chronic neck pain was defined as lasting more than 6 months	n=10,000 sent questionnaire, 77% (n=7,643) response rate	18–76	13,800/100,000	10,000/100,000	19,000/100,000
Brattberg et al. 1989[2]	Survey, PSAQ	General population, random sample, Sweden	Any pain, or obvious pain > 6 months	n=1,009, 82 % (n=827) response rate	18–84	Point prevalence any pain > 6 months: 19,300/100,000 obvious pain > 6 months: 12,700/100,000		

Table 5: Continued.

Côté *et al.* 1998[28]	Prospective survey, PSAQ	General population, random selection of residents Saskatchewan province	Acute and chronic, neck pain described as pain between occiput and 3rd thoracic vertebra Chronic neck pain questionnaire used to classify severity of pain	n=2,184 recruited, 55% (n=1,420) response rate	20–69	High-intensity/low disability 10,100/ 100,000 (8,200 to 11,900) significantly disabling neck pain 4,600/100,000 (3,300 to 5,800) 5.4 % had pain lasting 90 to 180 days in last 6 months	10,000/100,000
Jacobsson *et al.* 1989[29]	Prospective survey, questionnaire and physical exam	General population, random selection, residents of Malmo, Sweden	Neck pain with/ without brachalgia > 6 weeks	n=552, 81% (n=445) response rate	50–70	1 year period prevalence: 6,500/ 100,000 (4,200–8,800)	3,000/100,000
Mäkelä *et al.* 1991[30]	Prospective survey, questionnaire and clinical exam	General population, random selection, residents of Finland	Current or previous neck pain for > 3 months with physical signs	n=8,000, 90% (n=7,217) response rate	over 30	Point prevalence chronic neck syndrome: 9,500/100,000	Point prevalence chronic neck syndrome: 13,500/100,000
Takala *et al.* 1982[31]	Retrospective survey, PSAQ and clinical exam	General population, random selection residents, Finland	Neck ache, stiffness, soreness and frequency of symptoms	n=2,439, 93% (n=2,268) response rate	40–64	1 year period prevalence: < 50 years 13,000/100,000 > 50 years 20,000/100,000	1 year period prevalence: < 50 years 13,000/100,000 > 50 years 22,000/100,000

Polymyalgia rheumatica

The incidence and prevalence of polymyalgia rheumatica (PMR) has been determined in several hospital- or clinic-based prospective studies from Scandinavia, North America and Southern Europe, all using similar diagnostic criteria (**Table 6**). All of the studies concluded that PMR is a common disease of the elderly, rarely occurring under the age of 50. Prevalence and incidence figures vary rather a lot. For instance, prevalence estimates ranged from 30/100 000 for all ages to 2000/100 000 in an over-65 population. Incidence was also age-related. In a primary care trust population of 100 000 people there would be about 50 new cases a year, and about 500 at any one time.

Fibromyalgia

Fibromyalgia (chronic widespread pain) is a poorly defined complex pain syndrome characterised by chronic widespread pain and multiple tender points. It is the third commonest rheumatic complaint in Canada (23% of new patient rheumatology referrals).[43]

Four studies using American College of Rheumatology (ACR) criteria have been conducted to determine the prevalence of fibromyalgia in the general population (**Table 7**). All of the studies used a two stage screening process, an initial self-assessed questionnaire followed by interview, and clinical examination of tender points for those reporting chronic widespread pain. Chronic widespread pain appears to affect about 10 000/100 000 adults, though fibromyalgia may be diagnosed in 5–10% of those with chronic widespread pain. Trigger points are, however, poor indicators of fibromyalgia,[44] and trigger point numbers are unchanged by effective treatments.[45] It is perhaps better to think of the condition as a spectrum of musculoskeletal disorders, some of which will be severe.

In a primary care trust population of 100 000 people there would be about 10 000 cases of chronic widespread pain, with perhaps 200–1000 being defined as fibromyalgia by current criteria.

Cancer pain

Of every 100 patients with cancer some 60 will have moderate or severe pain. Most, some 80%, of these 60 will obtain at least moderate relief of their pain with appropriate use of the oral drugs on the pain 'ladder' (**Figure 1**), starting with simple analgesics and non-steroidal anti-inflammatory drugs (NSAIDs) and then using oral opioids, usually oral morphine.

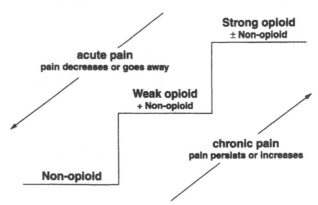

Figure 1: Pain treatment 'ladder'.

Table 6: Chronic pain due to polymyalgic rheumatica.

Reference	Type of study	Sample source	Disease definition	Sample size	Age range (years)	Incidence (per 100,000 95% CI)			Prevalence (per 100,000 population 95% CI)
						Overall	Men	Women	
Bengtsson and Malmvall 1981[35]	Retrospective review of medical records, 1973–75	Residents of a Swedish city referred to clinic or hospital	Diagnostic criteria: 1. Pain and/or stiffness affecting proximal muscle groups without evidence of inflammatory arthritis 2. ESR elevated 3. No evidence of other inflammatory or malignant disease 4. Prompt and persistent response to steroid therapy	n=126 patients identified and reported upon	51–87	PMR alone: 6.7/100,000 for all ages PMR plus GCA: 29/ 100 000 over 50s	PMR alone: 3.4/100,000 for all ages PMR plus GCA 20/ 100,000 over 50s	PMR alone: 9.8/100,000 for all ages PMR plus GCA: 35/ 100,000 over 50s	
Boesen and Sorensen 1987[36]	Prospective study, 1982–85	Residents of a Danish county, diagnosed with PMR referred to the study cohort, GP or hospital referrals	Diagnostic criteria: 1. Pain and/or stiffness affecting proximal muscle groups > 2 weeks 2. ESR > 40 mm/hour 3. Age > 50 years 4. No evidence of other inflammatory disease 5. Prompt and persistent response to steroid therapy	n=31 PMR alone n=10 PMR + temporal arteritis (TA) total population approx. 200,000	50+	19/100,000 for all ages 68/100,000 over 50s	7.4/100,000 for all ages 28/100,000 over 50s	32/100,000 for all ages 108/100,000 over 50s	30/100,000 for all ages 104/100,000 over 50s
Elling et al. 1996[37]	Prospective, longitudinal study, 1982–94 using medical record data	Residents of 13 counties in Sweden, all incident cases of PMR recorded in 2 general hospitals reported to national patient register	States diagnosed using established criteria	n=10,818 analysed	50+	41/100,000 (30 to 67)			

Table 6: Continued.

Reference	Type of study	Sample source	Disease definition	Sample size	Age range (years)	Incidence (per 100,000 95% CI)			Prevalence (per 100,000 population 95% CI)
						Overall	Men	Women	
Gran and Myklebust 1997[38]	Prospective, longitudinal survey, 1987–94, retrospective review of medical records of referrals to different hospital departments	Residents of Aust Agder county, Norway that were referred to regional hospital suspected of having PMR	PMR defined as: 1. Age > 50 years, bilateral aching and morning stiffness (> 30 min) for at least 1 month 2. Involving 2 of the following areas: neck or torso, shoulders or proximal regions of the arms and hips or proximal aspects of the thighs 3. ESR > 40 mm/hour Patients who met two of the three criteria and who had a prompt response to corticosteroid therapy also included	n=256, all patients reported on Includes 32 patients retrospectively included following initiation of drug treatment Prospective patients included in study before treatment started	50+	113/100,000	83/100,000	138/100,000	
Kyle et al. 1985[39]	Prospective study, questionnaire, interview and clinical exam	All patients > 65 years registered with GP practice, Cambridge, UK	Diagnostic criteria: 1. Shoulder and pelvic girdle pain, primarily muscular 2. Morning stiffness 3. Duration > 2 months 4. ESR > 30 mm or C reactive protein > 6 μ/ml 5. Absence of inflammatory or muscle disease 6. Prompt and dramatic response to steroid therapy	n=5,500 patients registered, n=650 ± 65 years recruited, 89% (579) responded, n=32 studied further	± 65	About 230 per 100,000			Prevalence about 2,000 per 100,000

Table 6: Continued.

Northridge and Hill, 1995[40]	Retrospective review of medical records	UK general practice	Patients with presumptive diagnosis treated with steroids	13,600 in one practice 72,400 in other practices	All ages	35–70/100,000 in one practice 55/100,000 in other practices		550/100,000 in one practice 457/100,000 in other practices	
Salvarani et al. 1991[41]	Longitudinal study (1980–88), by medical record review	All residents of Reggio Emilia metropolitan area (Italy) referred to the regional hospital	PMR defined as: 1. Age > 50 years, bilateral aching and morning stiffness (> 30 min) for at least 1 month 2. Involving two of the following areas: neck or torso, shoulders or proximal regions of the arms and hips or proximal aspects of the thighs 3. Erythrocyte sedimentation rate (ESR) > 40 mm/hour Included patients met two of the three criteria or had a prompt response to corticosteroid therapy	n=76 residents identified, all included in incidence data	All ages	4.9/100,000 all ages 12.7/100,000 over 50s	3.4/100,000 all ages 9.7/100,000 over 50s	6.4/100,000 all ages 14.9/100,000 over 50s	
Salvarani et al. 1995[42]	Longitudinal study (1970–91), medical record review (Mayo clinic)	Clinic-based population, all residents of Olmsted County, Minnesota, USA seeking medical care	PMR defined as: 1. Age > 50 years, bilateral aching and morning stiffness (> 30 min) for at least 1 month 2. Involving two of the following areas: neck or torso, shoulders or proximal regions of the arms and hips or proximal aspects of the thighs 3. ESR (Westergren) > 40 mm/hour Included patients met two of the three criteria or those that had a prompt response to corticosteroid therapy	n=245 residents met diagnostic criteria, all reported on and included in incidence data	50+	53/100,000 (46 to 59) in over 50s	40/100,000 (31 to 49) in over 50s	62/100,000 (52 to 71) in over 50s	Prevalence among persons > 50 years (1/1/92) = 627 (527 to 726)

Abbreviations: ESR = erythrocyte sedimentation rate; PMR = polymyalgia rheumatica.

Table 7: Chronic pain due to fibromyalgia.

Reference	Type of study	Sample source	Disease definition	Sample size	Age range (years)	Prevalence (%)	Men	Women
Croft et al. 1993[46]	Cross-sectional survey, SAQ	General population, two general practices in Cheshire, England	ACR definition of chronic widespread pain more than 3 months	n=2,034, 66% response rate (1,340)	18–85	Age- and sex-adjusted point prevalence: 11,200/100,000	Crude point prevalence: 9,400/100,000	Crude point prevalence: 15,600/100,000
Forseth and Gran 1992[47]	Survey, SAQ and clinical exam	General population, random selection female residents in Arendal, Norway	ACR diagnostic criteria; widespread pain, and tenderness in at least 11/18 sites	n=2,498 women, response rate 81.5% (2038) 217 agreed to clinical exam	20–49			Point prevalence of fibromyalgia 10,500/100,000 (95% CI 6,400 to 14,600)
Prescott et al. 1993[48]	National Health Interview Survey, interview and clinical exam	General population, random selection, Denmark	ACR diagnostic criteria; widespread pain, and tenderness in at least 11/18 sites	n=1,595, 1,219 interviewed, (76% response rate)	18–79	Point prevalence fibromyalgia: 660/100,000 (95% CI, 280 to 1290)		
Wolfe et al. 1995[12]	Prospective survey, PSAQ, sub-sample interviewed and examined	General population, random selection residents of Wichita, Kansas, USA	ACR diagnostic criteria; widespread pain, and tenderness in at least 11/18 sites	n=2,582 households, 74.8% response rate, n=3,006 persons n=392 categorised as having chronic, widespread pain	over 18	Point prevalence chronic widespread pain: 10,600 (95% CI 9,500 to 11,700) Point prevalence fibromyalgia (age- and sex-adjusted): 200/100,000 (96% CI 140 to 270)	Point prevalence fibromyalgia: 50/100,000 (95% CI 0 to 100)	Point prevalence fibromyalgia: 340/100,000 (95% CI 230 to 460)

Abbreviations: ACR = American College of Rheumatology, SAQ = self-assessed questionnaire.

Particular problems in the 20% who do not achieve relief with this regime are found with neuropathic (nerve damage) pain, and with incident pain. Incident pain is a bad term, but encompasses movement-related and neuropathic pain. Even more confusing is the American term 'breakthrough pain', which is used both to describe incident pain and pain in patients whose oral morphine dosing is inadequate.

Breakthrough cancer pain

There are relatively few studies describing this phenomenon. On the whole these studies report the number of patients experiencing breakthrough pain, but it has either not been evaluated as a primary outcome, or it has not been defined in detail. Two studies provide the most reliable evidence for the occurrence of breakthrough pain in cancer patients (**Table 8**).[49,50] The first, a prospective study, reports on 63 adult patients admitted to a hospital pain service. On admission to the study, all patients had well-controlled baseline pain (moderate intensity or less). Breakthrough pain that occurred in the previous 24 hours, defined as temporary flares of severe or excruciating pain with stable opioid dose, was reported by 63% (41) patients. In a later study by the same authors, a cross-sectional survey of 178 in-patients with cancer was conducted.[50] Of the 164 who met the inclusion criteria for controlled background pain, 51% (84) experienced breakthrough pain during the previous day. In both studies the characteristics of the breakthrough pains were varied, and were experienced many times during the day (median 6; range 1–60) lasting from seconds to hours. Precipitating factors were often identified, but pains occurred without warning half of the time. Bruera *et al.* described observations on the occurrence and nature of incident pain in 118 cancer patients enrolled in an open uncontrolled trial.[51] They identified 19% (23) with severe incident pain defined as spontaneous or provoked acute exacerbations of pain occurring against a background of good opioid pain control. Movement was the precipitating factor in all of the cases.

Face or head pain

Migraine

Numerous epidemiological studies have been published reporting prevalence rates of migraine headache. These rates vary widely from study to study depending on the disease definition used and the age and gender composition of the study population.[52] Only population-based studies that met standard International Headache Society (IHS) diagnostic criteria for migraine headache, were conducted in European or North American adults, and that reported prevalence rates of migraine for men and women separately, were included here.

Twelve studies meeting these criteria were identified, none in the UK (**Table 9**). Ten reported prevalence and two incidence. Migraine prevalence was higher in women (14 000 to 22 000/100 000) than in men (5000 to 8000/100 000, though one small study of older adults in Italy recorded no men with migraine). In five studies investigating a range of age groups, migraine prevalence was highest in 30–45 year old women and men. These findings are consistent with those reported in a meta-analysis of 18 studies of all ages and from all countries.[53]

The incidence of migraine headache has been estimated from two large population-based surveys in the USA. Medical records of 6478 patients with a diagnosis of headache were surveyed to determine the incidence of clinically detected migraine (IHS criteria) in 629 patients.[54] Age-adjusted incidence was 137 per 100 000 per person-years in men, and 294 per 100 000 per person-years in women. Incidence of migraine peaked in women (20–24 years) later than in men (10–14 years). Using a cross-sectional telephone interview of 10 169 subjects and estimated migraine incidence using reported age of onset, migraine with aura peaked in men at around five years of age, and without aura between 10 and 11 years.[55]

Table 8: Breakthrough pain in cancer patients.

Reference	Type of study	Sample source	Disease definition	Sample size	Age range	Occurrence
Bruera et al. 1992[51]	Open, uncontrolled trial, pain assessment	Cancer patients admitted to a palliative care unit, Canada	Incident pain defined as pain under good control with opiate analgesics while resting, and severe acute exacerbations that occurred spontaneously or on movement	118 patients admitted	63 ± 8 years	23/118 (19%) reported incident pain
Portenoy and Hagen 1990[49]	Prospective survey, questionnaire	Cancer patients attending pain service at a cancer hospital, USA	Breakthrough defined as pain > moderate intensity following pain of moderate or less intensity for > 12 hours/day in previous 24 hours, and stable opioid dose for > 2 days. Pain intensity rated on 5 point categorical scale (none, slight, moderate, severe, excruciating)	63, all patients reported on	15–81 years	Occurrence of breakthrough pain 41 (63%) in 24 hours preceding the interview. Tables in paper report pain frequency, type of onset and duration. Gives data on incident and spontaneous pain
Portenoy et al. 1999[50]	Cross-sectional survey, questionnaire and interview	Hospital inpatients with cancer, randomly selected, USA	Breakthrough pain defined as one or more episodes of severe or excruciating pain in patients with controlled background pain. The number of breakthrough pain episodes was recorded in addition to location, quality, and precipitating factors	178, 92% (164) included in analysis, 14 (7.8%) excluded due to uncontrolled background pain	26–77	84 (51%) reported breakthrough pain on preceding day

Table 9: Migraine.

Reference	Type of study	Sample source	Disease definition	Sample size	Age range	Prevalence per 100 000		
						Men	**Women**	**Overall**
Breslau et al. 1991[57]	Survey, face-to-face interview	HMO population, random sample, USA	IHS	1,200 84% (1007) response rate	21–30	Lifetime prevalence: 7,000/100,000 1 year period prevalence: 3,400/100,000	Lifetime prevalence: 16,300/100,000 1 year period prevalence: 12,900/100,000	Lifetime prevalence: 12,800/100,000
Franceschi et al. 1997[58]	Longitudinal study, clinical exam	Elderly population, random sample, Italy	IHS	312	65–84	1 year period prevalence: 0/100,000	1 year period prevalence: 2,000/100,000	
Göbel et al. 1994[59]	Survey, face-to-face interview	General population, random sample, Germany	IHS	5,000 8,1% (4,062) response rate	18 +	1 year period prevalence: 7,000 (6,000 to 9,000)	1 year period prevalence: 15,000/100,000 (13,000–17,000)	1 year period prevalence: 11,000/100,000 (10,000–13,000)
Henry et al. 1992[60]	Survey, face-to-face interview	General population, stratified quota with random element, France	IHS	4,204	15 +	Lifetime prevalence: 4,000/100,000	Lifetime prevalence: 11,900/100,000	Lifetime prevalence: 8,100/100,000 (6,200–10,000)
Linet et al. 1989[61]	Survey, telephone interview	General population, residents of Washington County, Maryland USA	IHS	10,000	12–29	1 year period prevalence: 5,300/100,000	1 year period prevalence: 14,000/100,000	
Michel et al. 1996[62]	Survey, PSAQ	General population, France	IHS	6,000 households 80% (n=9,411) response rate	18 +	3 month period prevalence: 8,000/100,000	3 month period prevalence: 18,000/100,000	3 month period prevalence: 15,000/100,000 (12,000–14,000)
O'Brien et al. 1994[63]	Survey, telephone interview	General population, random sample, Canada	IHS	4,235 66% (2,922) response rate	18 +	Lifetime prevalence: 7,800/100,000 1 year prevalence: 7,400/100,000	Lifetime prevalence: 24,900/100,000 1 year prevalence: 21,900/100,000	

Table 9: Continued.

Reference	Type of study	Sample source	Disease definition	Sample size	Age range	Prevalence per 100 000			Incidence per 100 000 person-years		
						Men	Women	Overall	Men	Women	Overall
Rasmussen et al. 1991[64]	Prospective survey, clinical exam	General population, random sample, Denmark	IHS	1,000 75.9% (740) response rate	25–64	Lifetime prevalence: 8,000/100,000 1 year period prevalence: 6,000/100,000 (4,000–9,000)	Lifetime prevalence: 25,000/100,000 1 year period prevalence: 15,000/100,000 (12,000–19,000)	Lifetime prevalence: 16,000/100,000 1 year period prevalence: 10,000/100,000 (8,000–13,000)			
Stewart et al. 1992[65]	Survey, PSAQ	General population, random sample, USA	IHS	20,468 63.4% response rate	12–80	1 year period prevalence: 5,700/100,000	1 year period prevalence: 17,600/100,000				
Stewart et al. 1996[66]	Survey, telephone interview	General population, USA	IHS	12,000	18–65	1 year period prevalence: 8,200/100,000	1 year period prevalence: 19,000/100,000				
Rozen et al. 1999[56]	Retrospective survey, medical record review, 1989–90	General population with medically recognised migrainous disorder, Olmsted County, Minnesota, USA	IHS		All ages				194/100,000	482/100,000	
Stang et al. 1992[54]	Retrospective survey, medical record review, 1979–81	General population with medically recognised migrainous disorder, Olmsted County, Minnesota, USA	IHS	6,476 records reviewed	All ages				137/100,000	294/100,000	216/100,000

In women, migraine incidence with aura peaked between ages 12 and 13 and migraine without aura between 14 and 17, giving a higher migraine incidence peaking at a lower age. The difference may be due to the different data collection methods. A recent report showed an increase in the incidence of migraine in the USA in women of reproductive age.[56]

A primary care trust of 100 000 people will have about 10 000 women and 2000 men who suffer from migraine. Only about one in five or six will seek medical care, the remainder using analgesics available off prescription, or no treatment at all.[67]

Headache

Based on five UK population-based studies in adults, the one year period prevalence of headache ranged from 70–83% in men and 78–90% in women.[68–72] These studies all used disparate, and in many cases unclear, headache definitions, and therefore do not provide reliable prevalence estimates.

When a more restricted headache definition was used, such as frequent headache as defined by IHS criteria, five population-based studies in adults from North America and Europe were found (**Table 10**). All of the studies used validated methods such as clinical examination, telephone interview or self-assessed questionnaires. In four studies, the one year prevalence of chronic tension-type headache (CTTH) was 1000 to 3000/100 000, and was reported more frequently by women than men.[58,73–75] One German study reported a lifetime prevalence of CTTH of 1% for women. There were no cases of CTTH reported by men in this study.[59]

The incidence of cluster headaches[76] was 10/100 000.

Trigeminal neuralgia

Incidence and prevalence of trigeminal neuralgia are difficult to estimate due to the lack of epidemiological studies with clear diagnostic criteria. Only two large population-based studies reported incidence rates for the UK[77] and USA,[78] respectively (**Table 11**).

From the medical records of the 70 000 residents of Carlisle between the years 1955–6 an incidence of 2.1/100 000 was derived.[77] The authors stated that the true incidence might have been higher because local ENT hospitals were not included. A retrospective review of the medical records of the 60 000 residents of Rochester county, Minnesota gave an annual incidence for the first episode of trigeminal neuralgia of 4.7 per 100 000 (95% CI 3.6 to 5.8).[78] Incidence rates increased with age, and were not significantly different between men and women. The authors also reported a crude prevalence rate by multiplying the annual incidence by the median survival time in years. They estimated that the prevalence of a current or recent attack of trigeminal neuralgia in a population aged 50–70 years would be < 1 in 250 or 400 per 100 000.

Only one direct estimate of trigeminal neuralgia prevalence was found.[79] In a survey of 1144 residents of a French village, 86% of the residents completed a neurological questionnaire, and three months later 261 were followed up with a neurological examination. One man was diagnosed with trigeminal neuralgia, diagnostic criteria not stated, to provide a prevalence estimate of 100/100 000.

Atypical facial pain

No studies providing reliable prevalence and incidence data for atypical facial pain were found.

Table 10: Headache.

Reference	Type of study	Sample source	Disease definition	Sample size	Age range (years)	Prevalence per 100,000		
						Men	**Women**	**Overall**
Franceschi et al. 1997[58]	Longitudinal study, clinical exam	Elderly population, random sample, Italy	IHS criteria for headache classification	n=312	65–84	1 year period prevalence CTTH: 1,200/100,000	1 year period prevalence CTTH: 4,000/100,000	1 year period prevalence CTTH: 2,600/100,000
Gobel et al. 1994[59]	Survey, face-to-face interview	General population, randomly selected, Germany	IHS criteria for headache classification	n=1,200, 8,4% (n=1,007) response rate	21–30	Lifetime prevalence CTTH: 0/100,000	Lifetime prevalence CTTH: 1,000/100,000	Lifetime prevalence CTTH: 1,000/100,000
Rasmussen 1995[73]	Survey, recruitment by telephone followed by examination and interview by a physician	General population, randomly selected residents Copenhagen county, Denmark	IHS criteria for headache classification	n=1,000 selected, 25 unattainable, 75.9% (n=790) response rate	25–64	1 year period prevalence: Tension-type headache: 63,000/100,000 ETTH: 56,000/100,000 CTTH: 2,000/100,000	1 year period prevalence: Tension-type headache: 86,000/100,000 ETTH: 71,000/100,000 CTTH: 5,000/100,000	

Table 10: Continued.

						Incidence per 100000		
						Men	**Women**	**Overall**
Scher et al. 1998[75] and Schwartz et al. 1998[74]	Survey, telephone interview	General population, randomly selected households, Baltimore County, USA	19,840 households selected, 6.7% could not be contacted Interview completed on 13,343 (77.4%) eligible subjects	18–65	Type of headache per IHS criteria, either migraine or frequent headache Frequent headache defined as > 180 headaches/year and further subclassified: chronic tension-type headache (CTTH), frequent headache with migrainous features (FH/M) and other frequent headache (FH/O)	1 year period prevalence: ETTH: 36,000/100,000 Frequent headache: 2,800/100,000 CTTH: 1,600/100,000 FH/M: 700/100,000 FH/O: 500/100,000	1 year period prevalence: ETTH: 42,000/100,000 Frequent headache: 5,000/100,000 CTTH: 2,600/100,000 FH/M: 1,700/100,000 FH/O: 800/100,000	1 year period prevalence: ETTH: 38,000/100,000 Frequent headache: 4,100/100,000 CTTH: 2,200/100,000 FH/M: 1,300/100,000 FH/O.: 600/100,000
Swanson et al. 1994[76]	Case ascertainment from population	Olmsted County, Minnesota, USA	6,476 respondents in migraine and headache survey	Adults	Cluster headaches, IH definition with minor variations	15.6/100,000 (8.9–22.3)	4.0/100,000 (0.4–7.6)	9.8/100,000 (6.0–13.6)

Abbreviations: IHS = International Headache Society; CTTH = chronic tension type headache; ETTH = Episodic tension type headache.

Table 11: Trigeminal neuralgia.

Reference	Type of study	Sample source	Disease definition	Sample size	Age range (years)	Incidence per 100 000 population			Prevalence	Natural history
						Overall	Men	Women		
Brewis et al. 1966[77]	Retrospective review of medical records	General population, residents of Carlisle, UK	Disease definition not given, but states that diagnosis by consultant physician was accepted, cases where diagnosis not clear further investigated, most excluded	n =70,000	0–85+	Annual age adjusted incidence 1955–61: 2/100,000				
Katusic et al. 1990[78]	Retrospective review of medical records 1945–84 with diagnosis confirmed by a neurologist by clinical examination	General population, all residents of Rochester County, Minnesota, USA	Diagnosis of trigeminal neuralgia per Rushton and Olafson, briefly: 1. Brief paroxysms of severe pain of trigeminal nerve 2. Unpredictable remissions and exacerbations of pain 3. No evidence of sensory or motor deficit of involved nerve 4. Occurrence of trigger zones	n=222 medical records identified with diagnosis of trigeminal neuralgia, 147 excluded from study due to not meeting diagnosis criteria, not meeting residency requirements or onset outside of study time period	24–93	Annual incidence of first episode of trigeminal neuralgia 1945–84: 4.7/100,000 (3.6–5.8)	Annual incidence of first episode of trigeminal neuralgia 1945–84: 3.4/100,000 (1.9–4.9)	Annual incidence of first episode of trigeminal neuralgia 1945–84: 5.9/100,000 (4.3–7.5)	Prevalence may be derived by multiplying the annual incidence by the median survival measured in years, providing that incidence does not change with time. An estimate of the prevalence of a current or recent attack of trigeminal neuralgia in a population aged 50–70 years would be < 1:250 or 400:100,000	Median number of episodes = 3 (range 1–11), 29% had 1 episode, 19% had 2, 24% had 3, 28% had 4–11 episodes Median length of an episode was 49 days, mean 116 days (range 1–1,462 days) 65% patients were estimated to have a second episode within 5 years, 77% within 10 years Among the 53 patients with 2 or more episodes, 66% experienced a third episode within 5 years of the second episode, 79% had a third episode within 10 years The 10 year survival from onset of trigeminal neuralgia to death was 46% (n=75)

Neuropathic pain

Diabetic neuropathy

Two large population-based studies have been conducted to determine the occurrence of diabetic neuropathy (**Table 12**). The first, in the UK, involved 97 034 adult patients registered with 10 general practices covering both urban and rural areas. According to strict diagnostic criteria, the occurrence of sensory neuropathy in all diabetics was 16% (95% CI 15 to 19%). There were no significant differences between prevalence rates for type I and II diabetes, or men and women.[80] There was no specific mention of painful neuropathy. In an American survey of a random sample of 84 572 adults there were 2405 diagnosed diabetics, and 99% completed a postal self-assessed questionnaire.[81] The occurrence of at least one symptom of sensory neuropathy in all diabetics was 38%, and pain or tingling in 23%.

These findings broadly agree with those from four clinic or hospital-based studies that determined the prevalence of sensory neuropathy in diabetic subjects having treatment (**Table 12**). The occurrence of painful neuropathy was 11% in type I diabetics with strict diagnostic criteria[82] and 25% in all diabetics using a pain questionnaire.[83] Nabarro[84] found 16% painful neuropathy and O'Hare et al.[85] found 13%.

These studies showed that sensory neuropathy becomes more prevalent at older ages, but occurs with similar frequency in men and women. There was no significant difference between the prevalence rates for type I and type II diabetes. A primary care trust of 100 000 people will have about 2000 diabetics. About one in five will have painful neuropathy at some stage

Postherpetic neuralgia

Herpes zoster occurs in the general population at a rate of about 340/100 000 per year,[86,87] with 195 000 new cases a year. Following primary infection with the varicella zoster virus, the virus becomes dormant in dorsal root ganglia. Postherpetic neuralgia (PHN) is a common complication of herpes zoster, occurring in about 13–26% of cases, and including persistent pain after the onset of zoster. In the over-60s particularly, pain is common.

A summary of the occurrence of PHN is in **Table 13**, though Edmunds et al. also have a detailed review of the epidemiology.[86,87] The occurrence of painful neuropathy depended upon populations studied because of the large age-dependency. Painful neuropathy in over 40% of people aged over 50 was a common finding (**Table 13**). One incidence study[88] indicated that a primary care group of 100 000 people could expect to see 34 new cases a year.

Multiple sclerosis

Multiple sclerosis has a crude prevalence of about 100/100 000 in England and Wales, but rates about double that in Scotland.[95] A number of studies have examined the occurrence of chronic pain in patients with multiple sclerosis, and they are summarised in **Table 14**. Whatever definition of pain used, pain was common, occurring in about half of multiple sclerosis patients. A primary care trust of about 100 000 people in England or Wales could expect to have about 50 patients with multiple sclerosis and chronic pain. There would be about twice as many in Scotland.

Table 12: Chronic pain due to diabetic neuropathy.

Reference	Type of study	Sample source	Disease definition	Sample size	Age range (years)	Occurrence
Boulton et al. 1985[82]	Prospective study, clinical exam	IDDM subjects attending diabetic clinic, Sheffield, UK	Definition of sensory polyneuropathy by strict criteria requiring presence of symptoms and signs of nerve dysfunction in the absence of peripheral vascular disease. Pain sensations for at least 1 year	387 approached, 99% (n=382) agreed to participate	16–59	Painful neuropathy in 10.7%
Chan et al. 1990[83]	Case-controlled survey, questionnaire	Patients attending a diabetic clinic, case-matched with non-diabetic control group (visitors of relatives in hospital), UK	Diabetes > 3 months duration. Chronic pain defined as pain present most of the time. Patients used diagram to indicate site and radiation of pain, pain descriptors include aching, burning, and stabbing/ shooting. Duration of pain also sought	Diabetics n=974 98% response rate (n=962)	adults – mean age all diabetics 58.1 ± 17.5	Chronic pain in 25.2% Burning and stabbing or shooting pain in 7.4%
Harris et al. 1993[81]	Cross-sectional survey, part of National Health Interview survey 1989, interview and questionnaire	General population, NIDDM adults identified from households, USA	Questions asked 'During the last 3 months have you experienced: 1. Numbness or loss of feeling in hands and feet 2. Painful sensation or tingling in hands and feet 3. Decreased ability to feel hot or cold in things you touch IDDM defined in paper'	84,572 surveyed 2,405 diagnosed diabetics, of these 99.3% (2,405) questioned further	± 18	In all diabetics over 3 months: numbness: 28.2% pain or tingling: 26.8% decreased sensation to hot or cold: 9.8% ± 1 of above symptoms: 37.9%. In type I diabetics over 3 months: numbness: 15.7% pain or tingling: 22.8% decreased sensation to hot or cold: 9.9% ± 1 of above symptoms: 30.2%.

Table 12: Continued.

Reference	Type of study	Sample source	Disease definition	Sample size	Age range (years)	Occurrence
Nabarro 1991[84]	Prospective survey, interview and questionnaire	Type I and type II diabetic outpatients attending diabetic clinic, 1954–88, London, UK	Type I and type II diabetes as per WHO criteria. Neuropathy recorded if considered to be clinically important, DNS diagnostic criteria	n=1,410 type I diabetes, n=4,962 Type II diabetes, data on all patients	DNS	In Type I: Painful neuropathy in 16.3% with neuropathy and 2.8% of all type I. In type II: Painful neuropathy in 5.4% with neuropathy and 0.6% of all type II
O'Hare et al. 1994[85]	Prospective survey, interview and questionnaire	Type I and type II diabetics attending outpatient diabetic clinic over 1 year, UK	Type I and type II diabetes per standard criteria neuropathy criteria not defined, pain intensity not defined	n=800, type I = 336, type II = 464, data on all patients	16–84	1 year period prevalence pain/paraesthesia: All diabetics: 13.3% Type I: 12.5% Type II: 13.8%
Walters et al. 1992[80]	Case-controlled survey, interview and clinical exam	All diabetics registered with 10 GP practices, case-matched with non-diabetic controls, UK	Diabetes defined per WHO criteria. Neuropathy defined as: 1. Presence of symptoms: numbness, burning, prickling, deep aching, tenderness or tingling present bilaterally, ± 1 year, at rest and included in the feet 2. Loss of light touch 3. Impairment of pain perception 4. Absent ankle jerks in subjects < 70 years 5. Abnormal vibration perception thresholds	n=97,034 patients registered in 10 practices n=1,150 diabetics (93.7% reviewed)	Diabetics all ages	Occurrence of neuropathy: All diabetics 16.3% (14.6–19.0) Type I diabetes 12.7% (8.0–17.6) Type II diabetes 17.2% (15.9–18.5)

Table 13: Chronic pain due to post-herpetic neuralgia (PHN).

Reference	Type of study	Sample source	Disease definition	Sample size	Age range (years)	Occurrence
Brown 1976[89]	Retrospective review of medical records	Patients attending dermatology outpatients, 10 year period 1963–72, USA	PHN defined as pain > 6 weeks after initial eruption of herpes zoster	140, all reported	Not stated	All ages: pain occurred in 34% Less than 50 years: pain occurred in 6% More than 50 years: pain occurred in 43%
de Moragas and Kierland 1957[90]	Retrospective review of medical records	Patients diagnosed with herpes zoster or PHN 1939–45, USA	PHN not defined	916 records reviewed, all reported	Less than 20 to more than 70	Pain occurred in 49% beyond 1 month Pain lasted 1–6 months in 21% Pain lasted 6–12 months in 4% Pain lasted more than 12 months in 25%
Helgason et al. 2000[91]	Prospective cohort study	January 1990 to June 1999 in 100,000 general practice population in Iceland	Single investigator diagnosis and questions about pain at 1, 3, 6 and 12 months	421 patients with complete ascertainment	All ages	In under-60s, 2% had pain at 3 months In over-60s, 7% had pain at 3 months and < 3% at 12 months
Lancaster et al. 1995[92]	Meta-analysis of randomised trials of acute interventions to prevent long-term pain	Any randomised trial measuring pain at (at least) 1 month	Treatment of acute zoster Pain (not defined)	617 patients treated with placebo and with at least 6 months' follow-up	Adults	94/617 patients had pain at 6 months (15%)

Table 13: Continued.

						Incidence
Meister et al. 1998[93]	Prospective documentation of all cases of zoster by random selection of German physicians	Patients recruited September 1994–March 1995 486 physicians contributed patients	Pain at 4–5 weeks	2,063 patients with zoster	Less than 10 to more than 70	Pain in afflicted dermatome at 4–5 weeks in 28%
Rogers and Tindall 1971[94]	Retrospective review of medical records	Patients attending a medical centre and diagnosed with HZ or post-zoster complications, 1939–68, USA	PHN defined as pain persisting > 4 weeks after HZ infection	n=576 patients with HZ or complications n=243 age 60+ (results presented for these patients)		Pain occurred in 47% of over-60s Pain occurred in 16% of under-60s Pain lasted longer than 6 months in 58% of over-60s
Cockerell et al. 1996[88]	Prospective 1 year study, clinical exam	Patients attending two GP surgeries, UK	Neurological disease as diagnosed by clinician	n=25,000 registered with 2 GPs	DNS	34/100,000

Table 14: Chronic pain due to multiple sclerosis.

Reference	Type of study	Sample source	Disease definition	Sample size	Age range (years)	Occurrence of pain
Archibald et al. 1994[96]	Prospective examination of consecutively referred outpatients with MS in a clinic	Clinic patients, Nova Scotia, Canada	Clinically definite MS Pain measured in a structured interview for severity, type and duration	85 of 94 approached	19–75	Pain occurred in 53%
Brochet et al. 1992[97]	Prospective study, questionnaire	Multiple sclerosis patients attending outpatients, Group 1 = pain reported at least once; Group 2 = no pain, France	Pain syndromes reported: painful paraesthesias or dysaesthesias; electric shocks; lightning pain; painful leg spasms; articular and myofascial pain, also location, duration and frequency of pain	108	DNS	Pain occurred in 41%
Clifford and Trotter 1984[98]	Retrospective medical record survey	Attendees at MS clinic between 1977 and 1983, in St Louis, Missouri, USA	Pain was defined as a major complaint that lasted at least 2 weeks	317	15–70	Pain occurred in 29%
Moulin et al. 1988[99]	Retrospective review of medical records, PSAQ and telephone interview	MS patients who attended outpatient clinic between 1973 and 1985, Canada	MS by Rose criteria, 62% definite MS, 38% probable or possible MS Clinically significant pain defined as: 1. Paroxysmal stereotyped pain syndrome regarded as characteristic for MS 2. Chronic pain present intermittently or continuously over 1 month	167 patients approached, 159 responded	20 to over 60	Occurrence of any clinically significant pain in 55% Occurrence of chronic pain in 48%

Table 14: Continued.

Stenager *et al.* 1991[100]	Prospective survey, questionnaire and interview	Random selection of patients with MS attending neurology clinic, Denmark	Chronic pain defined as constant or intermittent pain lasting more than 1 month. Acute syndromes included transient symptoms lasting < 1 month. Headaches and minor pain syndromes excluded	117, all patients interviewed	25–55 years	Occurrence of pain at any time in 65% Occurrence of pain at interview in 45%
Vermote *et al.* 1986[101]	Consecutive prospective survey of MS patients	Patients with MS attending MS clinic in Belgium	MS by Schumacher criteria Pain measured by Dutch equivalent of MPQ	83	not given	Pain occurred in 54%
Warnell 1991[102]	Prospective survey, PSAQ	MS patients attending outpatient clinic, Canada	Painful symptoms reported, including their frequency and intensity PIVAS scale	500, 73% (n=364) responders	19–74	Pain occurred in 64%

Chronic post-stroke pain

Only one prospective study of chronic post-stroke pain has been reported.[103] Two hundred and sixty seven adult patients were recruited to a Danish study after admission to hospital following an acute stroke. At six months, 78% had survived and the occurrence of chronic post-stroke pain, according to strict criteria, was 6.5% at six months and 8.4% at one year. The incidence of chronic post-stroke pain during the first year after stroke was 8%, of which 10/16 patients reported pain of moderate to severe intensity. In a retrospective survey of 400 cases of stroke in the UK, 2% were reported to have chronic post-stroke pain.[104] The median time for onset of pain was three months from stroke, and could be as long as 24 months. In a primary care trust of 100 000 people there could be as many as 10 to 50 people with chronic post-stroke pain.

Vascular pain

There is substantial information on the incidence and prevalence of cardiovascular disease due to its high mortality and morbidity. There is limited information about the incidence and prevalence of painful symptoms.

Intermittent claudication

Accurate estimates of intermittent claudication can only be obtained from population surveys, as most subjects with claudication are not referred to hospital unless symptoms are severe enough to warrant surgery. Larger studies published since 1990 are summarised in **Table 15**. Most studies are conducted in an older adult population because this is primarily a disorder of older adults. In older adults the prevalence of intermittent claudication is of the order of 1000/100 000 to 2000/100 000, according to a review.[105] When the age range involves mainly people in their seventh decade and older, higher prevalence rates are found.[106,107]

The incidence, again in older adults, is 400–1600/100 000. A typical primary care trust of 100 000 people might expect to have 400–800 people with intermittent claudication, and see 200 new cases a year.

Raynaud's phenomenon

One of the problems with prevalence estimates of Raynaud's phenomenon is that of knowing the degree of chronic pain experienced. The four population surveys identified (**Table 16**) record quite high figures for prevalence, though reducing with more exacting definitions of disorder.[112] It is likely that even the prevalence of a clear edge between pale and normal colour overstates the prevalence of painful Raynaud's.

Angina

Many UK epidemiological studies estimating prevalence of coronary heart disease are in specific occupational groups only (Whitehall and UK heart disease prevention study),[116] or use methods other than the standard Rose chest pain questionnaire and ECG to estimate prevalence rates.[117] The Speedwell and Caerphilly survey,[118] Scottish Heart Health Study,[119] Grampian survey[6] and the Maidstone and Dewsbury survey[106] provide reliable estimates of prevalence rates of angina in the UK (**Table 17**). Prevalence is age-dependent, because almost no angina occurs until the sixth decade of life. In all adults the prevalence is about 5000/100 000, but is about double this at 10 000/100 000 in over-50s. A US study suggests an incidence in adults between 30 and 74 years of about 1000/100 000.

A primary care trust with a population of 100 000 might expect to have about 4000 cases of angina, with about a third of them severe. There would be about 500 new cases a year.

Table 15: Claudication.

Reference	Type of study	Sample source	Disease definition	Sample size	Age range (years)	Prevalence per 100,000			Incidence per 100,000
						Overall	Men	Women	
Bainton et al. 1994[108]	Prospective, longitudinal study, part of Speedwell heart disease study, Q and clinical exam	Male patients registered with 16 GPs, Bristol, UK	Claudication defined as: 1. pain on walking in one or both calves 2. no pain on rest 3. relieved within 10 min resting 4. never disappears when walking continued 5. pain causes subject to stop or slow down	2,550 men selected, 92% attended clinic for first visit	45–59		Prevalence 1,200/100,000 at baseline rising to 2,800/100,000 after 10 years		Annual incidence of new cases 400/100,000
Bowlin et al. 1994[109]	Prospective study and follow-up of Israeli men	Male government employees	London School of Hygiene cardiovascular disease questionnaire	8,343 men free of coronary heart disease	40–65		baseline prevalence 2,700/100,000		Annual incidence of new cases 860/100,000
Leng et al. 1996[110]	Prospective, longitudinal study, SAQ and exam	Patients randomly selected from 10 GP practices, UK	Criteria for IC per Rose/WHO questionnaire, ankle brachial pressure index and reactive hyperaemia test. Grade 1 = calf pain when walking uphill or hurrying Grade 2 = pain upon walking ordinary pace on level Probable = calf pain present on exercise but not at rest	1,592 selected 65% responded	55–74	Prevalence at 5 years in those that completed WHO questionnaire: 7,100/100,000			Annual incidence 1,550/100,000

Table 15: Continued.

Reference	Type of study	Sample source	Disease definition	Sample size	Age range (years)	Prevalence per 100,000			Incidence per 100,000
						Overall	Men	Women	
Leng et al. 2000[106]	Prospective survey of random sample of men and women	Dewsbury and Maidstone, UK	Leg pain typical of intermittent claudication if pain on walking relieved within 10 minutes	417 of 481 men and 367 of 441 women attended for ultrasound examination	56–77		6,400/100,000 (2,100–10,700) in men without femoral plaque 17,200/100,000 (12,600 to 21,800 with femoral plaque) Plaque present in 64%	6,700/100,000 (2,500–10,900) in women without femoral plaque 5,600/100,000 (2,400 to 8,800 with femoral plaque) Plaque present in 64%	
Meijer et al. 1998[105]	Prospective follow-up study	Individuals aged 55 and over in Rotterdam, Holland	WHO/Rose questionnaire	10,275 invited, 7,983 responded (78%)	over 54	Prevalence 1,600/100,000	2,200/100,000	1,200/100,000	
Menotti et al. 2001[107]	Prospective longitudinal study of men in three European countries	Men aged 65 to 84 years in 1985 from previous longitudinal study	Rose leg pain questionnaire	2,285 men	65–84		Finland 11,000/100,000 Holland 7,600/100,000 Italy 8,400/100,000		
Smith et al. 1990[111]	Prospective longitudinal study of government employees	Large prospective study	Questionnaire	18,388	40–64	Probably intermittent claudication 800/100,000 Possible intermittent claudication 1,000/100,000			

Abbreviations: IC = intermittent claudication; Q = questionnaire; SAQ = self-assessed questionnaire; PSAQ = postal self-assessed questionnaire; ECG = electrocardiogram.

Table 16: Raynaud's phenomenon.

Reference	Type of study	Sample source	Disease definition	Sample size	Age range (years)	Prevalence per 100,000		
						Overall	Men	Women
Brand et al. 1997[113]	Longitudinal 16 year study, questionnaire and clinical exam	General population, 2nd generation participants in Framingham Heart study (offspring and their spouses of the original participants), USA	Evidence of Raynaud's phenomenon: 1. sensitivity to cold 2. blanching of fingers when exposed to cold, with numbness followed by cyanosis, then redness and tingling or pain.	4,182 selected DNS response rate	over 20	Prevalence: 8,800/100,000	Prevalence: 8,100/100,000	Prevalence: 9,600/100,000
Maricq et al. 1986[114]	Carolina Health Survey, interviewer administered questionnaire	General population, random selection residents of South Carolina, USA	Prevalence estimates given for several different criteria: 1. reported cold sensitivity of fingers or toes 2. cold sensitivity combined with blanching and/or cyanosis 3. cold sensitivity severe enough to lead to physician consultation	1,752 subjects interviewed	over 18	Lifetime prevalence: criteria 1: 10,000/100,000 criteria 2: 4,600/100,000 criteria 3: 3,000/100,000 criteria 2 + 3: 2,000/100,000		
Palmer et al. 2000[112]	Random sample of adults of working age	Randomly selected adult patients from 34 selected general practices across England, Wales and Scotland, plus members of armed forces	Prevalence estimates given for several different criteria: 1. Reported cold, numb and blanched fingers 2. Brought on by cold 3. Clear edge between pale and normal colour	22,194 questionnaires, 12,907 replies (58%)	16–64	Any blanching about 15,000/ 100,000 Cold induced blanching 12,000/100,000 Clear edge 4,800/100,000	Clear edge between 1,800/ 100,000 at 16–24 up to 7,200/100,000 at 55–65	Clear edge between 3,500/ 100,000 at 16–24 up to 5,100/100,000 at 55–65

Table 16: Continued.

Reference	Type of study	Sample source	Disease definition	Sample size	Age range (years)	Prevalence per 100,000		
						Overall	Men	Women
Silman *et al.* 1990[115]	Two questionnaire surveys: 1. SAQ clinic population 2. PSAQ	Two populations studied: 1. All new patients attending 5 GP practices 2. Random sample, patients registered with above 5 GPs, UK	Raynaud's phenomenon defined by presence of all 3 criteria: 1. Episodes of finger blanching 2. Precipitated by cold 3. Sensory sensations (pins and needles and numbness) Interview and clinical exam of the positive patients	1. n=1,119 (response rate not recorded) 2. n=600 69% (n=413) response rate	over 15	Prevalence: clinic attendees 19,000/100,000 postal sample 15,000/100,000	Lifetime prevalence: clinic attendees: 16,000/100,000 postal sample: 11,000/100,000	Lifetime prevalence: clinic attendees: 21,000/100,000 postal sample: 19,000/100,000

Abbreviations: IC = intermittent claudication; Q = questionnaire; SAQ = self-assessed questionnaire; PSAQ = postal self-assessed questionnaire; ECG = electrocardiogram.

Table 17: Angina.

Reference	Type of study	Sample source	Disease definition	Sample size	Age range (years)	Prevalence per 100,000 Overall	Men	Women	Incidence per 100,000
Bainton et al. 1988[118]	Two surveys: 1. Caerphilly and, 2. Speedwell surveys Rose chest pain questionnaire and 12 lead ECG	Both surveys general population: 1. selection middle-aged men, Caerphilly, UK 2. Selection men registered with 16 GPs, Speedwell, UK	Angina defined as: grade 1 (chest pain only on walking uphill or hurrying) grade 2 (chest pain on walking at an ordinary pace on the level)	1. n=2,818 selected 89% (n=2,512) examined 2. n=2,550 selected, 92% (n=2,348) examined	45–59		Prevalence of angina 8,200/ 100,000 About 30% was more severe grade 2		
Elliott et al. 1999[6]	Random sample of the general population	Adults aged over 25 in 29 general practices in Grampian Region, Scotland	Angina defined by patient in questionnaire, with instructions and after piloting	4,611 contacted, 3,605 responses	25 and over	Prevalence of angina 4,500/100,000, almost wholly in over-55s where prevalence was 10,100/100,000	4,900/100,000	4,100/100,000	
Leng et al. 2000[106]	Prospective survey of random sample of men and women	Dewsbury and Maidstone, UK	Rose chest pain questionnaire	417 of 481 men and 367 of 441 women attended for ultrasound examination	56–77	9,600/100,000 (6,100 to 13,100) without femoral plaque 15,400/100,000 (12,100–18,700 with femoral plaque) Plaque present in 64%			
McGovern et al. 2001[120]	Retrospective survey of hospital discharges for a population	All patients discharged from metropolitan hospitals, Twin Cities, Minnesota for 1985, 1990 and 1995	From hospital notes of signs, symptoms, medical history, enzymes, complications, therapy and ECGs	For 1995, 3,615 discharge records examined	30–74				Age-adjusted incidence of angina with or without MI in 1995 was 1,357/ 100,000 for men and 495/100,000 for women

Table 17: Continued.

Reference	Type of study	Sample source	Disease definition	Sample size	Age range (years)	Prevalence per 100,000			Incidence per 100,000
						Overall	Men	Women	
Menotti et al. 2001[107]	Prospective longitudinal study of men in three European countries	Men aged 65 to 84 years in 1985 from previous longitudinal study	Rose chest pain questionnaire	2,285 men	65–84		Finland 19,700/100,000 Holland 10,300/100,000 Italy 9,500/ 100,000		
Shaper et al. 1984[117]	British Regional Heart Study, administered questionnaire, 3 lead ECG	General population, random selection middle aged men, UK	Angina defined as chest pain or discomfort with exertion plus: 1. Area of pain confirmed on diagram 2. Pain causes subject to slow down or stop 3. Pain goes away if stops exertion 4. Takes < 10 minutes for pain to go away	n=7,735 selected, 78% (n=6,033) response rate	40–59		Prevalence: 8,000/100,000		
Smith et al. 1990[119]	Scottish Heart Health study, prospective survey, SAQ and physical examination with 12 lead ECG	General population, random selection from 22 GP districts, UK	Angina defined as: grade 1 (less severe) grade 2 (more severe) criteria as per Rose chest pain questionnaire	74% response rate, n=10,359 analysed	40–59		Prevalence angina 6,300/ 100,000 (3,900 to 14,800) About 30% more severe grade 2	Prevalence angina: 8,500/ 100,000 (4,300 to 17,600) About 30% more severe grade 2	

Chronic postoperative pain

The contribution of surgery to the prevalence of chronic pain has been systematically studied among outpatients attending specialist pain clinics[121] and studies have been published investigating chronic pain after particular operations.[122] In the systematic review of published studies reporting the prevalence of chronic postoperative pain after a range of common surgical operations,[122] the methodological quality of the majority of studies was poor.

In a large survey of 10 pain clinics in the UK, information was collected about 5130 adult patients by a questionnaire filled out by the physician.[121] Chronic pain due to surgery was reported by 23% of patients. The pain had lasted longer than 24 months in 59% of these, was of moderate to severe intensity in 76%, and significantly disabling in 44%. The sites of pain most frequently reported were: abdominal (47%), anal, perineal and genital (38%) and lower limb (35%). These estimates may be higher than expected for the general population as this survey represents a selective group of patients, but it does indicate that chronic postoperative pain can be a significant part of the work of pain clinics.

In another systematic review[123] which included studies with information about pain 12 weeks or longer after surgery, and excluded studies smaller than 50–100 patients (apart from amputation studies with 25 patients), chronic pain after surgery was common. Many studies had information to one year or longer, and many compared different surgical approaches, or anaesthesia. Phantom limb pain was common (up to 80%), but high rates of chronic pain were reported for all surgery. Even with hernia repair, which had the lowest incidence, rates varied from 0% to 29%. Predictive factors included pre-operative pain, repeat surgery, a surgical approach with risk of nerve damage, acute and severe postoperative pain, radiation, chemotherapy and a variety of psychological and depressive symptoms.

The focus here is on the best studied areas, of phantom limb and stump pain after amputation,[124,125] of chronic postoperative pain, and breast surgery[126,127] and thoracotomy.[128,129] Detailed information on pain after hernia repair can be found in Bay-Nielsen *et al.*[130] They surveyed all repairs in Denmark over two months in 1998; 29% reported having pain in the area of the hernia within the past month, and 11% reported that the pain impaired work or leisure activities. Only 4.5% (1 in 6) had sought medical advice or received treatment for the pain.

Pain after amputation

To determine the occurrence of phantom limb pain accurately, studies must differentiate between phantom limb sensation, phantom limb pain and stump pain. This section considers the studies where phantom limb pain was described distinctly (**Table 18**). Phantom limb pain occurred in half to three quarters of amputees, persisting at seven years post-amputation.

Pain characteristics were reported in most of the studies. In the 53% of amputees reporting phantom limb pain one year following amputation, pain intensity was rated as of mild or moderate intensity by all.[131] In three other studies, mean pain intensity ranged from 5.3 to 6.9 out of a maximum of 10.[124,125,132] Five years after limb amputation, pain was reported by 73%, in 65% pain was experienced frequently to occasionally, and 7.5% experienced constant pain in the phantom limb.[133] Most prevalence estimates are potentially biased because of small sample sizes and low response rates.

High rates of stump pain were reported in prospective surveys of military veterans, with at least half of amputees having stump pain. Rates were 49%,[134] 57%[125] and 62%[124] respectively.

There are perhaps 17–20 amputees per 100 000 population in Holland,[135,136] and 28/100 000 in Finland.[137] In a typical primary care trust, about 25/100 000 may be expected, most of whom will have chronic pain problems, either phantom limb pain, or stump pain, or both.

Table 18: Phantom limb pain.

Reference	Type of study	Sample source	Disease definition	Sample size	Age range	Occurrence of pain
Buchanan and Mandel 1986[138]	Retrospective review of medical records and interview by a technician	Amputees attending prosthetic clinic 1979–80, Canada	Presence of pain asked and recorded yes/no	716 respondents, in 93 (13%) of these some data missing but not specified	< 19 to 60+	Phantom limb pain in 63%
Houghton et al. 1994[139]	Retrospective survey, SAQ	Amputees at single centre	Pain intensity 0–10 scale	212 selected, 176 responded	Adults	Phantom limb pain in 78%
Kooijman et al. 2000[134]	Prospective survey with questionnaire	Amputees at a single orthopaedic centre	Not clearly stated	127 subjects of whom 99 filled in a questionnaire; 27 had congenital problems, so data on 72 with acquired defects	Adults	Phantom limb pain in 51% Stump pain in 49% Phantom sensations in 76%
Jensen et al. 1984[140]	Prospective hospital-based study April 1980 to March 1982 Interview, standard questionnaire and examination 8 days, 6 months and 2 years after limb amputation	Patients undergoing limb amputation, Denmark	Phantom pain defined as painful sensations referred to the lost body part, except stump pain	All 58 patients agreed to participate, 24 (42%) died	24–91	Patients with painful phantom limb: 8 days after amputation: 72%; 6 months: 65%; 2 years: 59%
Krebs et al. 1985[141]	Retrospective survey, interview	Patients with limb amputation 1970–77, random selection in 1983	Not stated	Of 624 amputees, 86 of 95 alive in 1983	Adults	Phantom limb pain in 52%
Pohjolainen et al. 1991[131]	Retrospective survey, clinical exam and interview	Amputees attending prosthetic factory	Pain intensity cat scale (mild, moderate, severe)	155 selected, 124 assessed 1 year later	Adults	1 year after amputation phantom limb pain in 53%; mostly mild or moderate intensity

Table 18: Continued.

Sherman et al. 1983[132]	Retrospective survey, PSAQ	Military veteran amputees, randomly selected, USA	Pain intensity 0–100 scale	764 of 1,321 members		Phantom limb pain in 85%
Sherman et al. 1984[124]	Retrospective survey, PSAQ	Military veteran amputees, randomly selected, USA	Stump pain and phantom pain both reported PI on 0–10 scale 0 = no pain, 10 = unbearable pain	55% responded 2,694/5,000		Phantom limb pain in 78% average PI = 5.3 ± 4.9 Stump pain in 62%
Steinbach et al. 1982[133]	Retrospective survey, interview	War veterans, traumatic amputees	Frequency of phantom limb pain assessed	75 survivors, 43 assessed	Adults	5 years after amputation phantom limb pain in 73% Pain frequency: constant 7.5% occasional 45% frequent 20%
Wartan et al. 1997[125]	Retrospective survey, PSAQ	Military veteran male amputees, randomly selected, UK	Pain intensity using 10 point cat scale (0 = no pain, 10 = unbearable pain) Phantom pain and stump pain evaluated Frequency, site and type of pain reported	526/590 (89%) response rate	median age 73	Phantom limb pain in 55%; Stump pain in 57% mean PI 5.6 16% complained of daily pain 16% pain always present

Chronic postoperative breast pain

Eight studies reported the occurrence of chronic post-mastectomy pain (**Table 19**). Different categories of pain were reported, including phantom breast, scar pain and pain in the ipsilateral arm. Time after operation was important, as there was a trend for some reduction in occurrence after two years or longer.[142] While most operations were partial or total mastectomy for cancer, pain occurred after augmentation and reduction operations, and after mastectomy with reconstruction.[143]

There was some variation because of time after surgery, but typically 25 to 35% of the patients reported pain more than a year after operation, and about half at one year.

Chronic postoperative thoracotomy pain

Surgical aspects of post-thoracotomy pain have been reviewed, together with reports on its occurrence.[149] **Table 20** gives results from six studies in the last ten years, all of which showed that chronic pain after thoracotomy was common, and that severe pain requiring treatment is also common, occurring in 15%–25% of patients undergoing thoracotomy. Results from surveys are supported by results from randomised trials; half of the patients reported long-term pain at one and half years.[150] The precise relationship between pain before, during, and after surgery, and the development of chronic pain, remains contentious.

Chronic postoperative cholecystectomy pain

Two prospective studies reported the occurrence of chronic scar pain following open cholecystectomy. At 12 months occurrence of chronic pain at the incision site was 27%,[155] and at 24 months 21%.[156] Two studies have attempted to compare the occurrence of chronic pain after open with the incidence after laparoscopic cholecystectomy. Stiff *et al.* reported a occurrence of 3.4% after laparoscopic compared with 9.7% after open procedure.[157] Wilson and Macintyre found a similar occurrence of 7% in both groups.[158]

Conclusion: prevalence and burden

Health care needs for chronic pain obviously extend from community through to hospital care. Patients with some chronic pain conditions, migraine for instance, may manage with over the counter medications, others will require prescription medication and some will need other interventions. **Figure 2** summarises prevalence data for some of the conditions mentioned above.

The prevalence data contains some surprises, and shows how biased a hospital view can be, omitting as it does those conditions which trouble patients but which they manage themselves (e.g. migraine), and those conditions which are managed largely in the community (e.g. polymyalgia rheumatica). A second facet of the prevalence data is that it does not capture, and indeed it cannot capture, the burden of the pain, nor the burden of the disability which goes with the pain in many of these conditions. Much of the 'repeat business' in secondary care pain management is for conditions for which there is no certain remedy. Health care needs therefore not only have to have to consider prevalence, but also the burden of the pain (and disability), and the 'treatability' of the pain.

The disease impact of some of the conditions mentioned above, compared with other conditions, was studied in about 15 000 Dutch patients. All research groups known to examine chronic diseases in the Netherlands were contacted to see what datasets were available.[159] Studies had to use a standardised quality of life instrument, have full coverage of quality of life domains, include a range of chronic diseases, be big (at least 200 patients), have medically confirmed diagnoses, be obtained since 1992 and be geographically broad. Eight datasets broadly fulfilling these categories were obtained, with information on about 15 000

Table 19: Mastectomy.

Reference	Type of study	Sample source	Disease definition	Sample size	Age range	Occurrence
Ivens et al. 1992[142]	Survey	Outpatient attending breast clinic	Not stated	126	28–80	Pain at 1 year 45 %, 1–2 years 37%, 2–4 years 28 %, > 4 years 20% Mostly mild, less than 20% of patients with at least moderate pain
Kroner et al. 1992[144]	Prospective 6 year survey	Patients attending oncology and radiotherapy department	Standard questionnaire	120, 110 at 1 year, 69 at 6 years	less than 69	Phantom breast pain at 1 year = 13 % Scar pain at 1 year = 23% Phantom breast pain at 6 year = 17% Scar pain at 6 year = 31%
Polinsky 1994[145]	Survey	Patients attending support group, post-mastectomy 16 months to 32 years	Pain intensity, categorical scale	314, 251 responded, 223 analysed	31–76	Pain 22–32 %
Smith et al. 1999[146]	Retrospective consecutive cohort	All surviving women having mastectomy from 1990 to 1995 in Aberdeen, Scotland	Character, location and timing of pain	511 questionnaires sent, 457 returned and 408 fully completed	32–93	Post-mastectomy pain in 43%, and 40% had pain related to operation site Highest rate in younger women
Stevens et al. 1995[147]	Survey	Oncology outpatients	Cancer pain questionnaire and McGill questionnaire	95	over 18	Post-mastectomy pain in 20%
Tasmuth et al. 1995[126]	Retrospective study, PSAQ	Patients with breast cancer treated by surgery between 1988–91 Types of surgery: modified radical mastectomy with axillary evacuation (MRM) or breast resection with axillary evacuation (BCT), Finland	PI VAS 10-cm scale, Finnish McGill pain questionnaire, Effect of chronic pain on daily lives 5 point cat scale (none, slight, mod., considerable, great), analgesic consumption	569, response rate 92%, 467 included in analysis	29–92	49% reported pain and about a quarter reported moderate or severe pain

Table 19: Continued.

Reference	Type of study	Sample source	Disease definition	Sample size	Age range	Occurrence
Tasmuth et al. 1996[127]	Prospective, 1 year study 1993–4. Patients assessed pre-op, 1 month, 6 months and 1 year after surgery. Patients assessed by a researcher by examination and questions	Patients with non-metastasised breast cancer. Types of surgery: modified radical mastectomy with axillary evacuation (MRM) or breast resection with axillary evacuation (BCT), Finland	PI VAS 10-cm scale: Activities of daily living that increase pain assessed. Pain in breast region or ipsilateral arm assessed	105 patients recruited, all agreed to participate, 93 (89%) included in final analysis 12 excluded due to disease complications	29 years	Chronic pain 1 year post-op in breast in 24% and in ipsilateral arm in 17%
Tasmuth et al. 1999[148]	Prospective survey in an oncology department	Consecutive women from January to June 1996, Helsinki, Finland	VAS and McGill questionnaire. Pain, chronic, and with at least a considerable effect on daily life	265 questionnaires sent, 221 responded (83%)	less than 70	Chronic pain in 56% in women operated on in high volume units, compared with 43% in those from low volume units.
Wallace et al. 1996[143]	Retrospective survey	Breast cancer patients attending medical centre	Pain intensity VAS, McGill pain questionnaire	n=429 recruited, 282 responded		Pain at 1 year follow-up: post-mastectomy = 31% mastectomy/reconstruction = 49% breast augmentation = 38% breast reduction = 22%

Table 20: Post-thoracotomy pain.

Reference	Type of study	Sample source	Disease definition	Sample size	Age range	Occurrence
Dajczman et al. 1991[151]	Retrospective cohort study of patients who had undergone thoracic surgery between 1982–87 by one particular surgeon were reviewed, then interviewed and questionnaire completed	Post-thoracotomy patients, disease-free without metastases and at least 2 months post-op, Quebec, Canada	PIVAS 10 cm scale, shoulder pain and aggravating factors assessed	206 patients identified, 59 interview and questionnaire, 56 analysed	35–79	54% had pain at thoracotomy site, moderate or severe in about half, between 5 months and 5 years after operation
Kalso et al. 1992[128]	Retrospective review of medical records, pain questionnaire sent to surviving patients	Patients who underwent a thoracotomy during 1986–88, Finland	Patients asked to describe pain as ache, burning, or tenderness and numbness, and state the duration and if analgesic required Patients asked to state if pain is associated with thoracotomy site	214 medical records reviewed, 150 surviving patients questioned further with pain questionnaire, 89% response rate	less than 70	44% persistent thoracotomy pain lasting longer than 6 months. 66% received treatment for pain.
Landreneau et al. 1994[152]	Postal questionnaire of an identified patient population	Post-thoracotomy patients > 3 months post-operation Patients had either pulmonary resection by lateral thoracotomy or video-assisted thoracic surgery (VATS) Divided into cohorts on basis of operation < 1 year or more than a year from this questionnaire contact None of patients had local recurrence of malignancy, USA	Post-thoracotomy pain defined as persistent pain along the thoracotomy scar and/or its intercostal dermatomal distribution lasting more than 2 months after operation	391, 343 (88%) responded, 165 thoracotomy, 178 VATS	mean age 59	Postoperative pain 3 months to 1 year after surgery in 44% with thoracotomy (18% treated), and 30% with VATS (11% treated) Postoperative pain more than 1 year after surgery in 29% with thoracotomy (16% treated), and 22% with VATS (6% treated)

Table 20: Continued.

Reference	Type of study	Sample source	Disease definition	Sample size	Age range	Occurrence
Matsunaga et al. 1990[153]	Retrospective survey, surgical records	Patients of one surgeon		n=90 contacted, 77 responded		Pain in 67% 6 to 18 months post-thoracotomy, 20% required analgesics
Perttunen et al. 1999[154]	Prospective cohort	Patients undergoing thoracotomy in Helsinki, Finland	Patients interviewed with standard letter at 3, 6 and 12 months	110 patients entered, with information on 62 at 1 year	19–77	Moderate or severe pain in 16% and mild pain in 45% at 1 year
Richardson et al. 1994[129]	Retrospective analysis of medical records of patients between January 1980 and December 1991 at a general hospital	Patients had undergone a thoracotomy, UK	Post-thoracotomy neuralgia defined as chest wall pain unrelated to recurrent tumour or infection at least 2 months post-operation Unilateral chest wall pain on the side of the thoracotomy 2 months after operation taken as positive presence of neuralgia	n=1,000 patient records reviewed, n=883 records evaluated	range 1–84 years, mean 55 years	Post-thoracotomy neuralgia in 14% at 12 months; 15% had pain sufficient for clinic referral in first year

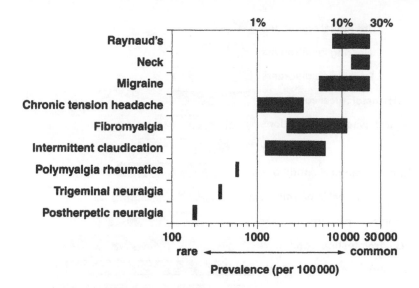

Figure 2: Prevalence of some chronic pain conditions.

people. They all used SF-36 or SF-24. These were analysed by quality of life dimension (physical functioning, physical role functioning, bodily pain, general health, vitality, social functioning and mental health) according to disease clusters (e.g. musculoskeletal conditions of osteoarthritis, joint complaints, rheumatoid arthritis and back impairments), disease categories (ranking the individual diseases within the cluster) and patient characteristics (sociodemographic variables, like age, gender, education).

The method used was the ranking of mean scores. Thus if three diseases scored (say) 5, 10 and 15 (with 5 the 'best' score), then they would be ranked 1, 2 and 3. This was done for all quality of life domains, and the ranks for individual domains added together. This summed rank produces low scores for the diseases or disease clusters causing the least distress, and high scores for those causing the most problems. The summed rank scores for chronic disease clusters are shown in **Figure 3**.

Musculoskeletal conditions, renal disease, cerebrovascular/neurological conditions and gastrointestinal conditions had the most severe impact on quality of life. In musculoskeletal conditions, osteoarthritis had more adverse impact than back impairments, which scored higher (worse) than rheumatoid arthritis. The method used for measuring quality of life, in this case SF-36, may not be perfect, but this analysis is thought-provoking for any consideration of health care needs in chronic pain, and highlights a research agenda.

The impact of the increasing age of the population, the higher prevalence of arthritis in older people and the 'worst' disease burden of musculoskeletal problems is a likely escalation of demand for pain management of arthritic problems. Co-morbidity, and treatment for that co-morbidity, can make pain management tricky in this patient group.

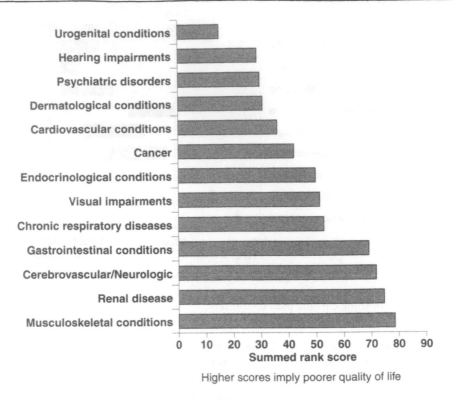

Figure 3: Summed rank scores for disease clusters.[159]

5 Services available and their costs

This section outlines current interventions available to treat pain, how these interventions are provided and used (the service as a whole) and the costs of providing a chronic pain service

Interventions

There are many interventions, pharmacological, non-pharmacological, invasive and non-invasive, from which to choose to treat chronic pain. These are outlined in **Figure 4**.

Analgesics

By far the majority of acute pain is managed with analgesics alone. Most chronic pain is also managed initially with analgesics, but in contrast with acute pain, more commonly involves nerve transmission block and alternative methods. **Figure 1** (the pain treatment ladder) showed a simple plan. As acute pain wanes, weaker analgesics are used. If chronic pain increases, stronger ones are used. The same analgesics,

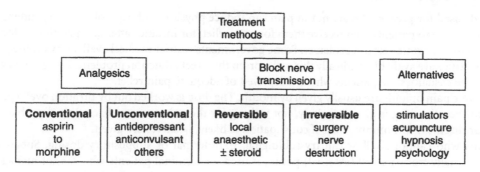

Figure 4: Treatment methods for chronic pain.

from paracetamol to NSAIDs through to opioids, are used in chronic as in acute pain. If analgesics relieve the pain to an adequate extent, and with tolerable or controllable adverse effects, then there is little reason to use other interventions. If analgesics are ineffective, other methods have to be considered. If analgesics are effective but cause intolerable or uncontrollable adverse effects then again other methods should be considered. The effectiveness and the adverse effects of the analgesics are critical.

It is known from work with cancer pain that using analgesics according to the WHO pain ladder (**Figure 1**) can relieve pain for 80% of patients. For most of the 80% the relief will be good, for a minority it will only be moderate. This presumes that the pain is managed optimally, but it is known from audit that this is often not the case. Optimal management requires that the correct drugs are available, and that they are given in the correct dose by the correct route and at the correct time. This needs staff who are well versed in the problems, and who are available to care for the patient. The second problem is the 20% of patients whose pain is not well managed by intelligent use of analgesic guidelines. The other treatment methods outlined in **Figure 4** are necessary to manage those for whom analgesics fail.

Non-opioid analgesics

Oral simple analgesics, combinations and NSAIDs

There is an old adage that if patients can swallow it is best to take drugs by mouth. Effective relief of nociceptive pain (as opposed to nerve damage pain) can be achieved with oral paracetamol, paracetamol/opioid combinations and oral NSAIDs. Paracetamol at doses of 4 gm or less per day is the safest analgesic, contrasting with NSAIDs which carry a small but finite chance of gastric bleed within the therapeutic dose range,[160] and risks of renal and cardiac problems.[161,162]

Topical NSAIDs

Many doctors are sceptical about the efficacy of topical NSAIDs. This may not be correct, however, with topical NSAIDs, like paracetamol, having a first-line role.

Opioids

In chronic pain there are two particular problems with opioids. The first is that adequate doses are often not available or are not given, primarily because of fears of addiction.[163] The second is that some (rarer) chronic pain states, particularly when the nervous system is damaged, may not respond fully to opioids.

Opioids used for people who are not in pain can induce physical and psychological dependence. This does not happen to patients who receive them for pain relief, for instance after an operation or for severe pain from osteoporotic vertebral collapse. Some governments restrict medical availability on the grounds that if the drugs are available medically this will worsen the street addiction problem. There is no evidence for this. The casualties are patients who are deprived of adequate pain relief.

In chronic pain opioids are usually given by mouth. The dose is worked out by titration over a period of days, and then the drug is given regularly, not waiting for the pain to come back. Initial problems with nausea or dizziness commonly settle. If constipation is likely, laxatives are given.

Patients who cannot swallow can try sublingual, transdermal or suppository dosing. Subcutaneous infusion, usually from a small (external) pump, is used for terminal patients who cannot manage these other routes. Rarely the epidural route is used for combination infusion of opioid and local anaesthetic.

If patients' pain starts to increase the dose is increased. If sensible dose increases do not produce pain relief, or if increasing the opioid dose provokes intolerable or unmanageable adverse effects, then other methods have to be considered, either as well as the opioid or instead of it. A working rule is that if the pain is in a numb area, which is a marker for a damaged nervous system, you should be less confident that opioids would necessarily produce pain relief,[164] and the threshold for using other strategies would be lower.

Unconventional analgesics

Unconventional analgesics[165] are drugs which have other indications in other medical settings, and are not normally thought of as analgesics. Treating chronic pain in a tertiary hospital setting these drugs are used for about one third of patients. The hall-mark is pain in a numb area, neuropathic pain.

When the patient has symptoms and signs of nervous system damage in the area of their pain it is expected that the response to conventional analgesics will be reduced. Conventional analgesics have often failed already, which is why the patient has been referred. If not, they should be tried, before empirical testing is embarked upon, to see if any of the unconventional analgesics can provide relief.

Antidepressants

Antidepressants work on the nervous system to relieve depression. They are used in much lower dosage (about half) to relieve pain.[166] Classically they were used to relieve pain that was burning rather than shooting in character, and anticonvulsants were used for shooting pains. Now antidepressants are used as first line for both types of pain, because greater success has been achieved and because it is believed that antidepressants cause fewer adverse effects.

Lower doses (median 75 mg amitriptyline nocte, maximum 150 mg) are used compared with those used to control depression. The pain-relieving effect happens, if it is going to happen, well within a week, whereas 10 days is the minimum often quoted for an antidepressant effect. The older (tricyclic) antidepressants seem to be better than the selective serotonin reuptake inhibitors as analgesics. The simplest analogy is that these older drugs are like shotguns, acting on multiple transmitter pathways, whereas the newer ones are more like rifles, designed as they are to be more selective and affect only one pathway.

Anticonvulsants

Anticonvulsants have been used for many years to treat the shooting pains of trigeminal neuralgia, painful diabetic neuropathy and postherpetic neuralgia. The catch-all explanation was that they stabilised nerve membranes, preventing them carrying spurious messages. Precisely how these channel blocking drugs work as analgesics in neuropathic pain remains unclear.

In the UK antidepressants are first choice drug therapy in neuropathic pain, supplemented or replaced by anticonvulsants if antidepressants alone provide inadequate analgesia or intolerable or unmanageable adverse effects.

Others

Clonidine and other alpha-2 adrenergic agonists have analgesic effects, both in conventional pain and in neuropathic pain. They extend the duration of local anaesthetic effect and have a synergistic effect with opioids. Their clinical utility is limited by the adverse effects of sedation and hypotension. Epidural clonidine is used in neuropathic cancer pain. Baclofen is used by intrathecal pump to treat the painful spasms of cerebral palsy. Ketamine and dextromethorphan, both drugs with NMDA antagonist action, are being used in severe neuropathic pain.

Block nerve transmission

Reversible

Local anaesthetics

Local anaesthetics block nerve conduction reversibly. When the local anaesthetic wears off the pain returns. That is the pharmacologically correct statement, but another old saying, that a series of local anaesthetic blocks can be used to 'break the cycle' of pain and effect a cure, now has some empirical support,[167] even if the mechanism is not understood. Arner and colleagues showed that the duration of pain relief could far outlast the duration of local anaesthetic action, and that prolonged relief could result from a series of blocks.[167] Local anaesthetic blocks can thus be diagnostic and therapeutic. Diagnosis of pain for instance from a 'trapped' lateral cutaneous nerve of thigh can be confirmed by local anaesthetic block, and a series of blocks may prevent pain recurring.

Pain clinics use such blocks commonly, for shoulder pain (suprascapular nerve block[168,169]), for intercostal neuralgia, for rectus sheath nerve entrapment, postoperative scar pains and other peripheral neuralgias (**Table 21**). What is not clear is the extent to which adding steroid to the local anaesthetic makes a difference, either prolonging the duration of effect of a particular procedure or increasing the chance of success of a series of blocks.

Fibromyalgia

Similar injections are done for the trigger points of fibromyalgia, but there do not appear to be any controlled comparisons of injections with other treatments. Antidepressants remain one of the few remedies of proven benefit.

Intravenous regional sympathectomy

Intravenous regional sympathetic blocks (IRSBs) are used in patients with reflex sympathetic dystrophy (complex regional pain syndrome). The blocks are useful if they facilitate mobility.

Table 21: Common nerve blocks.

Nerve block	Common indications
Trigger point	focal pain (e.g. in muscle)

Peripheral: intercostal
        sacral nerves
        rectus sheath
	pain in dermatomal distribution

Extradural (midline perineal pain)	Uni or bilateral pain (lumbosacral, cervical, thoracic etc.)
Intrathecal (midline perineal pain)	Unilateral pain (neurolytic injection for pain due to malignancy, limbs, chest etc.)
Autonomic Intravenous regional sympathectomy Stellate ganglion	reflex sympathetic dystrophy reflex sympathetic dystrophy arm pain brachial plexus nerve compression
Lumbar sympathetic	reflex sympathetic dystrophy lumbosacral plexus nerve compression vascular insufficiency lower limb perineal pain
Coeliac plexus	abdominal pain

Epidural steroids and facet joint blocks

Two other common pain clinic procedures particularly for back pain are epidural steroid injection and facet nerve blocks. However, there is considerable current controversy about the potential for epidural steroid to produce long-term neurological sequelae. Intrathecal injection of steroid can produce neurological sequelae. It is therefore important that intrathecal injection is avoided.

Classically facet joint injection with local anaesthetic and steroid is indicated when pain is worse when sitting, and pain is provoked by lateral rotation and spine extension. Recent studies suggest that whether or not the injection is actually in the facet joint makes little difference,[170] and indeed cast some doubt on long-term utility.[171] Short-lived success (less than six weeks) with local anaesthetic and steroid is said to be improved by use of cryoanalgesia or radiofrequency blocks to the nerves to the joints.

Irreversible

The destructive procedures are aimed at cutting, burning or damaging (**Table 21**) the nerve fibres carrying the pain signals. The flaw in the logic is that the nervous system can all too often rewire, finding a way around the lesion. If that happens, and the pain returns, then it may be even more difficult to manage – severe neuropathic pain can result. In general neurolytic blocks in non-malignant pain are not recommended, because they do not last forever, and recurrent pain may be more difficult to manage, and because of the morbidity. In cancer pain these neurolytic block procedures do have a place, when there is a short (less than three month) prognosis, or where alternatives such as meticulous drug control or long-term epidural infusion are not possible. Similar distinction between cancer and non-cancer pain holds for coeliac plexus block in pancreatic pain.

The limitation is the potential for motor and sphincter damage. This risk is higher with bilateral and repeat procedures, and higher the lower the cord level of the block. Extradural neurolytics have limited efficacy. While claims have been made that the paravertebral approach is preferable, patchy results may be attributed to unpredictable injectate spread. Results of spinal infusion of a combination of local anaesthetic and opioid are superior to neurolytic blocks, providing good analgesia with minimal irreversible morbidity.

Surgery

The relevant neurosurgical interventions for orthopaedic pain include dorsal column stimulation, rhizotomy, cordotomy and dorsal root entry zone (DREZ) lesions. The indications are usually non-malignant neuropathic pain which has failed to respond to pharmacological measures.

Alternatives

TENS and acupuncture

The rationale for transcutaneous nerve stimulation (TENS) is the gate theory.[172] If the spinal cord is bombarded with impulses from the TENS machine then it is distracted from transmitting the pathological pain signal. Acupuncture is another alternative method used to address chronic pain.

Physiotherapy and variants

Pain clinics keep a very open mind about other interventions such as physiotherapy. If patients benefit from alternatives they are encouraged to continue with these methods.

Behavioural management

Back schools through to behavioural management programmes offer a range of help for patients to cope with their (usually back) pain problems. Making decisions about the benefits of psychologically-based treatments of medical problems is not easy, and especially difficult to compare with other treatments and to measure relative benefit and cost. Patients whose pain has proved intractable to all reasonable medical and other interventions are chronic consumers of health care – GP or hospital clinic time, analgesic and psychotropic drugs, repeated admissions and sometimes surgery. If rehabilitation treatment enables these patients to carry on more satisfying lives with minimum medical help, how can it be most effectively and economically offered?

Chronic pain service provision and use

Clinical Standards Advisory Group Report

A report from the Clinical Standards Advisory Group (CSAG) on services for patients with pain analysed data collected in 1997 from a national survey (238 NHS Trusts) and 12 sample sites.[173] Of the 250 Trusts surveyed 215 (85%) provided a chronic pain service.

Activity data from the sample sites showed that only a minority (5 or 6 of 12) had activity data, and that there was wide variation in the activity levels for inpatient cases (6.4 to 35 inpatient cases annually per 100 000), day cases (72 to 155), new outpatients (67 to 158) and repeat outpatients (301 to 531).

Consultant weekly sessions per 100 000 population served varied nationally from 0 to 2.9, considerably below the recommended provision of 10 sessions per 100 000 population.[174]

The national survey showed wide variation in the level of service offered (defined as particular treatments offered), and this was reflected in the data from the 12 sample sites. Only one of the sample sites offered all the 15 treatments,* but the majority did offer injection treatments, transcutaneous nerve stimulation (TENS), single shot epidurals, and supervised opioid therapy for non-cancer pain. The reasons that all sites did not offer all 15 treatments may include the fact that it was a pretty eclectic list, including interventions such as acupuncture and hypnotherapy, which clinics might not offer because of lack of efficacy evidence. For some smaller clinics single-handed consultants might not have the skill mix to offer all the treatments.

Oxford Study

The use of chronic non-malignant pain services was estimated for the Oxford Region for the Summer of 1982.[175] The population served, 2.3 million, had a Regional Pain Relief Unit with 1115 'actively maintained records' of patients with non-malignant pain, records which had not been archived, excluding those who had died or not returned to the unit for 18 months. This gives an overall prevalence of 485 patients per million population. However, the Unit treated patients from outside the region, and adjusting for that the prevalence would be lower, at 325 patients per million.

Referrals in 1982

Referral patterns for 1982 are shown in the **Table 22**.

Changes since 1982

No documented evidence of change exists. Present patterns of referral and perceived changes include both patient-related and service-related factors. The patient-related factors include changes in the types of patient referred. More treatment now occurs in primary care,[176] particularly in Oxfordshire. For example, antidepressants for postherpetic neuralgia will often now be initiated by GPs. More difficult patients are being referred, and in greater numbers. The service factors are that overall workloads have increased since 1982. Medical staffing has increased from one consultant and senior registrar to two consultants and a 0.5 FTE honorary consultant running what is essentially a consultant-only service, with two psychology sessions per week. Joint clinics are run with psychiatry, neurology, neurosurgery and oral surgery. There are more specialist pain centres in the UK, and in the former Oxford Region there are consultants (especially anaesthetists) specialising in pain relief.

Chronic pain services – costs

Clinical Standards Advisory Group Report

Half of the 12 sample site Health Authorities in the CSAG report provided data on tariffs charged. For first outpatient consultation these varied from £54 to £171, for repeat outpatient from £54 to £134, for elective inpatient from £553 to £1471, and for day care from £75 to £384. The more than threefold variation shows that accurate costs are not available.

---

* Nerve blockade, TENS, X-ray assisted treatment, one-shot epidural, acupuncture, physiotherapy, supervised opioid therapy for non-cancer pain, continuous epidural, drug delivery systems: subcutaneous, psychology, drug delivery systems: intravenous, radiofrequency lesions, pain management programme, spinal cord stimulation, hypnotherapy.

Table 22: Prevalence, treatability and burden of chronic pain syndromes.

Condition	Percent	per 100,000		Treatability	Burden
Low back pain	6	6,000		variable	low to high
Ankylosing spondylitis	1.5	1,500		fair	low to high
Neck pain	15	15,000		fair	low to high
Whiplash	0.028	28		variable	low to high
Polymyalgia rheumatica	0.627	627		good	low to medium
Fibromyalgia	2	2,000		fair	low to medium
Migraine	15	15,000		good	low to medium
Headache (CTTH)	1	1,000		poor	low to medium
Trigeminal neuralgia	0.4	400		fair	low to high
Diabetic neuropathy	0.4	400		fair	low to high
Postherpetic neuralgia	0.03	34 (incidence)		fair	low to high
Multiple sclerosis	0.05	50	50% pain prev – how many MS?	variable	low to high
Central post stroke pain	0.01–0.05	10–50	8% of strokes	poor	high
Phantom limb pain	0.025	25	75% of amputees	poor	low to high
Stump pain	0.025	25		poor	low to high
Claudication	1	1,000		variable	low to high
Raynaud's	2–19			variable	low to medium
Angina	4	4,000		variable	low to high
Postop			say 10% of all?	variable	low to medium
post-mastectomy pain				variable	low to medium
thoracotomy				variable	low to medium
cholecystectomy				variable	low to medium

Treatability; poor, fair or good. Variable if variable.
Burden; low, medium or high.

Using the professional recommendation of 10 sessions per 100 000 population the requirements will be a consultant's salary, secretarial support, sessional nursing, psychology and physiotherapy, bed costs for inpatients and procedure costs for treatments. Using the CSAG activity data and tariffs yields annual costs per 100 000 population of £29 000 (lowest activity, lowest tariffs) and £210 000 (highest activity, highest tariffs). Thus a primary care trust covering 100 000 patients should be budgeting between £100 000 and £200 000 per year for chronic pain services.

As previously referred to in the section on prevalence and incidence, the burden of chronic pain seen at pain clinics has increased substantially in the last decade. Patients are usually in the sixth and seventh decade of life, so demographic imperatives will increase prevalence still further until at least about 2020. Some foresee increasing problems in recruiting and retaining staff to work in chronic pain, and this may make adequate provision more difficult.[177]

Canadian study on costs

A detailed Canadian study of the costs incurred by users of speciality pain clinic services[178] showed that users of the services incur less direct health care expenditure than non-users with similar conditions. This conclusion is important and in an ideal world this study would be repeated in the UK to show the financial benefit of the service.

Of 626 patients referred to the chronic pain clinic in Hamilton, Ontario, between January 1986 and April 1988, 210 did not attend the clinic (non-attender), 180 had a consultation appointment only (consultation only), 98 had an incomplete treatment programme (incomplete treatment) and 83 had a complete treatment programme. A sample of 222 of 626 patients was used to compute the use of different types of health services and other costs. This was done by asking patients about their use of five categories of direct health services – primary care, emergency room and specialists, hospital episodes and days, and the use of seven types of other health professionals. Other direct and indirect costs for the patient and associated with their use of health care were also estimated. Money values in the paper are given in 1991 dollars, but whether these are Canadian or US dollars is not stated.

There was no demographic or condition diagnosed difference between the four groups. The results showed that the direct health care costs were lower for users of chronic pain services than for non-users. Broken down by type of cost for one year these are shown in **Table 23**.

Table 23: Annual per patient direct health care costs for patients referred to a chronic pain unit using different levels of service (1991 dollars).

Service used	Non-attender	Consult only	Incomplete treatment	Complete treatment
Number surveyed	57	80	44	41
Primary care visits	477	422	412	462
Specialists	548	642	862	817
Emergency room	206	439	266	191
Hospital stay	3,116	2,017	462	1,290
Health professional	833	396	226	237
Total	5,181	3,917	2,229	2,996

The total annual direct health costs were much lower for users of chronic pain services (even if it was only a consultation), and the savings were clearly derived mostly from reduced costs of days spent in hospital. This is shown graphically in **Figure 5**.

The 74% of the chronic pain referrals who actually used some chronic pain services had only 64% of the total costs for the referred patients. The 'saving' that came from using chronic pain services derived mainly from the intensive users of the service who had treatments, rather than those who had only a consultation.

The average direct health care cost of a patient using chronic pain services, even if that was a single consultation, was $2947. Referred patients who did not use the service cost more, an average of $5181. The difference between these averages was $2234.

Using the most conservative estimate – that is, no cost inflation since 1991 and assuming that the currency was Canadian dollars with an exchange rate of about $2/£ – the average difference amounts to a saving in direct health care costs of about £1117 per patient. Using this figure with the 1982 figure of 1115 patients with non-malignant pain on the Oxford Pain Relief Unit books translates to health care savings of £1 250 000.

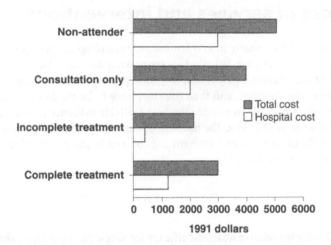

Figure 5: Total per patient direct health care costs and cost of hospital stay for patients referred to a chronic pain unit using different levels of service (1991 dollars).

This compares with the running costs (labour, consumables, estates, overheads) of the Pain Relief Unit in Oxford (with a larger workload) of £500 000 (see **Figure 6**).

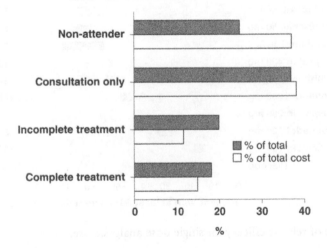

Figure 6: Percentage of total number and total direct health care costs for patients referred to a chronic pain unit using different levels of service.

6 Effectiveness of services and interventions

As mentioned previously there are many interventions, pharmacological, non-pharmacological, invasive and non-invasive, from which to choose. Whether we are making decisions for our own patients or for our service or for national or international guidelines, the same principles should apply. The relative efficacy and safety of the possible interventions, and then the cost, have to be the key determinants. This section uses systematic reviews when possible to provide the best available evidence for the various interventions, with the number-needed-to-treat (NNT) as the measure of clinical significance from quantitative systematic reviews. The arguments about best choice treatment are covered in greater detail in a Health Technology Assessment report[179] and in book form.[180]

Analgesics

Figure 7 shows a league table for relative analgesic efficacy for single dose use and **Table 24** shows the NNT for some analgesic interventions. Paracetamol 1 g will produce at least 50% relief of pain for one out of four patients, ibuprofen 400 mg (and other NSAIDs analysed) for one out of two patients. The efficacy evidence thus leads to the advice to start with paracetamol, and move to combination and then to NSAID if greater efficacy is needed. This is inherently a safer strategy than leaping in with the greater efficacy NSAID, because it carries greater risk than paracetamol. (A I-1)

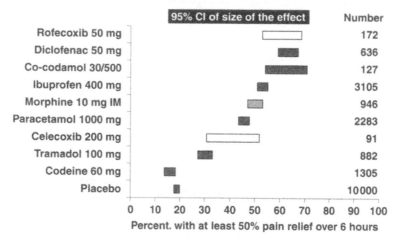

Figure 7: League table of relative efficacy for single dose analgesic use.

This philosophy is used in the American College of Rheumatologists Guidelines for arthritic pain. Two early studies suggested that there is little advantage in osteoarthritis of either NSAIDs over paracetamol[189] or weak opioids in combination with paracetamol over paracetamol alone,[190] but recent trials do show the expected superiority of NSAID over paracetamol.

No single-dose trial has shown any efficacy advantage of one NSAID over another.[191] This does not fit well with patients' reports on multiple dosing of increased efficacy from NSAIDs with greater anti-inflammatory action. The efficacy dose-response curve for NSAIDs is flat compared with the dose-response for adverse effects such as gastrointestinal symptoms, dizziness and drowsiness.[192] Increasing the dose to improve analgesia is therefore more likely to increase adverse effects than to improve analgesia.

Table 24: Number-needed-to-treat (NNT) for some analgesic interventions.

Condition	Intervention	Outcome	NNT	Reference
Postoperative pain	(good) ibuprofen 400 mg	> 50% pain relief	2	Moore, McQuay et al. 1996[181]
	paracetamol 1 g	> 50% pain relief	4	Moore, McQuay et al. 1996[181]
	(poor) codeine 60 mg oral	> 50% pain relief	> 10	Moore and McQuay 1997[182]
Back pain	epidural steroid	> 75% relief at 60 days	> 6	Watts and Silagy 1995, McQuay and Moore 1996[183,184]
Acute sprains etc.	topical NSAID (good)	> 50% pain relief	2+	Moore, Tramèr et al. 1998[185]
Trigeminal neuralgia	anticonvulsants	> 50% pain relief	2.5	McQuay, Carroll et al.[186]
Diabetic neuropathy	anticonvulsants	> 50% pain relief	2.5	McQuay, Carroll et al.[186]
	topical capsaicin	> 50% pain relief	4.2	Zhang and Li 1994[187]
Neuropathic pain	antidepressants	> 50% pain relief	2.5	McQuay, Tramer et al. 1996[188]

NSAIDs alone produced as good analgesia as single or multiple doses of weak opioids alone or in combination with non-opioid analgesics.[192] Adverse effect incidence and patient dropout rates were the same for multiple doses of NSAIDs or weak opioids in combination with non-opioid analgesics.[192]

In contrast to efficacy, where we see little difference between NSAIDs, the risk of NSAID-induced gastric bleeding is lowest with ibuprofen, and increases with increasing age.[193] Prophylactic misoprostol should be considered for preventing NSAID-associated gastrointestinal complications when age is greater than 75 years, cardiovascular disease, history of peptic ulcer or of gastrointestinal bleeding (NNTs to prevent one serious GI complication in one year 105, 58, 11 and 7 respectively).[194,195] The alternative to COX1 NSAID used with gastric protection is the COX2 specific inhibitors (COXIBs), which show similar efficacy to their forebears but with decreased risk of peptic ulceration or bleeding,[196] which has economic consequences.[197] Cardiac risk with NSAIDs does not appear to be improved by COXIBs.

Topical NSAIDs

Published RCTs on chronic pain conditions (mainly knee osteoarthritis) studied over 800 subjects treated with topical NSAIDs and 322 subjects who received placebo. The analgesic response for combined placebo treatment was 30%, and for combined topical non-steroidal anti-inflammatory preparations it was 63%. For analgesic effects the odds ratio was 3.6 (2.6–4.8) and the number-needed-to-treat was 3.2 (2.6–4.1).[185] (A I-1)

Opioids

There is little strong evidence to support the intrathecal pump administration of opioid in preference to the oral route.[198] (C I-1)

1 **Antidepressant drugs:** Antidepressants can provide good relief in neuropathic pain (NNT of 2–3, **Table 24**).[188] For fibromyalgia as in more classic neuropathic pain, antidepressants are one of the few remedies of proven benefit.[45] (A I-1)

2 **Anticonvulsant drugs:** Anticonvulsants can provide good relief in neuropathic pain (NNT of 2–3, **Table 24**).[186] Doses required for analgesic effect are close to the anticonvulsant dosing range, and carry an adverse effect burden. This systematic review suggests that there is little difference in the number of adverse effects seen with antidepressant and anticonvulsant used in neuropathic pain, but that may conceal a difference in severity (which was not reported). (A I-1)

3 **Others – Alpha-2 adrenergic agonists and NMDA antagonists:** Epidural clonidine is effective in neuropathic cancer pain[199](A I-2). Ketamine is used in severe neuropathic pain, with scientific rationale but little strong evidence yet of good benefit.[200] (C I-1)

4 **Reversible block nerve transmission:**

Epidural injections for back pain and sciatica: Epidural steroids in back pain have been studied in two systematic reviews.[183,201] Overall the combined data showed statistically significant (odds ratios) improvement for both short-term (1–60 days) and long-term (12 weeks up to one year). The clinical significance is that the NNT for short-term (1–60 days) greater than 75% pain relief from the ten trials with short-term outcomes combined, was just under 6, with 95% confidence intervals from 4 to 12.[184] This means that for 6 patients treated with epidural steroid, one will obtain more than 75% pain relief short-term. (A I-1)

The NNT for long-term (12 weeks up to one year) improvement from the five trials combined, was about 11, with 95% confidence intervals from 6 to 90. This means that for 11 patients treated with epidural steroid, one will obtain more pain relief over this longer-term period. There is still the interesting question of whether local anaesthetic alone could achieve these results (breaking the cycle), or whether the steroid is an essential component. (A I-1)

Intravenous regional sympathetic blockade: A systematic review of seven RCTs of IRSBs found that none of the four guanethidine trials showed significant analgesic effect. Two reports, one using ketanserin and one bretylium, with 17 patients in total, showed some advantage of IRSBs over control.[202] Adding guanethidine in IRSBs does not appear to be more effective than local anaesthetic alone. (D I-1)

5 **Irreversible block nerve transmission:** Pain associated with pancreatic cancer responds well to coeliac plexus block,[203] and it may also help those with abdominal or perineal pain from tumour in the pelvis. In chronic pancreatitis results are much less convincing. (A I-1)

6 **Surgery:** The difficulties of trials of uncommon surgical procedures are well known. These procedures are usually documented by glowing case series. Longer-term outcomes may not be so good.[204] (D II-2)

7 **TENS:** A systematic review shows that TENS has limited efficacy in chronic pain.[205] (D I-1)

8 **Acupuncture:** Several systematic reviews discuss acupuncture in chronic non-malignant pain.[206–9] These show limited effect on pain outcomes. Any effect on well-being is often short-lived (three days), and is therefore expensive in time. It is difficult to know what is the real place of acupuncture, like other complementary interventions, because of the lack of trials comparing complementary with mainstream procedures.[210] (D I-1)

9 **Physiotherapy:** The evidence from back pain, however, suggests that on rigorous outcome measures physiotherapy and other forms of manipulation have but limited success. Such analyses often did not include any measure of quality of life. If they make the patient feel better and they are cheap then it is a decision for the third party payer whether or not these physiotherapy manoeuvres should be offered. A number of systematic reviews are published on this subject.[211–19] (D I-1)

10 **Behavioural management:** Randomised comparison of the St Thomas' four-week inpatient treatment with eight-week half-day outpatient treatment, with fitness training, planned increases in activity, activity scheduling, drug reduction, relaxation and cognitive therapy as the pain management methods taught by the same staff team,[220] showed that for every three patients treated as inpatients rather than outpatients, one patient fewer was taking analgesic or psychotropic drugs. For every four patients treated as inpatients rather than outpatients, one patient fewer sought additional medical advice in the year after treatment. For every five patients treated as inpatients rather than outpatients, one patient more had a ten-minute walking distance improved by more than 50%. For every six patients treated as inpatients rather than outpatients, one patient fewer was depressed.[221] A number of systematic reviews exist in this area[222–9] (and see McQuay *et al.*[179] for evidence of efficacy of psychological interventions). (B I-1)

Effective service provision

Once the effectiveness of an intervention is known the next step must be to check whether the interventions used in pain clinics reflect these known levels of efficacy. **Table 25** shows the attempt the Audit Commission made to make a matrix of treatment efficacy, determine the percentage of clinics in their sample which offer particular treatments, and to put the percentage offering a particular treatment on the matrix.[230] The CSAG report on pain focused more on provision and process, but has interesting data on variation in provision of services (discussed above).[173]

Table 25: Chronic pain treatments classified by evidence of effectiveness and risk of side-effects, degree of invasiveness and cost of the procedure.[230]

Clinical risk and/ or cost:*	Evidence of effectiveness					
	Effective**		Thought to be effective, but with little formal evidence***		Ineffective****	
Low	Some minor oral analgesics (e.g. ibuprofen, paracetamol)		TENS provided for use at home	90%	Some minor oral analgesics (e.g. codeine alone)	
	Topical NSAIDs in rheumatological conditions (e.g. single arthritic joint pain)	90%	Relaxation therapy			
	Topical capsaicin in diabetic neuropathy, psoriasis	95%				
Medium	Antidepressant drugs (for e.g. neuropathic pain, post-herpetic neuralgia, diabetic neuropathy)	95%	Outpatient TENS courses	60%	Injection of corticosteroids in or around shoulder joints for shoulder pain	89%
	Anticonvulsant drugs (for e.g. trigeminal neuralgia)	100%	Outpatient psychological intervention programmes	70%		
	Systematic local anaesthetic drugs for nerve injury pain	60%	Acupuncture courses by nurse or therapist	50%		
			Manipulation for back pain	50%		
			Epidural given once, but abandoned if ineffective			
			Long-term, low-rate opioids			
			Surgical intervention for back pain when surgery has not yet been tried (e.g. laminectomy for sciatica with positive neurological signs and MRI)			
			Orthopaedic corsets, neck collars used for long periods			
			Sclerosis injection for low back pain	21%		

Table 25: Continued.

Clinical risk and/ or cost:*	Evidence of effectiveness						
	Effective**		Thought to be effective, but with little formal evidence***		Ineffective****		
High	Epidural for back pain and sciatica (effects for first 60 days)		Acupuncture courses provided by doctors (higher salary costs)	65%	Epidural for back pain and sciatica (effects beyond 3 months)		
	Inpatient psychological intervention programmes	25%	Trigeminal neuralgia treatments using specialised/ expensive equipment (e.g. radio frequency block kit)	30%	IRSB guanethidine	90%	
			Lignocaine infusion as inpatient	45%			
			Epidural left in-situ for several weeks as inpatient	84%			
			Long-term, high doses of a cocktail of opioids and other drugs				
			Repeated back pain surgery				
			Cordotomy	11%			
			Spinal cord implanted stimulators	25%			
			Destructive nerve burning, freezing, phenol injections	95%			

* Clinical risks could include side-effects, the degree of invasiveness of the procedure, and whether the effects on the body are reversible. Treatments have been placed into a category according to the professional judgement of consulted practitioners.

** Treatments proved to be effective are those with a sufficient number of randomised controlled trials available to calculate a statistic called the 'number needed to treat' (NNT), and, in this context, which have values of NNT between 2 and 4.

*** Many treatments have not been subjected to enough randomised controlled trials to make a statistical judgement about their effectiveness.

**** Treatments shown to be without effect in this context are those with NNTs greater than 4.

% = percentage of 20 Trusts providing each treatment is listed where known; some treatments may be provided via referral to another clinic.

Source: Audit Commission; evidence of effectiveness is drawn from previous chapters; relative risk/cost from discussion with practitioners

While all of us may disagree with the particular judgements made about efficacy and safety in **Table 25**, the approach is the same approach we all use (covertly) in our professional life. What might be perceived as threatening clinical freedom, in that those paying for health care might choose to pay only for treatments in the upper left sections of **Table 25**, is in reality a matter of judging relative efficacy, safety and cost.

Primary care prescribing

Another approach is to use the national prescribing data to see to what extent the prescribing of oral analgesics in primary care matches the efficacy league table for oral analgesics.[180] Using the Government Statistical Service Prescription cost analysis for England 2001,[231] which provides data on the number of prescriptions for particular categories of drug (**Table 26**), we then produced a simple scattergram of the number of prescriptions for the different drugs against the NNT for single dose analgesia[180] (**Figure 8**).

Table 26: UK oral analgesic prescribing and efficacy.

Analgesic studied	NNT	Prescriptions (thousands)
Codeine	17.7	1,324
Dihydrocodeine	9.7	2,460
Tramadol	4.7	1,815
Paracetamol	4.6	7,814
Dextropropoxyphene HCl 65 mg/paracetamol 650 mg	4.4	8,775
Ibuprofen	2.7	5,300
Diclofenac	2.3	7,040
Co-codamol 30 mg codeine/500 mg paracetamol	1.9	3,938

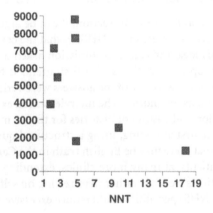

Figure 8: UK oral analgesic prescribing and efficacy (2001).

The graph shows that prescribing in primary care does a good job – there are more prescriptions for the more effective drugs. Prescribing advice will be a factor, as will cost, but most analgesics are cheap, so that efficacy should be the primary determinant. Given that there are differences between the single-dose efficacy of the different analgesics, safety issues now need to be brought into focus. A problem here is that while there may be differences in minor adverse effect incidence on single dosing, with opioids alone or in combination being the worst offenders, the real safety issues are about what happens with multiple or chronic dosing. For somebody with arthritic pain which requires months or years of analgesic use, which is the best choice, paracetamol or NSAID? At recommended doses paracetamol has minimal safety problems. Using data from four randomised trials, taking NSAIDs for more than two months carries a risk of bleeding or perforating gastroduodenal ulcer of 1 in 228 (150–479), RR 2.8 (1.2–6.2), absolute risk

0.69%.[160] We estimate that there is a 1 in 8.3 (12%) risk that these patients with bleed or perforation will die. Using a control event (death) rate of 0.0002% with this experimental death rate of 0.69%/8.3 = 0.083%, we calculate[160] that the average number-needed-to-kill (NNK) for a patient receiving chronic oral NSAIDs for at least two months is 1/(0.083%–0.002%) = 1/0.081% = 1235. This shows the complexity of what appears at first glance to be a simple choice between NSAID and paracetamol.

Cost-effectiveness

There is little information about the costs and benefits of chronic pain services, and what little there is barely constitutes evidence. Two possible approaches were looked at. Costs may be determined by contrasting, for instance, two or more different types of treatment for a condition and working out the costs and benefits for each. This method was precluded by lack of sufficient evidence, for instance the fact that we have no real evidence that TENS works in chronic pain. Evidence of effectiveness must come first. Rational assessment of cost–benefit needs evidence of effectiveness. Irrational assessment might just compare the cost of one ineffective therapy with another.

Another way to cost the service is to use an approach in which the disease burden is examined, changes are estimated, and judgement is made as to whether pain clinics add to costs or reduce them. Here at least there is some evidence, but not very much, and not very recent.

Do chronic pain clinics reduce other NHS expenditure? A case study

From the Canadian study described in the previous section, it can be argued that attendance at a chronic pain clinic could reduce expenditure elsewhere in the NHS, so that the cost of the clinics would more than be covered by savings. To test this idea, the Audit Commission asked a pain clinic to carry out a small study.[230] A randomly-selected group of 21 patients who first attended the clinic in October 1996 were asked to take part in a telephone interview. Some of the answers were verified from clinical case notes, but mostly the results relied on the patients' memories. The interviewer (an experienced research nurse) asked the patients about their consultation and treatment histories for the six months before attending the pain clinic, and for the six months since first attending, using a structured questionnaire.

The results (**Table 27**) suggest that there may be English truth in the Canadian study, but to be sure one would need a larger sample of patients, at many more clinics, extending the period before and after the clinics, and preferably tracing patients' records rather than relying on self-report. The implication is that close liaison between the different NHS specialities could reduce excessive referral/treatment and provide a better service for patients.

These data suggest that chronic pain services not only benefit patients, but are also an efficient way of dealing with chronic pain in the community.

Table 27: Do chronic pain clinics reduce other NHS expenditure? A case study.[230]

Average number per patient		In the six months		
		Before attending the pain clinic	**After attending the pain clinic**	**Change** + = increase − = reduction
Outpatient attendances:	NHS pain clinic	0.05	1.6	+97%*
	Other NHS medical specialities**	2.8	0.9	−222%*
	Total	2.8	2.5	−13%
	NHS treatments (e.g. TENS, physio, surgery)	1.0	0.9	−17%
	Days in hospital	0.2	0.5	+50%
	A/E attendances	0.1	0.05	−100%
	Different types of drug for pain	2	2.2	11%
	Visits to the GP about pain	5.0	3.0	−64%*
	Home visits by GP	0.1	0.1	−
	Other NHS home visits	0	0	−
	Private treatments	0.4	0.2	−125%*
	% of patients	**Before**	**After**	
Attending outpatient clinics	NHS pain clinic	5%	100%	
	Other NHS medical specialities**	81%	38%	
	Either	86%	100%	
Having NHS treatment	Relatively high cost treatments (e.g. surgery)	10%	5%	
	Medium cost (e.g. physio, nerve block)	62%	43%	
	Low cost (e.g. X-ray)	24%	38%	
	Any treatment	67%	62%	
Hospital inpatient		5%	10%	
Attending A/E		5%	5%	
Taking drugs for pain:	Opiates	14%	16%	
	Antidepressants, tranquillisers, etc.	24%	47%	
	NSAIDs	48%	63%	
	Minor analgesics	71%	74%	
	Any type of drug	90%	90%	
Visiting the GP about pain:	For repeat prescriptions	67%	52%	
	For consultant/advice about pain	62%	24%	
	Any reason to do with pain	86%	71%	
	Having a home visit by GP	5%	5%	
	Other NHS home visits	0	0	
Having private treatment		33%	19%	

* Significant change (paired sample t-test, 1-tailed, 5% level).
** Other NHS specialities include orthopaedics, neurology, vascular surgery, gynaecology, urology, rehabilitation medicine, nephrology.

7 Models of care and recommendations

The provision of chronic pain services clearly should not be taken in isolation, and **Figure 9** shows a simple view of some major service relationships. Many treatments, drug or procedures, are common to the different service providers; the additional expertise found in the pain service is the ability to do particular invasive procedures. The ideal promoted widely in the developed world is chronic pain services which are multidisciplinary. The medical components of such multidisciplinary services are the rehabilitation, neurology, orthopaedic and psychiatric services shown in **Figure 9**, together with clinical psychology, physiotherapy and pharmacy inputs as integral to the chronic pain service.

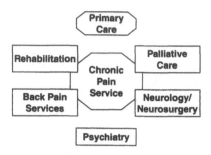

Figure 9: Chronic pain: service relationships.

The historic pattern in the UK has been a District General Hospital (DGH) service with a more comprehensive service regionally, often in the University Hospital. The size of the DGH service varies widely, and none of those sampled by CSAG came near to the 10 consultant sessions per 100 000 population recommended by the Pain Society.[174] There are two clear advantages to local service provision: the geographical proximity for the patient and the ability to interact easily with primary care and the other local specialities. The regional service would then provide the other speciality input or interventions not available at the DGH. The disadvantage of a small DGH service is the burden on a single-handed consultant, and lack of critical mass. It is hard to be precise about the minimum size of an effective service, but there would be few single-handed consultants if the 10 consultant sessions per 100 000 population recommendation were to be followed. Examples of a speciality intervention not usually available at a DGH would include a pain management programme.

The second level of decision in the model of care is determining which interventions a service should provide. We need to know whether the various components of the service (interventions) are effective, how much they cost, and examine whether their delivery is efficient. There are also the difficult issues of how treatable the pain syndrome is, and how big the burden is for the patient. As discussed above, in general the efficacy evidence for drug treatments (and pain management programmes) is as strong as the evidence for injection procedures is weak, but this weakness is sometimes a lack of evidence rather than evidence of lack of efficacy.

The evidence presented in the effectiveness section enables us to determine which effective treatments should be used and which ineffective interventions should be avoided:

Effective interventions

- Minor analgesics
- Combinations of different analgesics
- Anticonvulsant drugs

- Antidepressant drugs
- Systemic local anaesthetic-type drugs for nerve damage pain
- Topical NSAIDs in rheumatological conditions
- Topical capsaicin in diabetic neuropathy
- Epidural injections for back pain and sciatica.

Interventions where evidence is lacking

- Transcutaneous electrical nerve stimulation in chronic pain
- Relaxation
- Spinal cord stimulator.

Ineffective interventions

- Intravenous regional sympathetic blockade
- Injections of corticosteroids in or around shoulder joints for shoulder pain.

One clear recommendation is that if paracetamol is sufficient to control the pain then the choice should be paracetamol, because of its good long-term safety at recommended doses. Taking NSAIDs for more than two months carries a risk of bleed or perforation, and in turn a risk of death. Long-term harm has important financial implications. For example, the cost of NSAID gastrointestinal adverse effects, combining hospital admission and the cost of co-prescribing gastro-protective agents, was estimated as costing the NHS a conservative £250 million in 1997/8.[197] And NSAID-related gastrointestinal adverse effects account for about one-third of the long-term harm. With congestive heart failure and renal failure, NSAID prescribing can result in 50 hospital admissions each year for a primary care trust of 100 000 people.[232]

Difficult commissioning decisions will emerge on a case-by-case basis, with desperate patients seeking novel treatments. Different but also difficult is the complementary and alternative medicine lobby. Acupuncture, for instance, appeared on the CSAG checklist of interventions in chronic pain. There is no credible evidence of analgesic efficacy of acupuncture in chronic pain, but acupuncture, in common with other complementary and alternative interventions, may make patients feel better even if it does not alter the pain. One way to deal with these conundrums is to fund the unproven treatments only in the context of a randomised trial.

The fact that 85% of Trusts surveyed had a chronic pain clinic is evidence that there is a perceived need for the service. There is little evidence as to what constitutes the optimal form of the service, and very little evidence on resource use and benefit gained. The current satellite and hub model of DGH and regional centre works to an extent, but there has been a dearth of organisational research into service provision.

It is foolish to be didactic about service arrangements in this area, because there is overlap between the different services which make up the provision for chronic disease and pain. A strong rehabilitation service in a district, for example, might mean that other services could be less strong. What is clear is the need, and the ageing population means that this will become more and more apparent. The pain clinic should offer a mix of drug treatment, injection treatment, devices and psychological input, and the availability of this skill mix is the important principle rather than under which service banner it appears.

One pain consultant per 100 000 of the population seems a sensible estimate for available pain expertise. Precisely how this fits into the other service provision will vary. The current hub and spoke arrangements for chronic pain may be optimal for some regions. The need for good liaison with other specialities favours decentralised rather than centralised arrangements.

8 Information and research requirements

Information requirements

In order to organise the treatment of chronic pain better, we recommend the following information is gathered, organised and made available:

- A single electronic source of high quality evidence on the *diagnosis* of various pain conditions for use in primary care.
- A single electronic source of high quality evidence on the *treatment* of various pain conditions for use in primary care. This will involve predominantly systematic reviews of randomised trials, but will also summarise where evidence does not exist (like TENS in chronic pain) and especially where treatments are known not to be effective (acupuncture).
- A single electronic source of high quality evidence about the management of chronic pain in primary and secondary care.
- Regular training courses plus distance learning to encourage lifetime learning for developing professional pain specialists in primary care.
- Referral protocols.

Research requirements

The evidence base in pain relief is one of the best in medicine. Most of the interventions commonly used in chronic pain treatment can be shown to be very effective. Some have been shown not to be effective, and their use is less common than it was. While these findings buttress much of current practice in chronic pain treatment, a common theme is that we still need to know more. In particular, information on which to base economic analysis is missing. Such information as is available indicates that pain clinics result in direct health care savings of over £1000 per patient per year, and that total savings may be twice the cost of the chronic pain service. Knowing that major demographic changes will affect the NHS over the next several decades, and that ageing populations will demand more chronic (and cancer) pain therapy, providing more information on economic as well as humanitarian benefits will be important.

Appendix 1: Methods

Studies reporting prevalence or incidence of chronic pain were sought systematically. Chronic pain is usually as defined by authors, though a minimum requirement was duration of three months or more. Several different search strategies were used to identify reports from MEDLINE (1966 to July 2001), EMBASE (1980 to January 2001), PubMed (July 2001) and the Oxford Pain Relief Database (1950 to 1994),[233] and our own extensive literature collection in pain topics. Reference lists of retrieved reports were searched for additional studies. Abstracts and narrative review articles were not considered.

Inclusion criteria

Studies were included when they were full journal publications, studying adult community or clinic-based populations in Europe or North America, used clear and established diagnostic criteria for disease/pain conditions of interest, presented prevalence and/or incidence data for the disease/pain condition of interest and reported survey/study response rates.

Exclusion criteria

Studies were excluded if they were of occupational-based populations, used invalid or unclear diagnostic criteria, had a low response rate (below 60%) without an analysis of non-responders, or with an analysis which produced a biased result.

Data extraction

From each eligible report we extracted study design, sample source, disease/pain definition, sample size and response rate, age range, incidence and/or prevalence data. Gender and age specific rates were extracted if given, together with information on pain severity and disability.

Incidence was converted to annual incidence per 100 000 population with 95% confidence intervals (CI) where possible. Prevalence was converted to prevalence per 100 000 population with 95% CI where possible. Where pain within a condition was examined, we report the prevalence *within* the condition as occurrence, and then use prevalence information for the condition to calculate the prevalence of the *painful* condition.

References

1 Andersson HI, Ejlertsson G, Leden I, Rosenberg C. Chronic pain in a geographically defined general population: studies in differences in age, gender, social class, and pain localization. *Clin J Pain* 1993; **9**: 174–82.

2 Brattberg G, Thorslund M, Wikman A. The prevalence of pain in a general population. The results of a postal survey in a county of Sweden. *Pain* 1989; **37**: 215–22.

3 Birse TM, Lander J. Prevalence of chronic pain. *Canadian Journal of Public Health* 1998; **89**(2): 129–31.

4 Bowsher D, Rigge M, Sopp L. Prevalence of chronic pain in the British population: a telephone survey of 1037 households. *Pain Clinic* 1991; **4**: 223–30.

5 Chrubasik S, Junck H, Zappe HA, Stutzke O. A survey on pain complaints and health care utilization in a German population sample. *Eur J Anaesthesiol* 1998; **15**: 397–408.

6 Wall P. *Pain: the science of suffering.* London: Weidenfeld and Nicolson, 1999.

7 Brochet B, Michel P, Barberger-Gateau P *et al.* Pain in the elderly: an epidemiological study in south-western France. *Pain Clinic* 1991; **5**(2): 73–9.

8 Clinical Standards Advisory Group. *Back Pain.* London: HMSO, 1994.

9 Clarke CE, MacMillan L, Sondhi S, Wells NEJ. Economic and social impact of migraine. *QJM Monthly Journal of the Association of Physicians* 1996; **89**(1): 77–84.

10 Crombie IK, Croft PR, Linton SJ, LeResche L, VonKorff M (eds). *Epidemiology of pain.* Seattle: IASP Press, 1999.

11 Croft P, Papageorgious A, McNally R. Low Back Pain. In: Stevens A, Raftery J (eds). *Health care needs assessment.* Oxford and New York: Radcliffe Medical Press, 1997: 129–81.

12 Wolfe F, Ross K, Anderson J, Russell IJ, Hebert L. The prevalence and characteristics of fibromyalgia in the general population. *Arthritis Rheum* 1995; **38**: 19–28.

13 Magni G, Marchetti M, Moreschi C, Merskey H, Luchini SR. Chronic musculoskeletal pain and depressive symptoms in the National Health and Nutrition Examination. I. Epidemiologic follow-up study. *Pain* 1993; **53**(2): 163–8.

14 Higginson I. Palliative and Terminal Care. In: Stevens A, Raftery J (eds). *Health care needs assessment.* Oxford and New York: Radcliffe Medical Press, 1997: 183–260.

15 Smith BH, Elliott AM, Chambers WA *et al.* The impact of chronic pain in the community. *Fam Pract* 2001; **18**(3): 292–9.

16 Fox PL, Raina P, Jadad AR. Prevalence and treatment of pain in older adults in nursing homes and other long-term care institutions: a systematic review. *CMA* 1999; **160**: 329–33.

17 Cassidy JD, Carroll LJ, Côté P. The Saskatchewan health and back pain survey. *Spine* 1998; **23**(17): 1860–6.

18 Davies HTO, Crombie IK, Macrae WA. Back pain in the pain clinic: nature and management. *Pain Clinic* 1995; **8**(2): 191–9.

19 Thomas E, Silman AJ, Croft PR, Papageorgiou AC, Jayson MI, Macfarlane GJ. Predicting who develops chronic low back pain in primary care: a prospective study. *Br Med J* 1999; **318**(7199): 1662–7.

20 Calin A, Fries JF. Striking prevalence of ankylosing spondylitis in 'healthy' w27 positive males and females. *N Engl J Med* 1975; **293**(17): 835–9.

21 Gran JT, Husby G, Hordvik M. Prevalence of ankylosing spondylitis in males and females in a young middle-aged population of Tromsø, Northern Norway. *Annals of Rheumatic Diseases* 1985; **44**: 359–67.

22 Braun J, Bollow M, Remlinger G *et al.* Prevalence of spondylarthropathies in HLA-B27 positive and negative blood donors. *Arthritis Rheum* 1998; **41**(1): 58–67.

23 Carbone LD, Cooper C, Michet CJ, Atkinson EJ, O'Fallon WM, Melton LJ III. Ankylosing spondylitis in Rochester, Minnesota, 1935–1989: Is the epidemiology changing? *Arthritis Rheum* 1992; **35**(12): 1476–82.

24 Julkunen H, Korpi J. Ankylosing spondylitis in three Finnish population samples. Prostatovesiculitis and salpingo-oophoritis as aetiological factors. *Scand J Rheumatol* 1984; **12**(suppl. 52): 16–8.

25 Underwood MR, Dawes PD. Inflammatory back pain in primary care. *Br J Rheumatol* 1995; **34**: 1074–7.

26 Gran JT, Skomsvoll JF. The outcome of ankylosing spondylitis: A study of 100 patients. *Br J Rheumatol* 1997; **36**(7): 766–71.

27 Bovim G, Schrader H, Sand T. Neck pain in general population. *Spine* 1994; **19**: 1307–9.

28 Côté P, Cassidy JD, Carroll L. The Saskatchewan Health and Back Pain survey. *Spine* 1998; **23**: 1689–98.

29 Jacobsson L, Lindgärde F, Manthorpe R. The commonest rheumatic complaints of over six weeks' duration in a twelve-month period in a defined Swedish population. *Scand J Rheumatol* 1989; **18**: 353–60.

30 Mäkelä M, Heliövaara M, Sievers K *et al.* Prevalence, determinants, and consequences of chronic neck pain in Finland. *Am J Epidemiol* 1991; **134**: 1356–67.

31 Takala J, Sievers K, Klaukka T. Rheumatic symptoms in the middle-aged population in southwestern Finland. *Scand J Rheumatol* 1982; **47**: 15–29.

32 Galasko CSB, Murray PM, Pitcher M *et al.* Neck sprains after road traffic accidents: a modern epidemic. *Injury* 1993; **24**(3): 155–7.

33 Versteegen GJ, Kingma J, Meijler WJ, Ten Duis HJ. Neck sprain in patients injured in car accidents: A retrospective study covering the period 1970–1994. *Eur Spine J* 1998; **7**(3): 195–200.

34 Versteegen GJ, Kingma J, Meijler WJ, Ten Duis HJ. Neck sprain not arising from car accidents: A retrospective study covering 25 years. *Eur Spine J* 1998; **7**(3): 201–5.

35 Bengtsson BA, Malmvall BE. The epidemiology of giant cell arteritis including temporal arteritis and polymyalgia rheumatica. Incidences of different clinical presentations and eye complications. *Arthritis Rheum* 1981; **24**(7): 899–904.

36 Boesen P, Sorensen SF. Giant cell arteritis, temporal arteritis, and polymyalgia rheumatica in a Danish county. A prospective investigation, 1982–1985. *Arthritis Rheum* 1987; **30**(3): 294–9.

37 Elling P, Olsson AT, Elling H. Synchronous variations of the incidence of temporal arteritis and polymyalgia rheumatica in different regions of Denmark; association with epidemics of Mycoplasma pneumoniae infection. *J Rheumatol* 1996; **23**(1): 112–9.

38 Gran JT, Myklebust G. The incidence of polymyalgia rheumatica and temporal arteritis in the county of Aust Agder, south Norway: a prospective study 1987–94. *J Rheumatol* 1997; **24**(9): 1739–43.

39 Kyle V, Silverman B, Silman A *et al.* Polymyalgia rheumatica/giant cell arteritis in a Cambridge general practice. *Br Med J* 1985; **291**: 385–6s.

40 Northridge J, Hill SG. Polymyalgia rheumatica and giant cell arteritis in general practice. *Musculoskeletal Medicine* 1995; **2**: 13–7.

41 Salvarani C, Macchioni P, Zizzi F *et al.* Epidemiologic and immunogenetic aspects of polymyalgia rheumatica and giant cell arteritis in northern Italy. *Arthritis Rheum* 1991; 34/3(351–356).

42 Salvarani C, Gabriel SE, O'Fallon M, Hunder GG. Epidemiology of polymyalgia rheumatica in Olmsted County, Minnesota, 1970–1991. *Arthritis Rheum* 1995; **38**(5): 369–73.

43 White KP, Speechley M, Harth M, Østbye T. Fibromyalgia in rheumatology practice: a survey of Canadian Rheumatologists. *J Rheumatol* 1995; **22**: 722–6.

44 Croft P, Schollum J, Silman A. Population study of tender point counts and pain as evidence of fibromyalgia. *Br Med J* 1994; 309/6956(696–699).

45 O'Malley PG, Balden E, Tomkins G. *et al.* Treatment of fibromyalgia with antidepressants. A meta-analysis. *J Gen Intern Med* 2000; **15**: 659–66.

46 Croft P, Rigby AS, Boswell R *et al.* The prevalence of widespread pain in the general population. *J Rheumatol* 1993; **20**(4): 710–3.

47 Forseth KØ, Gran JT. The prevalence of fibromyalgia among women aged 20–49 years in Arendal, Norway. *Scand J Rheumatol* 1992; **21**: 74–8.

48 Prescott E, Kjøller M, Jacobsen S *et al.* Fibromyalgia in the adult Danish population: 1. A prevalence study. *Scand J Rheumatol* 1993; **22**: 233–7.

49 Portenoy RK, Hagen NA. Breakthrough pain: definition, prevalence and characteristics. *Pain* 1990; **41**: 273–81.

50 Portenoy RK, Payne D, Jacobsen P. Breakthrough pain: characteristics and impact in patients with cancer pain. *Pain* 1999; 81(1–2): 129–34.

51 Bruera E, Fainsinger R, MacEachern T, Hanson J. The use of methylphenidate in patients with incident cancer pain receiving regular opiates. A preliminary report. *Pain* 1992; **50**: 75–7.

52 Stewart WF, Simon D, Shechter A, Lipton RB. Population variation in migraine prevalence: a meta-analysis. *J Clin Epidemiol* 1995; **48**(2): 269–80.

53 Scher A I, Stewart W F, Lipton R B. Migraine and Headache: A meta-analytic approach. In: Crombie IK (ed). *Epidemiology of pain.* Seattle: IASP Press, 1999: 159–70.

54 Stang PE, Yanagihara T, Swanson JW *et al.* Incidence of migraine headache: a population-based study in Olmsted County, Minnesota. *Neurology* 1992; **42**: 1657–62.

55 Stewart WF, Linet MS, Celentano DD *et al.* Age- and sex-specific incidence rates of migraine with and without visual aura. *Am J Epidemiol* 1991; **134**: 1111–20.

56 Rozen TD, Swanson JW, Stang PE, McDonnell SK, Rocca WA. Increasing incidence of medically recognized migraine headache in a United States population. *Neurology* 1999; **53**(7): 1468–73.

57 Breslau N, Davis GC, Andreski P. Migraine, psychiatric disorders, and suicide attempts: an epidemiologic study of young adults. *Psychiatry Res* 1991; **37**: 11–23.

58 Franceschi M, Colombo B, Rossi P, Canal N. Headache in a population-based elderly cohort – an ancillary study to the Italian Longitudinal Study of Aging (ILSA). *Headache* 1997; **37**(2): 79–82.

59 Göbel H, Petersen-Braun M, Soyka D. The epidemiology of headache in Germany: a nationwide survey of a representative sample on the basis of the headache classification of the International Headache Society. *Cephalalgia* 1994; **14**: 97–106.

60 Henry P, Michel P, Brochet B *et al.* A nationwide survey of migraine in France: prevalence and clinical features in adults. *Cephalalgia* 1992; **12**: 229–37s.

61 Linet MS, Stewart WF, Celantano DD *et al.* An epidemiologic study of headache among adolescents and young adults. *JAMA* 1989; **261**(15): 2211–6.

62 Michel P, Pariente P, Duru G *et al.* MIG ACCESS: a population based, nationwide, comparative survey of access to care in migraine in France. *Cephalalgia* 1996; **16**: 50–5.

63 O'Brien B, Goeree R, Streiner D. Prevalence of migraine headache in Canada: a population based survey. *Int J Epidemiol* 1994; **23**(5): 1020–6.

64 Rasmussen BK, Jensen R, Schroll M, Olesen J. Epidemiology of headache in a general population-a prevalence study. *J Clin Epidemiol* 1991; **44**(11): 1147–57.

65 Stewart WF, Lipton RB, Celentano DD, Reed ML. Prevalence of migraine headache in the United States. Relation to age, income, race, and other sociodemographic factors. *JAMA* 1992; **267**(1): 64–9.

66 Stewart WF, Lipton RB, Liberman J. Variation in migraine prevalence by race. *Neurology* 1996; **47**: 52–9.

67 Hu XH, Markson LE, Lipton RB *et al.* Burden of migraine in the United States. *Arch Intern Med* 1999; **159**: 813–8.

68 Waters WE. Controlled clinical trial of ergotamine tartrate. *Br Med J* 1970; **1**(5705): 325–7.

69 Waters WE, O'Connor PJ. Epidemiology of headache and migraine in women. *J Neurol Neurosurg Psychiatry* 1971; **34**(2): 148–53.

70 Clarke GJR, Waters WE. Headache and migraine in a London general practice. In: Waters WE (ed). *The epidemiology of migraine.* Bracknell: Boehringer Ingelheim Ltd, 1974: 14–22.

71 Mills CH, Waters WE. Headache and migraine on the isles of Scilly. In: Waters W E (ed). *The epidemiology of migraine.* Bracknell: Boehringer Ingelheim Ltd, 1974: 49–58.

72 Newland CA, Illis LS, Robinson PK, Batchelor BG, Waters WE. A survey of headache in an English city. *Res Clin Stud Headache* 1978; **5**: 1–20.

73 Rasmussen BK. Epidemiology of headache. *Cephalalgia* 1995; **15**(1): 45–68.

74 Schwartz BS, Stewart WF, Simon D, Lipton RB. Epidemiology of tension-type head ache. *JAMA* 1998; **279**(5): 381–3.

75 Scher AI, Stewart WF, Liberman J, Lipton RB. Prevalence of frequent headache in a population sample. *Headache* 1998; **38**: 497–506.

76 Swanson JW, Yanagihara T, Stang PE *et al.* Incidence of cluster headaches: a population based study in Olmsted County, Minnesota. *Neurology* 1994; **44**: 433–7.

77 Brewis M, Poskanzer DC, Rolland C, Miller H. Neurological disease in an English city. *Acta Neurol Scand* 1966; **42**(suppl 24): 1–89.

78 Katusic S, Beard CM, Bergstralh E, Kurland LT. Incidence and clinical features of trigeminal neuralgia, Rochester, Minnesota, 1945–1984. *Ann Neurol* 1990; **27**: 89–95.

79 Munoz M, Dumas M, Boutros-Toni F *et al.* Neuro-epidemiological study of a small Limousin town. *Rev Neurol (Paris)* 1988; **144**(4): 266–71.

80 Walters DP, Gatling W, Mullee MA, Hill RD. The prevalence of diabetic distal sensory neuropathy in an English community. *Diabet Med* 1992; **9**(4): 349–53.

81 Harris M, Cowie C, Eastman R. Symptoms of sensory neuropathy in adults with NIDDM in the U.S. population. *Diabetes Care* 1993; **16**(11): 1446–52.

82 Boulton AJM, Knight G, Drury J, Ward JD. The prevalence of symptomatic, diabetic neuropathy in an insulin-treated population. *Diabetes Care* 1985; **8**(2): 125–8.

83 Chan AW, Macfarlane IA, Bowsher D *et al.* Chronic pain in patients with diabetes mellitus: comparison with a non-diabetic population. *Pain Clinic* 1990; **3**(3): 147–59.

84 Nabarro JDN. Diabetes in the United Kingdom: a personal series. *Diabet Med* 1991; **8**: 59–68.

85 O'Hare JA, Abuaisha F, Geoghegan M. Prevalence and forms of neuropathic morbidity in 800 diabetics. *Ir J Med Sci* 1994; **163**(3): 132–5.

86 Edmunds WJ, Brisson M, Rose JD. The epidemiology of herpes zoster and potential cost-effectiveness of vaccination in England and Wales. *Vaccine* 2001; **19**: 3076–90.

87 Hope-Simpson R. The nature of herpes zoster: a long-term study and a new hypothesis. *J R Soc Med* 1965; **58**: 9–20.

88 Cockerell OC, Goodridge DMG, Brodie D *et al.* Neurological disease in a defined population: the results of a pilot study in two general practices. *Neuroepidemiology* 1996; **15**: 73–82.

89 Brown GR. Herpes zoster: correlation of age, sex, distribution, neuralgia, and associated disorders. *South Med J* 1976; **69**(5): 576–8.

90 de Moragas J, Kierland R. The outcome of patients with herpes zoster. *Arch Dermatol* 1957; **75**: 193–5.

91 Helgason S, Petursson G, Gudmundsson S, Sigurdsson JA. Prevalence of postherpetic neuralgia after a single episode of herpes zoster: prospective study with long term follow up. *Br Med J* 2000; **321**: 1–4.

92 Lancaster T, Silagy C, Gray S. Primary care management of acute herpes zoster: systematic review of evidence from randomized controlled trials. *Br J Gen Pract* 1995; **45**(390): 39–45.

93 Meister W, Neiss A, Gross G *et al.* Demography, symptomatology, and course of disease in ambulatory zoster patients. *Intervirology* 1998; **41**: 272–7.

94 Rogers RS, Tindall JP. Geriatric herpes zoster. *J Am Geriatr Soc* 1971; **19**(6): 495–503.

95 Rothwell PM, Charlton D. High incidence and prevalence of multiple sclerosis in south east Scotland: evidence of a genetic predisposition. *J Neurol Neurosurg Psychiatry* 1998; **64**: 730–5.

96 Archibald CJ, McGrath PJ, Ritvo PG *et al.* Pain prevalence, severity and impact in a clinic sample of multiple sclerosis patients. *Pain* 1994; **58**(1): 89–93.

97 Brochet B, Michel P, Henry P. Pain complaints in outpatients with multiple sclerosis: description and consequences on disability. *Pain Clinic* 1992; **5**(3): 157–64.

98 Clifford DR, Trotter JI. Pain in multiple sclerosis. *Arch Neurol* 1984; **41**: 1270–3.

99 Moulin DE, Foley KM, Ebers GC. Pain syndromes in multiple sclerosis. *Neurology* 1988; **38**: 1830–4.

100 Stenager E, Knudsden L, Jensen K. Acute and chronic pain syndromes in multiple sclerosis. *Acta Neurol Scand* 1991; **84**: 197–200.

101 Vermote R, Ketelaer P, Carton H. Pain in multiple sclerosis patients. *Clin Neurol Neurosurg* 1986; **88**: 87–93.

102 Warnell P. The pain experience of a multiple sclerosis population: a descriptive study. *Axon* 1991; **13**(1): 26–8.

103 Anderson IM, Tomenson BM. Treatment discontinuation with selective serotonin reuptake inhibitors compared with tricylic antidepressants: a meta-analysis. *Br Med J* 1995; **310**: 1433–8.

104 Bowsher D. Cerebrovascular disease. *The Lancet* 1993; **341**: 156.

105 Meijer WT, Hoes AW, Rutgers D *et al.* Peripheral arterial disease in the elderly. The Rotterdam Study. *Arterioscler Thromb Vasc Biol* 1998; **18**: 185–92.

106 Leng GC, Papacosta O, Whincup P *et al.* Femoral atherosclerosis in an older British population: prevalence and risk factors. *Atherosclerosis* 2000; **152**: 167–74.

107 Menotti A, Mulder I, Nissinen A *et al.* Prevalence of morbidity and multimorbidity in the elderly male populations and their impact on 10-year all-cause mortality: The FINE study (Finland Italy, Netherlands, Elderly). *J Clin Epidemiol* 2001; **54**: 680–6.

108 Bainton D, Swetnam P, Baker I, Elwood P. Peripheral vascular disease: consequence for survival and association with risk factors in the Speedwell prospective heart disease study. *Br Heart J* 1994; **72**: 128–32.

109 Bowlin SJ, Medalie JH, Flocke SA *et al.* Epidemiology of intermittent claudication in middle-aged men. *Am J Epidemiol* 1994; **140**(5): 418–30.

110 Leng GC, Lee AJ, Fowkes FG *et al.* Incidence, natural history and cardiovascular events in symptomatic and asymptomatic peripheral arterial disease in the general population. *Int J Epidemiol* 1996; **25**: 1172–81.

111 Smith GD, Shipley MJ, Rose G. Intermittent claudication, heart disease risk factors, and mortality. The Whitehall Study. *Circulation* 1990; **82**(6): 1925–31.

112 Palmer KT, Griffin MJ, Syddall H *et al.* Prevalence of Raynaud's phenomenon in Great Britain and its relation to hand transmitted vibration: a national postal survey. *Occup Environ Med* 2000; **57**: 448–52.

113 Brand FN, Larson MG, Kannel WB, McGuirk JM. The occurrence of Raynaud's phenomenon in a general population: The Framingham Study. *Vasc Med* 1997; **2**: 296–301.

114 Maricq HR, Weinrich MC, Keil JE, LeRoy EC. Prevalence of Raynaud's phenomenon in the general population. *J Chronic Dis* 1986; **39**(6): 423–7s.

115 Silman A, Holligan S, Brennan P, Maddison P. Prevalence of symptoms of Raynaud's phenomenon in general practice. *Br Med J* 1990; **301**(6752): 590–2.

116 Reid DD, Brett GZ, Hamilton PJ, Jarrett RJ, Keen H, Rose G. Cardiorespiratory disease and diabetes among middle-aged male Civil Servants. A study of screening and intervention. *The Lancet* 1974; **1**(7856): 469–73.

117 Shaper AG, Cook DG, Walker M, Macfarlane PW. Prevalence of ischaemic heart disease in middle aged men. *Br Heart J* 1984; **51**: 595–605.

118 Bainton D, Baker IA, Sweetnam PM *et al.* Prevalence of ischaemic heart disease: the Caerphilly and Speedwell surveys. *Br Heart J* 1988; **59**: 201–6.

119 Smith WCS, Kenicer MB, Tunstall-Pedoe H *et al.* Prevalence of coronary heart disease in Scotland: Scottish Heart Health Study. *Br Heart J* 1990; **64**: 295–8.

120 McGovern PG, Jacobs DR, Shahar E *et al.* Trends in acute coronary heart disease mortality, morbidity, and medical care from 1985 through 1997. The Minnesota Heart Survey. *Circulation* 2001; **104**: 19–24.

121 Crombie IK, Davies HTO, Macrae WA. Cut and thrust: Antecedent surgery and trauma among patients attending a chronic pain clinic. *Pain* 1998; **76**(1–2): 167–71.

122 Macrae W A, Davies H T O. Chronic Postsurgical Pain. In: Crombie IK (ed). *Epidemiology of Pain.* Seattle: IASP Press, 1999: 125–42.

123 Perkins FM, Kehlet H. Chronic pain as an outcome of surgery. *Anesthesiology* 2000; **93**: 1123–33.

124 Sherman R, Sherman C, Parker L. Chronic phantom and stump pain among American Veterans: results of a survey. *Pain* 1984; **18**: 83–95.

125 Wartan SW, Hamann W, Wedley JR, McColl I. Phantom pain and sensation among British war amputees. *Br J Anaesth* 1997; **78**: 652–9.

126 Tasmuth T, Von Smitten KiP *et al.* Pain and other symptoms after different treatment modalities of breast cancer. *Ann Oncol* 1995; **6**: 453–9.

127 Tasmuth T, von Smitten K, Kalso E. Pain and other symptoms during the first year after radical and conservative surgery for breast cancer. *Br J Cancer* 1996; **74**: 2024–31.

128 Kalso E, Perttunen K, Kassinen S. Pain after thoracic surgery. *Acta Anaesthesiol Scand* 1992; **36**: 96–100.

129 Richardson J, Sabanathan S, Mearns AJ *et al.* Post-thoracotomy neuralgia. *Pain Clinic* 1994; **7**(2): 87–97.

130 Bay-Nielsen M, Perkins FM, Kehlet H. Pain and functional impairment 1 year after inguinal herniorraphy: a nationwide questionnaire study. *Ann Surg* 2001; **233**(1): 1–7.

131 Pohjolainen T. A clinical evaluation of stumps in lower limb amputees. *Prosthet Orthot Int* 1991; **15**: 178–84.

132 Sherman RA, Sherman CJ. Prevalence and characteristics of chronic phantom limb pain among American veterans. *Am J Phys Med* 1983; **62**(5): 227–38.

133 Steinbach TV, Nadvorna H, Arazi D. A five year follow-up study of phantom limb pain in post traumatic amputees. *Scand J Rehabil Med* 1982; **14**: 203–7.

134 Kooijman CM, Dijkstra PU, Geertzen JHB *et al.* Phantom pain and phantom sensations in upper limit amputees: an epidemiological study. *Pain* 2000; **87**: 33–41.

135 Pernot HF, Winnubst GM, Cluitmans JJ, De Witter. Amputees in Limburg: incidence, morbidity and mortality, prosthetic supply, care utilisation and functional level after one year. *Prosthet Orthot Int* 2000; **24**(2): 90–6.

136 Rommers GM, Vos LD, Groothof JW *et al.* Epidemiology of lower limb amputees in the north of The Netherlands: aetiology, discharge destination and prosthetic use. *Prosthet Orthot Int* 1997; **21**(2): 92–9.

137 Pohjolainen T, Alaranta H. Epidemiology of lower limb amputees in Southern Finland in 1995 and trends since 1984. *Prosthet Orthot Int* 1999; **23**(2): 88–92.

138 Buchanan DC, Mandel AR. The prevalence of phantom limb experience in amputees. *Rehabilitation Psychology* 1986; **31**(3): 183–8.

139 Houghton AD, Nicholls G, Houghton AL *et al.* Phantom pain: natural history and association with rehabilitation. *Ann R Coll Surg Engl* 1994; **76**: 22–5.

140 Jensen TS, Krebs B, Nielsen J, Rasmussen P. Non-painful phantom limb phenomena in amputees: incidence, clinical characteristics and temporal course. *Acta Neurol Scand* 1984; **70**: 407–14.

141 Krebs B, Jensen TS, Kroner K, Nielsen J, Jorgensen HS. Phantom limb phenomena in amputees 7 years after limb amputation. In: Fields HL, Dubner R, Cervero F (eds). *Advances in Pain Research and Therapy.* Vol 9 edition. New York: Raven Press, 1985: 425–9.

142 Ivens D, Hoe Al, Podd TJ *et al.* Assessment of morbidity from complete axillary dissection. *Br J Cancer* 1992; **66**: 136–8.

143 Wallace MS, Wallace AM, Lee J, Dobke MK. Pain after breast surgery: a survey of 282 women. *Pain* 1996; **66**: 195–205.

144 Kroner K, Knudsen UB, Lundby L, Hvid H. Long-term phantom breast syndrome after mastectomy. *Clin J Pain* 1992; **8**(4): 346–50.

145 Polinsky ML. Functional status of long-term breast cancer. *Health Soc Work* 1994; **19**(3): 165–73.

146 Smith WCS, Bourne D, Squair J *et al.* A retrospective cohort study of post mastectomy pain syndrome. *Pain* 1999; **83**: 91–5.

147 Stevens PE, Dibble SL, Miaskowski C. Prevalence, characteristics, and impact of post-mastectomy pain syndrome: an investigation of women's experiences. *Pain* 1995; **61**: 61–8.

148 Tasmuth T, Blomqvist C, Kalso E. Chronic post-treatment symptoms in patients with breast cancer operated in different surgical units. *Eur J Surg Oncol* 1999; **25**: 38–43.

149 Rogers ML, Duffy JP. Surgical aspects of chronic post-thoractomy pain. *Eur J Cardiothorac Surg* 2000; **18**: 711–6.

150 Katz J, Jackson M, Kavanagh BP, Sandler A. Acute pain after thoracic surgery predicts long-term post-thoracotomy pain. *Clin J Pain* 1996; **12**(1): 50–5.

151 Dajczman E, Gordon A, Kreisman H, Wolkove N. Long-term postthoractomy pain. *Chest* 1991; **99**: 270–4.

152 Landreneau RJ, Mack MJ, Hazelrigg SR *et al.* Prevalence of chronic pain after pulmonary resection by thoractomy or video-assisted thoracic surgery. *J Thorac Cardiovasc Surg* 1994; **107**: 1079–86.

153 Matsunaga M, Dan K, Manabe FY. Residual pain of thoracotomy patients with malignancy and non-malignancy. *Pain* 1990; suppl 5: S148.

154 Perttunen K, Tasmuth T, Kalso E. Chronic pain after thoracic surgery: a follow-up study. *Acta Anaesth Scand* 1999; **43**: 563–7.

155 Bates T, Mercer JC, Harrison M. Symptomatic gall stone disease: before and after cholecystectomy. *Gut* 1984; **24**: 579–50.

156 Ros E, Zambon D. Postcholecystectomy symptoms. A prospective study of gall stone patients before and two years after surgery. *Gut* 1987; **28**(11): 1500–4.

157 Stiff G, Rhodes M, Kelly A, Telford K, Armstrong CP, Rees BI. Long-term pain: Less common after laparoscopic than open cholecystectomy. *Br J Surg* 1994; **81**(9): 1368–70.

158 Wilson RG, Macintyre IMC. Symptomatic outcome after laparoscopic cholecystectomy. *Br J Surg* 1993; **80**(4): 439–41.

159 Sprangers MAG, de Regt EB, Andries F *et al.* Which chronic conditions are associated with better or poorer quality of life? *J Clin Epidemiol* 2000; **53**: 895–907.

160 Tramer MR, Moore RA, Reynolds DJ, McQuay HJ. Quantitative estimation of rare adverse events which follow a biological progression: a new model applied to chronic NSAID use. *Pain* 2000; **85**(1–2): 169–82.

161 Page J, Henry D. Consumption of NSAIDs and the development of congestive heart failure in elderly patients. *Arch Intern Med* 2000; **160**: 777–84.

162 Merlo J, Broms K, Lindblad U *et al.* Association of outpatient utilisation of non-steroidal anti-inflammatory drugs and hospitalised heart failure in the entire Swedish population. *Eur J Clin Pharmacol* 2001; **57**: 71–5.

163 McQuay H. Opioids in chronic non-malignant pain. There's too little information on which drugs are effective and when. *Br Med J* 2001; **322**(7295): 1134–5.

164 Jadad AR, Carroll D, Glynn CJ, Moore RA, McQuay HJ. Morphine responsiveness of chronic pain: double-blind randomised crossover study with patient-controlled analgesia. *The Lancet* 1992; **339**(8806): 1367–71.

165 McQuay HJ. Pharmacological treatment of neuralgic and neuropathic pain. *Cancer Surv* 1988; **7**(1): 141–59.

166 McQuay HJ, Moore RA. Antidepressants and chronic pain. *Br Med J* 1997; **314**(7083): 763–4.

167 Arner S, Lindblom U, Meyerson BA, Molander C. Prolonged relief of neuralgia after regional anesthetic blocks. A call for further experimental and systematic clinical studies. *Pain* 1990; **43**(3): 287–97.

168 Emery P, Bowman S, Wedderburn L, Grahame R. Suprascapular nerve block for chronic shoulder pain in rheumatoid arthritis. *Br Med J* 1989; **299**: 1079–80.

169 van der Heijden CJMG, van der Windt DAWM, Kleijnen J, Koes BW, Bouter LM. Steroid injections for shoulder disorders: a systematic review of randomized clinical trials. *Br J Gen Pract* 1996; **46**: 309–16.

170 Lilius G, Laasonen EM, Myllynen P, Harilainen A, Grönlund G. Lumbar facet joint syndrome. *J Bone Joint Surg Am* 1989; **71**: 681–4.

171 Carette S, Marcoux S, Truchon R et al. A controlled trial of corticosteroid injections into facet joints for chronic low back pain. *N Engl J Med* 1991; **325**: 1002–7.

172 Melzack R, Wall PD. Pain mechanisms: a new theory. *Science* 1965; **150**: 971–8.

173 Clinical Standards Advisory Group. *Services for patients with pain.* London: HMSO, 2000.

174 Pain Society. *Provision of pain services.* The Association of Anaesthetists of Great Britain and Ireland, 1997; 1–20.

175 McQuay HJ, Machin L, Moore RA. Chronic non-malignant pain: a population prevalence study. *Practitioner* 1985; **229**(1410): 1109–11.

176 Barsky AJ, Borus JF. Somatization and medicalization in the era of managed care. *JAMA* 1995; **274**: 1931–4.

177 Charlton JE. Two for the price of one – is it worth it? *Anaesthesia* 2002; **57**(1): 1–3.

178 Weir R, Browne GB, Tunks E, Gafni A, Roberts J. A profile of users of speciality pain clinic services: predictors of use and cost estimates. *J Clin Epidemiol* 1992; **45**: 1399–11415.

179 McQuay HJ, Moore RA, Eccleston C, Morley S, de C Williams AC. Systematic review of outpatient services for chronic pain control. *Health Technol Assessment* 1997; **1**(6).

180 McQuay HJ, Moore RA. *An evidence-based resource for pain relief.* Oxford: Oxford University Press, 1998.

181 Moore A, McQuay H, Gavaghan D. Deriving dichotomous outcome measures from continuous data in randomised controlled trials of analgesics. *Pain* 1996; **66**: 229–37.

182 Moore RA, McQuay HJ. Single-patient data meta-analysis of 3453 postoperative patients: Oral tramadol versus placebo, codeine and combination analgesics. *Pain* 1997; **69**(3): 287–94.

183 Watts RW, Silagy CA. A meta-analysis on the efficacy of epidural corticosteroids in the treatment of sciatica. *Anaesth Intensive Care* 1995; **23**: 564–9.

184 McQuay H, Moore RA. Epidural steroids (letter). *Anaesth Intensive Care* 1996; **24**: 284–6.

185 Moore RA, Tramèr MR, Carroll D, Wiffen PJ, McQuay HJ. Quantitive systematic review of topically-applied non-steroidal anti-inflammatory drugs. *Br Med J* 1998; **316**: 333–8.

186 McQuay H, Carroll D, Jadad AR, Wiffen P, Moore A. Anticonvulsant drugs for management of pain: a systematic review. *Br Med J* 1995; **311**(7012): 1047–52.

187 Zhang WY, Li WPA. The effectiveness of topically applied capsaicin. A meta-analysis. *Eur J Clin Pharmacol* 1994; **46**(6): 517–22.

188 McQuay HJ, Tramer M, Nye BA, Carroll D, Wiffen PJ, Moore RA. A systematic review of antidepressants in neuropathic pain. *Pain* 1996; **68**(2–3): 217–27.

189 March L, Irwig L, Schwarz J, Simpson J, Chock C, Brooks P. N of 1 trials comparing a non-steroidal anti-inflammatory drug with paracetamol in osteoarthritis. *Br Med J* 1994; **309**: 1041–6.

190 Kjærsgaard-Andersen P, Nafei A, Skov O *et al.* Codeine plus paracetamol versus paracetamol in longer-term treatment of chronic pain due to osteoarthritis of the hip. *Pain* 1990; **43**: 309–18.

191 Gøtzsche PC. Patients' preference in indomethacin trials: an overview. *The Lancet* 1989; **1**(8629): 88–91.

192 Eisenberg E, Berkey CS, Carr DB, Mosteller F, Chalmers TC. Efficacy and safety of nonsteroidal antiinflammatory drugs for cancer pain: a meta-analysis. *J Clin Oncol* 1994; **12**(12): 2756–65.

193 Henry D, Lim LL-Y, Rodriguez LAG *et al.* Variability in risk of gastrointestinal complications with individual non-steroidal anti-inflammatory drugs: results of a collaborative meta-analysis. *Br Med J* 1996; **312**: 1563–6.

194 Silverstein FE, Graham DY, Senior JR *et al.* Misoprostol reduces serious gastrointestinal complications in patients with rheumatoid arthritis receiving nonsteroidal anti-inflammatory drugs. *Ann Intern Med* 1995; **123**(4): 241–9.

195 Shield MJ, Morant SV. Misoprostol in patients taking non-steroidal anti-inflammatory drugs. *Br Med J* 1996; **312**: 846.

196 Bombardier C, Laine L, Reicin A *et al.* Comparison of Upper Gastrointestinal Toxicity of Rofecoxib and Naproxen in Patients with Rheumatoid Arthritis. *N Engl J Med* 2000; **343**(21): 1520–8.

197 Moore RA, Phillips CJ. Cost of NSAID adverse effects to the UK National Health Service. *Journal of Medical Economics* 1999; **2**: 45–55.

198 Williams J, Louw G, Towlerton G. Intrathecal pumps for giving opioids in chronic pain: a systematic review. *Health Technol Assess* 2000; **4**(32).

199 Eisenach JC, DuPen S, Dubois M, Miguel R, Allin D. Epidural clonidine analgesia for intractable cancer pain. The Epidural Clonidine Study Group. *Pain* 1995; **61**(3): 391–9.

200 Bell R, Eccleston C, Kalso E. Ketamine as an adjuvant to opioids for cancer pain. *Cochrane Database Syst Rev* 2003; (1): CD003351.

201 Koes BW, Scholten RPM, Mens JMA, Bouter LM. Efficacy of epidural steroid injections for low-back pain and sciatica: a systematic review of randomized clinical trials. *Pain* 1995; **63**: 279–88.

202 Jadad AR, Carroll D, Glynn CJ, McQuay HJ. Intravenous regional sympathetic blockade for pain relief in reflex sympathetic dystrophy: a systematic review and a randomized, double-blind crossover study. *J Pain Symptom Manage* 1995; **10**(1): 13–20.

203 Eisenberg E, Carr DB, Chalmers TC. Neurolytic celiac plexus block for treatment of cancer pain: a meta-analysis. *Anesth Analg* 1995; **80**(2): 290–5.

204 Abram SE. 1992 Bonica Lecture. Advances in chronic pain management since gate control. *Reg Anesth* 1993; **18**(2): 66–81.

205 Reeve J, Menon D, Corabian P. Transcutaneous electrical nerve stimulation (TENS): a technology assessment. *Int J Technol Assess Health Care* 1996; **12**: 299–324.

206 Patel M, Gutzwiller F, Paccaud F, Marazzi A. A meta-analysis of acupuncture for chronic pain. *Int J Epidemiol* 1989; **18**(4): 900–6.

207 ter Riet G, Kleijnen J, Knipschild P. Acupuncture and chronic pain: a criteria-based meta-analysis. *J Clin Epidemiol* 1990; **43**(11): 1191–9.

208 Bhatt Sanders D. Acupuncture for rheumatoid arthritis: an analysis of the literature. *Semin Arthritis Rheum* 1985; **14**(4): 225–31.

209 Smith LA, Oldman AD, McQuay HJ, Moore RA. Teasing apart quality and validity in systematic reviews: an example from acupuncture trials in chronic neck and back pain. *Pain* 2000; **86**: 119–32.

210 Puett DW, Griffin MR. Published trials of nonmedicinal and noninvasive therapies for hip and knee osteoarthritis. *Ann Intern Med* 1994; **121**(2): 133–40.

211 Abenhaim L, Bergeron AM. Twenty years of randomized clinical trials of manipulative therapy for back pain: a review. *Clin Invest Med* 1992; **15**(6): 527–35.

212 Anderson R, Meeker WC, Wirick BE, Mootz RD, Kirk DH, Adams A. A meta-analysis of clinical trials of spinal manipulation. *J Manipulative Physiol Ther* 1992; **15**(3): 181–94.

213 Assendelft WJ, Koes BW, Van der Heijden GJ, Bouter LM. The efficacy of chiropractic manipulation for back pain: blinded review of relevant randomized clinical trials. *J Manipulative Physiol Ther* 1992; **15**(8): 487–94.

214 Brunarski DJ. Clinical trials of spinal manipulation: a critical appraisal and review of the literature. *J Manipulative Physiol Ther* 1984; **7**(4): 243–9.

215 Koes BW, Assendelft WJ, van der Heijden GJ, Bouter LM, Knipschild PG. Spinal manipulation and mobilisation for back and neck pain: a blinded review. *Br Med J* 1991; **303**(6813): 1298–303.

216 Koes BW, Bouter LM, Beckerman H, van der Heijden GJ, Knipschild PG. Physiotherapy exercises and back pain: a blinded review. *Br Med J* 1991; **302**(6792): 1572–6.

217 Ottenbacher K, DiFabio RP. Efficacy of spinal manipulation/mobilization therapy. A meta analysis. *Spine* 1985; **10**(9): 833–7.

218 Powell FC, Hanigan WC, Olivero WC. A risk/benefit analysis of spinal manipulation therapy for relief of lumbar or cervical pain. *Neurosurgery* 1993; **33**(1): 73–8; discussion 78–9.

219 Shekelle PG, Adams AH, Chassin MR, Hurwitz EL, Brook RH. Spinal manipulation for low-back pain. *Ann Intern Med* 1992; **117**(7): 590–8.

220 Pither CE, Nicholas MK. Psychological approaches in chronic pain management. *Br Med J* 1991; **47**: 743–61.

221 Williams AC. NNTs used in decision-making in chronic pain management. *Bandolier* 1995; **22** (Dec).

222 Cohen JE, Goel V, Frank JW, Bombardier C, Peloso P, Guillemin F. Group education interventions for people with low back pain. An overview of the literature. *Spine* 1994; **19**(11): 1214–22.

223 Cutler RB, Fishbain DA, Rosomoff HL, Abdel-Moty E, Khalil TM, Rosomoff RS. Does nonsurgical pain center treatment of chronic pain return patients to work? A review and meta-analysis of the literature. *Spine* 1994; **19**(6): 643–52.

224 Fernandez E, Turk DC. The utility of cognitive coping strategies for altering pain perception: a meta analysis. *Pain* 1989; **38**(2): 123–35.

225 Gebhardt WA. Effectiveness of training to prevent job-related back pain: a meta-analysis. *Br J Clin Psychol* 1994; **33**: 571–4.

226 Hyman RB, Feldman HR, Harris RB, Levin RF, Malloy GB. The effects of relaxation training on clinical symptoms: a meta analysis. *Nurs Res* 1989; **38**(4): 216–20.

227 Malone MD, Strube MJ, Scogin FR. Meta analysis of non medical treatments for chronic pain. *Pain* 1988; **34**(3): 231–44.

228 Mullen PD, Laville EA, Biddle AK, Lorig K. Efficacy of psychoeducational interventions on pain, depression, and disability in people with arthritis: a meta analysis. *J Rheumatol* 1987; **14**(suppl 15): 33–9.

229 Suls J, Fletcher B. The relative efficacy of avoidant and nonavoidant coping strategies: a meta analysis. *Health Psychol* 1985; **4**(3): 249–88.

230 Audit Commission. *No feeling, no pain.* London: Audit Commission, 1997.

231 Government Statistical Service. *Prescription cost analysis, England 2001.* London: Department of Health NHSE, 2001.

232 Bandolier. More on NSAID adverse effects [Web Page]. September 2000; Available at http://www.jr2.ox.ac.uk/bandolier/band79/b79–6.html. (Accessed 10 Jan 2002)

233 Jadad AR, Carroll D, Moore A, McQuay H. Developing a database of published reports of randomised clinical trials in pain research. *Pain* 1996; **66**: 239–46.

8 Mental Ill Health in Primary Care

Siân Rees, Jo Paton, Chris Thompson, Tony Kendrick and Paul Lelliott

1 Summary

Statement of the problem

Mental ill health is common. However, whilst the risk of developing any disorder is high, the type and severity of disorder varies. Most mental health is mild and self-limiting, a significant proportion is chronic and causes moderate disability and a small proportion of people suffer life-long, severely disabling illness. Whatever the type and severity, the majority of mental ill health seen by health services initially presents to, and is managed by, primary care practitioners.

Mental health policy has, until recently, focused heavily on the need to provide a range of services for those with the most severe mental illness. However, the National Service Framework for Mental Health makes primary mental health care of central importance by setting two standards that relate directly to the delivery of mental health care by primary care practitioners. There is also a requirement to develop local referral protocols and for mental health promotion to be implemented. In addition, *The NHS Plan* makes reference to primary care mental health by creating new graduate primary care mental health workers.

The effect of mental ill health on the individual, their relatives and society is profound. For the individual it can affect quality of life, the ability to work and maintain social relationships and even to live an independent life. Mental illness also makes a significant contribution to premature mortality. For families and carers, mental ill health can be a significant burden. For society, the cost of mental ill health is significant as is its impact on employment.

Sub-categories

Mental ill health in primary care ranges from symptoms that don't reach case definition for a disorder, to clear cases of mental disorder which range significantly in severity and the disability they cause. It is this wide spectrum that makes it hard to categorise mental ill health in primary care into simple groupings for service planning. Levels of care as described by Goldberg and Huxley and the ICD-10 PC (primary care) diagnosis will be used in this chapter to help group the issues under consideration.

Prevalence and incidence

Two national UK prevalence surveys have been carried out. These surveys suggest that at any one point in time approximately 16% of the general population may be suffering from a diagnosable neurotic disorder and 0.4% from a psychotic illness. There are significant differences in prevalence in sub-sections of the population. It is well known that indicators of social deprivation, such as unemployment and homelessness, are associated with an increased prevalence of mental ill health. The burden of illness in any particular general practice will therefore reflect the socio-demographics of the geographical area served by that practice. Risk factors for development of mental disorder include relationship difficulties, learning disabilities, ethnicity, pregnancy and the postnatal period, bereavement and social isolation. Many of these factors are more prevalent in inner city populations. The co-existence of mental ill health with physical disorder, other mental disorders, substance misuse and social problems is also common.

The number of cases seen by any given primary care team will reflect both the population served and practice-related factors. The actual numbers of cases that are detected, diagnosed and treated reflect a complex interplay of attitudes, behaviours and knowledge and the resultant nature of the interaction between the patient and the health professional.

Service provision

Primary care is diverse in terms of its organisation, the services offered and the professionals involved. The services for patients with mental ill health that can be provided by primary care practitioners include health promotion; assessment and detection/diagnosis; management, advice and information, treatment including medication, psychological interventions or complementary therapies and referral; follow-up and continuing care of chronic and recurring disease; rehabilitation after illness; and co-ordination of services.

Professionals working in general practice relevant to mental ill health include general practitioners, practice nurses, health visitors, midwives, community psychiatric nurses, clinical psychologists, psychiatrists, psychiatric social workers and psychotherapists. Various agencies outside the practice are also involved, including voluntary organisations and self-help groups.

A variety of models of joint working between specialist mental health, social services and primary health care teams (PHCTs) have been described, although these models describe innovative schemes that are not widely distributed. In many areas links between PHCTs and specialist mental health services are only through referral. These routes may be heavily congested, or even blocked, for those that do not have severe mental illness. The availability of explicit referral criteria or of shared care arrangements, at least in relation to depression, is sparse. Primary care, specialist mental health services and the voluntary sector may work in relative isolation from each other, particularly in the management of less severe mental health problems.

Effectiveness

Determination of the effectiveness of interventions and service models for primary care mental health provision can be difficult and mainly focuses on the severe end of the spectrum of mental health problems. Caution is required in extrapolating the evidence for efficacy in populations in contact with specialist mental health services to patients seen in primary care. In addition, there is relatively little published on the views of people using primary care mental health services, which are an important source of information to help judge the effectiveness of services.

This section summarises the evidence of effectiveness of: health promotion interventions and prevention of mental ill health; the assessment, detection and diagnosis of mental ill health; and the management of mental ill health (including GP care, pharmacological interventions, psychological interventions, self-help and complementary therapies). It also considers improving the assessment, detections and management of mental illness in primary care.

Models of care

There is a consensus that the provision of primary mental health care could be improved but how improvements should be brought about cannot be agreed. The reality is that that there is no one model that will suit all practices and all patients equally, given the diverse nature of primary care and primary care practitioners. The most appropriate model for any particular PHCT is likely to be determined by a number of factors including local demography and prevalence of mental ill health; current organisation of specialist mental health services and the interest of local psychiatrists in primary care issues; the type and local availability of psychological interventions; alternative resource availability; the PHCT's interest in mental health issues and their willingness to extend their roles; and time availability of members of the PHCT to extend their role.

There are some basic questions that need to be addressed by PCTs and individual practices in developing a model of care: which mental health services they wish to provide in the primary care setting; what mix of skills they require to do so and which services they wish to obtain from external agencies. In order to help answer these questions, basic needs assessment must take place at the practice level. This information should be used in conjunction with wider needs assessment work, and mapping of local resource availability (money, people, skills and services). In order for local needs assessment to be useful it should take a holistic, multidisciplinary approach, recognising that many people with mental ill health identify their most pressing needs as employment, housing and personal relationships.

Areas that need to be addressed by a model of care for mental ill health in primary care include the effective assessment of patients, improved detection levels of mental ill health, effective management of those patients identified, the roles of relevant members of the PHCT, the interface between primary and specialist care and the involvement of the voluntary sector and community groups.

2 Introduction and statement of the problem

Introduction

Mental ill health is common and comprises disorders that range in severity from transient reactions to life events to enduring conditions affecting many aspects of psychological and social functioning. Types of disorder include mental illness, personality disorders and substance misuse. Community surveys suggest that at any point in time 23% of the population have psychological symptoms and 14–18% suffer from a mental disorder.[1,2] Over the period of a year this rises to up to 30% of the population. Lifetime risks are significantly higher. Mental ill health will therefore affect all of us at some time; if not ourselves directly, then friends, family or work colleagues.

Whilst the risk of developing any disorder is high, the type and severity of disorder varies enormously. Most mental ill health is mild and self-limiting, much of it not reaching caseness for diagnosis of disorder. A significant proportion is chronic and causes moderate disability, whilst a small number of people suffer life-long, severely disabling illness. Anxiety and depression affect the largest number of people, often occurring in conjunction with relationship and social problems, substance misuse or physical illness.

The majority of all mental ill health seen by health services presents to, and is managed by, primary care practitioners. As with all disorders seen in primary care, some will be dealt with entirely within the primary care setting, for example the majority of cases of depression, whilst others, such as the most severe cases of depression and many cases of schizophrenia, will also involve care provided by specialist mental health services. Inevitably, there is overlap between this chapter and the severe mental illness chapter (HCNA First series, Second edition, 2004 – chapter by John Wing). This chapter concentrates on non-psychotic disorders. Primary care provision for severe mental illness is addressed in the severe mental illness chapter, and is not repeated here. This chapter also does not cover child and adolescent disorders, learning disabilities, substance misuse (drug and alcohol) or the elderly. Most of these groups are discussed in other chapters published in *Health Care Needs Assessment: The epidemiologically based needs assessment reviews*, First series, Second edition, 2004 edited by Andrew Stevens, James Raftery, Jonathan Mant and Sue Simpson (Oxford: Radcliffe Publishing).

Policy context

Mental health policy has, until recently, focused heavily on the need to provide a range of community and inpatient services for those with the most severe illness. Specialist mental health and social services therefore prioritise these patients. The Department of Health's *Health of the Nation Key Area Handbook for Mental Illness* suggests that the role of primary care should be to help with the detection and monitoring of severe disorders and to take responsibility for the care and treatment of those with less severe illness.[3] It also suggests that primary care professionals have a role in preventive activities such as education and advice giving. *Modernising Mental Health Services* highlights the need for primary care to provide mental health services and to collaborate with specialist services.[4] This reinforces the significant emphasis of recent NHS policy on partnership.[5] The *National Service Framework (NSF) for Mental Health* makes primary mental health care of central importance by setting two standards that relate directly to the delivery of mental health care by primary care practitioners.[6]

Standard two says that any service user who contacts their primary health care team with a common mental health problem should have their mental health needs identified and addressed, be offered effective treatments, including referral to specialist services for further assessment, treatment and care if they require it. Standard three says that any individual with a common mental health problem should be able to make contact around the clock with the local service necessary to meet their needs and receive adequate care, and be able to use NHS Direct for first level advice and referral on to specialist helplines or to local services.

The responsibility for implementing standards two and three is with Primary Care Trust (PCT) chief executives. There is also a requirement to develop local referral protocols for depression, eating disorders, anxiety, postnatal depression, schizophrenia, those requiring psychological therapies and drug and alcohol dependence. The standard set for mental health promotion has further implications for primary care practitioners.

The NHS Plan makes specific reference to primary care mental health by creating new graduate primary care mental health workers.[7] One thousand will be trained in brief therapy techniques of proven effectiveness and employed to help GPs manage and treat mental health problems. The Plan also states that there should be a significant increase (500 across the country by 2004) in community mental health staff (now called gateway workers). These staff may work with primary care teams, NHS Direct and/or accident and emergency departments to respond to people who need immediate help.[8]

Suicide reduction remains a national priority; standard seven in the *Mental Health NSF* relates solely to it and a Suicide Prevention Strategy for England was published by the Department of Health in September 2002.

The needs of carers, including those that care for people with mental ill health, is covered in *Caring about carers – national strategy for carers*, and is also a specific standard area within the *Mental Health NSF*.[9] The *NHS Plan* pledges to employ 700 more staff nationally to increase breaks for carers and to strengthen carer networks.

Commissioning

The majority of patients with mental ill health in primary care do not have severe disorders. This can create tension between primary care practitioner's need for advice and support in managing this group and local specialist mental health and social services that prioritise those with severe mental illness. Balancing these competing demands presents both commissioners and providers with a considerable challenge.

A minority of PCTs have taken on community mental health services in contrast to other community services.[10] Evaluation of extended and total fundholding suggested that priorities for primary care commissioning were to:

- increase the number of mental health professionals attached to primary care
- increase the number of outreach clinics provided by mental health practitioners
- improve communication and information exchange with secondary care services.[11]

User involvement, systematic approaches to needs assessment and focusing on the severely mentally ill were lower priorities in most sites analysed. Analysis of the commissioning arrangements in primary care groups in 2000 suggested that the requisite management structures and skills were in relatively short supply.[12] Evaluation of new commissioning arrangements, particularly impact on those with severe mental illness, will be essential. The way in which strategic health authorities and PCTs work together to ensure adequate services for the relatively small numbers of the most severely ill will also need to be assessed.

The burden of disease

The effect of mental ill health on the individual, their relatives and society is profound. International assessment of the extent of mortality and disability caused by different diseases suggests that depression is the greatest burden of disease for women and alcohol misuse the leading cause of disability amongst men in developed regions.[13]

Impact on the individual

Mental ill health may affect all aspects of an individual's life, producing diminution in quality of life, inability to work, maintain social relationships or live an independent life. People with chronic mental health problems, particularly mood disorders, suffer more impairment in their quality of life than individuals with chronic physical conditions such as arthritis, diabetes and back pain and there are clear inter-relationships[14,15] (*see* 'Comorbidity' in section 4).[16]

The functional disabilities experienced by people with different disorders may vary. The UK Psychiatric Morbidity Surveys suggest that people with psychotic illness are most disabled with respect to activities of daily living, particularly activities that require systematic thinking, such as managing money.[17] About half of those with depression, phobias and obsessive compulsive disorders suffer significant interference with the ability to care for themselves, hold down a job or maintain family relationships. People with mixed anxiety and depression are also affected, but to a lesser degree.

Mortality

Mental illness makes a significant contribution to premature mortality. It shortens lives by increasing the risk of suicide and of premature death from physical causes. Overall, the number of excess deaths from natural causes is as great as that from suicide. People with eating disorders or substance misuse are at highest risk, followed by people with schizophrenia and depression.

The majority of people who commit suicide have some form of mental disorder, most frequently depression, at the time of death. It is as yet unclear why there is an association between mental illness and increased mortality from physical conditions.[18] A number of factors are likely to be involved; increased risk behaviours (e.g. smoking), self-neglect, adverse environments, poor professional monitoring of physical health and/or a causal association between mental and physical ill health.[19] The way in which the latter can be explained is not well understood, but in depression for example, there has been shown to be an association between coronary artery disease than cannot be easily explained by other factors.[20] In the US Epidemiological Catchment Area Studies this held true for sub-syndromal depression, as well as major depression.[21] There is an increasing body of evidence linking emotional stress to changes in the functioning of the immune system that may then have an impact on physical health.[22]

Impact on families and carers

Caring for people with mental ill health can be a significant source of strain on individual carers and their families.[23] The total extent of informal care provided by families and friends is significant, but unquantified. Analysis of a group of people who had started antidepressant medication for major depressive disorder suggested that at least 15% of them received help from family and friends with household activity, at an average of 8.5 hours/week.[24]

Impact on society

Financial

The monetary cost of mental disorder is significant in terms of time off work, social security payments, consultations and drug costs. The calculation of the total cost of mental ill health is complex, given the wide range of services that may be utilised, the impact on all aspects of social functioning and on the lives of carers and families. One attempt to calculate the total cost for England and Wales, gave a figure of £32.1 billion/year, £11.8 billion due to lost productivity and employment and NHS services costing £4.1 billion (1996/7 prices).[25] The authors acknowledge that this is likely to be a lower bound estimate as some costs, such as housing benefit claims or elements of the criminal justice system, were not included. Primary care expenditure, from the Department of Health programme budget costing exercise, has been estimated at 3.6% of total NHS expenditure on all mental illness categories (1996).[26]

Other costing exercises have tended to concentrate on specific diagnostic categories. In 1991, the direct costs for the treatment of depression were estimated at £420 million annually for England and Wales. Of that cost, 40% was accounted for by inpatient admission and drug costs were estimated at 11%.[27] The indirect cost of lost productivity was estimated to exceed £3 billion. In 1992, estimates suggested that the overall cost of schizophrenia was £2.6 billion. The health/social care costs for England were £810 million. Although the proportion is decreasing, this represented more than 5% of the total NHS inpatient costs.[28]

Employment

The effect of mental illness on the ability to maintain normal work activities is particularly pronounced.[29] Up to 40–50% of days off work are thought to be secondary to stress-related problems.[30] The CBI and Department of Health estimate that 80 million working days are lost every year as a result of anxiety and depression.[31] The OPCS Psychiatric Morbidity Surveys quantified the number of people out of work or permanently unable to work who had a mental illness (**Table 1**). The figures show the significant impact of both neurotic and psychotic disorders on the ability to maintain work, 10–20% of people in private households being permanently out of work irrespective of diagnosis.

Table 1: Mental ill health and work.

Disorder	Percentage of people in work	Percentage of people permanently unable to work
No disorder	71	2
Any neurosis	56	12
Obsessive/compulsive disorders	50	20
Psychosis living in private households – i.e. 82% of people with psychosis	39	21
Phobias	36	20
Suicidal thoughts	27	16
Psychosis living in long-term accommodation for those with mental illness	14	63
Neurosis living in long-term accommodation for those with mental illness	13	52

Source: OPCS survey[1]

3 Sub-categories

Emotional symptoms are very common in primary care, but do not necessarily mean that the sufferer has a mental disorder. Mental ill health in primary care ranges from sub-syndromal symptoms, i.e. not reaching case definition for disorder, to clear cases of mental disorder which range significantly in severity and the disability they cause. It is the existence of this spectrum that makes it hard to categorise mental ill health in primary care into simple groupings for service planning. At its simplest this is demonstrated by the difficulties in determination of prevalence figures. Determination of the prevalence of disorder is obviously fundamentally determined by the way in which disorder is defined. Studies often use psychiatric classification systems, DSM or ICD, to establish diagnosis, or a severity rating scale to dichotomise individuals into those above or below a threshold. This is problematic, as there is considerable evidence that less severe psychiatric morbidity, commonly seen in primary care, seldom separates out into discrete diagnostic entities.[32,33] It may be better to imagine a continuum where anxiety and depression, for example, behave as highly correlated aspects of the same disorder.[34,35] This view is strengthened by the evidence that the health and social burden of less severe, sub-syndromal, symptoms is considerable.[36–39]

This is acknowledged through the development of the ICD-10 PC (primary care) which uses a new nosology for mental ill health in primary care under 24 condition headings.[40]

Alternate approaches to diagnostic groupings might be to look at levels of care, as described by Goldberg and Huxley.[41] This model shows the relationship between prevalence of disorder and movement through levels of care; the individual recognising their ill health, consulting their GP and the action taken. Estimates of the proportion of individuals found at each tier are shown in **Figure 1**.

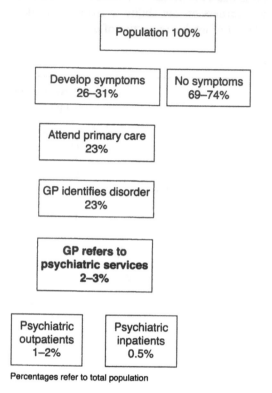

Percentages refer to total population

Source: adapted from Goldberg & Huxley.[41]

Figure 1: Patient flows for adult mental ill health

This provides a useful way of understanding the key relationships within the system of care, but again does not provide categories that easily inform service planning. Both levels of care and ICD-10 PC diagnosis will be used in this chapter to help group the issues under consideration. The main body of the text will address the community and primary care levels and filters of care, discussing mental ill health broadly. Some of the major groups from ICD-10 PC – depression, unexplained somatic complaints, anxiety, adjustment and eating disorders – are discussed in the appendices with cross-references in the main text.

4 Prevalence and incidence

Population prevalence is determined by community-based surveys. The majority of cases of mental illness detected in community surveys are unknown to specialist mental health services, although many will present to primary care (**Figure 1**).

Two national UK prevalence surveys have been carried out.[1,42] Prevalence figures for various diagnoses are shown in **Table 2**. Estimates of the numbers of individuals in an average general practice list of 1800 patients are also shown.

Table 2: Population and estimated general practice prevalence of mental disorder.

Diagnosis	Weekly prevalence per 1,000 adults aged 16–64	Number of patients aged 16–64 on GP list of 1,800 (assumes 63% of GP list is aged 16–64)
Mixed anxiety and depression	77	87
Generalised anxiety	31	36
Depressive episode	21	24
All phobias	11	13
Obsessive-compulsive disorder	12	14
Panic disorder	8	9
All neuroses	160	182
Functional psychoses	4.4	5
Eating disorders	100	

Source: OPCS survey[1]

These surveys suggest that at any one point in time approximately 16% of the general population may be suffering from a diagnosable neurotic disorder and 0.4% from a psychotic illness. Some commentators suggest the figures for neurotic disorder is high as sub-syndromal illness is included. There are significant differences in prevalence in sub-sections of the population. The major factors that affect prevalence are discussed in the following sections.

Factors affecting prevalence

The number of psychiatric cases in a population is strongly associated with the general characteristics of the population from which they are drawn.[43] It is well known that indicators of social deprivation, such as unemployment and homelessness, are associated with an increased prevalence of mental ill health.[44] The burden of illness in any particular general practice will therefore reflect the socio-demographics of the geographical area served by that practice. At its most gross, this is reflected in the differences between urban and rural areas (**Table 3**).

Table 3: Variations in prevalence of mental disorder in adults aged 16–64 living in private households in Great Britain between rural and urban areas in the UK (prevalence per 1000 adults).

Disorder		Urban	Semi-rural	Rural
Neuroses	Women	216	156	150
	Men	133	117	78
Psychoses	Women	5	5	1
	Men	6	5	3

Source: OPCS survey[1]

Socio-demographic factors

There are many variables that are associated with an increased risk of an individual developing mental ill health. At a population and practice level this may help to identify high-risk groups. Some of the characteristics of adults at high risk of developing mental disorder are shown in **Table 4.**

Table 4: Risk factors for development of mental disorder.

- Relationship difficulties; divorce/separation
- Unemployment
- Learning disabilities
- Membership of certain ethnic groups
- Refugees/asylum seekers
- Pregnancy and the postnatal period
- Single parenthood
- Bereavement
- Long-term caring
- Substance misuse
- Social isolation
- Chronic, painful or life-threatening conditions
- Disabilities, especially visual/hearing impairment
- History of sexual/physical abuse
- Homelessness

Source: adapted from Mental health promotion in high risk groups[83]

Many of the characteristics highlighted are more prevalent in inner city populations, explaining some of the increased morbidity. These and other variables are reflected in composite measures of deprivation, such as the Jarman index, which also correlate with high levels of mental ill health.[45]

Comorbidity

The co-existence of mental ill health with physical disorder, other mental disorders, substance misuse and social problems is common. There is a strong, and not yet fully understood, relationship between mental ill health and physical illness (*see* 'Impact on the individual'). Forty percent of those with psychotic disorders and half those with neurotic disorders suffer long-standing physical complaints.[46] People with chronic physical illness also suffer from high rates of mental ill health, particularly depression; the rates reported vary from 25 to 50%.[47] The prevalence of psychiatric disorder in medical patients has been estimated to be in the region of 20%.[48] Surveys also suggest that about 40% of new medical outpatients have symptoms that cannot be easily explained by physical illness.[49] At the extreme end of the spectrum are those with somatiform disorder who may attend a variety of specialists, with multiple complaints (*see* Appendix 3).

Prevalence in primary care populations

Up to 20% of the general population may have a neurotic disorder, whereas 25–50% of the people in a GP's waiting room do.[50,51] Frequent attenders in particular show high levels of disorder.[52] Other estimates suggest that up to 50% of those attending show at least some symptoms of depression, even if not amounting to disorder.[53] This contrasts with the figures reported in the UK GP Morbidity Surveys, which are much lower, around 7% of registered patients consulted for a mental illness within a survey year.[54] The majority of these consultations are for depressive illness. This highlights the relatively low detection/diagnosis and reporting rates from primary care (*see* 'Assessment, detection and diagnosis'). One in five new consultations in primary care are for somatic symptoms for which no specific cause can be found.[55]

Factors affecting prevalence in primary care

The number of cases seen by any given primary care team will reflect both the population served (*see* 'Factors affecting prevalence' above) and practice-related factors. The actual number of cases that are detected, diagnosed and treated reflect a complex interplay of attitudes, behaviours and knowledge and the resultant nature of the interaction between the patient and the health professional (*see* 'Assessment, detection and diagnosis' and 'Management' in section 6).

Practice-related factors

There are a number of practice-related factors that are known to influence the numbers of patients with mental ill health attending a particular general practice.[56] The practice:

- is in a socially deprived area
- is near to group homes for people with mental illness or shelters for people who are homeless
- has partners with an interest in mental disorder
- has a significant refugee or homeless population
- is close to a psychiatric hospital that is closing.

This can lead to a skewed spread of morbidity; in one part of Central London, 32% of psychiatric service users with the most severe illness were registered with 4% of the GPs.[57]

5 Services available

Introduction

Primary care is diverse in terms of its organisation, the services offered and the professionals involved. The services for patients that can be provided by primary care practitioners include:

- health promotion
- assessment and detection/diagnosis
- management, which may include follow-up and 'watchful waiting', advice and information, for example on self-help (sign posting), treatment including medication, psychological interventions or complementary therapies and referral
- follow-up and continuing care of chronic and recurring disease
- rehabilitation after illness
- co-ordination of services.

The Royal College of General Practitioners defines the core primary health care team (PHCT) as comprising general practitioners, practice nurses, community nurses, health visitors, practice managers and administrative staff. It is acknowledged that it may also be appropriate to define other staff, such as counsellors, as part of the team depending on the circumstances.[58]

This section describes the professional groups that may be involved in providing primary care mental health services, the interface between primary care and specialist mental health services and voluntary sector services.

Professional groups

The number of staff working in general practice rose by 20% between 1992 and 1997.[59] A survey of representative practices in England and Wales in 1992 showed the following professionals (in addition to general practitioners, GPs) to be working on site in general practices: practice nurses (97% of practices), health visitors (83%), community psychiatric nurses (CPNs, 34%), clinical psychologists (12%), psychiatrists (9%), psychiatric social workers (6%), psychotherapists (3%).[60] A study of 82 practices in West and East Surrey reported that professionals who provided mental health services in primary care included health visitors, midwives, practice nurses and counsellors, as well as GPs. Various agencies outside the practice are also involved, including voluntary organisations and self-help groups.[61] Receptionists may also have a role in mental health provision, as they are often the first point of contact between the public and the primary health care team.

Generic primary care practitioners

General practitioners

In 1999, there were approximately 33 000 GPs in England and Wales. An increase across the whole UK of 17% since 1985.[62] The number of female GPs and female GP registrars increased significantly. In 1999, 57% of GP registrars were female.

There is an increasing trend towards multi-partner practices. In 1997, there were approximately 9500 partnerships in England and Wales. Only 10% of practices were single-handed in England and 23% in

Wales.[63] In 1991/2, GPs across the country saw approximately 78% of the population at least once during the year. The proportion of the population consulting had risen by 7% since 1981/2.[64]

The role of the GP includes illness detection, diagnosis, prescribing, support, advocacy, information giving, monitoring health status, referral to other services and providing continuing care.

GPs vary greatly in how much training relating to mental ill health they have received. Studies consistently show a low uptake by GPs of education related to mental health/illness. A survey of 190 randomly selected GPs from 95 Health Authorities in England and Wales showed that only 35% had undertaken any course on mental health in the last three years.[65] Recent courses undertaken are often related to severe mental illness.[66] Only half of all GP trainees have completed a psychiatric training post. Many report that their training was a little value in helping them to meet the mental health needs of patients in a primary care setting. Training in psychological therapies and counselling has been highlighted as a gap.[67]

Primary care nurses

Primary care nurses include practice nurses, health visitors, district and school nurses (the term 'community nurse' is being increasingly used to refer to district nurses). The provision of mental health education for primary care nurses is sparse, with the exception of training health visitors in detecting and managing postnatal depression.

- **Practice nurses:** There are approximately 40 000 practice nurse posts in the UK, a whole-time equivalent number of between 25 000 and 30 000, approximately the same as the number of GPs. Their role usually includes health promotion activities, new registration checks, assisting with immunisations and some disease-specific clinics. In some practices they may also be involved in supervising computer-administered psychological treatment. Practice nurse work patterns vary tremendously, but between 13% and 43% state that early identification of anxiety and depression is a routine task.[68,69] They are asked for and offer advice and support, but report inadequate training for this aspect of their role. The gaps identified related to depression, anxiety and psychotropic medication.[70,71] Many practice nurses administer depot antipsychotic medication, a role for which many have no appropriate training.[72] A small minority have received formal mental health training.[73]
- **Health visitors:** In 1996, there were approximately 9600 health visitors in England and Wales.[74] They provide health promotion advice and education, particularly for families with children under 5. A Scottish survey showed that 69% of health visitors had some training in mental health, most frequently relating to postnatal depression and the use of the Edinburgh postnatal depression scale, but also in anxiety management, counselling and bereavement. The majority said that they had a role in detecting mental ill health. This was mainly postnatal depression, but depression in general, assessment of the elderly, bereavement and marital problems were also mentioned.[75]
- **District nurses:** In 1994, there were approximately 8500 district nurses in England.[76] Their role includes looking after the chronically ill, frail and those discharged from hospital. As a consequence they see many patients who are at risk of mental ill health, particularly arising from disability, chronic ill health or bereavement. They rarely receive mental health related training.

Pharmacists

Pharmacists can work as part of the PHCT or as community practitioners. They can help with prescribing advice for both other practitioners and patients.

Mental health practitioners

The closure of large psychiatric hospitals has contributed to the increase in community working by mental health professionals, including the increasing numbers working in primary care settings. This movement into primary care has been described as the 'silent growth of a new service'.[77] The impact on primary care workload is difficult to estimate, although there are some suggestions that, at least for some practices, it has led to an increase.[78,79] Links between general practices and mental health professionals are now common, but unevenly spread across the country. Some practices, often large, innovative ones, have multiple links with several types of professional, while others have no links at all.[80] It has been suggested that the frequency of links relate more to a GP's interest in mental health and/or the physical capacity of the premises than to local need.[81]

Community psychiatric nurses (CPNs)

National policy has encouraged CPNs to target people with severe mental illness. Many, however, work with less severe disorders.[82] A growing number of CPNs have been trained in assertive community treatment and psychosocial interventions for people with schizophrenia. Few have formal training in methods suitable for non-psychotic patients. One survey suggested that 41% of CPNs engaged in counselling in general practice had no formal qualifications in counselling, problem solving, cognitive/behavioural approaches or other psychotherapies.[83]

Psychiatrists

The numbers of psychiatrists nationally rose by a factor of 3.5 between 1966 and 1995. The ratio of psychiatrists to GPs consequently changed over the same period from 1:32.2 to 1:12.5.[84]

The current training of psychiatrists rarely includes formal attachments in primary care, or training in consultation, liaison and supervision skills that may assist in relating to and advising primary care staff.

Psychologists, counsellors and psychotherapists

The way in which these professional groups are employed in primary care varies enormously. They may be directly employed by the practice, be self-employed with contracts that are held by individual practices or be part of managed services. Alternatively, individuals may be part of specialist mental health services providing services to PHCTs.

The number of professionals employed, particularly counsellors, has increased rapidly since GP fundholding. Access to psychological therapies across the country, however, remains very varied with significant waiting lists in many areas.[85] Counsellors and psychologists are more often found in large, multi-partner, ex-fundholding practices. This distribution is likely to change with the growth of PCTs. Space availability within practices may, however, remain a limiting factor. Approximately half the practices in England employ some type of counsellor, the most commonly employed provider of primary care psychological interventions.

The experience and training of professionals providing psychological interventions is varied. Consequently, so are the types of interventions. An early study of a small number of counsellors suggested that a significant minority did not have appropriate formal training.[86] Research that is more recent suggests that the majority are appropriately trained and supervised.[87]

Occupational therapists (OTs)

The work of OTs is increasingly based in the community. It is likely that GPs welcome this, although there may be lack of clarity over the nature of interventions that OTs can provide.[88] Generally OTs in primary care focus on the ability of individuals to execute activities of daily living effectively, efficiently and meaningfully. This might include helping reduce social and environmental stressors by improving coping strategies, input into employment training or enhancing social skills and networks.[89,90]

The primary/specialist care interface

A variety of models of joint working between specialist mental health, social services and PHCTs have been described (**Table 5**).[91] By and large, however, these models describe innovative schemes that are not widely distributed. In many areas, links between PHCTs and specialist mental health services are only through referral. These routes may be heavily congested, or even blocked, for those that do not have severe mental illness. The formal liaison schemes that do exist often focus on the provision of shared care for the most severely ill.[92]

The availability of explicit referral criteria or of shared care arrangements, at least in relation to depression, is sparse.[93] Primary care, specialist mental health services and the voluntary sector may work in relative isolation from each other, particularly in the management of less severe mental health problems.[94]

Community and voluntary groups

There are a variety of self-help groups for people with mental ill health and their carers. *Saneline* maintains an extensive database that provides information about local resources. They also operate a national mental health helpline which offers practical information to anyone coping with mental illness whether a sufferer, carer, family member or professional. The *Help for Health Trust* is another national source of information on self-help groups. *NHS Direct* also gives out mental health information. The *National Council for Voluntary Organisations* publishes an annual Voluntary Agencies Directory. Most national voluntary organisations are listed, indexed by subject, and those with local groups are clearly marked. The computer-held version of ICD-10-PC includes national organisations; primary care workers can add information on local self-help and voluntary sector agencies under each condition heading.

Positive examples of close partnership working between individual general practices and community organisations or volunteer members of the practice population do exist, but are relatively unusual.[95]

Some voluntary organisations have developed schemes combining mutual support and educational programmes based on psychological interventions of known effectiveness, although the actual programmes may not have been evaluated. **Table 6** describes some of these.

Table 5: Summary of the models of joint working between secondary mental health and social services and GPs.[238,432–3]

Model	Description
Model 1: Secondary care-based CMHTs liaise with primary care	Mechanisms for doing this include: • The regular liaison meeting: A senior mental health professional attends the PHCT's meeting. Discussion focuses mostly on the management of individual patients. • The relocation of outpatient clinics from hospital to community sites. Most widely used by psychiatrists, who see both new and follow-up patients. Treatment may be relatively independent of the GP (shifted outpatient model). • The 'attached mental health professional': Professionals attached to primary care, but still employed by secondary care services. The opportunity exists for the attached professionals to be used for consultation rather than direct patient care, but this seems to be the exception rather than the norm.
Model 2: The integrated 'consultation liaison' model	Specialised services are provided through secondary care with the express aim of improving the quality of the PHCT-CMHT relationship and developing the capacity of the PHCT to work effectively with people with less severe mental health problems. Components may include: joint case registers of the long-term mentally ill, development of good practice protocols, liaison practitioners attached to practices, joint audit of care, and CMHTs sectorised around practice lists rather than geographical areas.
Model 3: The 'specialist function' approach	The CMHT divides into specialist teams providing specific functions. These typically include crisis intervention and support, assertive outreach, continuing care, primary care liaison and psychological therapies. This latter team has the responsibility for leading the development of the relationship with PHCTs and providing services within primary care settings for people with non-severe mental illness.
Model 4: The integrated model within primary care	A primary care-led model which involves most aspects of community mental health care being integrated within the primary care team. Characteristics of this model include a key worker (usually a CPN) who, although part of the CMHT, is integrated into the primary care team. This person usually acts as key worker for patients in the practice, and has a role in other aspects of care, e.g. continuing education of generalist nurses. CMHTs are aligned to practice lists and there is sessional psychologist and/or counsellor time provided within the practice for the management of people with less severe mental disorders.

Table 6: Voluntary and community groups offering self-help programmes.

Group	Description
Manic Depression Fellowship	With the aim of helping people prevent relapse, the Fellowship has recently developed a structured, evaluated, 10-session training programme (available for purchase) to train trainers in the self-management of manic depression. It covers awareness, coping strategies and self-medication.
Triumph over Phobia	Provide a national network of structured self-help groups using self-exposure (behaviour therapy) techniques with the aim of turning members into ex-members. People with phobias and obsessive-compulsive disorders learn, in a supportive group environment, how to measure, monitor and reduce their anxiety levels.
No Panic	Telephone helpline (01952 590545), self-help groups and telephone groups for sufferers of phobias, obsessive-compulsive disorders and other anxiety disorders, including tranquilliser withdrawal. Self-help techniques are based on cognitive-behavioural therapy.
Hearing Voices Network	There is some evidence that self-help coping methods can help users in dealing with their voices; this is particularly relevant for the large minority of people for whom medication is not effective in this respect. Details of Hearing Voices groups and of training packages for professionals who work with people who hear voices. Hearing Voices Network. Dale House, 35 Dale Street, Manchester M1. Tel: 0161 228 3896.
Eating Disorders Association	Provide a 10-week telephone self-help programme to bulimic women under the medical supervision of their GP. Participants must be normal weight for height and not abusing alcohol or drugs. The bulimic patient contacts the EDA and pays £150, which covers 45 minutes of targeted counselling by telephone weekly for 10 weeks, plus follow-up calls after one month and then three-monthly for two years. The patient agrees to eat three meals a day, keep a diary to record food and feelings, attend the GP surgery weekly to be weighed and write the weight in the diary before sending it to the EDA counsellor. GPs can suggest to suitable patients that they consider entering the scheme and may fund their programme. Contact with EDA must be made by the patient on 01603 621414 (helpline). Sackville Place, 44 Magdalen Street, Norwich NR3 1JU.

6 Effectiveness

Introduction

The limitations of research evidence

Determination of the effectiveness of interventions and service models for primary care mental health provision faces a number of difficulties that are outlined below.

- Most research is of treatments for definable, single, psychiatric conditions in inpatient or outpatient populations. Patients with less severe, mixed presentations and comorbid conditions, the kind most frequently seen in primary care, are often excluded.[96]
- The typical patient taking part in research may be better motivated than a primary care patient, who may be more reluctant to accept a psychiatric diagnosis and may be less inclined to concur with suggested treatment plans.
- The nature and duration of consultations in primary and specialist mental health care differ. The average general practice consultation is nine minutes. The usual assessment consultation in a psychiatric outpatient clinic is significantly longer. In addition, in an outpatient clinic the patient has already been assessed as likely to have a psychiatric problem, at an initial appointment in primary care this has to be determined.
- The extent of morbidity in primary care suggests that interventions should be targeted at those most likely to benefit. There is still a relative paucity of research to inform prediction of poor outcome for an individual presenting with mental ill health, particularly depression and anxiety (*see* 'The outcome of disorder' below). The capacity to target interventions effectively is thus limited.

Considerable caution is therefore required in extrapolating the evidence for efficacy in populations in contact with specialist mental health services as against patients seen in primary care. For instance, it is known that antidepressants are effective in 60–70% of people who are treated for major depression in inpatient and outpatient settings. There is less research on the effectiveness of the same antidepressants in primary care settings.[97] It is likely that, to achieve similar rates of efficacy in this population, it would be necessary to mimic some of the characteristics of outpatient populations. This would include selecting for treatment only those patients with depression of sufficient severity (excluding those with mild depression), coupled with follow-up appointments to ensure that the medication is acceptable to the patient and actually being taken by them. Similar issues arise with respect to evidence for the effectiveness of psychological and other interventions.

The outcome of disorder

The evaluation of interventions in primary care requires some understanding of the natural history of the disorders that commonly present. Although still poorly understood, research suggests that half of all mental disorders seen in primary care are mild and transient. The other half of the common disorders (depression and anxiety) are chronic, recurrent and last longer than a year.[98] Research suggests a number of factors that may predict the resolution of disorder. Follow-up of 100 patients in Warwickshire, who were identified by their GPs as having psychiatric illness and who scored highly on the general health questionnaire (GHQ), showed 49% not to be cases at one year. Overall severity at entry was the best predictor of caseness at the end of the year. Other factors associated with continued disorder included reduced social support, previous psychiatric history, the presence of physical illness and increasing age.[99]

An understanding of the chronic and relapsing nature of mental ill health in primary care, particularly depression, is important. Control groups are essential in order to take into account the proportion of illness that resolves spontaneously. Follow-up and treatment maintenance periods need to be adequate given the chronicity often seen.

The views of people with mental ill health

There is relatively little published research on the views of people using primary care mental health services. An understanding of their views is, however, an important source of information to help judge service effectiveness.[100,101] A study in Scotland elicited the views of members of general practice populations about the care that they expect and receive from primary care for less severe mental health problems.[102] The following was found:

- most people in distress want someone to listen to them and give them time
- people derive benefit from mutual support, given by others in similar situations, although a sizeable proportion of individuals, particularly men, are reluctant to join groups
- people want a combination of different kinds of help
- men are less likely than women to look to their GP for help with emotional problems
- people expect their GP to provide a sympathetic ear and to be able to give advice
- medication is regarded with considerable caution
- people are widely aware of counselling, but are unlikely to seek it unless suggested by someone like their GP.

Published effectiveness research rarely includes consideration of these sorts of issues even at the simplest of levels, for example, giving gender breakdown.

Health promotion and prevention

The percentage of people in low-risk groups who develop mental disorder is significantly smaller than that in high-risk groups, but there are many more of them. A health promotion strategy that is targeted solely at high-risk individuals will therefore be limited in its capacity to reduce the overall prevalence of common mental disorders.[103,104]

Strategies for the general population

Little research has been carried out in the general population. Successful preventive strategies often seek to increase the capacity of individuals to control their own lives and make maximum use of natural community support.[105]

Some approaches have been shown to have beneficial effects.

- Promoting good social relationships, e.g. through social skills training. Relationship skills training for couples has been shown to reduce the rate of break-up and divorce.[106]
- Developing effective coping skills, e.g. problem solving and parenting skills.[107]
- Providing social support and making social changes, e.g. changing attitudes to bullying in schools. Multi-faceted, school-based programmes are suggested to reduce levels of bullying, vandalism, theft and truancy.[108]
- Encouraging aerobic exercise may help mild to moderate depression and increase the capacity to deal effectively with stress[109] (see Appendix 1).

Strategies for high-risk groups

The evidence for effective interventions is better in high-risk groups. The following interventions have been shown to have benefits.[110]

- Antenatal and postnatal support groups have been shown to reduce postnatal depression significantly in first-time, vulnerable mothers.
- Widow to widow self-help groups have been shown to accelerate progress through stages of normal grieving.
- Promoting coping skills and offering respite care has been shown to reduce levels of strain in people caring for highly dependent relatives.
- Job search and problem-solving skills have been shown to benefit depressed, financially strained, unemployed adults with low assertiveness.
- Teaching specific parenting skills to parents of 7–8-year-old boys, identified as disruptive in school, has been shown to reduce the number of subsequent problems.

However, a population-based approach of social interventions targeted at high-risk individuals has been less successful at producing a decrease in prevalence in common mental disorders.[111]

Suicide prevention

The average GP only sees one case of suicide every 4–5 years.[112] Early studies showed that most people who committed suicide had seen their GP in the preceding four weeks.[113] Research that is more recent suggests that this proportion may have dropped to under half, 20% seeing their GP in the previous week.[114,115] This may relate to the number of suicides in young men, who visit their GP less frequently than other groups.

Approximately 25% of people who commit suicide in England and Wales have been in contact with mental health services in the previous year.[116] It was judged that 85% were at little immediate risk at the time of their final contact with those services, highlighting the difficulties inherent in accurate clinical quantification of suicide risk.

A small, uncontrolled, study in Gotland, Sweden suggested that improving recognition and management of depression in general practice could reduce the suicide rate.[117] However, at follow-up these effects appeared transient. A much larger British study was unable to demonstrate any connection between training GPs in recognition and management of depression and suicide rates[118] (*see* 'Staff training and education' below).

Evidence on the effectiveness of GPs in preventing suicide is thus contradictory. Solely providing training for GPs in identifying people at risk of suicide is unlikely to have a significant impact on the suicide rate.

Physical health of people with mental illness

The effectiveness of the delivery of physical health care for people with mental illness by primary care practitioners is not well researched. It is, however, recognised that much physical illness in psychiatric patients is unrecognised and assessment and monitoring of physical health by specialist mental health services is generally unsatisfactory.[119] A US study suggests that using a structured approach can be effective in detecting physical illness in patients with schizophrenia. However, the subsequent impact on outcome is unclear.[120] Primary care practitioners are well placed to provide physical health monitoring and continuing care.

Assessment, detection and diagnosis

Studies suggest that, on average, GPs detect about half of the people with mental disorder (according to screening questionnaire) who present to them.[121,122] What in actuality 'detection' represents is complex and related to both GP and patient factors (*see* below). Average detection rates hide wide variations between individual doctors and rates improve over time, with repeat consultations.[123] There is relatively less research on detection by other primary care practitioners. The rate of detection of depression by practice nurses has been reported as 23% and by health visitors 50%; the rate for district nurses is unknown.[124,125]

GP-related factors

Case definition

Most patients seen in primary care do not have a neat constellation of symptoms that conform to case definitions. GPs have identified inadequate nosology as a factor influencing the apparent low detection of mental disorder.[126] Some authors suggest that variance in detection relates primarily to GPs differing attitudes to ascribing a psychological component to illness aetiology.[127] GPs may be reluctant to label patients, fearing rejection by the patient, given the inevitable stigma associated with a psychiatric diagnosis.[128,129] In addition, multiple visits and assessments mean that diagnosis and management strategies are not determined at a single point in time. It may be that it is the severity of symptomatology, rather than a diagnosis, which determines management.

GP attributes and behaviour

Certain behaviours on the part of the GP are more likely to elicit symptomatology, both somatic and psychological, than are others. The factors associated with the accurate detection of mental disorder include, establishing eye contact, clarifying the presenting complaint, direct questioning about psychosocial matters and making frequent empathetic responses.[130] Doctors who are good detectors also seem to be better at giving information and advice.[131] Poor interviewing skills, in conjunction with short consultations, may reduce the rate of detection of psychosocial problems.[132,133]

GP knowledge and training

It has been suggested that both post-graduate training in psychiatry and an interest in psychiatry improve the capacity of GPs to detect mental ill health. Doctors with high levels of psychological sensitivity, however, also score better in tests of factual knowledge of medicine, suggesting a generalised, rather than specific, competence.[134,135]

Patient-related factors

Presentation

Detection is affected by the way in which patients present their problems. Generally, the combination of physical complaints and mental ill health impedes recognition of the latter.[136–139] In one study GPs recognised half of the patients who complained of somatic symptoms who could be persuaded to reframe them in psychological terms, but only 19% of those who complained of somatic symptoms who were highly resistant to recognising the psychological component. Only 11% of those who presented with physical illness and coincidental mental health problems were recognised.[140]

Other aspects of presentation are also important. Patients who tend to normalise their symptoms, i.e. minimise their importance, are common in general practice and are less likely to have their depression and anxiety diagnosed.[141]

Other factors

Higher rates of identification of psychological disorder have been reported in women, the middle age groups and the unemployed.[142–146] Severe disorders tend to be recognised more frequently.[147–154]

Doctor/patient interaction

The interaction between doctor and patient is clearly important in the detection and management of disorder. It has been suggested that patients give more cues to the doctor when the doctor uses an open interview style, good eye contact etc.[155]

It is also possible that patients self-impose restraints on the length of consultations that could impede recognition of mental ill health.[156]

Management

General practitioner care

Given the transitory nature of most mental ill health in primary care, the most appropriate management strategy in cases where there is no clear-cut disorder may well be to continue to provide good quality 'treatment as usual'. This may include listening, reassurance, information giving, negotiating the causes of symptoms, advising about coping strategies, homework diaries and follow-up visits. This sort of follow-up approach is sometimes referred to as 'watchful waiting'. Whilst this area is relatively under-researched, one study suggests that this approach may be effective for about half the people with 'minor affective disorders'.[157]

'Treatment as usual' is often used as a control group for studies of mental health interventions in primary care (*see* 'Psychological interventions' below). A meta-analysis of studies comparing treatment (including counselling, behavioural therapy and general psychiatry) by mental health professionals in general practice surgeries with 'treatment as usual' has suggested that mental health professionals of all kinds have a 10% greater success rate than the 'treatment as usual' group.[158] Further research in this area is needed.

Pharmacological interventions

The effectiveness (shown in RCTs) of the major groups of drugs used in the treatment of mental ill health in general practice is summarised below.

- Antidepressants are effective, at least when used in recommended doses, although there remains controversy over the relative cost-effectiveness of different classes of drugs. Antidepressants are most effective in severe episodes of depression. Concern over the adequacy of primary care prescribing with respect to both dose and duration is regularly highlighted in research.[159] Some practitioners advocate low-dose prescribing. However, robust evidence for its effectiveness is lacking (*see* Appendix 1).[160]

- Antipsychotic drugs are effective for the treatment of initial episodes of psychosis, for maintenance of remission and for the treatment of relapse.
- Mood stabilising drugs, such as lithium and carbamazepine, are effective in bipolar disorder.
- Anxiolytics, predominantly benzodiazepines, are useful in the very short-term treatment of anxiety disorders or as short-term hypnotics (*see* Appendix 2).

Primary care nurses and pharmacotherapy

Primary care nurses are often involved in depot neuroleptic administration. Their current effectiveness in this role must be questioned as it has been found that they may not be actively involved in monitoring symptomatology or drug side effects. In addition, in many cases, their knowledge of schizophrenia, its treatment and of drug side effects may be limited. This suggests the need for training, if they are to provide this function.[161,162]

Practice nurses may also be involved in follow-up of patients on antidepressants. Some studies have suggested that there is little difference in adherence to medication and outcome in patients followed-up by nurses and GPs.[163,164] However, an RCT has suggested that nurse-led drug counselling and information leaflets can improve outcome for those with major depression.[165] Trained practice nurses can also increase the proportion of patients who receive psychotherapy or pharmacotherapy for major depression.[166]

Psychological interventions

A wide range of psychological interventions is available, and clear evidence for the effectiveness of some.[167,168] The short-term effectiveness of cognitive/behavioural techniques, problem solving, inter-personal therapy and counselling in eating disorders, depression and anxiety disorders has been shown (*see* relevant appendices). Cognitive approaches may also be effective in the prevention of relapse, as well as an initial treatment for mild to moderate depression.[169] Longer-term outcomes for effective therapies in primary care are, however, less clear.

The effectiveness of counselling in primary care has received considerable attention and continues to provoke debate, although there is now more research in the field. Research has suggested the following.

- Counselling without additional interventions such as practical help, mutual self-help or training in coping skills has not been shown to produce sustained benefits in high-risk groups.[170]
- Brief counselling compared with routine GP care in an RCT found that GPs were as effective as counselling. Patients, however, preferred the counselling.[171]
- CPNs providing unstructured, supportive counselling to patients in primary care showed no benefit over routine GP care and intervention was costly.[172]
- Brief counselling by an experienced mental health professional compared with antidepressant use in primary care showed no significant differences in effectiveness between the two groups (RCT).[173]
- Similarly, a brief problem-solving approach has been suggested to be as effective as pharmacotherapy for major depression in primary care at 12-week follow-up (RCT).[174]
- More rigorously applied non-directive counselling compared to cognitive-behavioural counselling (in combination with antidepressants if prescribed by the GP) and usual GP care showed better self-reported outcomes for both therapy groups at four months, but not at 12, with no significant increase in cost.[175]

The apparent effectiveness of brief therapy approaches is important because of their potential to be widely applied in the primary care setting. Further work is needed on the impact of patient preference, (usually for counselling, which can reduce randomisation in published trials), the impact of severity on outcome, comparison of generic counselling with more standardised specific approaches, long-term outcomes, cost-effectiveness and primary care practitioners as therapists.

Therapist characteristics

Although there is clear evidence for the effectiveness of some psychological therapies, this is in part determined by their being delivered by appropriately trained and supported professionals. **Table 7** summarises the key characteristics of effective therapists. Research suggests that the single best predictor of a positive outcome is the establishment of a good 'therapeutic alliance' or working relationship between therapist and client.

Table 7: The factors that make psychological therapists effective.

Factor	Comments
Effective intervention is used	The effectiveness of different types of mental health professional depends not on the professional group to which they belong but on whether they are trained to provide interventions of proven effectiveness.
Quality of delivery of the intervention	Effectiveness is linked to the training and experience of the practitioner in the therapies used. It is not linked to the possession or otherwise of a professional mental health qualification.
Therapist and patient able to make a 'therapeutic alliance'	Not all therapists can work with all patients. There is some evidence that better outcomes are achieved where patient and therapist come from similar backgrounds. This has particular implications for therapy for people from minority ethnic communities.
Patient characteristics and preferences taken into account	Matching patients to their preferred treatment results in fewer treatment drop-outs and better clinical outcomes. Patients may prefer a shorter treatment or may be more of less willing to explore their life experiences.

Self-help

Some voluntary self-help groups have developed self-help programmes, others are available for use on computers or are taught in classes in general practice. Research is still at an early stage, but promising results include:

* Interactive, CD-ROM cognitive behavioural therapy and assisted bibliography for anxiety have been developed and piloted in GP surgeries. A small amount of staff supervision is required. A similar approach, BT Steps, uses the telephone to provide computerised help for people with obsessive-compulsive disorder.[176,177]
* Use of a self-help manual is an effective first step in the treatment of bulimia. In a study comparing individual cognitive/behavioural therapy, the use of a self-help manual and a waiting list control group, almost as many people using the self-help manual obtained full remission as the therapy group (*see* Appendix 5).[178]
* Teaching self-care skills (relaxation, stress management, meditation, nutrition and exercise) to people with anxiety and medical conditions thought to have a psychological basis may lead to significant improvements. These were maintained at one-year follow-up (*see* Appendix 2).[179]

Self-help approaches appear to be popular with patients and can extend clinician capacity. They are not, however, a substitute for professional help. Further evaluation of their use in primary care is required, using larger study numbers and examining their cost-effectiveness.[180]

Complementary therapies

Research, policy and practice in relation to the use of complementary and alternative therapies for a wide range of mental health problems was reviewed in 1998.[181] The strongest effectiveness evidence currently available is for hypericum or St John's Wort (which has monoamine oxidase inhibitor properties), with some evidence for exercise and transcendental meditation (see **Table 8**).[182,183] More robust research, with larger sample sizes and longer follow-up periods, is needed to confirm reported findings.

Table 8: The effectiveness of complementary therapies.

Type of therapy	Disorder	Outcomes	Type of research
Transcendental meditation	Anxiety and distress, including PTSD	Reduction of anxiety, significantly more effective than relaxation methods	Case reports and clinical trials
Acupuncture	Anxiety and depression	Claimed as effective as amitriptyline	RCTs, but doubts expressed as results of Chinese research are said to be always positive
Hypericum (St John's Wort)	Mild to moderate depression	As effective as antidepressants, fewer side effects	Review of RCTs
Healing	Chronic anxiety and depression	Improved scores on quality-of-life questionnaire	Small outcome study, no control group
Massage	Anxiety and depression	Lower anxiety and depression scores	Small, controlled trials
Aromatherapy – citrus oils	Severe depression	Replaced antidepressants in sample group	Small, controlled but not blind trial
Reflexology	Anxiety	Drop in self-rated anxiety	Small, controlled trial
Hypnotherapy	Bulimia	As effective as CBT	Small, controlled trial
Exercise and yoga	Anxiety and depression	Reduced depression using BDI, reduced stress	Review of RCT, but methodological limitations

Improving assessment, detection and management in primary care

Current approaches to reducing the individual and public health burden of mental ill health depend largely on attempts to increase recognition rates and apply treatments more effectively through primary care.[184,185] Improving detection is only a valid activity if it can be shown that outcome is also improved. There is some evidence that this is the case, although it is disputed.[186] A European, naturalistic study on the impact of detection and treatment of depression in primary care showed that at one year follow-up 60% of those treated were still cases, as were 50% of those that were not detected, although these cases were less severe.[187] A smaller study suggested that patients with major depressive disorder, who were not recognised, had a worse outcome at three months than those prescribed moderate doses of antidepressants.[188] Similarly, patients whose GPs were optimistic about their outcome and did not prescribe antidepressants fared worse than those who were treated.[189]

Studies looking at methods for changing clinical practice consistently indicate that a range of different methods are likely to have more effect than any one intervention on its own.[190] There are many approaches to changing practice including: educational materials, conferences, outreach visits, utilising local opinion leaders, patient-mediated interventions, reminders, marketing, local consensus processes, guidelines, audit and feedback. Evaluation of different approaches suggests that the effectiveness of interventions may be improved by:

- using the practice premises as the venue for continuing education, so that activities can focus on using practitioners' own experience[191]
- ongoing training schemes, with learning reinforced at intervals[192]
- ensuring that education is 'owned' and desired by the learner, is connected to any changes in service provision and is accepted by the team as a whole
- delivering training to the whole PHCT, rather than individuals.[193]

Attempts to improve detection and treatment of mental ill health have adopted a number of approaches:

- screening
- training and education, particularly education from 'experts' using educational materials such as consensus statements or clinical practice guidelines[194,195]
- consultation/liaison by specialist mental health practitioners[196]
- audit and feedback[197]
- multi-faceted interventions.

The following sections address some of these approaches in greater detail.

Screening

Many opportunities exist in primary care to screen for mental ill health, for example at new patient, well woman, well man, elderly and antenatal checks and during child health surveillance. Research suggests the following:

- few GPs use formal screening tools for depression or assessment of suicide risk[198]
- screening for risk factors for depression and anxiety during, for example, new patient interviews is acceptable to both patients and practitioners[199]
- however, case finding for depression and anxiety, using screening questionnaires such as the GHQ or HAD, followed by GP treatment of identified cases, has not been shown to lead to improved outcome when used routinely[200,201]
- the Edinburgh postnatal depression scale is widely used by health visitors and community midwives and it offers a reliable method of detecting clinically significant depression in postnatal women.[202,203]

The lack of demonstrable effectiveness for routine, unselected screening is likely to be the result of a number of factors.[204]

- Recognition by clinicians of the high rate of false positives produced by screening questionnaires and their consequent reluctance to use them.

- Clinicians may be unsure how to manage cases identified. Feedback on cases found by screening is found to be most effective when accompanied by an educational programme and another agency taking responsibility for management.
- There may be methodological issues of cross-contamination, i.e. because the clinician is aware that they will receive screening information feedback on some patients they may manage all patients differently, thus diluting any benefit.

Despite these negative findings some suggest that screening questionnaires may be useful by helping GPs confirm a diagnosis, agree that diagnosis with the patient and for monitoring progress.[205,206]

Staff training and education

Research suggests that improvements can be made in clinicians' ability to detect disorder. This is at least true for selected groups of doctors, undergoing intensive packages of education, which have acquisition of skills as their foundation.

- Before and after evaluation of intensive video feedback education with small groups of GPs and GP trainees shows that psychiatric skills can be improved. Improvement in clinical outcome has also been shown for patients with depression and anxiety. Patients felt that their problems were better understood.[207] The length of interviews apparently does not differ between the trained and untrained groups.[208]
- Training GPs in re-attribution skills, i.e. helping patients recognise the psychological causes of apparently physical problems, can result in significant improvements in both the symptoms and social functioning of patients. Reduction in health care expenditure can also be achieved through reduction in referrals of nearly a quarter, without corresponding increases in primary care costs.[209]
- Skills to improve the assessment and management of suicide risk can be taught, and GP confidence increase.[210]

It is unclear, however, whether these approaches can be generalised to less motivated practitioners and to larger groups. Experience with more didactic approaches to education has, despite initial optimism, not been shown to have lasting effects. Some uncontrolled studies have suggested that it might be possible to deliver effective educational programmes to larger groups.

- In Sweden, all GPs on the island of Gotland (n=18, population 60 000) were educated using a didactic seminar approach delivered by a psychiatrist.[211] A reduction in sick leave for depression, hospital referrals and suicide rates was shown compared to the mainland. There was also an increase in antidepressant prescribing which was maintained over four years.
- In the UK, a nurse-led, practice-based educational programme was been shown to produce a 7% increase in the recognition of the psychological nature of illnesses by GPs.[212]

The results of the Hampshire Depression Project have not been so promising.[213] The project covered 60 practices in Hampshire and aimed to increase adherence to a depression management protocol. After participation in the seminars 80% of GPs agreed that they would change their management of depression. No differences between educated and control groups in the GP's recognition of depression were found. The group of patients who were recognised as depressed by the GPs were more likely to have improved six weeks later if their GP had recently completed the seminar education, but at one year there was no difference between groups. Similar negative findings have been reported from the US.[214]

These findings emphasise that the production of guidelines and didactic teaching are unlikely to be sufficient to make a significant impact on the outcomes of mental ill health in primary care. Future educational programmes might usefully concentrate on skill acquisition and better management rather than detection alone (*see* 'Consultation/liaison' below). Other issues that need to be addressed are the reliance of many training courses on the enthusiasm of a particular researcher/trainer delivering training to a motivated, self-selected group of participants. This has implications for further dissemination by less motivated trainers and to less motivated learners.[215]

Consultation/liaison

In contrast to the educational model of improving care there have been good outcomes from two randomised-controlled studies in Seattle using a multidisciplinary model; intensive patient education, behavioural interventions from a psychologist, medication adherence counselling and alternating visits between primary care physician and psychiatrist.[216,217] The outcome of major depressive disorder was clearly improved up to seven months later. The same research team has also shown, in a randomised trial, that systematic follow-up and care management advice by telephone can significantly improve outcomes in GP treatment of depression (intensity of antidepressant treatment and in clinical outcomes). Simple monitoring and feedback about cases did not produce this effect.[218] The cost-effectiveness of such models for the UK is unclear. Despite improved outcomes, it is unlikely that the intensive mental health professional model would be routinely affordable. Treatment costs have been estimated to increase from £187.50 to £375 per patient.[219,220] Care manager support by telephone is, however, significantly less costly (approximately £50 per patient) and may therefore be more generally applicable.

Multi-faceted interventions

It seems that models that target several aspects of disease management, at least for depression, may prove most beneficial.[221]

Training in psychological interventions

Primary care practitioners can be trained to deliver effective, specific, brief psychological therapies effectively. The capacity to develop primary care practitioners to deliver appropriate psychological interventions is important given the pressure on specialist mental health services.

General practitioners

GPs have been trained to use behavioural and educational interventions successfully in depression, somatisation and obsessive/compulsive disorder.[222,223] GPs receiving extensive instruction in cognitive/behavioural approaches have been shown to produce good patient outcomes. However, GPs receiving only brief training have been shown not to be more effective in helping patients with depression.[224]

Practice and community nurses

The following interventions have been reported to be effective when delivered by nursing staff:

- assessment and management of patients with generalised anxiety, phobia and panic attacks using a range of anxiety management skills[225]
- structured problem-solving treatment for major depression in primary care (delivered by practice nurses)[226]

- nurse-administered behaviour therapy, which been shown to be significantly more effective in primary care for phobic and obsessive compulsive disorders than 'care as usual', with gains still apparent at one-year follow-up[227]
- non-directive counselling leading to significant improvement in the mental health of mothers at three months compared with controls, using trained health visitors and the Edinburgh postnatal depression score.[228]

The primary/specialist care interface

There are many evaluations of particular service models of primary/specialist care mental health working, but no comparative evaluations. It is probable that the success of a particular model will depend on factors such as local ownership and leadership. Particular models may not, therefore, be transferable in their entirety. The process of involving all parties and reaching agreement on the model to be adopted is therefore important. One clear and important finding, from a review of a large variety of models of organisation at the interface undertaken in Seattle, is that links must be both personal, involving face-to-face communication between clinicians, and maintained over a prolonged period.[229] No 'one shot' intervention is successful, as gains are lost once the intervention ends.

Evaluation of various models suggests the following.

- Psychiatrists tend to favour the consultation/liaison model, whereas GPs and PHCTs rate provision within primary care as more satisfactory than services provided elsewhere.[230]
- GPs' attitudes to shared care models have probably become less favourable over time.[231]
- Moving the base of community mental health teams to primary care may be associated with an increase in the caseload of specialist mental health workers, both in the long-term mentally ill and patients with less severe disorder.[232]
- Introduction of a link worker system between a community mental health trust (CMHT) and practices in inner London showed no improvement in staff morale in comparison to a non-integrated service.[233]
- Basing CPNs in general practice (retaining strong links with the CMHT) and employing nurse behavioural therapists (who provided specific treatments mainly for patients with severe neurotic illnesses) resulted in the majority of CPN visits being to patients with major psychosis. It is not clear if the focus of the CPNs on the severely mentally ill was facilitated more by their relationship with the CMHT or by the existence of the alternative resource provided by the nurse behaviour therapists.[234]

Community and voluntary groups

It is likely that the growing number of volunteer schemes in general practice contributes positively to the mental health of the practice population, but this has not been formally studied. This is particularly likely given the interest of patients in mutual support. There is some evidence from an RCT that the voluntary sector can benefit those with psychosocial problems who present to primary care.[235]

Specific disorders

Table 9 outlines the effectiveness of interventions for depression, anxiety disorders, eating disorders and unexplained somatic complaints. Further detail is in the relevant appendices.

Table 9: Summary of the effectiveness of interventions for specific disorders.

Diagnosis	Prevalence	Efficacy of drug treatment	Efficacy of non-drug treatments
Anxious depression	High	A I-1	A I-1
Pure depression	Medium	B I-2	A I-1
Generalised anxiety	Medium	B II-1	A I-1
Panic disorder	Low	A I-1	A I-1
Obsessive compulsive disorder	Very low	A I-1	A I-1
Phobias	High	C IV	A I-1
Unexplained medical symptoms	High	A I-1 (if depressed)	A I-1
Eating disorder – mild	High	C IV	A I-2
Eating disorder – severe	Very high	C IV	B III
Adjustment disorder	High	None	None
Bereavement	Low	None	BIII

Source: adapted from Goldberg and Gourney (1997)[84]

7 Models of care and recommendations

Introduction

There is a consensus that the provision of primary mental health care could be improved. There is, however, often disagreement about how that improvement should be brought about. It is somewhat simplistic, but not inaccurate, to say that the view of many primary care staff has been that improvements should come via more staff in primary care, whether counsellors, clinical psychologists or CPNs, and the view of some secondary care professionals and some academics is that improvement should come about via training primary care professionals in mental health care. The rationale for the latter approach has been the mathematics of the numbers of mental health professionals compared to the number of people with mental ill health. The reality is that that there is no one model that will suit all practices and all patients equally, given the diverse nature of primary care and primary care practitioners. The most appropriate model for any particular PHCT is likely to be determined by a number of factors:

- local demography and prevalence of mental ill health, including the numbers with serious mental illness, which may be affected by factors such as the number of nursing homes or institutions
- current organisation of specialist mental health services and the interest of local psychiatrists in primary care issues
- the type and local availability of psychological interventions
- alternative resource availability, including local voluntary sector provision, self-help groups etc.
- the PHCT's interest in mental health issues and their willingness to extend their roles
- time availability, i.e. the reality that members of the PHCT could extend their role.

Local discussion of these issues is essential in order to develop primary mental health care.

PCT/practice activities

Essential PCT and practice-based activities to develop mental health services include:*

- needs assessment
- team working, communication and networking both with PHCT members and other agencies
- supervision, teaching and professional development
- developing guidelines and protocols, information management and developing and maintaining patient resources.

Irrespective of the model of care that may exist or be desired, there are some basic questions that need to be addressed by PCTs and individual practices: which mental health services they wish to provide in the primary care setting; what mix of skills they require to do so; and which services they wish to obtain from external agencies. In order to help answer these questions, basic needs assessment must take place at the practice level. This should include:

- analysis of current prescribing of psychotropic drugs
- analysis of referrals to specialist and other mental health services
- analysis of CPA data
- mapping of current mental health caseloads of primary care practitioners
- reviewing information on patients known to have severe and enduring mental illness (prescribing information, CPA data, review of caseloads, mental illness diagnosis from practice computer etc.)
- ensuring that there is an accurate register of patients under the care of specialist mental health services
- reviewing the roles, skills and training needs of the PHCT in relation to mental health issues.

This information should be used in conjunction with wider needs assessment work and mapping of local resource availability (money, people, skills and services). In order for local needs assessment to be useful it should take a holistic, multidisciplinary approach, recognising that many people with mental ill health identify that their most pressing needs are employment, housing and personal relationships.[236,237]

Assessment, detection and management

Research that might guide redesigning services in primary care is, as yet, at an early stage. Studies on training have focused on improving recognition and prescribing for depression or on the feasibility of primary care staff extending their role to provide particular, time-limited, short-term psychological interventions. The factors already outlined, as well as resource availability, will dictate the extent to which these may be adopted. There is some evidence to suggest that developing the PHCT's understanding of caseload management and exploring the potential for referrals within the team can create better use of resources.[238] Equally, the involvement of the whole practice team in managing common mental disorders may lead to improved patient outcomes and an increased sense that mental health care is 'under control' and therefore less stressful. Local skill-based courses on common mental disorders may therefore be appropriate. Using a chronic disease management model may improve management for those with severe illness, although motivation and resources within the practice are likely to have an impact on how effective this can be.[239]

Generally, the management of service change in primary care can learn from generic approaches to change management. For example, implementation of multi-agency change is assisted by the use of

---

* NatPaCT has been established to assist PCTs in becoming 'fit for purpose'.

external facilitators; time out for planning meetings; drawing up detailed action plans; commitment from senior management and effective communication.[240]

The detection and management of physical ill health in those with severe and enduring mental illness should be addressed. Opportunistic health promotion is possible given the relatively high consultation rate for this group of patients.[241] The development of special health promotion clinics addressing a range of issues such as exercise, screening for physical ill health, smoking and medication side effects is an alternative approach.

General practitioners

It is clear that no matter how specialist mental health care is organised, a significant amount of general practitioner time will be spent in dealing with mental ill health. It is therefore reasonable to suggest that all GPs have training in the detection and management of those disorders, such as anxiety, depression and somatisation, that they will see commonly. Skill-based approaches seem to show the most promise with respect to training and changing practice. It may also be reasonable to offer longer consultations to people with psychological or social problems; patients appreciate longer booking intervals.[242] Given that consultation length, open consulting style and continuity of care may all contribute to improvements in detection and management, methods of developing and monitoring them should be discussed. GPs with a special interest in mental health could also be employed within multi-partner practices and/or across PCTs.

Primary care nurses

There have been many suggestions for the role that primary care nurses could usefully play in mental health care, for example using problem-solving techniques and monitoring medication. However, a recent Scottish study showed that, with few exceptions, GPs do not favour practice nurses taking on a further mental health role. In addition, whilst district nurses are aware of, and sympathetic towards, mental health ill health, they too are under time pressures and their caseload often requires that priority is given to physical procedures. Health visitors may be better placed to expand their mental health role, as some already have training in mental health issues and many would like to extend their mental health role.

In order that changing/extending the role of primary care nurses is a valid endeavour, further research is needed. So far only training health visitors in the use of the Edinburgh postnatal depression scale and non-directive counselling has been shown to definitely improve patient outcomes.

Whilst extending roles may be desirable it is also clearly important to support nurses in the roles they already carry out, in particular practice nurses that are engaged in giving depot injections and assessing those with less severe mental illness.[243]

Some have advocated the development of primary mental health nurses who have a unique set of skills and expertise.

Psychological therapies

Overall, it is clear that there is a need to increase the availability of psychological interventions for patients in primary care.

The research literature suggests that there are a number of recommendations that can be made with respect to the provision of psychological interventions in primary care.

- No one therapist is likely to be able to deal with the full range of problems and disorders seen in primary care. A service needs to offer a variety of types of intervention and a variety of gender and background of practitioner. Taking account of the client's view is an important part of the decision to treat.

- Therapists working as individuals in primary care need to be trained in a variety of types of intervention and be able to adapt their approach to the patients' needs.
- Skilled assessment at the point of referral is crucial to a successful outcome.
- The range of therapies available locally should include cognitive/behavioural and problem-solving approaches.
- Counsellors and therapists need to be appropriately trained and accredited and with regular ongoing clinical supervision.
- Special arrangements or services may be required for members of ethnic minorities.
- Skilled therapists should treat complex conditions.
- Clinical audit and service evaluation should be integral parts of service provision. The development of a core outcome measure for psychological therapies should aid this.[244]

General Practitioners

GPs can provide effective interventions with appropriate training. However, competing priorities/interests and the need for training may mean that this will only be appropriate for some.

Counsellors

With appropriate training and supervision counsellors can provide specific psychological interventions to people with disorders such as chronic fatigue, drug and alcohol misuse, milder eating disorders, somatisation and phobias. They could also play a role in education and support of other PHCT members.

Graduate mental health care workers

The precise role of the new graduate mental health care workers is currently being defined.[245] The potential for these workers to provide effective interventions may offer one avenue for expanding services for individuals suffering mild or moderate mental ill health caused by emotional, social and domestic difficulties. Befriending, support groups and the provision of practical and emotional support to people who are elderly, socially isolated, bereaved or recently unemployed might prove more cost-effective than specialist mental health care. There may also be a role for them in helping practice team work such as audit, maintenance of registers and outcome measurement. They could also help to develop wider mental health networks with other organisations and agencies.

A new professional organisation for counsellors, Counsellors in Primary Care, is currently setting standards (see www.cpc-online.co.uk).

The primary/specialist care interface

The varied nature of both general practice and of CMHTs means that the key word in ensuring adequate liaison and good working practices is flexibility. Teams at both primary and secondary care levels will have to find the most appropriate ways to work together. It is possible to make some generalisations about where certain disorders may be managed (**Table 10**), but the specifics will need to be agreed locally.

Table 10: Disorder, treatment effectiveness and management settings.

Group of disorders	Types of disorder	Chance of spontaneous remission	Primary/secondary care management
Severe mental illness for which a range of treatments is appropriate	Schizophrenia, bipolar, severe eating and organic disorders	Unlikely to remit spontaneously and associated with major disability	Care should usually involve both primary and secondary care practitioners, family involvement and other agencies
Well defined disorder – effective pharmacological and psychological treatments available	Depression ± anxiety, some anxiety disorder	May remit, but relapse common, associated with disability and some cases become chronic	Primary care management usually sufficient, chronic or treatment resistant cases should be reviewed by the CMHT
Defined disorder where psychological therapies may be effective, but drugs have a more limited role	Unexplained somatic complaints, panic disorder with agoraphobia, fatigue states	Spontaneous remission can occur with all these disorders, but chronicity develops in a substantial proportion	Rarely treated in primary care, a small proportion treated by CMHTs Increased availability of psychological therapies in primary care would allow many to be effectively managed
Specific mental health interventions not necessary	Adjustment disorders, bereavement reactions	Usually resolve spontaneously	Supportive help from primary care/self-help groups/voluntary sector usually sufficient

Source: adapted from Goldberg and Gourney (1997)[84]

A number of practical activities have been found, in practice, to improve liaison, communication and clinical care.[246] These include:

- liaison workers operating between primary and specialist mental health care: clear job descriptions, identified time to carry out the liaison role and support systems are essential
- joint strategies for improving communication between the teams
- jointly agreed referral criteria
- shared care protocols for specific conditions (similar to those developed for diabetes), including jointly agreed strategies for responding to crisis situations
- joint case registers of people receiving care from both teams
- provision of advice to GPs about patients whose care remains with the GP
- provision of training to primary care staff in the recognition and management of mental disorders
- joint health promotion between practice nurse and CPN
- service directories to assist in identifying local sources of help.

Models of working can be combined, for example, link workers and separate function community mental health teams. Others provide psychological therapies and support to the PHCTs in the use of psychological interventions for less severe mental ill health. Where CMHTs have developed separate functions, there is a danger of the team providing psychological and social therapies to primary care patients becoming overwhelmed. It should therefore be combined with clear referral protocols, plus a programme of support and education to the PHCTs.

The PHCT and social work

A responsive working relationship between primary care and social services may be facilitated by:[247]

- care managers being attached to PHCTs
- coterminosity of boundaries
- a local 24-hour mental health officer service
- a rapid response to requests for help in crises or breakdown of care packages
- a contact telephone number in every care plan.

Where social workers are fully integrated into CMHTs, GPs may relate to social workers as key workers for their patients.

Non-specialist social workers are often involved with families where less severe mental ill health is present. In these cases there is unlikely to be any formal mechanisms for communication and liaison with GPs. Consequently local discussion should take place to determine how best to facilitate information exchange.

Voluntary and community groups

Improving links between primary care and the voluntary sector may also be of benefit for those with less severe mental ill health. It is likely that there would need to be an attitudinal shift and greater availability of information about the effectiveness of local services to enable GPs to make best use of such resources. Establishing personal contacts may be helpful as a starting point to overcoming barriers.*

8 Outcome measures

Much has been written about quality in primary health care and the approaches that can be taken to improving it.[248] PCTs have a role in defining, accounting for and improving the quality of mental health provision under clinical governance, whether provided by primary care or by specialist mental health services. Fundamental to the success of clinical governance will be the extent to which there is sharing of beliefs and values, appropriate training to ensure that practitioners can undertake this work and the establishing of structures and processes needed to monitor and co-ordinate quality.[249] The generation and monitoring of standards of care is clearly a key part of this agenda. Given that no one model of care can be recommended, it is likely that this process will concentrate on process and outcome rather than structure. The measurement of quality for primary care mental health interventions and services is still in its infancy.[250] Attitudes to appropriate measures differ between different stakeholders. A recent Delphi Survey found agreement on only 26% of measures. However, some measures could be used to form the basis for local discussion.[251] A number of approaches to developing primary care mental health services have been published recently.**

---

* *How to work with self-help groups: Guidelines for professionals* by Judy Wilson (1996) is a useful resource.

** Primary care mental health education (PriMHE), Dr Chris Manning (www.primhe.org).

Whilst all issues need to be addressed at a local level, it may be helpful for the following areas to be considered for quality monitoring.

Needs assessment

- Local needs assessment, including incorporation of the views of users and carers.
- Availability of a directory of local services.

Assessment, detection and management

- Consultation length and content.
- Continuity of care, patients being followed up by the same GP for at least an episode of illness.
- Benzodiazepine prescribing.
- Lithium prescribing and monitoring.
- Antidepressant prescribing, including dosage.
- Repeat prescriptions of antipsychotic medication and recording if no new assessment has taken place.
- Protocols and training for practice nurses administering depot injection.
- Protocols and training for HVs in postnatal depression.
- Physical heath checks for patients with long-term mental ill health.
- Patients with mental ill health for whom social issues have not been addressed (relationships, housing, employment etc.).
- Shared care plans with specialist mental health services.
- Proportion of primary care staff with training in interviewing techniques, e.g. problem-based interviewing.
- Proportion of GPs and other primary care practitioners with recent training in the detection and management of depression, anxiety, unexplained somatic complaints or eating disorders.
- PHCT involvement in Mental Health Act assessment and CPA.
- Training for reception staff in mental health awareness/dealing with bizarre/aggressive behaviour.
- Psychological interventions – the proportion of primary care practitioners who:
  - provide psychological interventions and have had accredited training in a modality that has shown to be effective for their client group
  - receive regular supervision
  - are members of relevant professional bodies.
- Access to a range of psychological interventions in primary care/the community.

The primary/specialist care interface

- Proportion of patients with severe and/or long-term mental ill health not known to mental health services.
- Availability of locally agreed policies and procedures.
- Development of local management guidelines.
- Existence of shared care registers.

9 Information and research requirements

The extent to which mental health research has been undertaken in a primary care setting has increased in recent years, but there are still considerable gaps in knowledge. Broad areas for further research include the following.

Prevalence

- Improved understanding of clinical constructs for conditions to inform epidemiological research.
- Longitudinal studies to give a clearer picture on clinical course of disorder.
- Comparison of patients between primary and secondary care.

Assessment, detection and management

- Improved understanding of the impact of iatrogenic, social, financial and legal constraints on patient behaviour and clinical decision making.
- Evaluation of education and training on the behaviours of practitioners.
- Interventions suitable for mild and mixed disorders as they present in clinical practice.
- The components of 'as usual care' that make it effective.
- The cost-effectiveness of medical and non-medical interventions.
- The efficacy of low dosage antidepressants.
- The management of depression secondary to physical illness.
- The management of chronic disorder.
- The patient perspective on effectiveness, and how to increase concordance between patient and clinician views.
- The effectiveness of alternative and complementary therapies that patients report to be helpful.

The primary/specialist care interface

- Effectiveness of different skill mix and models of mental health provision in primary care and their interface with specialist mental health care.

Appendix 1: Depression

Introduction

The high prevalence and chronicity of depression is a major public health problem in all countries, not just the industrialised west.[252] Depression is consequently a costly disorder.[253] In the US high health care costs have been shown for depressed patients two to three years after identification by screening, $1500 per person more than non-depressed patients.[254] Antidepressant prescribing alone costs the National Health Service approximately £88 million per annum, increasing by 116% between 1990 and 1995.[255]

In the UK at least 80% of patients identified with depression are treated entirely in primary care.[256] The commonest presentation is of mixed anxiety and depression, with many patients also having alcohol problems.

There is continued concern at the relatively low levels of recognition and treatment received by patients, despite major national campaigns such as the Defeat Depression Campaign.[257]

Terminology and classification

'Depression' and 'anxiety' are words with such everyday usage that it is particularly important to be clear about what is meant when discussing epidemiology and related issues. The ICD-10 for primary care includes:

- depression – F32
- mixed anxiety and depression – F41.2.

There has been a shift in terminology over recent years away from reactive and endogenous depression to categories based on severity. The term 'major depression' refers to depression complying with diagnostic criteria that usually warrants specific treatment, often with medication. 'Dysthymia' refers to long-term, low-grade depressed mood (minor depression, sub-syndromal depression). The terms 'unipolar' and 'bipolar' are also used, the latter referring to depression that occurs in conjunction with manic episodes. Diagnosis should always be thought of in conjunction with disability and chronicity, which are major determinants of quality of life for the individual.

Aetiology

There is an extensive literature on the aetiology of depression, particularly in women. Psychosocial variables and the impact of life events are particularly important. There is an important genetic component for major depression.

Life event research suggests that the following factors are important in the generation of depression.[258]

- **Vulnerability factors:** Loss of mother before the age of 11, three or more children at home, lack of an intimate confidant, lack of outside employment and childhood adversity are all considered important. Internal vulnerability factors, such as low self-esteem, are also important and may be generated by early life experiences.
- **Provoking agents:** For example, major life events that are severe in terms of long-term contextual threat and unpleasantness. These events often involve the experience of loss.
- **Coping styles:** These may mediate the impact of a life event, despite the existence of vulnerability factors.

Other factors that may be important in the aetiology of depression are co-existing medical conditions, particularly those that are chronic and painful. Other psychiatric disorders such as learning disabilities or dementia may also increase the risk of depression.

Understanding aetiology can highlight groups that are at risk and therefore require extra vigilance and thought with respect to detection and preventive activities.

Epidemiology

The prevalence of disorder must be understood within the context of the difficulties inherent in fitting most primary care mental ill health into categorical grouping (*see* section 2) and the consequent importance of sub-syndromal cases.

Prevalence

Depression is the most prevalent form of mental disorder in primary care patients throughout the world.[259] In surveys of general practice as many as 25–30% of attendees have been found to have anxiety or depressive symptoms severe enough to interfere with day-to-day functioning. The UK OPCS Surveys show a prevalence of 7.7% for mixed anxiety and depression and 2.1% for depressive episodes. This translates into an average GP having at any one point in time (**Table A1.1**):

- 180 working age adults with an anxiety disorder, non-psychotic depression or both[260]
- 40 older people with depression.

Bipolar disorder is considerably less common. Estimates of lifetime prevalence are in the order of 1%.

Table A1.1: The prevalence of depression and anxiety in the average general practice.

Diagnosis	Weekly prevalence per 1,000 adults aged 16–64	Number of patients aged 16–64 on GP list of 1,800*
Mixed anxiety and depression	77	87
Depressive episode	21	24

*Assumes 63% of GP list is aged 16–64.
Source: OPCS survey[9]

Factors affecting prevalence

Gender

Most research shows that depression is twice as prevalent in women as in men (**Table A1.2**).[261]

Table A1.2: The prevalence of depression and anxiety in men and women.

Diagnosis	Prevalence per 1,000 women	Prevalence per 1,000 men
Mixed anxiety and depression	99	54
Depressive episode	25	17

Source: OPCS survey[9]

Ethnicity

There is some evidence to suggest differential rates in minority ethnic groups, but study numbers are small.[262]

Socio-economic variables

There are many socio-economic variables, particularly those relating to deprivation, such as unemployment, homelessness and urban living, that are associated with depression. About half the variance in prevalence in any general practice can be related to indices of deprivation.[263]

Mortality

Depression is associated with considerable excess mortality, especially suicide; approximately 15% of people with major depression will commit suicide.

Effectiveness of services and interventions

The proportion of patients with depression who are accurately identified and who receive appropriate treatment and care is a reasonable comment on the overall effectiveness of service provision. If the findings of some studies are generalisable then the picture is dismal: for instance, only 25% of all cases of depression and 9% of cases of anxiety and depression were receiving any intervention.[264] It must be borne in mind that, given the rate of spontaneous remission, not all cases should be receiving intervention, other than appropriate follow-up/'watchful waiting'.[265]

The outcome of disorder

Understanding the natural history of depression is important in determining whether interventions are effective or not. Overall, it is estimated that up to 10–25% of those with major depression will develop chronic depression (at least two years' duration).[266] The US Medical Outcomes Study of outpatients showed that those with dysthymia 54% had a major depressive episode during the two-year follow-up period.[267] Lower relapse rates might be expected in primary care given that the overall severity of depression is less than that seen in psychiatric outpatients. Functional impairment in dysthymia is, however, comparable to that in major depressive disorder, although symptom severity is less.[268]

Detection and diagnosis

Recognition rates for GPs varies from 7–70%; most studies report rates between 30% and 40%.[269] Practice nurses average 23% recognition in cases of depression and health visitors, compared to GHQ scores, average 50%.[270,271] Comorbid anxiety seems to increase the likelihood that depression will be diagnosed.[272,273] Physical problems appear to impede recognition.[274–276]

A study of 18 414 consecutive attenders to a representative group of GPs found that the doctors missed one case of clinically significant depression in every 28 consultations.[277] In most of these cases, they were aware of emotional disturbance, but they did not think it to be clinically significant. In about one third of all the missed cases the patient scored only 1 point above the threshold for case definition. Considering the absence of a gold standard diagnostic definition of depression, the general practitioners in this study did not appear to perform as badly as other studies suggest. A significant proportion of the missed cases however may be people who suffer from chronic and disabling illness.

As with all mental ill health, the reason for depression not being diagnosed reflects a complex interplay of factors; some that reside in the patient, some in the practitioner and some in their interaction (*see* 'Prevalence in primary care populations' in section 4).

Management

Table A1.3 outlines the effectiveness of specific interventions available for the treatment of depression. Appropriate management also involves follow-up, advice giving etc. (*see* 'Prevalence in primary care populations' in section 4). In many cases depression should be treated as a chronic disease, with appropriate chronic disease management such as management protocols and disease registers.

Table A1.3: The effectiveness of interventions in the management of depression.

Disorder	Interventions of known effectiveness	Interventions requiring more research
Acute	• Antidepressants for severe and moderate depression, but unclear evidence of effectiveness of medication in acute mild depression (A I-1, op mainly, some primary care research) • Cognitive/behavioural therapy, interpersonal therapy, structured problem-solving (A I-1 primary care research) • Better evidence for mixed anxiety and depression than pure depression	• Targeted counselling (where the client group and technique are specific) for mild and moderate depression, some RCT evidence • Less evidence for non-specific, untargeted counselling • Extracts of hypericum for mild and moderate depression: a meta-analysis of randomised controlled trials (RCTs) showed that extracts of hypericum are significantly superior to placebo and similarly effective to standard antidepressants in mild and moderate depression (A I-1)
Maintenance	• Maintenance drug therapy or cognitive/behavioural therapy (B I-1)	• Exercise: better quality research required (C I-2) • Further work on relapse prevention and the relative roles of CBT and drug therapy
Dysthymia (mild depression lasting 2 years)	• Cognitive/behavioural therapy; interpersonal therapy; structured problem solving (B I-2) • Antidepressants in outpatient populations (B II-1)	• Chronic disease management approaches

Pharmacological interventions

There are four main groups of antidepressants:

- tricyclic antidepressants (TCAs), e.g. amitryptyline, imipramine and lofepramine (a modified tricyclic)
- selective serotonin re-uptake inhibitors (SSRIs), e.g. fluoxetine (Prozac)
- monoamine oxidase inhibitors (now seldom used)
- newer, expensive, mixed action drugs such as venlafaxine and mirtazapine.

Tricyclics and SSRIs are the most widely prescribed. There are a number of factors that need to be understood when considering the effectiveness and cost-effectiveness literature.

- The two groups have different dosage schedules. Tricyclics have to be titrated up to a known therapeutic dose, usually above 100 mgs per day, whilst SSRIs can be started at a therapeutic dose.
- They have different side effects. Tricyclics have a range of receptor blocking actions, commonly causing dry mouth, constipation, postural hypotension and sedation. SSRIs induce nausea and headache.
- They have different costs. The older tricyclics are much cheaper to prescribe. Generic imipramine is the cheapest, a typical new tricyclic costing eight times as much, and the least expensive SSRI being twice as expensive again.
- They have different toxicities. Tricyclics are associated with 4% of all suicides, in overdose causing cardiac arrythmias, with the exception of lofepramine, which appears relatively safer in overdose. SSRIs are also relatively safer in overdose.

Prescribing guidelines

There is good consensus about some aspects of prescribing antidepressants. Several guidelines concur about the diagnostic indications for antidepressants and the need for correct dosage and duration of treatment.[278] It is thus possible to construct general comments on prescribing in primary care.

- Treatment should be given for episodes of moderate depression. The presence of four symptoms lasting more than two weeks appears to be a useful rule of thumb to identify those who will respond to a tricyclic better than a placebo.[279,280]
- This applies to antidepressants given in full therapeutic dose. The dose for which there is evidence from clinical trials of superiority over placebo is more than 100 mgs of a tricyclic.[281] The SSRIs all have evidence for efficacy in secondary care patients at or below the lowest tableted dose.
- The dose that is effective for an individual patient should be continued for four to six months after recovery from a first episode. If there has been a history of recurrence, it should be continued for significantly longer.

Randomised controlled trials have shown that adequate treatment according to established guidelines gives a clinical outcome for major depression that is superior to usual treatment.[282,283]

The role of low dose prescribing is unclear. The usual dose of tricyclics in general practice is 50 mgs, GPs report improvements at these low doses and meta-analysis suggests that high and low doses do not confer altered effectiveness, although drop-out rates increase with dose. Clearly further research is needed.[284]

Cost-effectiveness

There is little consensus about the merits of different classes of drug as first line treatment. There have been a large number of studies comparing the SSRIs and tricyclics. However, there have been relatively few in primary care, using a representative sample of depressed patients or addressing health economic outcomes. Meta-analyses cannot overcome the methodological limitations of these original studies but may be used to estimate differential efficacy and compliance under relatively ideal prescribing conditions. Bearing in mind the pitfalls of extrapolation from such data to routine practice, meta-analyses suggest that the SSRIs and tricyclics are of roughly equal efficacy when the latter are given in full dose.[285,286] Translating this to routine clinical practice, however, is far from simple; where variable adherence has a significant impact, drop-out rates for SSRIs are 3–4% lower than for tricyclics.

It has consequently been difficult to demonstrate a clear cost-effectiveness advantage to either SSRIs or tricyclics, once all NHS costs are taken into account. A US HMO-based study compared fluoxetine with desipramine or imipramine and found that those randomised to fluoxetine had fewer adverse effects, but no greater quality of life.[287] The extra prescribing costs of fluoxetine were offset by fewer outpatient visits. It has therefore been suggested that the more expensive SSRIs are cost-effective because they have a higher rate of treatment success, which leads to a reduction in the non-medication costs of disproportionately expensive specialist care.[288] It also seems the case, however, that differences in outcome between active drug and placebo are reduced in less severe depression, which is commonly seen in primary care.[289] Meta-analyses of published randomised controlled trials suggest that the modified tricyclic, lofepramine, may be a safe and cost-effective alternative to the SSRIs.

Further information from RCTs is likely to be available in the next few years. Furthermore, some SSRIs have lost their patent protection and generic versions will be available at a lower cost. This is likely to make the use of tricyclics as first line treatment less cost-effective and attractive.

Treatment adherence

The extent to which any course of treatment is adhered to is probably determined predominantly by the health beliefs of the public and their doctors. After five years of a national public education campaign only 24% of the public thought someone with depression should be offered antidepressants and 74% thought they were addictive.[290] Fears of dependence are therefore common.[291,292] Similarly, despite the campaign antidepressants are often prescribed at a dosage and for a duration that does not comply with guidelines.

Follow-up sessions by a nurse may improve continuation with medication, outcomes and patient satisfaction, as can the use of telephone care manager support in conjunction with follow-up[293,294] (*see* section 6).

Psychological therapies

There is growing evidence for the effectiveness of cognitive-behavioural, interpersonal and problem-solving approaches in primary care. There is relatively less evidence for non-directive counselling. Other psychotherapeutic approaches do not have sufficient empirical data to either prove or disprove their effectiveness. These approaches can all be used over a relatively short period (less than 20 sessions) and therefore lend themselves well to the primary care setting. There is evidence showing that patients often prefer psychological treatments to drugs, this presenting difficulty for randomisation in some trials.[295]

There is increasing evidence from RCTs of the effectiveness for cognitive approaches for major depression in primary care, although the evidence for benefit is not as clear-cut as it is for outpatient populations.[296,297] Meta-analysis has suggested that cognitive therapy is equivalent to either behavioural therapy or antidepressants for mild to moderate depression.[298] The impact of cognitive approaches on relapse prevention is not clear. Meta-analysis has suggested that five out of the eight trials included showed a preventative effect of cognitive therapy on relapse rate.[299] Most studies show a higher response rate and some reduction in relapse when cognitive approaches were used in combination with pharmacotherapy, at least in outpatient populations.[300,301]

In a small number of studies, interpersonal therapy has been shown to be effective, but it is far less prevalent as a clinical intervention than cognitive behavioural approaches.[302,303] Meta-analyses suggest that cognitive-behavioural approaches and interpersonal therapy show superiority over psychodynamically oriented therapies.[304]

Brief problem-solving approaches have also been evaluated in primary care. A study comparing outcomes between a psychiatrist and a trained GP treating patients with major depression suggested that outcomes were as good as those produced by adequate antidepressant treatment and twice as effective as placebo.[305] A further study by the same group suggested that the combination of problem solving with antidepressant medication was no more effective than either treatment alone.[306] In both studies a significant number of referred patients were excluded, as their depression was not severe enough. An international trial showed problem solving to reduce caseness and improve subjective functioning in comparison to a control group at four months (in individuals with depression or adjustment disorders, identified by a community survey).[307] At 12 months, however, difference only remained for subjective improvement.

The effectiveness of non-directive counselling remains contentious. Some studies have suggested that it is no more effective than 'as usual' GP care.[308] However, more recently, comparison of non-directive counselling, cognitive/behavioural therapy and 'as usual' GP care suggested benefit for both psychological therapies at four months (approximately 30% were also being prescribed antidepressants, approximately half those in the 'as usual' care group), but no difference in self-reported outcome at one year for those with moderately severe depression.[309] Economic evaluation in this study suggested short-term cost-effectiveness, but no long-term difference in cost between the three groups.[310] A recent study comparing generic counselling with antidepressants in primary care for mild to moderate depression, suggested that counselling was as effective, although those taking antidepressants got better more quickly.[311] However, as many patients expressed a preference for one treatment or the other, sample sizes were small and there may be longer-term outcomes that are different between the groups.

St John's Wort (Hypericum)

Hypericum has received increasing publicity as an over the counter preparation with antidepressant action. It has monoamine oxidase inhibitor qualities. A meta-analysis of randomised controlled trials showed that extracts of hypericum are significantly superior to placebo and similarly effective to standard antidepressants in mild and moderate depression.[312,313] A recent German randomised, double blind, placebo-controlled trial with eight week follow-up showed that a standardised dose of hypericum extract was more effective than placebo and as effective as 100 mgs imipramine (reduction in self-rated and standardised rating scores) for treating moderate depression in general practice.[314] Further research has shown equivalence with imipramine at 150 mgs dose.[315] This study suggested that patients tolerate hypericum better. Further research comparing higher doses of antidepressants over longer periods taking into account patient preference is clearly needed.

Exercise

There is some research to suggest that exercise may be helpful as an adjunct in the treatment of depression.[316–318] However, meta-analysis of RCTs up until 1999 concluded that the effectiveness of exercise in reducing the symptoms of depression could not be definitely determined because of a lack of good quality research.[319]

Summary

- Depression is very common in primary care populations, particularly in women.
- It is often associated with physical illness and other mental disorders, particularly anxiety.
- It is a long-term, relapsing condition for many sufferers and should be treated as a chronic disease.
- It can be effectively treated with both pharmacological and psychological interventions, but is often missed and un-/under-treated.
- Alternative approaches to management exist, with increasing evidence for the effectiveness of hypericum and equivocal literature for exercise.

Appendix 2: Anxiety disorders

Introduction

The symptoms of anxiety, such as worry, restlessness, reduced concentration and poor memory are extremely widespread and may be presenting symptoms for a wide range of disorders, both physical and psychological. These symptoms represent the action of the autonomic nervous system on the body and can therefore affect all aspects of physiology. People with anxiety disorders also have specific and recurring psychological symptoms, fears that they recognise as being irrational or unrealistic and intrusive.

Symptoms of anxiety are commonly short-term and self-limiting in reaction to a stressful event. For a significant number of people, however, anxiety disorders are long-term and cause significant disability.

The majority of sufferers can be managed in general practice and do not require referral to specialist services.

Terminology and classification

Anxiety disorders include generalised anxiety disorder (GAD), phobias, panic, obsessive compulsive disorder and somatoform disorders. ICD-10 for primary care covers these disorders in the following categories:

- phobic disorder – F40
- panic disorder – F 41.0
- generalised anxiety disorder – F 41.1.

It is unclear how useful specific categories are for those patients presenting to primary care, as comorbidity of two or more anxiety disorders is common, as is the co-existence of anxiety and depression.[320]

Other disorders such as post-traumatic stress disorder (PTSD) and adjustment disorder are important parts of the spectrum of anxiety disorders. The latter term is used for the group of patients who present with an acute anxiety reaction who, prior to the provoking event, were in good mental health.

Aetiology

Risk factors for anxiety and related problems include personality type, cognitive, behavioural, familial and social variables. Environmental issues are also important, for example the fear of crime, particularly when in conjunction with other factors.

There is no clear genetic component to anxiety disorders, although ways of responding to events may be learnt by exposure to negative responses by family/social group members. As with depression, life events have been linked to the onset of anxiety. It is thought that events associated with threat, rather than loss as in depression, are of particularly relevance for anxiety disorders, for example in PTSD. In comorbid depression and anxiety, it seems that anxiety has an earlier onset and thus may predispose to depression.[321]

Epidemiology

Prevalence

The assessment of prevalence is problematic given the high levels of comorbidity, particularly with depressive illness and between different types of anxiety disorders. In addition, many studies have not used reliable measures. The OPCS Surveys give prevalence rates for the community (**Table A2.1**). The numbers seen in general practice will, as with all disorders, be higher: around a sixth of patients consulting their GP are 'generally anxious'.[322] The prevalence of specific disorder is lower: an international multi-centre study suggests rates of GAD of 8.5%, agoraphobia 1.5% and panic disorder 2.2%. This gives an overall prevalence of 12.2% for defined anxiety disorders, only a minority of whom actually present complaining of anxiety.[323] Some estimates suggest that one in every 20 people will develop GAD at some point in their lives.[324]

Table A2.1: The prevalence of anxiety disorders in the average general practice.

Diagnosis	Weekly prevalence per 1,000 adults aged 16–64	Number of patients aged 16–64 on GP list of 1,800*
Generalised anxiety	31	36
All phobias	11	13
Obsessive-compulsive disorder	12	14
Panic disorder	8	9

* Assumes 63% of GP list is aged 16–64.
Source: OPCS survey[9]

Comorbidity

Studies suggest that depression is associated with anxiety disorders in approximately half of cases.[325,326] Severity and disability are increased significantly when GAD or panic are associated with depression, similarly for panic and agoraphobia.

Effectiveness of services and interventions

The outcome of disorder

Anxiety disorders are mainly chronic, almost by definition, as short-lived anxiety reactions to life events are categorised as adjustment disorders. Follow-up in the US Epidemiological Catchment Area Study suggests that their chronicity is somewhat less than schizophrenia and the same as affective disorders.[327,328] Severity may be a reasonable predictor of prognosis. In a study of a spectrum of non-severe mental ill health, symptoms were likely to be still present at six months if they remained severe one month after initial consultation with the GP.[329]

Detection and diagnosis

The WHO international study already quoted found that patients with GAD plus depression and patients with agoraphobia plus panic were more likely to seek medical help and be recognised by GPs as having psychiatric problems than other forms of anxiety.[330] In an earlier study, GPs diagnosed an anxiety disorder in 7.8% of normal controls, 39% of people with sub-threshold GAD, 33% of people with GAD, 47.9% of patients with GAD plus depression; 38.7% of patients with agoraphobia, 53.3% of patients with panic disorder and 64.3% of patients with agoraphobia and panic.[331] It seems that GPs are more likely to detect those with greater severity and disability.

The reasons for such findings are speculative, but must include patients presenting with physical symptoms and the common mixed presentation of ill-defined anxiety syndromes and social problems (*see* Appendix 3).

Management

There are well proven treatments for anxiety disorders using medication and psychological interventions. However, these treatments have not been well studied, or not studied at all, in primary care settings. It is therefore not possible to be sure of their effectiveness for the majority of the mixed presentation anxiety seen in primary care. An overview of effective interventions is found in **Table A2.2**.

Table A2.2: The effectiveness of interventions in the management of anxiety disorders.

Disorder	Interventions of known effectiveness	Interventions requiring more research
Panic, with or without agoraphobia	• Some antidepressants: B I-1 • Short-term use of anxiolytics (but relapse common on discontinuing medication): A I-1	• Targeted counselling for specific related psycho-social problems: evidence is variable
Generalised anxiety	• Cognitive/behavioural therapies: A I-1	• Non-specific, untargeted counselling: evidence is unfavourable • Non-specific relaxation
Obsessive-compulsive disorder	• Some antidepressants • Behaviour/cognitive therapies: A I-1	

Pharmacological interventions

• **Benzodiazepines:** A systematic review of RCTs of benzodiazepines showed that they are an effective and rapid treatment for GAD.[332] In a primary care setting, however, anxiolytic drugs such as the benzodiazepines seem no more effective in the management of less severe disorders, some of which will be anxiety disorders, than psychological approaches.[333] The potential for benzodiazepine dependence and tolerance over time is now well recognised. These drugs therefore have a role in the short-term management of acute anxiety, prescribed for a limited number of days, but are not appropriate for long-term use.

• **Antidepressants:** RCTs show antidepressants, particularly those working on the 5-HT system, e.g. SSRIs, to be effective to some extent in panic disorder and GAD, at least in secondary care populations.[334,335] Tricyclics, SSRIs, monamine oxidase inhibitors and benzodiazepines are thought to have roughly comparable efficacy in the short term (8–12 weeks). Side effects of tricyclics may, however, prove problematic. Short-term use of medication commonly results in relapse. Longer-term use is recommended (12–18 months), after which period the relapse rate is not known. The best evidence for effectiveness is for imipramine, clomipramine, paroxetine and citalopram. However, this is not proven in primary care populations.[336]

- The role of antidepressants for the treatment of phobias is less clear. For social phobia, treatment with paroxetine may result in symptom improvement in the short term. Again, relapse rates are very high after discontinuation and after longer-term treatment are not known.[337,338] Psychotherapeutic interventions have been shown more effective than medication (*see* below).
- **Buspirone:** A meta-analysis of drug studies suggests that in GAD buspirone had a much lower effect size than either benzodiazepines or antidepressants and its onset is slow (up to four weeks). Problems with dependence and withdrawal are minimal compared to benzodiazepines.[339]
- **Beta-blockers:** Beta-blockers, which negate the effects of the autonomic nervous system and hence ameliorate the physical symptoms of anxiety, may be helpful in the management of event specific anxiety, e.g. exam nerves.[340] There is, however, no good RCT looking at use in GAD.

Psychological therapies

The effectiveness of cognitive/behavioural approaches in the management of a wide range of anxiety disorders has been well established by RCTs.[341]

In GAD, cognitive-behavioural therapy (CBT) and anxiety management have been found the most effective of psychological treatments. Medication and psychological therapies were found equally effective in the short-term, but the gains of CBT and anxiety management were maintained at six months.[342]

In panic disorder an overview of the literature concluded that 85% of chronic patients stay well at between one- and two-year follow-up after treatment with CBT.[343] In addition, where agoraphobic fear and avoidance is present along with panic, exposure (a behavioural treatment) proved to be twice as effective as alprazolam.[344] There is also some evidence that treatment for panic disorder can be used effectively in primary care.[345]

Exposure plus cognitive therapy has been shown to be effective for social phobia and exposure plus CBT for agoraphobia.[346]

Structured problem-solving methods can help patients to manage current life problems or stresses which contribute to anxiety symptoms.[347] Simple problem-solving counselling has been shown to be effective in primary care for a range of less severe mental ill health.[348]

Self-help

Consensus plus some – usually small – trials suggest that there are several self-help approaches that may be effective. A review of studies suggests that they show promise as first-line interventions for anxiety disorders in primary care, although more severely ill patients will require more specialist interventions.[349] For example, giving an audiotape and booklet to patients with chronic anxiety can lead to reduced scores for depression as well as anxiety.[350] Similarly, patients with GAD and panic disorder can be helped by receiving literature on anxiety in addition to the usual care from their GP[351] Learning self-help skills through reading, supported by contact with a clinician, may lead to significant symptom improvement. Increasing clinician contact led to greater numbers improving.[352] Computer-aided and telephone-guided programmes are also becoming available.

Patients with phobias may benefit from self-administered behavioural treatments, involving gradual exposure to feared objects or situations.

A controlled trial of a general practice based class teaching self-care skills, relaxation, stress management, medication, nutrition and exercise has also showed improvements for individuals, which were maintained at one year.[353]

Social support

Improving social supports by training informal providers (e.g. former clients) may be a cost-effective strategy for creating access to a range of services.[354] This is the approach taken by self-help groups such as No Panic, Triumph over Phobia and the National Phobics Society.

Hypnosis and relaxation therapies

These complementary approaches are often reported as being of help in dealing with anxiety disorders.[355] The evidence base is not well developed, although there is some evidence from small RCTs that suggests that they can reduce anxiety in response to stressful situations or for treating panic disorders in combination with cognitive approaches. Further good quality research is needed.[356,357]

Summary

- Anxiety symptoms are very common and usually resolve spontaneously.
- Anxiety disorders are less common and may be associated with significant disability.
- Good evidence exists for the effectiveness of psychotherapeutic interventions, particularly cognitive-behavioural approaches.
- Some evidence exists for the effectiveness of drug therapies, complementary approaches, such as relaxation techniques and self-help.
- More research in primary care populations is needed.

Appendix 3: Unexplained somatic complaints

Introduction

Some people tend to present and explain psychosocial distress in terms of physical complaints and bodily dysfunction. Hence the use of the term 'somatisation', derived from the Greek word *soma* – the body. The fact that mental disorder may commonly present in this way in primary care is one explanation for the relative under-detection of frank psychiatric disorder.

The impact of unexplained somatic complaints on the use of health care resources is significant.[358-360] For the NHS, estimates suggest that 'signs, symptoms and ill defined conditions' (some of which will be somatisation) are the fifth highest reason for consultation with general practitioners, the third largest category of hospital expenditure and the highest single source of outpatient expenditure.[361]

Terminology and classification

Within ICD-10, somatoform disorders are in the F40 chapter, with other neurotic and stress-related disorders. Primary care ICD-10 contains the chapter 'unexplained somatic complaints' (F45).

In many clinical and research situations, it is difficult to distinguish between health-related anxiety (hypochondriasis), medically unexplained symptoms, actual somatoform disorder and those with physical symptoms and comorbid depression/anxiety, who present with somatisation.

There is a poorly understood overlap between somatoform disorders and medically unexplained symptoms, they are diagnoses of exclusion. There are many patients for whom no conventional diagnosis can be made for persistent symptoms or clusters of symptoms. Clearly, some will have disorder presenting in an unconventional way, some have disorder as yet undescribed, some a psychological cause for their symptoms and some will have both a physical and a psychological disorder.

It is also difficult to adequately categorise patients with unexplained medical symptoms. Many specialties have a category of functional illness to describe those conditions where it is thought that there is a significant psychological component, e.g. irritable bowel syndrome or fibromyalgia. Although there have been attempts to operationalise some of these conditions, there is often difficulty in describing a defining set of symptoms and consequently there is often overlap with other conditions.[362]

These difficulties have led to the questioning of the clinical validity of these disorders. It is likely that a mixed group of patients is being described as clinical course; outcome and utilisation of resources may be significantly different for individuals with the same label.

Epidemiology

A precise estimate of prevalence is hard to find given the definitional/classification difficulties described and the fact that research setting and ascertainment methodologies vary greatly.

The majority of patients with psychosocial problems in primary care present, at least initially, with physical symptoms.[363,364] Some of these patients may also have co-existing physical illness, which, however, may not be the explanation for the symptoms presented. A Canadian study described the presentation of patients in primary care.[365] Just under a third had a high score on a research depression scale, indicating significant depression or anxiety; of these only 15% could be classified as psychosocial presenters, i.e. this is how they initially presented their problem to the doctor. A further 34% described psychosocial causes for their physical symptoms and 26% accepted a psychosocial explanation for their problems when asked directly. The remaining 25% rejected the possibility that there could be a psychosocial cause to their illness, i.e. true somatisers. True somatisers did not differ markedly in their socio-demographic characteristics, except that there were more men in the somatisation group. UK research has also shown high scores for depression and anxiety in a majority of patients identified by GPs as having long-standing medically unexplained symptoms. More women than men were identified in this study. This suggests that men's symptoms may not become chronic, they stop consulting their GPs, or that GPs have a bias towards identification of women.[366]

Appropriately, many general practice consultations do not result in a diagnosis. It is likely that many of these patients do not return and recover.[367] Estimates for truly unexplained medical symptoms in general practice vary, but may be in the region of 20–25% of consultations.[368] Up to 5% of patients in general practice are estimated to be frequent attenders with somatising symptoms.[369] A proportion of these will have undiagnosed psychiatric disorder. A study from the Netherlands suggested that 45% of frequent somatising attenders had a depressive or anxiety disorder, often unrecognised.[370] A US study of 55 patients with panic disorder referred by family doctors psychiatrists suggested that most had presented with somatic complaints, which had been misdiagnosed for months or years. Cardiac, gastrointestinal and neurological symptoms were the most common.[371]

There is a high prevalence of medically unexplained symptoms in settings outside general practice such as gastroenterology, cardiology or gynecology outpatient clinics. Estimates of prevalence vary, but figures of 25% of attendees are not uncommon.[372] A proportion of these patients will have a predominantly psychosocial cause for their symptomatology or undiagnosed psychiatric disorder.

Effectiveness of services and interventions

The outcome of disorder

The terminological difficulties described have an impact on both ascertaining the outcome of disorder and the effectiveness of interventions. It is currently hard to identify individuals that will respond to conservative treatment and those who will go on to develop enduring difficulties. If identifiable, the latter group could be subject to early intervention, which could prevent the inappropriate and costly use of what may be unnecessary investigations and other resources.

Management

Explanation/information

Communication skills are of central importance for all health professionals: being able to listen, show an understanding of a patient's concerns and give information about health, illness and treatment in terms that can be understood. These skills are of particular importance when physical and mental ill health overlap. However, in one study patients with long-standing medically unexplained symptoms reported finding their GP's explanations of little help in understanding their condition.[373] Most explanations were seen as a rejection of the patient's suffering. Explanations that were found to be empowering shared some features of cognitive treatment approaches, such as reattribution.

There is some evidence to suggest that improvements in management can be made. One study showed that GPs given advice (via a letter) on how to deal with people who somatise referred nearly a third fewer patients to secondary medical and surgical specialties.[374] It is unclear, however, whether there was improved outcome for the patients.

Well-described advice on how best to manage these patients in primary care, using a mixture of understanding, advice and management plans, has been formulated.[375–377] Primary care professionals can be taught to improve recognition and management by using a reattribution model for symptoms.[378,379] Four key stages have been identified:

- provide clear information about the negative physical examination and investigations, whilst acknowledging the reality of the physical symptoms
- state the relevant mood and associated symptoms and refer to the psychosocial factors identified
- explain the relationship between mood and physical symptoms/pain
- emphasise the positive aspects of treatment and provide reality-based reassurance.[380]

Evaluation of this approach suggests that training can decrease referral costs by 23% with no corresponding increase in primary care costs. Better outcomes in those patients, at least those who were prepared to consider a psychological explanation for their symptoms, have also been described.[381,382]

Psychological therapies

Brief psychological therapies using cognitive or dynamic approaches may be effective in the management of somatisation.[383,384] Problem-solving approaches may also be of use in primary care, but further effectiveness studies are needed.[385] It is likely that patients with a very long history of symptoms and marked abnormal illness behaviour are unlikely to respond to brief intervention.

Pharmacological treatments

Antidepressant therapy should be tried in patients who have medically unexplained symptoms and who are depressed, if they will accept it. There is some evidence of the value of antidepressants, particularly tricyclics, in some patients with 'psychogenic' pain.[386] A systematic review of randomised, controlled trials of the use of antidepressants in patients who were depressed with a range of coexisting physical illness also suggests that antidepressants are effective in relieving depression in this group.[387]

Summary

- Mental ill health commonly presents in general practice with physical complaints or somatisation.
- Some patients will then accept that there is a psychological problem, whilst others will not and a small number suffer from true somatoform disorder.
- This group of disorders is ill defined and consequently is difficult to research.
- Primary care practitioners can be taught to help patients to deal with their symptoms through a process of reattribution.
- Cognitive/behavioural and problem-solving interventions may be effective in some individuals.
- Antidepressants are appropriate in those who are depressed and will accept treatment.

Appendix 4: Adjustment disorder

Introduction

The term 'adjustment disorder' refers to a short-lived (a few weeks or months) episode of anxiety in reaction to a stressful event. A range of relatively non-specific symptoms are experienced, such as feeling overwhelmed, unable to cope, depressed, anxious, worried, having difficulty sleeping and interference with performance of usual daily routines. Symptoms may also be primarily somatic, e.g. headaches, gastro-intestinal symptoms, chest pain and/or palpitations. In order to make a diagnosis of adjustment disorder there should be evidence that the symptoms would not have developed without the stressful event, i.e. the individual does not normally have symptoms of anxiety.

Terminology and classification

Clearly not everyone reacts to adverse life events in this way. However, the distinction between normality and disorder may be difficult to make. In fact, if the symptoms last over six months, then alternative diagnoses should be considered, such as depression, generalised anxiety disorder or panic disorder. Abnormal or traumatic grief reactions are a special form of adjustment disorder.

ICD-10 for primary care includes adjustment disorder under F43.

Epidemiology

Prevalence

Most cases of adjustment disorder will be seen in primary care, and prevalence rates are high. There is some evidence that different understandings of adjustment disorder contribute to misunderstandings between primary and secondary care clinicians. In a large primary care study, psychiatrists agreed with GPs that mental disorder was present in approximately 50% of cases. The other patients identified by GPs as having a disorder were mainly suffering from anxiety, worries, marital difficulties and other adjustment reactions, but whose symptoms were not of sufficient severity or duration to meet psychiatric diagnostic criteria.[388]

Effectiveness of services and interventions

The outcome of disorder

People undergoing certain kinds of stressful life events, such as divorce, unemployment or bereavement are at increased risk of developing a mental disorder and may also be vulnerable to developing physical illness.[389,390]

People with adjustment disorder may experience high levels of distress in the short term. A US study examined the relationship between self-reported distress and mood disturbance in a primary care population.[391] It found that, in the primary care sample, most distressed patients did not have a mood disturbance of more than short-term duration and that distress without mood disturbance was associated with little impairment. It concluded that, for this group of people, it might be very difficult to show an advantage for active treatment over no intervention.

A small US follow-up study carried out in the 1970s reported the five-year outcome for 48 adults given a diagnosis of adjustment disorder in an outpatient setting: 71% (34) were completely well and had suffered no further complications during the five years and 8% (4) were well, but had suffered depression or alcoholism in the intervening period. The remaining 22% (10) were found to be suffering from a specific disorder, usually major depression plus alcohol misuse and 4% (2) had committed suicide.[392] The outcome for adjustment disorder in primary care is likely to be significantly better, given that this study was of psychiatric outpatients. For a minority, however, symptoms may become chronic and future assessment for depression and/or alcohol misuse is likely to be important.

There are few studies that address how to identify those individuals who will go on to develop depression or anxiety disorders. The US study quoted above found that those who went on to develop major depression and had poorer outcomes at five years had more chronic symptoms at initial presentation.

There is good evidence from longitudinal studies on those individuals who are at risk of developing abnormal grief reactions. The factors, which increase risk, include:

- a history of mental disorder
- unexpected or violent death of a loved one, especially homicide or suicide or where the body is not present
- death of spouse or child
- ambivalence in the relationship between the dead person and the bereaved person
- lack of social support.[393]

Signs that the grief is becoming abnormal include severe depressive symptoms of retardation, guilt, feelings of worthlessness, hopelessness or suicidal ideation of a severity or duration that significantly interferes with daily living.

Management

Interventions for adjustment disorder have not been extensively studied, either in primary or secondary care. Most recommendations for management of adjustment disorder are therefore based on the experience of clinicians.

The management advised by a consensus of experienced clinicians comprises support and advice in primary care. A combination of education (e.g. about how anxiety can manifest itself physically), reassurance, advice on coping or problem solving, targeted supportive and practical help (e.g. welfare advice, relationship counselling) and passage of time is recommended. An invitation to return for a second consultation with the GP or nurse in a few weeks 'to see how things are going' may also help individuals get through the period of stress.[394,395]

Not many primary care studies exist to either support or challenge this advice. It is likely that in the majority of cases specialist mental health service intervention does not confer additional advantage over care as usual in primary care.

Medication should be reserved for severe anxiety symptoms, when anxiolytics can be used for a few days, or if the individual meets the criteria for major depression, in which case they should be treated appropriately.

Self-help and the community/voluntary sector

Many organisations provide supportive help and information for people experiencing particular problems of living, such as bereavement and relationship problems.

Coping strategy advice, targeted supportive and practical help (e.g. welfare advice, relationship counselling) and the passage of time may all be helpful.

Management of bereavement

Approaches to supporting bereaved individuals in primary care are based on professional consensus. This would include ensuring that the individual had access to a confiding and supportive relationship with the opportunity to cry and talk about their loss and feelings. Avoiding prescribing benzodiazepines is also important, unless on a short-term basis where the individual is very distressed by severe insomnia. GPs or other members of the primary care team can also have a role in preparing the individual for a forthcoming bereavement.

There is some evidence from small, uncontrolled trial to suggest that, in high-risk groups, focused bereavement counselling may improve long-term outcome.[396]

Organisations such as Cruse can provide advice and focused bereavement counselling.

Summary

- Adjustment disorders are common, but not well researched.
- Supportive advice and follow-up may be of benefit.
- Appropriate treatment interventions should be provided for those that develop depressive or anxiety disorders.

Appendix 5: Eating disorders

Introduction

Eating disorders are common and include the conditions of bulimia nervosa, anorexia nervosa and binge-eating disorder. Obesity alone is not included in psychiatric diagnostic systems. At any one point in time up to 10% of the female population may be affected by some eating difficulties. There is a spectrum of severity from mild, self-limiting difficulty or disorder amenable to self-help to severe debilitating illness with significant mortality. Anorexia has the highest mortality of any single psychiatric illness, including deaths from medical complications, starvation and suicide.

Classification and terminology

Eating disorders, anorexia and bulimia, are included in both DSM-IV and ICD-10, although the criteria for diagnosis are somewhat different. DSM-IV also describes research criteria for binge-eating disorder. Eating disorders are included in the ICD-10 for primary care under F50.
  The key components for diagnosis are described in the following sections.

Bulimia nervosa

Recurrent episodes of binge eating and compensatory behaviours to combat weight gain such as fasting, use of laxatives, self-induced vomiting or excessive exercise. The individual has an undue preoccupation with body shape and weight. Low self-esteem and low self-confidence are integral parts of the disorder.

Anorexia nervosa

Individuals typically avoid high calorie foods and are very preoccupied with food and meal preparation, leading to significant loss of body weight. Vomiting, the use of laxatives and obsessive exercise may all be part of the condition. Despite severe emaciation, individuals may continue to feel well, having a distorted body image.

Binge-eating disorder

This is a newer diagnostic concept included in the appendix of DSM-IV and as atypical disorder in ICD-10. It consists of recurrent episodes of binge eating not associated with inappropriate compensatory behaviours or occurring during an episode of anorexia or bulimia.

Epidemiology

Prevalence and incidence

Bulimia nervosa

The incidence rate varies with age. The average age of onset is 18 years with 25% developing disorder under age 16. In young women incidence rates of 52/100 000 have been found, 13/100 000 for the general population.[397] The overall prevalence is approximately 1–3% of women or over 5% if partial syndromes are included.[398,399] Figures of 0.25% have been found in young men.[400] Women with a history of dieting are at significantly greater risk of developing the disorder.

Anorexia nervosa

In Britain, the incidence of disorder is 7/100 000, or 4000 new cases per year.[401] The prevalence in young women ranges from 0.1–1%.[402]

Binge-eating disorder

2% of community samples meet the criteria for BED.[403]

Factors affecting prevalence

Time trends

Bulimia nervosa was first described in 1979. During the period 1988 to 1993, there was an apparent threefold increase in cases presenting to primary care. It is difficult to know how much of this reflects increased recognition rather than changes in underlying incidence.[404]

There have also been reports that there has been an increase in incidence of anorexia, but again changes in recognition must be taken into account.

Socio-demographic factors

Ninety percent of cases of anorexia and bulimia are in women with a typical age of onset in the late teens. Cases are more prevalent in occupations where slimness is valued, e.g. dancers, models and performers. Binge-eating disorder (BED) shows a male to female ratio in occurrence of 3:2.

Anorexia has been found more commonly in lower social classes and bulimia has an even class distribution.[405,406] Bulimia is more prevalent in large cities over other urban areas and rural communities.[407]

Comorbidity

Other psychiatric disorders are commonly associated with eating disorders. In bulimia there is a 36–70% lifetime risk of major depression; anxiety is similarly common.[408] Approximately 30% of those with bulimia have a history of PTSD.[409] Similar proportions have a history of anorexia. Depression is found in approximately 50% of those with anorexia.

Comorbidity is more likely in clinic than in community samples, with personality disorder, substance misuse and self-injury commonly found.[410]

Physical complications affecting the gastro-intestinal, cardiovascular and gynaecological systems are also commonly found in both bulimia and anorexia.

Binge-eating disorder commonly occurs with obesity.

Effectiveness of services and interventions

Key issues in assessing the effectiveness literature are:

- compliance with treatment of all modalities may be low, with high drop-out rates, particularly for medication and some inpatient regimens
- some of the most severely affected may be excluded from treatment trials
- most trials are not in primary care populations
- follow-up times are often short.

Outcome of disorder

Bulimia nervosa

For those that receive treatment, 50–70% are symptom-free at 5–10 years, the median length of illness being 3–6 years. Mortality rates are between 0.3% and 1.1%.[411] Poor outcomes are associated with the severity of bingeing, associated personality disorder and depression. A small number, 3–4%, develop anorexia or other eating disorders.

Anorexia nervosa

The median length of illness is six years. Thirty percent have a poor prognosis. Abnormally low serum albumin levels and a low body weight (60% of average) are predictors of poor outcome. Mortality rates are between 3% and 4%.

Binge-eating disorder

Little is known about outcomes. There is some suggestion that, of those treated, most have no disorder at six years.[412]

Detection and diagnosis

As with other mental ill health, detection in primary care is low – primary care physicians detect between 12% and 50% of cases.[413,414] The SCOFF questionnaire is a short tool designed to detect eating disorders and aid treatment. It has been shown to be efficient at detection of adult eating disorders in primary care.[415]

Management

Bulimia nervosa

Cognitive behavioural therapy (CBT) is the most widely used treatment. It has been evaluated in both RCTs and systemic reviews.[416,417] A usual course consists of between 16 and 20 sessions. At completion 40–60% of patients are symptom-free, with gains maintained at five years.[418] Self-help with some therapist support has also been found to effective.[419] Interpersonal therapy has been shown to be as effective as cognitive behavioural therapy at one-year follow-up, although CBT showed earlier gains.[420] Early studies using motivational enhancement suggest short-term outcomes similar to CBT.[421]

Randomised controlled trials of medication, varying from appetite suppressants to opioid antagonists, antidepressants and mood stabilisers, have been undertaken. Systematic reviews of RCTs suggest that antidepressants may decrease bingeing and depressive symptoms in the short term, although long-term effects are less clear.[422,423] The combination of CBT and antidepressants is more effective than antidepressants or placebo and probably equivalent to CBT alone.[424]

Complex cases with significant co-morbidity and/or histories of abuse are less likely to respond to simple treatment approaches as described and these cases are often excluded from treatment trials. More prolonged psychological interventions may be appropriate here, as with those who do not respond to short-term intervention. The role of day-care and inpatient care needs further evaluation, as do other psychological therapies such as dialectical behavioural and cognitive analytic therapies.

Anorexia nervosa

There are few RCTs to assess effectiveness. The age of the patient and the severity of disorder will usually determine which treatment is most appropriate. Brief, focused outpatient psychotherapy can be effective and prevent relapse for those less severely affected.[425] Family therapy is often recommended for younger patients.[426] Inpatient care may be necessary for those with severe weight loss. Regimes have changed significantly over the past 15 years with a move away from the more punishing approaches. Less punitive regimes are thought to be as effective as the older more coercive ones.[427] Day care has also shown promising results. A small randomised trial of intensive inpatient treatment versus day care with CBT showed, at three-year follow-up, fewer relapses, more stable weight and fewer admissions in the day care group.[428]

Binge-eating disorder

CBT can help to reduce bingeing and is effective in pure self-help and therapist-guided programmes.[429] Medication, including antidepressants, anorectic agents and opiate antagonists may also reduce bingeing in the short-term.

Models of service delivery

Large areas of the country have no access to dedicated NHS eating disorder services.[430,431] This is reflected in significant private sector provision.

Different models of service provision exist, including local comprehensive community-based services to highly specialist treatment centres. A range of services is required, given the range of disorder. Specialisation is likely to be required for some patients, such as those with complex disorder or those who do not respond to initial treatment. There is a significant role for primary care, albeit with appropriately skilled practitioners and with support from specialist services.

Summary

- Eating disorders are common in the female population; they are much less common in the male population.
- CBT is an effective treatment for less severe cases of bulimia.
- Evidence for the effectiveness of treatments for anorexia and severe bulimia is more limited.

References

1 Singleton N, Bumpstead K, O'Brien M *et al. Psychiatric morbidity among adults living in private households 2000.* London: Stationery Office, 2001.

2 Goldberg D, Huxley P. *Common mental disorders: a biosocial model.* London: Routledge, 1992.

3 Department of Health. *Health of the Nation: mental illness key area handbook.* (2e). London: HMSO, 1994.

4 Department of Health. *Modernising Mental Health Services: safe, sound and supportive.* London: Department of Health, 1998.

5 Department of Health. *The New NHS: modern, dependable.* London: Department of Health, 1997.

6 National Health Service. *National Service Framework Mental Health: modern standards ad service models.* London: NHSE, 1999.

7 National Health Service. *The NHS Plan: a plan for investment: a plan for reform.* Cm 4818-I. London: HMSO, 2000.

8 Department of Health. *Fast-forwarding Primary Care Mental Health: Gateway workers.* London: Department of Health, 2002.

9 HM Government. *Caring About Carers: a national strategy for carers.* London: HMSO, 1999.

10 Gask L, Croft J. Methods of working in primary care. *Adv Psyche Treatment* 2000; **6**: 442–9.

11 Lee J, Gask L, Roland M, Donnan S. *National Evaluation of total purchasing pilot projects.* London: King's Fund, 1999.

12 Sainsbury Centre for Mental Health/Royal College of General Practitioners. *Setting the Standard: the new agenda for primary care organisations commissioning mental health services.* London: SCMH, 2001.

13 Murray C, Lopex A (eds). *A comprehensive assessment of mortality and disability from diseases; injury and risk factors in 1990 and projected to 2020. The global burden of disease and injury series.* Boston: Harvard University Press, 1996.

14 Spitzer RL, Kroenke K, Linzer M *et al.* Health related quality of life in primary care patients with mental disorders. Results from the PRIME MD 1000 Study. *JAMA* 1995; **274(10)**: 1511–7.

15 Kisley, Gater R, Goldberg D. Results from the Manchester Centre. In: Ustun TB, Sartorius N (eds). *Mental illness in general health care: an international study.* Chichester: Wiley, 1996.

16 Stewart-Brown S. Emotional wellbeing and its relation to health. Editorial. *BMJ* 1998; **317**: 1608–9.

17 Meltzer H, Gill B, Petticrew M, Hinks K. *Economic activity and social functioning of adults with psychiatric disorders. OPCS surveys of psychiatric morbidity in Great Britain Report 3.* London: HMSO, 1995.

18 Harris EC, Barraclough B. Excess mortality and mental disorder. *Brit J Psyche* 1998; **173**: 11–53.

19 Hemingway H, Marmot M. Psychosocial factors in the aetiology and prognosis of coronary heart disease: systematic review of prospective cohort studies. *BMJ* 1999; **318**: 1460–7.

20 Dinan TG. The physical consequences of depressive illness. Editorial. *BMJ* 1999; **318**: 826.

21 Pratt LA, Ford LE, Crum RM *et al.* Depression, psychotropic medication, and the risk of myocardial infarction: prospective data from the Baltimore ECA follow-up. *Circulation* 1999; **94**: 123–9.

22 Stewart-Brown S. Emotional wellbeing and its relation to health. Editorial. *BMJ* 1998; **317**: 1608–9.

23 Knight BG, Lutzky SM, Macofsky-Urban F. A meta-analysis of interventions for caregiver distress: recommendations for future research. *Gerontologist* 1993; **33**: 240–8.

24 Kavanagh S, Fenyo A. Informal care and depression. *Mental Health Research Review* 1998; **5**: 56–8.

25 Patel A, Knapp M. Costs of mental illness in England. *Mental Health Research Review* 1998; **5**: 4–10.

26 NHS Executive. *Burdens of disease.* Leeds: NHSE, 1996.

27 Kind P, Sorensen J. The cost of depression. *Int Clin Psychopharm* 1993; **7**: 191–5.

28 Knapp MRJ. Costs of schizophrenia. *Brit J Psyche* 1997; **171(6)**: 509–18.

29 Meltzer H, Gill B, Petticrew M, Hinks K. *Economic activity and social functioning of adults with psychiatric disorders. OPCS surveys of psychiatric morbidity in Great Britain Report 3.* London: HMSO, 1995.

30 Cooper C, Cartwright S. *Mental health and stress in the workplace, a guide for employers.* London: HMSO, 1996.

31 Confederation of British Industry/Department of Health. *Promoting mental health at work.* London: CBI/DoH, 1992.

32 Goldberg D, Huxley P. *Common mental disorders: a biosocial model.* London: Routledge, 1992.

33 Goldberg DP, Bridges K, Duncan-Jones P, Grayson D. Dimensions of neuroses seen in primary care settings. *Psychol Med* 1997; **17**: 461–70.

34 Sartorius N, Ustun TB, Lecrubier Y, Wittchen H. Depression comorbid with anxiety: Results from the WHO study on psychological disorders in primary health care. *Brit J Psych* 1996; **168**: 38–43.

35 Lewis G. Dimensions of neurosis. *Psychol Med* 1992; **22**: 1011–18.

36 Spitzer RL, Kroenke K, Linzer M *et al.* Health related quality of life in primary care patients with mental disorders. Results from the PRIME MD 1000 Study. *JAMA* 1995; **274(10)**: 1511–7.

37 Wells KB, Stewart A, Hays RD *et al.* The functioning and well-being of depressed patients. Results from the Medical Outcomes Study. *JAMA* 1989; **262**: 914–19.

38 Broadhead WE, Blazer DG, George LK, Tse CK. Depression, disability days and days lost from work in a prospective epidemiologic survey. *JAMA* 1990; **264**: 2524–8.

39 Wohlfarth TD, Van Den Brink W, Ormel J, Koeter MWJ. The relationship between social dysfunctioning and psychopathology among primary care attenders. *Brit J Psych* 1993; **163**: 37–44.

40 Ustun TB, Goldberg D, Cooper J *et al.* New classification of mental disorders with management guidelines for use in primary care. *Brit J Gen Pract* 1995; **45**: 211–15.

41 Goldberg D, Huxley P. *Common mental disorders: a biosocial model.* London: Routledge, 1992.

42 OPCS Social Survey Division. *OPCS Surveys of Psychiatric Morbidity: Private Household Survey.* London: HMSO, 1993.

43 Anderson J, Huppert F, Rose G. Normality, deviance and minor psychiatric morbidity in the community; a population-based approach to General Health Questionnaire data in the health and lifestyle survey. *Psychol Med* 1993; **23**: 478–85.

44 Lewis G, Booth M. Regional differences in mental health in Great Britain. *J Epidem Comm Health* 1992; **46**: 608–11.

45 Jarman B, Hirsch S. Statistical models to predict district psychiatric morbidity. In: Thorncroft G, Brewin C, Wing JK (eds). *Measuring mental health need.* London: Royal College of Psychiatrists, Gaskel, 1992.

46 Meltzer H, Gill B, Petticrew M, Hinks K. *Physical complaints, service use and treatment of adults with psychiatric disorders. OPCS surveys of psychiatric morbidity in Great Britain Report 2.* London: HMSO, 1995.

47 Francisco GS. An overview of post stroke depression. *NEJM* 1993; **90**: 686–9.

48 Mayou RA. *Consultation liaison psychiatry: an international perspective.* Psychiatry Clinical Update. Crawley: Upjohn, 1988.

49 Creed F, Marks B. Liaison psychiatry in general practice: a comparison of the liaison attachment scheme and shifted outpatient clinic model. *J Royal Coll Gen Pract* 1989; **39**: 514–17.

50 Meltzer H, Gill B, Petticrew M, Hinks K. *Physical complaints, service use and treatment of adults with psychiatric disorders. OPCS surveys of psychiatric morbidity in Great Britain Report 2.* London: HMSO, 1995.

51 National Mental Health Strategy. Royal College of Australian General Practitioners/Royal College of Australian & New Zealand Psychiatrists. *Primary care psychiatry: the last frontier. A report of the joint*

consultative committee in psychiatry. Royal College of Australian General Practitioners/Royal College of Australian & New Zealand Psychiatrists, 1998.

52 Bowers PJ. Selections from current literature: psychiatric disorders in primary care. *Fam Pract* 1993; **10**(2): 231–7.

53 Freeling P, Tylee A. Depression in general practice. In: Paykel ES (ed). *Handbook of affective disorders.* (2e). Edinburgh: Churchill Livingstone, 1992.

54 Office of National Statistics. *Key Health Statistics from general practice 1998*. London: National Statistics, 2000.

55 Bridges KW, Goldberg DP. Somatic presentation of DSM-III psychiatric disorders in primary care. *J Psychosom Res* 1985; **29**: 563–9.

56 Kendrick A. The role of general practitioners in the care of the long term mentally ill. *BMJ* 1991; **302**: 508–10.

57 Chelsea and Westminster Health Authority. *Better Services for Mental Health.* Newsletter Primary Care Led Purchasing of Mental Health Services Project. May 1998.

58 Royal College of General Practitioners. *The primary health care team.* RCGP Information Sheet No 21. London: Royal College of General Practitioners, 1998.

59 Royal College of General Practitioners. *Profile of UK Practices.* RCGP Information Sheet No 2. London: Royal College of General Practitioners, 1999.

60 Kendrick T, Sibbald B, Addington-Hall J, *et al. Distribution of mental health professionals working onsite within English and Welsh general practices. BMJ* 1993; **307**: 544–6.

61 Onyett S, Pidd F, Cohen A, Peck E. Mental health service provision and the primary health care team. *Mental Health Review* 1997; **1**(3).

62 Royal College of General Practitioners. *Profile of UK general practitioners.* RCGP Information Sheet No 1. London: RCGP, 2000.

63 Royal College of General Practitioners. *Profile of UK general practitioners.* RCGP Information Sheet No 1. London: RCGP, 2000.

64 Office of Health Economics. *Compendium of health statistics.* (2e). London: OHE, 1995.

65 Turton P, Tylee A, Kerry S. Mental health training needs in general practice. *Primary Care Psych* 1995; **1**: 197–9.

66 Clinical Standards Advisory Group. *Services for patients with depression.* London: Stationery Office, 1999.

67 Turton P, Tylee A, Kerry S. Mental health training needs in general practice. *Primary Care Psych* 1995; **1**: 197–9.

68 Greenfield S, Stilwell B, Drury M. Practice nurses: social and occupational characteristics. *J Royal College GP* 1987; **37**: 341–5.

69 Thomas R, Corney R. The role of the practice nurse in mental health: a survey. *J Mental Health UK* 1993; **2**: 65–72.

70 Crossland A, Kai J. They think they can talk to nurses: practice nurses' views of their roles in caring for mental health problems. *Brit J GP* 1998; **48**: 1383–6.

71 Gray R, Parr, Plummer S *et al.* A national survey of practice nurse involvement in mental health interventions. *J Adv Nursing* 1999; **30**(4): 901–6.

72 Kendrick T, Millar E, Burns T, Ross F. Practice nurse involvement in giving depot neuroleptic injections: development of patient assessment and monitoring checklist. *Primary Care Psyche* 1998; **4**(3): 149–54.

73 Sainsbury Centre for Mental Health. *An executive briefing on primary care mental health services.* Briefing 19. SCMH/NHS Alliance: London, 2002.

74 Department of Health. *Health and personal social services statistics for England.* London: Stationery Office 1999.

75 Jones L, Sheehan C. Mental health and primary care: needs assessment research for the Health Education Board for Scotland. Final report 1999 (unpublished seeking permission to quote).

76 Department of Health. *Health and personal social services statistics for England.* London: Stationery Office, 1999.

77 Strathdee G, Williams P. A survey of psychiatrists in primary care. *J Royal Coll GP* 1984; **34**: 615–18.

78 Chisholm D. Use and cost of primary care services by people in residential mental health care. *Mental Health Research Review* 1998; **5**: 23–5.

79 Kendrick A. The role of general practitioners in the care of the long term mentally ill. *BMJ* 1991; **302**: 508–10.

80 Kendrick T, Sibbald B, Addington-Hall J *et al.* Distribution of mental health professionals working on-site within English and Welsh general practices. *BMJ* 1993; **307**: 544–6.

81 Thomas R, Corney R. A survey of links between mental health professionals and general practice in six district health authorities. *Brit J Gen Pract* Spt 1992.

82 Filson P, Kendrick T. Survey of roles of community psychiatric nurses and occupational therapists. *Psych Bull* 1997; **21**: 70–3.

83 Sibbald B, Addington Hall J. *The role of counsellors in general practice.* RCGP Occasional Paper No 74. London: RCGP, 1996.

84 Goldberg D, Gournay K: *The general practitioner, the psychiatrist and the burden of mental health care.* Maudsley discussion paper no. 1. London: Institute of Psychiatry, 1997.

85 Clinical Standards Advisory Group. *Services for patients with depression.* London: Stationery Office, 1999.

86 Kendrick T, Sibbald B, Addington-Hall J *et al.* Distribution of mental health professionals working on-site within English and Welsh general practices. *BMJ* 1993; **307**: 544–6.

87 Mellor-Clark J, Simms-Ellis R, Burton M. *National survey of counsellors in primary care; evidence for growing professionalism.* London: RCGP, 2001.

88 Sparling E, Clark N, Laidlaw J. Assessment of the demands by general practitioners for a community psychiatric occupational therapy service. *Brit J Occ Therapy* 1992; **55(5)**: 193–6.

89 de Witt P, de Luca PM. Occupational therapy and primary care: the mental health perspective. *S African J Occ Therapy* 1995; **Nov**: 34–40.

90 Brewer P, Gadsen V, Scrimshaw K. The community group network in mental health: a model for social support and community integration. *Brit J Occ Therapy* 1994; **579(12)**: 467–70.

91 Department of Health. *Fast-forwarding primary care mental health: Gateway workers.* London: Department of Health, 2002.

92 Clinical Standards Advisory Group. *Services for patients with depression.* London: Stationery Office, 1999.

93 Clinical Standards Advisory Group. *Services for patients with depression.* London: Stationery Office, 1999.

94 Jones L, Sheehan C. Mental health and primary care: needs assessment research for the Health Education Board for Scotland. Final report 1999 (unpublished).

95 Goodrick I, Nisbett M, White D. *Goodwill in practice: the GP volunteer handbook.* London: Royal College of General Practitioners, 1997.

96 Ormel J, Tiemens BG. Recognition and treatment of mental illness in primary care: Towards a better understanding of a multi-faceted problem. *Gen Hosp Psyche* 1995; **17**: 160–4.

97 MacGillivray S, Arroll B, Hatcher S *et al.* Efficacy and tolerability of selective serotonin re uptake inhibitors compared with tricyclic antidepressants in depression treated in primary care: systematic review and meta-analysis. *BMJ* 2003; **326**: 1014–7.

98 Mann A, Jenkins R, Besley E. The twelve-month outcome of patients with neurotic illness in general practice. *Psychol Med* 1981; **11**: 535–50.

99 Lloyd KR, Jenkins R, Mann A. Long term outcome of patients with neurotic illness in general practice. *BMJ* 1996; **313**: 26–8.

100 Faulkner A. *Strategies for liking*. London: Mental Health Foundation, 2000.

101 Rogers A, Pilgrim D. *Experiencing psychiatry: Users views of services*. London: MacMillan Press Ltd, 1993.

102 Jones L, Sheehan C. Mental health and primary care: needs assessment research for the Health Education Board for Scotland. Final report 1999 (unpublished).

103 Weich S. Prevention of the common mental disorders: a public health perspective. *Psychol Med* 1997; **27**: 757–64.

104 Weich S, Churchill R, Lewis G, Mann A. Strategies for the prevention of psychiatric disorder in primary care in south London. *J Epidem Comm Health* 1997; **51**: 304–9.

105 Newton J. *Preventing mental illness in practice*. London: Routledge, 1992.

106 Markman HJ, Renick MJ, Floyd FJ, Stanley SM *et al.* Preventing marital distress through communication and conflict management training: a 4 and 5 year follow up. *J Consul Clin Psychol* 1993; **61**: 70–77.

107 Health Education Authority. *Mental health promotion: a quality framework*. London: HEA, 1997.

108 Olweus D. Bully/victim problems among school children: basic facts and effects of an intervention programme. In: Ruben KH, Pepler DJ (eds). *The development and treatment of childhood aggression*. Hillsdale NH: Lawrence Erlbaum Associates, 1989.

109 Health Education Authority. *Mental health promotion: a quality framework*. London: HEA, 1997.

110 NHS Centre for Reviews & Dissemination. Mental health promotion in high risk groups. *Effective Health Care Bulletin* 1997; **3(3)**.

111 Weich S, Churchill R, Lewis G, Mann A. Strategies for the prevention of psychiatric disorder in primary care in south London. *J Epidem Comm Health* 1997; **51**: 304–9.

112 Tylee A, Priest R, Roberts A. *Depression in general practice*. London: Martin Dunitz Ltd, 1996.

113 Barraclough GM, Bunch J, Nelson B, Sainsbury P. A hundred cases of suicide: clinical aspects. *Brit J Psych* 1974; **125**: 355–73.

114 Vassilas D, Morgan G. General practitioners' contact with victims of suicide. *BMJ* 1993; **307**: 300–1.

115 Gunnell D. Recent studies of contacts with services prior to suicide. In: Jenkins R, Griffiths S, Wylie I, Hawton K *et al.* (eds). *The prevention of suicide*. London: HMSO, 1994.

116 Department of Health. *Safety first: Five-year report of the national inquiry into suicide and homicide by people with mental illness*. London: Department of Health, 2001.

117 Rutz W, von Knorring L, Walinder J. Long term effects of an educational program for general practitioners given by the Swedish committee for the prevention and treatment of depression. *Acta Psychiatr Scand* 1992; **85**: 83–8.

118 Thompson C, Kinmouth AL, Stevens L, Peveler R *et al.* Effects of a clinical practice guideline and practice based education on detection and outcome of depression in primary care: Hampshire depression project randomised control trial. *The Lancet* 1999; **355**: 185–91.

119 Phelan M, Stradins L, Morrison S. Physical health of people with severe mental illness. *BMJ* 2001; **322**: 443–4.

120 Jeste DV, Gladsjo JA, Lindamer LA, Lacro JP. Medical comorbidity in schizophrenia. *Schizophrenia Bulletin* 1996; **22**: 413–27.

121 Freeling P, Rao BM, Paykel ES, Sireling L *et al.* Unrecognized depression in general practice. *BMJ* 1985; **290**: 1880–3.

122 Tylee A, Freeling P, Kerry S. Why do general practitioners recognise depression in one woman patient yet miss it in another? *Brit J Gen Pract* 1993; **43**: 327–30.

123 Kessler D, Bennemith O, Lewis G, Sharp D. Detection of depression and anxiety in primary care: a follow-up study. *BMJ* 2002; **325**; 508–10.

124 Plummer S, Ritter S, Leach R *et al.* A controlled comparison of the abilities of practice nurses to detect psychological distress in patients who attend their clinics. *J Psych Mental Health Nursing* 1997; **4**: 221–3.

125 Briscoe M. Identification of emotional problems in postpartum women by health visitors. *BMJ* 1986; **292**: 1245–7.

126 Eisenberg L. Treating depression and anxiety in primary care. Closing the gap between knowledge and practice. *NEJM* 1992; **326**: 1080–4.

127 Shepherd M, Cooper B, Brown AC, Kalton GW. *Psychiatric illness in general practice.* Oxford: Oxford University Press, 1966.

128 Rost K, Smith GR, Mathews DB, Guise B. The deliberate misdiagnosis of major depression in primary care. *Arch Fam Med* 1994; **3**: 330–7.

129 Susman JL, Crabtree BF, Essink G. Depression in rural family practice: easy to recognise, difficult to diagnose. *Arch Fam Med* 1995; **4**: 427–31.

130 Goldberg DP, Jenkins L, Millar T, Faragher EB. The ability of trainee general practitioners to identify distress among their patients. *Psychol Med* 1993; **23**: 185–93.

131 Millar T, Goldberg DP. Link between the ability to detect and manage emotional disorders; a study of general practitioner trainees. *Brit J Gen Pract* 1991; **41**: 357–9.

132 Gask L, Sibbald B, Creed F. Evaluating models of working at the interface between mental health services and primary care. *Brit J Psych* 1997; **170**: 6–11.

133 Howie JGR, Porter AMD, Forbes JF. Quality and the use of time in general practice: widening the discussion. *BMJ* 1989; **298**: 1008–10.

134 Marks J, Goldberg D, Hillier V. Determinants of the ability of general practitioners to detect psychiatric illness. *Psychol Med* 1979; **9**: 337–53.

135 Joukammaa M, Lehtinen V, Karlsson H. The ability of general practitioners to detect mental disorders in primary health care. *Acta Psych Scand* 1995; **91**: 52–6.

136 Sartorius N, Ustun TB, Lecrubier Y, Wittchen H. Depression comorbid with anxiety: Results from the WHO study on psychological disorders in primary health care. *Brit J Psych* 1996; **168**: 38–43.

137 Bridges KW, Goldberg DP. Somatic presentation of DSM III psychiatric disorders in primary care. *J Psychosom Res* 1985; **29**: 563–9.

138 Badger LW, DeGruy FV, Hartman J *et al.* Patient presentation, interview content and the detection of depression by primary care physicians. *Psychosom Med* 1994; **56**: 128–35.

139 Odell SM, Surtees PG, Wainwright NWJ *et al.* Determinants of general practitioner recognition of psychological problems in a multi-ethnic inner-city health district. *Brit J Psyche* 1997; **171**: 537–41.

140 Kessler D, Lloyd K, Lewis G, Pereira Gray D. Cross sectional survey of symptom attribution and recognition of depression and anxiety in primary care. *BMJ* 1999; **318**: 436–9.

141 Weich S, Lewis G, Donmall R, Mann A. Somatic presentation of psychiatric morbidity in general practice. *Brit J Gen Pract* 1995; **45**: 143–7.

142 Hoeper EW, Ncyz, Kessler LG *et al.* The usefulness of screening for mental illness. *Lancet* 1984; **Jan 7** 1(8367): 33–5.

143 Marks JN, Goldberg DP, Hillier VF. Determinants of the ability of general practitioners to detect psychiatric illness. *Psychol Med* 1979; **9**: 337–53.

144 Boardman AP. The General Health Questionnaire and the detection of emotional disorder by general practitioners. A replicated study. *Brit J Psyche* 1987; **151**: 373–81.

145 Kirmayer LJ, Robbins JM, Dworkind M, Yaffe MJ. Somatization and the recognition of depression and anxiety in primary care. *Am J Psyche* 1993; **150**: 734–41.

146 Simon GE, Von Korff M. Recognition, management and outcomes of depression in primary care. *Arch Fam Med* 1995; **4**: 99–105.

147 Von Korff M, Shapiro S, Burke JD *et al.* Anxiety and depression in a primary care clinic. Comparison of diagnostic interview schedule, General Health Questionnaire and practitioner assessments. *Arch Gen Psych* 1987; **44**: 152–6.

148 Rand EH, Badger LW, Coggins DR. Towards a resolution of contradictions: utility of feedback from the GHQ. *Gen Hosp Psych* 1988; **10**: 189–96.

149 Gerber PD, Barrett J, Manheimer E *et al.* Recognition of depression by internists in primary care: a comparison of internist and 'gold standard' psychiatric assessments. *J Gen Intern Med* 1989; **4**: 7–13.

150 Coyne JC, Schwenck TL, Fechner-Bates S. Non-detection of depression by primary care physicians reconsidered. *Gen Hosp Psych* 1995; **7**: 3–12.

151 Tiemens BG, Ormel J, Simon GE. Occurrence, recognition and outcome of psychological disorders in primary care. *Am J Psych* 1996; **153**: 636–44.

152 Ronalds C, Creed F, Stone K *et al.* Outcome of anxiety and depressive disorders in primary care. *Brit J Psyche* 1997; **171**: 427–33.

153 Coyne JC, Klinkman MS, Gallo SM, Schwenck TL. Short-term outcomes of detected and undetected depressed primary care patients and depressed psychiatric patients. *Gen Hosp Psyche* 1997; **19**: 333–43.

154 Dowrick CF. Case or continuum? Analysing general practitioners' ability to detect depression. *Primary Care Psychiatry* 1997; **1**: 255–7.

155 Goldberg DP, Jenkins L, Millar T, Faragher EB. The ability of trainee general practitioners to identify distress among their patients. *Psychol Med* 1993; **23**: 185–93.

156 Pollock K, Grime J. Patients perception of entitlement to time in general practice consultations for depression: quantitative study. *BMJ* 2002; **325**: 687–9.

157 Catalan J, Gath D, Edmonds G, Ennis J. The effects of non-prescribing of anxiolytics in general practice. *Brit J Psyche* 1984; **144**: 593–602.

158 Balestrieri M, Williams P, Wilkinson G. Specialist mental health treatment in general practice: a meta-analysis. *Psychol Med* 1988; **18**: 711–17.

159 Dunn RL, Donoghue JM, Ozminski RJ *et al.* Longditundinal prescribing of antidepressants in primary care in the UK: comparison with treatment guidelines. *J Psychopharmacol* 1999; **13**: 136–43.

160 Simon G, Lin EHB, Katon W, Saunders K *et al.* Outcomes of 'inadequate' antidepressant treatment in primary care. *J Gen Int Med* 1995; **10**: 663–70.

161 Gray R, Parr, Plummer S *et al.* A national survey of practice nurse involvement in mental health interventions. *J Adv Nursing* 1999; **30**(4): 901–6.

162 Kendrick T, Millar E, Burns T, Ross F. Practice nurse involvement in giving depot neuroleptic injections: development of patient assessment and monitoring checklist. *Primary Care Psyche* 1998; **4**(3): 149–54.

163 Wilkinson G. The role of the practice nurse in the management of depression. *Int Rev Psych* 1992; **4**: 311–16.

164 Mann A, Blizaed R, Murray J *et al.* An evaluation of practice nurses working with GPs to treat people with depression. *Brit J Gen Pract* 1998; **48**: 875–9.

165 Peveler R, George C, Kinmouth A-L *et al.* Effect of antidepressant drug counseling and information leaflets on adherence to drug treatment in primary care: randomised controlled trial. *BMJ* 1999; **319**: 612–5.

166 Root K, Nutting P, Smith JL *et al.* Managing depression as a chronic disease: a randomised trial of ongoing treatment in primary care. *BMJ* 2002; **325**: 934–7.

167 Roth A, Fonagy P. *What works for whom? A critical review of psychotherapy research.* New York: Guilford Press, 1996.

168 DoH Psychol therapies.

169 Gloaguen V, Cottraux J, Cucherat M, Blackburn IM. A meta-analysis of the effects of cognitive therapy in depressed patients. *J Affect Dis* 1998; **49**: 59–72.

170 NHS Centre for Reviews & Dissemination. Mental health promotion in high risk groups *Effective Health Care Bulletin* 1997; **3(3)**.

171 Friedli K, King MB, Lloyd M, Horder J. Randomised controlled assessment of non-directive psychotherapy versus routine general practitioner care. *The Lancet* 1997; **350**: 1662–5.

172 Gournay K, Brooking J. Community psychiatric nurses in primary health care. *Brit J Psyche* 1994; **165**: 231–8.

173 Chilvers C, Dewey M, Fielding K *et al.* Antidepressant drugs and generic counselling for the treatment of major depression in primary care: randomised trial with patient preference arms. *BMJ* 2001; **322**: 722–5.

174 Mynors-Wallis LM, Gath DH, Day A, Baker F. Randomised controlled trial of problem solving treatment, antidepressant medication, and combined treatment for major depression in primary care. *BMJ* 2000; **320**: 26–30.

175 Ward E, King M, Lloyd M *et al.* Randomised control trial of non-directive counselling, cognitive behavioural therapy, and usual general practitioner care for patients with depression. 1. Clinical effectiveness. *BMJ* 2000; **321**: 1383–8.

176 Kupshik G, Fischer C. Assisted bibliographics: effective, efficient treatment for moderate anxiety problems. *Brit J Gen Pract* 1999.

177 Marks I. Computer aids to self-treatment of anxiety. *Progress in Neurology and Psychiatry* 1988: 35–7.

178 Treasure J, Schmidt U, Troop N *et al.* First step in managing bulimia nervosa. Controlled trial of therapeutic manual. *BMJ* 1994; **308**: 686–9.

179 McLean J, Pietroni P. Self Care – Who does best? *Soc Sci Med* 1990; **30(5)**: 591–6.

180 Bower P, Richards D, Lovell K. The clinical and cost-effectiveness of self-help treatments for anxiety and depressive disorders in primary care: a systematic review. *Brit J Gen Pract* 2001; **51**: 838–45.

181 Wallcraft J. *Healing Minds.* Mental Health Foundation: London, 1998.

182 Linde K, Mulrow CD. St John's Wort for depression. In: *Cochrane Collaboration.* Oxford: The Cochrane Library, Update, 2001.

183 Lawlor DA, Hopker SW. The effectiveness of exercise in the management of depression: systematic review and meta-analysis of randomised controlled trials. *BMJ* 2001; **322**: 763–7.

184 Weich S. Prevention of the common mental disorders: a public health perspective. *Psychol Med* 27: 757–64.

185 Simon GE, Von Korff M. Recognition, management and outcomes of depression in primary care. *Arch Fam Med* 1995; **4**: 99–105.

186 Dowrick C, Buchan I. Twelve month outcome of depression in general practice: does detection or disclosure make a difference? *BMJ* 1995; **311**: 1274–6.

187 Goldberg D, Privett M, Ustun B *et al.* The effects of detection and treatment on the outcome of major depression in primary care. A naturalistic study in 15 cities. *Brit J Gen Pract* 1998; **48**: 1840–4.

188 Freeling P, Rao BM, Paykel ES, Sireling L *et al.* Unrecognized depression in general practice. *BMJ* 1985; 290, 1880–3.

189 Zung WW, Magill M, Moore J, George DT. Recognition and treatment of depression in a family medicine practice. *J Clin Psyche* 1985; **44**: 3–6.

190 Oxman, Thomson, Davis, Haynes. No magic bullets: a systematic review of 102 trials of interventions to improve professional practice. *Can Med Ass J* 1995; **153(10)**: 1423–31.

191 Kerwick SH, Jones RH. Educational interventions in primary care psychiatry: a review. *Primary Care Psyche* 1996; **2**: 107–17.

192 Rutz W, von Knorring L, Walinder J. Long term effects of an educational program for general practitioners given by the Swedish committee for the prevention and treatment of depression. *Acta Psychiatr Scand* 1992; **85**: 83–8.

193 Tylee A. Training the whole primary care team. In: Tonsella M, Thornicoft G (eds). *Common mental disorders in primary care.* Routledge: London, 1999.

194 Paykel ES, Priest RG. Recognition and management of depression in general practice: consensus statement. *BMJ* 1992; **305**: 1198–202.

195 Stevens L, Thompson C. Consensus statement on the treatment of depression in primary care. *Primary Care Psych* 1995; **1**: 45–6.

196 Katon W, Robinson P, Von Korff M *et al.* A multi-faceted intervention to improve treatment of depression in general practice. *Arch Gen Psyche* 1996; **53**: 924–32.

197 Armstrong A. *The primary mental health care toolkit.* London: NHS Executive, 1997.

198 Clinical Standards Advisory Group. *Services for patients with depression.* London: Stationery Office, 1999.

199 Armstrong E. Screening and assessment measures for the primary care team. *Int Rev Psych* 1998; **10**: 110–13.

200 Gilbody S, House AO, Sheldon TA. Routinely administered questionnaire for depression and anxiety: a systematic review. *BMJ* 2001; **322**: 406–8.

201 Lewis G: Case finding in primary care. In: Jenkins R, Ustun TB (eds). *Preventing mental illness: mental health promotion in primary care.* Chichester: Wiley, 1998.

202 Clinical Standards Advisory Group. *Services for patients with depression.* London: Stationery Office, 1999.

203 Cox JL, Holden JM, Sagovsky R. Detection of postnatal depression. Development of the 10 item Edinburgh Postnatal Depression Scale. *Brit J Psyche* 1987; **150**: 782–6.

204 Gilbody S, House AO, Sheldon TA. Routinely administered questionnaire for depression and anxiety: a systematic review. *BMJ* 2001; **322**: 406–8.

205 Freeman, Gillam S, Shearin, Plamping D. *Community oriented primary care, depression and anxiety intervention guide.* London: King's Fund, 1997.

206 WHO.

207 Gask L, Goldberg D. Impact on patients care, satisfaction and clinical outcome of improving the psychiatric skills of general practitioners *Euro J Psyche* 1993; **7**: 203–18.

208 Scott J, Jennings T, Standart S *et al.* The impact of training in problem based interviewing on the detection and management of psychological problems presenting in primary care. *Brit J Gen Pract* 1999; **49**: 441–5.

209 Morriss R, Gask L, Ronalds C *et al.* Cost effectiveness of a new treatment for somatised mental disorder taught to general practitioners. *Fam Pract* 1998; **15**: 19–25.

210 Appleby L, Morriss R, Gask L *et al.* An educational intervention for frontline staff in the assessment and management of suicidal patients (the STORM project) *Psychol Med* 2000; **30**: 805–12.

211 Rutz W, von Knorring L, Walinder J. Long term effects of an educational program for general practitioners given by the Swedish committee for the prevention and treatment of depression. *Acta Psychiatr Scand* 1992; **85**: 83–8.

212 Hannaford PC, Thompson C, Simpson M. Evaluation of an educational programme to improve the recognition of psychological illness by general practitioners. *Br J Gen Pract* 1996; **46**: 333–7.

213 Thompson C, Kinmouth AL, Stevens L, Peveler R *et al.* Effects of a clinical practice guideline and practice based education on detection and outcome of depression in primary care: Hampshire depression project randomised control trial. *The Lancet* 1999; **355**: 185–91.

214 Lin E, Katon WJ, Simon GE, Von Korff M *et al.* Achieving guidelines for the treatment of depression in primary care. *Medical Care* 1997; **35**: 831–42.

215 Tylee A. Training the whole primary care team. In: Tonsella M, Thornicoft G (eds). *Common mental disorders in primary care.* London: Routledge, 1999.

216 Katon W, Robinson P, Von Korff M *et al.* A multi-faceted intervention to improve treatment of depression in general practice. *Arch Gen Psyche* 1996; **53**: 924–32.

217 Katon W, Von Korff M, Lin E, Walker E *et al.* Collaborative management to achieve treatment guidelines. Impact on depression in primary care. *JAMA* 1995; **273**: 1026–31.

218 Simon GE, Von Korff M, Rutter C, Wagner E. Randomised trial of monitoring, feedback and management of care by telephone to improve treatment of depression in primary care. *BMJ* 2000; **320**: 550–4.

219 Lave J, Frank R, Schulberg H, Kamlet M. Cost effectiveness of treatments for major depression in primary care. *Arch Gen Psyche* 1998; **55**: 645–51.

220 Von Korff M, Katon W, Bush T, Lin EHB *et al.* Treatment costs, cost offset, and cost effectiveness of collaborative management of depression. *Psychosom Med* 1998; **60**: 143–9.

221 Katon W, von Korff M, Lin E, Simons G. Rethinking practitioners role in chronic illness: the specialist, primary care physician and the practice nurse. *Gen Hosp Psyche* 2001; **23**: 138–44.

222 Mynors Wallis L, Gath D. Brief psychological treatments. *Int Rev Psyche* 1992; **4**: 301–5.

223 Gedenk M, Nepps P. Obsessive compulsive disorder diagnosis and treatment in the primary care setting. *J Am Board Fam Pract* 1997; **10**: 349–56.

224 King M, Davidson D, Taylor FD *et al.* Effectiveness of teaching general practitioners skills in brief cognitive behaviour therapy to treat patients with depression: randomised controlled trial. *BMJ* 2002; **324**.

225 Morris R, Gask L, Smith C, Battersby L. *Training practice nurses to assess and manage anxiety disorders.* Report to the NHSE, 1996.

226 Mynors-Wallis LM, Gath DH, Day A, Baker F. Randomised controlled trial of problem solving treatment, antidepressant medication, and combined treatment for major depression in primary care. *BMJ* 2000; **320**: 26–30.

227 Marks I. *Psychiatric nurse therapy in primary care: Research monographs in nursing series.* London: Royal College of Nursing, 1996.

228 Holden J, Sagovsky R, Cox J. Counselling in a general practice setting: a controlled study of health visitor intervention in treatment of postnatal depression. *BMJ* 1989; **298**: 223–6.

229 Katon W, Robinson P, Von Korff M *et al.* A multi-faceted intervention to improve treatment of depression in general practice. *Arch Gen Psyche* 1996; **53**: 924–32.

230 Onyett S. *The South Thames study: executive summary.* London: Centre for Mental Health Services Development, 1997.

231 Brown J *et al.* GPs responses to a primary care project aimed to integrate primary care and specialist mental health services. Submitted for publication.

232 Jackson G, Gater R, Goldberg D. A new community mental health team based in primary care: a description of the service and its effects on service use in the first year. *Brit J Psyche* 1993; **162**: 375–84.

233 Roberts T, Amonsah S, Downes-Grainger E *et al.* Integrating mental health services in Inner London: effects on staff.

234 Tyrer P, Hawksworth, Hobbs, Jackson. The role of the CPN. *Brit J Hosp Med* 1990; **43**: 439–42.

235 Grant C, Goodenough T, Haney I, Hine C. A randomised controlled trial and economic evaluation of a referral and facilitator between primary care and the voluntary sector. *BMJ* 2000; **320**: 419–23.

236 Murray S. Experiences with 'rapid appraisal' in primary care involving the public in assessing health needs, orientating staff, and educating medical students. *BMJ* 1999; **318**: 441–5.

237 Murray SA, Chick J, Perry B. Mental health, alcohol and drugs: constructing a neighbourhood profile. *Prim Care Psyche* 1996; **2**: 237–43.

238 Peck E. *Mental health service provision and the primary care team: emerging trends and critical questions.* CCMP 5(3): Pavilion Publications, 1997.

239 Scott J, Thorne H, Horn P. Effect of a multifaceted approach to detecting and managing depression in primary care. *BMJ* 2002; **325**: 951–4.

240 Sloper P, Mukherjee S, Beresford B *et al. Real change not rhetoric: putting research into practice in multi-agency services.* Policy Press 1999.

241 Cohen A, Phelan M. The physical health of patients with mental illness: a neglected area. *Mental Health Promotion Update.* London: Department of Health, Dec 2001.

242 Howie JGR, Porter AMD, Heaney DJ, Hopton JL. Long to short consultation ratio: a proxy measure of quality of care for general practice *Brit J Gen Pract* 1991; **41**: 48–54.

243 Mead, Bower, Gask L. Emotional problems in primary care: what is the potential for increasing the role of nurses? *J Adv Nurs* 1997; **26**: 869–90.

244 Barkham M, Margison F, Leacu C *et al.* Service profiling and outcome benchmarking using CORE-OM. Towards practice-based evidence in the psychological therapies. *J Con Clin Psychol;* **69(2)**: 184–96.

245 Department of Health. *Fast-forwarding primary care mental health: the role of graduate workers.* London: Department of Health, 2003.

246 Thompson, Strathdee G, Kelly (eds). *Mental health services development workbook.* London: Sainsbury Centre for Mental Health, 1996.

247 Department of Health. *Bridging the gap: a resource pack for successful joint working* London: Department of Health, 1998.

248 Rosen R. Improving quality in the changing world of primary care. *BMJ* 2000; **321**: 551–4.

249 Huntington J, Gillam S, Rosen R. Organisational development for clinical governance. *BMJ* 2000; **321**: 679–82.

250 Mann A, Tylee E. Evaluation of change in primary care practice. *Int Rev Psyche* 1998; **10**: 148–53.

251 Shield T, Campbell S, Rogers A *et al.* Quality indicators for primary care mental health services. *Qual Saf Health Care* 2003; **12**: 100–6.

252 Ustun TB, Sartorius N. *Mental illness in general health care.* Chichester: Wiley, 1995.

253 Stoudemire A, Frank R, Hedemark N *et al.* The economic burden of depression. *Gen Hosp Psych* 1986; **8**: 387–94.

254 Henk HJ, Katzelnick DJ, Kobak *et al.* Medical costs attributed to depression among patients with a history of high medical expenses in an HMO. *Arch Gen Psych* 1996; **53**: 899–904.

255 Martin RM, Hilton SR, Kerry SM, Richards NM. General practitioners perceptions of the tolerability of antidepressant drugs: a comparison of selective serotonin inhibitors and tricyclic antidepressants. *BMJ* 1997; **314**: 646–51.

256 Goldberg D, Huxley P. *Common mental disorders. A biosocial model.* London: Routledge, 1992.

257 Clinical Standards Advisory Group. *Services for patients with depression.* London: Stationery Office, 1999.

258 Brown GW, Bifulco A, Harris TO. Life events, vulnerability and onset of depression: some refinements. *Brit J Psych* 1987; **150**: 30–42.

259 Goldberg DP, Lecrubier Y. *Mental illness in general health care: an international study.* John Wiley & Sons, 1995.

260 Meltzer H, Gill B, Petticrew M, Hinks K. The prevalence of psychiatric morbidity among *adults living in private households. OPCS surveys of psychiatric morbidity in Great Britain Report 1.* London: HMSO, 1995.

261 Bebbington P. The origin of sex differences in depressive disorder: bridging the gap. *Int Rev Psych* 1996; **8**: 295–332.

262 Nazroo JY. Rethinking the relationship between ethnicity and mental health: the British Fourth National Survey of Ethnic Minorities. *Social Psychiatry & Psychiatric Epidemiology.* 1998; **33(4)**: 145–8.

263 Ostler K, Thompson C, Kinmonth AL, Peveler RC, Stevens L, Stevens A. Influence of socio-economic deprivation on the prevalence and outcome of depression in primary care: the Hampshire Depression Project. *British Journal of Psychiatry* 2001; **178(1):** 12–17.

264 Meltzer H, Gill B, Petticrew M, Hinks K. The prevalence of psychiatric morbidity among *adults living in private households. OPCS surveys of psychiatric morbidity in Great Britain Report 1.* London: HMSO, 1995.

265 Kendrick T. Prescribing antidepressants in general practice: watchful waiting for minor depression and full dose treatment for major depression. Editorial. *BMJ* 1996; **313:** 829–70.

266 Angst J. A regular review of the long-term follow-up of depression. *BMJ* 1997; **315:** 1143–6.

267 Wells KB, Burman MA, Rogers W *et al.* The course of depression in medical out patients. Results from the medical outcome study. *Arch Gen Psych* 1992; **49:** 788–94.

268 Howland RH. General health, health care utilization and medical co-morbidity in dysthymia. *Int Rev Psych* 1993; **23:** 211–38.

269 Docherty JD. Barriers to the diagnosis of depression in primary care. *J Clin Psych* 1997; **58:** 5–10.

270 Plummer S, Ritter S, Leach R *et al.* A controlled comparison of the abilities of practice nurses to detect psychological distress in patients who attend their clinics. *J Psych Mental Health Nursing* 1997; **4:** 221–3.

271 Briscoe M. Identification of emotional problems in postpartum women by health visitors. *BMJ* 1986; **292:** 1245–7.

272 Coyne JC, Schwenk TL, Fechner-Bates S. non-detection of depression by primary care physicians reconsidered. *Gen Hosp Psych* 1995; **17:** 3012.

273 Sartorius N, Ustun TB, Lecrubier Y, Wittchen H. Depression comorbid with anxiety: results from the WHO study on psychological distress in primary health care. *Brit J Psych* 1996; **168:** 38–43.

274 Bridges KW, Goldberg DP. Somatic presentation of DSM III psychiatric disorders in primary care. *J Psychosom Res* 1985; **29:** 563–9.

275 Badger LW, DeGruy FV, Hartman J *et al.* Patient presentation, interview content and the detection of depression by primary care physicians. *Psychosomatic Med* 1994; **56:** 128–35.

276 Odell SM, Surtees PG, Wainwright NWJ *et al.* Determinants of general practitioner recognition of psychological problems in a multi-ethnic inner city health district. *Brit J Psych* 1997; **171:** 537–41.

277 Thompson C, Kinmouth AL, Stevens L, Peveler R *et al.* Effects of a clinical practice guideline and practice based education on detection and outcome of depression in primary care: Hampshire depression project randomised control trial. *The Lancet* 1999; **355:** 185–91.

278 Stevens L, Thompson C. Consensus statement on the treatment of depression in general practice. *Primary Care Psych* 1995; **1:** 45–6.

279 Hollyman JA, Freeling P, Paykel ES. Double blind controlled trial of amitryptyline among depressed patients in general practice. *J Royal Coll GPs* 1988; **38:** 393–7.

280 Paykel ES, Hollyman JA, Freeling P, Sedgewick P. Predictors of therapeutic benefit from amitriptyline in mild depression: a general practice placebo controlled study. *J Affect Disorders* 1988; **14:** 83–95.

281 Thompson C, Thompson CM. The prescription of antidepressants in general practice I: a critical review. *Human Psychopharmacology* 1989; **4:** 91–102.

282 Schulberg HC, Block MR, Madonia MJ *et al.* Treating major depression in primary care practice, eight month clinical outcomes. *Arch Gen Psych* 1996; **53:** 913–19.

283 Katon W, Robinson P Von Korff M *et al.* A multi-faceted intervention to improve treatment of depression in primary care. *Arch Gen Psych* 1996; **53:** 924–32.

284 Bollin P, Pampallona S, Tibaldi G *et al.* Effectiveness of antidepressants. Meta-analysis of dose-effect relationships in randomised controlled trials. *Brit J Psyche* 1999; **174:** 297–303.

285 Song F, Freemantle N, Sheldon TA *et al.* Selective serotonin reuptake inhibitors: a meta-analysis of efficacy and acceptability. *BMJ* 1993; **306:** 683–7.

286 Hotopf M, Hardy R, Lewis G. Discontinuation rates of SSRIs and tricyclic antidepressants: a meta-analysis and investigation of heterogeneity. *Brit J Psych* 1997; **170**: 120–7.

287 Simon G, Von Korff M, Heiligenstein J *et al.* Initial antidepressant choice in primary care: effectiveness and cost of fluoxetine vs. tricyclic antidepressants. *JAMA* 1996; **275**: 1897–902.

288 Jonsson B, Bebbington P. Economic studies of the treatment of depressive illness. In: Jonsson B, Rosenbaum B (eds). *Health economics of depression.* Chichester: Wiley, 1993.

289 US Dept Health Human Services, Agency for Health Care Policy & Research.: *Depression in primary care. Treatment of major depression.* Clinical Practice Guideline no 5 1993. AHCPR publication 93–0551.

290 Paykel ES, Hart D, Priest R. Changes in public attitudes to depression during the defeat depression campaign. *Brit J Psych* 1998; **173**: 519–22.

291 MORI Poll, conducted for Defeat Depression Campaign. London: MORI, 1992.

292 MORI Poll, conducted for Defeat Depression Campaign, London: MORI, 1995.

293 Peveler R, George C, Kinmouth A-L, Campbell M *et al.* Effect of antidepressant drug counseling and information leaflets on adherence to drug treatment in primary care: randomised controlled trial. *BMJ* 1999; **319**: 612–5.

294 Simon GE, Von Korff M, Rutter C, Wagner E. Randomised trial of monitoring, feedback and management of care by telephone to improve treatment of depression in primary care. *BMJ* 2000; **320**: 550–4.

295 Paykel ES, Hart D, Priest R. Changes in public attitudes to depression during the defeat depression campaign. *Brit J Psych* 1998; **173**: 519–22.

296 Sheldon T, Freemantle N, House A *et al.* Examining the effectiveness of treatments for depression in general practice. *J Mental Health* 1993; **2**: 141–56.

297 Scott C, Tacchi MJ, Jones R, Scott J. Acute and one year outcomes of a randomised controlled trial of brief cognitive therapy for major depressive disorder in primary care. *Brit J Psych* 1997; **171**: 131–4.

298 Gloaguen V, Cottraux J, Cucherat M, Blackburn IM. A meta-analysis of the effects of cognitive therapy in depressed patients. *J Affect Dis* 1998; **49**: 59–72.

299 Gloaguen V, Cottraux J, Cucherat M *et al.* A meta-analysis of the effects of cognitive therapy in depressed patients. *J Affect Dis* 1998; **49**: 59–72.

300 Fava GA, Rafanelli C, Grandi S *et al. Arch Gen Psych* 1998; **55**: 816–20.

301 Paykel ES, Scott J, Teasdale JD *et al.* Prevention of relapse in residual depression by cognitive therapy. A controlled trial *Arch Gen Psyche* 1999; **56**: 829–35.

302 Schulberg HC, Block MR, Madonia MJ *et al.* Treating major depression in primary care practice. eight month clinical outcomes. *Arch Gen Psych* 1996; **52**: 913–19.

303 Kupfer DJ, Frank E, Perel JM *et al.* Five year outcome for maintenance therapies in recurrent depression. *Arch Gen Psych* 1992; **49**: 769–73.

304 US Dept Health Human Services, Agency for Health Care Policy & Research.: *Depression in primary care. Treatment of major depression.* Clinical Practice Guideline no 5 1993. AHCPR publication 93–0551.

305 Mynors-Wallis LM, Gath DH *et al.* Randomised controlled trial comparing problem solving treatment with amitryptyline and placebo for major depression in primary care. *BMJ* 1995; **310**: 441–5.

306 Mynors-Wallis LM, Gath DH, Day A, Baker F. Randomised controlled trial of problem solving treatment, antidepressant medication and combination treatment for major depression in primary care. *BMJ* 2000; **320**: 26–30.

307 Dowrick C, Dunn G, Ayuso-Mateos JL *et al.* Problem solving treatment and group psychoeduction for depression: multicentre randomised controlled trial. *BMJ* 2000; **321**: 1450–4.

308 Freidli K, King M, Lloyd M, Horder J. Randomised controlled assessment of non-directive psychotherapy versus routine general practitioner care. *The Lancet* 1997; **350**: 1662–5.

309 Ward E, King M, Lloyd M *et al.* Randomised controlled trial of non-directive counselling, cognitive-behaviour therapy and usual general practitioner care for patients with depression. I Clinical effectiveness. *BMJ* 2000; **321**: 1383–8.

310 Bower P, Byford S, Sibbald B *et al.* Randomised controlled trial of non-directive counselling, cognitive-behaviour therapy and usual general practitioner care for patients with depression. I Cost effectiveness. *BMJ* 2000; **321**: 1389–92.

311 Chilvers C, Dewey M, Fielding K *et al.* Antidepressant drugs and generic counselling for treatment of major depression in primary care: randomised trial with patient preference arms. *BMJ* 2001; **322**: 772–5.

312 Linde K, Mulrow CD. *St John's Wort for Depression.* Cochrane Review. Oxford: the Cochrane Library, 2001.

313 Thiede HM, Walper A. Inhibition of MAO and CoMT by hypericum extracts and hypericin. *Journal of Geriatric Psychiatry and Neurology* 1994; **7** (Suppl 1): S54–6.

314 Phillip M, Kohnen R, Karl-O H. Hypericum extract versus imipramine or placebo in patients with moderate depression: randomised multi-centre study of treatment for eight weeks. *BMJ* 1999; **319**: 1534–9.

315 Woelk H for the Remotiv/Imipramine Study Group. Comparison of St John's Wort and imipramine for treating depression: randomised controlled trial. *BMJ* 2000; **321**: 536–9.

316 Glenister D. Exercise and mental health: a review. *J Royal Soc Health* 1996; **Feb**: 7–13.

317 McCann L, Holmes D. Influence of aerobic exercise on depression. *J Pers Soc Psychol* 1984; **46**: 1142–7.

318 Health Education Authority. Physical activity and mental health: national consensus statements and guideline for practice. London: HEA, 2000.

319 Lawlor DA, Hopker SW. The effectiveness of exercise as an intervention in the management of depression: systematic review and meta-analysis of randomised controlled trials. *BMJ* 2001; **322**: 763–6.

320 Shear MD, Schulberg HC. Anxiety disorders in primary care. *Bulletin of the Menninger Clinic.* 1995; **59**: 2 (suppl A).

321 Reiger DA, Rae DS, Narrow WE *et al.* Prevalence of anxiety disorders and their co-morbidity with mood and addictive disorders. *Brit J Psych* 1998; **173** (Suppl 34): 24–8.

322 Lader MH. Guidelines for the management of patients with generalised anxiety. *Bull Royal Coll Psych* 1992; **16**: 560–5.

323 Weiller E, Bisserbe JC, Maier W, Lecrubier Y. Prevalence and recognition of anxiety symptoms in five European primary care settings: a report from the WHO study on psychological problems in general health care. *Brit J Psych* 1998; **173** (Suppl 34): 18–23.

324 Kessler RC, McGonagle KA, Zhao S *et al.* Lifetime and 12 month prevalence of DSM-II-R psychiatric disorders in the Untied States: results from the national comorbidity study. *Arch Gen Psyche* 1992; **51**: 8–19.

325 Sartorius N, Ustun TB, Lecrubier Y, Wittchen H. Depression comorbid with anxiety: results from the WHO study on psychological distress in primary health care. *Brit J Psych* 1996; **168**: 38–43.

326 Reiger DA, Rae DS, Narrow WE *et al.* Prevalence of anxiety disorders and their co-morbidity with mood and addictive disorders. *Brit J Psych* 1998; **173** (Suppl 34): 24–8.

327 Reiger DA, Rae DS, Narrow WE *et al.* Prevalence of anxiety disorders and their co-morbidity with mood and addictive disorders. *Brit J Psych* 1998; **173** (Suppl 34): 24–8.

328 Kessler RC, McGonagle KA, Zhao S *et al.* Lifetime and 12 month prevalence of DSM-II-R psychiatric disorders in the United States: results from the national comorbidity study. *Arch Gen Psyche* 1992; **51**: 8–19.

329 Catalan P, Gath DH *et al.* The effects of not prescribing anxiolytics in general practice. *Brit J Psyche* 1984; **144**: 593–602.

330 Sartorius N, Ustun TB, Lecrubier Y, Wittchen H. Depression comorbid with anxiety: results from the WHO study on psychological distress in primary health care. *Brit J Psych* 1996; **168**: 38–43.

331 Fifer SD, Mathias SD, Patrick DL *et al.* Untreated anxiety among adult primary care patients in a health maintenance organisation. *Arch Gen Psych* 1994; **51**: 740–50.

332 Gould RA, Otto MW, Pollack MH, Yap L. Cognitive behavioural and pharmacological treatment of generalised anxiety disorder: a preliminary meta-analysis. *Behav Ther* 1997; **28**: 285–305.

333 Catalan P, Gath DH *et al.* The effects of not prescribing anxiolytics in general practice. *Brit J Psyche* 1984; **144**: 593–602.

334 Kahn R, Mcnair D, Lipman R *et al.* Imipramine and chlordiazepoxide in depressive and anxiety disorders II Efficacy in anxious outpatients. *Arch Gen Psych* 1986; **43**: 79–85.

335 Rocca P, Fonzo V, Scotta M *et al.* Paroxetine efficacy in the treatment of generalised anxiety disorder. *Acta Psych Scand* 1997; **95**: 444–50.

336 American Psychiatric Association. Practice guideline for the treatment of patients with panic disorder. *Am J Psych* 1998; **155**: 5 (May suppl).

337 Stein MB, Chartier MJ, Hazen Al *et al.* Paroxetine in the treatment of generalised social phobia: open-label treatment and double-blind, placebo-controlled discontinuation. *J Clin Psychopharm.* 1996; **16**: 218–22.

338 Murray B, Stein M, Michael R *et al.* Paroxetine treatment of generalized social phobia (social anxiety disorder): a randomised controlled trial. *JAMA* 1998; **280**: 8.

339 Gould RA, Otto MW, Pollack MH, Yap L. Cognitive behavioural and pharmacological treatment of generalised anxiety disorder: a preliminary meta-analysis. *Behav Ther* 1997; **28**: 285–305.

340 Tyrer P. Use of beta blocking drugs in psychiatry and neurology. *Drugs* 1980; **20**: 300–8.

341 Roth A, Fonagy P. *What works for whom? A critical review of psychotherapy research.* New York: Guilford, 1996.

342 Gould RA, Otto MW, Pollack MH, Yap L. Cognitive behavioural and pharmacological treatment of generalised anxiety disorder: a preliminary meta-analysis. *Behav Ther* 1997; **28**: 285–305.

343 Roth A, Fonagy P. *What works for whom? A critical review of psychotherapy research.* New York: Guilford, 1996.

344 Marks I, Swinson RP. Alprazolam and exposure for panic disorder with agoraphobia; summary of London/Toronto results. *J Psych Res* 1990; **24**: 100–1.

345 Wade WA, Treat TA, Stuart GL. Transporting an empirically supported treatment for panic disorder to a service clinic setting; a benchmarking strategy. *J Con Clin Psychol* 1998; **66**: 231–9.

346 De Rubeis RJ, Crits-Cristoph P. Empirically supported individual and group psychological treatments for adult mental disorders. *J Con Clin Psychol* 1998; **66**(1): 37–52.

347 Hawton K, Kirk J Problem-solving. In: Hawton K, Salkovskis PM, Kirk J, Clark DM (eds). *Cognitive therapy for psychiatric problems.* Oxford: Oxford Medical Publications, 1989.

348 Catalan P, Gath E. Benzodiazepines in general practice a time for decision. *BMJ* 1985; **290**: 375–6.

349 Shear MD, Schulberg HC. Anxiety disorders in primary care. *Bulletin of the Menninger Clinic.* 1995; **59**: 2 (suppl A).

350 Donnan P, Hutchinson A, Paxton R *et al.* Self help materials for anxiety: a randomised controlled trial in general practice. *Brit J GP* 1990; **Dec.**

351 Sorby NGD, Reavley W, Huber JW. Self-help programmes for anxiety in general practice: controlled trial of an anxiety management booklet. *Brit J GP* 1991; **41**: 417–20.

352 Kupshik G, Fisher C. Assisted bibliotherapy: effective, efficient treatment for moderate anxiety problems. *Brit J GP* 1999; **Jan**.

353 McLean B, Pietroni R. Self care – Who does best? *Soc Sci Med* 1990; **30**(5): 591–6.

354 Milne DL, Jones RQ, Walters P. Anxiety management in the community: a social support model and preliminary evaluation. *Beh Psychotherapy* 1989; **17**: 221–6 – quoted in Shear & Schulberg.

355 Vickers A, Zollman C. ABC of complementary therapies: hypnosis and relaxation. *BMJ* 1999; **319**: 1346–8.

356 Kirsch I, Montgomery G, Sapirstein G. Hypnosis as an adjunct to cognitive-behavioural psychotherapy. *J Con Clin Psychol* 1995; **63**: 214–20.

357 NIH Technology Assessment Panel on integration of behavioural and relaxation approaches into the treatment of chronic pain and insomnia. *JAMA* 1996; **276**: 313–8.

358 Smith GR. The course of somatisation and it effects on the use of health care resources. *Psychosomatics* 1994; **35**: 263–7.

359 Speckens A, van Hemert A, Bolk J, Rooijmans H, Hengeveld M. Unexplained physical symptoms: outcome and utilisation of medical care and associated factors. *Psychol Med* 1996; 45–52.

360 Reid S, Wessely S, Crayford T, Hotope M. Frequent attenders with medically unexplained symptoms: service use and costs in secondary care. *Brit J Psyche* 2002; **280**: 248–53.

361 NHS Executive. *Burdens of disease: a discussion document.* London: Department of Health, 1996.

362 Peveler R. Understanding medically unexplained symptoms: more progress in the next century than in this? *J Psychsom Res* 1998; **45**: 93–7.

363 Ustun TB, Privett, Costa de Silva. *Mental disorders in primary care: an executive summary of the WHO collaborative study on psychological problems in general health care.* Geneva: WHO, 1998.

364 Ustun TB (ed). *Mental disorders in primary care a World Health Organisation training package.* Geneva: WHO, 1998.

365 Kirmayer LJ, Robbins JM. Patients who somatize in primary care: a longitudinal study of cognitive and social characteristics. *Psychol Med* 1996; **26**: 937–51.

366 Salmon P, Peters S, Stanley I. Patients' perceptions of medical explanations for somatisation disorders: qualitative analysis. *BMJ* 1999; **318**: 372–6.

367 Thomas KB. Temporarily dependent patents in general practice. *BMJ* 1974; **268**: 625–6.

368 Peveler RC, Kilkenny L, Kinmouth AL. Medically unexplained physical symptoms in primary care: a comparison of self-report screening questionnaires and clinical opinion. *J Psychosom Res* 1997; **42**: 245–52.

369 Schilte AF, Portegijis PJM, Blankenstein AH *et al.* Randomised controlled trial of disclosure of emotionally important events in primary care. *BMJ* 2001; **323**: 86–9.

370 Schilte AF, Portegijis PJM, Blankenstein AH *et al.* Randomised controlled trial of disclosure of emotionally important events in primary care. *BMJ* 2001; **323**: 86–9.

371 Katon W. Panic disorder and somatisation: review of 55 cases. *Am J Med* 1984; **77**: 101–6.

372 Creed F, Mayou R, Hopkins A. *Medical symptoms not explained by organic disease.* London: Royal College of Psychiatrists and Royal College of Physicians, 1992.

373 Salmon P, Peters S, Stanley I. Patients' perceptions of medical explanations for somatisation disorders: qualitative analysis. *BMJ* 1999; **318**: 372–6.

374 Smith GR Jnr *et al.* A trial of the effect of a standardised psychiatric consultation on health outcomes and costs in somatising patients. *Arch Gen Psych* 1995; **52**: 238–43.

375 O'Dowd T. Five years of heartsink patients in general practice. *BMJ* 1988; **297**: 528–30.

376 Heartsink *BJGP* 1999; **49**: 230–3.

377 Gask L, Morriss R, Goldberg D. *Managing somatic presentation of emotional distress (reattribution; 2nd edition) videotape.* Manchester: University of Manchester, 1999.

378 Gask L, Goldberg D, Porter R, Creed F. The treatment of somatisation: evaluation of a training package with general practice trainees. *J Psycvhosom Res* 1989; **33**: 697–703.

379 Goldberg D, Ask l, O'Dowd T. The treatment of somatisation: teaching the skills of reattribution. *J Psychosom Res* 1989; **33**: 689–95.

380 Goldberg D, Benjamin S, Creed F. Abnormal illness behaviour In: *Psychiatry in medical practice.* London: Routledge, 1994.

381 Morris R, Gask L, Ronalds C *et al.* Cost-effectiveness of a new treatment for somatised mental disorder taught to general practitioners. *Fam Pract* 1998; **15**: 19–25.

382 Morris R, Gask L, Ronalds C *et al.* Clinical and patient satisfaction outcome of a new treatment for somatised mental disorder taught to general practitioners. *Brit J Gen Pract* 1999; **49**: 263–7.

383 Guthrie E. Psychotherapy of somatization disorders. *Current Opinion in Psyche* 1997; **9(3)**: 182–7.

384 Speckens A, van Hemert A, Spinhoven P *et al.* Cognitive behavioural therapy for medically unexplained symptoms: a randomised controlled trial. *BMJ* 1995; **311**: 1328–32.

385 Wilkinson PB, Mynors-Wallis L. Problem solving in the treatment of unexplained physical symptoms in primary care: a preliminary study. *J Psychosom Res* 1994; **38**: 591–8.

386 Pilowsky I, Barrow CG. A controlled study of psychotherapy and amitriptyline used individually and in combination in the treatment of chronic intractable 'psychogenic' pain. *Pain* 1990; **40**: 3–19.

387 Gill D, Hatcher S. *A systematic review of the treatment of depression with antidepressant drugs in patients who also have physical illness.* Cochrane Review. Oxford: Cochrane Library, 2001.

388 Ustun TB, Privett, Costa de Silva. *Mental disorders in primary care: an executive summary of the WHO collaborative study on psychological problems in general health care.* Geneva: WHO, 1998.

389 NHS Centre for Reviews & Dissemination. Mental health promotion in high risk groups *Effective Health Care Bulletin* 1997; **3(3)**.

390 Parkes CM. *Bereavement: studies of grief in adult life.* London: Tavistock and Pelican, New York, International Universities Press, 1986.

391 Coyne J, Schwenk T. The relationship of distress to mood disturbance in primary care and psychiatric populations. *J Consul Clin Psychol* 1997; **65(1)**: 161–8.

392 Andreasen N, Hoenk P. The predictive value of adjustment disorders: a follow up study. *Am J Psych* 1982; **139**: 5.

393 Parkes CM. *Bereavement: studies of grief in adult life.* London: Tavistock and Pelican; New York: International Universities Press, 1986.

394 Treatment protocol project. *Management of mental disorders.* (Vol 1, 2e). Geneva: WHO Collaborating Centre for Mental Health and Substance Abuse, 1997.

395 Ustun TB, Privett, Costa de Silva. *Mental disorders in primary care: an executive summary of the WHO collaborative study on psychological problems in general health care.* Geneva: WHO, 1998.

396 Raphael B. Preventative intervention with the recently bereaved. *Arch Gen Psych* 1979; **34**: 1450–4.

397 Turnbull S, Ward A, Treasure J *et al.* The demand for eating disorder care: an epidemiological study using the general practice research database. *Brit J Psych* 1996; **169**: 705–12.

398 Whitehouse AM, Cooper PJ, Vize CV *et al.* The prevalence of eating disorders in three Cambridge general practices; hidden and conspicuous morbidity. *Brit J Gen Pract* 1992; **42**: 57–60.

399 Von Hoeken D, Lucas AR, Hoek HW. Epidemiology. In: Hoek HW, Treasure JL, Katzman MA (eds). Neurobiology in the treatment of eating disorders. Chichester: John Wiley and Sons, 1998.

400 Carlat DJ, Camargo CA. Review of bulimia nervosa in males. *Am J Psych* 1991; **154**: 1127–32.

401 Turnbull S, Ward A, Treasure J *et al.* The demand for eating disorder care: an epidemiological study using the general practice research database. *Brit J Psych* 1996; **169**: 705–12.

402 Von Hoeken D, Lucas AR, Hoek HW. Epidemiology. In: Hoek HW, Treasure JL, Katzman MA (eds). *Neurobiology in the treatment of eating disorders.* Chichester: John Wiley and Sons, 1998.

403 BED prevalence.

404 Turnbull S, Ward A, Treasure J *et al.* The demand for eating disorder care: an epidemiological study using the general practice research database. *Brit J Psych* 1996; **169**: 705–12.

405 Gard MCE, Freeman CP. The dismantling of a myth: a review of eating disorders and socioeconomic status. *Int J Eating Dis* 1996; **20**: 1–12.

406 Hay PJ, Bacaltchuk J. Bulimia nervosa. *BMJ* 2001; **323**: 33–7.

407 Hoek HW, Bartelds AI, Bosveld J *et al.* Impact of urbanisation on detection of eating disorders. *Am J Psych* 1995; **152**: 1272–8.

408 Herzog DB, Nussbaum KM, Marmor AK. Comorbidity and outcome in eating disorders. *The Psychiatric Clinics of America* 1996; **19**: 843–59.

409 Dansky BS, Brewerton TD, Kilpatrick DG, O'Neil PM. The national women's study: relationship of victimisation and post traumatic stress disorder to bulimia nervosa. *Int J Eating Dis* 1997; **21**: 213–28.

410 Favaro A, Santonastaso P. Suicidality in eating disorders; clinical and psychological correlates. *Acta Psych Scand* 1997; **95**: 508–14.

411 Keller MB, Herzog DB, Lavori PW *et al.* The naturalistic history of bulimia nervosa: extraordinarily high rates of chronicity, relapse, recurrence and psychosocial morbidity. *Int J Eating Dis* 1992; **12**: 1–9.

412 Fichter MM, Quadflieg N, Gnutzmann A. Binge eating disorder: treatment and outcome over a six-year course. *J Psychosom Res* 1998; **44**: 385–405.

413 Welch SL, Fairburn CG. *Sampling bias and bulimia nervosa.* Paper presented at the 5th International Conference on Eating Disorders. Abstract 161. New York, 1992.

414 Whitehouse AM, Cooper PJ, Vize CV *et al.* The prevalence of eating disorders in three Cambridge general practices; hidden and conspicuous morbidity. *Brit J Gen Pract* 1992; **42**: 57–60.

415 Luck AS, Morgan F, Reid F *et al.* The SCOFF questionnaire and clinical interview for eating disorders in general practice: compartative study. *BMJ* 2002; **325**: 755–6.

416 Schmidt U. Treatment of Bulimia nervosa. In: Hoek HW, Treasure JL, Katzman MA (eds). *Neurobiology in the treatment of eating disorders.* Chichester: John Wiley and Sons, 1998.

417 Hay PJ, Bacaltchuk J. *Psychotherapy for bulimia nervosa and bingeing.* Cochrane Database. Oxford: Cochrane Collaboration 2001.

418 Fairburn CG, Welch SL, Doll HA *et al.* A prospective study of the outcome of bulimia nervosa and the long-term effects of three psychological treatments. *Arch Gen Psych* 1995; **54**: 509–17.

419 Thiels C, Schmidt U, Treasure J *et al.* Guided self-change for bulimia nervosa incorporating a self-treatment manual. *Am J Psych* 1998; **2155**: 947–53.

420 Agras WS, Walsh BT, Fairburn CG. A multi-centre comparison of cognitive-behavioural therapy and interpersonal psychotherapy. *Arch Gen Psych* 2000; **54**: 459–65.

421 Treasure JL, Katzman M, Schmidt U. Engagement and outcome in the treatment of bulimia nervosa: first stage of a sequential design comparing motivational enhancement therapy and cognitive behavioural therapy. *J Behav Res Ther* 1999; **37**: 405–18.

422 Mayer LES, Walsh BT. Pharmacotherapy of eating disorders. In: Hoek HW, Treasure JL, Katzman MA (eds). *Neurobiology in the treatment of eating disorders.* Chichester: John Wiley and Sons, 1998.

423 Bacaltchuk J, Hay P, Mari JJ. Antidepressants versus placebo for the treatment of bulimia nervosa: a systematic review. *Aust NZ J Psych* 2000; **34**: 310–17.

424 Schmidt U. Treatment of Bulimia nervosa. In: Hoek HW, Treasure JL, Katzman MA (eds). *Neurobiology in the treatment of eating disorders.* Chichester: John Wiley and Sons, 1998.

425 Treasure JL, Todd G, Brolly M *et al.* A pilot study of randomised trial of cognitive analytic therapy versus educational behavioural therapy for adult anorexia nervosa. *Beh Res Ther* 1995; **33**: 363–7.

426 Russell GFM, Szmukler G, Dare C, Eisler I. An evaluation of family therapy in anorexia and bulimia nervosa. *Arch Gen Psych* 1987; **44**: 1047–56.

427 Touyz SW, Beaumont PJ, Dunn SM. Behaviour therapy in the management of patients with anorexia nervosa. A lenient flexible approach. *Psychotherapy and psychosomatics* 1987; **48**: 151–6.

428 Freeman C. Cognitive therapy. In: Schmuckler G, Dare C, Treasure J (eds). *Handbook of eating disorders. Theory, treatment and research.* Chichester: John Wiley and Sons, 1995.

429 Levine MD, Marcus MD. The treatment of binge eating disorder. In: Hoek HW, Treasure JL, Katzman MA (eds). *Neurobiology in the treatment of eating disorders.* Chichester: John Wiley and Sons, 1998.

430 Royal College of Psychiatrists. *Eating disorders.* Council report CR15. London: RCO Psych, 1992.

431 Eating Disorders Association. *Eating disorders a guide to purchasing and providing services.* EDA, 1997.

432 Gask L, Sibbald B, Creed F. Evaluating models of working at the interface between mental health services and primary care. *Brit J Psych* 1997; **170**: 6–11.

433 Strathdee G, Sutherby K. *Review of the literature relevant to the development of a primary care strategy for mental health.* Report for Lambeth, Southwark and Lewisham Health Authority. Available from Health Service Research Unit, Institute of Psychiatry, 1993.

9 Peripheral Vascular Disease

Gerald Fowkes

1 Summary

Introduction and statement of problem

This chapter is concerned with two peripheral vascular diseases:

- peripheral arterial disease, defined as atherosclerosis of the distal aorta and/or lower limb arteries causing arterial narrowing and disruption of blood flow to the legs
- abdominal aortic aneurysm defined as abnormal dilatation of the aorta distal to the renal arteries.

Peripheral arterial disease commonly presents as intermittent claudication, which is pain in the calf that occurs on walking and which is relieved by rest. More severe forms of peripheral arterial disease present as rest pain, gangrene or ulceration, occasionally leading to amputation.

Abdominal aortic aneurysms commonly remain asymptomatic but sometimes rupture with a high risk of death. Symptomatic aneurysms and large asymptomatic aneurysms require surgical repair because of an increased risk of rupture.

Health service issues that are currently important in meeting the needs of patients with these peripheral vascular diseases are, in primary care, the appropriate management of cardiovascular risk factors and referral of patients with intermittent claudication. In secondary care, key issues are the centralisation of services around major vascular units at regional and supra-district level and the minimum facilities that should be provided in these units. In the clinical management of patients, the diagnosis and treatment of claudication, the use of interventional radiology and reconstruction surgery, and the management of asymptomatic aneurysms are important. Also, the value of screening, particularly for asymptomatic aneurysms, has been debated in recent years.

A key problem for purchasers at present is the specification of the minimum requirements for providing a vascular service at secondary care level. Whether or not to screen for aortic aneurysms is another important issue.

Sub-categories

The sub-categories of disease used throughout this chapter are:

- peripheral arterial disease
    - intermittent claudication
    - critical limb ischaemia
    - asymptomatic peripheral arterial disease

- abdominal aortic aneurysm
  - ruptured aneurysm
  - asymptomatic aneurysm.

Prevalence and incidence

Intermittent claudication occurs rarely in men and women under 55 years of age but affects 5% of those aged 55 to 74 years. Prevalence increases rapidly with age and it is slightly more common in men than women. It is more frequent in the lower social classes, mostly due to higher levels of smoking. Only one quarter of claudicants have a deterioration in symptoms. The main risk for claudicants is a two to threefold higher mortality than non-claudicants, mostly due to associated coronary heart disease. The time trends in claudication are unknown.

Critical limb ischaemia is rare, with an estimated incidence of 500–1000 per million population per year. Twenty-five percent have an amputation and 50% are dead within 5 years.

Asymptomatic peripheral arterial disease causing a major disruption to blood flow in the legs is common, affecting 8% of 55- to 74-year-olds; a further 17% have minor asymptomatic disease. These individuals are also at increased risk of acute coronary events and stroke.

The most important form of symptomatic aneurysm is rupture. The annual incidence is about 17 per 100 000. The death rate due to aortic aneurysm in 1996 was 24.1 per 100 000 in men and 13.8 per 100 000 in women.

The prevalence of asymptomatic aneurysm is about 5% in men aged 65 to 74 years. The male:female ratio is about 3:1 and the prevalence increases steeply with age.

Services available and their costs

For peripheral arterial disease the consultation rate in general practice is low, accounting for only 1 in 420 of total consultations, and thus specific services are not provided at that level. The services available at secondary level have been documented in detail in Scotland, and less so in England, and show that around 80% of vascular work is performed outside specialist units and that two thirds of 'vascular surgeons' are general surgeons with a special interest in vascular surgery. Access to intensive care units and vascular laboratory support is not available in 50% of hospitals providing vascular surgery.

In 1995/96, the number of patients discharged in England with a primary diagnosis of peripheral atherosclerosis was 36 000, mostly from general surgical units. Diagnostic angiography was performed on 39 000 occasions; 10 600 patients had an arterial bypass operation and 4400 had a vascular amputation. Relatively few angiographies and angioplasties were carried out as day cases. Since the mid-1980s, a steep increase has occurred in the use of angioplasty, but the effects on amputation and reconstruction rates are unclear. The mean hospital cost of amputation is about £6000 and of reconstructive surgery about £5000, whereas angioplasty costs about £1500.

Over 11 000 discharges in 1995/96 were due to aortic aneurysms. More than 5000 aortic aneurysm repairs were carried out, with around one quarter performed as emergencies. The hospital cost of an aneurysm repair is about £4500. Operations per head of population showed little regional variation. Screening for abdominal aortic aneurysms in the community is not carried out routinely in the UK.

Effectiveness of services and interventions

Smoking cessation in patients with intermittent claudication is associated with better results following surgery, lower amputation rates and improved survival. The most effective health service methods to achieve smoking cessation are advice from a health professional and nicotine replacement therapy. Exercise can improve walking distance by 150%, but lipid-lowering therapy has an inconsistent effect on symptoms. Most patients with peripheral arterial disease can benefit from treatment with statins. Good control of blood pressure and glycaemia are also appropriate in relevant patients.

Antiplatelet therapy is important in reducing cardiovascular risk in claudicants. Cilostazol and naftidrofuryl are the only specific drugs that can be recommended to possibly improve walking distance. Percutaneous transluminal angioplasty may have a short-term benefit but this is unlikely to be sustained by 2 years. Likewise, the long-term results of bypass grafting are quite variable, depending greatly on the location and extent of disease and type of intervention.

For critical limb ischaemia, the success of arterial reconstruction is also variable with 2-year patency rates between 30% and 70%. For below-knee amputation, 80% of patients achieve reasonable mobility compared to only 40% having above-knee amputations.

For ruptured abdominal aortic aneurysms, the peri-operative mortality is between 40% and 60%. On the other hand, almost 100% would die without surgery. Asymptomatic aneurysms of diameter > 6 cm are generally operated on but the latest evidence, from the recently published UK Small Aneurysm Trial, indicates that aneurysms < 5.5 cm should simply be observed using ultrasound surveillance. The mortality of elective surgery is 5.8%. Trials are currently in progress investigating the effectiveness of endovascular repair and have recently shown benefits of aneurysm screening in the general population.

Models of care/recommendations

National guidelines are required on the management and referral of patients with intermittent claudication in primary care. Several recent reports in the UK have indicated that vascular services at secondary care level need to be centralised in major vascular units serving populations of at least 500 000. Minimum staffing requirements and facilities can be specified to ensure that such a unit can provide a high-quality vascular service round the clock. This specification includes provision of at least three full-time vascular surgeons and an equivalent number of full/part-time interventional radiologists, a 30-bed vascular unit plus 10 beds for rehabilitation of amputees, a fully equipped vascular laboratory, appropriate radiological facilities and access to intensive care beds on site.

This major vascular unit should be the focus for an integrated regional or supra-district vascular service in which some services are provided in other hospitals in a 'hub and spoke' arrangement. Hospitals on the 'spoke' would provide outpatient clinics, some diagnostic facilities including Duplex scanning, pre-operative assessment, day surgery, post-acute care and rehabilitation. In a few geographically remote areas, smaller hospitals may require to provide a more substantial range of vascular services, including emergency surgery and more straightforward elective procedures.

2 Introduction and statement of the problem

Definition of peripheral vascular diseases

The term peripheral vascular disease does not have a precise and agreed meaning. When used in the plural, peripheral vascular diseases normally refers to all diseases that affect the arteries, veins and lymphatics of the peripheral vasculature.[1] When used in the singular, peripheral vascular disease normally refers to only those diseases that affect arteries; these include atherosclerosis, aortic aneurysm, Buerger's disease, Raynaud's syndrome and others.[1] The most common is atherosclerosis, in which lipid is deposited in the arterial wall; sometimes peripheral vascular disease refers to this condition only. 'Peripheral' refers to the location of disease. Usually peripheral vascular disease includes conditions that affect the arteries serving the lower limbs, sometimes the upper limbs, and less commonly the carotid, renal and other extra coronary arteries.

In this chapter, two peripheral vascular diseases will be evaluated. These are atherosclerosis that affects the lower limb, which will be referred to as 'peripheral arterial disease', and aneurysms of the lower abdominal aorta, referred to as 'abdominal aortic aneurysm'. These conditions have been chosen because they are common and have a major impact on the use of health service resources. Precise definitions of these conditions are as follows:

- Peripheral arterial disease: atherosclerosis of the distal aorta and/or lower limb arteries causing arterial narrowing and disruption of blood flow in the legs.
- Abdominal aortic aneurysm: abnormal dilatation of the aorta distal to the renal arteries.

Aetiology and pathology

In peripheral arterial disease, the pathological condition of atherosclerosis is identical to that which occurs in the coronary arteries, causing ischaemic heart disease. The deposition of atheroma, comprising mostly lipid in the media of the arterial wall, may begin in childhood, and by late middle age most adults have evidence of atheroma in their peripheral arteries.[2] Atheroma has a predilection for certain sites in the arterial tree, notably at bifurcations and bends, and may lead to stenosis (narrowing) or occlusion (complete blockage) of the artery. The pattern, severity and effects of the disease vary greatly, so that some individuals remain asymptomatic while in others, the arterial narrowing leads to inadequate muscle blood flow (ischaemia) with resulting pain.

As the underlying pathology of peripheral arterial disease and coronary heart disease are the same, it is not surprising that the aetiological risk factors for the two conditions are similar.[3] The classic cardio-vascular risk factors of cigarette smoking, hypercholesterolaemia and hypertension are implicated in peripheral arterial disease. Likewise, more recently investigated risk factors for coronary heart disease, such as lack of physical exercise, alcohol consumption, diabetes mellitus, low high density lipoprotein (HDL) cholesterol, hyperhomocysteinaemia, thrombophilia and hypercoagulable states, are also associated with an increased risk of peripheral arterial disease.[4] Cigarette smoking would appear to be a more important risk factor for peripheral arterial disease than coronary heart disease, with over 90% of patients with intermittent claudication stating that they are current or ex-smokers.[5] Diabetes mellitus is often believed to be a more important risk factor for peripheral arterial disease than coronary heart disease but the evidence for this is inconsistent. There is no doubt that diabetes mellitus is very important in the later stages of peripheral arterial disease in which diabetic neuropathy and small vessel disease, as well as atherosclerosis in large vessels, may cause gangrene and ulceration.[6]

Aortic aneurysm affecting the lower abdominal aorta is the result of a weakening and thinning of the aortic wall leading to dilatation and ballooning of the aorta.[7] It is believed to result from a change in the composition of the collagen and elastin matrix in the media of the arterial wall. This matrix is affected by the activity of certain enzymes, including the metalloproteinases. The presence of an aneurysm often coincides with the occurrence of significant atherosclerosis in the aortic wall, and population studies have shown the two conditions to be inter-related. However, the extent to which atherosclerosis may be involved in the pathogenesis of aneurysms is not well established.[8]

The only risk factor that has been shown conclusively to be involved in the aetiology of aortic aneurysm is cigarette smoking, with some smokers having a two- to threefold increased risk compared with non-smokers.[9] Aneurysms have been shown in some studies to occur more frequently in the close relatives of cases,[10] but to date, a mode of inheritance has not been demonstrated.[5] Nor has a specific gene affecting, for example, enzyme activity in the arterial wall been identified. However, future research is likely to lead to greater understanding of the role of inheritance and genes in the aetiology of this condition.

Clinical presentation, diagnosis and treatment

The most common clinical presentation of peripheral arterial disease is intermittent claudication, in which pain occurs in the calf on exercise and is relieved by rest. The diagnosis can often be made on the clinical history alone but may be confirmed by measurement of the ankle brachial pressure index (ABPI). This is the ratio of the ankle to brachial systolic pressure and can be measured easily using a sphygmomanometer and Doppler ultrasound machine. In the presence of symptoms, a ratio of < 0.9 is over 90% sensitive and specific in identifying peripheral arterial disease.[11] A treadmill exercise test may be useful to document pain-free walking distance and a Duplex scan may be used to locate significant atherosclerotic lesions. Angiography, which involves injection of an opaque dye into the arterial system, may be required for the accurate identification of lesions, pending interventional treatment.

The clinical course of patients with intermittent claudication is very variable. Most patients either improve or stay about the same; deterioration leading to amputation is uncommon.[12,13] In mild claudication, 'stop smoking and keep walking' is standard advice;[14] drug therapy is of limited value.[15] Interventional treatment may be warranted when patients perceive the handicap as severely limiting their quality of life. In such cases, balloon angioplasty or bypass surgery may be carried out, although there have been few controlled trials examining the cost-effectiveness of these procedures. Balloon angioplasty involves passing a catheter through the skin into the artery and inflating a balloon to crack and obliterate the atheromatous plaque. Bypass operations, which are the main type of reconstructive surgery, involve the insertion of a graft comprising vein or synthetic material, such as Dacron. This graft allows blood to bypass the narrowed or obstructed artery. In most cases of intermittent claudication, risk factor management and antiplatelet therapy is also warranted.

The intermittent pain may worsen and be present when the patient is stationary (rest pain). Gangrene and ulceration of the foot may also occur. In such severe forms of peripheral arterial disease (critical limb ischaemia), bypass surgery, angioplasty or amputation are usually required.

An aortic aneurysm may present either as an emergency following rupture or with symptoms such as a pulsating abdominal mass or back pain.[1,7] The diagnosis can rarely be made on clinical examination alone and usually requires confirmation by ultrasound or computed tomography (CT) scanning of the abdomen. Sometimes asymptomatic aortic aneurysms are found when an abdomen is being scanned for other purposes or as part of an aneurysm screening programme.

Treatment of an aneurysm is highly dependent on the presenting features. Ruptured aneurysms require emergency surgical repair, which is associated with a high mortality of 40–60%.[16] Symptomatic aneurysms also require surgical treatment, usually elective, to relieve the symptoms and reduce risk of rupture. Management of asymptomatic aneurysms is dependent on their size – larger aneurysms are operated on while smaller aneurysms, in which the risk of rupture is low, are surveilled routinely using ultrasound, and only operated on if the aneurysm grows substantially and is at increased risk of rupture.

Diagnostic and treatment codes

The International Classification of Diseases (ICD-10), Office of Population Censuses and Surveys (OPCS-4) operation codes, and Healthcare Resource Group (HRG-3) codes relevant to peripheral arterial disease and aortic aneurysm are shown in Table 1.

As a general rule, the diagnostic codes for peripheral arterial disease are not very helpful because they are not specific enough to identify individual clinical conditions, and the same condition may occur under different codes. For example, a patient with intermittent claudication may be categorised as 170.2, 170.8, 170.9 or 173.9 (Table 1). The codes for aortic aneurysm are probably more accurate, although there may be misclassification of ruptured/non-ruptured. The operation codes are more precise, although under-reporting is likely, particularly of more minor procedures such as diagnostic angiography and angioplasty.

In addition to the HRGs as shown in Table 1, the National Casemix Office set up in 1998 a process of developing Health Benefit Groups (HBGs). These are groups of people: (a) with similar healthcare need; (b) who require similar healthcare interventions; and (c) who, given those interventions, would have a similar range of outcomes. For any condition, HBGs are classified within four stages of the natural history: 1, at risk of the condition; 2, presenting with the condition; 3, confirmed disease requiring initial care; and 4, consequences of disease requiring continuing care and/or rehabilitation. Each of these HBG categories is placed together with relevant HRG categories, such as prevention and promotion, investigation and diagnosis, into a matrix format. These matrices enable disease morbidity, health service activity and finance data to be turned into information on a condition-specific and a case group basis.

Health service issues

In primary care, the appropriate indications and threshold for referral of patients with peripheral arterial disease are not well established. Practice undoubtedly varies between different parts of the UK and it is likely that many referrals to vascular units do not benefit from additional investigations or receive more effective treatment than was advised in general practice. Another important issue for primary care is that it has become increasingly recognised that patients with peripheral arterial disease are at greatly increased risk of cardiovascular and cerebrovascular events and that risk-factor management in such patients is often lacking.

In secondary care, a major issue that has been of concern in recent years is the appropriate location and organisation of vascular units so that a comprehensive vascular service can be provided with adequate emergency cover, technological facilities and ancillary services. In considering the organisation of services, an important issue is the minimum specification required for a vascular unit in order to provide a high-quality service. Such a specification will include the required surgical, radiological, anaesthetic and other staff per head of population, number of inpatient beds, range of diagnostic facilities, intensive care and high dependency units, rehabilitation and other services.

Another issue relevant to secondary care is that the diagnosis and management of patients with intermittent claudication referred to hospital is extremely variable. The appropriate sequence of investigations and indications for treatment, particularly angioplasty or surgery, is not well specified. Precise guidelines are required on the most cost-effective strategies. In particular, indications for appropriate diagnostic

Table 1: International Classification of Diseases (ICD-10), Office of Population Census and Surveys (OPCS-4) operation codes, and Healthcare Resource Groups (HRG-3) for peripheral arterial disease and aortic aneurysm.

ICD-10	
I70.2	Atherosclerosis of arteries of extremities
I71.3	Abdominal aortic aneurysm, ruptured
I71.4	Abdominal aortic aneurysm, without mention of rupture
I71.8	Aortic aneurysm of unspecified site, ruptured
I71.9	Aortic aneurysm of unspecified site, without mention of rupture
I73.9	Peripheral vascular disease, unspecified (includes intermittent claudication)

I70.0 atherosclerosis of aorta, I70.8 atherosclerosis of other arteries, I70.9 generalised and unspecified atherosclerosis, and E10-E14 diabetes with .5 (peripheral circulatory complications) may also include some cases of peripheral arterial disease.

OPCS-4	
L16.-, L18.-, L19.-, L25.4	Aortic aneurysm repairs*
L50.-, L51.-, L52.-, L53.2, L58.-	Iliac and femoral bypass/
L59.-, L60.1, .2, L62.2	endarterectomy/embolectomy
X09.3, .4, .5, X11.-	Amputations – knee/toe**
L26.1, .2, .3, .8, .9, L31.1, .8, .9	
L39.1, .2, .3, .8, .9, L43.1, .2, .3, .8, .9	Transluminal operations
L47.1, .2, .8, .9, L54.1, .2, .8, .9	including angioplasty
L63.1, .2, .3, .8, .9, L71.-	
L26.4, L31.2, L39.4, L43.4, L47.3	Diagnostic angiography
L54.3, L63.4, L72.1	

* Includes only those cases that have diagnosis of abdominal aortic aneurysm (in any position).
** Includes only those cases that have diagnosis of atherosclerosis or peripheral vascular disease (in any position).

HRG-3	
Q01	Emergency aortic surgery
Q02	Elective abdominal vascular surgery
Q03	Lower limb arterial surgery
Q04	Bypasses to tibial arteries
Q12	Therapeutic endovascular procedures
Q13	Diagnostic radiology – arteries or lymphatics with comorbidity/complications
Q14	Diagnostic radiology – arteries or lymphatics without comorbidity/complications
Q15	Amputations
Q16	Foot procedures for diabetes or arterial disease, and procedures to amputation
Q17	Peripheral vascular disease > 69 years or with comorbidity/complications
Q18	Peripheral vascular disease < 70 years without comorbidity/complications

imaging need to be specified. Also, interventional radiological techniques, such as balloon angioplasty and stenting, are being widely used and undergoing continuing development and refinement, so that ongoing guidance on their use is required.

For patients with severe peripheral arterial disease requiring surgery, the indications for when arterial reconstruction, especially bypass grafting, or amputation should be performed are not clear-cut. Decisions are affected by the availability of resources, because reconstructive surgery is often more time-consuming and demanding than amputation. Appropriate organisation of services and adoption of surgical guidelines would ensure more uniform practice and higher rates of limb salvage in patients with severe peripheral arterial disease. Also, for patients having amputation, the availability of rehabilitation services varies greatly. It is well known that early rehabilitation has a major effect on outcome for amputees, but unfortunately limb-fitting services are not always easily accessible.

The management strategy of aortic aneurysms is generally straightforward, except that some doubt exists as to the appropriate treatment for smaller, asymptomatic aneurysms, with a choice of elective aneurysm repair or routine ultrasound surveillance in which the size and growth of the aneurysm is monitored. The recently published results of the UK Small Aneurysm Trial, however, indicate that it is generally not cost-effective to operate on aneurysms < 5.5 cm diameter, and that Trusts would be better to invest in ultrasound surveillance.

In the prevention of peripheral vascular disease, the value of screening for aortic aneurysms is currently under consideration by the Department of Health following a recommendation by the National Screening Committee. The costs and organisation of a district-based screening service are considerable although trials have shown that screening and then management of aneurysms, either by surgery or surveillance, is cost-effective. For the prevention of peripheral arterial disease, the risk factors, such as cigarette smoking and hyperlipidaemia, are essentially the same as for coronary heart disease, although smoking appears to be more important. Primary prevention programmes for coronary heart disease are therefore applicable to peripheral arterial disease and separate initiatives are not required.

Key problems for purchasers

The key problems currently facing purchasers are first, to ensure that the minimum service requirements for the management of peripheral vascular diseases are in place at secondary care level in order to ensure provision of a high-quality service. Also, methods of monitoring need to be established to ensure that the process and outcome of care is satisfactory. The second key problem concerns screening for aortic aneurysms, an area in which professional groups have put pressure on authorities but on which national guidance is awaited. Finally, purchasers need to try and ensure that an efficient and consistent programme exists for the management of intermittent claudication in both primary and secondary care.

3 Sub-categories

The following sub-categories of peripheral arterial disease and aortic aneurysm are used in this chapter because they reflect different severities of disease and approaches to management.

Peripheral arterial disease

(a) *Intermittent claudication* is the most common condition and the only condition that many patients experience. Mild symptoms are likely to be treated conservatively, whereas more severe symptoms might be treated with angioplasty or bypass surgery.
(b) *Critical limb ischaemia* is a more severe form of peripheral arterial disease in which the patient has rest pain, gangrene or ulceration. These patients normally require urgent hospital admission and are treated by means of surgical reconstruction, amputation or, occasionally, angioplasty in the first instance.
(c) *Asymptomatic peripheral arterial disease* is now being increasingly recognised as a high-risk group for future cardiovascular and cerebrovascular events, requiring appropriate risk factor management.

Abdominal aortic aneurysm

(a) *Ruptured aneurysm* is managed by surgical repair where appropriate. This will be carried out as an emergency procedure and requires that a skilled vascular team is available out of hours.
(b) *Asymptomatic aneurysm*, on the other hand, may be managed either using an elective surgical repair or by ultrasound surveillance. Population screening for asymptomatic aneurysms may also be carried out.

4 Prevalence and incidence

Intermittent claudication

The prevalence of intermittent claudication in the general population has been measured by questionnaire. Table 2 shows the prevalence by age and sex found in three population surveys[17-19] carried out in the UK during the 1980s and 1990s using the WHO/Rose questionnaire on intermittent claudication.[20] These studies came to broadly the same conclusions. Under the age of 55 years intermittent claudication is uncommon, affecting less than 1% of men and women. Over the age of 55 years, the prevalence increases steeply with age and overall in 55- to 74-year-old men and women the prevalence is almost 5%.[17] At younger ages the prevalence of claudication is almost twice as high in men as in women, but at older ages the sex difference narrows, in keeping with the findings in other forms of atherosclerotic disease. The WHO/Rose questionnaire is known to lack sensitivity (60–70%)[21-22] and more recent adaptations, such as the Edinburgh Claudication Questionnaire,[23] are now recommended for use. However, despite the low sensitivity of the WHO/Rose questionnaire, the prevalence figures in Table 2 are probably only a slight underestimate because of the inclusion of false positives. In the Scottish Health Survey,[24] which used the Edinburgh questionnaire, the prevalence was measured over a wide range from 16 to 64 years. In men, the prevalence at age 16–24 years was 0.4% rising consistently to 1.9% at age 45–54 years and 5.0% at age 55–64.

Reliable information on the geographical variation in prevalence of intermittent claudication in the UK is not available, but the distribution by social class and the strong relationship with cigarette smoking would suggest that there is a north–south divide as is found for coronary heart disease. In the Edinburgh Artery Study of 55- to 74-year-old men and women[17] a consistently increasing trend in the prevalence of claudication was found with lower social class (3.6% in Class I to 5.9% in Classes IV+V). Likewise, an

Table 2: Prevalence (%) of intermittent claudication by age in general population surveys in the UK in the 1980 and 1990s.

Age group	Men			Women	
	SHHS	**SS**	**EAS**	**SHHS**	**EAS**
40–44	0.4			0.2	
45–49	1.0			0.4	
50–54	0.8	0.8		0.4	
55–59	2.2	1.8	2.2	1.0	2.3
60–64		2.4	4.6		5.0
65–69		3.9 (65–72)	3.6		5.5
70–74			8.4		6.6

EAS: Edinburgh Artery Study.[17]
SS: Speedwell Study.[18]
SHHS: Scottish Heart Health Study.[19]
EAS, SS and SHHS used WHO/Rose questionnaire[20] and included Grades I and II claudication.
EAS also included 'probable' claudication (increasing figures by around one quarter).
SS included men only.

inverse trend occurred with educational attainment: those who left school and did not proceed to further education had a twofold higher prevalence than those entering college or university. Also, using the Carstairs deprivation score, which classifies households in postcode sectors according to a combination of four variables (men unemployed, overcrowded housing of more than one person per room, households without a car and household heads in semi- or unskilled/manual occupations), a higher prevalence of peripheral arterial disease was associated with greater deprivation, especially in men.[25] Although peripheral arterial disease in this analysis[25] was measured using hospital discharge data and the ABPI, it would be very surprising if the relationship did not also hold true for intermittent claudication. In the Edinburgh Artery Study, much of the association with deprivation appeared to be related to cigarette smoking.[25]

Limited information is available on the incidence of intermittent claudication in the UK. In the Speedwell Study, 4% of men aged 45–63 years developed claudication during 10 years of follow-up, with the incidence increasing consistently with age.[18] In the Edinburgh Artery Study among men and women aged 55 to 74 years, 9% developed claudication during 5 years of follow-up – a figure equivalent to 1.8% per annum or 15.5 per 1000 person years.[26] Overall, the 5-year incidence was higher among men (8.7%) than among women (6.6%). The higher incidence rate in the Edinburgh Artery Study compared to the Speedwell Study was due to the older population and inclusion of 'probable' claudicants.

Since atherosclerosis is the cause of peripheral arterial disease, coronary heart disease and ischaemic stroke, it is not surprising that concomitant heart disease and a history of stroke occurs commonly in subjects with intermittent claudication. In the general population, around 40% of claudicants have angina.[17] The prevalence of concurrent coronary heart disease in claudicants is between two and four times that in non-claudicants.[27] In patients presenting to hospital, between 38% and 58% have evidence of coronary heart disease diagnosed by history and electrocardiogram (ECG), but if patients are investigated intensively by, for example, coronary angiography, 90% have evidence of coronary atherosclerosis.[12] A history of stroke occurs in about 15% of claudicants but depends on the age, sex and other features of the population studied.[27] This high prevalence of other manifestations of atherosclerosis in claudicants emphasises the importance of total patient management and not just treatment of the claudication in these patients.

In patients developing intermittent claudication, the natural history of their leg ischaemia is relatively good.[12] In claudicants referred to hospital, around one third will become symptom-free during their lifetime without intervention; around one third to one half remain about the same; and in only one quarter will the symptoms deteriorate, resulting in a lifetime amputation rate for hospital referrals of less than 7%.[28] This prognosis is even better among claudicants identified in community surveys. In the Edinburgh Artery Study, 50% of claudicants became symptom-free during 5 years of follow-up,[26] and the lifetime incidence of amputation in claudicants in the general population, as shown in the Framingham Study in the USA, is only about 1–2%.[29]

However, a major concern in patients with intermittent claudication is the high risk of mortality. The 5-year mortality among claudicants referred to hospital is around 25–50%[12] and the relative risk of dying is two to three times that of individuals without claudication.[13] Similar relative risks occur in claudicants in the general population.[26,30] Given that many individuals with peripheral arterial disease in the legs have evidence of widespread vascular disease, not surprisingly over 60% of deaths are due to coronary heart disease and about 10% are due to stroke.[31] Very few deaths are due directly to complications of leg ischaemia.

Patients with intermittent claudication are also at greatly increased risk of major non-fatal cardiovascular and cerebrovascular events. Long-term follow-up studies of claudicants in the general population in Scotland,[26] USA,[30] Sweden[32] and other Western countries have found a twofold relative risk of non-fatal myocardial infarction compared with non-claudicants. In typical claudicants referred to hospital, roughly 15% will have a non-fatal coronary event within 5 years.[12] Likewise, non-fatal stroke occurs more commonly in claudicants than in healthy subjects. In the Edinburgh Artery Study the 5-year incidence of stroke or transient ischaemic attack (TIA) in claudicants was 6.8% with a twofold increased relative risk compared to non-claudicants.[26] Even when adjusted to take account of the higher levels of cardiovascular risk factors in claudicants (cigarette smoking, hypercholesterolaemia and elevated blood pressure), the increased risks of future coronary heart disease and stroke were reduced only slightly.[26,30,32]

Valid information on time trends in the prevalence of intermittent claudication in the UK would need to be based on repeated large cross-sectional surveys in the general population. Such repeat surveys have not been carried out. Data on trends in claudication, however, are available from the Reykjavik Study in Iceland.[33] Between 1970 and 1986, both the prevalence and incidence of claudication decreased in men at all ages between 40 and 70 years. The decline in prevalence was about 55% and in incidence 66%. No data were collected for women. Interestingly, the decline in claudication was greater than that for coronary heart disease in men during the same period and started a few years earlier.[34] In the UK, claudication has been measured sequentially in two cohort studies, the Speedwell Study[18] and the Edinburgh Artery Study.[17,26] The numbers within the specified age groups were small but neither study suggested that there had been a decline in prevalence of claudication. Results for the Speedwell Study are shown in Table 3.

The trends in prevalence and incidence of intermittent claudication in the UK are thus unknown. The expectation would be that trends in claudication would closely mirror those for coronary heart disease and, as was found in the Reykjavik Study, be influenced particularly by trends in cigarette smoking in the general population.[33] The decline in the incidence of coronary heart disease[35] and smoking prevalence[36] would point to a decreasing frequency of claudication. On the other hand, a possible lower case fatality rate for myocardial infarction[37] would lead to increasing survival of those with severe atherosclerotic disease and perhaps an increased occurrence of chronic manifestations such as intermittent claudication.

Table 3: Age specific prevalence of intermittent claudication at baseline and at subsequent examinations in the Speedwell Study.

	Sample number and % prevalence claudication							
	50–54 yrs		55–59 yrs		60–64 yrs		≥ 65 yrs	
Examination								
Baseline	727	1.0	852	1.8	318	2.2	–	–
3-year	598	0.8	686	1.2	695	3.5	45	2.2
6-year	205	0	639	1.6	646	2.9	472	3.8
9–10-year	–	–	440	1.4	575	2.4	741	3.9

Baseline examination conducted in 1979–82.
Source: adapted from Bainton *et al.*[18]

Critical limb ischaemia

The frequency of critical limb ischaemia in the general population is difficult to estimate because it is too rare to measure reliably in population surveys. Although most patients are admitted to hospital, diagnostic coding is too imprecise to identify such patients reliably. However, in a multicentre study in the UK in the mid-1980s, of 409 patients with critical limb ischaemia, 25% had major amputations within 12 months.[38] An expert European consensus group utilised this information, together with reasonably valid data on the frequency of amputation and knowing that the vast majority of these amputations were for ischaemia, to calculate an overall incidence of critical limb ischaemia in the range 500–1000 per million population per year.[39]

The natural history and survival of patients with critical limb ischaemia is poor. The UK Joint Vascular Research Group found that 1 year after presentation with critical ischaemia 20% of patients were dead and only 53% were alive with both legs intact.[38] Of the 25% having major amputation, the 5-year survival rate was less than 50%.[40] As might be expected, amputation or reconstructive surgery on the ischaemic leg has little effect on survival. In one study of patients with rest pain who did not have surgery, the 5-year mortality was over 50%.[41] The poor survival in patients with critical limb ischaemia is undoubtedly related to the widespread atherosclerotic disease which is invariably present.

Asymptomatic peripheral arterial disease

Asymptomatic peripheral arterial disease causing a severe disruption to blood flow occurs commonly in the general population. In the Edinburgh Artery Study, 8.0% had evidence of major asymptomatic disease (Figure 1) and the results of Duplex scanning indicated that at least one third of these subjects had occlusion of a major artery.[17] A further 16.6% were classified as having minor asymptomatic disease. Asymptomatic disease has not been investigated in other population studies in the UK, but comparable findings have been reported in surveys overseas. In the Basle Study, conducted some years ago on workers in the pharmaceutical industry, the prevalence of occlusion confirmed by arteriography was 0.4% at age 20–24 years, increasing to 7.5% at age 60–64 years.[41] Surveys in Denmark[42] and Israel[43] found that 14% and 5% respectively had low ankle brachial systolic pressure ratios (< 0.9). The Lipid Research Clinics study in the USA used a combination of non-invasive tests and found that the prevalence of large vessel disease

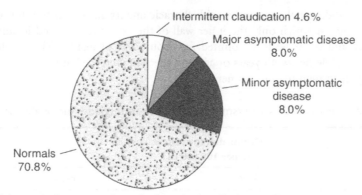

Intermittent claudication 4.6%

Major asymptomatic disease
8.0%

Minor asymptomatic
disease
8.0%

Normals
70.8%

Major and minor asymptomatic disease classified according to results
of ankle brachial pressure index and reactive hyperaemia test.

Figure 1: Prevalence of symptomatic and asymptomatic peripheral arterial diseases in the general population aged 55 to 74 years: Edinburgh Artery Study.

affecting the lower limb increased progressively with age from 3% at less than 60 years to more than 20% in those aged 75 years and over.[44]

Individuals in the general population with demonstrable asymptomatic peripheral arterial disease are at increased risk of developing intermittent claudication. In the Edinburgh Artery Study, over a 5-year follow-up period, 15.2% with major asymptomatic disease developed claudication, compared with 7.1% of those with minor asymptomatic disease and 3.2% of normals.[26] A low ABPI, irrespective of the presence of ischaemic symptoms, is indicative of a higher prevalence of concomitant coronary heart disease, history of stroke or TIA, and carotid stenosis.[45] It is not surprising therefore that subjects with lower limb arterial disease, as measured by a low ABPI, have an increased mortality mostly due to coronary heart disease and stroke. There is a two- to threefold increased risk of cardiovascular mortality in both men and women without symptoms of any vascular disease but an ABPI < 0.9 compared with those with an ABPI ≥ 0.9.[26,30,32,46] Also, those with a low ABPI are at increased risk of non-fatal myocardial infarction and stroke.[26,32] Interestingly, these risks associated with a low ABPI occur independently of those due to risk factors such as cigarette smoking, hypercholesterolaemia and hypertension,[47] so that the ABPI may be a useful marker of vascular risk in supposedly healthy individuals.

Ruptured aneurysm

Aneurysms may cause minor symptoms such as backache, but the most important symptomatic phenomena are those due to rupture. Rupture is often catastrophic and causes sudden death before the patient is admitted to hospital. The incidence of rupture in the population therefore requires tracing of all ruptures causing sudden death in the community as well as those in patients admitted to hospital. In a study in Swansea in 1983, the annual incidence was found to be 17 per 100 000 population, and of these, 60% died outside hospital.[48] Of those admitted to hospital well over half die during that admission. As the mortality rate from rupture is extremely high and because there are no valid figures on incidence of rupture per se, mortality rates from aortic aneurysm are the best routine measure of community burden.

In England and Wales in 1996, 6163 men and 3663 women died due to an aortic aneurysm[49] resulting in a mortality rate of 24.1 and 13.8 per 100 000 men and women respectively (Table 4). The majority of the deaths were due to abdominal aneurysms, with thoracic aneurysm accounting for about 7% of deaths. Dissecting aneurysms, in which only the inner wall of the artery is ruptured leading to blood flowing between the inner and outer walls, accounted for about 20% of deaths. The death rate due to aortic aneurysms was negligible below 45 years of age and the rate increased at successive ages. At all ages the mortality was higher in men than in women.

Table 4: Mortality due to aortic aneurysm by age and sex in England and Wales, 1996.

Age group (yrs)	Deaths due to aortic aneurysm Rate per 100,000 (n)	
	Male	Female
0–14	0.0 (1)	0.0 (1)
15–44	0.4 (40)	0.1 (14)
45–64	10.9 (644)	2.5 (148)
65–74	103.3 (2,128)	34.4 (835)
75+	254.7 (3,350)	108.6 (2,665)
Total	24.1 (6,163)	13.8 (3,663)

Deaths due to aortic aneurysm include thoracic ($n \sim 700$) and dissecting ($n \sim 2,000$) aneurysms.
Source: Office for National Statistics[49]

Asymptomatic aneurysm

The population prevalence of abdominal aortic aneurysms (which are mostly asymptomatic) can be determined only from community surveys using ultrasound screening. Table 5 shows the results of four such surveys carried out in the UK.[50–53] The prevalence figures are affected by the population studied, definition of aneurysm according to diameter and measurement technique. Overall, roughly 5% of men aged 65–74 years would appear to have an aneurysm ≥ 3.0 cm in diameter. The prevalence of aneurysms in females is much lower, with a male:female ratio of about 3:1. Although comprehensive data on prevalence by age are not obtainable from screening studies, it would seem from the limited data available and from mortality and hospital admission statistics that aneurysms are relatively uncommon below the age of 50 years. The prevalence would appear to rise steeply with age in older subjects, and may be up to 10-fold higher in those over 85 compared to those aged 55.[7,54,55]

As aneurysms may, in part, be genetically determined[7] and would appear to occur more often in the presence of aortic atherosclerosis,[7–9], the prevalence of aneurysms has been shown to be higher in close family relatives of those affected and also in those with various manifestations of cardiovascular disease.[55] Also the prevalence has been found to be higher in those with cardiovascular risk factors, such as cigarette smoking, hypertension and hypercholesterolaemia. The prevalence of aneurysm in these risk categories varies greatly with the exception perhaps of cigarette smokers, in whom prevalences between 10% and 14% have been reported.[55]

Table 5: Population prevalence of abdominal aortic aneurysms in community surveys in the UK.

Author	Location	Age and sex	Number	Aneurysm diameter (cm)	Prevalence (%)
Collin et al.[50]	Oxford	65–74 men	824	≥ 3	4.0
O'Reilly & Heather[51]	Gloucester	65–74 men	1,195	≥ 2.5	7.8
Scott et al.[52]	Chichester	65–80 men	2,342	≥ 3	7.6
		65–80 women	3,052	≥ 3	1.3
Smith et al.[53]	Birmingham	65–75 men	2,669	≥ 2.9	8.2

Magnitude of disease in a UK district

The figures on prevalence and incidence of the different manifestations of peripheral vascular disease are mostly based on the results of ad hoc surveys in different populations in the UK. The following extrapolation of these figures to a typical UK district population must therefore be interpreted with caution.

In a district of 500 000 population with the age and sex distribution of the estimated 1996 population in England and Wales, there would be about 9500 claudicants and around 1000 individuals would develop intermittent claudication each year. (The total number of claudicants in the UK is about 1 million.) Each year around 375 individuals in this district would develop critical limb ischaemia. In addition to the claudicants, almost 20 000 would have major asymptomatic peripheral arterial disease causing severe disruption to blood flow in the legs. About 120 males and 70 females would die each year due to an aortic aneurysm, the majority being caused by rupture of an abdominal aneurysm. Also, the population at large would contain around 4500 individuals with an asymptomatic abdominal aneurysm.

5 Services available and their costs

Peripheral arterial disease

Primary care

In primary care, the main service requirement is to provide adequate diagnosis, referral and risk factor management in patients with intermittent claudication. This is normally part of routine general practice. In the diagnosis of peripheral arterial disease, measurement of the ABPI is a simple, inexpensive and useful test to perform but few GPs have the equipment or skill to perform this test. Otherwise, providing a proper service at primary care level does not require any special facilities or expertise.

Table 6 shows the consultation rates in general practice for the major peripheral vascular disease diagnostic groups in England and Wales in 1991–92. The number of patients consulting and total number of consultations per head of population per year for peripheral arterial disease and aortic aneurysm was extremely low, particularly as many in the 'other peripheral vascular diseases' group would have had neither of these categories of disease. The number of consultations per 10 000 people per annum was 82 and accounted for only 0.24% (1 in 420) of total consultations in general practice. Data from the Continuous

Morbidity Recording system in general practice in Scotland indicates that in 1997 there were 8404 new consultations for peripheral arterial disease in Scotland. This consultation rate is equivalent to 17 per 10 000 person years at risk, a figure comparable to the 25 per 10 000 found in England and Wales (Table 6).

Table 6: Consultation rates for peripheral vascular diseases in general practice in England and Wales, 1991–92.

Diagnostic group (ICD-9)	Rate per 10,000 person years at risk		
	New and first ever episodes*	Patients consulting**	Consultations with doctor
Atherosclerosis (440)	1	2	4
Aortic aneurysm (441)	2	3	6
Other aneurysm (442)	0	0	1
Other peripheral vascular diseases (443)	24	40	71
All diseases and conditions	n.a.	7,803	34,785

* Episodes: single or sequence of consultations covering the duration of a continuing illness. A new episode is an episode for a condition for which the patient has previously consulted.
** Patients consulting at least once during the year.
Source: Office of Population Consensus and Surveys. *Morbidity Statistics from General Practice. Fourth national study 1991–1992*. London: Her Majesty's Stationery Office, 1995

Secondary care: availability of services

The services available for the secondary care of peripheral arterial disease in the UK are not comprehensively documented. However, an unpublished survey of vascular services in hospital trusts in Scotland for the recent Acute Services Review[56] revealed a diversity of provision. This survey found the following.

Location

- The vascular service in most hospitals was part of the general surgery service. Three out of 18 hospitals had a unit dedicated to vascular disease only.
- A large number of general hospitals, including teaching hospitals, did not provide any vascular service.

Staffing

- One third of 'vascular surgeons' performed vascular surgery only, whereas two thirds of 'vascular surgeons' were general surgeons with a principal specialty interest of vascular surgery.
- All hospitals providing a vascular service had anaesthetists with a special interest in vascular cases but not all elective vascular lists were covered by vascular anaesthetists.
- Among radiologists performing vascular interventions, less than one third specialised, i.e. 50% or more of their work was in interventional radiology.
- Three out of 18 vascular services were supported by physicians specialising in vascular medicine.
- Four out of 18 vascular services had nursing staff with specialist training in the management of vascular disease.

Facilities

- A vascular laboratory was not available in 50% of hospitals providing a vascular service.
- All vascular units had access to intensive therapy unit beds and two thirds had access to high dependency unit beds and on-site renal dialysis.

Organisation

- Emergency rotas varied greatly from a 1 in 4 rota of specialist vascular surgeons to rotas in which non-vascular general surgeons participated. Occasionally single-handed vascular surgeons were continuously on call for vascular emergencies.
- About 90% of hospitals providing a vascular service had a separate vascular waiting list and around one third had a dedicated vascular theatre.

A previous survey of Trusts in Scotland in 1992 produced very similar findings.[57] Also, the results of a 1995 survey of vascular surgeons in the UK, carried out by the Vascular Surgeons Society of Great Britain and Ireland, suggested that the situation in Scotland was not atypical of the UK as a whole.[58] This latter survey found that around half the surgeons were working in hospitals servicing populations of 250 000–500 000, 40% in hospitals serving 100 000–250 000 and 20% in hospitals serving over 500 000. Around one third of surgeons had specifically allocated vascular beds and about one third had a dedicated vascular list. Half had no access to intensive therapy unit beds. The National Confidential Enquiry into Perioperative Deaths (1994/95) in England and Wales found that one third of cases admitted with vascular emergencies were treated by consultants with no vascular interest.[59] Therefore, the overall picture in the UK is that the majority of vascular surgery is being carried out in general surgery units in district general hospitals and not in tertiary specialist referral centres.

Some limited information is available on the costs of providing a vascular service for the diagnosis and treatment of peripheral arterial disease. Hospital costs for HRGs relevant to peripheral arterial disease obtained from an ongoing survey of a sample of NHS Trusts in 1997/98 are shown in Table 7. The highest mean cost was for amputations (£5994), whereas a bypass to tibial arteries cost £5378. In contrast, a therapeutic endovascular procedure, which would comprise mostly angioplasty, had a mean cost of only £1519. In recent years, costs have been estimated separately in some hospitals. For example, in a survey of patients followed up for one year in one centre, the costs of arterial reconstruction at 1988/89 prices ranged from £6590 per patient for proximal grafts to £11 000 for distal grafts.[60] These included costs of revision of failed grafts, secondary amputation and treatment of the other leg. In contrast, the cost of primary amputation ranged from £10 400–£10 850 per patient. In another hospital, a report published in 1995 indicated that the median inpatient cost of primary amputation was £8000 and for a successful bypass graft was £5300.[61] The average total health and social service costs consumed during, and up to 6 months following, surgery were £12 500 for amputation and £6000 for bypass surgery. Thus the results of these studies show that amputation is, on average, a more costly procedure than reconstructive surgery.

Capital costs for providing a vascular service may be substantial, particularly the equipment required for vascular radiology. A Duplex scanning machine costs £100 000, spiral CT £350 000, digital subtraction angiography (DSA) £500 000 and a fixed theatre C arm £500 000. Magnetic resonance angiography (MRA), which is available in a few centres but is currently not essential for routine practice, costs £500 000–£1 000 000.

Table 7: Reference costs for peripheral arterial disease Health Related Groups (HRGs) in NHS Trusts in 1997/98.

HRG No.	HRG label*	Mean average cost (£)**	Range for 50% of NHS Trusts***	
			Minimum (£)	Maximum (£)
Q03	Lower limb art. surg.	4,024	3,011	4,724
Q04	Bypass to tibial art.	5,378	3,765	6,613
Q12	Therap. endovasc. proced.	1,519	910	1,766
Q13	Diag. radiol. with comorb/complic	2,032	1,377	2,510
Q14	Diag. radiol. w.o. comorb/complic	1,019	651	1,123
Q15	Amputations	5,994	4,449	6,615
Q16	Foot proced. diab. arter.	2,709	1,720	3,516
Q17	PVD > 69 yrs or comorb/complic	1,363	967	1,549
Q18	PVD < 70 yrs w.o. comorb/complic	1,087	642	1,175

* See Table 1 for full text of labels.

** Mean of the average cost of HRG in 249 NHS Trusts.

*** Range from the minimum average cost to maximum average cost of the mid 50% of Trusts, i.e. from bottom of 2nd to top of 3rd percentiles.

Source: The National Schedule for Reference Costs. London: Department of Health, 1998

Secondary care: use of services

The use of secondary vascular services in hospitals in England in 1995/96 for the diagnosis and treatment of peripheral arterial disease is shown in Tables 8–10. The number of patients discharged with a primary diagnosis of peripheral atherosclerosis was about 36 000 and, of these, the great majority were in general surgical units (which included specialist vascular centres) (Table 8). Almost an equal number of cases were given a secondary diagnosis of peripheral atherosclerosis. The precise nature of these cases is difficult to determine given the generality of the diagnostic group.

Table 9 shows the number of procedures performed in 1995/96. The commonest was diagnostic angiography (nearly 40 000). Transluminal procedures, which would have been mostly angioplasties, comprised the most frequent interventional treatment, while iliac/femoral bypass was the most common major surgical operation. The number of amputations was about half that of bypass procedures but the mean length of stay of amputations was the highest, at 27.7 days. Most amputations were carried out in general surgery or vascular units (rather than orthopaedic units). The accuracy of this data on number of procedures carried out is not precisely known but is probably an underestimate of the true vascular workload. A recent report comparing the OPCS and local audit figures in five hospitals in England and Wales in 1994/95 found considerable under-reporting.[62] For example, 31% of arterial reconstructions were not reported, ranging from 13% to 68% under-reported in the five hospitals. The figure for angioplasties not reported was 58%.

The number of discharges and mean lengths of stay for the HRGs relevant to peripheral vascular disease are shown in Table 10. The lengths of stay for lower limb arterial surgery (Q03) and amputations (Q15) are comparable to those in Table 9. The mean length of stay for bypass to tibial artery (Q04) was considerably higher than for lower limb arterial surgery as a whole (Q03), 23.1 compared with 14.3 days. As expected, the lengths of stay for peripheral vascular disease in those < 70 years with no complications or comorbidities (Q18) were less than those for peripheral vascular disease in older patients with complications or comorbidities (Q17).

Table 8: Discharges with primary or secondary diagnosis of peripheral vascular disease in England in 1995/96.

	Primary diagnosis			Secondary diagnosis		
	n	% general* surgery	population** rate	n	% general* surgery	population** rate
Peripheral atherosclerosis (ICD 170.2 or 173.9)	35,860	88	73.3	34,182	24	69.9
Ruptured aneurysm (ICD 171.3 or 171.8)	3,644	75	7.5	342	34	0.1
Non-ruptured aneurysm (ICD 171.4 or 171.9)	7,656	83	15.7	7,107	31	0.1

* Percentage of vascular discharges that were from general surgical units, including vascular surgery.
** Crude number of discharges per 100 000 population
Source: Hospital Episode Statistics. National Casemix Office, 1997.

Table 9: Peripheral vascular procedures and mean lengths of stay in hospitals in England in 1995/96.

Surgical procedure	Number primary or secondary	Population rate*	% General surgery**	Length of stay***
Iliac/femoral bypass	10,636	20.6	95	16.6
Amputation (vascular)	4,458	9.1	93	27.7
Transluminal procedure	15,972	32.7	85	5.4
Diagnostic angiography	39,160	80.1	71	4.9
Aortic aneurysm repair	5,164	10.6	95	12.2

* Crude number of procedures per 100 000 population.
** Percentage of vascular procedures that were carried out in general surgical units, including vascular surgery.
*** Mean length of stay in general surgical units trimming the data at 100 days and weighting day cases as zero length of stay.
Source: Hospital Episode Statistics. National Casemix Office, 1997

In England in 1996/97, approximately 10% of diagnostic angiographies and less than 3% of transluminal procedures were performed as day cases (Hospital Episode Statistics, unpublished information). By contrast, in Scotland in 1995, 34% of angiographies and 13% of transluminal procedures were carried out as day cases (ISD, Scottish Office, unpublished information). However, these differences between England and Scotland could be due to differences in recording practices. Linkage of hospital discharge records for individuals in Scotland also permit readmission rates to be calculated. For the period 1989–95, the proportion of patients readmitted within 28 days following an iliac/femoral procedure was 9.8%, amputation 9.6% and transluminal procedure 5.4% (ISD, Scottish Office, unpublished information).

Table 11 shows regional variations in the population rates for major vascular procedures.[63] Femoral reconstructions varied over twofold between 3.2 per 100 000 in South Thames Region to 7.0 per 100 000 in North West Region. The North West Region also had the highest rate of amputations (14.6) and North Thames Region had the lowest rate (9.6). Consistent regional differences in the incidence of femoral

Table 10: Health Related Group (HRGs) for diagnoses of peripheral vascular diseases: number of discharges and mean length of stay for hospitals in England 1995/96.

HRG number	HRG label*	Number discharges with primary PVD diagnoses**	Mean length of stay (days)***	Number discharges with any diagnoses†	Mean length of stay (days)***
Q01	Emergency aortic surgery	1,488	10.4	1,660	10.4
Q02	Elective abdom. vasc.surg.	4,011	12.7	4,973	12.8
Q03	Lower limb art. surg.	4,067	14.3	9,319	14.1
Q04	Bypass to tibial art.	517	23.1	1,038	23.2
Q12	Therap. endovasc. proced.	6,099	3.0	12,270	3.6
Q13	Diag. radiol. with comorb/complic				
Q14	Diag. radiol. w.o. comorb/complic	10,312	1.7	18,535	2.0
Q15	Amputations	2,330	29.8	6,290	27.3
Q16	Foot proced. diab. arter.	267	13.4	1,279	12.0
Q17	PVD > 69 yrs or comorb/complic	5,303	5.8	7,253	6.0
Q18	PVD < 70 yrs w.o. comorb/complic	2,281	3.9	3,584	4.2

* See Table 1 for full text of labels.
** Number of discharges in general surgery only with primary peripheral vascular disease diagnosis (I70.2, I71.3, –.4, –.8, –.9, I73.9). Majority of discharges for these diagnoses (> 95%) were in general surgery except for Q17 and Q18 in which discharges were also from general medicine, geriatric medicine and other specialties.
*** Mean based on length of stay trimmed at 100 days, day cases weighted as zero length of stay.
† Number of discharges in general surgery only with any diagnosis. This category will include both primary and secondary peripheral vascular disease diagnoses.
Source: Hospital Episode Statistics. National Casemix Office, 1997

reconstruction and amputation were not apparent. The variations probably reflected a combination of many factors including differences in the age, sex, disease and behavioural characteristics of the populations, the accuracy of reporting and differing surgical practices.

An increase in the use of reconstructive surgery since the 1980s has frequently been associated with some reduction in amputation rates, but the extent to which this might be causally related is unclear.[64] More recently, there has been considerable interest in the increasing trends in the use of angioplasty in the NHS and how this might affect the rate of bypass procedures and amputations carried out. Figure 2 shows that in Scotland from 1989 to 1995, there was a steep increase in the rate of performance of transluminal procedures (angioplasty). There was a less marked rise in the rate of iliac and femoral bypass operations and amputations (and a reduction in all three procedures in 1995, with the fall in amputations beginning in 1994). In England, an increase in the rate of transluminal procedures from 1993 to 1996 was accompanied by a very slight reduction in the amputation rate and no change in the rate of bypass procedures (Figure 3). These rates would have been influenced by changing disease incidence, referral threshold and surgical practice, and it is difficult to know the extent to which angioplasty has reduced the need for surgery.

Table 11: Selected peripheral vascular procedures per population carried out in hospitals in England by region in 1994/95.

	Operations per 100,000 population		
	Abdominal aortic aneurysm repair (L184–186) (L194–196)	Femoral reconstruction (L294–295)	Amputation (X093–95)
Northern & Yorks	9.2	5.4	13.1
Trent	9.3	3.8	12.3
Anglia & Oxford	9.1	3.3	11.8
North Thames	10.3	4.7	9.6
South Thames	10.2	3.2	11.4
South & West	12.8	6.7	10.4
West Midlands	10.2	4.2	13.6
North West	9.9	7.0	14.6

Source: Hospital Episode Statistics. Office of National Statistics 1994/95. Adapted from Darke[63]

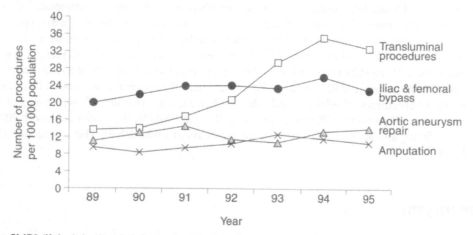

Source: SMRI (linked database), Information Services Division, Scottish Office

Figure 2: Trends in selected peripheral vascular surgical procedures per population in Scotland, 1989–95.

Rehabilitation services

The provision of appropriate and accessible artificial limb and appliance fitting is the main rehabilitation service required for patients with peripheral arterial disease. Although amputation is relatively uncommon in such patients, over 80% of amputations are due to vascular disease.[65] The provision of artificial limb and appliance services in England was reviewed by a Department of Health working party in 1986[66] and, following this, most district health authorities established a local service. In most parts of the country, the local service is complemented by a supra-district or regional service providing more complex needs, such as non-standard electronic control systems. In Wales, there are three centres and in Scotland, there are six centres covering the country with satellite clinics held in local hospitals.[67]

Table 9 shows that in England in 1995/96, 4458 amputations for vascular disease were carried out, giving a population rate of 9.1 per 100 000. An audit of amputations carried out in hospitals in Scotland, found

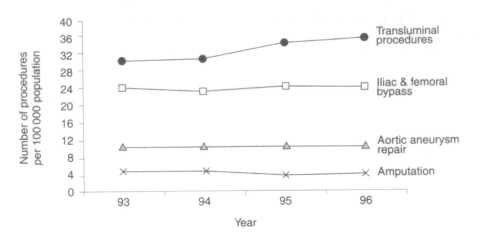

Source: Hospital Episodes Statistics

Figure 3: Trends in selected peripheral vascular surgical procedures per population in England, 1993–96.

that in 1995/96, 60% of lower limb amputations were transtibial and 37% were transfemoral.[65] Fourteen percent of amputees died before discharge, 60% received a prosthesis and 26% did not receive a prosthesis before discharge to home or long-term care. Of those referred to limb fitting centres, 45% were seen within 4 weeks of amputation and 75% within 8 weeks.[68] These referrals comprised 15% < 55 years of age, 55% aged 55–74 years and 20% aged 75 years and over. Among the referrals, 83% received a prosthesis.[68] The total cost of providing the artificial limb and appliance service in the six centres in Scotland in 1995/96, including the cost of prostheses, wheelchairs and other appliances, was £14 million,[67] which is equivalent to a cost of over £160 million for the UK as a whole. In Scotland in 1995/96, the service dealt with 700 new referrals for limb fitting and about 15 000 referrals for provision of a wheelchair. There were also 17 000 other attendances.[67]

Aortic aneurysm

In primary care, the diagnosis of abdominal aortic aneurysm is very rare and the consultation rate is so low (Table 6) that a typical GP is likely to see a patient with this condition only about once per year.

From Table 8, it can be seen that around 4000 ruptured aneurysms were diagnosed in hospitals in England in 1995/96 and that nearly twice that number of primary diagnoses of non-ruptured aneurysms were made. Over 5000 aortic aneurysm repairs were carried out and the mean length of stay for these patients was 12.2 days (Table 9). The figures for emergency aortic surgery (Q01) and elective abdominal vascular surgery (Q02) in Table 10 suggest that around one quarter of the aortic aneurysm repairs were carried out as emergencies. With the exception of South and West Region, which had a high aneurysm repair rate of 12.8 per 100 000 population, there was surprisingly little variation in repair rates between the different regions of England (range 9.1 to 10.3 per 100 000). Figure 2 shows that there has been a slight upward trend in aortic aneurysm repair rates in Scotland in recent years (1989–95) contrasting with a more rapid two- to threefold increase in the 1970s and early 1980s.[68] The same is likely to have been true in England and Wales, where there was also a substantial increase between 1968 and 1983.[54]

The costs of carrying out elective aneurysm repair in the UK have been studied in detail[69] as part of the UK Small Aneurysm Trial. The average cost of carrying out an elective aneurysm repair in the UK in 1996 was estimated to be about £5000. One third of costs were attributable to duration of stay in a standard surgical ward, about 27% to use of intensive care or high dependency beds and about 20% to the cost of the operation. As part of this costing exercise, a survey of over 100 vascular surgeons in the UK indicated that there was considerable variation in the use of these resources between centres, for example mean length of stay in a standard ward varying between 8 and 12 days. It was estimated that the cost of an aneurysm repair for a typical patient in the UK might vary between ± 50% of the national average. Indeed, the HRG mean average reference cost for aneurysm surgery (elective and emergency) was about £4300 in 1997/98 with the average cost for the middle 50% of Trusts varying between about £2800 to £5300.

Screening for abdominal aortic aneurysms is not carried out routinely in the UK. A recommendation from the National Screening Committee that screening should be implemented is under consideration by the Department of Health. Some data are currently available from some local initiatives[50–53] showing that the likely uptake of screening in men aged 65–80 years is likely to be between about 50% and 70%[51,52] depending on the social class, location and targeting of the catchment population. It was estimated that the cost of detecting an asymptomatic aneurysm in a screening programme in the UK would have been about £100 in 1990.[70]

6 Effectiveness of services and interventions

Intermittent claudication

Physical examination

Clinicians have over the years used many different physical signs as aids to the diagnosis of peripheral arterial disease. The clinical utility of these signs has been assessed recently in a systematic review of published studies.[71] Although a statistical meta-analysis was not conducted, the following positive findings were considered to be helpful in diagnosing the presence of peripheral arterial disease: abnormal pedal pulses, unilateral cool extremity and a femoral bruit. Table 12 shows the sensitivities, specificities and likelihood ratios for these tests in the largest study. This was carried out in general practices in Holland.[72] Another test, the venous filling time, was found to be useful in the identification of more severe peripheral arterial disease.[71]

Diagnostic tests

In the diagnosis of intermittent claudication, measurement of the ratio of the ankle to brachial systolic blood pressure, that is the ABPI, using Doppler ultrasound and a sphygmomanometer is the simplest and most commonly used test. In symptomatic patients, the sensitivity and specificity of identifying angiogram-positive disease is up to 95% and almost 100% respectively,[73] and the ABPI is related inversely to the severity of disease. The variability is comparable to that of routine arm blood pressure and a difference of less than 0.15 between sequential readings in a patient is not considered to be clinically significant.[74] The sensitivity of the test may be increased to 97% by conducting an exercise test, usually on a treadmill, in which significant arterial disease invariably results in a fall in ankle pressure.[73]

The severity of intermittent claudication may be assessed by a standard treadmill test in which the maximum distance to claudication and the maximum walking distance may be measured. However, results must be interpreted with caution because of considerable intra-patient variability and the many different ways in which vascular laboratories carry out the investigation.[75] Also many patients are not physically able to be assessed on the treadmill.

Table 12: Sensitivities, specificities and likelihood ratios for abnormal physical findings in detecting peripheral arterial disease diagnosed as ankle brachial pressure index < 0.9.

Physical finding	Sensitivity	Specificity	Likelihood ratio	
			Positive	Negative
Pedal pulse absent or weak	0.73	0.92	9.0	0.3
Femoral bruit	0.29	0.95	5.7	0.7
Unilateral cool extremity	0.10	0.98	5.8	0.9

Pedal pulse comprises pulse at either posterior tibial artery or dorsalis pedis artery.
Study based in general practice. n=2,455.
Source: Stoffers *et al.*[72]

The main non-invasive test now used commonly to assess the location of disease is Duplex scanning. The test is good at identifying occlusions and discriminating between large (> 50%) and small (< 50%) stenoses. In a review of evidence comparing Duplex with arteriography, Duplex was found to be 71–98% sensitive and 91–100% specific in discriminating stenoses of greater or less than 50%.[76] Discrimination of more precise degrees of stenosis is less good but may improve with technological developments. In practice, the advent of Duplex scanning has reduced but not eliminated the need for arteriography in the management of patients requiring an interventional procedure.

Angiography (arteriography) is considered to be the gold standard of investigations for peripheral arterial disease, although it is prone to considerable observer variability.[73] DSA has now replaced conventional arteriography in most centres because less contrast is used, radiation dosage is reduced and more detailed images are obtained. Newer imaging modalities, such as MRA, CT, including helical or spiral CT, angioscopy and intravascular ultrasonography are used in a few centres but have not been sufficiently developed or evaluated for widespread routine use in the investigation of peripheral arterial disease.

Risk factor management

The management of cardiovascular risk factors in peripheral arterial disease is an important issue for the NHS because it has become recognised only recently that a high priority must be given to this aspect of patient care.

Smoking cessation

Cigarette smoking is related to the development of peripheral arterial disease and to a worse prognosis[13] and thus smoking cessation would be expected to be beneficial.[14] Randomised controlled trials of the effectiveness of smoking cessation are not available because of the difficulties of ensuring patient compliance. However, two large follow-up studies of patients with intermittent claudication referred to hospital indicate probable benefits.[77,78] In one of these[77] 11% and in the other[78] 27% of the patients complied with the advice to stop smoking. Within 3 years of stopping smoking there was no reduction in limb-threatening complications of the vascular disease. After 7 years, however, rest pain had developed in 16% of persistent smokers, but in none of those who had stopped smoking.[77] After 10 years 53% of persistent smokers suffered a myocardial infarction compared with only 11% of stopped smokers; 54% of persistent smokers died compared with 18% of stopped smokers.[77] In a recent comprehensive review of the literature, abstinence from smoking was found to be associated consistently with better outcomes following revascularisation, lower amputation rates and improved survival.[79] However, smoking cessation had probably only a minimal effect in improving walking distance in claudicants.[79]

The NHS Centre for Review and Dissemination has recently produced a brief report on smoking cessation and concluded that the most effective interventions the health service can provide are advice from a health professional and nicotine replacement therapy.[80] This accords with findings of the US Agency for Health Care Policy and Research.[81] Brief advice to stop smoking given by health professionals, and taking around 3 minutes, achieves a 2% reduction in the number of smokers. This may be increased to up to 5% by lengthening the duration of advice and follow-up.[81,82] Meta-analysis of trials on the efficacy of nicotine replacement therapies indicate that, when accompanied by advice or counselling, a quit rate of around 20% over a minimum period of 6 months can be achieved.[83] All modes of nicotine replacement therapy (gum, patches, sprays and inhalers) appear to be effective, although there is some evidence that higher-dose gum may be more effective in heavily dependent smokers – a common category of smoker in those with peripheral arterial disease.[84] Such smoking cessation interventions are considered to be cost-effective in saving lives and reducing morbidity, and hence a good use of NHS resources.[80]

Little information is available on the effectiveness of smoking cessation programmes in patients with peripheral arterial disease[79] but the assumption is that the measures shown to be effective in the general population also work in the diseased population, although the level of effectiveness may differ. Fortunately, nicotine replacement therapy has been shown to be safe in patients with cardiovascular disease.[85,86] An increase in angina, palpitations or adverse events was not found in patients with coronary heart disease. In these studies, about one third of patients had peripheral arterial disease, but no acceleration of adverse limb events or worsening of symptoms was found.[85,86] Thus, nicotine replacement therapy, along with advice on smoking cessation, can be recommended for patients with peripheral arterial disease.

Exercise

The effectiveness of exercise programmes in the treatment of intermittent claudication has been investigated in a Cochrane systematic review.[87] Exercise therapy significantly improved maximal walking distance by approximately 150% and in one study produced a better result than angioplasty at 6-month follow-up.[88] In another systematic review investigating the components of exercise rehabilitation programmes that were most effective, the optimal programme used intermittent walking to near maximal pain for a minimum period of 6 months.[89] There was also some evidence to suggest that the exercise sessions should be carried out at least three times per week and that each should last a minimum of 30 minutes.[89] However, the cost-effectiveness of different exercise regimens needs to be evaluated.

The long-term effects of exercise in patients with peripheral arterial disease on the incidence of fatal and non-fatal cardiovascular events has not been investigated. In the population as a whole, those who exercise on a regular basis have half the cardiovascular mortality of those who are inactive, and the benefits occur in those who take either moderate or intense exercise.[90] The National Institutes of Health Consensus Conference on physical activity and health concluded that individuals should ideally have 30 minutes of moderate exercise, such as walking, each day.[91] It is likely that patients with peripheral arterial disease would also enjoy longer-term benefits from regular exercise.

Lipid lowering

A Cochrane systematic review has been carried out of lipid-lowering therapy in peripheral arterial disease.[92] In two trials in which disease progression was measured in the femoral artery using angiography,[93,94] there was a significant overall reduction in disease progression in the groups receiving lipid-lowering therapy (OR 0.47, 95% CI 0.29 to 0.76) (Figure 4). In all seven trials, however, the changes in walking distance were inconsistent, although a general improvement in symptoms, which could not be combined in a statistical meta-analysis, was found.[92] The conclusion of the review was that lipid lowering may improve symptoms but the variation in the trials was such that firm conclusions could not be drawn.

	Disease progression on angiogram / number in group				
Study	Lipid lowering therapy	Control	Peto OR (95% CI Fixed)	Weight %	Peto OR (95% CI Fixed)
CLAS	21/77	30/76		51.3	0.58 [0.30, 1.13]
St Thomas' trial	10/144	27/156		48.7	0.38 [0.19, 0.77]
Total (95% CI) Chi-square 0.70 (df=1) Z = 3.04	31/221	57/232		100.0	100.0 [0.29, 0.77]

.1 .2 1 5 10

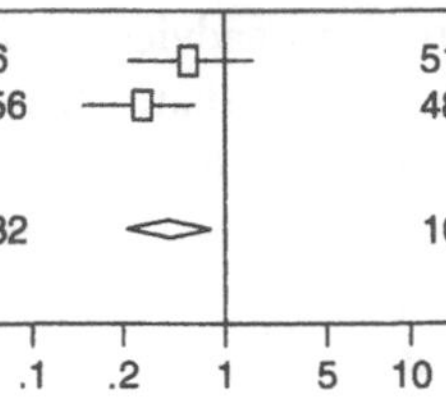

Figure 4: Effect of lipid lowering on angiographic progression of peripheral arterial disease: meta-analysis.

The review also found evidence that lipid-lowering therapy might reduce mortality in patients with peripheral arterial disease (OR 0.21, 95% CI 0.03 to 1.17), but with little change in non-fatal cardiovascular events (OR 1.21, 95% CI 0.80 to 1.83).[92] However, these results need to be interpreted with caution because of the relatively small numbers of events in the studies. On the other hand, the benefits of lipid-lowering therapy, especially with the statin group of drugs, in the secondary prevention of cardiovascular events have been demonstrated in large randomised controlled trials.[95,96] Statins result in a risk reduction of about one third for fatal and non-fatal myocardial infarction and total mortality in patients with coronary heart disease.[95,96] The relative risk reductions are consistent, irrespective of baseline cholesterol, so that the largest absolute benefits are in patients with high risk of cardiovascular events. Since patients with peripheral arterial disease are at high risk, the case for treating such patients with a statin is as strong as the case for treating survivors of myocardial infarction.[97] In the light of this evidence, key messages on lipid lowering in claudicants have been proposed by an expert group in the UK (Davies *et al.*, unpublished information).

- Measure non-fasting serum cholesterol.
- Provide dietary advice if cholesterol > 5.2 mmol/l.
- Prescribe statin if < 70 years of age and cholesterol > 5.2 mmol/l despite dietary measures.

Blood pressure control

Randomised controlled trials have demonstrated that in patients with hypertension, reducing blood pressure decreases morbidity and mortality from cardiovascular and cerebrovascular disease. Guidelines based on the best available evidence on the management of hypertension are readily available.[98,99] Trials on the long-term cardiovascular effects of controlling blood pressure in patients with peripheral arterial disease have not been carried out. However, the control of blood pressure, including the use of anti-hypertensive drugs, is considered to be more beneficial in patients at high risk of future cardiovascular events than in low-risk patients.[98] Indeed the cost-effectiveness of treatment is greater in elderly patients and in those with established cardiovascular disease.[98]

Although control of blood pressure in patients with peripheral arterial disease is warranted, the treatment requires special care because lowering systolic pressure can decrease local perfusion pressure and blood flow to ischaemic muscle and skin. The type of antihypertensive drug used may be important[100] and the reduction in blood pressure needs to be carried out slowly and monitored carefully, particularly in patients with critical ischaemia.[100]

Diabetes control

There is limited evidence from follow-up studies of patients with peripheral arterial disease that those with diabetes have a higher amputation rate and higher mortality.[3,13] However, the extent to which glycaemic control in patients with peripheral arterial disease affects prognosis has not been determined. In diabetics as a whole, good control is likely to reduce the development of microvascular complications, especially retinopathy[101] and nephropathy.[102] However, only borderline support exists for a comparable reduction in macrovascular outcomes, such as myocardial infarction, in both type I diabetes[103] and type II (as shown in the UK Prospective Diabetes Study[104]). There is no reason to believe that these findings would not be relevant to diabetics with peripheral arterial disease. Thus, despite the lack of firm evidence in peripheral arterial disease, good diabetic control, at least to prevent microvascular complications, can be recommended, as specified in European guidelines based on expert consensus.[105]

Drug therapy

For many years there has been considerable debate about the value of drug therapy for intermittent claudication. Four oral drugs have been licensed for use in the treatment of intermittent claudication in the UK: naftidrofuryl, oxpentifylline, inositol and cinnarizine. An expert group of the Scottish Intercollegiate Guideline Network (SIGN) produced an authoritative guideline on drug therapy for peripheral arterial disease in which the recommendations were graded according to the level of evidence.[106]

Naftidrofuryl (Praxilene)

In nine double-blind, placebo-controlled trials of naftidrofuryl in the treatment of intermittent claudication, the placebo response produced an average improvement in pain-free walking distance of 25%, but an additional 30% was achieved with naftidrofuryl at 3 and 6 months post-treatment. These results were confirmed in two meta-analyses.[107,108] The group recommend that: 'Naftidrofuryl may be considered for symptomatic benefit in patients suffering moderate disease but it is not known if it has any effect on the outcome of the disease'.[106]

Oxpentifylline (Trental)

The expert group referred in particular to a meta-analysis of 10 randomised controlled trials which concluded that the limited amount and quality of data precluded an overall reliable estimate of oxpentifylline efficacy.[109] The guideline stated that: 'In the absence of consistent evidence from clinical trials, it is not possible to make any recommendation on the use of oxpentifylline as a treatment for intermittent claudication'.[106]

Inositol nicotinate (Hexopal)

Four double-blind, randomised controlled trials showed no clear evidence of benefit of this drug over placebo. The guideline therefore stated that: 'Inositol nicotinate is not recommended for treatment of intermittent claudication'.[106]

Cinnarizine (Stugeron Forte)

The expert group did not find any studies that were of adequate quality to assess clinical effect and concluded that: 'It is not possible to make a recommendation on the use of cinnarizine in the treatment of intermittent claudication'.[106]

The SIGN guidelines have recently been updated and now include a recommendation that the newly developed drug, cilostazol, be considered as a first line treatment for intermittent claudication.

Antiplatelet drugs

A comprehensive meta-analysis of the effect of aspirin, and other antiplatelet drugs, in reducing the risk of fatal and non-fatal vascular events in patients with various manifestations of atherosclerosis was published in 2002 by the Antithrombotic Trialists' Collaboration.[110] Overall, antiplatelets reduced the risk of myocardial infarction, stroke and death by about 25%. In patients with intermittent claudication, the reduction was similar. The SIGN expert group concluded that: 'Patients with intermittent claudication should receive aspirin long term as prophylaxis against cardiovascular events'.[106] A large multinational trial has shown that clopidogrel, a new antiplatelet agent, has a significant improvement (8.7%) over aspirin in overall efficacy and has fewer side effects, but with a higher treatment cost.[111]

Percutaneous transluminal angioplasty

Dilatation and recannalisation of an artery by percutaneous means (percutaneous transluminal angioplasty) may be carried out as a treatment for intermittent claudication for those with relatively mild symptoms. Its effectiveness needs to be compared with conventional medical treatment, such as smoking cessation, exercise programmes and low-dose aspirin.[112] A Cochrane systematic review[113] of the two completed trials found that at 6-month follow-up, walking distances in the angioplasty group in one trial were greater than in the control group, but in the other trial were no better than an exercise programme. After a minimum of 2 years of follow-up, walking distances and quality of life were no better in the angioplasty groups. The conclusion of the review was that, although angioplasty may have a short-term benefit, it is unlikely to be sustained, and widespread use of angioplasty for mild to moderate claudication cannot be recommended.[113] However, these trials were small and could not examine possible differential effects for lesions at different arterial sites.

In patients with more severe claudication, angioplasty may be used instead of a surgical operation such as thromboendarterectomy or bypass grafting. A well-conducted randomised controlled trial was carried out in the early 1990s in which angioplasty was compared with bypass surgery.[114] Patency rates did not differ significantly between the angioplasty and surgical groups; 4-year patencies were 64.1% and 68.1% respectively (Figure 5). Also limb survival, that is the retention of the treated leg without a major amputation or death, was similar between the two groups. There were, however, three operative deaths (2.3%) in the surgical group and none in the angioplasty group. A formal cost-effectiveness study has not been carried out, but since the cost of angioplasty is in the region of £1500 and of surgery around £5000 (see Table 7), in patients with a lesion amenable to angioplasty, this may be the preferred option.

Reconstructive surgery

The treatment of intermittent claudication by means of bypass surgery using a vein or prosthetic graft is a well-established practice in patients who have severe claudication which causes a major disruption in quality of life.[115] It is generally assumed that in such severe cases, conservative treatment is inadequate,

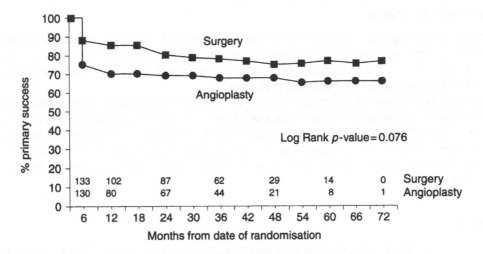

Figure 5: Life-table analysis of primary patency, angioplasty versus surgery.

therefore few randomised controlled trials comparing surgery and conservative therapy have been carried out. In one small trial in which patients were followed up for 1 year, exercise training produced a mean improvement in pain-free walking distance of 120 metres, reconstruction 320 metres, and a combination of reconstruction and training produced an improvement of 489 metres.[116] However, the medium- to long-term patency rates, which vary greatly depending on the location and extent of disease and type of surgical intervention, may be quite poor, for example only about 50% at 4 years for a prosthetic below-knee bypass.[116] Thus, graft surveillance programmes are common and a further surgical intervention is often required. Although the costs of revascularisation procedures have been estimated, formal estimates of the costs per added quality of life are not available.

Critical limb ischaemia

Diagnostic tests

In the diagnosis and assessment of critical limb ischaemia, the validity and variability of Doppler ultrasound measurement of ankle pressures, Duplex scanning and arteriography are comparable to the use of these procedures in severe claudication. A very low ankle pressure (< 40 mmHg) was considered indicative of severe ischaemia and increased risk of limb loss, but this has now been criticised because many patients with critical limb ischaemia have non-compliant vessels resulting in falsely elevated ankle pressures.[39]

Transcutaneous measurement of the oxygen tension in the skin ($TcPO_2$) is used in some centres to assess the degree of ischaemia. It is time-consuming and considerable experience is required to produce reproducible results. However, in combination with other tests $TcPO_2$ measurements can reliably determine the severity of limb ischaemia[118] and may be of use in selection of amputation sites.

Reconstructive surgery

In patients presenting with critical limb ischaemia, around one half undergo arterial reconstructive surgery, one quarter have a major amputation and the remainder are treated conservatively.[119] Partly due to the diverse nature of the presentation of critical limb ischaemia, randomised controlled trials of the effects of these interventions have not been performed.

Observational studies indicate that, as is the case in patients with intermittent claudication, the success rate of arterial reconstruction in patients with critical limb ischaemia is variable with 2-year patency rates varying between 30% and 70%, depending on the procedure carried out.[115] Also technical failures in up to 20% at operation may lead to secondary amputation. The overall effect, as has been shown in Sweden, is that around one third of vascular surgery may be concerned with re-operations, redo surgery and other interventions.[120]

Amputation

Major amputation may be carried out as a primary procedure or secondary to a failed reconstruction. The success of amputation depends especially on the level of surgery: 80% of patients with below-knee amputations end up having reasonable mobility compared with only 40% of those with above-knee amputations.[121] However, only 5% will never require a wheelchair. The long-term survival in such patients is nevertheless poor, with only about 50% alive 5 years after amputation.

Reconstruction or amputation?

Evidence comparing the cost-effectiveness of arterial reconstruction or primary amputation for critical limb ischaemia is limited. In a restrospective survey of patients having amputation or reconstruction for critical limb ischaemia, it was estimated that proximal reconstruction (i.e. surgery involving large arteries only, such as the iliac, femoral and popliteal) resulted in a net saving at 1989/90 prices of £3791 per person compared with amputation, with a net gain of 0.14 quality-adjusted life years per person.[60] On the other hand, distal reconstruction (i.e. surgery involving small arteries in the lower leg, such as the crural) resulted in a net cost of £143 per person compared with amputation and a net gain of 0.10 quality-adjusted life years per person, so that the net cost per quality-adjusted life year gained by distal reconstruction was £1430.

The clinical indications defining which patients with critical limb ischaemia should have arterial reconstruction or primary amputation have not been clear-cut and have partly depended on surgical preference. The Scottish and Northern Vascular Audit Groups reached a consensus using a modified Delphi method on which procedures were appropriate for specified clinical presentations (Table 13),[122] but a subsequent audit of practice found that around one quarter of amputations did not conform to the agreed indications. A decision to amputate or reconstruct may be based on other factors, such as operating resources. It is likely that a higher proportion of legs could be saved,[119] in keeping with some specialist centres, which can achieve success rates of over 80% patency at 5 years following reconstruction.[123]

Percutaneous transluminal angioplasty

Instead of proceeding directly to surgery for the treatment of critical limb ischaemia, in some centres, angioplasty is attempted in the first instance for patients with suitable lesions. A multicentre, randomised controlled trial comparing these two approaches in the UK found little short-term difference between the two approaches. Information from uncontrolled trials and observational studies has produced mixed results. Evaluation of long-term cost-effectiveness is important because many patients having angioplasty

Table 13: Arterial reconstruction or amputation agreed as appropriate for categories of clinical presentation of critical limb ischaemia.

Angiographic findings	Degree of gangrene	Appropriate procedure
SFA or more proximal occlusion	None	Arterial reconstruction
with patient popliteal and distal vessels	Digital	Arterial reconstruction
	Forefoot	Arterial reconstruction
	Midfoot or heel	Arterial reconstruction in most cases
Patent SFA and proximal vessels.	None	Major amputation in most cases
Complete occlusion of tibial, ankle	Digital	Major amputation in most cases
and foot vessels	Forefoot	Major amputation in most cases
	Midfoot or heel	Major amputation
SFA and all distal vessels occluded	None	Major amputation in most cases
	Digital	Major amputation in most cases
	Forefoot	Major amputation
	Midfoot or heel	Major amputation
Inflow and distal vessels occluded,	None	Arterial reconstruction
SFA and PFA patent	Digital	Arterial reconstruction
	Forefoot	Arterial reconstruction
	Midfoot or heel	Arterial reconstruction in most cases
Tibial vessels occluded but	None	Arterial reconstruction (if vein available)
patent segment(s) at ankle or foot	Digital	Arterial reconstruction (if vein available)
	Forefoot	Arterial reconstruction (if vein available)
	Midfoot or heel	Arterial reconstruction (if vein available)

SFA = superficial femoral artery; PFA = profunda femoral artery.
Source: Pell *et al.* on behalf of Scottish and Northern Vascular Groups[121]

are likely to have surgery at a later stage. Recently the new technique of subintimal angioplasty has been carried out in a few centres with apparently impressive outcomes.

Drug therapy

In around 10% of patients with critical limb ischaemia, surgery is not feasible and pharmacological agents have been tried, particularly infusions of vasodilators such as inositol nicotinate and prostanoids.[15] However, evidence on the effectiveness of these preparations in critical limb ischaemia is sparse and stronger evidence is required before they can be recommended for widespread use.[115]

Asymptomatic peripheral arterial disease

Since there is good evidence that a low ABPI measured on subjects in the community is a marker of an increased risk of fatal and non-fatal cardiovascular events, the possibility exists of screening the population in an attempt to detect low ABPI and thus prevent vascular events in previously healthy individuals.[124] In addition to management of cardiovascular risk factors, antiplatelet therapy might be justified, given the benefits in individuals with symptomatic atherosclerotic disease.[110] A randomised controlled trial, the

Aspirin for Asymptomatic Atherosclerosis (AAA) trial, is currently in progress in the UK to test this hypothesis. It will report in 2009.

Ruptured aneurysm

In patients with aneurysms that are symptomatic, whether due to rupture or pressure on surrounding tissues or tenderness on palpation, surgical repair of the aneurysm is warranted in those fit for surgery. This will usually be performed as an emergency or urgent operation. The peri-operative mortality for emergency repair of a ruptured aneurysm ranges between about 40% and 60%.[125] On the other hand, the mortality rate without surgery is for all practical purposes 100%. If surgery is successful, the long-term survival approaches that of the normal population,[126] although it is slightly worse due to a relatively high prevalence of concomitant coronary heart disease and hypertension in patients with aneurysms. The quality of life of survivors following surgery is also good.[125]

Asymptomatic aneurysm

Diagnostic tests

The principal test used to identify and measure the diameter of an abdominal aortic aneurysm is B-mode ultrasound. This examination is easy to perform, and a maximum variation in the diameter measured both between and within observers of ± 0.2 cm can be achieved.[127,128] However, the most sensitive investigation is a CT scan, which also allows improved visualisation of renal artery origins and can more precisely delineate the relation of the aneurysm to nearby structures.[129] Spiral CT, which provides a three-dimensional reconstruction of an aneurysm, is indispensable prior to endovascular treatment and for postoperative surveillance.

Surgery or surveillance?

In patients with asymptomatic abdominal aortic aneurysms, the risk of rupture rises with increasing aortic diameter. In the UK, surgeons generally recommend prophylactic repair of aneurysms of more than 6 cm diameter and routine surveillance by means of ultrasound of aneurysms < 4 cm diameter. The results of the recent UK Small Aneurysm Trial indicate that aneurysms of 4–5.5 cm diameter should also have routine ultrasound surveillance rather than early surgery.[128] Although 61% of those assigned to surveillance eventually had surgery, there was no difference in mortality after 6 months of follow-up between the early surgery and surveillance groups (Figure 6). The 30-day operative mortality in the early elective surgery group was 5.8%. Furthermore, the mean cost in those allocated surveillance (£4000), was less than those allocated to early surgery (£5000).[130] Health-related quality of life was generally similar in the two groups 1 year post-treatment, but early surgery patients reported positive improvement in current health perceptions and less negative change in bodily pain.[130]

The use of endovascular repair of aortic aneurysms has been introduced in recent years but has been associated with several problems.[131] Like many minimally invasive techniques, it may fail and require conversion to open surgery. This conversion may be associated with a high complication rate such that major complications occur in 10–25% of endovascular repairs. Furthermore, the mortality is surprisingly high, normally around 6–10%.[131] However, there does appear to be a learning curve as centres become more experienced and achieve better results. At present, the overall costs of endovascular repair appear to be no cheaper than open surgery.[132] Randomised controlled trials have been conducted comparing

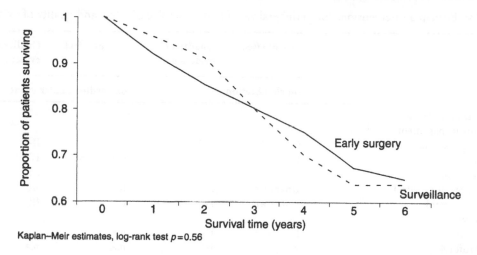

Kaplan–Meir estimates, log-rank test $p = 0.56$

Figure 6: Survival following surgery or ultrasound surveillance for small asymptomatic abdominal aortic aneurysms.[128]

endovascular and conventional aneurysm repair and the National Institute for Clinical Excellence (NICE) has recommended recently that endovascular repair should normally be pursued in the first instance.

Screening

Several pilot studies of screening for asymptomatic abdominal aortic aneurysms have been set up in the UK[49–52] and some health authorities have been encouraged to set up programmes. Although these pilot studies have provided information on uptake and detection rates, they have not provided information on effectiveness compared to no screening. However, the results of the Multicentre Aneurysm Screening Study (MASS) and other trials has led to a recommendation by the National Screening Committee that screening be implemented.

A summary of the size of effects of interventions in the treatment of critical limb ischaemia and aneurysms is shown in Table 14.

Table 14: Principal interventions for peripheral vascular disease: size of effect and quality of evidence.

	Size of effect	Quality of evidence	Size of effect	Quality of evidence
	on claudication		on cardiovascular events	
Intermittent claudication				
Risk factor management				
smoking cessation	C	II-1	A	II-I
exercise	C	I-1	Unknown	IV
lipid lowering	C	I-1	A	III
blood pressure control	Unknown	IV	B	III
diabetes control	Unknown	IV	C	III
Drug therapy				
cilostazol	B	I-1	n.a.	n.a.
naftidrofuryl	B	I-1	n.a.	n.a.
oxpentifylline	Unknown	IV	n.a.	n.a.
inositol	D	I-1	n.a.	n.a.
cinnarizine	Unknown	IV	n.a.	n.a.
antiplatelets	n.a.	n.a.	A	I-1
Percutaneous transluminal angioplasty	C	I-2	n.a.	n.a.
Reconstructive surgery	B	I-2	n.a.	n.a.
Critical limb ischaemia	*on critical limb ischaemia*			
Reconstructive surgery	B	II-2	n.a.	n.a.
Amputation	B	II-2	n.a.	n.a.
Percutaneous transluminal angioplasty	C	II-2	n.a.	n.a.
Ruptured aneurysm	*on mortality*			
Surgery	B	II-2	n.a.	n.a.
Asymptomatic aneurysm				
Surgery ≤ 5.5 cm diameter	D	I-1	n.a.	n.a.
> 5.5 cm diameter	B	III	n.a.	n.a.
Screening	B	I-1	n.a.	n.a.

n.a. = not applicable.

7 Models of care and recommendations

In recommending models of care for peripheral arterial disease and aortic aneurysm, the two diseases can be considered together because they comprise the bulk of the work covered by a vascular service. This section considers the service required in (i) primary care, (ii) secondary care and (iii) screening, although the major component is at secondary care level.

Primary care

At primary care level, good-quality care requires appropriate diagnosis and referral of patients with peripheral arterial disease and aortic aneurysm. For intermittent claudication, diagnosis is relatively straightforward but clear indications are required for when it is appropriate to refer patients for a specialist opinion. Anecdotal evidence suggests that many patients are referred inappropriately. Furthermore, the management of risk factors and antiplatelet therapy is haphazard in these patients and requires to be standardised. National guidelines are required for the management and referral of patients with intermittent claudication in primary care. Such guidelines might encompass the following.

- Diagnosis: key history including, walking ability and cigarette smoking; clinical examination, including peripheral pulses and blood pressure; investigations, including ABPI, serum cholesterol and urinalysis.
- Treatment: smoking cessation, including advice and nicotine replacement therapy; exercise advice; antiplatelet therapy; management of risk factors such as hypertension, hypercholesterolaemia and diabetes mellitus.
- Referral: minimum duration of claudication, say 3 months; degree of impairment of quality of life; level of diagnostic uncertainty; need for investigation and treatment of hypertension, hypercholesterolaemia and diabetes mellitus; minor injuries to foot, such as abrasions that do not heal.

Although the long-term care of claudicants and management of risk factors should ideally be carried out in general practice, in some districts, a shared care approach between primary and secondary care may be appropriate.

In patients with abdominal aortic aneurysm presenting either with symptoms or rupture in primary care, the main problem is awareness of the diagnosis because of its rarity in the primary care setting. Reinforcement of the existence of the condition in postgraduate education and in shared care arrangements for the management of peripheral vascular disease may be adequate to heighten awareness.

Secondary care: minimum specification for a major vascular unit

As demonstrated in Section 5, there are serious shortcomings in the provision of a 24-hour specialist vascular service throughout the UK. The two key issues that need to be addressed are first, the minimum specification for a major vascular unit, and second, how services should be organised to ensure best possible access by the whole population to this service.

In recent years in the UK, these issues have been addressed by three specialist working groups, which have published the following reports: 'Vascular surgery services' by a Working Group of the National Medical Advisory Committee in Scotland[57]; 'The provision of vascular services' by the Vascular Advisory Committee of the Vascular Surgical Society of Great Britain and Ireland[63]; and 'Vascular services in Scotland' by a subcommittee of the Acute Services Review.[56] In addition, relevant recommendations on surgery as a whole have been made in The Royal College of Surgeons of England report on the 'Provision of emergency surgical services'[133] and the Senate of Surgery of Great Britain and Ireland report on 'Consultant surgical practice and training in the UK'.[134] These reports have been used, in addition to the evidence already described, to make recommendations on the provision of secondary care services for the management of peripheral vascular disease.

These reports recommend that the minimum catchment population required to provide a specialist vascular service is between 450 000 and 600 000. This is based primarily on the necessity to provide 24-hour emergency cover by full-time specialist vascular surgeons in an on-call rota of 1 in 3 or 1 in 4, with 1 in 3 being the minimum considered acceptable in present surgical practice. Since around one third of admissions to a vascular unit require major emergency or urgent surgery,[56,63] the provision of a high-quality emergency service is extremely important.

Audits in the UK,[135] Ireland[63] and Sweden[136] have shown that a population of 100 000 generates approximately 70–80 arterial operations per annum (excluding major amputations) plus a large number of venous procedures. These figures are higher than the national data for England (Tables 9 and 10) probably due to under-reporting.[62] A surgeon would normally be able to perform an average of two major elective arterial reconstructions per week, a similar number of emergency operations and several lesser procedures. From these figures, it has been estimated that a minimum population of 150 000 is required to generate an appropriate workload for one consultant surgeon practising full-time vascular surgery.[56,57,63] For a 1-in-4 rota to operate, a catchment population of at least 600 000 is required. A 1-in-3 rota would require a population of about 500 000.

The minimum staffing requirements for a major vascular unit serving a population of 500 000 are described in Box 1. The number of beds, theatre sessions, support services and other facilities are described in Box 2.

Box 1:　Major vascular unit: staffing

Consultant vascular surgeons

Three fte (full-time equivalent) surgeons devoting all of their time to vascular work are required. This enables a 1-in-3 specialist rota to operate. It also assumes that these surgeons, in addition to performing surgery for peripheral arterial disease and aneurysms, including amputations, carry out complicated venous surgery, carotid surgery and renal dialysis access. A larger consultant complement is required if they have other responsibilities, such as teaching. Also, any trend towards a consultant-led service with consultants providing more direct patient care, particularly in emergency work, would require an increase in the number of consultants.

Specialist registrars and senior house officers in vascular surgery

Two of these middle grade staff are required to provide adequate support in the unit. In addition, two junior house officers are required, while accepting that cross-cover for out-of-hours work is required from house officers working in other units.

Interventional radiologists

The scope and volume of vascular interventional radiology is increasing greatly, both in the provision of diagnostic services and endovascular treatments. The Royal College of Radiologists has stated that specialised emergency procedures should be performed only by those who routinely undertake such procedures as part of their normal working day.[137] Thus at least three specialist radiologists need to be available to provide an on-call rota. The extent to which these radiologists work full time or part time on vascular cases depends on current practice in a unit, but the work is likely to increase with the technological advances in transluminal approaches.

Vascular physicians

Although there is not currently a recognised specialty of vascular medicine/angiology in the UK, the importance of the contribution of vascular physicians to the management of patients with peripheral arterial disease is being recognised increasingly. Despite the fact that the majority of patients referred to vascular outpatient clinics do not have surgery and that most outpatients and inpatients have cardiovascular problems requiring medical management, very few units at present have a dedicated vascular physician. The recent reports on vascular services[56,57,63] are unanimous in recommending that physicians with a special interest in vascular disease be integral members of the vascular team with recommendations ranging from 0.5 to 1.5 fte. This depends very much on the extent to which the vascular physicians have responsibility for the initial assessment of outpatient referrals.

Anaesthetists

For complex vascular cases, consultant anaesthetists with a specialist expertise are required to ensure optimal results, not only for elective operations but especially for emergency operations, including ruptured aneurysms. The number of anaesthetists required is about 1.5–2.0 fte, although it is likely that this will comprise 3–4 half-time in order that they can provide a dedicated on-call service for emergencies.

Nurses/professions allied to medicine

Consideration should be given to having a greater nursing complement than in a general surgical unit to take into account the high proportion of dependent elderly patients and amputees. Specialist support is also required from physiotherapists, occupational therapists, pharmacists and chiropodists with special expertise in the management of vascular patients, particularly the rehabilitation of amputees.

Vascular technologists

A major vascular unit will have a dedicated vascular laboratory for the purpose of performing appropriate diagnostic tests. This needs to be staffed by one fte vascular technologist/nurse who has had special training in the conduct of the diagnostic tests.

These recommendations on staffing complement depend very much on local circumstances, for example, on the provision of outreach clinics, the staffing of intensive care and high dependency beds, and the presence of other specialties in a hospital. What is important, however, is that a major vascular unit has an integrated vascular team comprising all of the above professions working jointly in the care of vascular patients.

Box 2: Major vascular unit: facilities

Surgical beds

The number of acute surgical beds required in the vascular unit is about 30 and varies depending on whether amputations are carried out in the vascular or orthopaedic unit. If the early rehabilitation of amputees takes place in the vascular unit, a further 10 beds are required. These figures, recommended by specialist working groups,[57,63] are based on requirements specified currently by major vascular units.

Intensive therapy unit (ITU)/high dependency unit (HDU)

An ITU with specialist nursing care, clinical monitoring and facilities for ventilation are essential and must be available on the same site as the vascular unit. An HDU is also desirable as this may relieve demand on the more costly ITU. It has been estimated that a total of 1.5–5 intensive care/high dependency beds are required,[57,59] but this depends on the definition of 'high dependency' and on surgical and anaesthetic practice.

Operating theatre

Given a consultant's overall workload, which includes operating, outpatient sessions, pre- and postoperative inpatient care, and emergency work, about four elective operating sessions per week per consultant is appropriate. Additional theatre time for emergency work is required. Also it should be recognised that many vascular operations are complex and time-consuming with the possibility of sessions frequently running over time. In the theatre, there has to be provision for on-table angiography, invasive monitoring and microvascular repair.

Radiology

A dedicated angiography room with high-quality image intensification, digital subtraction angiography and C-arm function is required. Also the ability to carry out ultrasound scanning including colour flow and spectral Doppler is essential. In addition, spiral CT is desirable. MRA is currently available in only a few centres in the UK, but this may well become standard equipment for a major vascular unit in the future. It has been estimated that the capital cost of providing the appropriate radiological equipment, including that in the operating theatre, would be about £2.5 million with recurrent running costs of about £150 000.[56]

Vascular laboratory

In the vascular unit, a well-equipped vascular laboratory for performing diagnostic tests and postoperative surveillance of patients is essential. The equipment should include a treadmill, colour flow Duplex ultrasound and equipment for assessing microvascular circulation.

Day-care facilities

Day-care beds are becoming required increasingly for vascular diagnosis and treatment, particularly for angiography and percutaneous transluminal angioplasty.

Limb fitting and rehabilitation

This service should be provided in association with the vascular unit and should be sited within the geographical area of the vascular unit. Close proximity enhances the team approach to rehabilitation and makes it easier for limb fitting and rehabilitation to begin soon after amputation. The rehabilitation service also has to provide longer-term follow-up for patients, including those who live at some distance from the vascular unit.

Access to other specialties

In a small proportion of vascular patients, renal dialysis is required. Ideally, this is provided on the same site as the vascular unit, but in almost all cases patients can be transferred if necessary. Furthermore, for surgery and angioplasty of the renal artery, a close relationship with renal medicine and the provision of renal support is important. For many specialties it is desirable, although not essential, that they are on the same site as the vascular surgery unit in order to aid combined management of some patients. For patients with peripheral arterial disease and aortic aneurysm these specialties include cardiology, diabetic medicine, haematology and renal medicine.

Secondary care: organisation of vascular services

The provision of secondary care vascular services in the UK is currently not organised around major vascular units in all areas. There has been debate in recent years on whether vascular services should be centralised in specialist centres at regional or supra-district level or provided locally within districts as part of a general surgery service. Health service trials have not been carried out. However, some evidence on differing clinical outcomes can be obtained from: (i) observational studies or audits comparing outcomes in specialist and general surgical units; (ii) studies on outcome in relation to volume of activity; and (iii) the extent to which emergency transfer of patients from local to specialist centres is hazardous.

(i) In one of the first major audits of surgical practice in the UK, conducted in Edinburgh, the results of arterial surgery were found to be better in units in which surgeons specialised in vascular surgery than in units where vascular surgery formed a small proportion of the work.[138] This led to the concentration of services into one specialist vascular unit. Subsequent studies investigating outcomes before and after formation of the unit showed an improvement in survival of patients with a ruptured aneurysm from 42% to 68%.[139] For patients with acute limb ischaemia, the overall limb salvage rate improved, although no change was observed in mortality.[140] The authors of these reports thought it unlikely that other factors, such as change in surgical techniques, could fully explain the improved outcomes.

   Comparisons between specialist and generalist centres in other parts of the UK have found similar differences to those found in Edinburgh. In the Northern Region, the mortality rate for elective aneurysm repair was 3.9% in teaching hospitals and 12.0% in district general hospitals, although there was no difference in mortality of emergency repair between the two categories of hospital.[141] In Glasgow, the overall case fatality for aneurysm repair was 7.9% in the specialist centre with full-time vascular surgeons and 19.7% in the other non-specialist hospitals.[142] The case fatalities for emergency repairs of ruptured aneurysm were 40.5% and 58.8%, respectively. Although some differences in casemix might explain the differences in outcome between specialist and generalist centres, there is some evidence to support the commonly held belief that specialist centres produce better outcomes than generalist units. Indeed the National Confidential Enquiry into Peri-operative Deaths has commented on the large number of deaths in vascular patients occurring under the care of non-specialists in vascular surgery.[143] Research in other countries has also produced similar findings and conclusions.[63]

(ii) One possible explanation for improved outcomes in specialist compared to generalist units is that the volume of work in generalist units may be too low to permit the maintenance of expertise or provision of specialist facilities. An extensive literature review of the evidence relating volume of activity and clinical outcome was published by the NHS Centre for Reviews and Dissemination in 1996.[144] Overall, the studies generally reported that outcomes were worse with decreasing levels of activity and that this relationship was most apparent at low levels of activity. There may also have been a minimum threshold effect above which outcome was not affected significantly by volume. However, many of the studies did not adequately adjust for casemix differences, emergency elective ratios and degree of specialisation, and did not distinguish between volumes per hospital and per clinician. When these are taken into account, the evidence suggests that overall 'there is no general relationship between volume and quality'.[144]

   In some specialties, however, increased volume has been related to improved outcomes, and this includes peripheral vascular surgery. In this specialty, four better-quality studies[145–148] were identified in the review[144] in which age, severity of disease, comorbidities and other factors were adjusted. These studies investigated repair of abdominal aortic aneurysms and one also examined lower limb amputations, which were predominantly vascular.[145] No studies of adequate quality were found for reconstructive surgery or angioplasty. The conclusions of each of the better-quality studies[145–148] were summarised in the review as follows.[144]

- Standardised mortality ratio (SMR) for in-hospital mortality was 30% higher in hospitals treating < 14 aneurysm patients per annum, but no relationship was found between mortality and volume per surgeon.[145]
- Mortality for low-volume hospitals (< six aneurysm repairs per annum) was 12% compared with 5% for high-volume hospitals (> 38 repairs per annum). The mortality for low-volume surgeons (< six repairs per annum) was 9% compared with 4% for high volume surgeons (> 26 repairs per annum).[146]
- In-hospital mortality for aneurysm repair was inversely correlated with hospital volume but no correlation was found with number of repairs performed by surgeons.[147]
- A 2% increased risk of death occurred in hospitals performing < 21 aneurysm repairs per annum compared with those performing > 21. The risk difference was greater for ruptured aneurysms and was related to surgeon volume.[148]
- For lower-limb amputations, the SMR was 16% higher in hospitals with below the average annual volume of 10.5 amputations per annum.[145]

Although these studies[145–148] were conducted in the USA, the results may be relevant to practice in the UK. Some consistency of effect was found, at least for hospital volume and mortality related to aneurysm repair, and the results imply that volume is a consideration in relation to the organisation of services. However, the evidence is not sufficiently comprehensive or robust to indicate the minimum volume required to ensure the best outcomes.

(iii) Centralisation of vascular services into specialist units inevitably requires that emergency patients may need to travel greater distances to be admitted and that some transfer of emergency patients from generalist to specialist units may be required. These situations would arise principally for patients with ruptured abdominal aneurysms and, in a population of 250 000, would, in theory, affect fewer than 20 patients per annum (*see* Table 8). Currently, around 60% of patients with ruptured aneurysms do not reach hospital alive. A requirement for urgent surgery is obvious but the extent to which transportation and its duration affects survival is not clear. Most of the studies have investigated only patients who actually reached the specialist centre. The numbers were small in most studies and confounding factors were not always accounted for. In one study in the UK, for example, postoperative mortality was around 50% for patients transported < 5 miles and 40% for patients transported > 5 miles.[149] The patients travelling longer distances might have been less severely ill. In studies in Norway and the USA, transportation time had no independent effect on hospital mortality.[150,151] Although the duration between rupture and operation is likely to have an effect on survival, the maximal time undoubtedly varies greatly depending on many patient factors, such as duration of hypotension and co-existing cardiac disease,[152] so that it is not possible to identify a critical time for the purposes of organising vascular services.

Major specialist units versus district general service

The arguments for and against centralisation were summarised in one of the recent reports on vascular services.[57]

The case for centralisation

1 Audit has shown that specialist vascular units achieve better outcomes for patients.
2 Centralisation of services achieves economies in this 'high-tech', high-cost specialty.
3 Satisfactory training is possible only in units with a high throughput of patients with vascular disease.

4   Research is facilitated by centralisation of clinical cases, medical personnel and technical resources.
5   Centralisation permits appropriate specialist staff cover in a specialty with a particularly high emergency on-call component.
6   Centralisation enables collaboration with a wide range of other specialties, including access to special laboratory facilities and a blood bank.
7   Centralisation, with the need for transfer of emergency patients, does not prejudice survival.

The case against centralisation

1   Some general surgeons currently performing vascular operations may be excluded from such work.
2   Patients and their relatives would have to travel longer distances in order to consult vascular surgeons.
3   Fewer hospitals would have a vascular surgeon so that 'on-the-spot' diagnoses and treatment might suffer.
4   There would be no experience of vascular surgery for middle-grade surgical staff except in the centralised units.

In each of the reports published recently on the future of vascular and surgical services,[56,57,63] emphatic recommendations have been made on the desirability of centralisation and that implementation of such a service should be a high priority in the UK. This service should be centred around major vascular units as specified above.

However, each of the reports differed slightly on how services should be provided for substantial populations that fall short of the minimum catchment population of 500 000 for a major unit. Such populations might be urban and comprise about 250 000 people. One recommendation was that intermediate vascular units be formed.[57,63] These would not have the same high specification as a major unit but would provide a specialist on-call rota of surgeons with a special interest in vascular disease and would have many of the basic facilities of a major unit. However, such a recommendation was made partly in recognition of the current distribution and provision of services in the UK and recognised that an intermediate unit could not provide an ideal service to the populations in those areas.

Integrated regional/supra-district vascular service

A more attractive model has been suggested for providing a vascular service in which urban populations of insufficient size can have access to a major vascular unit. This model of an integrated regional or supra-district vascular service would have a centralised major vascular unit but would also provide certain services in local district general hospitals with smaller catchment populations.[56] Complex vascular work would be carried out in the major vascular unit. The outreach service in the local hospital would include the provision of outpatient clinics, some diagnostic facilities including Duplex scanning, pre-operative assessment, day surgery, post-acute care and rehabilitation. Also, vascular advice would be provided to other specialties in the hospital.

Such an arrangement would require split working by some staff but would allow good patient access to local outpatient and other facilities while allowing optimum provision of high-quality services for emergency and major elective surgery. The occasional transfer of emergency patients would not be problematic given the good transport links in most parts of the UK. This model has also been referred to as a 'hub and spoke' arrangement, with the major vascular unit sitting at the hub of the service.[63]

An alternative model has been proposed for certain areas of the country in which there are currently several small vascular units or individual surgeons providing a service in areas that are contiguous. This model does not envisage establishment of a major vascular unit but rather that smaller units provide cross-cover for each other, and that surgeons work together in a 'virtual' unit. This, however, is unsatisfactory because it leads to a fragmented service preventing the concentration of clinical activity. It inhibits the development of a 'comprehensive team approach with all the advantages of economies of scale, patient care, training and professional satisfaction'.[63]

Remote vascular units

There are, within the UK, a few small, geographically isolated hospitals, which do not easily fit into a conventional integrated vascular service and which serve a diffuse and sparse population. Transfer to major vascular units for such patients might involve unacceptable delay and might not be easily carried out. Under these circumstances, the local hospital would need to provide a more substantial range of vascular services, including emergency surgery and straightforward elective procedures. In such a hospital, there should be a minimum of one surgeon with a special interest in vascular surgery as well as other general surgeons on the on-call rota with some training and experience in vascular surgery. The number of beds required per head of population would be only slightly less than that specified for a major vascular unit. A radiologist with a special interest in vascular work would also be required, but it would have to be accepted that the care of patients by other specialists and professions would be provided by generalists rather than those with a special interest in vascular disease. Although such a remote unit would operate independently, close clinical and professional links would need to be established with a major vascular unit and arrangements made for the occasional transfer of particularly complex cases.

There are economic and resource implications of establishing integrated regional/supra-district vascular services in the UK. In terms of workload, beds and staffing, much of the rationalisation would require redeployment of existing resources within a region. Some capital expenditure might be required at the site of the major vascular unit unless some of the less severely ill patients currently managed at that site could be managed at the local 'spoke' hospital. Also, additional operating facilities might well be required at the site of the major vascular unit. On the other hand, centralisation might create savings in the provision of equipment and facilities by not having a requirement for 'duplicate' facilities in the local hospitals. The provision of vascular experts in the various specialties and professions associated with a major unit might be accommodated by slowly changing the responsibilities of staff within the institution rather than having to take on additional manpower. Overall, the economic implications will depend very much on local circumstances, but creation of an integrated vascular service will inevitably require additional resources.

Screening programmes

Screening for peripheral arterial disease and asymptomatic abdominal aortic aneurysms are currently not taking place in the UK and, until screening has been approved by the Department of Health, models of care cannot be recommended. If programmes are to be established, it would make sense for these to be part of an integrated vascular service with involvement of both the primary and secondary care sectors.

8 Outcome measures

Outcome measures

In assessing the quality of a peripheral vascular disease service, the 'outcome' measures should include structure, process and outcome criteria. The facilities provided and the procedures undertaken, as well as the end results of care, are important indicators of quality.

Primary care

Process criteria

In primary care, the key element of process that needs to be assessed is the risk factor management of patients with intermittent claudication. Such process criteria would include:

- smoking history taken in all patients
- serum cholesterol measured
- blood pressure measured
- antiplatelet therapy prescribed.

If necessary, the following treatment is given:

- smoking cessation advice
- nicotine replacement therapy
- lipid-lowering diet and/or therapy
- antihypertensives.

Outcome criteria

These would essentially comprise 'healthy' levels of the risk factors:

- smoking abstinence
- serum cholesterol < 5.2 mmol/l
- systolic pressure < 160 mmHg; diastolic pressure < 90 mmHg.

In assessing the clinical management of intermittent claudication, the most important outcome criteria measurable in the primary care setting are:

- walking distance (measured using the Walking Impairment Questionnaire,[153] which has been shown to be reasonably valid[154])
- quality of life (measured using standard generic questionnaire, such as the EuroQol or SF-36[155]).

There are no absolute desirable levels of the above two criteria but the effects of treatment should be to improve or maintain baseline levels. Therefore *change* in these criteria can be monitored. Other outcome measures, such as treadmill walking distance, are not feasible to assess in the primary care setting and the ABPI is insufficiently sensitive to detect change in disease status in the early stages.

Secondary care

Structure criteria

At secondary care level, criteria on structure are very important for ensuring that adequate facilities are in place. These criteria relate closely to the minimum specification of a major vascular unit as described in Section 7 above.

- 24-hour emergency cover is provided by full-time vascular surgeons.
- Minimum number of full-time consultant vascular surgeons is three.
- Number of full-time or part-time vascular interventional radiologists is equivalent to number of vascular surgeons.
- A physician with expertise in vascular medicine is a member of the vascular team.
- Anaesthetists have special expertise in the management of vascular cases.
- Number of vascular beds is 30 to serve population of 500 000.
- Intensive therapy unit is available on site.
- Specified radiological equipment is available in theatre and in the radiology department.
- Vascular diagnostic laboratory is part of the unit.
- Limb-fitting service is provided in association with the unit.

Process criteria

An assessment of the overall efficiency and appropriateness of care can be obtained by examining indicators of process. These are not necessarily valid indicators of actual quality, but may be screening criteria that are pointers to potential problems when targets are not achieved.

- Waiting time from referral to outpatient appointment is < 13 weeks.
- Waiting time on list for elective surgery is < 13 weeks.
- Angioplasty is performed as a day case.
- Length of stay for elective aneurysm repair is < 12 days.
- Ratio of arterial reconstruction to amputation is > 2:1 (a crude measure of a unit's practice to reconstruct instead of amputate).
- Amputations performed by non-vascular surgeon to occur after assessment for limb salvage by vascular specialist.

The above waiting-time criteria are derived from the Patient's Charter[156] and lengths of stay and surgical ratios from published norms (Tables 9 and 10).

Outcome criteria

The criteria that are the most important measures of the success of secondary care are those following the major treatments of reconstructive surgery, amputation and angioplasty for peripheral arterial disease, and elective and emergency repair of abdominal aortic aneurysms.

- Mortality, usually quoted within 30 days of surgery, for:
  - major arterial reconstruction
  - major amputation
  - emergency aneurysm repair
  - elective aneurysm repair.
- Limb survival at 4 years:
  - post-arterial reconstruction
  - post-angioplasty.

- Mobile post-major amputation.

These criteria cover some principal outcome measures but criteria covering other procedures and other outcomes can be set.

Audit methods

At primary care level, the most appropriate method of audit is by internal, or occasionally external, peer review of the management of individual patients with intermittent claudication. Routine GP and prescription records, despite some doubts on accuracy, are the most appropriate source of data because prospective collection of data when patients are being managed would undoubtedly influence practice.

At the present time none of the above criteria concerning secondary care has been set nationally, therefore it is important that such criteria are agreed locally, probably at regional level. Furthermore, an important principle of audit is that criteria are agreed before data on current practice are analysed. The data can be collected from routine hospital statistics, if available. If such data are not available, special ad hoc surveys may be required, mostly of hospital records. Rarely, special ad hoc surveys of patients may be required.

Targets

As national targets for the above criteria concerning vascular services have not been established, targets must be set locally. These will undoubtedly be based on perceived optimum levels and be influenced by current levels of practice. Targets are normally expressed as a percentage in relation to the criteria, e.g. the national waiting time standard for any condition states that 90% of patients waiting for an outpatient appointment can expect to be seen within 13 weeks and that all should be seen in 26 weeks.[156] For inpatient admissions, 100% should take place within 18 months of referral.[156]

In secondary care, the structural criteria above are essentially the minimum requirement, and therefore the target should be 100%. Targets for the process criteria are partly dependent on local circumstances and therefore it is more difficult to be prescriptive. Targets for the outcome criteria can be set in accordance with the results from research studies, as described in Section 6.

- 30-day mortality:
  - major arterial reconstruction < 5%
  - major amputation < 15%
  - emergency aneurysm repair < 50%
  - elective aneurysm repair < 6%.
- Limb survival at 4 years:
  - post-arterial reconstruction > 80%
  - post-angioplasty > 85%.
- Mobile post-major amputation (survivors):
  - > 40% (above knee)
  - > 80% (below knee).

For such criteria, terms such as patency and mobility must be defined precisely. Also, it should be recognised that case mix and other factors have a profound effect on these outcome indicators so that a unit not operating at an appropriate target level may still be providing high-quality care.

9 Information and research requirements

Further information

Current data systems can provide much information for successful audit and monitoring of vascular services, for example on waiting times and length of stay. However, the accuracy of some clinical discharge information has been shown to be lacking, with considerable under-reporting,[62] so that priority should be given more to improving the accuracy of current systems than collecting additional data. In Scotland, hospital discharges are now linked to mortality data, and this has proved useful in developing hospital outcome indicators. Nationally in the UK, availability of statistics on 30-day mortality figures following the major vascular operations might prove useful if adjustments could be made for case mix and comorbidities.

Further research

The chapter has highlighted many gaps in knowledge about the occurrence of peripheral vascular disease and its management. Further research in many areas would prove useful but the following should be given high priority.

- More information is required on the burden of peripheral vascular disease in the community. The impact of intermittent claudication on the quality of life and on patient and societal costs is required.
- Trends in peripheral arterial disease and aortic aneurysms need to be specified and more accurate predictors made of future incidence and prevalence, particularly as it is likely that an ageing population and increased survival from coronary heart disease will lead to an increased burden of disease and demand for services.
- In primary care, research is required on the management of intermittent claudication, particularly how to achieve smoking cessation in long-term older smokers. Also, cost-effectiveness studies are required of different approaches to increasing exercise in claudicants, including the value of different exercise programmes.
- Also, in claudicants, more specific trials are required on the management of risk factors. For example, the effects of combinations of antiplatelets such as aspirin and clopidogrel compared with aspirin alone need to be evaluated. Also, more information would be useful on the impact of good glycaemic control in peripheral arterial disease patients with diabetes.
- The interface between primary and secondary care needs to be studied, investigating differing thresholds for referral of claudicants, and the most appropriate strategies for long-term management of risk factors, including shared care.
- For patients referred to hospital, one-stop clinics need to be evaluated to determine which patients can be managed in this way, and the relative costs and effectiveness of this approach compared with routine outpatient referral.
- The initial management of claudicants referred to hospital also has to be evaluated to determine the optimum investigative strategies, the value of diagnostic technologies such as Duplex screening and the criteria for differing approaches to management, for example conservative therapy, angioplasty and reconstructive surgery.
- More research is required on angioplasty. In mild to moderate claudicant patients, a large trial to compare the cost-effectiveness of angioplasty versus conservative therapy is required, allowing for comparisons of lesions at different sites in the arterial tree. Further studies on the technological

advances in angioplasty, including adjuvant stenting, are warranted. Also the long-term effects of angioplasty on surgical rates in individuals and the community are of interest.

- The prognosis of claudication and the identification of factors that affect prognosis and treatment outcomes require further research with the eventual aim of being able to better predict the course of disease for an individual and to better target treatment.

- For patients with more severe peripheral arterial disease, more research is needed to better define the indications for arterial reconstruction versus amputation. Prognosis is very poor for such patients and the cost-effectiveness of different approaches needs to be specified, with more attention paid to quality of survival.

- In the treatment of aortic aneurysms, the upper size limit for conservative treatment is not well specified. Also, for aneurysm surgery, as well as for other elective procedures, there appears to be considerable differences between centres in lengths of stay and resource use, indicating a requirement for cost-efficiency studies.

- In terms of organisation of a vascular service, research on the impact of integrated regional networks would be helpful. A specific question, for example, might address the hazards of transferring emergency patients into regional centres.

- With the advent of clinical governance, research might be conducted on the sensitivity and appropriateness of performance indicators. More refined studies in the UK (rather than the USA) on the volume effect on quality and identifying a possible minimal threshold effect would be useful.

- Further research is required in prevention. The mortality from aortic aneurysm is high and surgery is the only effective treatment. Medical treatments to prevent growth and rupture will emerge only if there is greater understanding of the aetiology and natural history of aneurysms.

References

1 Young JR, Graor RA, Olin JW, Bartholomew JR. *Peripheral Vascular Diseases.* St Louis, MI: Mosby Year Book, 1991.

2 Mitchell JRA, Schwartz CJ. *Arterial Disease.* Oxford: Blackwell, 1965.

3 Fowkes FGR. Epidemiology of atherosclerotic arterial disease in the lower limbs. *Eur J Vasc Surg* 1988; **2**: 283–91.

4 Fowkes FGR (ed). *Epidemiology of Peripheral Vascular Disease.* London: Springer-Verlag, 1991.

5 Fowkes FGR, Housley E, Riemersma RA *et al.* Smoking, lipids, glucose intolerance and blood pressure as risk factors for peripheral atherosclerosis compared with ischaemic heart disease in the Edinburgh Artery Study. *Am J Epidemiol* 1992; **135**: 331–40.

6 Jarrett RJ. Diabetes mellitus. In Fowkes FGR (ed). *Epidemiology of Peripheral Vascular Disease.* London: Springer-Verlag, 1991: pp. 187–93.

7 Greenhalgh RM, Mannick JA. *The Cause and Management of Aneurysms.* London: WB Saunders, 1990.

8 Reed D, Reed C, Stemmermann G, Hayashi T. Are aortic aneurysms caused by atherosclerosis? *Circulation* 1992; **85**: 205–11.

9 Lee AJ, Fowkes FGR, Carson MN, Leng GC, Allan PL. Smoking, atherosclerosis and risk of abdominal aortic aneurysm. *Eur Heart J* 1997; **18**: 671–6.

10 Baird PA, Sadovnick AD, Yee IML, Cole CW, Cole L. Sibling risks of abdominal aortic aneurysm. *The Lancet* 1995; **346**: 601–4.

11 Bernstein EF, Fronek A. Current status of non-invasive tests in the diagnosis of peripheral arterial disease. *Surg Clin North Am* 1982; **62**: 473–87.

12 Dormandy J, Mahir M, Ascady E *et al.* Fate of the patient with chronic leg ischaemia. *J Cardiovasc Surg* 1989; **30**: 50–7.

13 Leng GC, Fowkes FGR. The epidemiology of peripheral arterial disease. *Vascular Medicine Review* 1993; **4**: 5–18.

14 Housley E. Treating claudication in five words. *Br Med J* 1988; **296**: 1483.

15 Lowe GDO. Drugs in cerebral and peripheral arterial disease. *Br Med J* 1990; **300**: 524–8.

16 Bradbury AW, Makhdoomi KR, Adam DJ, Murie JA, Jenkins AMcL, Ruckley CV. Twelve year experience of the management of ruptured abdominal aortic aneurysm. *Br J Surg* 1997; **84**: 1705–7.

17 Fowkes FGR, Housley E, Cawood EHH, Macintyre CCA, Ruckley CV, Prescott RJ. Edinburgh Artery Study: prevalence of asymptomatic and symptomatic peripheral arterial disease in the general population. *Int J Epidemiol* 1991; **20**: 384–92.

18 Bainton D, Sweetnam P, Baker I, Elwood P. Peripheral vascular disease: consequence for survival and association with risk factors in the Speedwell prospective heart disease study. *Br Heart J* 1994; **72**: 128–32.

19 Smith WCS, Woodward M, Tunstall-Pedoe H. Intermittent claudication in Scotland. In Fowkes FGR (ed). *Epidemiology of Peripheral Vascular Disease.* London: Springer-Verlag 1991: pp. 117–24.

20 Rose GA. The diagnosis of ischaemic heart pain and intermittent claudication in field surveys. *Bull WHO* 1962; **27**: 645–58.

21 Richard JL, Ducimetiere P, Elgrishi I *et al.* Depistage par questionnaire de l'insuffisance coronarienne et de la claudication intermittente. *Rev Epidemiol Med Soc Sante Publ* 1972; **20**: 735–55.

22 Criqui MH, Fronek A, Klauber MR *et al.* The sensitivity, specificity and predictive value of traditional clinical evaluation of peripheral arterial disease: results from non-invasive testing in a defined population. *Circulation* 1985; **71**: 516–22.

23 Leng GC, Fowkes FGR. The Edinburgh Claudication Questionnaire: an improved version of the WHO/Rose questionnaire for use in epidemiological surveys. *J Clin Epidemiol* 1992; **45**: 1101–9.

24 Dong W, Erens B (eds). *Scottish Health Survey*. Edinburgh: Stationery Office, 1997.

25 Macintyre CCA, Carstairs VDL. Social factors. In: Fowkes FGR (ed). *Epidemiology of Peripheral Vascular Disease*. London: Springer-Verlag, 1991: pp. 197–206.

26 Leng GC, Lee AJ, Fowkes FGR, Whiteman M, Dunbar J, Housley E, Ruckley CV. Incidence, natural history and cardiovascular events in symptomatic and asymptomatic peripheral arterial disease in the general population. *Int J Epidemiol* 1996; **25**: 1172–81.

27 Fowkes FGR. Epidemiology of atherosclerotic arterial disease in the lower limbs. *Eur J Vasc Surg* 1988; **2**: 283–91.

28 Jelnes R, Gaardsting O, Hougaard Jensen K, Baekgaard N, Townesen K, Schroeder T. Fate in intermittent claudication – outcome and risk factors. *Br Med J* 1986; **293**: 1137–40.

29 Kannel WB, Skinner JJ, Schwartz MJ, Shurtleff D. Intermittent claudication in the Framingham Study. *Circulation* 1970; **41**: 875–83.

30 Criqui MH, Langer RD, Fronek A, Feigelson H *et al*. Mortality over a period of 10 years in patients with peripheral vascular disease. *New Engl J Med* 1992; **326**: 381–6.

31 Smith GD, Shipley MJ, Rose G. Intermittent claudication, heart disease risk factors and mortality: the Whitehall Study. *Circulation* 1990; **82**: 1925–31.

32 Ogren M, Hedblad B, Isaccson S-O, Janzon L, Jungquist G, Lindele SE. Non-invasively detected carotid stenosis and ischaemic heart disease in men with leg arteriosclerosis. *The Lancet* 1993; **342**: 1138–41.

33 Ingolfsson IÖ, Sigurdsson G, Sigvaldason H, Thorgeirsson G, Sigfusson N. A marked decline in the prevalence and incidence of intermittent claudication in Icelandic men 1968–86: a strong relationship to smoking and serum cholesterol – the Reykjavik Study. *J Clin Epidemiol* 1994; **47**: 1237–43.

34 Sigfusson N, Sigvaldason H, Steingrimsdottir L, Gudmundsdottir H *et al*. Decline in ischaemic heart disease in Iceland and change in risk factor levels. *Br Med J* 1991; **302**: 1371–5.

35 Mayer M, Mockford C, Boaz A. *Coronary Heart Disease Statistics*. British Heart Foundation Statistics Database 1998. London: British Heart Foundation, 1998.

36 Office for National Statistics. Social Survey Division. *Living in Britain. Results from the 1996 General Household Survey*. London: The Stationery Office, 1998: pp. 151–78.

37 Scottish Needs Assessment Programme. *Coronary Heart Disease*. Glasgow: Scottish Forum for Public Health Medicine, 1998.

38 Wolfe JHN. Defining the outcome of critical ischaemia. A one year prospective study. *Br J Surg* 1986; **73**: 321.

39 Second European Consensus Document on Chronic Critical Limb Ischaemia. *Circulation* 1991; **84**(Suppl 3).

40 Dormandy JA, Thomas PRS. What is the natural history of a critically ischaemic patient with and without his leg? In: Greenhalgh RM (ed). *Limb Salvage and Amputation for Vascular Disease*. Philadelphia, PA: WB Saunders, 1988: pp. 11–26.

41 Widmer LK, Greensher A, Kannel WB. Occlusion of peripheral arteries: a study of 6400 working subjects. *Circulation* 1964; **30**: 836–42.

42 Schroll M, Munck O. Estimation of peripheral atherosclerotic disease by ankle blood pressure measurements in a population study of 60 year old men and women. *J Chron Dis* 1981; **34**: 261–9.

43 Gofin R, Kark JD, Friedlander Y *et al*. Peripheral vascular disease in a middle aged population sample. *Isr J Med Sci* 1987; **23**: 157–67.

44 Criqui MH, Fronek A, Barrett-Connor E. The prevalence of peripheral arterial disease in a defined population. *Circulation* 1985; **71**: 510–15.

45 Newman AS, Siscovick DS, Manolio TA *et al.* Ankle/arm index as a marker of atherosclerosis in the Cardiovascular Health Study. *Circulation* 1993; **88**: 837–45.

46 Kornitzer M, Dramaix M, Sobolski J, Degre S, de Backer G. Ankle/arm pressure index in asymptomatic middle aged males: an independent predictor of 10 year coronary heart disease mortality. *Angiology* 1995; **46**: 211–19.

47 Leng GC, Fowkes FGR, Lee AJ, Dunbar J, Housley E, Ruckley CV. Use of ankle brachial pressure index to predict cardiovascular events and death: a cohort study. *Br Med J* 1996; **313**: 1440–4.

48 Ingoldby CJH, Wujanto R, Mitchell JE. Impact of vascular surgery on community mortality from ruptured aortic aneurysms. *Br J Surg* 1986; **73**: 551–3.

49 Office for National Statistics. *Mortality Statistics 1996. Cause.* London: The Stationery Office, 1998.

50 Collin J, Araujo L, Walton J, Lindsell D. Oxford screening programme for abdominal aortic aneurysm in men aged 65 to 74 years. *The Lancet* 1988; **ii**: 613–5.

51 O'Kelly J, Heather P. General practice-based population screening for abdominal aortic aneurysms: a pilot study. *Br J Surg* 1989; **76**: 479–80.

52 Scott AP, Tisi PV, Ashton HA, Allen DR. Abdominal aortic aneurysm rupture rates: a 7 year follow-up of the entire abdominal aortic aneurysm population detected by screening. *J Vasc Surg* 1998; **28**: 124–8.

53 Smith FCT, Grimshaw GM, Patterson IS, Tsang GMK, Shearman CP, Hamer JD. Community based aortic aneurysm screening. *Br J Surg* 1992; **79** (Suppl):152.

54 Fowkes FGR, Macintyre CCA, Ruckley CV. Increasing incidence of aortic aneurysms in England and Wales. *Br Med J* 1989; **298**: 33–5.

55 Pleumeekers HJCM, Hoes AW, van der Does E, Urk HV, Groebbee DE. Epidemiology of abdominal aortic aneurysms. *Eur J Vasc Surg* 1994; **8**: 119–28.

56 The Scottish Office Department of Health. *Acute Services Review Report.* Edinburgh: The Stationery Office, 1998. (Subcommittee Report on Vascular Services in Scotland unpublished – available for reference in Scottish Office Library, Edinburgh.)

57 National Medical Advisory Committee. Scottish Office Home and Health Department. *Vascular Surgery Services.* Edinburgh: Her Majesty's Stationery Office, 1994.

58 Audit Committee of the VSS. *Registry 1995.* London: Vascular Surgical Society of Great Britain and Ireland, 1995.

59 *Report of the National Enquiry into Peri-operative Deaths 1994/95.* London: National CEPOD, 1997.

60 Davies L, Noone M, Drummond M, Cheshire N, Wolfe J. Technology assessment in the development of guidelines for vascularising the ischaemic leg. Discussion Paper No. 89. York: Centre for Health Economics, University of York, 1991.

61 Johnson BF, Evans L, Drury R *et al.* Surgery for limb threatening ischaemia: a reappraisal of the costs and benefits. *Eur J Vasc Endovasc Surg* 1995; **9**: 181–8.

62 Galland RB, Magee TR, Berridge DC *et al.* Accuracy of centrally recorded OPCS codes for vascular surgery in the United Kingdom. *Eur J Vasc Endovasc Surg* 1998; **16**: 415–8.

63 Darke SG. *The Provision of Vascular Services*, revised edn. London: Vascular Surgical Society of Great Britain and Ireland, 1998.

64 Pell J, Murray S, Boyd A. The impact of arterial reconstructive surgery on major amputation. *Critical Ischaemia* 1999; **9**: 29–32.

65 Treweek SP, Condie ME for Scottish Physiotherapy Amputee Research Group (SPARG). *A Survey of the Lower Limb Amputee Population in Scotland Between 1/10/95 and 30/9/96.* Glasgow: National Centre for Training and Education in Prosthetics and Orthotics, 1998.

66 Department of Health and Social Security. *Review of Artificial Limb and Appliance Centre Services.* (McColl Report). London: Department of Health and Social Security, 1986.

67 National Services Division. *Review of Artificial Limb and Appliance Centres.* Edinburgh: Common Services Agency, Scottish Health Service, 1996.

68 Naylor AR, Webb J, Fowkes FGR, Ruckley CV. Trends in abdominal aortic aneurysm surgery in Scotland (1971–1984). *Eur J Vasc Surg* 1988; **2**: 217–21.

69 Jepson RG, Forbes JF, Fowkes FGR. Resource use and costs of elective surgery for asymptomatic abdominal aortic aneurysm. *Eur J Vasc Endovasc Surg* 1997; **14**: 143–8.

70 Collin J. The value of screening for abdominal aortic aneurysm by ultrasound. In: Greenhalgh RM, Mannick JA. *The Cause and Management of Aneurysms.* London: WB Saunders Company, 1990: pp. 457–60.

71 McGee SR, Boyko EJ. Physical examination and chronic lower-extremity ischaemia. A critical review. *Arch Intern Med* 1998; **158**: 1357–64.

72 Stoffers HEJH, Kester ADM, Saiser V, Rindens PELM, Knotternus JA. Diagnostic value of signs and symptoms associated with peripheral arterial occlusive disease seen in general practice: a multivariable approach. *Med Decis Making* 1997; **17**: 61–70.

73 Fowkes FGR. The measurement of atherosclerotic peripheral arterial disease in epidemiological surveys. *Int J Epidemiol* 1988; **17**: 201–7.

74 Fowkes FGR, Housley E, Macintyre CCA, Prescott RJ, Ruckley CV. Variability of ankle and brachial systolic pressures in the measurement of atherosclerotic peripheral arterial disease. *J Epidemiol Commun Health* 1988; **42**: 128–33.

75 Hiatt WR, Hirsch AT, Regensteiner JG, Brass EP. Clinical trials for claudication. *Circulation* 1995; **92**: 614–21.

76 Jäger K, Frauchiger B, Eichlisberger R. Vascular ultrasound. In Tooke JE, Lowe GDO (eds). *A Textbook of Vascular Medicine.* London: Arnold, 1996.

77 Jonason T, Bergstrom R. Cessation of smoking in patients with intermittent claudication. *Acta Med Scand* 1987; **221**: 253–60.

78 Smith I, Franks PJ, Greenhalgh RM, Poulter NR, Powell JT. The influence of smoking cessation and hypertriglyceridaemia on the progression of peripheral arterial disease and the onset of critical ischaemia. *Eur J Vasc Endovasc Surg* 1996; **11**: 402–8.

79 Hirsch AT, Treat-Jacobson D, Lando HA, Hatsukami DK. The role of tobacco cessation, antiplatelet and lipid lowering therapies in the treatment of peripheral arterial disease. *Vasc Med* 1997; **2**: 243–51.

80 Effectiveness Matters. *Smoking Cessation: what the health service can do.* York: NHS Centre for Reviews and Dissemination, 1988.

81 Smoking Cessation Clinical Practice Guidelines Panel and Staff. Consensus statement: Agency for Health Care Policy and Research Smoking Cessation Clinical Practice Guidelines. *JAMA* 1996; **275**: 1270–80.

82 Law M, Ling Tang J. An analysis of the effectiveness of interventions intended to help people stop smoking. *Arch Intern Med* 1995; **155**: 1933–41.

83 Silagy C, Mant D, Fowler G, Lodge M. Meta-analysis on efficacy of nicotine replacement therapies in smoking cessation. *The Lancet* 1994; **343**: 139–42.

84 Ling Tang J, Law M, Wald N. How effective is nicotine replacement therapy in helping people to stop smoking. *Br Med J* 1994; **308**: 21–6.

85 Transdermal Nicotine Working Group. Nicotine replacement therapy for patients with coronary artery disease. *Arch Inter Med* 1994; **154**: 989–95.

86 Joseph AM, Norman S, Ferry L *et al.* Safety of transdermal nicotine therapy in patients with cardiac disease: a randomised controlled trial. *N Engl J Med* 1996; **335**: 1792–8.

87 Leng GC, Fowler N, Ernst E. Exercise for intermittent claudication (Cochrane Review). In: The Cochrane Library, Issue 4. Oxford: Update Software, 1998.

88 Creasy TS, McMillan PJ, Fletcher EWL, Collin J, Morris PJ. Is percutaneous transluminal angioplasty better than exercise for claudication? Preliminary results from a prospective randomised trial. *Eur J Vasc Surg* 1990; **4**: 135–40.

89 Gardener AW, Poehlman ET. Exercise rehabilitation programs for the treatment of claudication pain. *JAMA* 1995; **274**: 975–80.

90 Powell KE, Pratt M. Physical activity and health. *Br Med J* 1996; **313**: 126–7.

91 NIH Consensus Development Panel on Physical Activity and Cardiovascular Health. Physical activity and health. National Institutes of Health Consensus Conference. *JAMA* 1996; **267**: 241–6.

92 Leng GC, Price JF, Jepson RG. Lipid lowering therapy in lower limb atherosclerosis (Cochrane Review). In: The Cochrane Library, Issue 4. Oxford: Update Software, 1998.

93 Blankenhorn DH, Azen SP, Crawford DW *et al.* Effects of colestipolniacin therapy on human femoral atherosclerosis. *Circulation* 1991; **83**: 438–47.

94 Duffield RGM, Lewis B, Miller NE, Jamieson CW, Brunt JNH, Cochester ACF. Treatment of hyperlipidaemia retards progression of symptomatic femoral atherosclerosis. *The Lancet* 1983; **ii**: 639–42.

95 Sacks FM, Pfeffer MA, Moye LA *et al.* for Cholesterol and Recurrent Events Trial Investigators. The effect of pravastatin on coronary events after myocardial infarction in patients with average cholesterol levels. *N Engl J Med* 1996; **335**: 1001–9.

96 Scandinavian Simavastatin Survival Study Group. Randomised trial of cholesterol lowering in 4444 patients with coronary heart disease: the Scandinavian Simavastatin Survival Study (45). *The Lancet* 1994; **344**: 1383–9.

97 Haq IU, Yeo WW, Hackson PR, Ramsay LE. The case for cholesterol reduction in peripheral vascular disease. *Critical Ischaemia* 1997; **7**: 15–22.

98 Subcommittee of WHO/ISH Mild Hypertension Liaison Committee. Summary of 1993 World Health Organisation – International Society of Hypertension guidelines for the management of mild hypertension. *Br Med J* 1993; **307**: 1541–6.

99 Sever P, Beevers G, Bulpitt C *et al.* Management guidelines in essential hypertension: report of the second working party of the British Hypertension Society. *Br Med J* 1993; **306**: 983–7.

100 Clement DL, Verhaeghe R. Atherosclerosis and other occlusive arterial diseases. In Clement DL, Shepherd JT (eds). *Vascular Diseases in the Limbs. Mechanisms and Principles of Treatment.* St Louis, MI: Mosby Year Book, 1993: pp. 81–2.

101 Brinchmann-Hansen O, Dahl-Jorgensen K, Sandvik L, Hanssen KF. Blood glucose concentrations and progression of diabetic retinopathy: the seven year results of the Oslo study. *Br Med J* 1992; **304**: 19–22.

102 Feldt-Rasmussen B, Mathieson ER, Deckert T. Effect of two years strict metabolic control on progression of incipient nephthropathy in insulin-dependent diabetes. *The Lancet* 1986; **ii**: 1300–4.

103 DCCT Research Group. The effect of intensive diabetes treatment on the development and progression of long term complications in insulin-dependent diabetes mellitus. The Diabetes Control and Complications Trial. *N Engl J Med* 1993; **329**: 978–86.

104 UK Prospective Diabetes Study (UKPDS) Group. Intensive blood-glucose control with sulphonylureas or insulin compared with conventional treatment and risk of complications in patients with type 2 diabetes (UKPDS 33). *The Lancet* 1998; **352**: 837–53.

105 European IDDM Policy Group. Consensus guidelines for the management of insulin-dependent (Type 1) diabetes. *Diab Med* 1993; **10**: 990–1005.

106 Scottish Intercollegiate Guidelines Network. *Drug Therapy for Peripheral Vascular Disease.* SIGN Publication number 27. Edinburgh: SIGN Secretariat, 1998.

107 Lehert P, Riphagen FE, Gamand S. The effect of naftidrofuryl on intermittent claudication: a meta-analysis. *J Cardiovasc Pharmacol* 1990; **16**: 81–6.

108 Lehert P, Covate S, Gamand S, Brown TM. Naftidrofuryl in intermittent claudication: a retrospective analysis. *J Cardiovasc Pharmacol* 1994; **23**: 548–52.

109 Radak K, Wyderski RJ. Conservative management of intermittent claudication. *Ann Intern Med* 1990; **113**: 135–46.

110 Antithrombotic Trialists' Collaboration. Collaborative meta-analysis of randomised trials of anti-platelet therapy for prevention of death, myocardial infarction, and stroke in high risk patients. *Br Med J* 2002; **324**: 71–86.

111 CAPRIE Steering Committee. A randomised, blinded trial of clopidogrel versus aspirin in patients at risk of ischaemic events (CAPRIE). *The Lancet* 1996; **348**: 1329–39.

112 Price JF, Fowkes FGR. Effectiveness of percutaneous transluminal angioplasty for lower limb atherosclerosis. In: Greenhalgh RM, Fowkes FGR (eds). *Trials and Tribulations of Vascular Surgery.* London: WB Saunders, 1996: pp. 245–57.

113 Fowkes FGR, Gillespie IN. Angioplasty (versus non-surgical management) for intermittent claudication (Cochrane Review). The Cochrane Library. Issue 4. Oxford: Update Software, 1998.

114 Wolf GL, Wilson SE, Cross AP *et al.* Surgery or balloon angioplasty for peripheral vascular disease: a randomised controlled trial. *J Vasc Interven Radiol* 1993; **4**: 639–48.

115 Shearman CP, Beard JD, Gaines PA. Treatment of chronic lower limb ischaemia. In: Beard JD, Gaines PA (eds). *Vascular and Endovascular Surgery.* London: WB Saunders, 1998: pp. 47–81.

116 Lundgren F, Dahllöf A-G, Lundholm K, Schersten T, Volkmann R. Intermittent claudication – surgical reconstruction or physical training? *Ann Surg* 1989; **209**: 346–55.

117 Veith FJ, Gupta SK, Ascer E *et al.* Six year prospective multicentre randomised comparison of autologous saphenous vein and expanded PTFE grafts in infrainguinal arterial reconstruction. *J Vasc Surg* 1986; **3**: 104–14.

118 Ubbink DTh, Tulevski II, Hartog D den, Koelemay MJW, Legemate DA, Jacobs MJHM. The value of non-invasive techniques for the assessment of critical limb ischaemia. *Eur J Vasc Endovasc Surg* 1997; **13**: 296–300.

119 Anonymous. Amputation or arterial reconstruction? (Editorial). *The Lancet* 1992; **339**: 900–1.

120 Swedish Vascular Registry. Reoperations, redo surgery and other interventions constitute more than one third of vascular surgery. *Eur J Vasc Endovasc Surg* 1997; **14**: 244–51.

121 Houghton AD, Taylor PR, Thurlow S, Rootes E, McColl I. Success rates for rehabilitation of vascular amputees: implications for pre-operative assessment and amputation level. *Br J Surg* 1992; **79**: 753–5.

122 Pell JP, Fowkes FGR, Lee AJ on behalf of the Scottish and Northern Vascular Audit Groups. Indications for arterial reconstruction and amputation in the management of chronic critical lower limb ischaemia. *Eur J Vasc Endovasc Surg* 1997; **13**: 315–21.

123 Hickey NC, Thomson IA, Shearman CP, Simms MH. Aggressive arterial reconstruction for critical lower limb ischaemia. *Br J Surg* 1991; **78**: 1476–78.

124 Fowkes FGR, Price JF, Leng GC. Targeting subclinical atherosclerosis. *Br Med J* 1998; **316**: 1764.

125 Stonebridge PA, Ruckley CV. Abdominal aortic aneurysms. In: Tooke JE, Lowe GDO (eds). *A Textbook of Vascular Medicine.* London: Arnold, 1996: pp. 176–90.

126 Stonebridge PA, Callam MJ, Bradbury AW *et al.* Comparison of long-term survival following successful repair of ruptured and non-ruptured abdominal aortic aneurysm. *Br J Surg* 1993; **80**: 585–6.

127 Ellis M, Powell JT, Greenhalgh RM. The limitations of ultrasonography in surveillance of abdominal aortic aneurysms. *Br J Surg* 1991; **78**: 614–16.

128 The UK Small Aneurysm Trial Participants. Mortality results for randomised controlled trial of early elective surgery or ultrasonographic surveillance for small abdominal aortic aneurysms. *The Lancet* 1998; **352**: 1649–55.

129 Browse NL, Lea Thomas M. Abdominal aneurysms: the value of computerized axial tomography (CAT). In: Greenhalgh RM, Mannick JA. *The Cause and Management of Aneurysms.* London: WB Saunders, 1990.

130 The UK Small Aneurysm Trial Participants. Health service costs and quality of life for early elective surgery or ultrasonographic surveillance for small abdominal aortic aneurysms. *The Lancet* 1998; **352**: 1656–60.

131 Thompson MW, Sayers RD. Arterial aneurysms. In: Beard JD, Gaines PA. *Vascular and Endovascular Surgery.* London: WB Saunders, 1998.

132 Makaroun M, Zajko A, Orons P *et al.* The experience of an academic medical center with endovascular treatment of abdominal aortic aneurysms. *Am J Surg* 1998; **176**: 198–202.

133 The Royal College of Surgeons of England. *The Provision of Emergency Surgical Services. An Organisational Framework.* London: The Royal College of Surgeons of England, 1997.

134 The Senate of Surgery of Great Britain and Ireland. *Consultant Surgical Practice and Training in the UK.* London: Senate of Surgery Secretariat, Lincoln's Inn Field, 1997.

135 Michaels JA, Browse DJ, McWhinnie DL, Galland RB, Morris PJ. The provision of vascular surgical services in the Oxford Region. *Br J Surg* 1994; **81**: 377–81.

136 Vascular Registry on Southern Sweden. The vascular registry: a responsibility for all vascular surgeons. *Eur J Vasc Surg* 1987; **1**: 219–26.

137 Board of the Faculty of Clinical Radiology. *Advice to Clinical Radiology Members and Fellows with Regard to Out of Hours Working.* London: The Royal College of Radiologists, 1996.

138 Gruer R, Gordon RS, Gunn AA, Ruckley CV. Audit of surgical audit. *The Lancet* 1986; **1**: 23–5.

139 Jenkins AMcL, Ruckley CV, Nolan B. Ruptured abdominal aortic aneurysm. *Br J Surg* 1986; **73**: 395–8.

140 Clason AE, Stonebridge PA, Duncan AJ, Nolan B, Jenkins A McL, Ruckley CV. Acute ischaemia of the lower limb: the effect of centralising vascular surgical services on morbidity and mortality. *Br J Surg* 1989; **76**: 592–3.

141 Berridge DC, Chamberlain AJ, Guy AJ, Lambert D. Prospective audit of abdominal aortic aneurysm surgery in the northern region from 1988 to 1992. *Br J Surg* 1994; **82**: 906–10.

142 Samy AK, McBein G. Abdominal aortic aneurysm. Ten hospitals population study in the city of Glasgow. *Eur J Vasc Surg* 1993; **7**: 561–6.

143 *The Report of the National Confidential Enquiry into Peri-operative Deaths 1993/94.* London: National CEPOD, 1996.

144 NHS Centre for Reviews and Dissemination. Hospital volume and health care outcomes, costs and patient access. *Effective Health Care Bulletin* **2**(8). York: University of York, 1996.

145 Flood AB, Scott WR, Ewy W. Does practice make perfect? Part I. The relation between hospital volume and outcomes for selected diagnostic categories. *Med Care* 1984; **22**: 98–114.

146 Veith FJ, Goldmill J, Leather RP, Hannan EL. The need for quality assurance in vascular surgery. *J Vasc Surg* 1991; **13**: 523–6.

147 Kelly JV, Hellinger FJ. Physician and hospital factors associated with mortality of surgical patients. *Med Care* 1986; **24**: 785–800.

148 Katz DJ, Stanley JC, Zelenock GB. Operative mortality rates for intact and ruptured abdominal aortic aneurysms in Michigan: an eleven year statewide experience. *J Vasc Surg* 1994; **19**: 804–17.

149 Fielding JWL, Black J, Ashton F, Slaney G. Ruptured aortic aneurysm: post-operative complications and their aetiology. *Br J Surg* 1984; **71**: 487–91.

150 Amundsen S, Skjaeven R, Troppenstad A, Soreide O. Abdominal aortic aneurysm – a study of factors influencing post-operative mortality. *Eur J Vasc Surg* 1989; **3**: 405–9.

151 Farooq MM, Frieschlag JA, Seabrook GR *et al.* Effect of duration of symptoms, transport time, and length of emergency room stay on morbidity and mortality in patients with ruptured abdominal aortic aneurysms. *Surgery* 1996; **119**: 9–14.
152 Barros D'Sa AAB. Optimal travel distance before ruptured aortic aneurysm repair. In: Greenhalgh RM, Mannick JA, Powell JT (eds). *The Cause and Management of Aneurysms.* London: WB Saunders, 1990.
153 Regensteiner JG, Steiner JF, Panzer RJ, Hiatt WR. Evaluation of walking impairment by questionnaire in patients with peripheral arterial disease. *J Vasc Med Biol* 1990; **2**: 142–50.
154 McDermott MM, Liu K, Guralmik JM, Martin GJ, Criqui MH, Greenland P. Measurement of walking endurance and walking velocity with questionnaire: validation of the walking impairment questionnaire in men and women with peripheral arterial disease. *J Vasc Surg* 1998; **28**: 1072–81.
155 Brazier JAU, Jones NA, Kind P. Testing the validity of the EuroQol and comparing it with the SF-36 survey questionnaire. *Qual Life Res* 1993; **2**: 169–80.
156 Department of Health. *England: The Patient's Charter and You.* London: Department of Health, 1996.

10 Pregnancy and Childbirth

Jane Henderson, Leslie L Davidson, Jean Chapple, Jo Garcia and Stavros Petrou

1 Summary

Introduction

Pregnancy and childbirth are common and highly important aspects of women's lives. Government policy has affected maternity care through a number of policy documents, particularly *Changing Childbirth*, which aimed to provide more woman-centred care, offering choice, continuity of care and control. In the UK, NHS maternity care is provided in hospitals and the community by midwives, GPs, obstetricians and paediatricians.

The material in this chapter is primarily concerned with uncomplicated pregnancy and childbirth but also focuses on two other sub-groups: women with major obstetric complications and women in vulnerable social groups. Material for this chapter was researched in 2001 and sent to the editors in 2002.

Prevalence and incidence

Vital statistics

In 1999, 615 994 women in England and Wales had pregnancies ending in live or stillbirth and there were 57.7 live births per thousand women aged 15–44 years. The live birth rate ranged from 52 to 65 per 1000 women aged 15–44 years, and was slightly higher in London and Northern Ireland, and slightly lower in Scotland. Age-specific fertility rates show that many women are postponing childbearing into their 30s and 40s.

Perinatal and infant mortality rates declined steadily through the twentieth century but may now be plateauing, although the infant mortality rate in 2000 was the lowest ever at 5.6 per thousand live births in England and Wales. Families from lower social classes still experience greater perinatal and infant mortality than other groups and the incidence of low birthweight is also greatest in families from lower social classes. The percentage of low birthweight babies as a proportion of all births increased steadily over the last two decades. Over 7% of babies had a birthweight of less than 2500 g in England in 1999. This was partly a result of increases in number and survival of multiple births.

Pregnancy, labour and delivery

The Hospital Episode Statistics provide some information on complications in pregnancy and labour. They suggest that prolonged pregnancy and hypertension were the most common reasons for admission antenatally. Major complications, such as haemorrhage, occurred only rarely. Trauma to the perineum was the most common adverse outcome arising from labour.

Postnatal health

Adverse postnatal health problems such as incontinence, perineal pain and backache are common after childbirth. Postnatal depression affects between 10–15% of women in the first few months after childbirth but the proportion declines rapidly up to about 6 months. Breastfeeding rates in the UK compare unfavourably with other developed countries. Initiation of breastfeeding has remained about the same over the last decade at 68% in England and Wales, 55% in Scotland and 45% in Northern Ireland in 1995, compared to over 90% in Russia and Norway and over 70% in Italy. Six weeks after birth only 44% of women were breastfeeding in England and Wales.

Services currently available

Patterns of care

Many different patterns of care have been set up including 'shared care', 'midwife-led care', and 'caseload midwifery'. Such systems of care were established to provide more woman-centred care and involved midwives as primary carers. They were generally available only to women at low risk of complications, although some schemes were aimed at women at higher risk of complications. In general, women receiving these new models of care have been enthusiastic about them, as were midwives who had been involved in designing and setting up the schemes. Evaluation of these new systems of care has been limited and there is little reliable evidence about their impact on maternal or neonatal morbidity, their sustainability or the costs associated with them.

Hospital-based services

There is substantial variation geographically in provision of maternity beds and in the way they are organised into small and large units. Since the NHS was established, there has been a steady decline in numbers of maternity beds available and they have tended to become more concentrated in large units. In common with other specialties, durations of inpatient stay in maternity have declined considerably over the last decade. In 1997–98 (the most recent national data available) in England and Wales about 13% of women left hospital on the same day as delivery and three quarters within 3 days.

Elements of care

Women may receive an enormous range of care antenatally, intrapartum and postnatally. It is not possible to cover the whole range of services offered and the following is a partial summary. Pregnant women are generally offered tests for anaemia, blood group antibodies, rhesus type and certain infectious diseases (including rubella, hepatitis B, HIV, syphilis and asymptomatic bacteriuria). Blood pressure and fetal growth are monitored throughout pregnancy. Most maternity units offer screening for Down's syndrome using biochemical markers.

Data from the Hospital Episode Statistics give information on induction rates (22% in 1998–99 in England and Wales), method of delivery (caesarean section rate 19% in 1998–99 in England and Wales) and pain relief in labour (about half of women delivered by elective caesarean had a spinal anaesthetic in England and Wales in 1997–98).

The Infant Feeding Survey describes the type of support available to mothers when breastfeeding. The vast majority (86%) of mothers reported receiving help the first time they breastfed their baby. For subsequent feeding problems, mothers turned predominantly to midwives and health visitors for support. Postnatal depression is screened for in many areas using the Edinburgh Postnatal Depression Scale.

Costs of services

About three quarters of the total NHS budget goes to the hospital and community health services (HCHS) and about two thirds of this goes on staff salaries. Over half of the maternity budget goes to inpatient services. The programme budget for maternity and early childhood amounted to 5.6% of the total HCHS budget in 1997/98. There is insufficient information on costs for detailed planning of local maternity services.

Effectiveness and cost-effectiveness of services

Due to the breadth of the subject of maternity care it is not possible to cover clinical and cost-effectiveness comprehensively. Selected examples of relevance to commissioners of services are given in this section.

Interventions to reduce smoking in pregnancy have been systematically reviewed and published in the Cochrane Library. The most intensive smoking cessation programmes achieved significant reductions which reduced problems of low birthweight and prematurity. There were no differences in perinatal mortality, a much rarer outcome.

Ultrasound screening is carried out primarily to detect anomalies and can be used to screen for Down's syndrome. The most common test for Down's syndrome is a biochemical blood test (the triple test) which has 69% detection rate for a 5% false positive rate. The quadruple test has a 76% detection rate for a 5% false positive rate but is more costly.

Breech presentation at term occurs in 3–4% of pregnancies and good evidence exists that external cephalic version (ECV) is a safe and cost-effective method to increase the rate of vaginal delivery. However, if ECV is unsuccessful (approximately one third of cases), the evidence suggests that the safest method of delivery is by caesarean section.

Preterm birth (birth at less than 37 weeks of pregnancy) is strongly associated with poor perinatal and infant outcomes. The most common problem is respiratory distress syndrome (RDS). Although there have been no interventions demonstrated to prevent preterm labour, administration of corticosteroids has been shown to speed up maturation of the fetal lungs and reduce RDS and perinatal mortality.

Models of care and recommendations

Professional and governmental bodies recommend that various problems be routinely screened for in pregnancy and postnatally including HIV, hepatitis B, and Down's syndrome antenatally and domestic violence postnatally.

Various themes have also emerged as important principles in caring for women in the maternity service. For women with uncomplicated pregnancies and labour, the most important is woman-centred care, which permits women choice and control in their childbearing. Where complications or problems arise, it is important that appropriate referral procedures are in place, that staff communicate well between themselves and with the woman, and that policies consistent with national guidelines are in place which cover health professionals' training for emergencies, referral and audit of outcomes.

2 Introduction and statement of the problem

Pregnancy is an important part of the lives of the majority of women aged 15 to 44 years. It is not an illness, although in a minority of cases pregnancy-associated medical problems arise for the mother or the baby. In 1999, 615 994 women in England and Wales had pregnancies ending in live or stillbirth and there were 57.7 live births per thousand women aged 15–44 years. As the topic of pregnancy and childbirth is a very broad one, this needs assessment will focus on uncomplicated pregnancy and its outcome, although specific major complications experienced by some mothers and babies will be included. Rather than attempting to be comprehensive, the text will review antenatal, intrapartum and postnatal care of women and well babies and give directions to sources providing clear and up to date information on other aspects of maternity care, summarised in Appendix 1. A glossary of terms is given in Appendix 2.

The material included has been taken from a selective review of the worldwide literature (available in English), including Cochrane reviews where available. The Cochrane Database of Systematic Reviews includes over 400 regularly updated reviews in the area of pregnancy and childbirth. For this chapter, the epidemiological data and information on current services and costs relate primarily to England and Wales. Material from Scotland and Northern Ireland which is easily accessible has been incorporated into the relevant tables and mentioned in the text. Information on costs and cost-effectiveness has been included where available.

This review excludes services for the management of sub-fertility, early pregnancy loss and termination of pregnancy, which are covered in the chapter on gynaecology. This chapter does not review the neonatal care of acutely ill preterm or term babies. Clinical obstetric management is also not covered.

Maternity care is distinct from many other health areas in having a legal framework that governs parts of practice and service provision. Readers should bear in mind that the legal framework and guidance documents may be different in Scotland and Northern Ireland from those in England and Wales. The legal framework relating to maternity care in England and Wales is outlined in **Box 1** below.

Box 1: Summary of legal framework.

- Midwives are obliged to notify the UKCC of their intention to practice in the forthcoming year (Nurses, Midwives and Health Visitors Rules 1983; Nurses, Midwives and Health Visitors Act 1997).
- Notification of births and registration of stillbirths by attendant at birth (Notification of Births (Extension) Act 1915).
- Registration of births by nearest relative (Birth and Deaths Registration Act 1953; Stillbirth (Definition) Act 1992).
- It is no longer required that a GP be present at a home delivery. Maternity records need to be retained for a minimum of 25 years (HSC 1999/053).

In addition to laws specific to maternity care, normal legal requirements regarding healthcare also apply. Staff working in maternity care must be aware that personal data storage must be registered (Data Protection Act 1998) and that clients have a right of access to records pertaining to themselves (Access to Health Records Act 1990). Staff should also be aware of the Children Act (1989), the Human Rights Act (1998) and the Health and Social Care Act (2001). The Department of Health publication *Working together to safeguard children* brings together much of the relevant material relating to children.[1] Providing appropriate services for minority ethnic groups is also covered by legislation. Guidance for NHS Trusts is provided by the Commission for Racial Equality (website listed in Appendix 1).

In September 2001 a new Nursing and Midwifery Council responsible for professional self-regulation replaced the existing UK Central Council for Nursing, Midwifery and Health Visiting (UKCC) and the four National Boards. It is responsible for maintaining the professional register and regulating practice.

There are also minimum standards of care recommended by such bodies as the Royal College of Midwives (RCM) and the Royal College of Obstetricians and Gynaecologists (RCOG), such as those relating to the organisation of labour wards[2] and routine ultrasound screening in pregnancy.[3] Maternity care is unusual in having local Maternity Services Liaison Committees that advise Health Authorities, which include representatives of users of maternity services along with professionals in maternity care (website listed in Appendix 1).

Changing Childbirth (1993)[4] was a government policy document focused entirely on maternity services. It represented a change in approach to maternity care, moving the service from being a clinically driven one to focusing on the needs of women and their babies to have woman-centred care that offers choice, continuity of care and control to each pregnant woman.

Other recent government plans for health and health services have been less specific about maternity care. The White Paper *Saving Lives: Our Healthier Nation* (July 1999)[5] was an action plan to tackle poor health and required the setting of local targets for reducing health inequalities. The NHS Plan[6] published in July 2000 uses this emphasis on removing inequalities to set the agenda for improving the health of babies. It proposes national health inequalities targets to narrow the health gap in childhood and throughout life between socio-economic groups and between the most deprived areas and the rest of the country. Targets will be set to narrow the longstanding gap in infant and early childhood mortality and morbidity between socio-economic groups. It recognises that women's health in infancy can affect the health of their children. A National Service Framework is currently being drafted.

These government documents propose that targets to reduce inequalities will be achieved by a combination of specific health policies and broader government policies. These include abolishing child poverty, expanding Sure Start (a government programme which aims to improve the health and well-being of families and children – *see* Appendix 1 for website) to cover one third of children living in poverty, increasing support for breastfeeding and parenting and introducing effective and appropriate screening programmes for women and children. Screening programmes include a new national linked antenatal and neonatal screening programme for haemoglobinopathy and sickle cell disease. The national plan gives particular priority to reducing smoking. Specialist smoking cessation services are to be set up to try to reduce the prevalence of maternal smoking and the incidence of low birthweight. Midwives are also expected to develop their role in public health and family well-being, working with local doctors and nurses in developing maternity and child health services and Sure Start projects. *Making a Difference* (1999) introduced new nurse, midwife and health visitor consultant posts, extending pay scales and career structures for staff. An all party parliamentary group on maternity was set up in December 2000 to focus on maternity services and build on the success of *Changing Childbirth* in the modernised NHS.

3 Sub-categories

- The majority of pregnant women are in good health and have straightforward pregnancies, uncomplicated deliveries and healthy babies. They comprise the main sub-category in this chapter.
- The next sub-category includes women with major obstetric complications such as pregnancy-induced hypertension, multiple pregnancies or breech presentation.

- The final sub-category includes women in vulnerable social groups including teenagers, women who do not speak English, women experiencing domestic violence, and women with physical and mental health problems.

The following sections will give information primarily on the first group, with selected information on women with obstetric complications and on women in vulnerable social groups where available.

4 Prevalence and incidence

This section provides national information on birth rates, mortality, complication and intervention rates, low birthweight and postnatal problems. The sources for these data are given in the relevant tables. They include data from the Office for National Statistics (ONS), the Confidential Enquiry into Maternal Deaths (CEMD) published triennially, and the Confidential Enquiry into Stillbirth and Deaths in Infancy (CESDI) published annually. Many of the prevalence and incidence rates vary by social class, geographical area and ethnicity. Up to the year 2000, births and deaths were classified using the Registrar General's social classes, but in 2001, the Office for National Statistics introduced a new classification, the National Statistics Socio-economic Classification.[7,8]

Vital statistics

Fertility

Summary statistics for the UK by country and region are shown in **Table 1**. The general fertility rate was between 52 and 65 per 1000 women aged 15–44 years, slightly higher in Northern Ireland and London, slightly lower in Scotland. Fertility rates declined steadily through the 1980s and 1990s and age-specific fertility rates show that many women are continuing to postpone childbirth into their 30s and 40s. The crude birth rate (not shown in the table) was 1230 births per 100 000 total population in 1997. A typical Primary Care Group or Primary Care Trust (PCG/PCT) population of 100 000 might expect to have about 1200 births per year.

Variations in birthweight by country and region in 1999 are shown in **Table 2**. There is a substantial correlation between birthweight and infant and perinatal mortality rates (*see* **Table 1**). The proportion of babies born weighing less than 2500 g was lowest in Northern Ireland at 5.7% and highest in the West Midlands region at 8.5%. Mortality rates within each birthweight group have fallen since the 1960s, particularly among babies born at or below 1000 g.[9] As a result, the percentage of low birthweight babies as a proportion of all births increased steadily through the late 1980s and 1990s. This was due, in part, to the increase in survival of multiple births as well as improvements in care. The proportion of babies with birthweight of 4000 g and over also increased over the last two decades.[9]

Perinatal and infant mortality

Mortality rates generally have been declining steadily through the twentieth century but appeared to be levelling off during the 1990s, although the infant mortality rate in 2000 in England and Wales was the lowest ever recorded. The decline in postneonatal mortality (deaths from one month to one year of age) was attributed to the 'Back to sleep' campaign, launched in December 1991, which encouraged parents to place their babies to sleep on their backs, to avoid cigarette smoke and over-wrapping their babies.

Table 1: Summary statistics by Regional Office area, 1999.

	General fertility rate[1]	Stillbirth rate[2]	Perinatal mortality rate[3]	Neonatal mortality rate[4]	Infant mortality rate[5]
England	57.8	5.3	8.2	3.9	5.7
Wales	56.6	4.8	7.8	4.1	6.4
Scotland	52.9	5.6	8.7	3.6	5.6
Northern Ireland*	64.9	5.1	8.1	3.9	5.6
Regional Office areas					
Northern & Yorkshire	55.3	5.2	8.3	4.0	6.0
Trent	55.2	4.8	8.2	4.4	6.1
Eastern	57.5	4.9	7.1	3.0	4.6
London	63.2	5.9	8.9	4.0	6.0
South East	57.6	4.5	6.9	3.2	4.9
South West	55.0	5.3	7.8	3.2	4.6
West Midlands	59.2	6.1	9.9	4.8	6.9
North West	56.7	5.4	8.6	4.4	6.6

[1] Rate of live births per 1000 resident women aged 15–44 years.
[2] Rate per 1000 live and stillbirths.
[3] Stillbirths and deaths at 0–6 days, rate per 1000 live and stillbirths.
[4] Deaths at 0–27 days after birth, rate per 1000 live births.
[5] Deaths under the age of 1 year after live birth, rate per 1000 live births.
* Data for Northern Ireland relate to 1998.
Source: ONS VS5, ISD Scottish Health Statistics, Northern Ireland Statistics and Research Agency

Table 2: Birthweight (grams) by country and Regional Office area, 1999 (%).

	Under 1,000	1,000–1,499	1,500–1,999	2,000–2,499	2,500–2,999	3,000–3,499	3,500+	Not stated
England	0.5	0.8	1.5	4.8	16.8	35.8	39.5	0.3
Wales	0.5	0.8	1.6	4.4	16.3	35.7	40.5	0.1
Scotland	0.4	0.6	1.4	4.4	16.0	34.6	42.5	0.0
Northern Ireland*	0.5	0.6	1.1	3.5	13.9	34.9	45.4	0.0
Regional Office areas								
Northern & Yorkshire	0.4	0.8	1.7	5.2	17.3	35.9	38.3	0.3
Trent	0.6	0.8	1.8	5.0	17.1	35.5	39.2	0.2
Eastern	0.4	0.6	1.5	4.2	15.4	35.9	41.9	0.1
London	0.6	0.8	1.5	5.0	18.4	37.0	36.1	0.6
South East	0.4	0.8	1.4	4.2	15.4	35.0	42.4	0.5
South West	0.4	0.7	1.3	4.3	15.3	35.3	42.4	0.2
West Midlands	0.6	0.8	1.7	5.4	18.0	35.9	37.4	0.2
North West	0.5	0.8	1.6	5.0	17.1	35.7	39.2	0.2

* Data for Northern Ireland relate to 1996.
Source: ONS VS5, ISD Scottish Health Statistics, Northern Ireland Statistics and Research

However, the decline in postneonatal mortality began before the campaign was initiated. In 1999, stillbirth rates varied from 4.5 per 1000 live and stillbirths in the South East region to 6.1 in the West Midlands region. Perinatal mortality rates (PMR) showed a parallel pattern, as shown in **Table 1**. The PMR was 8.2 per 1000 live and stillbirths in England; rates in other parts of Europe varied from 5.4 in Sweden and Finland to 9.7 in Greece. However, these differences are probably partly due to differences in criteria for registration.[10] Neonatal and infant mortality rates show similar regional variation, again, with lowest rates in the South and East and highest in the West Midlands and Northern regions.

Pregnancy, labour and delivery

Health-related behaviour in pregnancy

The Infant Feeding Survey, conducted every 5 years, provides nationally representative information on feeding practices and also about women's use of folic acid, smoking habits and alcohol intake during pregnancy.[11]

There is strong evidence to support periconceptional supplementation with folic acid to reduce the rate of neural tube defects[12] (*see* 'Folic acid in pregnancy' in section 6). Approximately 75% of the women sampled in the Infant Feeding Survey knew that folic acid would be good for them in early pregnancy.[11] Most of these women had increased their intake of folic acid, half through changing their diet and half through folic acid supplements.

Smoking prevalence before pregnancy, in pregnancy, and between 6 and 10 weeks after birth is also reported in the Infant Feeding Survey,[11] based on maternal report. For the UK as a whole, 35% of mothers smoked before they became pregnant, decreasing to 24% during pregnancy and 26% postnatally. All these figures were higher for Scotland and Northern Ireland than for England and Wales. For example, the proportion of women who smoked during pregnancy in England and Wales, Scotland and Northern Ireland were 23%, 28% and 27%, respectively. In all countries, however, women reported that they smoked fewer cigarettes per day while they were pregnant than before their pregnancy.[11] There has been some decline in the prevalence of smoking over the last decade, both before pregnancy and during pregnancy. For example, in 1990 38% of mothers in the UK smoked prior to pregnancy and 33% during pregnancy compared to 35% and 27% respectively in 1995.[11]

Alcohol consumption in pregnancy is also reported in the Infant Feeding Survey.[11] In the UK in 1995, 86% of mothers drank alcohol before pregnancy and 66% drank alcohol during pregnancy. However, the amount was very low – 70% consumed less than one unit of alcohol per week. Only 3% drank more than 7 units per week. There was some variation by age: mothers older than 30 years were more likely to continue drinking in pregnancy and tended to drink more than younger mothers. Similarly, women in England and Wales were more likely to continue drinking in pregnancy than women in Scotland and Northern Ireland but were also more likely to reduce their consumption.[11] The survey found a reverse social class gradient for alcohol consumption; women whose partners were in non-manual occupations were more likely to have drunk alcohol in pregnancy than other women.

Common complications in pregnancy and labour

National data about complications in pregnancy and labour are derived from the Hospital Episode Statistics (HES). Only about two thirds of these data have diagnostic information. The most recent published data relate to 1997/98. HES report a standard list of complications, as shown in **Table 3**, for England, 1997–98.[13]

According to HES, in the delivery episode the most common conditions related to the pregnancy were prolonged pregnancy (7%) and preterm delivery (before 37 weeks' gestation) (4%)[13] (*see* **Table 3**). The most common complications of labour were long labour (9%), fetal distress (19%) and perineal laceration (31%).

Table 3: NHS hospital deliveries: deliveries with antenatal, delivery or postnatal complications, England, 1997–98.

ICD-10 condition code	Condition	1997–98	
		% of deliveries with mention of complication/ indication for care	Estimated number of cases
Oedema, proteinuria and hypertensive disorders in pregnancy, childbirth and the puerperium			
O10	Pre-existing hypertension complicating pregnancy, childbirth and the puerperium	0.2	1,400
O11	Pre-existing hypertensive disorder with superimposed proteinuria	0.0	200
O12	Gestational (pregnancy-induced) oedema and proteinuria without hypertension	0.6	3,500
O13	Gestational (pregnancy-induced) hypertension without significant proteinuria	2.5	14,700
O14	Gestational (pregnancy-induced) hypertension with significant proteinuria (pre-eclampsia)	1.8	10,600
O15	Eclampsia	0.1	500
O16	Unspecified maternal hypertension	1.7	10,100
Other maternal disorders predominantly related to pregnancy			
O20	Haemorrhage in early pregnancy	0.1	600
O21	Excessive vomiting in pregnancy	0.2	1,200
O22	Venous complications in pregnancy	0.2	1,400
O23	Infections of genitourinary tract in pregnancy	0.7	4,100
O24	Diabetes mellitus in pregnancy	0.9	5,500
O25	Malnutrition in pregnancy	0.0	0
O26	Maternal care for other conditions predominantly related to pregnancy	2.8	16,500
O28	Abnormal findings on antenatal screening of mother	0.2	1,200
O29	Complications of anaesthesia during pregnancy	0.0	0
Maternal care related to the fetus and amniotic cavity and possible delivery problems			
O30	Multiple gestation	0.7	4,100
O31	Complications specific to multiple gestation	0.0	200
O32	Maternal care for known or suspected malpresentation of fetus	4.9	28,700
O33	Maternal care for known or suspected disproportion	0.4	2,500
O34	Maternal care for known or suspected abnormality of pelvic organs	5.9	34,400
O342	Uterine scar from previous surgery (including previous caesarean section)	4.6	26,800
O35	Maternal care for known or suspected fetal abnormality and damage	0.2	1,300
O36	Maternal care for known or suspected fetal problems	7.3	42,300
O40	Polyhydramnios	0.4	2,100
O41	Other disorders of amniotic fluid and membranes	1.2	6,800
O42	Premature rupture of membranes	3.5	20,500

Table 3: Continued.

ICD-10 condition code	Condition	1997–98	
		% of deliveries with mention of complication/ indication for care	Estimated number of cases
O43	Placental disorders	1.2	7,300
O44	Placenta praevia	0.5	3,200
O45	Premature separation of placenta (abruptio placentae)	0.3	2,000
O46	Antepartum haemorrhage not elsewhere classified	1.4	8,400
O47	False labour	1.1	6,200
O48	Prolonged pregnancy	7.3	42,900
Complications of labour and delivery			
O60	Preterm delivery	4.2	24,600
O61	Failed induction of labour	0.7	4,000
O62	Abnormalities of forces of labour	2.5	14,700
O63	Long labour	9.5	55,400
O630	Prolonged first stage	2.0	11,800
O631	Prolonged second stage	6.6	38,700
O632	Delayed delivery of second twin, triplet, etc.	0.0	100
O64	Obstructed labour due to malposition and malpresentation of fetus	2.1	12,300
O65	Obstructed labour due to maternal pelvic abnormality	0.4	2,400
O66	Other obstructed labour	1.8	10,300
O67	Labour and delivery complicated by intrapartum haemorrhage, not elsewhere classified	0.4	2,300
O68	Labour and delivery complicated by fetal stress (distress)	19.4	113,300
O69	Labour and delivery complicated by umbilical cord complications	5.2	30,500
O70	Perineal laceration during delivery	30.9	180,700
O71	Other obstetric trauma	1.3	7,800
O72	Postpartum haemorrhage	5.1	29,700
O73	Retained placenta and membranes, without haemorrhage	1.0	6,100
O74	Complications of anaesthesia during labour and delivery	0.2	900
O75	Other complications of labour and delivery, not elsewhere classified	4.3	25,400
Complications predominantly related to the puerperium			
O85	Puerperal sepsis	0.0	200
O86	Other puerperal infections	0.9	5,400
O87	Venous complications in the puerperium	0.4	2,200
O88	Obstetric embolism	0.0	100
O89	Complications of anaesthesia during the puerperium	0.1	400
O90	Complications of the puerperium, not elsewhere classified	0.4	2,300
O91	Infections of breast associated with childbirth	0.0	200
O92	Other disorders of breast and lactation associated with childbirth	0.2	1,400
Other obstetric conditions complicating pregnancy, childbirth and the puerperium			
O98	Maternal infectious and parasitic diseases	0.3	1,900
O99	Other maternal diseases	8.6	50,500

Source: DoH Statistical Bulletin[13]

Postnatal health

We know much more now about women's physical and mental health in the postnatal period than we did 10 years ago. Recent studies have shown that problems like incontinence, perineal pain, backache, sexual problems, tiredness and depression are more common than previously supposed.[14-16] Some understanding of the factors related to this ill health is beginning to emerge, and interventions directed at the problems are being tested in randomised trials.[18,19] This chapter focuses on a few of the key areas of women's postnatal health.

Postnatal depression

Postnatal depression (PND) is thought to affect between 10–15% of women in the first few months after childbirth.[20] It usually disappears by 6 months but can occasionally lead to serious mental disorder in the mother and is related to cognitive and behavioural disturbances in the infant.[21] The condition becomes recurrent in about one third of cases.[20] It may continue for a year or more[22] but psychosis is rare. Depression also occurs antenatally and both antenatal and postnatal depression are associated with social adversity and the lack of a supportive partner.[20]

Breastfeeding

In 1995 about 68% of women in England and Wales initiated breastfeeding, 55% in Scotland and 45% in Northern Ireland.[11] This was a slight improvement over previous years but nevertheless contrasts poorly with the situation in Scandanavia and in Southern and Eastern Europe. For example, in 1994 in Russia 99% of women initiated breastfeeding and in Norway 98%.[23] In the UK there are enormous variations by social class, with 90% of women with partners in social class I starting breastfeeding compared to only 50% with partners in social class V. More women breastfed their first babies than second or later babies and women who were older and better educated were more likely to breastfeed.[11]

Breastfeeding rates decline sharply over time after birth: in England and Wales the proportion of women breastfeeding fell from 68% at birth to 58% at one week, 44% at 6 weeks, 28% at 4 months and 14% at 9 months.[11] The rate of decline was similar in the other countries of the UK and similar to previous surveys. The most common single reason given for stopping breastfeeding for all time periods up to 8 months was that the baby seemed hungry and a perception that insufficient milk was being produced. Other important reasons for giving up breastfeeding in the first few weeks were that the baby would not suck or rejected the breast, and that breasts or nipples were painful.[11]

Perineal problems

By far the most common adverse outcome of labour for women as reported in HES data was perineal trauma. Such injury, which is associated with pain, infection and delay in return to sexual activity,[24-26] was reported as a complication in a third of women. However, this is likely to be an under-estimate, as perineal trauma may not be noted as a complication and diagnostic information is available for only two thirds of episodes. A better estimate of the prevalence comes from a trial carried out amongst 5500 women who had spontaneous vaginal births in Southern England in the mid-1990s. It estimated that 85% of those women experienced some genital tract trauma, with two thirds having lacerations which involved the perineal skin (first degree trauma) or perineal skin and muscle (second degree trauma).[27] Perineal trauma involving the anal sphincter (third degree trauma) is associated with higher rates of episiotomy[27,28-30] and with instrumental delivery.[26,29,31] Such damage increases the risk of serious postnatal morbidity such as incontinence.[26,29]

Women with major obstetric complications

Multiple pregnancies

The multiple birth rate has been increasing steadily over the past 20 years. Numbers of triplet and higher order multiple births in England have increased from 96 in 1980 to 304 in 1998. This increase is thought to be primarily as a result of infertility treatment.[32] **Table 4** shows HES data on the incidence of multiple deliveries in England in 1997–98 and their gestational age at birth. It demonstrates the rarity of high order multiple deliveries; there were only 280 deliveries of triplets or higher order multiple births out of approximately 585 000 deliveries. Eighty-nine percent of higher order multiple births were born preterm compared to 7% of singletons and 47% of twins.

Table 4: NHS hospital deliveries: total, singleton, twin and higher order multiple deliveries by gestation, England, 1997–98.

Gestation (weeks)	Total deliveries		Singleton deliveries		Twin deliveries		Triplet and higher	
	Estimated number	%	Estimated number	%	Estimated number	%	Estimated number	%
Total	585,000	100.0	576,000	100.0	8,300	100.0	280	100
under 20	130	0.0	130	0.0	0	0.0	0	0
20–23	500	0.1	500	0.1	50	0.5	10	2
24–27	2,300	0.4	2,100	0.4	180	2.2	20	7
28–31	4,800	0.8	4,200	0.7	500	6.4	70	24
32–36	33,900	5.8	30,600	5.3	3,200	38.3	160	55
37–41	511,300	87.4	506,900	87.9	4,300	52.1	30	11
42 or over	32,100	5.5	32,100	5.6	40	0.4	0	0

Source: DoH Statistical Bulletin[13]

Similarly, rates of low birthweight are significantly higher among multiples than among singletons. National data for England and Wales for the years 1991–95 showed an 11-fold differential in birth rates between singletons and multiples in the lowest birthweight category, those less than 1000 grams.[9] In the 1000–1499 gram category, there was a 12-fold differential. In the 1500–1999 gram category, there was a 13-fold differential.[9] For all low birthweight infants, there was a 9-fold differential in birth rates between singletons and multiples.

In addition to the impact upon low birthweight, it has long been known that stillbirth rates and death rates in infancy are higher among multiples than among singletons. National data for England and Wales for the year 1996 showed a three-and-a-half-fold differential in the stillbirth rate, a seven fold differential in the neonatal mortality rate, a two-and-a-half-fold differential in the postneonatal mortality rate and a five-and-a-half-fold differential in the infant mortality rate.

Maternal mortality

The triennial report by the Confidential Enquiry into Maternal Deaths (CEMD) reported that maternal mortality between 1994–96 for the UK was 268 or 12.2 per 100 000 maternities.[33] The two most common causes of death were thrombosis and thromboembolism, which were the causes of 46 deaths. Thrombo-embolic disease (TED) is the most common single cause of maternal death in developed countries.[34] Eclampsia, though rare, is a serious disease associated with hypertension in pregnancy and it is still an important cause of maternal death. Between 1994–96 there were 22 deaths from hypertensive disease of pregnancy, 19 of which were due to pre-eclampsia and eclampsia in the UK.[33]

Haemorrhage is also an important cause of maternal mortality; in 1994–96 there were 12 maternal deaths directly due to haemorrhage.[33] About half of bleeding in the second half of pregnancy is associated with either placental abruption, in which the placenta begins to detach from the uterine wall, or placenta praevia, in which the placenta is located close to the cervix. Perinatal mortality due to placental abruption and placenta praevia is about one in three and morbidity is common. Postnatal haemorrhage may be due to trauma or failure of the uterus to contract. Four of the five deaths from postnatal haemorrhage reported in the most recent CEMD followed caesarean section; two of them were repeat sections, the fifth followed vacuum extraction.

Women in vulnerable social groups

Minority ethnic groups

The chapter by Gill *et al.* in this volume (Black and Minority Ethnic Groups) provides key information about health needs of minority ethnic groups. In relation to language needs, the survey of Infant Feeding Practices in Asian Families Living in England[35] asked a representative sample of Bangladeshi, Indian and Pakistani women about their infant feeding. Interpreters were needed for 44% of first interviews; 25% of interviews with Indian women, 44% with Pakistani and 68% with Bangladeshi mothers. Some information on pregnancy outcome is available from ONS by country of origin, but not by ethnic background of mothers born in the UK. Crude mortality rates and incidence of low birthweight were higher in babies born to mothers from the 'New Commonwealth', especially from Pakistan.[8] The association between birthweight and mortality is striking but not straightforward because birthweight distributions differ between populations; what is considered low birthweight for Europeans may still be a healthy weight for other populations.

A number of studies of antenatal care use by different ethnic groups showed that, after adjusting for parity, Pakistani and Indian women consumed fewer antenatal resources and initiated care later than other groups.[36–37] However, there is no evidence that these differences in use of services account for the differences in infant mortality rate. The chapter by Gill *et al.* in this volume (Black and Minority Ethnic Groups) suggests that, apart from South Asians, Chinese immigrants may be particularly in need of help in accessing care generally.

Teenage pregnancies

The rise in teenage pregnancies has been a cause of enormous concern. The UK has teenage birth rates which are much higher than those in Germany, France and the Netherlands.[38] A halving of the teenage pregnancy rate was one of the key health targets of the government.[5] Conceptions to girls under the age of 16 increased from 7.2/1000 in 1980 to 8.9/1000 in 1997 but the rate appears to have levelled off since then. Approximately half of these pregnancies were terminated.[9]

Social class variations

There are marked social class gradients in stillbirths and infant mortality. In 1997, stillbirths were about twice as likely to occur in babies born into social class V and babies of single mothers compared to those born into social classes I and II.[8] However, the new classification of social class reveals a slightly different pattern. Stillbirth rates were lowest among babies with fathers in higher managerial and professional occupations and also those whose fathers were small employers or self-employed.[8] There are also marked social class differences in low birthweight. A high proportion of low birthweights occurred in babies born with fathers in semi-skilled or unskilled occupations and in those registered by their mother alone.[8] There also remains the well-known association between social class and smoking; women in non-manual social classes were less likely to smoke and more likely to give up smoking in pregnancy.

Domestic violence

Domestic violence (defined as violence between current or former partners in an intimate relationship, wherever and whenever the violence occurs[6]) affects women in pregnancy as well as at other times. It is thought that between one in ten and one in three women experience domestic violence at some stage of their lives.[33] It is a common cause of injury and psychological distress to women and may have an impact on pregnancy outcome.[39–40] The high estimates of the prevalence of domestic violence make it one of the most common health-related problems suffered by pregnant women. Health consequences can range from psychological effects to physical injury and death. There is some evidence that domestic violence may be initiated or increase in severity around the time of pregnancy though this is not proven.[39–40]

5 Services available and their costs

Introduction

This section is organised into three main sub-sections dealing with (i) patterns of care; (ii) hospital-based services including beds, lengths of stay and staffing; and (iii) the different elements of care such as antenatal visits and screening.

Patterns of care

In general, maternity care is provided by GPs, by midwives working in the hospital or the community or both, and by specialist doctors working in hospital. Over the course of pregnancy, birth and the puerperium, almost all women receive some care from professionals in each category.[41] The majority of care, in terms of time spent with the woman, is usually provided by midwives. Detailed data about the proportion of care provided by each type of care-giver in each phase of care are not routinely available. Some of the different patterns of care are described in **Box 2**.

Box 2: Summary of different patterns of care.

- **Shared care:** Usually an arrangement between the GP and obstetrician but may also be between the midwife and obstetrician. The majority of the antenatal care takes place at the GP's surgery or health centre, where care is provided by the GP and a midwife. Women are booked to deliver at hospital.
- **Midwife-led care:** Where the midwife is the lead professional taking responsibility for planning and providing care antenatally, intrapartum and postnatally.

- **Community-led care:** Care provided by GPs and midwives where hospital visits are kept to a minimum.
- **Caseload midwifery:** A single midwife or a group of midwives with a specified number of women under their care.
- **Domino schemes (Domiciliary In and Out):** Care is provided by midwives working in the community throughout the antenatal, intrapartum and postpartum period. Women are usually discharged 6–24 hours after the birth.
- **GP care:** Care provided by the GP and midwife at the GP's surgery or health centre. The woman is usually booked to give birth at the hospital but the GP and midwife provide postnatal care.
- **GP unit:** Small maternity hospital run by GPs.
- **Planned home birth:** This occurs under the care of a midwife working in the community; usually two midwives are present at the birth.
- **Midwifery unit:** Units in which women give birth, staffed only by midwives and, sometimes, GPs. They may be separate or attached to a hospital.
- **Team midwifery:** A group of midwives working together to provide antenatal, intrapartum and postpartum care for a named group of women in both the hospital and community.

Taken from Green *et al.*, 1998[42]

A survey by the English National Board for Nursing, Midwifery and Health Visiting in 1999[43] found that 66% of maternity units in England offered midwife-led care but only 42% offered GP care (*see* **Table 5**). This ranged from 48% in North West region to 91% in South West region for midwife-led care, and from 23% in South East region to 65% in Trent region for GP care. These schemes are generally available only to women without major obstetric complications. In a survey of English maternity care carried out at the beginning of 2001, directors of midwifery services were asked about the organisation of midwife staffing in the maternity units within their Trusts (personal communication – Jacci Parsons). Of the 156 responding Trusts, 116 had some form of team or group practice midwifery operating. In total there were 687 teams within the 116 Trusts. There were 9 Trusts with one team, and one Trust with 19 teams. Most Trusts had between 4 and 8 teams. The mean number of teams was 5.9. Team size varied substantially, with teams as small as 2 and as large as 57 midwives. The most common team size was 6 midwives (in whole time equivalents).

Table 5: Percentage of units in each region offering specific aspects of care.

Region	Midwife-led care	GP care	Satellite consultant clinics	Fetal assessment day care	Early pregnancy unit care	High dependency care	Transitional care (neonatal)
Northern & Yorkshire	67	55	61	78	69	65	45
Trent	71	65	53	94	87	73	50
Eastern	75	43	80	35	50	55	37
London	81	28	47	87	80	73	53
South East	68	23	88	65	58	42	32
South West	91	59	76	30	38	20	23
West Midlands	58	50	55	75	60	65	60
North West	48	45	57	86	79	62	55
England	66	42	62	64	60	51	41

Source: ENB 2000

Hospital-based services

The majority of women attend a hospital for antenatal care at least once during their pregnancy, usually for an ultrasound scan and booking. Women with complications usually attend more frequently.

Maternity services are provided in different ways across England and Wales. In 1999, the majority were managed within 171 NHS Trusts providing acute services; an additional 5 were within community Trusts.[43] In some Trusts a single main consultant unit is affiliated with smaller GP or midwife-led units. In other Trusts there may be more than one consultant unit offering care. Mergers between Trusts are changing these patterns of service provision. The most up-to-date figures available to us come from a survey of English Trusts carried out at the beginning of 2001. At that time there were 183 eligible Trusts identified. Of the 156 that responded to the questionnaire, 83% included one maternity unit, 8% two and the rest more than two (personal communication – Jacci Parsons).

Units and beds

Table 6 shows the number of maternity units in the countries and regions of the UK in 1996 sub-divided by number of births. Overall there is a trend away from small maternity units towards larger ones. The majority of maternity units in England had between 2000 and 4000 births in 1996 although in the other countries of the UK there were still more small maternity units. Within England, only the South and West region still had significant numbers of small maternity units in 1996. The 75 units with fewer than 10 births in 1996 were probably where births took place unintentionally.[8]

Table 6: Distribution of maternity units by number of births, 1996.

	All units	Less than 10*	10–199	200–999	1,000–1,999	2,000–2,999	3,000–3,999	4,000 and over
England	341	75	45	22	43	63	62	31
Wales	31	3	12	1	7	6	2	0
Scotland	54	–	30	2	9	5	5	3
Northern Ireland	16	–	1	3	7	4	1	0
Regional office areas								
Northern & Yorkshire	49	12	5	4	13	7	4	4
Trent	32	6	6	1	4	7	5	3
Anglia and Oxford	32	5	5	2	3	5	7	5
North Thames	54	16	4	3	3	9	15	4
South Thames	41	7	2	1	7	13	11	0
South and West	59	12	17	8	6	6	5	5
West Midlands	37	10	5	3	1	7	5	6
North West	37	7	1	0	6	9	10	4

* Thought to be births taking place unintentionally at non-maternity units.
Source: Macfarlane *et al.*[8]

Average numbers of maternity beds available daily and beds per thousand maternities are shown for the countries and regions of the UK for 1999/2000 in **Table 7**. They do not include beds in delivery suites. There has been a marked decline in NHS maternity beds available, from 59 beds per 1000 maternities in 1949 to about 20/1000 maternities in 1999/2000.[8] Regional differences in provision are largely historical, with Scotland and the northern regions having greatest numbers of available beds.

Table 7: Average available beds by Regional Office area, 1999/2000.

	Average number available daily	Beds/thousand maternities
England	10,203	17.8
Wales	627	19.5
Scotland	1,220	22.2
Northern Ireland	466	20.1
Regional Office areas		
Northern & Yorkshire	1,358	19.3
Trent	930	16.4
Eastern	1,035	16.7
London	1,769	16.9
South East	1,607	16.1
South West	1,003	19.4
West Midlands	1,038	16.5
North West	1,463	19.3

Source: Macfarlane *et al.*[8]

Duration of antenatal and postnatal inpatient stay

There is an important relationship between number of available beds, lengths of stay and the costs of the service. Durations of antenatal and postnatal stay are shown in **Tables 8** and **9** for 1997–98 for the regions of England. About 56% of deliveries took place on the same day as admission and a further 33% on the next day. Only 3% of women were in hospital for 4 days or more prior to delivery. There was very little regional variation.

Table 8: NHS hospital deliveries: duration of antenatal stay by region, 1997–98.

	Days from start of episode to delivery (percentages)									
	total	same day	1	2	3	4 or more				
						total	4	5	6	7 or more
England	100	56	33	6	2	3	1	1	0	1
Regional Office area										
Northern & Yorkshire	100	54	35	6	2	3	1	1	0	2
Trent	100	59	31	6	2	3	1	0	0	1
Eastern	100	57	33	5	2	3	1	0	0	1
London	100	56	32	6	2	2	1	1	0	2
South East	100	54	35	7	2	3	1	0	0	1
South West	100	60	30	5	2	3	1	0	0	1
West Midlands	100	56	33	6	2	3	1	1	0	2
North West	100	53	35	6	2	3	1	1	0	2

Source: DoH Statistical Bulletin, 2001[13]

Table 9: NHS hospital deliveries: duration of postnatal stay by region, 1997–98.

| | Total | Total days from delivery to end of episode (percentages) | | | | | | | | | |
| | | 0 to 3 | | | | | 4 to 6 | | | | |
		total	same day	1	2	3	total	4	5	6	7 or more
England	100	79	13	31	21	13	19	11	6	2	3
Regional Office areas											
Northern & Yorkshire	100	76	12	26	21	16	21	12	6	2	4
Trent	100	81	13	32	22	13	17	11	5	2	2
Eastern	100	81	16	34	19	12	16	10	5	2	3
London	100	79	13	36	19	11	18	10	6	2	4
South East	100	78	13	32	20	13	19	10	6	2	3
South West	100	81	12	32	22	14	17	10	5	2	3
West Midlands	100	77	11	30	23	14	20	12	6	2	3
North West	100	75	10	27	23	15	21	11	8	3	3

Source: DoH Statistical Bulletin, 2001[13]

Following delivery, 13% of women left hospital on the same day as delivery and three quarters within 3 days of the birth. There has been a considerable decline in length of postnatal stay over the last 25 years. This reduction is driven, in part, by women's wishes to return home sooner, as well as by concerns over cost and service capacity. Given the increase in caesarean section rates over the same time period, which necessitate longer postnatal stays, it is perhaps surprising that overall lengths of stay have declined to such an extent. There were substantial differences between regions in duration of postnatal stay. In 1997–98 in the North West region, only 10% of women were discharged on the same day, compared to 16% in the Eastern region. A correspondingly higher proportion of women stayed more than 4 days in hospital in the North West. This tallies with the greater bed provision in the north described in the previous section.

Staffing

Table 10 shows the whole time equivalent (wte) number of hospital medical staff in obstetrics and gynaecology by grade, country and region in the UK in 1996. Numbers are highest in Northern & Yorkshire region and the North Thames region, both in terms of absolute number and as rate per 1000 maternities (*see* **Tables 11(a)** and **11(b)**). Between 20–30% of hospital medical staff were consultants, higher in Scotland and Northern Ireland and lower in Wales; around 40% were senior house officers, slightly more in Scotland, Wales and Northern Ireland. There were quite substantial differences in the proportions of staff at registrar and senior registrar level, 3% and 15% respectively in Trent region compared to 16% and 5% respectively in Northern Ireland.

Tables 11(a) and **11(b)** shows numbers of qualified and student midwives, nurses working in maternity and health visitors in countries and regions of the UK in 1998. Some figures are also expressed as rates per 1000 maternities. As expected, there were considerably fewer nurses working in maternity than midwives. The rate of qualified midwives ranged from 25.7 per 1000 maternities in the South Thames region to 52.7 in Scotland. In general, Scotland appeared to be better resourced than other countries in the UK.

Table 10: Hospital medical staff in obstetrics and gynaecology by grade, Regional Office areas, England, Wales, Scotland and Northern Ireland, 1996 (whole time equivalent).

	All staff	Consultant	Staff grade	Associate specialist	Senior registrar*	Registrar	Senior house officer	House officer	Other staff	Hospital practitioner	Clinical assistant
England	3,540.1	909.6	142.1	65.2	487.2	339.6	1,480.0	16.0	0.0	7.0	93.4
Regional Office areas											
Northern & Yorkshire	572.1	146.2	23.9	13.4	117.0	24.4	225.5	1.0	0.0	1.8	18.8
Trent	329.9	84.5	19.0	3.0	48.2	10.0	146.3	14.0	0.0	0.4	4.6
Anglia and Oxford	353.7	98.7	10.3	9.0	50.2	34.1	142.8	0.0	0.0	0.6	8.0
North Thames	595.1	137.5	13.7	9.2	66.1	99.1	245.8	1.0	0.0	0.5	22.2
South Thames	501.3	123.7	23.8	7.6	59.7	67.7	210.2	0.0	0.0	0.7	8.0
South and West	363.9	94.9	12.8	7.4	36.5	44.8	156.2	0.0	0.0	1.0	10.4
West Midlands	352.8	95.1	17.0	6.1	59.5	25.0	143.0	0.0	0.0	1.0	6.0
North West	471.3	129.0	21.6	9.5	50.0	34.5	210.2	0.0	0.0	1.0	15.4
Wales	231.5	52.6	17.7	3.0	20.0	20.0	113.5	0.0	4.7	0.0	0.0
Scotland	453.7	135.0	0.0	5.1	79.9	17.0	216.7	0.0	0.0	0.0	0.0
Northern Ireland	157.6	47.7	0.0	2.9	7.5	25.5	74.0	0.0	0.0	0.0	0.0

* For Wales and Scotland includes specialist registrar.

Source: Department of Health, Medical and Dental Workforce Census, Welsh Office, ISD Scotland, DHSS Northern Ireland

Table 11(a): Midwives, nursing staff working in maternity and health visitors by Regional Office area, 1998.

	Qualified midwives (wte)	Student midwives	Nurses working in maternity (wte)	Health visitors
England	18,479	3,263	7,869	10,068
Regional Office areas				
Northern & Yorkshire	2,375	391	1,129	1,288
Trent	1,845	345	757	1,046
Anglia and Oxford	1,820	207	865	1,004
North Thames	2,524	483	1,062	1,311
South Thames	2,249	570	1,287	1,536
South and West	2,416	374	811	1,234
West Midlands	2,266	441	790	1,105
North West	2,975	452	1,167	1,544
Wales[1]	1,764	39	–	644
Scotland	2,994.7	497	1,019.8[2]	1,459
Northern Ireland	1,002.7	57	–	434

Table 11(b): Rate of wte staff per thousand maternities.

	Hospital medical staff[3]	Qualified midwives	Nurses working in maternity
England	5.81	31.0	13.2
Regional Office areas			
Northern & Yorkshire	7.57	32.8	15.6
Trent	5.46	31.5	12.9
Anglia and Oxford	5.36	27.8	13.2
North Thames	6.13	26.1	11.0
South Thames	5.78	25.7	14.7
South and West	4.86	32.8	11.0
West Midlands	5.27	35.2	12.3
North West	5.80	38.3	15.0
Wales[1]	6.69	–	–
Scotland	7.74	52.7	17.3[2]
Northern Ireland	6.50	42.4	–

[1] Welsh data aggregates midwives and nursing staff working in maternity.

[2] Scottish data for nursing staff working in maternity relate to 1997.

[3] Data for hospital medical staff relate to 1996.

Source: English National Board of Nursing, Midwifery and Health Visiting, Department of Health, Non-Medical Workforce Census, Welsh Office, ISD Scotland, Personnel Information Management System, Northern Ireland; Department of Health, Medical and Dental Workforce Census

There is a statutory duty for midwifery care to be available to women for 10 days routinely and up to 28 days if needed. Clearly, as the length of postpartum hospital stay has decreased, the workload of midwives working in the community has increased. The health visitor takes over general responsibility for both women's postnatal care and care of the infant at the point at which the midwife discharges the woman, any time between 10 and 28 days.

Data on GPs working in maternity are derived from their claims for payment and the General Medical Register. **Table 12** shows the number of GPs on the 'obstetric list' and the rate per 1000 maternities in the Regional Office areas. A GP may be included on the 'obstetric list' on completion of 6 months' training in a department of obstetrics and gynaecology or on meeting other criteria. In 1997, 91% of GPs were on the obstetric list, although this does not necessarily mean that they undertook maternity care.[8] Numbers of GPs on the 'obstetric list' ranged from 37.9 per 1000 maternities in North Thames to 52.5 per 1000 maternities in the South and West.

Table 12: General medical practitioners on obstetric list, 1997, England, regional office areas and Wales.

	Principals on obstetric list	
	Number	Rate per 1,000 maternities
England	26,618	44.3
Regional Office areas		
Northern & Yorkshire	3,496	47.5
Trent	2,706	46.0
Anglia and Oxford	2,989	45.2
North Thames	3,657	37.9
South Thames	3,581	41.0
South and West	3,892	52.5
West Midlands	2,797	42.5
North West	3,500	44.3
Wales	1,731	50.7

Source: General Medical Services Statistics, England and Wales, May 1998.

Home births

Although the great majority of babies are born in hospital, numbers of women giving birth at home increased steadily during the last decade of the twentieth century. In 1999 in England and Wales 2.2% of births were at home.[44] This varied across the country from 1.2% in the North West and Northern & Yorkshire Regions to 3.6% in the South West Region. In Scotland, 0.9% of maternities were at home in 1999 (*see* **Table 13**). These figures include both planned and unplanned home births, which often have very different maternal and infant health outcomes (*see* 'Home birth' in section 6).

Table 13: Home births, numbers and percentages of maternities.

	Numbers of maternities at home				Percentage of maternities			
	1995	1996	1997	1998	1995	1996	1997	1998
England and Wales	12,487	13,460	14,412	13,815	1.9	2.1	2.3	2.2
England	11,752	12,719	13,621	13,104	1.9	2.1	2.3	2.2
Regional Office areas								
Northern & Yorkshire	780	867	976	947	1.0	1.1	1.3	1.3
Trent	920	965	1,030	1,085	1.5	1.6	1.7	1.9
Anglia and Oxford	1,459	1,495	1,712	1,662	2.2	2.3	2.6	2.5
North Thames	1,822	2,036	2,127	1,987	1.9	2.1	2.2	2.1
South Thames	2,741	2,825	3,124	3,007	3.2	3.3	3.6	3.4
South and West	2,085	2,475	2,527	2,490	2.8	3.3	3.4	3.4
West Midlands	955	1,014	1,033	949	1.4	1.5	1.6	1.5
North West	990	1,042	1,092	977	1.2	1.3	1.4	1.3
Wales	735	741	791	711	2.1	2.1	2.3	2.1
Scotland	541	476	543	502	0.9	0.8	0.9	0.9

	Number	%
	1999	
England and Wales	13,272	2.2
England	12,561	2.2
New Regional Office areas		
Northern & Yorkshire	873	1.2
Trent	1,088	1.9
Eastern	1,737	2.8
London	2,262	2.2
South East	2,881	2.9
South West	1,881	3.6
West Midlands	895	1.4
North West	945	1.2
Wales	710	2.2
Scotland	490	0.9

Source: ONS/OPCS Birth statistics, Series FM1; General Register Office, Scotland

Antenatal care

Antenatal visits

In the UK, women traditionally visit their GP or clinic once every four weeks between 12 and 28 weeks, fortnightly until 36 weeks and weekly thereafter, making 13 visits in total.[45] Some women see only their midwife on these visits, some see both midwife and GP and a few see only their GP (personal communication – Mary Renfrew). The randomised controlled trials which have evaluated a reduced antenatal visiting schedule are considered in 'Antenatal visits' in section 6.

It is generally recommended that women carry their own notes[46,47] but it is not clear to what extent this is carried out.

Antenatal screening

Antenatal screening is carried out to check the health and well-being of both the mother and fetus. Pregnant women are generally offered tests for anaemia, blood group antibodies, rhesus type and certain infectious diseases (including rubella, hepatitis B, HIV, syphilis and asymptomatic bacteriuria). Most maternity units offer screening for Down's syndrome using biochemical markers. Ultrasound scanning is used to test for multiple pregnancy, fetal growth and anomalies and to determine gestational age. At each routine antenatal consultation fundal height is assessed to estimate fetal growth, maternal blood pressure is measured and urine tests are carried out for proteinuria and glycosuria, which are signs of pre-eclampsia.

A recent survey of maternity units in the UK asked about policies for antenatal screening for Down's syndrome, neural tube defects (NTD), haemoglobinopathies and cystic fibrosis.[48] They found that 76% of units had local and regional policies for Down's syndrome screening, 66% for neural tube defects, 35% for haemoglobinopathies and 22% for cystic fibrosis. Written policies often differed widely from guidelines published by the RCOG. The National Screening Committee (NSC) sub-group on antenatal screening has responsibility for developing national screening policy and issuing recommendations. The website for the NSC is given in Appendix 1.

Labour and delivery

Induction

About 20% of women in England in 1994–95 had their labour induced. In 1998–99 this had increased slightly to 22%.[49] This was usually by oxytocic drugs, some by surgical procedure such as artificial rupture of the membranes, and some using a combination.[13] This is shown by Regional Office area for 1997–98 in **Table 14**. About 8% of deliveries were by elective caesarean section, part of an increasing trend in both emergency and elective caesarean section (*see* **Figure 1**). Induction rates, however, after peaking in the 1970s, have been around 20% since 1989–90. In 1997–98 there was some geographical variation in induction rates, ranging from 18% in London to 24% in West Midlands region.

Method of delivery

Just over two thirds of all births in 1995–98 occurred by spontaneous vaginal delivery, as shown in **Table 15**. The caesarean section rate has been increasing steadily, from under 3% in the 1950s to 10% in the early 1980s, 15% in 1994–95 and 19% in 1998–99[49] (*see* **Figure 1**). Instrumental deliveries accounted for about 10% of births in 1994–95 and 1998–99, of which an increasing proportion were ventouse. Geographically there was little variation, but the Northern & Yorkshire and North West regions had highest rates of spontaneous delivery (74%) and South East the lowest (68%).

Table 14: NHS hospital deliveries: method of onset of labour by region, 1997–98 (%).

	Total	Spontaneous	Caesarean section	Induction Total	Surgical induction	Oxytocic drugs	Surgical and drugs
England	100	70	8	21	3	13	5
Regional Office areas							
Northern & Yorkshire	100	72	7	21	3	12	5
Trent	100	72	7	21	2	11	5
Eastern	100	71	8	21	3	14	7
London	100	74	8	18	3	10	5
South East	100	69	9	22	4	13	5
South West	100	70	10	20	3	13	4
West Midlands	100	67	10	24	4	14	5
North West	100	68	8	23	3	15	5

Source: DoH Statistical Bulletin, 2001[13]

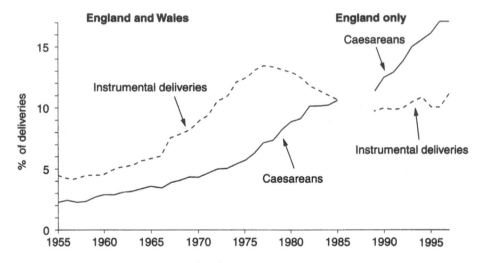

Figure 1: Operative delivery rates, 1955 to 1997/98.

Pain relief in labour

Table 16 shows type of pain relief used, sub-divided by method of delivery. Eighty-six percent of women having a spontaneous delivery used only gas and air or pethidine ('other' in the table) or no analgesic, 12% of them had an epidural. Over half of women having an instrumental delivery had an epidural or spinal anaesthetic. Among women having an elective caesarean section, the majority had a spinal anaesthetic; women having an emergency section generally had an epidural or general anaesthetic.

Continuous support in labour has been demonstrated to reduce the need for pain relief in labour as well as reducing the rate of operative deliveries (*see* 'Continuous support in labour' in section 6). At present nearly a third of maternity units are unable to give women in labour one-to-one care.[43]

Table 15: NHS hospital deliveries: method of delivery by region, 1997–98 (%).

	Total	Spontaneous		Forceps		Ventouse	Breech	Breech extraction	Caesarean			Other
		Vertex	Other	Low	Other				Total	Elective	Emergency	
England	100	69	1	2	2	7	1	0	18	8	10	1
Regional Office area	100	73	1	3	2	4	1	0	16	7	9	1
Northern & Yorkshire												
Trent	100	69	1	2	2	8	0	0	17	7	11	0
Eastern	100	68	1	3	2	7	0	0	19	8	11	0
London	100	68	1	2	2	7	0	0	19	7	12	1
South East	100	67	1	3	2	7	0	0	19	9	10	1
South West	100	68	1	2	2	8	1	0	18	8	10	1
West Midlands	100	69	1	2	2	5	0	0	20	9	11	0
North West	100	73	2	2	1	5	1	0	16	8	8	0

Source: DoH Statistical Bulletin, 2001[13]

Table 16: NHS hospital deliveries: anaesthetics used before or during delivery by method of onset of labour and method of delivery, 1997–98 (%).

Method of onset of labour	Method of delivery	Total number of cases	Type(s) of anaesthetic/analgesic used before or during delivery						
			General anaesthetic	Epidural	Spinal anaesthetic	General & epidural	General & spinal	Epidural & spinal	Other/none
Total all deliveries		585,000	4	20	7	0	0	1	67
Spontaneous	Spontaneous	325.7	1	12	0	0	0	0	86
	Instrumental	44.2	1	49	3	0	0	1	47
	Caesarean	40.0	22	31	24	3	1	3	16
Induced	Spontaneous	87.0	1	22	1	0	0	1	76
	Instrumental	17.3	1	59	2	0	0	2	37
	Caesarean	19.7	20	39	18	5	0	3	15
Caesarean	Caesarean	47.0	17	10	55	0	1	5	11

Source: DoH Statistical Bulletin, 2001[13]

Postnatal care

Breastfeeding support

There was little change in the proportion of women who initiated breastfeeding from 1980 to 1995. In 1995 the incidence of breastfeeding was 68% in England and Wales, 55% in Scotland and 45% in Northern Ireland.[11] Breastfeeding rates are described more fully in 'Breastfeeding' in section 4.

The vast majority of first-time mothers (86%) reported having been given help the first time they breastfed their baby. Mothers of subsequent children were less likely to receive help at this stage. Mothers who reported having problems breastfeeding after leaving hospital turned predominantly to midwives and health visitors for advice. A small proportion of women received help or advice from voluntary agencies such as La Leche League or National Childbirth Trust. These women were more likely to continue breastfeeding. However, they were also more likely to be in non-manual social classes and it is difficult to identify the separate effects of advice received.[11] In the survey carried out at the beginning of 2001, English Trusts were asked if they included maternity units accredited by the UNICEF UK Baby Friendly Initiative. Of the 154 Trusts that responded, 17 had an accredited unit. A further 47 Trusts had signed a certificate of commitment towards the Baby Friendly Initiative. Trusts that signed but were not yet accredited were also asked about which of the 10 Steps to Successful Breastfeeding had been implemented in their Trust. Seven of the ten steps had been implemented by over 89% of Trusts. The step that was least likely to be fulfilled was *'Give newborn infants no food or drink other than breastmilk, unless medically indicated'*, which was reported by 57% of these Trusts (personal communication – Jacci Parsons).

Screening for postnatal depression

As described in 'Postnatal depression' in section 4, postnatal depression (PND) is thought to affect between 10–15% of women in the first few months after childbirth.[20] Routine screening of women during the postnatal period has been advocated by the RCM. The Edinburgh Postnatal Depression Scale (EPDS) was developed as a screening tool for use in the community.[22] It has satisfactory sensitivity and specificity (86% and 78%, respectively) and is now used extensively by health visitors and some midwives working in the community.[50] A recent survey found that 94% of maternity units asked about psychological problems at booking, 25% screened for PND antenatally and 57% screened postnatally. Screening was most often done by health visitors using the EPDS (personal communication – Lucy Tully).

The expectation is that increased identification of cases and increases in referral and treatment will lead to reductions in incidence and duration of PND and improved infant outcomes. However, to date this has not been tested. In addition, adequate resources and effective interventions are needed for women with PND.

Well babies and neonatal screening

Although this chapter deals primarily with maternity, certain aspects of neonatal care fall within the remit of maternity care. There is a consensus that well babies should be checked prior to discharge to rule out congenital problems not apparent on physical inspection. This is currently done by paediatricians but consideration is currently being given to whether this could be done by specially trained midwives.[51]

Neonatal screening is carried out on the maternity wards to identify babies with particular disorders who may benefit from early diagnosis and treatment. It is also sometimes done even if there is no treatment available, to alert parents and their doctors to the risk to subsequent pregnancies. Though there are many disorders that *can* be screened for neonatally, the majority of them are not tested for routinely but only if there is a specific indication for doing so. They will not be reviewed in this chapter except to list those currently offered nationally. Current practice is described in **Box 3**.

Box 3: Neonatal screening/examinations.

- 'Guthrie' test – blood spot taken at 6 days – hypothyroidism and phenylketonuria (PKU) and, in some parts of the UK, cystic fibrosis and muscular dystrophy. There are plans for universal neonatal testing for haemoglobinopathies (sickle cell anaemia and thalassaemia).
- Congenital dislocation of the hip – there is some debate as to whether routine testing by the Barlow Ortolani test is effective.
- Routine examination at birth to check for obvious structural and neurological abnormalities such as congenital heart disease, cataracts.

Collaboration with the regional laboratories and paediatric services are essential to ensure rapid and complete notification and intervention where appropriate, as even a short delay can result in significant developmental impairment in the case of PKU or hypothyroidism.

Women with major obstetric complications

Antenatal conditions

Medical conditions in the mother, such as diabetes, thyroid disorders, congenital heart disease and epilepsy, may be affected or exacerbated by pregnancy and may cause health problems for mother and/or baby. As these occur relatively infrequently in the pregnant population, many units hold combined clinics between physicians and obstetricians to cut down on the number of visits for the woman and to pool knowledge and expertise on dealing with complications of medical conditions.

Multiple pregnancy, although increasing in prevalence, is also relatively infrequent and mothers expecting more than one child benefit from referral to a specialist centre.

High dependency care

Occasionally, women will have serious health problems during pregnancy either as a result of existing illness or a new pregnancy-related illness. Women with serious and/or rare disorders or fetal problems are generally cared for in a high dependency unit. Problems may include pre-existing conditions which may affect the pregnancy or be exacerbated by pregnancy, such as severe cardiac disease, or pregnancy-related problems such as severe pre-eclampsia. Where high dependency units also monitor severe fetal problems, it is usually in association with fetal medicine specialists and a neonatal intensive care unit because of the frequent need for preterm delivery. Nationally, about half of maternity units provide high dependency care (*see* **Table 5**), but this varies geographically from only 20% in the South West region to 73% in Trent and London regions.[43]

Women in vulnerable social groups

Minority ethnic groups

The chapter by Gill *et al.* in this volume (Black and Minority Ethnic Groups) provides detailed information about the health needs of black and minority ethnic groups and about the limited evidence on the effectiveness of interventions. The responsibilities of care providers are also discussed. Specific issues for maternity care include appropriate offers of prenatal screening and the challenge of providing advocacy or interpreter services for care that takes place in both community and hospital settings and at unpredictable hours. An annotated bibliography of studies relevant to maternity care for non-English speaking women is available[52] but no systematic reviews have been identified.

Routine questioning for domestic violence

Because almost all pregnant women access NHS maternity care in the UK, pregnancy is considered an opportune time at which to screen for domestic violence. Professional and governmental bodies (RCOG, RCM, DoH) have recommended that all pregnant women are seen unaccompanied at least once during antenatal care, and asked about their experience of violence. Provision of an interpreter, should that be needed, who is not the partner, a friend or family member, is also advocated (*see* 'Recommendations on screening and interventions' in section 7). Training of professionals and appropriate referral is essential[6] but often not in place.

A survey of all NHS Trusts in England and Wales was conducted in 1999 to measure the extent to which these guidelines were matched by practice in maternity units. Only 49% of units offered women an appointment without their partner and only 12% of units routinely asked women about violence.[53] Most pregnant women carry their own notes and this, clearly, has implications for confidentiality. The majority of units maintain a separate hospital record for women experiencing domestic violence. Although these measures are recommended by the CEMD, RCOG and BMA, this approach has not been tested in a randomised controlled trial. There may well be risks as well as benefits of such measures, particularly if introduced without appropriate training and resources.

Very little has been published on the costs of domestic violence. Health service costs in Hackney in 1996 amounted to £590 000 for injury and psychological care, but excluded hospitalisation and medication costs.[54] Other studies have documented the considerable additional health services resources used in treatment and care of women suffering domestic violence.[55–57]

Costs of maternity services

It is impossible to calculate the exact costs of maternity care. In 1997/98 a total of £44 billion was allocated to the NHS in the UK. Almost three quarters of this (74%) was spent on the hospital and community health services (HCHS). Of this, 65% was spent on staff salaries. The programme budget for maternity and early childhood amounted to 5.6% of the total HCHS budget in 1997/98.[9] Estimates for maternity budgets are shown in **Table 17** for the years 1988/89 to 1997/98 at 1997/98 prices. These exclude GP services and are consistently dominated by the cost of obstetric inpatient care, which accounted for over half of the total expenditure. Spending on hospital and community maternity care increased in real terms until 1991/92 but has declined thereafter. The Audit Commission estimated that maternity services cost £1.1 billion in 1997 or around £1700 per birth.[58]

GPs also provide some maternity care and get paid separately. GP maternity payments are shown in **Table 18,** along with the HCHS maternity budget. However, these figures should be interpreted cautiously given that there were changes in methods of data collection over this period.

Table 17: Hospital and community health services programme budget, 1988/89 to 1997/98, at 1997/98 prices.

	Obstetric inpatient	Obstetrics outpatient	Community maternity	Professional advice & support	All
	£ million				
1988/89	840	120	195	272	1,427
1989/90	805	109	209	294	1,417
1990/91	780	100	222	305	1,407
1991/92	854	161	165	351	1,531
1992/93	832	167	160	333	1,492
1993/94	777	151	161	336	1,425
1994/95	776	135	163	325	1,399
1995/96	751	129	176	329	1,385
1996/97	731	134	202	277	1,344
1997/98	730	137	210	266	1,343

Source: NHS Executive, Leeds, FPA PX-3

Table 18: Total expenditure on maternity services, 1992/93 to 1997/98.

Financial year	Total expenditure on HCHS maternity services (£ millions)	GP maternity payments (£ thousand)
1992/93	21,265	71,243
1993/94	22,096	72,465
1994/95	22,573	74,017
1995/96	23,890	73,148
1996/97	24,148	76,449
1997/98	25,329	80,381

Sources: Health and personal social services statistics for England, Table E3
GP maternity payments: NHS Executive FIS (FHS)

Since the introduction of the internal market in healthcare, information about costs of services, initially considered confidential, have been more widely disseminated. *The new NHS: reference costs* includes averages, ranges and variation in costs of certain maternity events as shown in **Table 19**. These data are provided by Trusts but it is not always clear how these costs are arrived at. The website for NHS reference costs is given in Appendix 1.

Intrapartum care costs are principally dependent on the duration of labour, provision of analgesia or anaesthesia, mode of delivery and staff present. A recent systematic review of costs associated with different methods of delivery has been conducted.[59] It found that, although there was considerable overlap in costs, complicated caesarean section costs were greater than those associated with instrumental delivery which, in turn, were greater than spontaneous vaginal delivery.

Postnatal care costs depend mainly on duration of inpatient stay. Community care costs are also important, particularly where women are discharged early. Some early discharge schemes used more resources than they saved due to the number of domiciliary visits made.[60]

Table 19: NHS reference costs for different methods of delivery.

HRG label	No. of trimmed* FCEs	Mean	Range for 50% of NHS Trusts		Range for all NHS Trusts	
			Minimum	Maximum	Minimum	Maximum
Elective inpatients						
Normal delivery with complications	80	795	795	795	795	795
Normal delivery without complications	7,376	883	547	1,183	352	1,886
Assisted delivery with complications	42	1,773	1,773	1,773	1,773	1,773
Assisted delivery without complications	535	1,024	767	1,272	684	1,362
Caesarean section with complications	168	2,556	1,773	3,339	1,593	4,039
Caesarean section without complications	1,523	1,649	1,222	2,065	1,034	2,370
Other maternity events	5,088	578	288	775	81	1,886
Non-elective inpatients						
Normal delivery with complications	1,036	901	770	1,088	232	1,797
Normal delivery without complications	26,115	720	500	855	171	1,673
Assisted delivery with complications	295	1,469	1,141	1,922	893	2,468
Assisted delivery without complications	3,645	1,162	886	1,362	741	1,875
Caesarean section with complications	860	2,284	2,055	2,403	1,788	3,092
Caesarean section without complications	5,727	1,577	1,393	2,040	227	2,370
Other maternity events	40,595	516	328	638	108	2,086

* 'Trimmed' means excluding outliers.

Multiple births are potentially very costly for the health service. We analysed the data for the former North West Thames Region in England (St Mary's Maternity Information System (SMMIS)) in order to estimate the cost of hospital obstetric care by multiplicity of birth. For this analysis, we attached unit costs, derived from primary and secondary sources, to each item of resource use, and built up a picture of the total cost of obstetric care. Mean obstetric costs per woman totalled £1360 for mothers of singletons, £2836 for mothers of twins, £6400 for mothers of triplets and £9514 for mothers of quadruplets (1998 prices) (Unpublished data). We also estimated the cost of neonatal care by attaching unit costs, derived from primary and secondary sources, to the neonatal experiences of each group of babies. We estimated neonatal costs at £167 for a singleton, £856 for a twin, £2395 for a triplet and £4424 for a quadruplet (1998 prices) (Unpublished data).

Litigation is an important issue in maternity care and contributes independently to overall NHS costs. There has been a steady rise in the rate of litigation from about 0.46 closed cases per 1000 finished consultant episodes in 1990 to 0.81 in 1998. This represents a growth rate of about 11% per year.[61] The most pronounced growth in litigation has occurred in obstetrics and gynaecology. Total costs nationally arising from clinical negligence claims have been estimated at between £32 million to £99 million per year across all specialties. This includes defence costs as well as costs from successful claims.[61]

6 Effectiveness of services and interventions

Introduction

Due to the breadth of the subject and the extent of the research that has been carried out, it is impossible to be comprehensive in this section. *Effective Care in Pregnancy and Childbirth*, published in 1989,[62] was one of the first major outputs of the evidence-based medicine movement. The second edition of *A Guide to Effective Care in Pregnancy and Childbirth*[63] provides comprehensive information as of 1995 and an updated edition will be available in the second half of 2001. There are now over 400 Cochrane reviews of randomised controlled trials in the area of pregnancy and childbirth, which provide excellent resources. There is consequently more material than could be covered in a chapter. We have therefore selected examples where there is compelling evidence in areas particularly relevant to PCTs and health authority commissioners.

Different patterns of care

'Patterns of care' in section 5 summarises the different elements and patterns of midwifery and maternity care that have been implemented. A range of different care schemes has been set up and some evaluated. All attempt to provide a service that is less fragmented and more user-friendly and women-centred, which minimises duplication of tasks and obstetric contact for women without obstetric problems whilst utilising midwives' skill. The five randomised controlled trials, two comparative studies, and four multi-scheme descriptive studies which attempted to evaluate the effects of women knowing their midwife, having midwife-only care and/or a homely care environment have been summarised by Green *et al.*[42] Some of the different schemes shared goals such as having the same carer throughout the antenatal, intrapartum and postpartum periods. Most were set up for women perceived to be at low risk of complications. Some were implemented by highly committed and motivated midwives and may not be generalisable to other settings; other schemes proved too consuming of midwives' family and social life to be workable. Midwives were also more motivated and enthusiastic about systems that they had chosen or developed. Users of these services perceived the majority of these schemes as better than the traditional hospital-based approaches. A consistent finding was that continuity of carer was at least as important for midwives as for the women they were caring for[42] (Grade B I-2).

There have been a limited number of economic evaluations comparing the costs of alternative models of maternity care.[14,64,65] These have varied in their findings from cost-saving to cost-generating depending on resource components included in the evaluation, the settings of the evaluations and the costing methodology. For example, epidural use was costed in a different way in each study.

Antenatal care

Information needs in antenatal care

Women often present very early in pregnancy at which stage many women want information. *The Pregnancy Book*, published by Health Promotion England, and given free to all women in their first pregnancy, can fill that need. The MIDIRS leaflets on Informed Choice also give clear information on various subjects. They are produced in pairs; the one for health professionals gives details of the research evidence, the one for women gives a summary. A recent evaluation of the MIDIRS leaflets found that, although they were considered helpful or very helpful by over 90% of the women who returned the questionnaires, they did not promote informed decision making.[66] This was thought to be partly due to the lack of coherent strategy for leaflet distribution (Grade D I-1).

Folic acid in pregnancy

The evidence for the beneficial effect of folic acid comes from a case-control study in the early 1980s[67] and a number of randomised controlled trials (*see* Cochrane review[12]) (Grade A I-1). Folic acid supplementation decreased the incidence of neural tube defects by at least half. On the basis of this, the government has planned to routinely supplement flour with folic acid. The Cochrane review suggested that there may be the possibility of increases in multiple births as a result of increased folic acid and subsequent perinatal loss.[12] The policy may therefore, on balance, be detrimental. The impact of this policy should be evaluated.

Smoking in pregnancy

Cigarette smoking in pregnancy is still common, as shown in 'Health-related behaviour in pregnancy' in section 4. It is associated with low birthweight, preterm birth, perinatal death and infant morbidity. A systematic review of interventions for promoting smoking cessation during pregnancy reviewed 44 trials including 16 916 women.[68] Interventions included information about the harmful effects of smoking, advice by health professional, reinforcement at antenatal visits, group counselling and peer support, a self-help manual, rewards and incentives, and others. The interventions achieved a significant reduction in smoking with absolute differences between the experimental and control groups of between 6.4% and 8.1% of women depending on the intensity of the intervention. As a result there was a reduction in low birthweight as well as in the proportion of babies born preterm but no difference in perinatal mortality[68] (Grade B I-1).

Several studies document increased neonatal hospital costs associated with maternal smoking.[69] The general conclusion of this body of literature is that neonatal costs could be reduced substantially by identifying family and social problems that mothers face antenatally and by delivering effective anti-smoking advice.

Antenatal visits

There have been six randomised controlled trials, which compared a reduced schedule of antenatal visits with a traditional schedule of visits, five of which were carried out in developed countries. All but the most recent randomised controlled trial[70] have been included in systematic reviews.[71] There was no significant difference in clinical outcomes but women's satisfaction with care was lower in those receiving fewer visits.

Most of the trials did not achieve a large reduction in number of visits and the lack of clear effect may be due to this (Grade C I-1). An economic evaluation of one of the trials showed that there would be no significant reduction in costs of care if a policy of reduced visits was implemented, partly because of non-significant but costly increases in admissions to neonatal care.[72]

Antenatal screening

One of the main purposes of antenatal care is screening for fetal and maternal disorders. The evidence for the effectiveness of some of these are summarised below. Detection of a problem will generally necessitate referral to a specialist.

Screening for Down's syndrome

Most maternity units provide some form of screening for Down's syndrome, although sometimes with age restrictions. There are a number of different serum markers that can be measured, including alpha feto-protein (AFP), human chorionic gonadotrophin (hCG) and unconjugated oestriol (uE$_3$), along with maternal age. These have various detection rates: AFP and hCG (the double test) with maternal age and a first trimester dating scan gives a detection rate of 59% with a 5% false positive rate. This rises to 69% for AFP, hCG and uE$_3$ (the triple test), and to 76% if inhibin A is added (the quadruple test)[73] (Grade B II-1). Ultrasound markers can also be used to detect Down's syndrome, and nuchal fold thickness and nuchal translucency show great potential but have not been subjected to randomised controlled trial.

If Down's syndrome is suspected then antenatal diagnosis is by amniocentesis or chorionic villus sampling with karyotyping of cultured cells. This allows the family either to plan for birth of an affected child or to terminate the pregnancy. The triple test appears to be the most cost-effective option in terms of cost per Down's syndrome birth avoided.[73] The NHS Executive plans to implement a national programme of screening for Down's syndrome but the particular approach is currently under discussion.

Ultrasound screening for anomalies, dates, multiple pregnancy and fetal well-being

A Cochrane review compared the use of routine ultrasound for detection of fetal anomalies with selective ultrasound prior to 24 weeks' gestation.[74] Routine ultrasound was associated with earlier detection of twins and a reduction in inductions for post-term pregnancies. There was no difference in perinatal mortality (Grade B I-1).

Another Cochrane review examined the evidence for third trimester scans for fetal well-being and intrauterine growth retardation in an unselected population. It included seven trials and found no benefit in terms of perinatal mortality although placental grading may be of value.

Labour and delivery

Method of delivery

As described in 'Method of delivery' in section 5, the majority of women have spontaneous vaginal deliveries. However, there is ongoing debate about the use of caesarean section. Proponents of caesarean section argue that it is now a safe operation, that perineal problems are avoided and that an elective caesarean section avoids the possibility of a long labour followed by emergency caesarean section.[75] Opponents of the more liberal use of caesarean section argue that it is associated with considerable maternal morbidity such as depression, difficulty with breastfeeding and ectopic pregnancy[76,77] (Grade IV). Caesarean section for breech presentation is discussed in 'Breech presentation' below. With regard to instrumental delivery, a Cochrane review suggests that ventouse has advantages over forceps, causing less maternal trauma,[78] (Grade B I-2) but in many regions forceps are still more commonly used (*see* **Table 15**).

Home birth

The debate about home birth has been characterised by a similar polarisation of views. In the 1960s and 1970s, improvements in perinatal mortality rates were taken, without evidence, as proof of the superiority of hospital birth.[79] However, such correlational inferences were challenged.[80] A review of the literature on place of birth concluded that there is some evidence, although not conclusive, that women and their babies do better and women are more satisfied with their care when cared for out of an institutional setting[79] (Grade II-2). It is important to differentiate between planned and unplanned home births. For women at low risk of complications, outcomes of planned home births are generally as good or better than hospital births.[69] Unplanned home births often occur when women don't get to hospital in time and are commonly associated with problems requiring transfer to hospital[81] (Grade II-1).

An economic evaluation was carried out as part of the National Birthday Trust Fund study of home birth in 1994. Planned hospital birth was compared with planned home birth and with unplanned home birth. Planned home birth was less costly to the health service than a planned hospital birth, although costs to the women were higher. For women who had an unplanned home birth, outcomes were significantly poorer, and costs consequently higher than for women who had either a planned home birth or a hospital birth.[82]

Continuous support in labour

The effects of having the continuous supportive presence of midwife or other trained person with a labouring woman have been analysed in 12 randomised controlled trials and summarised in a Cochrane review.[83] Continuous professional support reduces rates of instrumental delivery and, in some settings, rates of caesarean section. Duration of labour and use of epidural analgesia and other forms of pain relief are also reduced, while satisfaction with care is increased (Grade B I-1). In trials carried out in hospitals in developing countries, where friends or relatives are generally not permitted to attend women during labour, the additional support is often provided by lay helpers and the intervention has far greater effect.

The costs of a policy of continuous support by midwives would appear to be higher than the costs associated with current care, but this depends on the assumptions made about staffing patterns.[84] If midwives can work more flexibly, increasing their time with women in labour, it may be possible to provide continuous support without additional cost. This is the subject of ongoing research.

The maternal postnatal period

This is the time at which many women suffer health problems of shorter or longer duration, such as painful stitches, sore nipples, mastitis, other infections and bleeding and 'baby blues' or depression. In addition, women report the lowest levels of satisfaction with maternity care, particularly in hospital.[58] The section below concentrates on evidence of effectiveness in relation to some key aspects of care.

Breastfeeding

Babies who are not fully breastfed for the first three to four months of life are more likely to suffer health problems such as gastroenteritis, respiratory infection, otitis media, urinary tract infections and atopic disease if a family history of atopic disease is present.[23] There is also evidence of reduced mortality in preterm infants who are fed breast milk.[85] Breastfeeding is also beneficial to the mother's health, protecting against epithelial ovarian cancer and pre-menopausal breast cancer.[23] Breastfeeding is, however, contra-indicated if the mother is infected with HIV. The initiation and duration of breastfeeding is described in 'Breastfeeding' in section 4. These rates are disappointing considering the considerable short-term and long-term health benefits of breastfeeding.[23]

Interventions have been aimed at increasing the initiation as well as the duration of breastfeeding. Various strategies have been used, including health education programmes, media campaigns, peer support programmes and health service changes. Postnatal support from health professionals resulted in a modest increase in breastfeeding at 2 months. Where the support was provided face to face it was more effective than where it was provided by telephone[85] (Grade B I-1).

There are no economic evaluations in the English language literature of breastfeeding support. However, an increase in breastfeeding rates is likely to lead to a decrease in admissions for gastrointestinal, respiratory and other infections and thus reduce costs to the health service.[86,87]

There is very little evidence relating to effective support for women who bottlefeed their babies. Anecdotally, midwives and health visitors feel some difficulty in providing this support, fearing to undermine breastfeeding. Nevertheless, the dangers of over and under-concentrating formula milk, of poor hygiene and inappropriate feeds, are very real and need addressing.

Postnatal depression

There is evidence that women may not report their symptoms of depression to health professionals and that PND often goes undetected.[22] As a result, many professionals advocate screening for PND. The Edinburgh Postnatal Depression Scale (EPDS) has been validated as a screening tool for recognition of PND[22] and is being used widely by health visitors. On the other hand, there have not yet been any trials to test the effectiveness of routine screening for postnatal depression.

Small randomised controlled trials have shown beneficial effects of non-directive counselling and cognitive behavioural counselling in treatment of PND[21,88] (Grade B I-2). Anti-depressant drugs were also found to be an effective treatment, but women were less keen to take them[21] (Grade B I-2). Some hormonal therapy has been tested in randomised controlled trials with mixed results. Progestogens may have a role in causing depression but oestrogen therapy may be beneficial.[89]

A recent study of debriefing (a psychological treatment involving some form of emotional processing, catharsis or ventilation) following operative childbirth found no effect on rates of postnatal depression[18] (Grade D I-2). A randomised controlled trial of extra postnatal care in the form of home visits by support workers showed that this new model of care was welcomed by women. However, it was not effective in reducing rates of postnatal depression or improving well-being, as measured using the SF36[19] (Grade D I-2).

To date, there have been no economic evaluations of successful strategies for the prevention or treatment of postnatal depression in the English language literature. It is, however, likely that this condition has considerable cost consequences to the health service, women and their families and society at large.

Women with major obstetric complications

Multiple pregnancy

One of the purposes of the antenatal ultrasound scan is to determine fetal number. When a multiple pregnancy is found it is important to establish whether the fetuses share the same placenta and the same chorionic sac (di or mono-amniotic) because mono-chorionic fetuses share the same placenta and fetal blood circulation which may lead to problems. This may result in life-threatening haemodynamic imbalance as well as poor fetal growth and require closer monitoring than in other multiple pregnancies[90] (Grade B-III).

A greater proportion of multiple gestation pregnancies have adverse clinical outcomes than of singleton pregnancies. These will inevitably have significant resource implications for the health service and the wider economy. Multiple gestation pregnancies carry a significantly increased risk of maternal complications, including gestational diabetes, pregnancy-induced hypertension and caesarean delivery. They also carry a significantly increased risk of perinatal complications, including intrauterine growth restriction, premature delivery, intrauterine demise, low birthweight, and an increase in both short- and long-term medical and neurodevelopmental problems. In addition, multiple gestation pregnancies and births impose psychosocial and economic stresses on families. At the extreme end, this may lead to serious difficulties in daily living and marital discord and occasionally to child abuse, divorce and serious financial difficulties.

Hospitalisation and bed rest for multiple pregnancy has been evaluated in a systematic review of six trials.[91] Preterm birth and perinatal mortality were not reduced; indeed, for twin pregnancies the risk of very preterm birth was increased. Therefore routine hospitalisation and bed rest are not recommended (Grade E I-1).

Gestational diabetes

This is defined as 'carbohydrate intolerance of varying degrees of severity with onset or first recognition during pregnancy'.[92] There is diversity in opinions as to whether all pregnant women should be screened routinely. Gestational diabetes is associated with macrosomia (a birthweight in the upper centiles of the distribution). This, in turn, may lead to complications at birth, and women with gestational diabetes are commonly delivered by caesarean section.[93] Reasons for screening are to identify women at risk of developing diabetes mellitus in the future, and to prevent fetal malformations and macrosomia.[94] However, others argue that the glucose tolerance test is poorly reproducible and that the acquisition of a disease label and the increased risk of caesarean section are disadvantageous to women.[93] Moreover, there is no good evidence that diagnosis and treatment of gestational diabetes alter perinatal outcome[95,96] (Grade IV).

Breech presentation

Although the incidence of breech presentation at 28 weeks is about 20%, most of them turn spontaneously, so the incidence at term is only 3–4%. Babies in breech presentation suffer higher incidence of mortality and morbidity, due mainly to prematurity, congenital malformations and birth asphyxia or trauma.[97] External cephalic version (ECV) has been rigorously tested and found to reduce the risk of a caesarean section without any increased risk to the baby[98] (Grade A I-1).

A recent randomised controlled trial comparing vaginal breech delivery with elective caesarean section at term found that babies born vaginally were three times more likely to die or be injured than those born by elective caesarean section[99] (Grade A I-1). Management of preterm (<37 weeks) breech lacks good evidence on which to base recommendations. The decision about mode of delivery should therefore be made with the labouring woman and her partner.[97]

Adams *et al.*[100] examined the hospital clinic and Medicaid claims for 679 deliveries with breech presentation in a US inner city population. Based on the amounts that Medicaid was billed, attempting ECV reduced the use of resources by a little over US$3000 per birth of babies breech at term. Sensitivity analysis showed, however, that the savings may be as low as US$906.

Another American study aimed to determine the most cost-effective delivery management method of vertex and non-vertex twin pair gestations.[101] The investigators found that maternal and neonatal hospital charges were both significantly lower in the vaginal delivery and breech extraction group than in either the vaginal delivery and ECV group or the caesarean delivery group.

Preterm labour

Preterm birth is the most important predictor of infant outcome, both in terms of mortality and morbidity.[97] Preterm birth is defined as birth prior to 37 completed weeks, but it is babies born prior to 34 weeks who experience the worst outcomes.

The most common problem associated with preterm birth is respiratory distress syndrome (RDS), which affects 40–50% of babies born at less than 32 weeks.[97] Antenatal corticosteroids are associated with significant reduction in rates of RDS, neonatal death and intraventricular haemorrhage[97] (Grade A I-1). The cost and duration of neonatal intensive care is reduced following corticosteroid therapy.

Preterm uterine contractions can be suppressed by beta-agonists, which delay birth, but this is not reflected in improvements in perinatal mortality or morbidity. Beta-agonists do have side effects, occasionally serious, including maternal pulmonary oedema and myocardial ischaemia. Beta-agonists also cross the placenta and have a similar effect on the fetus[97] (Grade C I-1).

Eclampsia and pre-eclampsia

Eclampsia is a rare condition. Consequently, few medical staff have much experience of treating it. Specific continuing education of both medical and midwifery staff is therefore recommended.[32] It is also considered vital that such cases are managed in a delivery suite or high dependency unit by consultant obstetric and anaesthetic staff[97] (Grade A-III).

Prior to 1996, diazepam and phenytoin were the main treatments for eclampsia in the UK. A large randomised controlled trial found that magnesium sulphate produced significantly better results[102] (Grade A I-1). Pre-eclampsia, characterised by maternal hypertension and significant proteinuria, is much more common (*see* **Table 3**). It can lead to eclampsia and other significant health risks for the mother and baby, as well as the possibility of adverse neurodevelopmental outcome for the baby. The effectiveness of magnesium sulphate in the treatment of pre-eclampsia is currently under evaluation.

Shoulder dystocia

Shoulder dystocia is a rare and dangerous problem where the baby's emerging shoulders become stuck as the baby is delivered. It is more commonly a problem in large babies and can be associated with brachial plexus injury to the baby and perineal trauma to the mother. It may cause long-term disability or be fatal for the baby and calls for an emergency response by senior trained obstetric and paediatric staff.[103] There is reasonable consensus on the various manoeuvres that may be attempted to expedite delivery[103] (Grade III).

Training

In common with other specialities where emergency situations are encountered, the need for special training in obstetrics has been highlighted. The importance of 'fire drills', simulating real emergencies, to deal with rare but life-threatening obstetric emergencies has been stressed by the RCOG, RCM, CESDI and CEMD. The successful implementation of such training programmes should reduce perinatal and maternal mortality and morbidity and also reduce litigation to the NHS (Grade III). The Advanced Life Support in Obstetrics (ALSO) course is one such training programme for doctors and midwives. However, staff must also be recognised as having a role to play in reducing morbidity associated with obstetric emergency. With more obstetric care being provided in the community, GPs and paramedics also need to be trained in the basics of obstetric emergency care.[104] There have, however, been no trials to support this (Grade III). In the past, obstetric and neonatal flying squads were considered useful but they are not now recommended.

Women in vulnerable social groups

Teenage pregnancies

An Effective Health Care review noted that teenage pregnancy was associated with poorer health outcomes for both mother and baby.[105] This may be ameliorated by use of programmes promoting access to antenatal care, targeted support by health visitors, social workers or lay mothers and provision of social support and educational opportunities.[106] In one study from the USA special teen clinics were shown to have some potential for reducing low birthweight.[107] The recently launched government Teenage Pregnancy Strategy is being evaluated in a series of complementary studies.

Women living in poverty

Babies of women living in poverty are at higher risk of low birthweight and preterm birth. Various strategies have been tried, with the aim of increasing birthweight and reducing preterm birth. These have included home visiting, education, support, nutrition supplements and community links. Unfortunately, these have generally been unsuccessful.[108–110] The only positive outcome reported was in a study of home visiting by nurses, which helped to reduce pregnancy-related hypertension.[111]

7 Models of care and recommendations

General themes

For most women, pregnancy and birth are straightforward. However, they are life-changing events of enormous significance to the woman and her family. All too often in the past, and sometimes still, the importance of the latter was lost in the routine of the former by treating pregnancy and birth as a medical problem. The following principles have emerged as important themes in developing services for women in the maternity services.

Philosophy

- The majority of women have uncomplicated pregnancies and can be cared for in the community.
- Services should be 'women-centred', allowing women choice of models of care that best meet their needs.
- Providers and users of the service and MLSCs should have regular input into service development.
- Service development should reflect local case-mix, age structure of the population and ethnicity.

Structure of services

- Appropriate referral procedures are necessary to ensure that women at higher risk or those who develop problems receive specialist help.
- Combined clinics should be held where appropriate, to ensure integrated service delivery for women with medical problems or complications.

Information sharing

- Information services, including leaflets and access to interpreters, should be available to all women.
- Women should carry their own maternity notes and the National Maternity Record should be used.
- All provider units should send complete information for inclusion in HES.
- Routine data should be monitored to ensure implementation of the contract, to monitor quality and users' satisfaction.
- Translation and advocacy should be provided where necessary.

Process

- Good communication between staff and between staff and women and their families is essential.
- Women and their families should be treated with respect for privacy, confidentiality and informed consent.
- Women should be encouraged and facilitated to adopt healthy lifestyles.
- Policies should be in place, consistent with national guidelines, about antenatal screening, obstetric emergencies, training, referral and audit.
- Guidelines and recommendations from Department of Health (DoH) and professional bodies should be implemented.
- Models of care and interventions in pregnancy and childbirth should be evidenced-based as far as possible given current knowledge, and cost-effective.
- In particular, reducing rates of smoking in pregnancy and increasing rates of breastfeeding would have significant and far reaching benefits.

These recommendations may pose considerable challenges to health providers and commissioners. Planning and prioritising these different themes require that the different parts of the service work together. Some of the interventions and strategies highlighted may be costly to set up but be cost-saving in the longer term. For example, providing continuous support to women in labour reduces their need for pain relief and operative delivery, with long-term benefits.[82]

Recommendations on screening and interventions

Antenatal screening

Infectious diseases

Screening for the following infectious diseases is recommended by the RCOG[97] and/or the Department of Health:

- **Rubella:** Sero-negative women should be informed of their status and offered postnatal vaccination to protect future pregnancies.
- **Syphilis:** Antenatal serological screening should be offered to all pregnant women even though the incidence of the disease is now very low. This recommendation was made by the National Screening Committee because of the rising incidence of syphilis in Eastern Europe.
- **Hepatitis B:** Screening should be offered in early pregnancy, to allow for immunisation of babies born to infected mothers.
- **HIV:** An HIV test should be offered and recommended to all pregnant women as a routine part of their antenatal care. The test is highly sensitive (99.9%) and specific (99.7%). Arrangements for screening were to be in place by the end of 2000. A minimum take-up rate of 50% is expected by this date. By the end of 2002 take-up is expected to be at least 90%.
- **Asymptomatic bacteriuria:** Urine culture to detect asymptomatic bacteriuria should be offered to all women early in pregnancy to reduce the incidence of pyelonephritis, preterm birth and low birthweight babies. If a culture is positive, treatment with appropriate antibiotics should be offered.[97]
- **Toxoplasmosis, bacterial vaginosis and cytomegalovirus:** There is currently insufficient evidence to recommend screening for these infections.[97]

Other antenatal screening/interventions for pregnant women

- Screening for hypertension should be accompanied by a urine test for proteinuria. Blood pressure should be measured using standardised techniques and conditions (RCOG).[97]
- Symphisis-fundal height measurement (in centimetres) may have value in assessing uterine size. However, the interpretation is not straightforward. A randomised controlled trial (cited in RCOG[97]) detected no differences in any of the outcomes. Nevertheless, symphisis-fundal height measurement takes minimal equipment, training and time and may still have value.
- Screening for haemoglobinopathies is recommended for all people in whose racial background the haemoglobinopathies predominantly occur. In areas where greater than 15% of the population fulfil these criteria universal screening is recommended (RCOG).[112]
- Screening for rhesus negativity and provision of anti-D for those identified. This prevents RhD alloimmunisation (RCOG).[97]
- The UK National Screening Committee (website listed in Appendix 1) has recommended that there should be second trimester serum screening for Down's syndrome. This should be at least a double test but it would be desirable for laboratories to move to triple or quadruple tests in the future when possible. Screening in the first trimester and other screening modalities is being kept under review by the committee.
- All women should be offered an ultrasound scan between 18 and 22 weeks' gestation to look for major fetal anomalies (RCOG).[97]
- Identifying domestic violence in pregnancy. All pregnant women should be seen, unaccompanied, by a health professional at least once during antenatal care. All women should be asked about their experience of violence as part of the social history. Provision of an interpreter, should that be needed,

who is not the partner, a friend or family member, is also advocated. Training of professionals and appropriate referral is essential (DoH, RCOG, RCM).[6]

Interventions around the time of birth

- All women with an uncomplicated breech presentation at term should be offered ECV (RCOG).[97,98] Cardiotocography should be done; ultrasound and tocolysis can be helpful. Training and supervision of health professionals in carrying out ECV is an important consideration to avoid the loss of skills.
- Babies that are still in a breech position at term, who could not be turned by ECV, should be delivered by elective caesarean section (RCOG).[97]
- All women presenting in premature labour should be offered corticosteroids (RCOG).[97]
- The use of beta-agonists in preterm labour should be cautious, with careful monitoring. The time gained should be used actively to promote fetal maturation (RCOG).[97]
- Pregnant women should be made aware of the early symptoms of pre-eclampsia, its importance and the need to obtain formal assessment (DoH).[32] Because of the uncertainty in the efficacy of magnesium sulphate in treatment of pre-eclampsia and because magnesium sulphate is not without toxicity, units should develop local protocols for prophylaxis of seizures which may include the use of magnesium sulphate.
- It is essential that protocols are in place to deal with shoulder dystocia (CESDI).[103]
- All units should have a protocol for the management of massive haemorrhage. Regular 'fire drills' should be organised so that when these emergencies occur all members of staff know exactly what to do (DoH).[32]

Screening/interventions for women and babies after birth

- Identification of postnatal depression so that effective interventions can be offered.
- Vitamin K prophylaxis against haemorrhage.
- Hypothyroidism and phenylketonuria (PKU) (Guthrie) screening.
- BCG vaccination.
- Neonatal hearing screening.
- Support for breastfeeding.

Interventions for special groups at risk

- The recently launched Teenage Pregnancy Strategy calls on each Local and Health Authority area to jointly appoint a local co-ordinator. Their role is set out in guidance from the Teenage Pregnancy Unit in the Department of Health.
- Translation services and health information should be made available to non-English speakers.

8 Outcome measures

The Department of Health has published recommendations for health outcome indicators for normal pregnancy and childbirth.[113] These are tabulated by availability nationally and locally (**Table 20**). Many of these data items are not routinely collected or published and many are process rather than outcome measures. Data are available from routine systems for 11 of these data items, six have been piloted using data from the St Mary's Maternity Information System (SMMIS). They report a high level of completeness, although noting that SMMIS may be unrepresentative. They also note that there are some problems of definition and many indicators are associated more with social variables than hospital care.

Table 20: 'Candidate' outcome indicators for pregnancy and childbirth.

	Availability
Effective and safe care during pregnancy, labour, delivery and post-delivery:	
Maternal mortality rate	CEMD
Stillbirth, neonatal and post-neonatal mortality rate	CESDI
Incidence of eclampsia	No
Incidence of severe post-partum haemorrhage	HES
Perineal trauma and episiotomy	HES
Pain in labour and delivery	No
Incidence of postnatal urinary incontinence	No
Incidence of postnatal faecal incontinence	No
Gestational age	HES
Birthweight	ONS
Maternal admission to ICU	Locally
Use of antenatal corticosteroids to enhance pulmonary maturity	No
Mode of delivery rates	HES
Neonatal admissions to intensive care or special care	Locally
Emergency postnatal admission of mother	Locally
Well-being of mother and baby during and after pregnancy:	
General health status of mother after delivery	No
Incidence of postnatal depression	No
Smoking among pregnant women	Infant Feeding Survey
Weekly alcohol consumption among pregnant women	Infant Feeding Survey
Illicit drug use among pregnant women	No
Incidence of domestic violence associated with pregnancy and childbirth	No
Incidence and duration of breastfeeding	Infant Feeding Survey

HES contains diagnostic information on approximately two thirds of deliveries.

The Infant Feeding Survey is carried out approximately every 5 years on a sub-sample.

Some of these data may be available from local ad hoc surveys.

Source: Troop P, Goldacre M, Mason A, Cleary R. *Health outcome indicators: normal pregnancy and childbirth. Report of a working group to the Department of Health.* Oxford: National Centre for Health Outcomes Development, 1999

Other resources for audit include:

- **The Confidential Enquiry into Maternal Deaths:** This is an audit of all maternal deaths in the UK. It is carried out triennially, most recently covering the years 1994–96.[32] It reports causes of death and makes recommendations that it follows up in subsequent reports. The next volume will be issued at the end of 2001.
- **The Confidential Enquiry into Stillbirths and Deaths in Infancy:** This is carried out annually over the UK and aims to provide an overview of the numbers and causes of stillbirths and infant deaths, together with a detailed enquiry into specific subsets. Specific topics have included audits in three reports, on postmortem reporting (1993 and again in 1994–95), and CTG education (1999).[114]
- **Effective Procedures in Maternity Care Suitable for Audit:** This publication by the RCOG is available on the internet (*see* Appendix 1). It includes six sections: prevention of malformations, e.g. by appropriate management of diabetics; antenatal screening and diagnosis, e.g. Down's syndrome; antenatal management, e.g. of smoking; management of antenatal complications such as eclampsia; labour and birth such as fetal monitoring; and care after birth, including infant feeding. For each sub-section auditable standards are listed.
- **Sentinel audit:** A survey has been carried out by the RCOG of all caesarean sections in England and Wales. It collected information over a 3 month period in 2000. Data collected included type of section (elective/emergency), method of onset of labour, anaesthetic, the reason for the woman having a section and the birth outcome. Information on women's views was also collected for a sample. Information from the survey is now becoming available.
- **Perinatal Audit:** A report produced for the European Association of Perinatal Medicine in 1996.[115] This covers various approaches to audit of maternal mortality and morbidity and fetal and infant mortality and morbidity.
- **Women's views count:** This resource pack, published by the College of Health, aims to help health professionals and user representatives ask service users their views.[116] It includes copies of four validated questionnaires with directions on how to use them.
- **Evaluation through clinical audit (Ch. 9 in The Organization of Maternity Care: A Guide to Evaluation[121]):** This chapter describes the different stages in the audit process; setting standards, objectives, getting information, feeding back results and writing up. Other chapters in this book examine other methods of evaluation.
- **Assessing the needs and experiences of women using the maternity services who do not speak or write English:** A pamphlet that gives some of the reasons why it is important to assess the views of these women and looks at ways of doing so[51] (available from the NPEU).

9 Information and research requirements

Information requirements

The information collected about maternity care and its outcome falls well short of what is required to monitor the care given in pregnancy and birth and its outcome for mothers and babies.[8,117] Data are collected and aggregated in different ways in each of the four countries of the United Kingdom. Each has considerable deficiencies, even in Scotland, which has the best information systems.

In England, data about care given at birth are available at a national level for only about a two thirds of deliveries, despite the fact that the data items required and a wider range of information are recorded at a local level.[118] This is in part because some maternity units do not have computer systems and others have systems which are not linked to their hospital patient administration systems.[119] Even where such systems exist, there is a lack of linkage with other hospital systems, notably those in neonatal units and community systems, especially child health systems.[119] Child health systems exist in most districts. They were first designed as operational systems to schedule immunisation and screening programmes but they contain information on gestation and neonatal screening. Sometimes the software makes it difficult to extract data from them and in some places there are problems with the completeness of data.

These problems are well documented and it is hoped that a number of initiatives under way at the time of writing will lead to improvements. The NHS number programme (website listed in Appendix 1), to be implemented by 2002, will issue NHS numbers to babies at birth, instead of waiting for up to six weeks for the birth to be registered. The availability of NHS numbers to babies admitted to neonatal and intensive care will enable their records to be linked to those of their birth and hence their mothers' pregnancy. As a welcome by-product, the project will ensure that all maternity units have access to a computer system.

There are considerable inconsistencies between ways in which any given data item is recorded in maternity systems, thus making comparisons between units difficult. The Maternity Care Data Project (web site listed in Appendix 1) is working to compile a data dictionary with definitions agreed by representatives of clinicians. It is also working with system suppliers to ensure that they all use these common definitions. The Körner minimum dataset of items to be collected about birth was compiled in the early 1980s and so more up to date datasets are needed to reflect current concerns and practice. Although there is a minimum dataset associated with the allocation of NHS numbers at birth, it is very limited and so cannot, in its present form, replace the Körner minimum dataset. The Maternity Care Data Project is therefore inviting clinical groups to use the common dictionary, to define their own minimum datasets containing the items they need to monitor their practice.

As maternity care takes place in a variety of settings and usually involves two individuals, records need to be linked together to give a full picture of the care given antenatally, in labour, at birth and postnatally. In the longer term, this should be achieved through implementing electronic health records, due to be implemented in 2003. Linkage of records should also improve when babies receive NHS numbers at birth rather than at 6 weeks of age. However, it is likely that some years will elapse before these capture all the information related to any one pregnancy. Maternity care is an area where more resources are needed in terms of both infrastructure and skilled staff before the aims set out in policy documents are translated into reality.

Research requirements

Detailed lists of research topics cannot be accommodated in this chapter. Research in the area of pregnancy and childbirth benefits from being multidisciplinary and having user involvement. In addition to the ongoing work of assessing interventions, research is needed on the organisation of maternity care, on costs and benefits and on the views of patients and care-givers. Long-term follow-up of both mothers and babies will be needed to address key questions of effectiveness and cost-effectiveness. Priorities for R&D in primary care of mother and infant have also been evaluated in an NHS strategic review.[120]

Appendix 1: Sources of further information

Data sources

- *Cochrane Library* – includes Cochrane Database of Systematic Reviews, the Database of Abstracts of Reviews of Effectiveness, the Cochrane Controlled Trials Register, the NTA database, and the NHS economic evaluation database.
- *Birth Counts: statistics of pregnancy and childbirth* (Volumes 1 and 2)[8,9]
- National Guidelines Clearing House http://www.guidelines.gov
- *Effective Care in Pregnancy and Childbirth*[62] – tables on effective/ineffective care
- Maternity Data Project Data Dictionary http://www.nhsia.nhs.uk/mcd
- National Maternity Record http://www.nmrp.co.uk/demo
- NHS Number for babies http://www.nhsia.nhs.uk/nn4b
- Health Service Circulars http://www.open.gov.uk/doh/coinh.htm
- NHS Reference Costs http://www.doh.gov.uk/nhsexec/costing.htm
- Sure Start http://www.surestart.gov.uk

Professional bodies

- Royal College of Obstetricians and Gynaecologists http://www.rcog.org.uk
- Royal College of Midwives http://www.rcm.org.uk
- UK Central Council for Nursing, Midwifery and Health Visiting http://www.ukcc.org.uk/cms/content/home
- English National Board for Nursing, Midwifery and Health Visiting http://www.enb.org.uk
- Maternity Services Liaison Committee http://www.mslc.org
- Office for National Statistics http://www.statistics.gov.uk
- National Screening Committee http://www.doh.gov.uk/nsc/index.htm
- National Institute of Clinical Excellence http://www.nice.org.uk
- Sure Start http://www.surestart.gov.uk/home.cfm
- Commission for Racial Equality http://www.cre.gov.uk
- NHS Information Authority http://www.nhsia.nhs.uk

Appendix 2: Glossary of terms[8]

Readers should also check the Maternity Data Project Data Dictionary (*see* Appendix 1).

Abruptio placenta: condition in which the placenta detaches from the uterine wall.

Amniocentesis: withdrawal of fluid from the amniotic sac surrounding the fetus in the uterus for investigation of genetic constitution of fetus.

Anaemia: deficiency of haemoglobin in the red blood cells.

Anaesthesia: a state in which drugs are used to make the whole body, in general anaesthesia, or part of it, in local or regional anaesthesia, insensible to pain.

Analgesia: relief of pain by drugs or other means. May be general or local.

Antepartum: before delivery.

Booking: arranging where the baby will be born.

Caesarean section: delivery of the baby through an incision in the mother's abdominal wall and uterus.

Consultant obstetric maternity unit: a maternity unit in which women book with a consultant obstetrician to give birth under the supervision of midwives and obstetricians.

Domino: domiciliary in and out.

Down's syndrome: disorder caused by the presence of an extra chromosome.

Eclampsia: convulsions associated with hypertension in pregnancy.

Elective: a planned procedure, not undertaken as an emergency.

Epidural: a local anaesthetic injected into the space around the spinal cord, causing loss of sensation to the lower part of the body.

Episiotomy: surgical cut through the perineum performed at the end of labour immediately before a vaginal birth to facilitate delivery of the baby.

Fetal distress: changes in the condition of the fetus which might indicate a potentially harmful environment in the womb. The most common signs are abnormalities of fetal heart rate and rhythm and meconium staining of the amniotic fluid.

Forceps: instrument applied to the baby's head to assist in delivery.

Fundal height: distance between a pregnant woman's pubic bone and umbilicus.

General practitioner maternity unit: a maternity unit in which women book with a general practitioner to deliver under the supervision of midwives and general practitioners.

Glycosuria: the presence of glucose in the urine.

Haemorrhage: bleeding. Loss of blood either internally, when bleeding occurs into body cavity, organs or tissues, or externally onto the body surface.

High dependency care: care additional to usual routine care.

Hypertension: raised blood pressure.

Hysterectomy: operation to remove the uterus.

Induction: of labour or abortion. Process by which contractions of the womb are initiated artificially, either by breaking the membranous sac around the baby, or by drugs, or both.

Intrapartum: during labour.

Intrauterine: inside the uterus or womb.

Labour: the process of delivering a baby. It can be divided into three stages: dilatation of the cervix, delivery of the baby, and delivery of the placenta.

Midwife: a person who is qualified to supervise women in childbirth.

Neonatal: the period from birth to 28 days.

Neural tube defect: a defect of closure of the spinal canal or skull associated with failure of development, or an abnormal protrusion of brain or spinal cord tissue. Includes anencephaly, spina bifida and is often associated with hydrocephaly.

Oxytocin: drug commonly used in induction and acceleration of labour.

Parity: total number of previous live births and stillbirths. This does not include abortions or miscarriages.

Periconceptional: the period around conception.

Perineum: a woman's area of pelvic floor between the vagina and the anus.

Placenta praevia: condition in which the placenta is located close to the cervix.

Pre-eclampsia: complication of pregnancy including raised blood pressure and protein in urine, also known as toxaemia.

Prolonged pregnancy: a pregnancy that extends beyond the expected date of delivery.

Prostaglandin: hormone used in induction of labour or abortion, among other uses.

Proteinuria: the presence of protein in the urine.

Puerperium: time period after delivery during which the mother's body adjusts to the end of pregnancy.

Respiratory distress syndrome (RDS): condition occurring usually in preterm babies: can result from lack of surfactant, which is necessary for lung expansion of immature lungs.

Rubella: german measles.

Spina bifida: congenital defect of the spinal column.

Thalassaemia: a genetic blood disorder.

Trimester: approximately one third of pregnancy.

Ultrasound: high frequency sound waves used in obstetrics. They can be of two kinds. Doppler sound is used for measurement of fetal blood flow. Real time scanning ultrasound gives a picture of the area scanned, allowing assessment of fetal position, size and diagnosis of some malformations or of multiple pregnancy. Also used after birth for assessment of extent of neonatal brain damage caused by intracranial or intraventricular haemorrhage.

Vacuum extraction: method increasingly used as an alternative to forceps to assist delivery. Also known as ventouse delivery. Vacuum extraction may also refer to a method of induced abortion using suction, done early in pregnancy, before 12 weeks.

Ventouse: equipment used for vacuum extraction.

Appendix 3: Voluntary organisations

Action on Pre-Eclampsia (APEC)
Action for Sick Children
Arthrogryposis
Association for Community-based Maternity Care
Association for Improvements in the Maternity Services (AIMS)
Association for Spina Bifida and Hydrocephalus
BLISS
CERES
Caesarean Support Network
Child Bereavement Trust
Child and Adolescent Self-Harm in Europe
National Children's Bureau
Child Poverty Action Group (CPAG)
Contact at Family
Down's Syndrome Association (previously Down's Children's Association)
Foundation for the Study of Infant Deaths
Group B Strep Support
In Touch Trust
Maternity Alliance
MIND
Miscarriage Association
Multiple Births Foundation
National Childbirth Trust
National Children's Bureau
National Council for One-Parent Families
National Council of Voluntary Organisations (NCVO)
Parents in Partnership-Parent Infant Network (PIPPIN)
PETS
The Patients' Association
Royal Society for Mentally Handicapped Children and Adults (MENCAP)
SCOPE
STEPS
Stillbirths and Neonatal Death Association (SANDS)
Support Around Termination for Fetal Abnormality (SATFA)
Toxoplamosis Trust
Twins and Multiple Births Association (TAMBA)

References

1 Department of Health. *Working together to safeguard children: a guide to inter-agency working to safeguard and promote the welfare of children.* London: The Stationery Office, 1999.

2 Royal College of Obstetricians and Gynaecologists. *Towards Safer Childbirth – Minimum Standards for the Organisation of Labour Wards – Report of the RCOG/RCM Working Parties* [Web Page], 1999; available at http://www.rcog.org.uk/medical/saferbirth.html.

3 Royal College of Obstetricians and Gynaecologists. *Routine Ultrasound Screening in Pregnancy: Protocol, Standards and Training* [Web Page], 2000; available at http://rcog.org.uk/medical/ultrasound.html.

4 Department of Health. *Changing Childbirth. Part 1: Report of the Expert Maternity Group* (Chair: Baroness Cumberlege). London: HMSO, 1993.

5 Department of Health. *Saving Lives: Our Healthier Nation.* London: The Stationery Office, 1999.

6 Department of Health. *Domestic Violence: A Resource Manual for Health Care Professionals.* London: Department of Health, 2000; 67.

7 Rose D, O'Reilly K. *The ESRC Review of Government Social Classifications.* London: Office for National Statistics and the ESRC, 1998.

8 Macfarlane AJ, Mugford M. *Birth Counts: statistics of pregnancy and childbirth Volume 1.* (2e). London: The Stationery Office, 2000.

9 Macfarlane AJ, Mugford M, Henderson J, Furtado A, Stevens J, Dunn A. *Birth Counts: statistics of pregnancy and childbirth Volume 2: Tables.* (2e). London: The Stationery Office, 2000.

10 Graafmans WC, Richardus JH, Macfarlane A, Rebagliato M *et al.* Comparability of published perinatal mortality rates in Western Europe: the quantitative impact of differences in gestational age and birth weight criteria. *Br J Obstet Gynaecol* (in press).

11 Foster K, Lader D, Cheesbrough S. *Infant Feeding 1995.* London: The Stationery Office, 1997. OPCS Social survey reports; SS 1387.

12 Lumley J, Watson L, Watson M, Bower C. Periconceptional supplementation with folate and/or multivitamins for preventing neural tube defects. *The Cochrane Library.* Oxford: Update Software, 2000; 1–13.

13 Department of Health. *NHS Maternity Statistics, England: 1989–90 to 1994–95.* London: DoH, 1997; and Department of Health. *NHS Maternity Statistics, England: 1995–96 to 1997–98.* London: DoH, 2001.

14 Hundley V, Donaldson C, Lang GD *et al.* Costs of intrapartum care in a midwife-managed delivery unit and a consultant-led labour ward. *Midwifery* 1995; **11**(3): 103–9.

15 MacArthur C. What does postnatal care do for women's health? *The Lancet* 2000; **353**: 343–4.

16 Brown S, Lumley J. Physical health problems after childbirth and maternal depression at six to seven months postpartum. *Br J Obstet Gynaecol* 2000; **107**: 1194–201.

17 Saurel-Cubizolles M, Romito P, Lelong N, Ancel P. Women's health after childbirth: a longitudinal study in France and Italy. *Br J Obstet Gynaecol* 2000; **107**: 1202–9.

18 Small R, Lumley J, Donohue L, Potter A, Waldenstrom U. Randomised controlled trial of midwife led debriefing to reduce maternal depression after operative childbirth. *BMJ* 2000; **321**: 1043–7.

19 Morrell C, Spiby H, Stewart P, Waters S, Morgan A. Costs and effectiveness of community postnatal support workers: randomised controlled trial. *BMJ* 2000; **321**(7261): 593–8.

20 Appleby L, Koren G, Sharp D. Depression in pregnant and postnatal women: an evidence-based approach to treatment in primary care. *Br J Gen Pract* 1999; **49**: 780–2.

21 Appleby L, Warner R, Whitton A, Faragher B. A controlled study of fluoxetine and cognitive-behavioural counselling in the treatment of postnatal depression. *BMJ* 1997; **314**: 932–6.

22 Cox J, Holden J, Sagovsky R. Detection of postnatal depression: Development of the 10-item Edinburgh Postnatal Depression Scale. *Br J Psychiatry* 1987; **150**: 782–6.

23 Fairbank L, Lister-Sharpe D, Renfrew M, Woolridge M, Sowden A, O'Meara S. *Interventions* for Promoting the Initiation of Breastfeeding [protocol]. *The Cochrane Library.* Oxford: Update Software, 1999; 1–8.

24 Haddem K, Orlahnder S, Lingman G. Long-term ailments due to anal sphincter rupture caused by delivery – a hidden problem. *Eur J Curr Opin Obstet Gynaecol Reprod Biol* 1988; **27**: 27–32.

25 Sleep J. Perineal care: a series of five randomized controlled trials. In: Robinson S, Thomson A (eds). *Midwives, Research and Childbirth Vol 2.* London: Chapman & Hall, 1991; 199–251.

26 Sultan AH, Kamm MA, Hudson CN, Bartram CI. Third degree obstetric anal sphincter tears: risk factors and outcome of primary repair. *BMJ* 1994; **308**: 887–91.

27 Albers L, Garcia J, Renfrew M, McCandlish R, Elbourne D. Distribution of genital tract trauma in childbirth and related postnatal pain. *Birth* 1999; **26**(1): 11–5.

28 Carroli G, Belizan J. Episiotomy for vaginal birth (Cochrane Review). In: *The Cochrane Library*, Issue 2. Oxford: Update Software, 2001.

29 Fitzpatrick M, O'Herlihy C. The effects of labour and delivery on the pelvic floor. In: Drife J, Walker J (eds). *Best Practice & Research Clinical Obstetrics & Gynaecology* 2001; **15**(1): 63–79.

30 Sleep J, Grant A, Garcia J, Elbourne D, Spencer J, Chalmers I. West Berkshire perineal management trial. *Br J Midwifery* 1984; **289**: 587–90.

31 Donnelly V, Fynes M, Campbell D, Johnson H, O'Connell P, O'Herlihy C. Obstetric events leading to anal sphincter damage. *Curr Opin Obstet Gynaecol* 1998; **92**: 955–61.

32 Human Fertilisation and Embryology Authority. *Eighth annual report and accounts 1999.* London: The Stationery Office, 1999.

33 Department of Health, Welsh Office, Scottish Office Department of Health, Department of Health and Social Services Northern Ireland. *Why Mothers Die. Report on Confidential Enquiries into Maternal Deaths in the United Kingdom 1994–1996.* London: The Stationery Office, 1998.

34 Gates S. Thromboembolic disease in pregnancy. *Curr Opin Obstet Gynaecol* 2000; **12**: 117–22.

35 Thomas M, Avery V. *Infant Feeding in Asian Families: early feeding practices and growth.* London: HMSO, 1997. OPCS Social survey reports; SS 1366.

36 Knott PD, Penketh RJ, Lucas MK. Uptake of amniocentesis in women aged 38 years or more by the time of the expected date of delivery: a two-year retrospective study. *Br J Obstet Gynaecol* 1986; **93**(12): 1246–50.

37 Petrou S, Kupek E, Vause S, Maresh M. Clinical, provider and sociodemographic determinants of the number of antenatal visits in England and Wales. *Soc Sci Med* 2001; **52**(7): 1123–34.

38 *Teenage Pregnancy.* June 1999. Cm 4342.

39 Dye TD, Tollivert NJ, Lee RV, Kenney CJ. Violence, pregnancy and birth outcome in Appalachia. *Paediatr Perinat Epidemiol* 1995; **9**(1): 35–47.

40 Schei B, Bakkesteig LS. Gynaecological impact of sexual and physical abuse by spouse: a study of a random sample of Norwegian women. *Br J Obstet Gynaecol* 1989; **96**: 1379–83.

41 Garcia J, Redshaw M, Fitzimons B, Keene J. *First Class Delivery. A national survey of women's views of maternity care.* London: Audit Commission, 1998.

42 Green J, Curtis P, Price H, Renfrew M. *Continuing to care: The Organization of Midwifery Services in the UK: a structured review of the evidence.* Cheshire: Books for Midwives, 1998.

43 English National Board for Nursing Midwives and Health Visitors. *Report of the Board's Midwifery Practice Audit.* London: ENB, 1999–2000.

44 Office for National Statistics. *Birth Statistics.* London: The Stationery Office, 2000. FM1; No.28.

45 Sikorski J, Wilson J, Clement S, Das S, Smeeton N. A randomised controlled trial comparing two schedules of antenatal visits: the antenatal care project. *BMJ* 1996; **312**(7030): 546–53.

46 Elbourne D, Richardson M, Chalmers I, Waterhouse I, Holt E. The Newbury Maternity Care Study: a randomized controlled trial to assess a policy of women holding their own obstetric records. *Br J Obstet Gynaecol* 1987; **94**: 612–9.

47 Lovell A, Zander L, James C, Foot S, Swan A, Reynolds A. The St. Thomas's Hospital maternity case notes study: A randomised controlled trial to assess the effects of giving expectant mothers their own maternity care notes. *Paediatr Perinat Epidemiol* 1987; **1**: 57–66.

48 Lane B, Challen K, Harris H, Harris R. Existence and quality of written antenatal screening policies in the United Kingdom: postal survey. *BMJ* 2001; **322**: 22–3.

49 *Select Committee on Health.* Parliamentary report. 2000.

50 Clinical Standards Advisory Group. *Depression: Report of a CSAG Committee chaired by Professor Chris Thompson.* 1999.

51 Lomax A. Expanding the midwife's role in examining the newborn. *Br J Midwifery* 2001; **9**(2): 100–2.

52 Garcia J. *Assessing the needs and experiences of women using the maternity services who do not speak or write English.* Oxford: NPEU, 1999.

53 Marchant S, Davidson LL, Garcia J, Parsons JE. Addressing domestic violence through maternity services – policy and practice. *Midwifery* 2001; **17**: 164–70.

54 Stanko EA. *Taking Stock: what do we know about violence?* Uxbridge: ESRC Violence Research Programme, 1998.

55 Scottish Needs Assessment Programme. *Domestic Violence.* Glasgow: Scottish Forum for Public Health Medicine, 1997.

56 Bergman B, Brismar B, Nordin C. Utilisation of medical care by abused women. *BMJ* 1992; **305**(6844): 27–8.

57 Webster J, Chandler J, Battistutta D. Pregnancy outcomes and health care use: effects of abuse. *Am J Curr Opin Obstet Gynaecol* 1996; **174**(2): 760–7.

58 Audit Commission. *First Class Delivery: improving maternity services in England and Wales.* London: Audit Commission, 1997.

59 Henderson J, McCandlish R, Kumiega L, Petrou S. Systematic review of economic aspects of alternative modes of delivery. *Br J Obstet Gynaecol* 2001; **108**: 149–57.

60 Scott A. A cost analysis of early discharge and domiciliary visits versus standard hospital care for low-risk obstetric clients. *Aust J Public Health* 1994; **18**(1): 96–100.

61 Fenn P, Diacon S, Gray A, Hodges R, Rickman N. Current cost of medical negligence in NHS hospitals: analysis of claims database. *BMJ* 2000; **320**: 1567–71.

62 Chalmers I, Enkin M, Keirse MJNC. *Effective Care in Pregnancy and Childbirth.* Oxford: Oxford University Press, 1989.

63 Enkin M, Keirse MJNC, Renfrew MJ, Neilson J. *A Guide to Effective Care in Pregnancy and Childbirth.* (2e). Oxford: OUP, 1995.

64 Ratcliffe J, Ryan M, Tucker S. The costs of alternative types of routine antenatal care for low risk women: shared care vs. care by general practitioners and community midwives. *J Health Serv Res Policy* 1996; **1**: 135–40.

65 Young D, Lees A, Twaddle S. The costs to the NHS of maternity care: midwife managed vs. shared. *Br J Midwifery* 1997; **5**(8): 465–71.

66 Kirkham M, Stapleton H. *Informed choice in maternity care: an evaluation of evidence based leaflets.* York: NHS Centre for Reviews and Dissemination.

67 Smithells R, Sheppard S. Possible prevention of neural-tube defects by perioconceptional vitamin supplements. *The Lancet* 1980; **(i)**: 647.

68 Lumley J, Oliver S, Waters E. Interventions for promoting smoking cessation during pregnancy. *The Cochrane Library.* Oxford: Update Software, 2000; 1–23.

69 Li CQ, Windsor RA, Hassan M. Cost differences between low birthweight attributable to smoking and low birthweight for all causes. *Preventative Medicine* 1994; **23**(1): 28–34.

70 Jewell D, Sanders J, Sharp D. The views and anticipated needs of women in early pregnancy. *Br J Obstet Gynaecol* 2000; **107**: 1237–40.

71 Khan-Neelofur D, Gulmezoglu M, Villar J. Who should provide routine antenatal care for low-risk women, and how often? A systematic review of randomised controlled trials. *Paediatr Perinat Epidemiol* 1998; **12**(2): 7–26.

72 Henderson J, Roberts T, Sikorski J, Wilson J, Clement S. An economic evaluation comparing two schedules of antenatal visits. *J Health Serv Res Policy* 2000; **5**(2): 69–75.

73 Wald N, Kennard A, Hackshaw A, McGuire A. *Antenatal Screening for Down's Syndrome*. HTA report available at http://www.hta.nhsweb.nhs.uk

74. Neilson J. Ultrasound for fetal assessment in early pregnancy. In: *The Cochrane Library*, Issue 1. Oxford: Update Software, 2001.

75 Steer P. Caesarean section: an evolving procedure? *Br J Obstet Gynaecol* 1998; **105**: 1052–5.

76 Hemminki E. Impact of Caesarean section on future pregnancy – a review of cohort studies. *Paediatr Perinat Epidemiol* 1996; **10**: 366–79.

77 Hemminki E, Merilainen J. Long-term effects of cesarean sections: Ectopic pregnancies and placental problems. *Am J Obstet Gynecol* 1996; **174**: 1569–74.

78 Johanson R, Menon B. Vacuum extraction versus forceps for assisted vaginal delivery. In: *The Cochrane Library*, Issue 1. Oxford: Update Software, 2001.

79 Campbell R, Macfarlane A. *Where To Be Born? The Debate and the Evidence*. Oxford: National Perinatal Epidemiology Unit, 1987.

80 Tew M. The case against hospital deliveries: the statistical evidence. In: Kitzinger S, Davis JA (eds). *The Place of Birth*. Oxford: Oxford 1978.

81 Chamberlain G, Wraight A, Crowley P (eds). *Home Births. The report of the 1994 confidential enquiry by the National Birthday Trust Fund*. Carnforth: Parthenon Publishing Group, 1997.

82 Henderson J, Mugford M. An economic evaluation of home births. In: Chamberlain G, Wraight A, Crowley P (eds). *Home Births. The report of the 1994 confidential enquiry by the National Birthday Trust Fund*. Carnforth: Parthenon Publishing Group, 1997; 191–211.

83 Hodnett E. Caregiver support for women during childbirth. In: *The Cochrane Library*, Issue 1. Oxford: Update Softward, 2001.

84 Henderson J, Mugford M, Hodnett E. *Cost Consequences of Continuous Support During Labour: economic implications of the results of a systematic review of trials*. 8th International Conference of Maternity Care Researchers.

85 Sikorski J, Renfrew M. Support for breastfeeding mothers. *The Cochrane Library*. Oxford: Update Software, 2000; 1–11.

86 Howie P, Forsyth J, Ogston S, Clark A, Florey C. Protective effect of breastfeeding against infection. *BMJ* 1990; **300**: 11–6.

87 Tuttle C, Dewey K. Potential cost savings for Medi-Cal, AFDC, food stamps, and WIC programs associated with increasing breast-feeding among low-income women in California. *J Am Diet Assoc* 1996; **96**(9): 885–90.

88 Holden J, Sagovsky R, Cox J. Counselling in a general practice setting: controlled study of health visitor intervention in treatment of postnatal depression. *BMJ* 1989; **298**: 223–6.

89 Lawrie T, Herxheimer A, Dalton K. Oestrogens and progestogens for preventing and treating postnatal depression. *The Cochrane Library*. Oxford: Update Software, 2000; 1–9.

90 Bryan E. *Twins and Higher Multiple Births: A Guide to their Nature and Nurture*. London: Arnold, 1992.

91 Crowther C. Hospitalisation and bed rest for multiple pregnancy. *The Cochrane Library*. Oxford: Update Software, 2000; 1–9.

92 Metzger B, Coustan D. Summary and recommendations of the fourth international workshop-conference on gestational diabetes mellitus. *Diabetes Care* 1998; **21**(2): B1617.

93 Jarrett R. Should we screen for gestational diabetes? *BMJ* 1997; **315**: 736–9.

94 Soares J, Dornhorstt A, Beard RW. The case for screening for gestational diabetes. *BMJ* 1997; **315**: 737–9.

95 Walkinshaw S. Dietary regulation for 'gestational diabetes'. In: *The Cochrane Library*, Issue 1. Oxford: Update Software, 2001.

96 Canadian Task Force on the Periodic Health Examination. 1992 update 1: Screening for gestational diabetes mellitus. *Can Med Assoc J* 1992; **147**: 435–43.

97 Royal College of Obstetricians and Gynaecologists. *National Evidence-Based Clinical Guideline: Antenatal Care for the Healthy Woman – Draft Copy*. London: RCOG, 2001.

98 Hofmeyr G, Kulier R. External cephalic version of breech presentation at term. In: *The Cochrane Library*, Issue 1. Oxford: Update Software, 2001.

99 Hannah M, Hannah W, Hewson S, Hodnett E, Saigal S, *et al.* Planned caesarean section versus planned vaginal birth for breech presentation at term: a randomised multicentre trial. *The Lancet* 2000; **356**: 1375–83.

100 Adams E, Mauldin P, Mauldin J, Mayberry R. Determining cost savings from attempted cephalic version in an inner city delivering population. *Health Care Manag Sci* 2000; **3**(3): 185–92.

101 Mauldin J, Newman RMP. Cost-effective delivery management of the vertex and non-vertex twin gestation. *Am J Obstetr Gynaecol* 1998; **179**: 864–9.

102 The Eclampsia Trial Collaborative Group. Which anticonvulsant for women with eclampsia? Evidence from the Collaborative Eclampsia Trial. *The Lancet* 1995; **345**(8963): 1455–63.

103 *Confidential Enquiry into Stillbirths and Deaths in Infancy*. 5th Annual Report. London: CESDI

104 Chamberlain G, Steer P. ABC of labour care; obstetric emergencies. *BMJ* 1999; **318**(7194): 1342–5.

105 Effective Health Care. Preventing and reducing the adverse effects of unintended teenage pregnancies. *Effective Health Care* 1997; **3**(1).

106 Felice ME, Granados JL, Ances IG, Hebel R, Roeder LM, Heald FP. The young pregnant teenager. Impact of comprehensive prenatal care. *J Adolesc Health Care* 1981; **1**(3): 193–7.

107 Graham AV, Frank SH, Zyzanski SJ, Kitson GC, Reeb KG. A clinical trial to reduce the rate of low birth weight in an inner-city black population. *Fam Med* 1992; **24**(6): 439–46.

108 Widga AC, Lewis NM. Defined, in-home, prenatal nutrition intervention for low-income women. *J Am Diet Assoc* 1999; **99**(9): 1058–62.

109 Bryce RL, Stanley FJ, Garner JB. Randomized controlled trial of antenatal social support to prevent preterm birth. *Br J Obstet Gynaecol* 1991; **98**(10): 1001–8.

110 University of York, NHS Centre for Reviews and Dissemination. Preventing and reducing the adverse effects of unintended teenage pregnancy. *Effective Health Care* 1997; **3**(1): 1–12.

111 Kitzman H, Olds DL, Henderson CR Jr., *et al.* Effect of prenatal and infancy home visitation by nurses on pregnancy outcomes, childhood injuries, and repeated childbearing. A randomized controlled trial. *JAMA* 1997; **278**(8): 644–52.

112 Royal College of Obstetricians and Gynaecologists. *Effective Procedures in Maternity Care Suitable for Audit* [Web Page]; available at http://www.rcog.org.uk

113 National Centre for Health Outcomes Development. *Results of the Phase 3 Pilot Studies: Normal Pregnancy*. Oxford: NCHOD, 1999.

114 Confidential Enquiry into Stillbirths and Deaths in Infancy. *7th Annual Report*. London: Maternal and Child Health Research Consortium, 1998.

115 Dunn P, McIlwaine G. *Perinatal Audit: A Report Produced for The European Association of Perinatal Medicine.* 1996.

116 Craig G. *Women's Views Count: building responsive maternity services.* London: College of Health, 1998.

117 Radical Statistics Health Group. *The Unofficial Guide to Official Health Statistics.* (2e). London: Radical Statistics, 1981.

118 House of Commons Health Committee. *Maternity Services: second report* (Chair: N Winterton). London: HMSO, 1991. Session 1991–92. HC 29-I; Vol. I: Report.

119 Kenney N, Macfarlane A. Identifying problems with data collection at a local level: survey of NHS maternity units in England. *BMJ* 1999; **319**: 619–22.

120 Renfrew M, Davidson L, Zander L. NHS Strategic review of R&D. Priorities for R&D in primary care – mother and infant health. 1999.

121 Garcia J. Evaluation through clinical audit. In: Campbell R, Garcia J (eds) *The Organization of Maternity Care. A Guide to Evaluation.* Hochland & Hochland Ltd: Cheshire, 1997.

Acknowledgements

We would like to acknowledge the help of Rona McCandlish, Alison Macfarlane and Jane Thomas, who formed an advisory group to the authors. We also appreciated the help of Juliet Oerton, Elizabeth Bryan and Peter Brocklehurst in preparation of this chapter. Jane Henderson, Leslie Davidson, Jo Garcia and Stavros Petrou are funded by the Department of Health. Views expressed here are those of the authors and not necessarily those of the Department of Health.

11 Health Care in Prisons*

Tom Marshall, Sue Simpson and Andrew Stevens

1 Summary

Introduction

Providing health care for prisoners has historically been the responsibility of the prison service, not the NHS. Prison governors have been responsible for allocating resources to health care leading to considerable variation between prisons in the way in which health care services are provided. Prisons face many problems in the provision of health care, in particular relating to the need for security and inmates' isolation from their communities.

Describing the prison population

The prison population has three key features: it is largely young, overwhelmingly male and has a very high turnover. About 60% of inmates are under 30 years old. Fewer than one in twenty prisoners are female. New receptions per year amount to four times the prison population. Local prisons, which receive remand prisoners directly from the courts and prisoners on short sentences, have the highest turnover. Training prisons and high security prisons, which hold prisoners on longer sentences, have a lower turnover. About one in five prisoners are on remand, that is, they are awaiting legal proceedings or sentencing. Prisoners are drawn from lower socio-economic groups and have poor levels of education. Ten per cent of the prison population is black.

Prevalence and incidence of health problems

The range and frequency of physical health problems experienced by prisoners appears to be similar to that of young adults in the community. However, prisoners have a very high incidence of mental health problems, in particular neurotic disorders, compared to the general population. By ICD-10 criteria, in any week, almost half of prisoners are suffering from a neurotic disorder such as anxiety or depression. One in ten prisoners has suffered from a psychotic disorder in the past year.

* This chapter is an updated version of a report commissioned jointly by the Department of Health and the Directorate of Health Care of the Prison Service in England and Wales in 1998/9.

Suicide is about eight times more common among prisoners than in an equivalent community population. Suicides most frequently occur within the first weeks and months of imprisonment. Incidents of deliberate self-harm are reported in one in sixty prisoners a year.

Half of prisoners are heavy alcohol users and about one in twenty has a serious alcohol problem. About half of prisoners are dependent on drugs (principally opiates, cannabis and stimulants) and at least one quarter have injected drugs. A minority of prisoners continue to use drugs while in prison.

Services available

Opportunities for informal care and self-care are very limited in prisons. Per capita expenditure on formal health care services are higher than equivalent expenditure for young adults in the NHS.

Directly employed health care staff include health care officers (prison officers with some training in nursing), nursing staff (some whom may also be prison officers) and medical officers. Many prisons also contract with local general practitioners, hospital trusts, medical, dental and other specialists. In addition to access to NHS in-patient facilities, many prisons also have their own in-patient facilities.

A substantial part of the work of Prison Health Care Services involves routine medical examination at entry and prior to release and preparing medical reports for legal reasons.

Per year of imprisonment, prison inmates consult primary care doctors three times more frequently and other health care workers about 80 to 200 times more frequently than young adults in the community. Prison inmates are admitted to NHS hospitals as frequently as young adults in the community, but are also admitted to prison in-patient facilities two to sixteen times more frequently than this. Inmates are also heavy users of medical specialists and professions allied to medicine.

Effectiveness of services

There is little direct evidence of the effectiveness of health services in a prison setting. Relevant data are available from a range of sources of evidence-based reviews and guidelines.

It is known that screening prisoners at reception fails to identify many who are mentally ill. There are effective means of managing many of the health problems of prisoners. There is a range of effective treatments for minor illnesses, some of which are available without prescription. There is a range of medications and some psychological treatments (in particular cognitive behaviour therapy) which are effective for neurotic disorders and symptoms. For a range of health problems, the work of doctors can be successfully carried out by other professionals using clinical guidelines.

Recommendations

Planning of health care should be based on an understanding of health care needs. Planning of health care should not be primarily driven by a concern for demand (by patients or professionals) and historical precedent.

Efforts should be made to increase prisoners' ability to self-care and to reduce their dependence on the formal health care system. The recognition and management of neurotic disorders using effective pharmacological and psychological treatments should be given a high priority in the primary health care system. To achieve this, staff will need appropriate training. The provision of prison-based in-patient facilities should be reviewed. The management of chronic physical and mental illnesses should follow appropriate clinical guidelines.

2 Introduction and statement of the problem

Health care in prisons was for many years a matter of concern.[1] Prison medicine was said to be out of date, with a very 'medicalised' model of care, focusing on illness not health, and with little attention to prevention, guidelines, multidisciplinary work, audit, continuing professional development, or information.[2] HM Chief Inspector of Prisons, working independently of the Prison Service, reports directly to the Home Secretary on the treatment of prisoners and the conditions in which they are held. Adverse reports following inspections led to investigations into health care in prisons. In 1997 the Standing Health Advisory Committee to the Prison Service in its report *The Provision of Mental Health Care in Prisons* highlighted an uncoordinated approach to the delivery of mental health care.[3] More recent publications addressing the main issues of concern include *Patient or Prisoner?*[4] and the joint Prison Service and NHS Executive working group report, *The Future Organisation of Prison Health Care.*[5]

Both of these reports made recommendations for the restructuring of the Prison Health Care Service with a view to improving prison health care. Health care delivered in prisons was found rarely to be planned on the basis of need. Both reports also recommended that comprehensive health needs assessment of the prison population should be carried out.

Responsibility for the health care of prisoners

The health care of prisoners has until recently been funded and organised separately from the National Health Service (NHS), being the responsibility of HM Prison Service. The broad aim of the Prison Health Care Service was:

> to provide for prisoners, to the extent that constraints imposed by the prison environment and the facts of custody allow, a quality of care commensurate with that provided by the National Health Service for the general community, calling upon specialist services of the NHS as necessary and appropriate.
>
> Standing Order 13. Health Care. Home Office. HM Prison Service

From 1992 Governors were responsible for purchasing health care for their individual prisons, with the Directorate of Health Care providing advice on strategy, policy and standards.[1] This included the payment of staff; the provision of clinics for dentistry; opticians' services; genito-urinary medicine; and pharmacy.[4] The NHS was responsible for funding NHS (secondary) in-patient and outpatient care. The source of funding for NHS visiting consultants and for NHS services which reach into prisons (such as community mental health support) was less clear and varied from one prison to another. In 1996 annual health care expenditure by the prison service averaged approximately £1000 per prisoner (based on the Average Daily Population). However, this figure concealed wide variation in expenditure on health care, with some institutions spending as little as a few hundred pounds per inmate and others as much as £9000 or between 3% and 20% of their total budget on health care.[5]

In 1999 the establishment of a formal partnership between the Prison Service and the NHS was agreed. The partnership was lead by two national joint units – a policy unit and a task force – to help support and drive the reform of prison health care from the centre. The units formally came into being on 1 April 2000. In September 2002, Ministers announced the decision to transfer the budgetary responsibility for prison health from the Prison Service to the Department of Health. In addition a timetable of April 2006 was agreed for full devolution of commissioning responsibility to Primary Care Trusts (PCTs).

General features of the health care needs of prisoners

Prisoners have general health needs similar to those found in the general population. These are often overshadowed by health care needs related to offending behaviour such as substance misuse and mental health problems. Prisoners also have health care needs which are a consequence of imprisonment. Imprisonment restricts access to family networks, informal carers and over the counter medication; the prison environment can be overcrowded and may be violent; prisoners suffer emotional deprivation and may become drug abusers or develop mental health problems whilst incarcerated. Other health care needs may be made more complicated by imprisonment such as the management of chronic diseases like diabetes or epilepsy. Finally, certain health care needs are requirements of the prison system itself, for example health screening on arrival at prison and assessments carried out to determine a prisoner's fitness to appear in court.

Most health care in prisons is primary care. However, health care delivery in prisons faces a significant number of challenges not experienced by primary care in the wider community:

> *The primary purpose of prison is custody and rehabilitation and the need to provide primary health care in such a setting, places constraints and duties on doctors, nurses and other health care staff.*[5]

Providing health care in a custodial setting

There are particular challenges in maintaining a health care ethos to thrive in an environment where the highest priorities are maintaining order, control and discipline.[6] These include:

- Custody affects care in that it removes the opportunity for self-care and independent action; inmates have to ask staff for the most simple health care remedies.
- The health care teams' access to inmates may have to be curtailed in the interests of security.
- The proposed actions of medical staff may clash with security considerations.
- Nurses may be asked to carry out duties unrelated to health care.
- Some patients may be manipulative, try to obtain medication they do not require and create suspicion amongst health care staff of all prisoners.
- The health care centre is often seen as a sanctuary or 'social care' option for some prisoners, in particular those who are being bullied.

The prison estate in England and Wales

The prison estate is diverse, comprising small and large establishments, serving different roles and widely distributed geographically. There are currently 139 prison establishments in total.[7] Most prisons are managed directly by the Prison Service but a small number are managed on behalf of the Prison Service by the private sector.

Prisons are primarily classified by the age and sex of their inmates. There are prisons for male and female prisoners and separate institutions serve the needs of young offenders and adults. Prisons are further subdivided into local prisons, training prisons and high security prisons.

The total number of places in the prison estate is increasing, from around 60 000 in 1997 to 76 600 in 2005. It is planned to increase capacity to around 80 400 in 2007.[8]

Adult men's prisons

Local prisons and remand centres

Local prisons are institutions which hold prisoners when they are first sentenced. A number of local prisons are also designated as remand centres and therefore are used to hold prisoners who have been remanded in custody by the courts. Prisoners who are sentenced to a short term of imprisonment may spend their whole sentence in a local prison. Prisoners whose sentence is longer than a few months are usually transferred to training prisons. Because of the large numbers of remand prisoners and prisoners with short sentences, local prisons have a very high turnover. They contain a high proportion of prisoners who may be experiencing difficulties in adjusting to their recent incarceration or recent sentencing.

At any one time local prisons can hold 40% of the prison population. Because they act as reception and allocation centres they have a high throughput of prisoners. Local prisons usually have in-patient facilities and 24-hour cover for health care. The nature of the remand population will mean that it is likely to contain the highest percentage of seriously ill people with physical and mental disease.[9]

Training prisons

It is intended that training prisons are where all but very short sentence prisoners serve most of their sentences. Prisoners are categorised according to the level of security. They may have a high level of security (closed prisons) or lower levels of security (open prisons). Inmates in training prisons are allocated work.

The prison population is more static in training prisons. Since seriously ill prisoners normally have been detected at the initial receiving establishment, there is less need for medical assistance. In this population more physical disorders and fewer serious psychiatric disorders are present.[9]

High security prisons

Category A prisoners and those who are serving long sentences usually serve most of their sentence in high security prisons. For security reasons, prisoners are usually rotated between high security prisons every three years. High security prisons were previously known as dispersal prisons.

Because the prison population is older and present for longer, high security prisons tend to have the most comprehensive health care services in the prison service.[10]

Women's prisons

The female estate comprises 16 prisons in England and no prisons in Wales.[11] Women's prisons are divided into Young Offender Institutions, adult local prisons and adult training prisons (open and closed). The majority of women's prisons are entirely dedicated to the custody of women prisoners; however, some women prisoners are located in wings of adult male prisons, with separate sleeping and living areas. Despite an increase of more than 50%, since the early 1990s females comprise only 6% of the prison population.[12] The geographical spread of women's prisons means that many women may be imprisoned far away from their homes and families.

There are a number of health problems and needs that are specific to women in prison. These include maternity care, gynaecology and care of babies in prison, as well as a range of health education services such as family planning. Primary care consultation rates and admission rates to prison health care centres are high in women's prisons compared with other prison types and considerably higher than consultation rates for women in the community.[13]

Young Offender Institutions

Prisoners between the ages of 15 and 21 are held in designated establishments run under the Young Offender Institution Rules.[14] These institutions are further subdivided into those whose inmates are predominantly juveniles (aged 15 to 18) and those which hold inmates of all ages up to 21. Some Young Offender Institutions are designated as remand centres and therefore receive prisoners who are remanded in custody by the courts. Others are training prisons and, like their adult counterparts, may either be open (low security) or closed (secure).

In Young Offender Institutions there is often a small health care centre with a part-time medical officer and a few health care officers to provide day nursing cover.[9] Chronic physical illness is generally uncommon in this age group and serious mental illness, such as schizophrenia, is unusual. However, many offenders have temperamental, emotional and behavioural problems that manifest as self-harm and suicidal behaviour.

Models of health care provision in prisons

Within prisons, the way in which health care is managed and organised varies considerably. Following an investigation into a sample of 38 prisons in 1998,[13] models of health care were broadly classified into five types. These are listed in **Box 1**.

Box 1: The five main models of health care provision in prisons.

---

1 One or more directly employed full-time prison doctors supported by a mix of health care officers and nurses provide primary care. External NHS specialists provide specialist care. A variety of local contractual arrangements exist to support this requirement. The prison may have its own pharmacy service, or share with one or more others; in some cases pharmacy is provided under contract with external organisations either in the public or private sector. This is the model that is typical in most local and remand prisons.
2 Primary care is provided by NHS General Practitioners who are employed by the prison to work a set number of sessions within the prison, again supported by a mix of health care officers and nurses, with other services provided as at (1). This applies to predominantly smaller establishments.
3 Primary care contracted out to a local general practice who provide full-time medical services again supported as at (2).
4 The entire health care service in prison is met by an external organisation, for example a private sector provider or an NHS Trust. These examples are relatively few, mostly in contractually managed establishments, though there are some cases in the directly managed sector of the prison estate.
5 Primary care provided by clustering arrangements between several prisons.

Source: The Joint Prison Service and National Health Service Executive Working Group.[13]

These models serve as a general description, but there are prisons where elements of the models apply in different combinations or proportions. For example, general practitioners complementing and supporting the work of directly employed doctors, while some services are contracted out entirely. In addition the models of care have been described in relation to the medical composition of care rather than the nursing composition. In a few establishments health care is nurse-led, but this is not generally the case.

The models of care described highlight the range of personnel who may either be directly employed or contracted to deliver health care in prisons. The majority of prisons have a health care manager. The health care manager may be the most senior nurse by grade or a principal health care officer, with or without first level nurse registration. Most prisons either have a directly appointed full-time medical officer or a local GP appointed as a part-time medical officer. In the former case, the GP is an employee of the Home Office and is therefore classed as a civil servant.

During the period April 1996 to March 1997 staff providing health care in prisons handled over 2 million consultations with inmates. In around 30 000 cases prisoners received treatment in NHS hospitals as outpatients, in-patients or at accident and emergency departments.[13]

Describing the prison population

The prison population can be described numerically in a number of ways. The first of these is the Average Daily Population (ADP). This refers to the average number of prisoners in the prison at any one time. The second, New Receptions, refers to the number of new prisoners arriving in the prison in a given time period. In any one prison, the total number of new receptions is made up of newly sentenced or remanded prisoners (referred to as New New Receptions) and prisoners who have been transferred from other prisons. The relationship between these three statistics is shown in **Figure 1**. The significance of this is that the prison service is not just dealing with an average of around 73 000 people in prison at any one time but with the 150 000 who pass through prison each year.

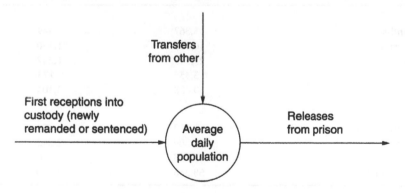

Figure 1: Throughput and average daily population of a prison.

Overall description of the prison population and trends

Between 1993 and 1997 the prison population increased by 37%.[15] The seasonally adjusted prison population rose to 66 000 in July 1998 and then decreased by around 2% (attributed to the Home Detention Curfew introduced in January 1999).[16] The ADP in England and Wales in 1998 was 65 299 and at the end of March 1999 was 64 200.[16] In 1998 the prison population rate in England and Wales (per 100 000 of the national population) was 125.[17] More recently the prison population has grown, reaching a population of 75 249 in March 2005, with a further 3375 prisoners under the Home Detention Curfew.[7]

Certified Normal Accommodation (CNA) is the capacity of the prison estate with no overcrowding. The CNA at the end of March 1999 was 61 900, i.e. the prison population exceeded the CNA by around 4%. Operational capacity is the maximum number of prisoners which can be accommodated in the prisons, albeit with some overcrowding. The number of prisoners held in March 2005 was 1400 below the operational capacity of 76 620.[7]

The total cost of the prison service in 2003–04 was over £2000 million, equivalent to approximately £27 000 per prisoner per year.[18]

Description of the prison population by category of prisoner

At the end of April 2005 the majority of inmates (67%) were sentenced adult male prisoners. The remainder was divided between male young offenders (12%), male remand prisoners (15%) and female prisoners (6%).

Sentenced prisoners

The commonest reason for imprisonment among sentenced females is drug offences (more than one-third) whereas among sentenced males the largest proportion (24%) were held for violence against the person. In April 2005, on average, 44% of sentenced male adults and 40% of sentenced adult females were serving terms of more than 4 years (excluding life) (see **Table 1**).

Table 1: Population of sentenced prisoners: April 2005.

Type of prisoner	Males	Females
Adults		
Less than 12 months	5,367	549
12 months to 4 years	16,259	1,130
4 years and over	23,348	1,247
Life	5,455	173
All adults*	50,488	3,104
Young offenders		
Less than 12 months	1,722	94
12 months and over	6,000	2,242
All young offenders*	7,728	336
All sentenced prisoners*	58,216	3,440

* Includes fine defaulters.

Lifers

Prison service statistics indicate that between 1987 and 1997 there was a 58% increase in the male, and an 85% increase in the female, life sentence population. On 30 April 2005 there were 5633 male lifers and 181 female lifers.

Reconvictions

Just over half (56%) of prisoners released from prison in 1994 were re-convicted of a standard list offence within two years. Reconviction rates are highest for male young offenders (76%). About half of sentenced adult males (49%) and females (51%) were reconvicted within two years.[15]

Prisoners on remand

Remand prisoners represent around 16% of the prison estate. The average time spent in custody for untried prisoners in 1997 was 51 days for males and 36 days for females. However, there were 200 untried prisoners who had been in prison for more than one year.[15]

Description of the prison population by category of prison

The health care needs of prisoners will to some extent depend on the primary function of the establishments where they are held. A description of the prison population by category of prison is therefore useful. In general terms the prison population is characterised by a high turnover: overall the number of new receptions is about four times larger than the Average Daily Population. However, the turnover of prisoners is considerably higher in local prisons and Young Offender Institutions and somewhat lower in closed training prisons, where prisoners are serving longer sentences (**Table 2**).

Table 2: Turnover of prisoners in different categories of prison in 1996/97.

Type of prison	Turnover: new receptions per year divided by ADP per year
Closed training prison (female)	4
Local prison (female)	8
Open training prison (female)	4
Young Offender Institution (female)	8
Closed training prison (male)	2
Local prison (male)	5
Open training prison (male)	3
Young Offender Institution (male)	4
All prisons	4

Source: Directorate of Health Care, Home Office.

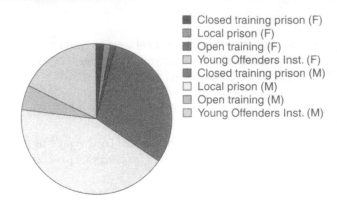

Source: Directorate of Health Care, Home Office.

Figure 2: Average Daily Population (ADP) by category of prison in 1996/97.

Description of the prison population by age

Males

A quarter of all male remand prisoners are aged 16 to 20 (young offenders) and 65% are under 30 years of age. The equivalent figures for sentenced male prisoners are 16% and 58%. The age structure of the male prison population is illustrated in Figures 3, 4 and 5 and **Table 3** below.

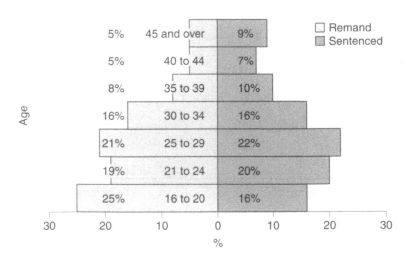

Source: Directorate of Health Care, Home Office.

Figure 3: Age structure of the male prison population: remand and sentenced prisoners.

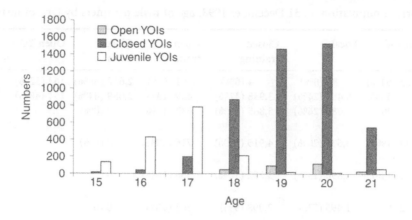

Source: Directorate of Health Care, Home Office.

Figure 4: The numbers and ages of male prisoners in Young Offender Institutions on 31 December 1998.

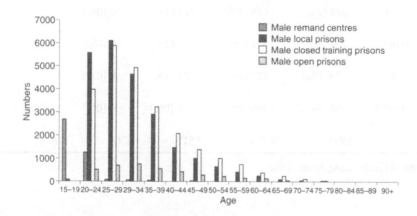

Source: Directorate of Health Care, Home Office.

Figure 5: The numbers and ages of male prisoners in adult prisons on 31st December 1998.

Table 3: The prison population on 31 December 1998: age of male prisoners by type of institution.

Age	Remand	Local	Closed training	Open training	Closed YOIs	Open YOIs	Juvenile
15–19	2,623 (64%)	88 (0%)	4 (0%)	1 (0%)	2,617 (56%)	163 (52%)	1,583 (96%)
20–24	1,307 (32%)	5,486 (24%)	3,938 (17%)	469 (13%)	2,089 (44%)	151 (48%)	64 (4%)
25–29	72 (2%)	6,089 (26%)	5,865 (25%)	682 (19%)	0 (0%)		
29–34	49 (1%)	4,627 (20%)	4,915 (21%)	716 (20%)	0 (0%)		
35–39	33 (1%)	2,890 (13%)	3,272 (14%)	556 (16%)	0 (0%)		
40–44	12 (0%)	1,495 (7%)	2,098 (9%)	365 (10%)	0 (0%)		
45–49	18 (0%)	963 (4%)	1,358 (6%)	277 (8%)	0 (0%)		
50–54	3 (0%)	633 (3%)	1,019 (4%)	235 (7%)	0 (0%)		
55–59	1 (0%)	368 (2%)	625 (3%)	113 (3%)	0 (0%)		
60–64	0 (0%)	206 (1%)	341 (1%)	71 (2%)	0 (0%)		
65–69	0 (0%)	88 (0%)	175 (1%)	24 (1%)	0 (0%)		
70+	0 (0%)	58 (0%)	103 (0%)	8 (0%)	0 (0%)		
Total	4,118	22,991	23,713	3,517	4,706	314	1,647

Source: Directorate of Health Care, Home Office.

Females

About one in seven of all female remand prisoners are aged 16 to 20 (young offenders) and 62% are under 30 years of age. The equivalent figures for sentenced female prisoners are 14% and 51%. The age structure of the female prison population is illustrated in the figures and the table below.

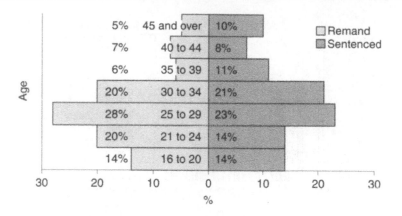

Source: Directorate of Health Care, Home Office.

Figure 6: Age structure of the female prison population: remand and sentenced prisoners.

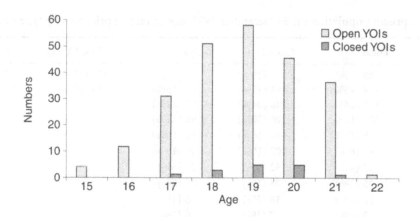

Source: Directorate of Health Care, Home Office.

Figure 7: The numbers and ages of female prisoners in Young Offender Institutions on 31 December 1998.

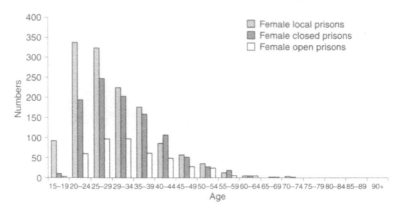

Source: Directorate of Health Care, Home Office.

Figure 8: The numbers and ages of female prisoners in adult prisons on 31 December 1998.

Table 4: The prison population on 31 December 1998: age of female prisoners by type of institution.

Age	Local	Closed	Open	Closed YOIs	Open YOIs
15–19	88 (7%)	13 (1%)	4 (1%)	155 (65%)	9 (60%)
20–24	337 (25%)	191 (19%)	64 (15%)	84 (35%)	6 (40%)
25–29	324 (24%)	246 (24%)	93 (22%)		
29–34	227 (17%)	206 (20%)	95 (22%)		
35–39	178 (13%)	161 (16%)	66 (15%)		
40–44	83 (6%)	107 (10%)	45 (10%)		
45–49	57 (4%)	52 (5%)	27 (6%)		
50–54	35 (3%)	28 (3%)	22 (5%)		
55–59	12 (1%)	18 (2%)	6 (1%)		
60–64	7 (1%)	7 (1%)	6 (1%)		
65–69	0 (0%)	1 (0%)	1 (0%)		
70+	3 (0%)	2 (0%)	0 (0%)		
Total	1,351	1,032	429	239	15

Source: Directorate of Health Care, Home Office.

Description of the prison population by ethnicity

Ethnic minority groups accounted for 18% of the male and 24% of the female prison population at the end of March 1999 compared with about 6% of the male and female general population of England and Wales.[16] However, of this ethnic minority population, 29% of males and 49% of females were foreign nationals. Given this, a more representative way to compare the data with the general population is to only describe prisoners who are British nationals (see **Table 5**).

Table 5: Ethnicity of the prison population who are British nationals and of the population of England & Wales aged 15 to 64.

Ethnicity	Males		Females	
	Prisoners	England & Wales	Prisoners	England & Wales
White	86%	95%	86%	95%
Black	10%	1%	11%	2%
South Asian (Bangladeshi, Indian, or Pakistani)	2%	3%	1%	2%
Chinese or other ethnic groups	2%	1%	2%	1%

Adapted from: White P *et al.*, *Prison Population Brief.*[9]

Other important factors describing the prison population

Socio-economic backgrounds of prisoners

Table 6 illustrates the employment and educational backgrounds of the prison population. The unemployed and undereducated are over-represented. Overall, a minority of prisoners are engaged in productive work (employed or bringing up a family), with a very high proportion either unemployed or long-term sick. Almost half of prisoners have no educational qualifications and only a small minority have been educated to A-level or beyond.

Table 6: The employment and educational characteristics of the prison population.

Economic activity	Male		Female	
	Remand	Sentenced	Remand	Sentenced
Working	36%	44%	26%	34%
Unemployed	34%	28%	24%	23%
Living off crime	15%	17%	14%	12%
Long-term sick	11%	7%	14%	8%
Bringing up family	0%	0%	13%	17%
Other	4%	3%	9%	6%
Educational qualifications	**Remand**	**Sentenced**	**Remand**	**Sentenced**
A-level or higher	12%	15%	13%	13%
GCSE	34%	37%	42%	36%
Other	3%	2%	1%	1%
None	52%	46%	44%	48%

Source: Psychiatric Morbidity among Prisoners in England and Wales.[34]

Table 7 illustrates that a significant minority of the prison population were homeless (in temporary accommodation, hostels or living on the streets) prior to incarceration and a similar proportion were in insecure forms of accommodation (bedsits or rooms with shared amenities).

Table 7: The prior accommodation arrangements of the prison population.

Type of accommodation	Males		Females	
	Remand	Sentenced	Remand	Sentenced
Privately owned	8%	15%	7%	14%
Rented (self-contained)	47%	48%	56%	61%
Bedsit/room (shared amenities)	7%	6%	8%	3%
Homeless (temporary accommodation, hostel, living on streets)	7%	5%	8%	4%
With parents/relatives	22%	20%	13%	13%
Other	9%	6%	8%	3%

Source: Psychiatric Morbidity among Prisoners in England and Wales.[34]

Childhood influences

Many prisoners have experienced various childhood influences relevant to their offending behaviour and health later in life. Compared to the wider community, a very high proportion have been in local authority care as children, spent time in an institution as a child or attended special school.

In relation to ethnicity and cultural background, it is of note that a significant minority of prisoners were born outside the UK (see **Table 8**).

Table 8: Childhood factors affecting prisoners.

Childhood factors	Males		Females	
	Remand	Sentenced	Remand	Sentenced
Born outside UK	11%	10%	17%	16%
In local authority care as a child	33%	26%	29%	25%
Spent time in an institution as a child	43%	35%	27%	25%
Attended special school	27%	23%	16%	11%

Source: Psychiatric Morbidity among Prisoners in England and Wales.[34]

Stressful life events affecting prisoners

The majority of prisoners have experienced three or more stressful life events at some time in their life. The commonest stressful events are bereavement, relationship breakdown, expulsion from school, running away from home, redundancy and money problems. Many prisoners (especially women prisoners) have experienced domestic violence (see **Table 9**).

Table 9: Types of stressful life events experienced by prisoners.

	Males		Females	
	Remand	Sentenced	Remand	Sentenced
Violence at home	28%	25%	51%	48%
Bullying	30%	30%	21%	26%
Sexual abuse	9%	8%	34%	31%
Serious illness/injury	18%	14%	16%	13%
Violence at work	6%	6%	3%	4%
Relationship breakdown	42%	45%	46%	46%
Death of close friend or relative	46%	47%	41%	47%
Death of parent or sibling	24%	29%	30%	30%
Death of spouse or child	6%	6%	17%	15%
Stillbirth of baby	8%	7%	10%	11%
Expelled from school	55%	49%	41%	33%
Running away from home	51%	47%	59%	50%
Homelessness	47%	37%	52%	34%
Serious money problems	55%	50%	50%	48%
Sacked or made redundant	44%	49%	26%	31%

Source: Psychiatric Morbidity among Prisoners in England and Wales.[34]

Adverse experiences in prison

Imprisonment entails a loss of privacy, living in a densely populated environment and isolation from everyday environments. Individual behaviour is restricted by institutional routines and low levels of stimulation can lead to boredom. This kind of environment has been shown to lead to maladaptive behaviour.[19]

Prisoners, in particular male prisoners, tend to organise themselves on the basis of a clearly defined hierarchy. At the top are professional criminals, in particular armed robbers, who may exercise considerable power in the prison. Most prisoners occupy a middle stratum. At the bottom are prisoners who are shunned by other inmates, often because of the nature of their offences (for example, sexual assaults on children). Because they are at risk of violence, these inmates are held in segregation units. The existence of this hierarchy has implications for the experience of victimisation.

Victimisation

Because of the nature of the prison population, it is not uncommon for prisoners to experience victimisation while imprisoned. The most common types of victimisation are threats of violence, theft of belongings and actual violence. Among women prisoners, unwanted sexual attention is also common (see **Table 10**).

Table 10: Prisoners' experience of victimisation while in prison.

Type of victimisation	Males		Females	
	Remand	Sentenced	Remand	Sentenced
Threatened with violence	22%	30%	13%	17%
Victim of violence	10%	14%	6%	8%
Belongings stolen	18%	30%	25%	36%
Intimidated to hand over belongings	6%	7%	4%	5%
Unwanted sexual attention	1%	4%	10%	11%
Victim of forced sexual attention	0%	1%	3%	1%

Source: Psychiatric Morbidity among Prisoners in England and Wales.[34]

3 Sub-categories

Sub-categories of health care needs are used to enable planners of health care services to recognise and manage the different requirements for services that sub-groups in a single population or disease group may present. There are a number of ways in which the health care needs of the prison population could be sub-categorised.

Categorisation by type of prison

The health care needs of establishments depend to some extent on their primary function, as this will affect the type and turnover of inmates and their general health problems. One method of sub-categorisation would be to categorise by the type of prison, i.e.:

- prisoners in Young Offender Institutions
- prisoners in women's prison
- prisoners in training establishments/open prisons
- prisoners in local prisons/remand centres
- prisoners in high security prisons.

Categorisation by type of health problem

Health care needs of prisoners could also usefully be sub-categorised by diseases and health problems. This is because many of the health problems found in a prison setting are common in all types of establishment regardless of age or sex. There are health problems that:

- are important in primary care outside of prisons: These include the commonest reasons for consultation in the (non-elderly) general population, for example epilepsy, asthma, diabetes, infectious diseases, dental health, minor and self-limiting diseases and neurotic disorders

- are risk factors for (or associated with) criminal behaviour: These health problems include mental disorders which appear to dominate the workload of the Prison Health Care Service despite official policy encouraging early diversion of mentally disordered offenders from custody to hospital, i.e. personality disorders, functional psychoses and substance misuse
- are associated with imprisonment: These are health problems that may arise because of imprisonment and include neurotic disorders, self-harm and suicide
- are a consequence of, or are associated with poverty: As described in the section 2, the unemployed and homeless are over-represented in the prison population. Therefore health problems that are more prevalent in these groups will be more prevalent in the prison population than in the community. These include epilepsy, asthma, ischaemic heart disease, dental health problems and infectious diseases
- are particularly difficult to handle in the prison environment: This particularly refers to maternity care.

Other sub-categories

The health care needs of prisoners could also be sub-categorised by length of stay (short, medium or long stay), category of prisoner (remand or sentenced) or the prisoners' external stability and support (i.e. access to family networks, social services, support groups etc.).

Sub-categorisation chosen for health care needs assessment of a prison population

In the sub-categories described above, a number of health problems could fit into more than one sub-category and would therefore make the process of data collection unnecessarily complicated. As a result of this the sub-categories that will be used through this report are based on type of health problem and, where necessary within these categories, the type of prisoner.

- Main sub-categories
  - minor and self-limiting illnesses
  - physical health problems
  - pregnancy and maternal health
  - mental disorders
  - substance misuse
  - health promotion.
- Secondary sub-categories:
  - age
  - sex
  - remand or sentenced.

Data on the prevalence of illness in the community is often available on the basis of age and sex. Where the prevalence of illness in the prison population has been estimated on the basis of its prevalence in the wider community, the figures have been broken down by age and sex. The sections of the document which are concerned with chronic physical illnesses generally report the age and sex specific prevalence and apply these to the average prison population.

Where the prevalence of illness in the prison population has been estimated from data collected from the prison population, inmates have generally been subdivided into male and female, and sentenced and remand prisoners. The sections of the document that are concerned with psychiatric illness generally report the prevalence of illness on the basis of whether prisoners are on remand or are sentenced.

4 Prevalence and incidence

One of the limitations of an approach to needs assessment which begins with the incidence and prevalence of health problems is that it can overlook the promotion of positive health. Because this section is concerned with identifying needs, it includes a sub-section on health promotion, although strictly speaking we cannot meaningfully talk about the prevalence of need for health promotion.

Health promotion

Health promotion is based on an assessment of needs and supported by evidence of effectiveness can help achieve three objectives. It can build the physical, mental and social health of prisoners and staff; prevent the deterioration of prisoners' health during or because of custody; and encourage prisoners to adopt healthy behaviours which can then be carried back into the community.[20]

The report of the Joint Working Group endorses the role of health promotion as a legitimate and integral part of the prison's activities. It states that: 'Good health care and health promotion in prisons should help enable individuals to function to their maximum potential on release, which may assist in reducing offending. It should also reduce morbidity in a high risk section of the general population with medium and long-term reduction in demands on the NHS.'[13]

Alongside the role of health care, five factors have been identified which affect the health of prisoners. These can all be considered under the heading of health promotion:

- the social demography of the prison population
- the built environment of the establishment
- the organisational culture in the prison
- relationships between prisoners, and with the external world
- specific medical issues facing the prison population.[21]

Health promotion needs of prisoners

It may be helpful to consider the health promotion needs of prisoners under three headings. Needs that all prisoners are likely to have, needs that many prisoners are likely to have and needs that some prisoners have. Examples each of these are illustrated in **Box 2**.

Box 2: Health promotion needs common to all prisoners.

All need:
- *advice on avoiding sexually transmitted diseases, HIV and hepatitis
- *hepatitis B immunisation
- advice on avoiding drug overdose on leaving prison (needed by all because staff cannot identify all at risk)
- protection against harm caused by smoking
- appropriate levels of physical activity
- a balanced diet
- adequate association time
- a meaningful occupation (work, education, artistic activity, physical education)
- contact with the outside world and help to maintain family ties.

*All prisoners can be considered to have these needs although not all prisoners are necessarily at high risk. This is because it is difficult for staff to identify all those who are at high risk, and because all prisoners need information in order to reduce fear and stigma.

Many need:
- psychological skills training
  - cognitive behavioural skills training
  - activities to improve self-esteem
  - thinking skills
  - anger management
- practical skills training
  - job search skills
  - parenting education
  - advice on selection and cooking of food
- health-related education
  - dietary advice, advice on exercise and smoking
- specific health promotion interventions
  - access to listeners or equivalent
  - support to give up drugs, alcohol or smoking.

Some need:
- immunisation against TB, pneumococcus or influenza
- advice on specific conditions, e.g. minor illnesses, diabetes, epilepsy, asthma, the menopause, sickle-cell disease
- access to equivalent cancer prevention and early detection advice and services.

Minor illness

The term 'minor illnesses' is used here to describe self-limiting conditions which occur frequently in the community. They include musculo-skeletal problems (such as minor injuries, back and neck pain), respiratory infections (such as coughs, colds and sore throats), gastro-intestinal complaints (such as indigestion, constipation and diarrhoea), neurological complaints (such as tension headaches and migraine), allergies (such as hayfever) and skin conditions (such as dermatitis, eczema and psoriasis).

In the community, respiratory conditions, injuries, infectious diseases and skin disorders are the most common reasons for consultations with general practitioners among males aged 16–44. In women of this age, by far the most common reasons for consultation are for preventive or other health-related reasons. This principally means services such as family planning and pregnancy care but also includes routine physical examination and cervical screening. After this, respiratory conditions, genito-urinary disorders, infectious diseases and skin conditions are the most common reasons for consultation. For most conditions, women in this age group consult a general practitioner more often than men. This information originates from the *Morbidity Statistics from General Practice Fourth National Study*[22] and is illustrated in **Table 11**, **Table 12** and **Table 13**.

Table 11: Principal reasons for GP consultation among persons in the community (adjusted to age of prison population).

Reason for consultation (ICD category)	Males		Females	
	Percentage of consultations	Consultations per person year	Percentage of consultations	Consultations per person year
Infectious and parasitic diseases	6%	0.1	6%	0.3
Neoplasms	1%	0.0	1%	0.0
Endocrine and metabolic	2%	0.0	1%	0.1
Blood diseases	0%	0.0	0%	0.0
Mental disorders	7%	0.1	6%	0.2
Neurological disorders	7%	0.1	5%	0.2
Circulatory disorders	3%	0.1	2%	0.1
Respiratory disorders	19%	0.4	14%	0.6
Digestive disorders	5%	0.1	3%	0.1
Genito-urinary disorders	2%	0.0	11%	0.5
Pregnancy-related	0%	0.0	2%	0.1
Skin disorders	9%	0.2	6%	0.3
Musculo-skeletal disorders	10%	0.2	6%	0.3
Congenital abnormalities	0%	0.0	0%	0.0
Perinatal conditions	0%	0.0	0%	0.0
Ill-defined symptoms	6%	0.1	6%	0.2
Injury and poisoning	11%	0.2	4%	0.2
Other (medical examination, maternity care, screening, contraception)	11%	0.2	26%	1.1
Total consultations per person year	100%	1.98	100%	4.30

Source: Morbidity Statistics from General Practice. Fourth national study, 1991–1992.[22]

Table 12: Commonest reasons for consultation by category (males, adjusted to age of prison population).

Reason for consultation (diagnosis)	Persons (per 10 000) who consult during the course of a year
Infectious and parasitic diseases	
Ill-defined intestinal infections (009)	238
Dermatophytosis (110)	188
Other diseases due to viruses and Chlamydiae (078)	158
Mental disorders	
Neurotic disorders (300)	228
Diseases of the nervous system and sense organs	
Disorders of external ear (380)	344
Disorders of conjunctiva (372)	181
Nonsuppurative otitis media and Eustachian tube disorders (381)	120
Diseases of the circulatory system	
Essential hypertension (401)	139
Diseases of the respiratory system	
Acute bronchitis and bronchiolitis (466)	397
Acute upper respiratory infections of multiple or unspecified site (465)	370
Acute pharyngitis (462)	339
Asthma (493)	305
Acute tonsillitis (463)	300
Allergic rhinitis (477)	288
Acute sinusitis (461)	195
Influenza (487)	191
Common cold (460)	115
Diseases of the digestive system	
Disorders of function of stomach (536)	126
Diseases of skin and subcutaneous tissue	
Diseases of sebaceous glands (706)	279
Atopic dermatitis and related conditions (691)	140
Contact dermatitis and other eczema (692)	136
Diseases of the musculo-skeletal system and connective tissue	
Other and unspecified disorders of back (724)	345
Other and unspecified disorder of joint (719)	196
Other disorders of soft tissues (729)	118
Symptoms, signs and ill-defined conditions	
Symptoms involving respiratory system and other chest symptoms (786)	201
Other symptoms involving abdomen and pelvis (789)	144
General symptoms (780)	140
Symptoms involving head and neck (784)	121
Injury and poisoning	
Sprains and strains of other and unspecified parts of the back (847)	234
Certain adverse effects not elsewhere classified (995)	204
Sprains and strains of knee and leg (844)	116
Sprains and strains of ankle and foot (845)	103

Table 12: Commonest reasons for consultation by category (males, adjusted to age of prison population).

Reason for consultation (diagnosis)	Persons (per 10 000) who consult during the course of a year
Supplementary classification: factors influencing health status and contact with health services	
Encounters for administrative purposes (V68)	641
Need for prophylactic vaccination and inoculation against bacterial diseases (V03)	387
Need for prophylactic vaccination and inoculation against certain viral diseases (V04)	272
General medical examination (V70)	262
Special screening for cardiovascular, respiratory and genito-urinary diseases (V81)	181
Special screening for endocrine, nutritional, metabolic and immunity disorders (V77)	115

Source: Morbidity Statistics from General Practice. Fourth national study, 1991–1992.[22]

Table 13: Commonest reasons for consultation by category (females, adjusted to age of prison population).

Commonest reasons for consultation (over 250 only): in categories and ranked	Persons (per 10 000) who consult during the course of a year
Infectious and parasitic diseases	
Candidiasis (112)	823
Ill-defined intestinal infections (009)	360
Endocrine, nutritional and metabolic disorders and immunity disorders	
Obesity and other hyperalimentation (278)	150
Mental disorders	
Neurotic disorders (300)	579
Diseases of the nervous system and sense organs	
Disorders of external ear (380)	356
Disorders of conjunctiva (372)	326
Diseases of the respiratory system	
Acute upper respiratory infections of multiple or unspecified site (465)	688
Acute bronchitis and bronchiolitis (466)	606
Acute pharyngitis (462)	603
Acute tonsillitis (463)	515
Acute sinusitis (461)	455
Allergic rhinitis (477)	407
Asthma (493)	374
Influenza (487)	257
Diseases of the digestive system	
Functional digestive disorders not elsewhere classified (564)	301
Diseases of the genito-urinary system	
Disorders of menstruation and other abnormal bleeding from female genital tract (626)	822
Pain and other symptoms associated with female genital organs (625)	492
Other disorders of urethra and urinary tract (599)	466

Table 13: Continued.

Commonest reasons for consultation (over 250 only): in categories and ranked	Persons (per 10 000) who consult during the course of a year
Diseases of skin and subcutaneous tissue	
Diseases of sebaceous glands (706)	351
Contact dermatitis and other eczema (692)	279
Atopic dermatitis and related conditions (691)	271
Diseases of the musculo-skeletal system and connective tissue	
Other and unspecified disorders of back (724)	454
Other and unspecified disorder of joint (719)	256
Symptoms, signs and ill defined conditions	
Other symptoms involving abdomen and pelvis (789)	401
General symptoms (780)	310
Symptoms involving respiratory system and other chest symptoms (786)	270
Injury and poisoning	
Certain adverse effects not elsewhere classified (995)	323
Supplementary classification of factors influencing health status and contact with health services	
Contraceptive management (V25)	3,002
Special screening for malignant neoplasms (V76)	1,259
Normal pregnancy (V22)	610
Encounters for administrative purposes (V68)	605
Need for prophylactic vaccination and inoculation against bacterial diseases (V03)	524
General medical examination (V70)	465
Postpartum care and examination (V24)	414
Need for prophylactic vaccination and inoculation against certain viral diseases (V04)	384
Special screening for cardiovascular, respiratory and genito-urinary diseases (V81)	285

Source: Morbidity Statistics from General Practice. Fourth national study, 1991–1992.[22]

Prevalence of minor illness in the prison population

The prevalence of minor illnesses in the prison population is likely to mirror the prevalence in the equivalent population in the community. Minor illnesses account for the bulk of consultations in community general practice and are likely to account for the bulk of consultations in the prison population. The OPCS survey of sentenced male prisoners[23] indicated that about one in ten had suffered from skin diseases, respiratory problems and allergies in the past year (see **Table 14**).

Table 14: Conditions reported as occurring within the past 12 months (sentenced male prisoners).

Condition	Age band				
	16–24	25–34	35–44	45+	Total
Skin diseases	8%	14%	11%	12%	12%
Respiratory (excluding asthma)	9%	10%	8%	17%	10%
Asthma	15%	10%	4%	10%	10%
Allergies	7%	5%	9%	7%	7%

Source: Survey of the Physical Health of Prisoners 1994: a survey of sentenced males.[23]

In a survey of women prisoners[24] (n=214), 48% reported menstrual complaints, 47% anxiety and depression, 45% musculo-skeletal complaints and 30% reported respiratory problems. A high proportion of women also reported minor conditions in the two weeks prior to the survey (see **Table 15**).

Table 15: Minor illnesses reported by women prisoners in the previous two weeks.

Mainly psychological or neurological symptoms	Percentage (n)	Mainly dermatological symptoms	Percentage (n)
Difficulty sleeping	64% (136)	Skin problems	41% (88)
Feeling tired	62% (133)		
Headache	57% (121)		

Mainly gastro-intestinal symptoms	Percentage (n)	Mainly respiratory or infectious symptoms	Percentage (n)
No appetite/off food	30% (64)	Persistent cold/flu	34% (73)
Constipation	26% (55)	Persistent cough	26% (55)
Diarrhoea or sickness	15% (33)	Sore throat	22% (46)
		High temperature	8% (17)

Source: Smith C, Assessing health needs in women's prisons.[24]

Physical health problems

A number of surveys, described below, indicate that, in general, the physical health of prisoners is worse than that of people of equivalent age in the general population.

Adult male prisoners

A survey of the physical health of sentenced male prisoners was carried out on a representative sample of sentenced prisoners in England and Wales in 1994.[23] Three-fifths of men rated their health as good or very good but 48% said they had a long-standing illness or disability. The most commonly reported long-standing conditions and a comparison between adult men aged 18–49 in the general population are listed in **Table 16**. Prisoners aged 18–49 were more likely than men of equivalent age in the general population to report a long-standing illness or disability. They were also more likely to have consulted a doctor in the last two weeks and to be taking prescribed medicines.

The survey also indicated that prisoners on average had a lower body mass index than men in the general population. Just over one-third of prisoners were classed as overweight or obese compared with just over a half of men of equivalent age in the general population.

Young prisoners

In a survey of the physical health of young prisoners (aged 16–24), 39% reported long-standing illness or disability, 21% reported respiratory problems (asthma in 15%) and 10% reported musculo-skeletal problems.[14] Many young prisoners were receiving treatment: 26% were taking medicines, an average of 1.6 medications each. Over half (55%) of all young prisoners had consulted their GP during the six months immediately prior to arrest. A separate survey of 500 young offenders[25] found that on entering prison 17% (n=82) of the respondents said they were currently receiving medical treatment. This included 9% who

Table 16: Comparison of the physical health of prisoners with the general population.

Condition group	Percentage reporting each condition	
	Prisoners (n=925)	General population (n=4407)
Musculo-skeletal complaints	16%	12%
Respiratory conditions	15%	8%
Digestive system	5%	3%
Nervous system	5%	3%
Mental disorders	5%	1%
Skin complaints	3%	1%

Source: Survey of the Physical Health of Prisoners 1994: a survey of sentenced males.[23]

were prescribed inhalers for asthma, 7% who were taking a short course of specific treatment (antibiotics) and 1% who were on long-term medical treatment for conditions such as diabetes, epilepsy and depression.

Women prisoners

Women prisoners have been found to report higher rates of various physical and psychological problems than women in the general population. These include asthma, epilepsy, high blood pressure, anxiety and depression, stomach complaints, period and menopausal problems, sight and hearing difficulties, and kidney and bladder problems.[26] A survey of the health care needs of women in prisons[24] indicated that 60% rated their own health as fair, poor or very poor.

Epilepsy

If the incidence and prevalence of epilepsy in the community is similar to that in prison inmates, we would expect about 0.4% of the prison population to suffer from epilepsy and 0.13% to become epileptic while in prison. **Table 17** shows the effects of applying these estimates to the prison population. Overall this implies that there would be about 250 prisoners with chronic epilepsy and 80 or 90 new epileptics each year.

Table 17: Estimated number of epileptics in the prison population based on community prevalence.

Age	Male prisoners					Female prisoners				
	Incidence	Prevalence	Prisoners	New	Chronic	Incidence	Prevalence	Prisoners	New	Chronic
16 to 24	0.19%	0.45%	20,583	39	93	0.15%	0.45%	697	1	3
25 to 44	0.09%	0.36%	33,736	30	121	0.11%	0.38%	1,831	2	7
45 to 64	0.10%	0.40%	6,231	6	25	0.08%	0.36%	277	0	1
65 to 74	0.16%	0.38%	396	1	2	0.16%	0.43%	7	0	0
75 to 84	0.18%	0.46%	58	0	0	0.16%	0.40%	0	0	0
85+	0.12%	0.30%	2	0	0	0.14%	0.35%	0	0	0
Total	0.13%	0.39%	61,006	76	241	0.01%	0.02%	2,812	3	11

Source: Morbidity Statistics from General Practice. Fourth national study, 1991–1992.[22]
Prison population: Home Office statistics for 31 December 1998.

However, direct estimates of the prevalence of epilepsy among prisoners are somewhat higher. In 1969, Gunn observed a prevalence of epilepsy among male British prisoners almost twice as high as in the general population.[27] These findings have been confirmed in subsequent surveys.[28] Gunn's figures (see **Table 18**) suggest that the prevalence of epilepsy in the prison population is almost twice that in the community, i.e., on 31 December 1998 an estimated 530 prison inmates (0.8% of prisoners) would have had epilepsy.

Table 18: Estimated number of epileptics in the prison population: based on prison estimate.

Age	Male prisoners			Female prisoners**		
	Prevalence	Prisoners	Numbers	Prevalence	Prisoners	Numbers
15–24	1.10%	20,583	226	1.10%	951	10
25–34	0.70%	23,015	161	0.70%	1,191	8
35–44	0.60%	10,721	64	0.60%	640	4
45–64*	0.80%	6,687	53	0.80%	284	2
Total	0.83%	61,006	505	0.81%	3,066	25

Source: Adapted from Gunn J.C. The prevalence of epilepsy among prisoners. *Proceedings of the Royal Society of Medicine* 1969; **62**: 60–3.
Prison population: Home Office statistics for 31 December 1998. * Includes those over 64. ** Male prevalence rates have been applied to female prisoners.

A direct estimate of the prevalence of epilepsy in male sentenced prisoners can also be made from the OPCS survey of the physical health of prisoners.[23] The survey recorded the percentage of male sentenced prisoners reporting 'fits' in the past 12 months (see **Table 19**). This is a broad case definition – not everyone who has a fit is epileptic – but the overall prevalence was 2%, which is closer to Gunn's estimate of the prevalence of epilepsy than estimates based on the general population.

Table 19: Percentage of male sentenced prisoners reporting 'fits' in the past 12 months.

Age	Percentage reporting 'fits' in past 12 months
15 to 24	1%
25 to 34	4%
35 to 44	1%
≥45	–
Total	2%

Source: Survey of the Physical Health of Prisoners 1994: a survey of sentenced males.[23]

Asthma

Table 20 shows the age-specific prevalence of wheezing in the past year, doctor-diagnosed asthma and treated asthma in the general population. The figures are based on the *Health Survey for England 1996*[29] and *Key Health Statistics from General Practice 1996*.[30] The table also shows the expected prevalence of asthma in the prison population. Asthma tends to be more common in the young. As the prison population is predominantly young, the overall prevalence of asthma is higher than that of the general population. Based on these figures, 13% of male and 14% of female prisoners have doctor-diagnosed asthma. Just under half of these will be receiving treatment; 5% and 6% respectively.

Table 20: Age-specific prevalence of wheezing in the past year, doctor-diagnosed asthma and treated asthma in the community and expected prevalence in the prison population.

Age	Males				Females			
	Prison population	Wheezing in the past year*	Diagnosed asthma*	Treated asthma[†]	Prison population	Wheezing in the past year*	Diagnosed asthma*	Treated asthma[†]
16–24	20,583	20%	19%	7%	951	23%	17%	8%
25–34	23,015	19%	12%	5%	1,191	19%	14%	6%
35–44	10,721	18%	11%	4%	640	17%	12%	5%
45+	6,687	19%	8%	4%	284	19%	11%	6%
Total prevalence in the prison population	61,006	19%	14%	5%	3,066	20%	14%	6%

Source: *Health Survey for England 1996.*[29] † *Key Health Statistics from General Practice 1996.*[30] (Prison population derived from Home Office statistics for 31 December 1998. NB: figures have been rounded to the nearest percentage point.)

In the information presented in **Table 20**, in the 16–24 year old age group the prevalence of diagnosed asthma was similar to the prevalence of wheezing symptoms, particularly for males. However, in the older age groups the prevalence of diagnosed asthma was much less than the prevalence of wheezing. The prevalence of wheezing recorded in the *Health Survey for England 1996*[29] showed a strong social-class gradient: 15% and 27% of men in socio-economic classes I and V respectively. The prevalence of diagnosed asthma did not show this social-class gradient: 13% and 11% of men in socio-economic classes I and V respectively. This suggests that asthma is under-diagnosed in the social classes from which the prison population is drawn. Since about one-fifth of prisoners will have experienced wheezing symptoms in the past year. It is likely that some of these have unrecognised asthma.

Diabetes

Table 21 shows the estimated prevalence of diabetes in the prison population. The figures have been extrapolated from the age-specific prevalence of diabetes in community populations. Based on these data we can expect diabetes to affect between 0.6% and 0.8% of the prison population. Because the prison population is predominantly young, insulin-dependent diabetes mellitus (IDDM) is much more common than non-insulin-dependent diabetes mellitus (NIDDM).

Table 21: The age-specific prevalence of diabetes in the community and the estimated prevalence in the prison population.

Age	Male			Female		
	Prison population	IDDM prevalence	NIDDM prevalence	Prison population	IDDM prevalence	NIDDM prevalence
16–24	20,583	0.3%	0.0%	951	0.3%	0.0%
25–34	23,015	0.5%	0.1%	1,191	0.4%	0.1%
35–44	10,721	0.6%	0.3%	640	0.5%	0.2%
45–54	4,506	0.6%	1.0%	221	0.5%	0.7%
55–64	1,725	0.9%	2.8%	56	0.8%	2.1%
>64	456	1.1%	4.2%	7	0.9%	3.1%
Total prevalence in the prison population	61,006	0.5%	0.3%	3,066	0.4%	0.2%

Source: Key Health Statistics from General Practice 1996.[30] Prison population: Home Office statistics for 31 December 1998.

There are few direct estimates of the prevalence of diabetes in prison. In one male prison, 35% of an eligible population of inmates attended a Well Man Clinic.[31] Attendees ranged in age from 21 to 62 (mean 32 years). Eight percent (95% CI 4.5–11.1%) were found to be diabetic, well above the expected prevalence in this age group. Even if it is assumed that all diabetic inmates in the eligible population selectively attended this clinic, this implies a prevalence of 2.7% (95% CI 1.6–3.9%). If this figure is representative of the whole prison population, it implies that diagnosed diabetes is two to eight times as common in prison inmates as in the community.

Ischaemic heart disease and cardiovascular risk factors

Prisoners with ischaemic heart disease

Patients with pre-existing cardiovascular (heart disease) or cerebrovascular disease (strokes) are at very high risk of further vascular events. Because of this they are the highest priority in the management of cardiovascular disease and its risk factors.

The prevalence of ischaemic heart disease is very dependent on the age of the population. **Table 22** shows the age-specific prevalence of ischaemic heart disease in the general population.[32] Based on these figures about 0.5% of male inmates and 0.3% of female inmates are likely to suffer from ischaemic heart disease.

However, because inmates are drawn largely from lower social classes, the above may be an underestimate. Heart disease is about half as common again among socio-economic class V as among the general population.[33] The adjusted prevalence estimate is shown in **Table 22**.

Table 22: Age-specific prevalence of ischaemic heart disease in the 1994 Health Survey for England.

Age band	Based on general population		Adjusted for social class of prisoners	
	Men	Women	Men	Women
16–24	0.0%	0.2%	0.0%	0.3%
25–34	0.3%	0.1%	0.5%	0.2%
35–44	0.5%	0.3%	0.8%	0.5%
45–54	3.0%	2.3%	4.5%	3.5%
55–64	10.3%	5.9%	15.5%	8.9%
Total prevalence in the prison population	0.5%	0.3%	0.7%	0.5%

Source: 1994 Health Survey for England.

Smoking

Smoking is highly prevalent among the prison population. Over three-quarters of all prisoners smoke and over half are moderate or heavy smokers[34] (see **Table 23**).

Table 23: Prevalence of smoking among the prison population.

Smoking behaviour	Male (%)		Female (%)	
	Remand	Sentenced	Remand	Sentenced
Heavy smoker	31	24	41	34
Moderate smoker	36	34	31	32
Light smoker	18	19	11	15
All smokers	85	77	82	82
Ex or non-smoker	15	23	18	18

Source: Psychiatric Morbidity among Prisoners in England and Wales.[34]

Raised blood pressure and raised serum cholesterol

The risk of heart disease increases with blood pressure and with cholesterol levels. However, risk of heart disease is also affected by a number of other factors, principally age and sex. Because of this it is not helpful simply to estimate the numbers of persons with raised blood pressure or raised cholesterol. Management of raised cholesterol and raised blood pressure are considered later in this document.

Infectious diseases

Bloodborne viruses: HIV, hepatitis B and hepatitis C

In 1997, a survey of eight prisons was carried out by the Public Health Laboratory Service and the Prison Service Directorate of Health Care, to find out about the prevalence of bloodborne virus infections and risk factors for bloodborne virus infections.[35] The total sample size was 3942 prisoners, 83% of those asked to participate.

Prevalence of risk factors

The survey found that about one in four adult prisoners have engaged in activities likely to put them at risk of infection with HIV, hepatitis B or hepatitis C. **Figure 9** shows the proportion who have injected drugs. One quarter of prisoners have injected drugs and more than half of these have done so recently: a significant minority have shared needles. These findings have been confirmed in a more recent prison-based survey.[36]

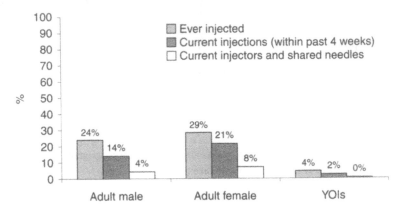

Source: Prevalence of HIV in England and Wales in 1997: Annual Report of the Unlinked Anonymous Prevalence Monitoring Programme.[35]

Figure 9: Injecting drug behaviour among the prison population in 1997.

High proportions of prisoners also engage in risky sexual behaviour. Over half of all male prisoners reported two or more sexual partners in the past year but had not consistently used condoms to reduce risk of infection (see **Figure 10**). Seventeen per cent of females and 15% of males had a sexually transmitted disease.

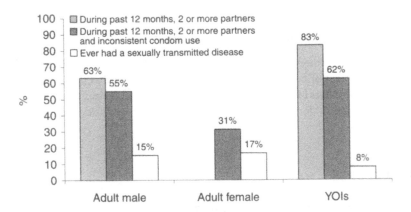

Source: Prevalence of HIV in England and Wales in 1997: Annual Report of the Unlinked Anonymous Prevalence Monitoring Programme.[35]

Figure 10: Sexual behaviour and risk factors for sexually transmitted diseases in the prison population in 1997.

A previous survey of behaviours, which might put prisoners at risk of HIV infection, was conducted among 1009 adult prisoners in 13 prisons in England and Wales.[37] This portrayed a similar situation, indicating that the male prison population showed higher levels of drug misuse and injecting behaviour than the general population and that there was a relationship between this behaviour and higher levels of criminal behaviour. Prisoners who continued to inject in prison were again likely to share needles. Male prisoners also showed more risky sexual behaviour and were more likely to have had sexual contact with women who were at increased risk of HIV, such as prostitutes. This survey suggested that between 1.6% and 3.4% of the adult male prison population engaged in homosexual activity.

More recent evidence confirms that risky behaviour is common among inmates of Young Offender Institutions: 20% of attendees at a genito-urinary clinic reported intravenous drug misuse and 2% were hepatitis C positive. These prevalences are much more frequent than in genito-urinary clinic attendees in the community.[38]

Prevalence of bloodborne viral infections

In 1997, about one in ten prisoners had antibodies to hepatitis B and hepatitis C (see **Figure 11**). This indicates previous exposure to infection. It also suggests that other inmates who share injecting equipment with these prisoners, their sexual partners within and outside of prison, and persons (including health care staff and prison officers) who come into contact with their blood or saliva are at risk of infection.

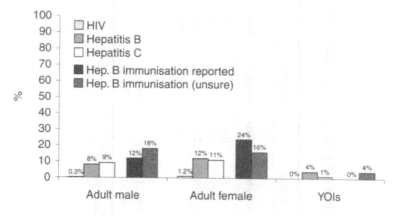

Source: *Prevalence of HIV in England and Wales in 1997: Annual Report of the Unlinked Anonymous Prevalence Monitoring Programme.*[35]

Figure 11: The prevalence of HIV, hepatitis B & C infection and immunisation against hepatitis B, among prisoners in 1997.

The numbers of new cases of acute and chronic viral hepatitis and HIV infection in the prison population between 1993/94 and 1997/98 are listed in **Table 24**.

Table 24: New cases of infectious diseases identified in the prison population: numbers and rate per 1000 prisoner years (1993/94 to 1997/98).

	1993/94		1994/95		1995/96		1996/97		1997/98		Average on 31 March 1998	
	Number	Rate	Number	Rate	Number	Rate	Number	Rate	Number	Rate	Number	Rate
Tuberculosis cases	32	0.7	31	0.6	29	0.6	22	0.4	50	0.8	6	–
Hepatitis B cases	146	3.2	175	3.5	202	3.9	161	2.8	246	3.9	70	–
Hepatitis C cases	0	0.0	102	2.1	543	10.5	760	13.4	916	14.6	317	–
HIV +ve	–	–	–	–	62	1.2	123	2.2	177	2.8	49	–
HIV +ve CD4 count <250	–	–	–	–	–	–	–	–	28	0.4	4	–
Total new receptions	–		196,212		198,441		200,500		233,202			
ADP	45,827		49,308		51,470		56,671		62,584			

Source: Annual Report of the Director of Health Care 1997–98.[48]

Sexually transmitted diseases

There are no direct estimates of the prevalence of other sexually transmitted diseases in the UK prison population. It is possible to make an indirect estimate of the prevalence from national data sources. All genito-urinary medicine (GUM) clinics in England submit KC60 statistical returns to the HIV & STD Division of the Public Health Laboratory Service. New diagnoses of a number of sexually transmitted conditions in 1998 are reported in **Table 25**. While these form a basis for estimates of the incidence of sexually transmitted diseases in the prison population, it is important to recognise that prisoners are likely to have a higher incidence of these infections than the general population.

Sexually transmitted diseases are more common in young people. In 1998, diagnoses of infectious syphilis, uncomplicated gonorrhoea, uncomplicated chlamydia, genital herpes and genital warts were highest among those aged 25–34 years in males. In females diagnoses of uncomplicated gonorrhoea were highest in 16–19 year olds, of uncomplicated chlamydia and first attack genital warts in 20–24 year olds, and of infectious syphilis and genital herpes in 25–34 year olds.

Sexually transmitted diseases (STDs) diagnosed at GUM clinics represent only the tip of the iceberg of sexually transmitted infections. The KC60 returns provide an estimate of the incidence and prevalence of symptomatic disease, but provide little information on the population incidence and prevalence of total infection (asymptomatic and symptomatic).[39] A very large proportion of sexually transmitted infections remain undiagnosed and asymptomatic – as many as 70% of women with genital chlamydial infection are asymptomatic,[40] as are 60% of cases of genital herpes.[41]

Tuberculosis

Tuberculosis is an important illness for a number of reasons. First, despite being treatable it has a significant mortality. Second, untreated cases may spread the illness to others including prison staff. Indeed, the British Thoracic Society recommends that all new prison staff are screened for tuberculosis.[42] Third, treatment is complicated by the requirement that patients take medications for many months. Interrupted courses of treatment may lead to the emergence of drug-resistant tuberculosis.

In the UK tuberculosis is more common among deprived groups[43] and is particularly common among the homeless. In London, 1.5% of residents in a shelter for the homeless were found to have tuberculosis following screening.[44] Tuberculosis is also more prevalent among immigrants, in particular those who have recently arrived in this country.[45] Since the socio-economic groups at risk of tuberculosis are represented in the prison population, prisoners are likely to be at risk of tuberculosis. In addition, since tuberculosis is transmitted from person to person by inhalation of infectious material, the crowded conditions found in prisons lend themselves to spread of the disease.

In the USA tuberculosis is highly prevalent in the prison population and as a result discharged prisoners have been known to spread tuberculosis to the wider community. Moreover, there is evidence that prison staff in the USA and Canada suffer from a higher prevalence of tuberculosis than the wider community, probably because they are exposed to infected prisoners.[46,47]

In view of this it seems encouraging that in England and Wales the reported prevalence of active tuberculosis in prisons to date remains low. Nevertheless, tuberculosis is more common in the prison population than in the wider community. Fifty new cases of tuberculosis were reported in prisoners in England and Wales from April 1997 to March 1998.[48] This is about 8 cases per 10 000 ADP or 2 cases per 10 000 new receptions in custody. In the general population, in the UK, there are about 6000 annual notifications. This is equivalent to 1.4 and 1.0 cases per 10 000 males and females. Adjusted to the prison population's age structure, the figures are 1.4 and 1.2 per 10 000 male and female prisoners respectively.

It is possible that not all cases of tuberculosis are detected among the prison population. Given that at least 5% of the prison population are homeless, a prevalence rate of 1.5% among the homeless implies that

Table 25: Numbers and rates of new diagnoses of selected sexually transmitted infections, by sex and age, England, 1998.

Condition	Infectious syphilis				Uncomplicated gonorrhoea				Uncomplicated chlamydia				Herpes simplex (first attack)				Genital warts (first attack)			
	Male		Female		All Males		Female		Male		Female		Male		Female		Male		Female	
Age/Sex																				
<16	0	0.0	0	0.0	36	0.1	155	0.3	53	0.1	552	1.1	11	0.0	93	0.2	91	0.2	425	0.8
16–19	6	0.1	4	0.0	982	7.9	1,435	12.2	2,335	18.7	8,290	70.5	313	2.5	1,798	15.3	2,718	21.8	8,284	70.5
20–24	4	0.0	13	0.1	2,094	10.8	1,202	6.5	6,136	31.7	8,997	49.0	1,197	6.2	2,602	14.2	100,076	52.1	9,909	53.9
25–34	37	0.1	26	0.1	3,475	8.3	930	2.3	7,860	18.8	5,945	14.7	2,697	6.4	3,469	8.6	12,705	30.4	7,527	18.7
35–44	22	0.1	4	0.0	1,327	3.8	241	0.7	2,083	6.0	1,123	3.3	1,255	3.6	1,088	3.2	3,691	10.7	1,961	5.7
45+	14	0.0	2	0.0	448	0.5	75	0.1	576	0.6	229	0.2	612	0.7	570	0.5	1,625	1.8	964	0.9
Total	83		49		8,362		4,038		19,043		25,136		6,085		9,620		30,906		29,070	

Source: PHLS (1999) Sexually transmitted infections. www.phls.co.uk/facts/std-t01.htm

among formerly homeless prisoners alone there are likely to be about 41 cases of tuberculosis at any one time. It also implies that 150 cases are likely to pass through prison a year. (These figures are estimated as follows: 5% of an ADP of 55 000 is 2750 homeless prisoners; 1.5% of this is 41. Similarly 5% of 200 000 new receptions is 10 000 new homeless prisoners; 1.5% of this is 150.)

Dental health

A number of measures are used to assess oral health. One of these is the DMFT index. This is simply a count of the total number of teeth which are decayed, missing or filled. Other key measures include the number of sound teeth (teeth which have no evidence of decay) and the number of standing teeth (at least a root is present). The prison population is drawn disproportionately from the lower socio-economic classes,[49] and it is therefore likely that the dental health of social classes IV and V most closely reflects that of the prison population.

The Office of Population Censuses and Surveys carries out a dental health survey every ten years. **Table 26** illustrates the proportion of adults in social classes IV and V in the 1988 survey[50] who are dentate. Prisoners are predominantly young adults and very few young adults are edentulous.

Table 26: Proportion of adults who are dentate in social classes IV and V.

Age	Males	Females
16–24	100%	100%
25–34	99%	93%
35–44	98%	91%
45–54	88%	74%
55–64	59%	49%
65–74	35%	27%
75+	–	7%

Source: Adult Dental Health 1988: United Kingdom.[50]

Table 27 illustrates a number of indicators of the dental health of adults in social classes IV and V. Significant numbers of adults in these social classes have substantial numbers of filled, decayed or unsound teeth.

In the survey of adult dental health, the prevalence of decayed or unsound teeth were estimated on the basis of visual examination. The prevalence following more thorough examination is likely to be higher. These figures are therefore likely to indicate the minimum number of persons who are in need of dental services. Overall the prevalence of decayed teeth is similar at all ages, with an average of one decayed or unsound tooth per adult. However, decayed or unsound teeth are unevenly distributed, with just over half of the population having none and a small minority having more than five (see **Table 28**).

Table 27: Indicators of the dental health of adults in social classes IV and V.

Age	Proportion of dentate adults in social classes IV and V with:			
	≥21 standing teeth	≥18 sound teeth	≥12 filled teeth	no decayed or unsound teeth
16–24	99%	80%	5%	57%
25–34	95%	38%	32%	42%
35–44	75%	28%	24%	41%
45–54	53%	14%	22%	46%
55–64	45%	26%	9%	54%
65+	25%	13%	5%	32%

Source: Adult Dental Health 1988: United Kingdom.[50]

Table 28: Numbers of decayed or unsound teeth among dentate adults: by age.

Age	Numbers of decayed or unsound teeth among dentate adults			
	0	1–5	>5	Mean
16–24	62%	35%	3%	0.9
25–34	57%	40%	4%	1.1
35–44	55%	42%	3%	1.0
45–54	50%	48%	3%	1.1
55+	54%	42%	4%	1.1

Source: Adult Dental Health 1988: United Kingdom.[50]

However, the adult dental health survey found the prevalence of decayed or unsound teeth to be higher in the lower social classes[50] (see **Table 29**).

Table 29: Numbers of decayed or unsound teeth among dentate adults in social classes IV and V.

Social class	Numbers of decayed or unsound teeth among dentate adults			
	0	1–5	>5	Mean
IV & V	47%	47%	· 6%	1.5

Source: Adult Dental Health 1988: United Kingdom.[50]

A survey of the dental health and attitudes of the Scottish prison population was commissioned by the Scottish Executive Health Department in 2002. The aim of the survey was to provide accurate and up-to-date information on the dental health of the Scottish prison population. The survey consisted of a structured interview followed by dental examinations of a random sample of the Scottish prison population. The survey protocol followed the 1998 UK Adult Dental Health Survey methodology, thus allowing direct comparison to the Scottish population. A total of 559 prisoners participated in the survey, a 75% response rate. The results showed that on average the prison population had more decayed but fewer filled teeth than the Scottish population. The severity of tooth decay was also considerably worse in the prison population, especially for female prisoners. Reported length of stay data showed that it took two years to improve the dental health of prisoners. No other more serious pathology (e.g. suspected malignancy) was found in any subject.[51]

Oral health of prisoners outside of the UK

A survey of the oral health of prisoners in a single prison in USA showed their dental health to be poor. The mean DMFT indices were 12.9, 16.4 and 22.1 for inmates aged respectively 20 to 34, 35 to 44 and 45 and older.[52] However, as patterns of oral health are rather different in the USA, it is difficult to draw conclusions for the UK prison population.

Special senses and disability

Disability

A survey of the number of prisoners known to have a physical disability was carried out in all 129 UK prisons (n=56 151) in July 1996 (Ingram L, Home Office internal report, 1997). In all, 118 prisons responded. It was estimated that approximately 0.6% (n=324) of the prison population were known to have a disability. Over 70% of prisoners known to have a disability had mobility problems, either alone or in combination with other problems (see **Figure 12**). About 17% were known to have hearing problems and 20% problems with personal care among their disabilities. As the survey only identified prisoners whose disabilities were known, it is therefore likely to have underestimated less visible impairments such as hearing problems. The projected number of prisoners with a hearing problem based on the total population on 28th November 1997 was 54. More recent information indicates that there are at least 70–100 deaf prisoners and many more who have a serious hearing difficulty which remains undetected.[53]

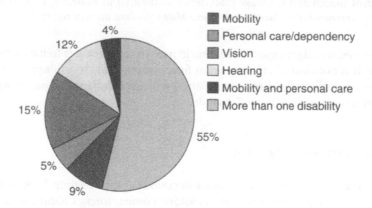

Source: Ingram L (1997) Home Office internal report, 1997.

Figure 12: Nature of prisoners' disabilities.

Speech, language and communication problems

The ability to communicate is important for three related reasons. First, it is essential for normal social functioning. Second, other types of health care are less likely to be effective if communication is impaired. This applies to simple interventions such as advice and reassurance as much as more complex interventions which rely on communication, such as cognitive therapy. Third, communication problems may be linked to some kinds of offending behaviour. Information on the prevalence of speech and language problems is far from complete.

The most comprehensive prevalence data comes from a survey of 20 years' experience in Polmont YOI in Scotland.[54] The majority of those serving sentences of three months or more underwent a screening assessment by the Speech and Language Therapist using an Initial Interview Questionnaire (see **Appendix 1**). Between 1973 and 1994, of almost 10 000 young offenders who were screened 11% needed treatment. More detailed information on the types of speech and language problems encountered is available from 1986 to 1994. This is illustrated in **Figure 13**. The commonest problems are with pragmatic communication, articulation and stammering. Pragmatic communication refers to the ability to interpret, synthesise and use verbal and non-verbal communication within a variety of contexts. Articulation refers to the ability to elicit specific phonemes and stammering refers to difficulties in maintaining fluency of speech.

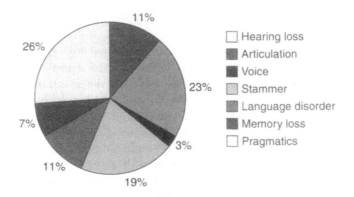

Figure 13: Types of speech and language disorders encountered in Polmont YOI, 1986–1994. *Source: A Review of Communication Therapy with Young Male Offenders: internal report.*[54]

Based on these figures, we might expect about one in nine young offenders to have a need for speech and language therapy. It is not clear whether a similar figure would apply to adult prisoners. However, adult inmates are unlikely to have received speech and language therapy and in the absence of specific prevalence data it is probably a reasonable estimate for adults.

Pregnancy and maternity care

There will always be a number of pregnant women in custody at any one time. Pregnant prisoners can be a vulnerable group, including adolescent and immature women, foreign nationals and women abusing drugs and alcohol.[26] The total number of diagnosed pregnancies, number of inmates admitted to hospitals for delivery, number of live births in hospital and number of inmates referred for termination between 1994/95 and 1997/98 are shown in **Table 30**. Around 1% of female prisoners have a baby when they are in a prison establishment, whilst around 6% of females coming into prison in a year (i.e. total new receptions) are pregnant.

Table 30: Information relating to pregnancies in prisons 1994/95–1997/98.

	1994/95		1995/96		1996/97		1997/98	
	Number	% of TNR*	Number	% of TNR*	Number	% of TNR*	Number	% of TNR*
Diagnosed pregnancies	480	6	494	6	477	6	440	5
Live births in hospital or establishment	63	0.8	80	1	88	1.1	72	0.8
Inmates referred for termination	–	–	–	–	15	0.2	17	0.2

* TNR (total new receptions) is based on the total female prison population being 4% of the total prison population from 1994/95 to 1997/98.
Source: Annual Report of the Director of Health Care 1997–98.[48]

Parenthood

On 21 November 1994 a survey of women prisoners was carried out to establish the number of prisoners who were mothers.[55] Motherhood was defined as having children under 18 or being pregnant at the time of the survey. Overall 3% of (a sample of 1766) women were pregnant. The majority of imprisoned women had dependent children (see **Table 31**).

Table 31: Female inmates with children.

Category	
Non-mothers	
No children	31%
All children >18	8%
Mothers	
Children <18	58%
Children <18 and pregnant	2%
No children but pregnant	1%

Source: Imprisoned Women and Mothers: Home Office Research Study 162.[55]

The preliminary results of more recent research on women prisoners provide further data on imprisoned mothers.[56] Five hundred and sixty seven sentenced women aged 18 to 40 (excluding Category A, lifers and foreign nationals) were studied. Of these, 66% of the sample had dependent children (see **Table 32**) and 3% were caring for children in prison.

Table 32: Results of a survey of 567 sentenced women prisoners aged 18–40.

Age of children	Percentage with dependent children of this age
0–4	34%
5–10	40%
11–18	26%

Number of children	Percentage with this number of dependent children
1	23%
2	22%
3 or more	21%

Source: Women prisoners: work experience and intentions, HM Prison Service 1999.

It is likely that the majority of male prisoners are also parents, as they are drawn from age groups when parenthood is common. However, as parental responsibility is in practice unequally distributed, it is also likely that a minority of male prisoners bear primary responsibility for their children. A review of young male offenders[14] found that almost a quarter were fathers or expectant fathers. However, in the majority of cases the young man was no longer in a relationship with the mother.

Mental disorders

The most comprehensive information on the prevalence of mental disorders is contained in the publication *Psychiatric Morbidity Among Prisoners in England and Wales* prepared by the Office of National Statistics.[34] Most of the information included in this section on mental disorders is based on this report.

Background

Intellectual functioning

Prisoners tend to have below average levels of intellectual functioning. Greater proportions of remand than sentenced prisoners have very low levels of intellectual functioning. Assessed by the Quick Test (a brief intelligence test of perceptual-verbal performance), one in ten male sentenced, one in twenty male remand and one in ten female prisoners had very low levels of intellectual functioning (a Quick Test score below 25 – the median QT score in the population would be expected to be 42, equivalent to an IQ of 100).[34]

Co-morbidity

Prisoners tend to suffer from more than one mental health problem. Those with more serious neurotic disorders are more likely to suffer from functional psychosis and personality disorders. Alcohol and drug misuse also tends to be associated with personality disorders. An estimated 3–11% of prison inmates have co-occurring mental health disorders and substance abuse disorders.[57]

Disciplinary problems

Prisoners with evidence of a personality disorder are more likely than others to have been held in cellular confinement or in strip cells.[34]

Social support

Compared to the general population, prisoners have low perceived levels of social support (see **Box 3** for information on how social support is assessed). This is particularly striking among those identified as probably suffering from psychosis, those exhibiting more neurotic symptoms, male prisoners and those with personality disorders (other than antisocial personality disorders).[34] These groups of prisoners are also more likely to have small primary support groups (i.e. close friends and relatives).

Box 3: Statements used in the assessment of perceived social support.

- There are people I know who do things to make me happy.
- There are people I know who make me feel loved.
- There are people I know who can be relied on no matter what happens.
- There are people I know who would see that I am taken care of if I needed to be.
- There are people who accept me just as I am.
- There are people I know who make me feel an important part of their lives.
- There are people I know who give me support and encouragement.

Individuals say if the statements are not true (score =1), partly true (score=2) or certainly true (score =3). A score of 21 indicates no lack of social support. Scores of 17 and below show that individuals perceived a severe lack of social support.

Source: Psychiatric Morbidity among Prisoners in England and Wales.[34]

Personality disorders

Personality disorder is defined as 'an enduring pattern of inner experience and behaviour that deviates markedly from the expectation of the individual's culture, is pervasive and inflexible, has an onset in adolescence or early adulthood, is stable over time, and leads to distress or impairment'.[58] Different categories of personality disorder have been defined, but there is no agreement about the usefulness of these categories. In the Office of National Statistics survey, during clinical interviews, the prevalence of personality disorder was assessed by Structured Clinical Interview for DSM-IV Personality Disorder (SCID-II).

Overall, the majority of prisoners have an identifiable personality disorder. The most common of these is antisocial personality disorder. It is not uncommon for prisoners to fulfil the diagnostic criteria for more than one personality disorder. The prevalence of personality disorder among the prison population is shown in **Figure 14** and in **Table 33**. Over half of male prisoners and almost a third of female prisoners have an antisocial personality disorder. In comparison, surveys of communities in the general population in New Zealand, Canada and the USA have identified antisocial personality disorder in only 3–7% of men and 1% of women.[34]

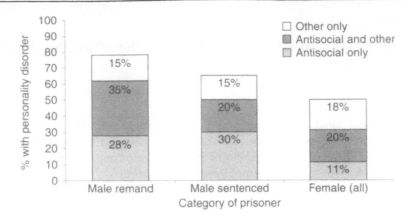

Source: Psychiatric Morbidity among Prisoners in England and Wales.[34]

Figure 14: The prevalence of personality disorder among prisoners: clinical interview.

Table 33: Percentage of prisoners with a personality disorder.

Type of personality disorder	Male remand	Male sentenced	Female (all)
Antisocial only	28%	30%	11%
Antisocial & other	35%	20%	20%
Other only	15%	15%	18%
Total (any personality disorder)	78%	64%	50%

Source: Psychiatric Morbidity among Prisoners in England and Wales.[34]

Functional psychoses

Functional psychoses include schizophrenic and other delusional disorders, mania and severe depression. However, in practice, the great majority of functional psychoses are schizophrenic and delusional disorders. In 1997, when assessed by clinical interview, 10% of male remand, 7% of male sentenced and 14% of female prisoners had suffered from functional psychosis in the past year (see **Table 34**). In the general population (the adult population resident in private households) the prevalence of functional psychosis is approximately 0.4%.[59]

In the Office of National Statistics survey, the presence of functional psychosis was assessed by lay interview. The findings were confirmed by a clinical interview using the Schedules for Clinical Assessment of Neuropsychiatry (SCAN) in a 1 in 5 sub-sample of respondents. About two-thirds of those identified as probably suffering from functional psychosis by lay interview were confirmed as having psychosis. The majority (96%) of those identified by lay interview as not suffering from psychosis were confirmed not to be suffering from functional psychosis. However, just over one-third were missed by lay assessment and just over a third of those judged ill by lay assessors were subsequently judged not to be ill (see **Table 35**).

Table 34: Prevalence of functional psychoses within the past year (clinical interview).

	Percentage within last year		
	Male remand	Male sentenced	Female (all)
Schizophrenia	2%	1%	3%
Other non-organic psychotic disorder	7%	4%	10%
Any schizophrenic/delusional disorder	**9%**	**5%**	**13%**
Manic episode	1%	1%	1%
Bipolar affective disorder	0%	0%	0%
Severe depression + psychosis	1%	0%	1%
Any affective disorder	**2%**	**1%**	**2%**
Any functional psychosis (Approximately 95% CI)	**10% (±4)**	**7% (±4)**	**14% (±6)**

Source: Psychiatric Morbidity among Prisoners in England and Wales.[34]

Table 35: Sensitivity and specificity of lay interview in detecting functional psychosis.

Lay interview	SCAN assessment	
	Functional psychosis	No functional psychosis
Probable psychosis	6%	4%
Probably no psychosis	4%	87%

Source: Psychiatric Morbidity among Prisoners in England and Wales.[34]

Assessed by lay interview, the prevalence of functional psychosis is similar to when it is assessed clinically. Functional psychosis seems to be twice as common in remand as in sentenced prisoners and twice as common in female as in male prisoners. Rates also appear to be higher in white than in black prisoners (see **Table 36** and **Figure 15**).

Table 36: Prevalence of probable psychotic disorder (lay interview).

	White	Black	Other	All
Male remand	10%	2%	8%	9%
Male sentenced	5%	3%	3%	5%
Female remand	25%	6%	17%	21%
Female sentenced	12%	4%	8%	10%

Source: Psychiatric Morbidity among Prisoners in England and Wales.[34]

Neurotic disorders

Neurotic disorders are a group of related problems, the most common of which is depression. Depression often co-exists with anxiety and the disorders are sometimes referred to as two sides of the same coin. Major depression is a syndrome of low mood or loss of interest along with a number of other symptoms

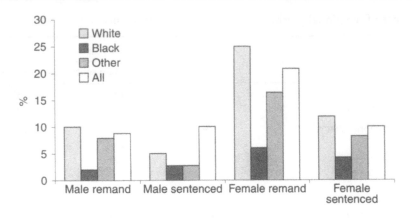

Source: Psychiatric Morbidity among Prisoners in England and Wales[34]

Figure 15: Prevalence of functional psychosis by ethnicity (lay interview).

(see **Box 4**). Many people have some of the symptoms of depression, such as sleep disturbance, lack of energy, loss of appetite, anxiety and worry about physical health.

Box 4: Diagnostic criteria for major depression.

Must have one of the following:

- depressed mood most of the day
- diminished interest or pleasure in almost all activities most of the day.

Must have four or more of the following:

- significant change in weight or appetite (increase or decrease)
- sleep disturbance (insomnia or excessive sleeping)
- agitation or retardation (sluggishness)
- fatigue or loss of energy
- feelings of worthlessness or guilt
- inability to concentrate
- suicidal thoughts or intentions.

Symptoms must have been present nearly every day for two weeks.

Source: Diagnostic and Statistical Manual of Mental Disorders (4e) (DSM IV).[58]

Risk factors for depression

It is useful to consider the risk factors for depression under three headings: predisposing factors, precipitating factors and maintaining factors. These are illustrated in **Table 37**. Apart from a genetic predisposition to depression, all of the predisposing factors are common among prisoners. Conviction and imprisonment are important social precipitating factors and helplessness, while a rational response to loss of liberty may also help precipitate depression. Unsupported and untreated, some individuals recover from depression. The frequency of depression is therefore likely to decline in long-term prisoners. However, lack of supportive social networks and low self-esteem each contribute to maintaining depression. Both factors are common in prisoners.

Table 37: Risk factors for depression.

Predisposing factors		
Biological	**Social**	**Psychological**
Genetic predisposition to depression	Emotional deprivation in childhood Childhood in care of local authority Bereavement or separation Work or marital difficulties Lack of supportive personal relationships Unemployment	Poor parental role models (e.g. violence, alcoholism or mental illness) Low self-esteem Learned helplessness
Precipitating factors		
Biological	**Social**	**Psychological**
Recent illness or injury Drug and alcohol misuse	Recent life events, especially involving loss: redundancy, unemployment, family illness, separation, divorce, loss of a supportive relationship. Conviction Imprisonment Inappropriate responses to precipitating factors, e.g. passivity	Inappropriate responses to precipitating factors, e.g. passivity Helplessness
Maintaining factors		
Biological	**Social**	**Psychological**
Chronic pain or disability Chronic illness Sensory impairment	Chronic social stresses (housing, work, family) Lack of an intimate confiding relationship at home Lack of practical information and help with social problems	Low self-esteem

Source: Adapted from Jenkins (1992).[231]

Neurotic symptoms

In the ONS survey, the prevalence of neurotic symptoms and of neurotic disorders was assessed by Clinical Interview Schedule (CIS-R).[34] The CIS-R has 14 different sections, each encompassing an area of neurotic symptoms. Respondents can score from zero to four on each section, depending on the occurrence of symptoms in the past week. Zero indicates that they have been absent and a high score indicates that they have been frequent and severe in the past week. Those with a score of 2 or more are considered to be suffering from neurotic symptoms.

Most neurotic symptoms are considerably more common among prisoners than in the community (see **Table 38**). Some neurotic symptoms, for example sleep problems, are reported by the majority of prisoners. By themselves, however, these do not necessarily warrant health care intervention.

Table 38: The prevalence of neurotic symptoms (CIS-R ≥2) in prisoners compared to the community.

Symptom	Male			Female		
	Remand	Sentenced	Prevalence in the community	Remand	Sentenced	Prevalence in the community
Sleep disorders	67%	54%	21%	81%	62%	28%
Worry	58%	42%	17%	67%	58%	23%
Fatigue	46%	35%	21%	64%	57%	33%
Depression	56%	33%	8%	64%	51%	11%
Irritability	43%	35%	19%	51%	43%	25%
Depressive ideas	38%	20%	7%	57%	39%	11%
Concentration/ forgetfulness	34%	23%	6%	53%	38%	10%
Anxiety	33%	21%	8%	42%	32%	11%
Obsessions	30%	22%	7%	35%	24%	12%
Somatic symptoms	24%	16%	5%	40%	30%	10%
Compulsions	24%	15%	5%	25%	18%	8%
Phobias	20%	13%	3%	31%	22%	7%
Worry about physical health	22%	16%	4%	25%	23%	5%
Panic	18%	8%	2%	26%	15%	3%

Source: Psychiatric Morbidity among Prisoners in England and Wales.[34]

Neurotic disorders

In the same survey, the prevalence of neurotic disorders was also assessed using the CIS-R. Diagnoses were obtained by looking at the answers to various sections and applying algorithms based on the ICD-10 diagnostic criteria for research.[60]

In male prisoners the prevalence of any neurotic disorder in the past week is 59% in remand and 40% in sentenced prisoners. In female prisoners, 76% and 63% respectively. Anxiety and depression either separately or in combination are by far the most common neurotic disorders.

As we would expect from the nature of the precipitating and maintaining factors which affect prisoners, the general pattern with neurotic symptoms and with neurotic disorders is that they are more common in remand than sentenced prisoners (see **Table 39** and **Figure 16**).

In prisons as in the community, neurotic symptoms and neurotic disorders are more common in female than male prisoners.

The prevalence of any neurotic disorder in the general population (the adult population resident in private households) is 12% for men and 20% for women. This means that neurotic disorders are three to five times more common in prisoners compared to the adult population in the community. This is particularly true for phobias and obsessive-compulsive disorder, which are common in prisoners but relatively rare in the general population.

Table 39: The prevalence of neurotic disorders in the last week.

Disorder	Male			Female		
	Remand	Sentenced	Community prevalence	Remand	Sentenced	Community prevalence
Mixed anxiety and depression	26%	19%	5%	36%	31%	10%
Generalised anxiety disorder	11%	8%	3%	11%	11%	3%
Depressive episode	17%	8%	2%	21%	15%	3%
Phobias	10%	6%	1%	18%	11%	1%
Obsessive-compulsive disorder	10%	7%	1%	12%	7%	2%
Panic disorder	6%	3%	1%	5%	4%	1%
Any neurotic disorder	59%	40%	12%	76%	63%	20%

Source: Psychiatric Morbidity among Prisoners in England and Wales.[34]

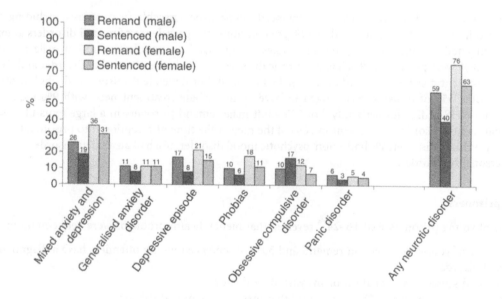

Source: Psychiatric Morbidity among Prisoners in England and Wales.[34]

Figure 16: The prevalence of neurotic disorders in prisoners. Proportion of the population with this disorder in the past week.

Post-traumatic stress disorder

Post-traumatic stress disorder (PTSD) is a diagnosis with the following features. Patients have been exposed to a stressful event or situation of exceptionally threatening or catastrophic nature which would be expected to cause pervasive distress in most people. The syndrome is characterised by persistent intrusive memories of the stressful event (such as flashbacks, vivid memories or dreams); partial memory loss; and avoidance of circumstances associated with the stressful event. Symptoms must have begun within six months of the stressful event.

Table 40 shows the prevalence of post-traumatic stress disorder in the prison population. It is more common in remand prisoners and in female prisoners although overall prevalence is low.

Table 40: The prevalence of all conditions defining post-traumatic stress disorder.

Type of prisoner	Male		Female	
	Remand	Sentenced	Remand	Sentenced
Percentage with PTSD	5%	3%	6%	5%

Source: Psychiatric Morbidity among Prisoners in England and Wales.[34]

Overview of mental health data from other sources

Adult male prisoners

About a third of all male prisoners who are sentenced can be given a psychiatric diagnosis, including 2% who are psychotic.[61] A study, published in 1996, to determine the prevalence of mental disorders among male unconvicted prisoners in England and Wales found that in a population of 750 male remand prisoners, 4.8% were psychotic, 18% had a neurotic disorder, 11.2% had a personality disorder and 7.6% had an adjustment disorder.[62] In addition, 38% had a harmful or dependent misuse of alcohol or other drugs. In total, 555 of inmates were judged to have an immediate treatment need with 9% requiring transfer to a NHS bed. A further study[63] of 569 adult male remand prisoners in a large remand prison found that mental disorder was present in 26% of the men at the time of reception into prison. Of these, 5% had a psychotic disorder, 4% had a non-psychotic mood disorder, 6% had an anxiety disorder and 7% had a personality disorder.

Young prisoners

A review of young prisoners aged 16–24[14] revealed that mental health problems were very common:

- over 50% of young prisoners on remand and 30% of sentenced young offenders have a diagnosable mental disorder
- 23% had discussed emotional problems with their doctor
- 37% of young women and 7% of men said that they had attempted suicide
- 15% of young women and 10% of men admitted to self-harm.

Most young prisoners with mental health problems do not meet the criteria under the Mental Health Act 1983 for transfer to the NHS and require treatment in prison.

Women prisoners

In England and Wales there is a significantly higher rate of mental disorder for women sentenced prisoners, compared to their male counterparts and in the remand population there is an even greater number of women identified as having a mental disorder.[26]

Self-harm and suicide

Self-harm and suicide in the community

In the community, self-harm accounts for 70 000 to 80 000 hospital admissions a year.[64] By contrast, suicides are relatively uncommon in the community. Suicide is more common in men than women and suicide in men is most common between the ages of 25 and 44 and in the very elderly (see **Table 41**). Although the overall suicide rate in England and Wales decreased between 1982 and 1996, suicides increased by 30% in men between the ages of 25 and 34 and by 16% in women aged 15 to 24. Further analysis suggests that the increase in the suicide rate for young men is accounted for by a large increase in the risk of suicide among young single men.[65]

Table 41: Annual suicide rates in the community (England and Wales 1993 to 1995) and expected numbers if this rate applied to the prison population.

Age	Males			Females		
	Rate per 100 000 in general population	Prison population 31 December 1998	Expected numbers of suicides in prison	Rate per 100 000 in general population	Prison population 31 December 1998	Expected numbers of suicides in prison
15–24	11	20,583	2	2	951	0
25–34	18	23,015	4	3	1,191	0
35–44	18	10,721	2	5	640	0
45–54	14	4,506	1	4	221	0
55–64	12	1,725	0	4	56	0
65–74	11	396	0	4	7	0
75–84	14	58	0	6	0	0
85 and over	23	2	0	5	0	0
Total for prison population	15	61,006	9	3	3,066	0

Source: Office for National Statistics. *Mortality statistics: general. England and Wales 1993, 1994 and 1995.* London: The Stationery Office.

Risk factors for suicide in the community

In the community the great majority of those who commit suicide have a previous history of some form of mental disorder. The most common diagnosis is depression, but histories of alcoholism and schizophrenia also occur more frequently in those who have committed suicide. In the community persons who self-harm are 100 times more likely to commit suicide than those who do not.[66]

Self-harm and suicide in the prison population

Direct comparisons between suicide rates in the prison population and the community are difficult to make, as it is not clear whether the Average Daily Population or the number of New Receptions should be used as a denominator. The more favourable interpretation is to use the number of new receptions. Even so the suicide rate is much higher than that in the community; in 1998 there were 42 self-inflicted deaths in custody for every 100 000 new receptions[66] compared to 15 per 100 000 in the community for males and 3 per 100 000 for females.

Table 42 shows the numbers of self-inflicted deaths in custody for the years 1996 to 1998; suicides are consistently higher among remand than among sentenced prisoners. Self-inflicted deaths in custody have more than doubled in the last sixteen years. In 1982 there were 54 per 100 000 Average Daily Population; by 1998 this figure had reached 127 per 100 000. Suicides may be less frequent in female than male prisoners, although the small numbers of female prisoners make this estimate uncertain.

Table 42: Self-inflicted deaths in custody 1996 to 1998.

Year	Legal status	Average Daily Population (ADP)	New Receptions	Number of self-inflicted deaths	Annual rate per 100 000 ADP	Annual rate per 100 000 New Receptions
1996	Sentenced	43,043	82,861	28	65	34
	Remand (untried)	8,374	58,888	31	370	53
	Convicted unsentenced	3,238	34,987	5	154	14
	1996 total	**54,655**	**176,736**	**64**	**117**	**36**
1997	Sentenced	48,412	87,168	34	70	39
	Remand (untried)	8,453	62,066	26	308	42
	Convicted unsentenced	3,678	36,424	8	218	22
	1997 total	**60,543**	**185,658**	**68**	**112**	**37**
1998	Sentenced	52,176	86,800	27	52	31
	Remand (untried)	8,157	64,600	40	490	62
	Convicted unsentenced	4,411	42,400	15	340	36
	1998 total	**64,744**	**193,800**	**82**	**127**	**42**

Adapted from: *Suicide is Everyone's Concern: a thematic review.*[66]

The risk of suicide in prisoners is similar at all ages (see **Table 43**). A disproportionate number of suicides are by prisoners charged with violent offences and sexual offences compared to those charged with acquisitive offences (burglary, robbery, theft), drugs offences or other offences (see **Table 44**). Suicides seem to be less common among non-white (particularly black) than white prisoners (see **Table 45**).

Table 43: Proportions of self-inflicted deaths in custody by age of prisoner (1998).

Age	Males			Females		
	ADP	Suicides	Rate per 100 000	ADP	Suicides	Rate per 100 000
15–17	2,167	3	138	73	0	0
18–20	7,715	11	143	302	0	0
21+	51,124	65	127	2,691	3	111
All prisoners	61,006	79	129	3,066	3	98

Adapted from: *Suicide is Everyone's Concern: a thematic review.*[66]

Table 44: Proportions of self-inflicted deaths in custody by type of offence (1996 to 1998).

Offence type	1996			1997			1998		
	Suicides	Population	% of average rate	Suicides	Population	% of average rate	Suicides	Population	% of average rate
Violence	30%	22%	136%	28%	21%	133%	34%	21%	162%
Acquisitive offences	34%	41%	83%	38%	42%	90%	38%	40%	95%
Sexual offences	12%	8%	150%	12%	8%	150%	10%	8%	125%
Drugs offences	8%	13%	62%	7%	14%	50%	8%	16%	50%
Other	16%	15%	107%	15%	15%	100%	10%	15%	67%

Adapted from: *Suicide is Everyone's Concern: a thematic review.*[66]

Table 45: Proportions of self-inflicted deaths in custody by ethnicity (1996 to 1998).

Ethnicity	1996			1997			1998		
	Suicides	Population	% of average rate	Suicides	Population	% of average rate	Suicides	Population	% of average rate
White	91%	81%	112%	93%	82%	113%	89%	82%	109%
Black	5%	13%	38%	6%	12%	50%	9%	12%	75%
Asian	2%	3%	67%	0%	3%	0%	2%	3%	67%
Other	0%	3%	0%	1%	3%	33%	0%	3%	0%
Not known	2%	0%	n/a	0%	n/a	n/a	0%	0%	n/a

Adapted from: *Suicide is Everyone's Concern: a thematic review.*[66]

The great majority of suicides in prison occur early during the period of custody. **Figure 17** shows the cumulative risk of suicide during the first year of custody (100% is the total number of suicides between 1994 and 1997 for which this data was available). Eight per cent of suicides take place in the first day of custody, 26% in the first week and 42% in the first 28 days of custody. After the first year of custody, the annual risk of suicide is similar to that of males in the community (i.e. 15 per 100 000).

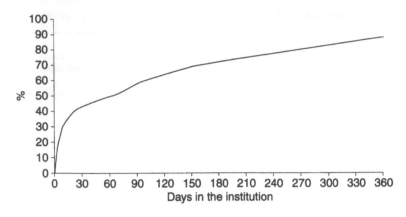

Adapted from: *Suicide is Everyone's Concern: a thematic review.*[66]

Figure 17: Cumulative proportion of suicides occurring in the first year in the institution (1994–1997).

Self harm and suicide

The incidence of self-harm is high in the prison population (about 1.6% per prisoner per year) and seems to be higher in prisoners under the age of 30 (see **Table 46**).

Table 46: Incidents of deliberate self-harm by age of prisoner and age-specific annual risk of self-harm (1996/97).

Age	Self-harm incidents	Percentage of self-harm incidents	Percentage of population this age (1997)	Age-specific annual risk of self-harm
15–17	73	4%	4%	1.5%
18–20	277	14%	12%	1.9%
21–29	960	48%	41%	1.9%
30–39	506	25%	27%	1.5%
40–49	114	6%	10%	0.9%
50–59	23	1%	5%	0.4%
60–69	2	0%	1%	0.2%
Not known	30	2%		
Total	1,985	100%	100%	1.6%

Adapted from: *Suicide is Everyone's Concern: a thematic review.*[66]

Self-harm incidents occur with greater frequency among the unsentenced (remand) population than among sentenced prisoners (see **Table 47**). Incidents of self-harm increased from 1996 to 1997, partly because of changes in reporting procedures (not all incidences of cutting or mutilation were recorded previously). Nevertheless the number of attempted hangings increased from about 400 to about 500.

Table 47: Incidents of self-harm by legal status of prisoner (1996/97).

Year	Legal status	Average Daily Population (ADP)	New receptions	Number of episodes of self-harm	Annual rate per ADP	Annual rate per new reception
1996	Sentenced	43,043	82,861	468	1.1%	0.6%
	Unsentenced	11,612	93,875	439	3.8%	0.5%
	Total	54,655	176,736	907	1.7%	0.5%
1997	Sentenced	48,412	87,168	807	1.7%	0.9%
	Unsentenced	12,131	98,490	784	6.5%	0.8%
	Total	60,543	185,658	1,591	2.6%	0.9%

Adapted from: *Suicide is Everyone's Concern: a thematic review.*[66]

About half of prisoners who commit suicide have previously self-harmed while in custody. In 1996/97, 72 suicides were in prisoners who had previously self-harmed (see **Table 48**). In the same period 2026 prisoners self-harmed, implying a ratio of about 4% between self-harming prisoners who go on to commit suicide and all self-harmers. For those who self-harm twice or more, the ratio is 6%. (NB: These calculations are estimates. It is impossible to say that the prisoners who self-harmed in 1996/97 were the same ones who committed suicide in these years. Nevertheless they form the basis of an estimate.)

Table 48: Suicides following self-harm in relation to the numbers of episodes of self-harm (1996/97).

Number of episodes of self-harm	Total number of prisoners who self-harmed	Number of suicides preceded by an episode of self-harm	Suicides preceded by self-harm divided by the number of prisoners who self-harmed
≥1 episode of self-harm	2,026	72	4%
≥2 episodes of self-harm	299	19	6%

Adapted from: *Suicide is Everyone's Concern: a thematic review.*[66]

There is also evidence that contact with others who self-harm makes young offenders more likely to self-harm themselves.[67]

Suicidal thoughts and attempts

The Office of National Statistics survey[34] found suicidal thoughts were more common in female than male prisoners. This also found that about three times as many remand as sentenced prisoners reported suicidal thoughts in the past week. More female than male prisoners reported suicide attempts. This is in contrast to the figures for completed suicides. The results of the survey are shown in **Table 49**.

Table 49: Prevalence of suicidal thoughts, suicide attempts and self-harm in prisoners.

	Male		Female	
	Remand	**Sentenced**	**Remand**	**Sentenced**
Suicidal thoughts				
In the past week	12%	4%	23%	8%
In the past year	35%	20%	50%	34%
Suicide attempts				
In the past week	2%	0%	2%	1%
In the past year	15%	7%	27%	16%
Self-harm (not suicide attempt) during current prison term	5%	7%	9%	10%

Source: Psychiatric Morbidity among Prisoners in England and Wales.[34]

Other risk factors for suicide in prisons

In 1996 and 1997, about 40% of those prisoners who committed suicide had a previous psychiatric history. Young offenders who commit suicide are more likely to have experienced multiple family breakdown, sexual abuse, frequent violence, local authority placement as a result of family problems, truancy as a result of bullying and short periods in the community between periods of custody. Once in prison they are more likely to be isolated, have no outside contacts, have difficulty expressing themselves to other prisoners or staff and are less likely to have a job or anything to occupy them during the day.[66]

Alcohol and drug misuse

Addictive behaviour is common in the prison population, with many inmates reporting use of or addiction to cigarettes, alcohol, and illicit or prescribed drugs. Addiction to smoking is considered earlier under the heading of 'Ischaemic heart disease and cardiovascular risk factors'.

Alcohol misuse

In the ONS survey,[34] alcohol misuse is measured by the Alcohol Use Disorders Identification Test (AUDIT). The AUDIT questionnaire assesses the presence of hazardous alcohol consumption, symptoms of dependence and harmful alcohol consumption. A higher score indicates more problems; over 8 indicates 'hazardous drinking'; over 32 is a very high score.

The AUDIT score was 8 or over in more than half of male prisoners and over a third of female prisoners. The differences between remand and sentenced prisoners are small (see **Table 50**). Seven per cent of male remand prisoners and 4% of male sentenced prisoners scored AUDIT scores of 32 or over. Figures for female prisoners were similar.

Table 50: Proportion of prisoners misusing alcohol in the year prior to imprisonment.

	Male		Female	
	Remand	Sentenced	Remand	Sentenced
AUDIT score >8	57%	63%	34%	39%
AUDIT score >32	7%	4%	8%	4%

Source: Psychiatric Morbidity among Prisoners in England and Wales[34]

Alcohol misuse is more common in younger prisoners (under 30), prisoners with fewer educational qualifications and among white than black prisoners. **Figure 18** compares the prevalence of alcohol misuse in prisoners to those in the community. Surveys of male outpatients in Belfast and unemployed men in Norway respectively found 27% and 30% to have an AUDIT score of 8 or over. The figures for women were 10% and 8% respectively. Compared to the community, hazardous drinking therefore seems to be about twice as common in male prisoners and about three times as common in female prisoners.

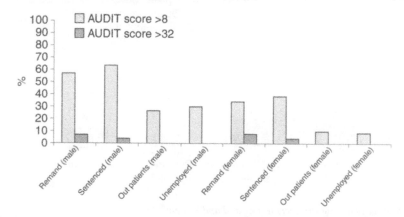

Source: Psychiatric Morbidity among Prisoners in England and Wales[34]

Figure 18: Prevalence of hazardous drinking in the year prior to imprisonment.

Use of alcohol may continue during imprisonment. In one survey of Category B prisoners in a single prison, 59% (95% CI 48–71%) admitted to using alcohol or hooch while in prison. This made it the second most commonly used drug (after cannabis).[68]

Drug misuse

Drug misuse has a direct impact on the health of an individual for a number of reasons. Users may suffer harm as a direct result of drug misuse (for example, intoxication and accidental overdose) and some users become dependent on drugs. Sustaining this dependency often contributes to their adverse socio-economic circumstances and their offending behaviour. There are also important health-damaging effects associated with some forms of drug use, in particular in relation to injecting and needle sharing.

About half of remand prisoners and 40% of sentenced prisoners have been dependent on drugs prior to imprisonment.[34] The majority of these are dependent on opiates, stimulants or a combination of both (**Figure 19** and **Table 51**). Drug dependence is more common in single or cohabiting prisoners than in married prisoners, more common in younger than older prisoners, more common in white than in black prisoners and more common in prisoners with lower levels of educational attainment.

Table 51: The prevalence of drug dependence in prisoners.

Prevalence of primary dependence on:	Male		Female	
	Remand	Sentenced	Remand	Sentenced
Cannabis only	9%	8%	2%	5%
Stimulants only	17%	16%	11%	12%
Opiates and stimulants	15%	10%	24%	13%
Opiates only	11%	8%	17%	10%
Dependence on any drug	52%	42%	54%	40%

Source: Psychiatric Morbidity among Prisoners in England and Wales.[34]

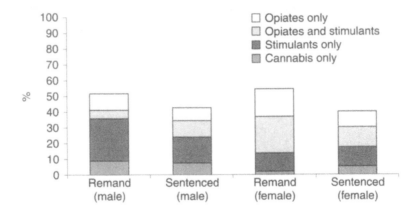

Source: Psychiatric Morbidity among Prisoners in England and Wales.[34]

Figure 19: Dependence on drugs in the year prior to imprisonment.

Prison-related drug misuse problems continue after release from prison; indeed, there may be a higher risk of drug-related death reported in first two weeks after release.[69]

Intravenous drug abuse is a particular concern because of the relationship between this and the spread of hepatitis C, hepatitis B and HIV. About one quarter of prisoners have injected drugs at some time and a small minority have injected in prison (see **Table 52**).

Table 52: Injecting drug use by prisoners.

Prisoners who have injected drugs:	Male		Female	
	Remand	Sentenced	Remand	Sentenced
At some time	28%	23%	40%	23%
While in prison	2%	1%	2%	2%

Source: Psychiatric Morbidity among Prisoners in England and Wales.[34]

A significant minority of prisoners use drugs while in prison (see **Figure 20** and **Table** 53). Because sentenced prisoners have been in prison for a longer period of time than remand prisoners, reported drug use during imprisonment is higher in sentenced than in remand prisoners. By far the most commonly used drug is cannabis, but heroin use is also common. About half of prisoners who inject drugs want help to give up; this figure is only one in ten for non-injecting prisoners.[70]

Table 53: The use of drugs during imprisonment.

Prevalence of drug use in prison	Male		Female	
	Remand	Sentenced	Remand	Sentenced
Cannabis	36%	46%	19%	31%
Heroin	12%	19%	17%	20%
Methadone (illicit)	1%	2%	2%	3%
Amphetamines	2%	4%	0%	3%
Crack cocaine	2%	5%	5%	8%
Cocaine	1%	4%	1%	2%
No drug use	62%	52%	75%	66%

Source: Psychiatric Morbidity among Prisoners in England and Wales.[34]

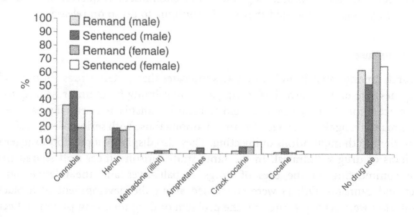

Source: Psychiatric Morbidity among Prisoners in England and Wales.[34]

Figure 20: The use of drugs during imprisonment.

Overview of other data sources

Young prisoners: male and female

Over three-quarters of young women prisoners and nine-tenths of young male prisoners report having used drugs or alcohol.[14] Pre-sentence reports stated that a quarter of male young offenders were under the influence of alcohol at the time of the offence and up to a quarter claim to have a current or past drink problem. Cannabis use is widespread among young prisoners, but the use of other drugs is limited.

Adult male prisoners

A survey of 1009 prisoners in 13 prisons in England and Wales found that three-quarters had used cannabis at sometime during their life, 62% had used the drug in prison at some time and 11% said that their first experience of using cannabis took place in a prison.[37]

Other drug use included illicit tranquillisers (22%), solvents (12.5%), hallucinogens (36.5%) and ecstasy (27%), in each case some prisoners reported use in prison. More than half of the sample had used opiates (mainly heroin) and/or stimulant drugs (amphetamines, cocaine and crack) at some time in their lives and 40% of these had injected drugs. Of those who used opiates, 24% reported their first time use in prison. Of those who inject drugs while in prison, more than half of these share injecting equipment.[37]

A survey among 548 newly remanded prisoners found that before remand 57% of men were using illicit drugs, 33% met DSM IV (Diagnostic and Statistical Manual of Mental Disorders, 4th edition) drug misuse or dependence criteria and 32% men met misuse or dependence criteria for alcohol.[71]

Adult female prisoners

In an interview of a random sample of women prisoners[26] two-thirds of the women reported having used illegal drugs at some point in their lives, and of these 40% reported heavy use or addiction, with over half using heroin and one-fifth intravenous drugs. Nearly 20% used amphetamines, with one in ten of these injecting. Ten per cent said they had been dependent on tranquillisers. A quarter of the drug dependent women still took drugs in prison and said they would continue to do so on release.

Attitudes to drug misuse

Qualitative research among inmates and ex-inmates indicates that certain drugs (in particular cannabis and benzodiazepines) are often regarded as serving a useful calming function or helping to alleviate the experience of incarceration.[72] Many inmates seem to regard cannabis as essentially harmless. Alongside these attitudes, inmates recognise a need for treatment among those with serious drug problems and were aware of some of the health implications of injecting. They also displayed a possibly exaggerated concern about the problems of drug withdrawal. In the same study, prison officer staff shared many of these attitudes, some commenting on the uses of drugs as palliatives and the relative harmlessness of benzodiazepines and cannabis. Others were concerned about the development of a black market in drugs. In general, staff were acutely aware that the problem of drug misuse in prisons reflected a similar problem in the community.

5 Services available and their costs

Introduction

In this section the range of health services available to prisoners are discussed. These vary from simple advice to specialist investigation and management. This section also considers the impact of other services on health, such as health promotion and informal systems of care, although they are not strictly health care services. Services available in prison are also compared in general terms with the services available to the general population in the community.

It should be noted that this is a very general overview. The provision of health care varies from one category of prison to another and within these categories from one prison to another. Services available in the community also vary from one region to another. The main aim of this document is to give an overview of the care available for common health problems. Rather than attempt to describe in detail the management of specialist problems, this section simply records the fact that the management of some disorders is usually the remit of a particular specialist service. It is beyond the scope of this document to review the full range of specialist services available for each specific disorder.

Overview of services available by type of prison

Adult men's prisons

Local prisons and remand centres

At any one time local prisons can hold 40% of the prison population. Because they act as reception and allocation centres they have a high throughput of prisoners. Local prisons usually have in-patient facilities and 24-hour cover for health care. Present rules dictate that each prisoner must have a medical assessment on reception and on leaving. The nature of the remand population will mean that this population is likely to contain the highest percentage of seriously ill people with physical and mental disease.[9]

Training prisons

The prison population is more static in training prisons. Health care staff are not usually present for 24 hours as the need for medical assistance is less. Seriously ill prisoners will normally have been detected at the initial receiving establishment. More physical disorders (such as sports injuries) and less serious psychiatric disorders would be expected in this prison population.[9] Health education and promotion services will be very relevant.

High security prisons

Primary care consultation rates and admission to prison health care centres are high in high security prisons. It is also a feature of prisons that the most comprehensive health care services are available in secure establishments.[10]

Women's prisons

There are a number of health problems and needs that are specific to women in prison. These include maternity care, gynaecology and care of babies in prison, as well as a range of health education services such as family planning. Primary care consultation rates and admission rates to prison health care centres are high in women's prisons compared with other prison types and considerably higher than consultation rates for women in the community.[13]

Young Offender Institutions

In Young Offender Institutions there is often a small health care centre with a part-time medical officer and a few health care officers to provide day nursing cover.[9] Chronic physical illness is generally uncommon in this age group and serious mental illness, such as schizophrenia, is unusual. However, many offenders have temperamental, emotional and behavioural problems that manifest as self-harm and suicidal behaviour.

Overview of models of health care provision in prisons

Health care services are not standard across the prison estate and it has been said that no two prisons are the same.[13] However, a number of broad models of health care exist. These have been classified into the five types listed earlier in **Box 1**.

These models serve as a general description, but there are prisons where elements of the models apply in different combinations or proportions, with, for example, General Practitioners complementing and supporting the work of directly employed doctors, while some services are contracted out entirely. In addition, the models of care have been described in relation to the medical composition of care rather than the nursing composition. In a few establishments health care is nurse-led, but this is not generally the case.

The models of care described highlight the range of personnel who may either be directly employed or contracted to deliver health care in prisons. However, the majority of prisons have a health care manager – who is usually the most senior nursing officer by grade – and either a directly appointed full-time medical officer or a local GP appointed as a part-time medical officer. In the former case, the GP is an employee of the Home Office and is therefore classed as a civil servant.

Levels of health care provision

Health care provision is currently organised around prison health care centres. Four categories according to the level of service provided have been identified:[13]

- day time cover, generally by part time staff
- day time cover, generally by full-time staff
- health care centre with in-patient facilities with 24 hour nurse cover
- health care centre within-patient facilities with 24 hour nurse cover, but also serving as a national or regional assessment centre.

Health care in the community

When deciding what to do about a possible health problem, an individual weighs up a number of factors. How serious could the problem be? Who can best deal with it? What are the costs (in the broadest sense) and inconveniences of accessing one or another type of health care?

In general the costs of accessing informal care are very low. However, although the NHS is free at the point of delivery, visiting the GP involves some inconvenience (time spent travelling and waiting, the cost of travelling to and from the surgery and so on). Most people prefer to make use of their time in ways other than sitting in a waiting room or travelling to and from the GP. In other words, even attending the GP means giving up the opportunity to do something else. Because of this, although patients do not incur a financial cost, the inconvenience of using formal services favours the use of informal care first.

In the community, a person with a health care problem has a number of possible routes to health care. These are summarised in **Figure 21**. They can be broadly sub-categorised as:

- **Self-care, informal and semiformal care:** These include care by family members, voluntary organisations, over the counter medication, advice from pharmacists and telephone advice services (such as NHS Direct).
- **Primary health care services:** These include the primary health care team, principally GPs, practice nurses and other community-based nursing services. They also include other direct access services, such as accident and emergency services, dentists, opticians, private services and so on.

- **Specialist care or secondary health care services:** These are generally accessed following referral by members of the primary health care team, but direct access (self-referral) is possible in some cases (e.g. genito-urinary medicine).

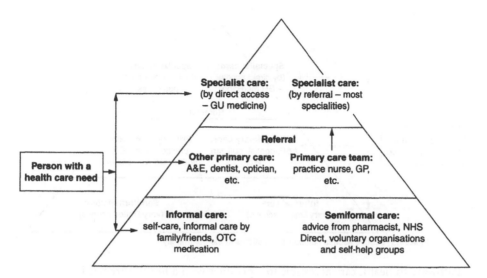

Figure 21: Pathways to health care accessible to a person in the community with a health care need.

Health care in prisons

The categories of services available to the prison population are broadly the same as those in the community, i.e. self-care and informal care, primary care (first contact care) and secondary care. Access to these is rather different to the situation in the community. In addition, two further categories need to be added: health promotion and specific prison-related health care. Because the main prison regime governs all aspects of a prisoner's life (accommodation, diet, exercise, occupation) it has control over many of the factors which affect prisoners' health. The prison therefore assumes a certain responsibility for health promotion. Prisons, rather than prisoners, also generate their own institutional needs for health services, such as the need for medical assessments to be carried out on reception, on transfer and prior to release.

For a prisoner, deciding what to do about a problem, some of the factors he weighs up are the same as a member of the public. How serious might the problem be? Who can best deal with it? What are the costs (in the broadest sense) and inconveniences of accessing one or another type of health care? However, some aspects of this equation differ.

In the first place many prisoners are worried about their physical health (see **Table 38**) and may have exaggerated concerns about the seriousness of the health problem. Second, some types of informal care are not available to prisoners (access to health information, the advice of family members, over the counter medication and so on) – see **Figure 22**. Third, there is little of the inconvenience normally associated with using formal care in the community. Some services (such as dentistry) may be more accessible than in the community; it may not be necessary to make an appointment; and health care is provided within the prison site. Finally, prisoners have little else to do with their time and time spent waiting in a waiting room or visiting a health care worker may (from the prisoner's perspective) be preferable to spending time in a cell. In other words, for prisoners, there are a number of factors which favour the use of formal care where informal health care services would have been used in the community.

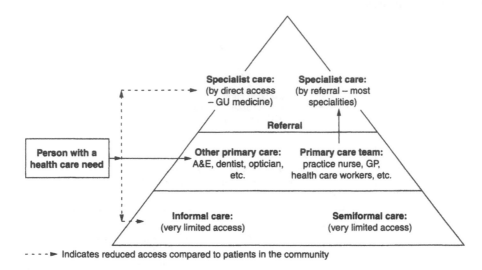

Figure 22: Pathways to health care accessible to a prisoner with a health care need.

Overview of health care services available in prisons

By focusing on the availability of services to address health problems, it is possible to overlook the characteristics of patients and of the services which affect the quality and effectiveness of care. In the context of prisons this includes ethnicity, which may create cultural or attitudinal barriers between staff and patients; language; educational background and the perceived relationship between health services and the main prison regime.

Self-care, informal and semiformal care

Self-care and informal care are not thought of as health services but availability of and access to informal care (such as 'over the counter' treatments) clearly has an effect on the demand for formal health care.

In general, health problems are common, but consultations with health professionals are relatively infrequent. The relationship between frequent health problems and relatively infrequent consultation has been described as an iceberg. Only the tip of the iceberg (usually, but not always, the more severe health problems) comes to the attention of the health services.

In the community most health care problems are dealt with through self-care, the use of over the counter medication and by consulting family members or friends – it has been reported that more than three-quarters of all symptoms are managed without medical consultation.[73]

Several factors restrict self-care in prisons. Prisoners have very restricted access to, and little disposable income for, over the counter medication. They are not generally knowledgeable about health or self-care and information may not be available. They may have health beliefs (such as fatalism) which will limit self-help. Prisoners are also necessarily isolated from their families and informal social networks. Finally, prisoners tend to become institutionalised. In other words, in prison the resources for a prisoner to manage his or her own problems are not available. This means that prisoners are more likely to turn to the primary care service. The result of this is that primary care in the prison system is likely to be burdened with more frequent consultation for less important medical conditions than in an equivalent community setting. This can cause significant problems. The health care system can become overstretched, thereby reducing the time available for the detection of important health problems (such as depression) and ultimately can lead to the deskilling of health professionals.

Primary care

Standards

The *Health Care Standards for Prisons in England and Wales*[74] specify that prisons should provide primary care services to a standard equivalent to that available from general practices in the community. This is expected to include medical consultations, referral to secondary care, continuing care, minor surgery and trauma care, contraceptive services, maternity care and counselling. It is also expected to include health promotion in accordance with Standard 6 (i.e. to provide clinical and related services to prisoners for preventing illness and disability, maintaining and improving their health, and enabling then to take informed decisions on matters affecting their health). The standards state that doctors providing these services should be general practitioners or have experience of general practice.

Unconvicted prisoners can also apply – under prison rule 17 (4) – to be treated by a doctor or dentist of their choice at their own expense. It is up to the Governor in consultation with the medical officer to decide if there are reasonable grounds for the application.

Prisoners are more likely to turn to primary care services because of restrictions on self-care and informal care. The Joint Prison Service and National Health Service Executive Working Group's report *The Future Organisation of Prison Health Care*[13] found that during the period April 1996 to March 1997 staff providing health care in prisons handled over 2 million consultations with inmates. About two-thirds of these involved contact with health care officers or nurses and 27% with prison doctors. Primary care consultation rates and admission to prison health care centres varied between different types of prison, with the rate in women's prisons and high security prisons being considerably higher. The primary care consultation rate is considerably higher than that found in the community.

Primary care activity rates in prison

Male prisoners consult doctors about 10 times per prisoner year. This is about five times more frequent than persons of equivalent age in the community (see **Table 54** and **Table 55**). However, these figures are difficult to interpret in view of the high throughput of prisoners; most prisoners are likely to consult at least once during any period in an institution, however brief. To account for consultations generated by the prison population's high throughput, an adjusted consultation rate has been calculated. This has been achieved by reducing the total number of consultations by one consultation for each new reception. This adjustment considerably reduces the consultation rate for male prisoners. Nevertheless, consultations remain about three times higher than those for equivalent community populations.

Female prisoners consult doctors about 20 times a year. This is also about five times more frequently than women of equivalent age in the community. The adjusted consultation rate for female prisoners is also three times higher than for equivalent community populations (see **Table 54** and **Table 55**).

Table 54: Consultation rates and adjusted consultation rates per ADP per year.

Sex	Male					Female				
Type of prison	Closed training	Local prisons	Open training	YOI	All male prisons	Closed training	Local prisons	Open training	YOI	All female prisons
Health care worker consultations	27	20	17	27	23	61	65	55	23	59
Doctor consultations	10	11	7	6	10	21	20	15	26	20
Doctor consultations (adjusted)	8	7	3	3	6	17	13	11	18	14

Source: Home Office statistics 1996/97 (unpublished).

Table 55: Age-specific general practitioner consultation rates (per person year) in the community and predicted consultation rates for the prison population.

Age	Males		Females	
	Age-specific consultation rate	Percentage of prison population of this age	Age-specific consultation rate	Percentage of prison population of this age
16–24	1.7	34%	4.3	31%
25–44	1.9	55%	4.3	60%
45–64	3.1	10%	4.3	9%
65–74	4.3	1%	4.7	0%
75–84	5.2	0%	5.4	0%
85+	5.8	0%	5.5	0%
All ages	2.0	100%	4.3	100%

Source: Morbidity Statistics from General Practice. Fourth national study, 1991–1992.[22]

Male prisoners consult health care workers twice as frequently as they consult doctors, with 23 consultations per prisoner-year. Female prisoners consult health care workers three times as frequently as they consult doctors, with 59 consultations per prisoner year. There are no directly comparable data on the use of health care workers in the community. However, in the community, consultations with nurses (practice nurses, health visitors, district nurses etc.) are much less frequent than consultations with doctors, running at about 0.3 per person-year for patients between the ages of 16 and 64.[22]

On the face of it, therefore, male prisoners consult other health care workers 77 times more frequently than patients in the community consult nurses. Female prisoners consult other health care workers 197 times more frequently than patients in the community consult nurses. However, nurse consultations in the community are not directly comparable to health care worker consultations by prisoners. The latter may substitute for lay consultation (for example asking family members' advice), consultation with pharmacists, nurses, physiotherapists and other health care workers. However, it is clear that prison populations make very frequent demands on health care workers in comparison to community-based populations.

Reasons for using primary care

Any attempt to reduce the burden on the primary care team will require increased use of informal care to deal with some of the problems usually addressed by the formal services. It is therefore important to identify the reasons for primary care consultation among the prison population. Unfortunately there are no national data on the diagnoses of prisoners who consult health care workers or primary care doctors. However, there are extensive data on the use of primary care in the community. Observations of a number of GP sessions in prisons have confirmed that the more common reasons for consultation in the community are also important in the prison population.

Table 11 gives a breakdown of the main categories of reasons for consultation in the community. Among men, respiratory conditions, musculo-skeletal disorders, injury and poisoning are the most common categories. Among women the category which includes maternity care, screening and contraception is the most common reason for consultation, followed by respiratory conditions and genito-urinary disorders. **Table 56** and **Table 57** show the ICD diagnostic codes for which GP consultations are most frequent. The data have been adjusted to the age of the prison population. Together these diagnoses account for almost half of all GP consultations. It is clear that even in community populations, many consultations are for administrative purposes. Various upper respiratory infections, back pain and neurotic disorders are all important reasons for consultation among men. Among women, contraceptive management and pregnancy are the most common reasons for consultation.

Not all of these services are also provided in prison. Female prisons do not all provide cervical screening and those that do, tend to have contracted with a local practice to provide primary care.[26] In some cases, the high rate of turnover of prisoners makes it difficult to communicate results and to arrange follow-up. However, prisoners are drawn from a group with many of the risk factors for cervical cancer.

Secondary care

Standards

The Health Care Standards for Prisons in England and Wales[74] state that specialist services should be provided within the prison, appropriate to the health care needs of the prisoners.

Rates of consultation with specialists

Direct comparisons between the use of secondary care by prisoners and community populations are not straightforward. Prison service data record the numbers of consultations, whereas health service data record the number of referrals, each of which can generate a number of consultations. In addition, health service data are not easily available for referrals to professions allied to medicine.

Because 68% of prisoners are under 34 and 96% are under 54, GP referral rates for these age groups give the most accurate indication of service use by an equivalent community population. To reflect the predominant socio-economic backgrounds of prisoners, ideally, comparison would be made between service use by prisoners and social classes IV and V. However, these data are not easily available. It is not clear how this adjustment would affect referral rates. Lower socio-economic classes have more morbidity, but they may also have poorer access to health care.

Table 56: Most frequent reasons for consultation by males in the general population (adjusted to the age of the prison population). All diagnoses accounting for ≥ 200 consultations per 10 000 person years.

Reason for consultation	Consultation rate per 10 000 person years
Infectious and parasitic diseases	
Ill-defined intestinal infections (009)	281
Other diseases due to viruses and chlamydiae (078)	224
Dermatophytosis (110), e.g. athlete's foot, ringworm	226
Mental disorders	
Neurotic disorders (300)	471
Diseases of the nervous system and sense organs	
Disorders of conjunctiva (372)	224
Disorders of external ear (380)	397
Diseases of the circulatory system	
Essential hypertension (401)	347
Diseases of the respiratory system	
Acute sinusitis (461)	243
Acute pharyngitis (462)	397
Acute tonsillitis (463)	374
Acute upper respiratory infections of multiple or unspecified site (465)	434
Acute bronchitis and bronchiolitis (466)	526
Allergic rhinitis (477)	331
Influenza (487)	218
Asthma (493)	544
Diseases of the skin	
Diseases of sebaceous glands (706)	424
Diseases of the musculoskeletal system and connective tissue	
Other and unspecified disorder of joint (719)	279
Other and unspecified disorders of back (724)	626
Peripheral enthesopathies and allied syndromes (726) e.g.: tendinitis	277
Symptoms, signs and ill-defined conditions	
Symptoms involving respiratory system and other chest symptoms (786)	248
Sprains and strains of other and unspecified parts of back (847)	351
Injury and poisoning	
Certain adverse effects not elsewhere classified (995)	221
Others: factors influencing health status and contact with health services	
Encounters for administrative purposes (V68)	1,365
Consultation rate for all the above reasons (percentage of total consultations)	9,030 (46%)
Total consultation rate (all reasons)	19,827

Source: Morbidity Statistics from General Practice. Fourth national study, 1991–1992.[22]

Table 57: Most frequent reasons for consultation by females in the general population (adjusted to the age of the prison population). All diagnoses accounting for ≥500 consultations per 10 000 person years.

Reason for consultation	Consultation rate per 10 000 person years
Infectious and parasitic diseases	
Candidiasis (112)	1,101
Mental disorders	
Neurotic disorders (300)	1,153
Diseases of the respiratory system	
Acute sinusitis (461)	586
Acute pharyngitis (462)	725
Acute tonsillitis (463)	662
Acute upper respiratory infections of multiple or unspecified site (465)	840
Acute bronchitis and bronchiolitis (466)	832
Asthma (493)	764
Diseases of the genito-urinary system	
Other disorders of urethra and urinary tract (599)	655
Pain and other symptoms associated with female genital organs (625)	697
Disorders of menstruation and other abnormal bleeding from female genital tract (626)	1,222
Diseases of the skin	
Diseases of sebaceous glands (706)	526
Diseases of the musculoskeletal system and connective tissue	
Other and unspecified disorders of back (724)	758
Symptoms, signs and ill-defined conditions	
Other symptoms involving abdomen and pelvis (789)	573
Others: factors influencing health status and contact with health services	
Normal pregnancy (V22)	2,244
Postpartum care and examination (V24)	551
Contraceptive management (V25)	4,668
Encounters for administrative purposes (V68)	1,198
Special screening for malignant neoplasms (V76)	693
Consultation rate for all the above reasons (percentage of total consultations)	20,445 (48%)
Total consultation rate (all reasons)	42,993

Source: Morbidity Statistics from General Practice. Fourth national study, 1991–1992.[22]

In the community, specialist outpatient referral rates are low in the age-group 16–54. The highest referral rates are for women – in particular referrals to gynaecology (**Table 58**). Because data are not directly equivalent, comparison should be made with caution, but it appears that total consultation rates by prisoners are higher than referral rates in the community (**Table 59**). This is particularly striking where direct speciality comparisons can be made such as referrals to psychiatry.

Table 58: Referral rates (per 1000 person years) among patients in the general population registered with a general practitioner.

Speciality	Male		Female	
	16–34	35–54	16–34	35–54
Gynaecology	0	0	52	48
General surgery	19	32	23	45
Dermatology	10	10	16	15
Orthopaedic	17	23	14	23
General medicine	9	20	12	23
Ear, nose & throat	10	14	12	15
Psychiatry	8	7	11	8
Ophthalmology	4	8	5	10
Neurology	3	4	4	6
Rheumatology	2	4	3	7
Total (all included specialities)	83	121	153	199

Source: Key Health Statistics from General Practice 1996.[30]

Table 59: Prisoner consultation rates (per 1000 prisoner-years) with medical specialists, dentists and professions allied to medicine.

Speciality	Specialist consultations per 1000 ADP
Medical and dental specialists	
Psychiatrist	468
Dentist	1,708
Radiologist	76
Genito-urinary medicine	241
Professions allied to medicine	
Optician	245
Physiotherapy	172
Chiropodist	190
Radiographer	144
Other	176

Source: Home Office statistics 1996/97.

In-patient care

Prisoners have access to the full range of NHS beds provided in the community. In addition, prisons have their own health care centre beds. These provide a less intensive level of care.

Numbers of beds and occupancy

In 1997/98, 1792 in-patient beds were provided within prisons.[48] This amounts to approximately 29 health care beds per 1000 of the prison population. In contrast, in the UK as a whole there are approximately 5 beds per 1000 population.[75]

In 1996/97, overall occupancy of health care centre beds in prisons was 75%, use by patients accounted for 66% of occupancy and other inmates accounted for an additional 9%. However, these figures conceal wide variations in bed usage. Because of the pressures of overcrowding, for example, health care centre beds are not always used for health care. Occupancy rates in open prisons were particularly low and when beds were occupied this was frequently not by patients (but by other inmates). At the other end of the spectrum, occupancy rates in local prisons were consistently high (see **Table 60** and **Figure 23**).

Table 60: In-patient beds and bed occupancy in prisons in 1996/97 (unpublished).

Type of prison	Number of in-patient beds	ADP occupying in-patient beds	ADP other inmates	Bed occupancy by patients	Bed occupancy by other inmates
Closed (female)	52	33	2	62%	4%
Local (female)	115	76	2	66%	1%
Open (female)	11	3	5	28%	45%
YOI (female)	5	5	0	104%	2%
Closed (male)	152	89	17	58%	11%
Local (male)	1,097	780	99	71%	9%
Open (male)	30	4	5	13%	18%
YOI (male)	271	146	24	54%	9%
Total	1,733	1,136	155	66%	9%

Source: Prison Service, Directorate of Health Care, statistics for 1996/97 (unpublished).

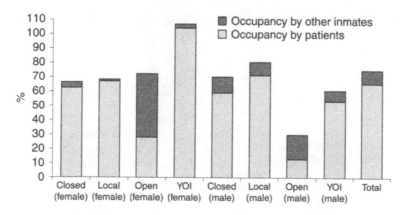

Source: Prison Service, Directorate of Health Care, statistics for 1996/97 (unpublished).

Figure 23: Bed occupancy in health care centre beds (1996/97).

Reasons for in-patient admission

In 1996/97, just over one-third of admissions to health care centre beds were for mental health reasons, one quarter for physical health problems and the remainder for self-harm, substance misuse and for sanctuary (see **Table 61**). Mental health admissions are particularly prominent in local prisons, physical health problems in training prisons and female prisons and self-harm in Young Offender Institutions. These data are illustrated in **Table 61** and **Figure 24**.

Table 61: Numbers of in-patient admissions and principal reasons for admission (1996/97).

| Type of prison | Total in-patient admissions to health care centre (HCC) beds by reason for admission | | | | | | | Admissions to hospital beds |
	Physical health	Mental health	Substance Misuse	Self-harm	Sanctuary	Overflow	Total admissions to HCC beds	
Female	2,116 (35%)	1,162 (19%)	1,329 (22%)	582 (10%)	330 (5%)	514 (9%)	6,033	327
Trainer	1,421 (46%)	993 (32%)	152 (5%)	281 (9%)	123 (4%)	136 (4%)	3,106	913
Local	5,957 (22%)	11,107 (41%)	3,667 (14%)	3,492 (13%)	837 (3%)	1,740 (6%)	26,800	1,004
YOI	1,750 (26%)	1,612 (24%)	483 (7%)	1,689 (25%)	429 (6%)	829 (12%)	6,792	226
All prisons	11,244 (26%)	14,874 (35%)	5,631 (13%)	6,044 (14%)	1,719 (4%)	3,219 (8%)	42,731	2,470

Source: Prison Service, Directorate of Health Care, statistics for 1996/97 (unpublished).

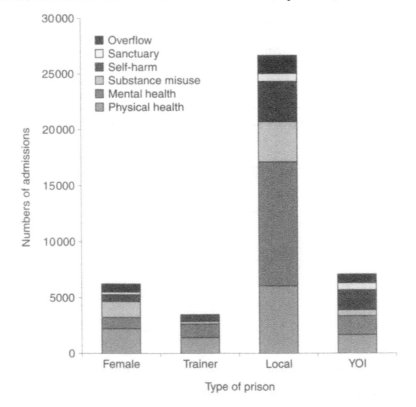

Source: Prison Service, Directorate of Health Care, statistics for 1996/97 (unpublished).

Figure 24: Numbers of admissions and principal reasons for admission (1996/97).

Admission rates

Overall there are about 7800 admissions to health care centre beds per 10 000 prisoner-years. Admissions to health care beds are particularly high in female prisons. The figures for female prisons, training prisons, local prisons and Young Offender Institutions are respectively 30 200, 1500, 11 400 and 7400. Admissions to NHS hospitals by prisoners are at a much lower rate, ranging from 1600 per 10 000 prisoner-years in female prisons to 250 per 10 000 prisoner-years in Young Offender Institutions (see **Table 62** and **Figure 25**).

Table 62: In-patient admission rate per 10,000 prisoner years and principal reasons for admission (1996/97).

Type of prison	Total in-patient admissions to health care centre beds per 10,000 population (by reason for admission) 1996/97							Admissions to hospital beds
	Physical health	Mental health	Substance misuse	Self-harm	Sanctuary	Overflow	Total admissions to HCC beds	
Female	10,578	5,809	6,644	2,909	1,650	2,569	30,159	1,635
Trainer	707	494	76	140	61	68	1,545	454
Local	2,541	4,738	1,564	1,490	357	742	11,432	428
YOI	1,895	1,746	523	1,829	465	898	7,356	245
All prisons	2,053	2,715	1,028	1,103	314	588	7,801	451

Source: Prison Service, Directorate of Health Care, statistics for 1996/97 (unpublished).

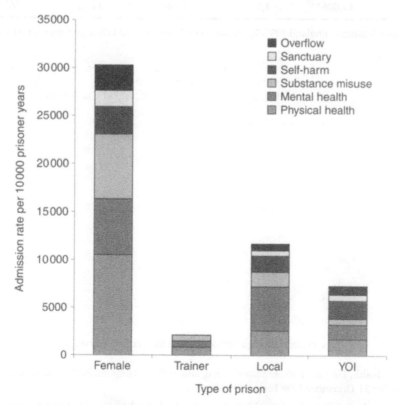

Source: Prison Service, Directorate of Health Care, statistics for 1996/97 (unpublished).

Figure 25: Admission rates per 10 000 prisoner-years and principal reasons for admission 1996/97.

Applying 1995/96 age- and sex-specific hospital admission rates for England to the prison population we would expect admission rates of 749 (per 10 000 person-years) for males and 1844 for females (see **Table 63**). Prisoners, particularly young offenders, are admitted less frequently to NHS (outside) hospitals than the general population, with standardised admissions ratios (compared to age and sex adjusted 1995/96 hospital admissions) of 0.9 for female prisons, 0.6 for trainer prisons, 0.6 for local prisons and 0.3 for Young Offender Institutions. However, apart from training prisons, admissions to health care centre beds are many times more frequent than hospital admissions in the general population. Standardised admission ratios are 16.4 for female prisons, 1.9 for trainer prisons, 14.3 for local prisons and 9.2 for Young Offender Institutions. These figures are illustrated in **Figure 26**.

Table 63: In-patient admission rates in the general population and expected admissions in a population of the same age as the prison population.

Age group	Males			Females		
	Admissions per 10,000	Prison population	Expected number of admissions	Admissions per 10,000	Prison population	Expected number of admissions
15–19	611	7,079	433	1,375	269	37
20–44	689	47,240	3,256	1,976	2,513	497
45–54	970	4,506	437	1,027	221	23
55–64	1,735	1,725	299	1,365	56	8
65–74	2,956	396	117	2,138	7	1
75–84	4,819	58	28	3,613	0	0
85+	6,830	2	1	5,056	0	0
Total	749	61,006	4,571	1,844	3,066	565

Source: Hospital Episode Statistics, England 1995/96. Prison population: Home Office statistics for 31 December 1998.

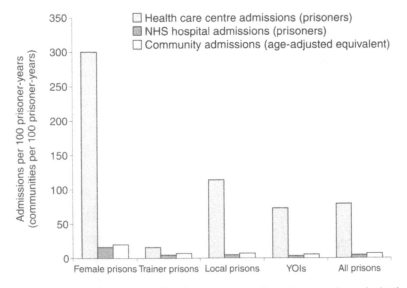

Source: Department of Health, *Hospital Episode Statistics*, England 1995/96 (unpublished). Prison population: Home Office statistics for 31 December 1998 (unpublished).

Figure 26: In-patient admission rates to health care centre beds and to outside hospitals compared to expected admission rates in a community population of equivalent age.

NHS hospital activity data

In 1997/98, prisoners made 3635 visits to accident and emergency. In the same year there were 25 690 NHS outpatient visits (410 per 1000 ADP). Of these 13% (3346) were surgical outpatient visits; 28% (7131) were medical outpatient visits and 59% (15 213) were for other reasons. The number of NHS in-patient admissions was 2475 (40 per 1000 ADP) in 1997/98. Of these 50% (1228) were medical admissions, 40% (986) surgical admissions and 10% (261) other admissions. The total number of escorts required to take prisoners to NHS hospitals was 25 770 and the total number of bed watch nights amounted to 6793.[48]

Cancelled NHS appointments

In 1997/98, 4243 appointments at NHS hospitals were cancelled (see **Table 64**).

Table 64: Cancelled Appointments at NHS hospitals.

Reasons for cancellations	Number of cancellations
Security implications	388
Staff shortages	1,721
Inmate transfers	584
Other	1,550
Total	4,243

Source: Annual Report of the Director of Health Care 1997–98.[48]

Health promotion

Health care and health promotion are complementary. They may be closely connected, for example in the prevention of communicable diseases, or offering specific advice on avoiding harmful behaviours such as smoking. However, to be effective health promotion must have a wider focus. WHO takes this approach, stating that: 'The target audience is not only prisoners, but also staff, prisoners' families, and local communities. Equally health promotion and disease prevention are not just the responsibility of the clinical professionals within the prison, but can, and to be effective should, be built into every branch of prison management to create a whole climate for improving health.'[76]

In seeking to address the wider issues of health promotion, a settings approach has recently been recommended for Scottish prisons.[77] The Chief Inspector of Prisons recommends a 'whole institution approach' as part of the business plan.[14] Some attempts have been made to measure institutional characteristics that are associated with a more health promoting environment.[78]

The prison environment is unique and in some ways – because of lack of privacy, stress, lack of normal social contact and support – potentially harmful to health. A 'settings' or 'whole institution' approach can address these problems through a three-pronged strategy: creation of 'healthy policy', health promotion and patient education.

The creation of 'healthy policy'

A healthy policy means that senior management team automatically consider health implications whenever they review existing policy and practice or intended policy changes and their implementation. The aim is to ensure that wider prison policy assist prisoners and staff in making healthy choices, as far as is possible, and limits any potential harm. The philosophy behind the settings approach will integrate the work so that ultimately prisons will routinely seek to be secure, safe, reformative and *health promoting*. Typically examples would be to consider and maximise the health improvement potential in a prison's Anti-bullying Policy or its Induction Programme. More proactive would be providing better education to enhance prisoners job skills, for example.

Health promotion

This involves many types of staff and possibly prisoners in, for example, campaigns to promote a particular health issue, or policy development in an area such as smoking or exercise, or the provision of preventive services (e.g. drugs harm minimisation.)

Patient education

The aim of patient education or health education is to promote a healthy lifestyle through planned interventions which enable prisoners/staff to examine their knowledge, attitudes and skills in relation to a relevant health issue. Health promotion is not solely the responsibility of health care staff. Many staff, from education staff to officers on the wing and many others, have a role to play. They can look to NHS colleagues in primary care trusts for planning and practical support.

Health promoting prisons

The World Health Organization (Regional Office for Europe) in collaboration with the Department of Health co-ordinates the Health in Prisons Project. The Project's aim is to promote health in its broadest sense within the prison community (see www.hipp-europe.org). Membership of the Project requires a commitment at ministerial level backed by an appropriate level of resources to promote health in prisons. In October 2004 the project had 28 member countries involved and seven international partner organisations including the World Federation for Mental Health and the International Committee of the Red Cross.

The Project's annual business meetings, and the member countries' annual reports and plans, have so far concentrated on three priority areas (communicable diseases, mental health and drug misuse). The 1990 project meeting in The Hague resulted in the publication of a Consensus Statement on Mental Health Promotion in Prisons, which was distributed to prisons in England and Wales for World Mental Health Day 1999. The Statement recognises the potential harm imprisonment may do to mental health, which is described as: 'important for everyone, and not only for those who have been diagnosed as suffering from mental disorders, because it underpins all health and well-being'. The Statement goes on to analyse the aspects of prison life which may be damaging to the mental health of prisoners and prison staff, and to suggest steps prison managers and staff may take to protect and promote the mental well-being of prisoners and of their colleagues.

Prisoner's self-perceived needs

There is evidence that some prisoners are themselves interested in factors which affect their health. A survey of two male prisons identified about half of prisoners as being interested in diet, exercise, stress and sleeping problems (see **Table 65**). The preferred methods of receiving health information were individual discussion (63%), group discussion (41%), leaflets (33%) and video (27%). In addition, the great majority of prisoners were interested in attending a well person clinic and of those who had not undertaken training in First Aid the great majority expressed an interest in First Aid training.[79]

Recent research using focus discussion groups with prisoners and a seminar with staff found that issues such as HIV or drugs were not overriding concerns, but rather basic health issues such as dental health, mental health and relationship.[77]

Table 65: Main topics of health interest among male prisoners.

Topic of health interest	Percentage of prisoners mentioning topic
Diet and nutrition	53%
Physical exercise	45%
Handling stress	44%
Sleeping problems	43%
Smoking	34%
Managing anger	30%

Source: Cassidy *et al.* (1979).[79]

A similar survey of female prisoners[24] indicated that women would also welcome health promotion services. The most popular perceived need was for advice about coping with stress (see **Table 66**).

Table 66: Perceived need for services among female prisoners.

Subject of interest	Would be some help/great help at the moment
Diet and nutrition	36%
Physical exercise	49%
Advice about coping with stress	64%
Advice about problems with children	40% (62% of those with children)
Advice about giving up smoking	34%
Coming off drugs (illegal/prescribed/alcohol)	23%/17%/15%

Source: Smith C, Assessing health needs in women's prisons.[24]

Examples of health promotion initiatives in practice

Much health promotion activity is already taking place in prisons. Some initiatives are listed in **Table 67**, information on other initiatives is available through the *Health in Prisons Project*.

Health care services specific to the prison service

In addition to the health care services provided in response to the health care needs and demands of the prison population, there are health-related services that are an inherent part of the prison system.

Health screening on arrival at prison

Health Care Standard 1 in *The Health Care Standards for Prisons in England and Wales*[74] requires all prisoners to undergo health screening on arrival at prison. Prisoners are also expected to be assessed when they are transferred between prisons or from an outside hospital for in-patient care. Prisoners are to be

Table 67: Examples of health promotion initiatives in prisons.

	Examples of initiatives
Healthy eating	Cookery, food hygiene and healthy eating classes; Heartbeat Awards; reduced levels of fat, salt and sugar in meals.
Smoking	Self-help no smoking group; smoking awareness sessions; interest paid on the savings of inmates who do not purchase tobacco.
Physical activity	Provision of additional competitive sports; PE linked with induction screening and the Well Person clinic.
Mental well-being	Suicide prevention policy; posters and leaflets on metal well-being; anti-bullying messages, self harm therapy group.
Life and social skills	Course on Enhanced Thinking Skills; course covering stress, dependency, parent-craft, assertiveness and self-esteem; inmates encouraged to produce poetry and art on drugs issues; inmates encouraged to work for NVQs.
Sexual health	Information on HIV, STDs and TSE given on induction, confidential counselling on all sexual matters, support of World AIDS day, information leaflets on HIV/AIDS, drama workshop.
Substance misuse including alcohol	Voluntary testing on reception; videos on induction programmes; drug-free landing; poetry and art sessions on drug issues; links with therapists including acupuncturists, a Zen meditation specialist and a stress management specialist; drug education and rehabilitation training programme (DEPART).
Cancer prevention and early detection	'Sun Know How' packages for staff; testicular self-examination (TSE) in HIV/AIDS awareness sessions, prosthetic aids for the teaching of TSE and breast self-examination.
Safety and cleanliness	Training in food hygiene and cleanliness, first aid training.

Source: HIPP Resources – good practice guide, www.hipp-europe.org/resources/internal/good-practice.

seen by a health care worker on the day of their arrival and by a doctor within 24 hours. In local prisons, in particular, the primary health service has to cope with the large numbers of prisoners received every day. Reports indicate that the screening service is often very rushed and inadequate at identifying some important health problems.[62,63,71] This situation is exacerbated by lack of access to previous medical records. In March 2003, the Home Office linked its suicide prevention strategy to new triage-based reception health screening arrangements and mental health in-reach services in some selected English prisons. The Under-Secretary of State announced that all English prisons would be implementing the new screening system in 2004 and by 2006 mental health in-reach services would be available in every prison.

Details from the medical examination are recorded in an Inmate Medical Record and will normally follow the prisoner from prison to prison during their remand and sentence period. Medical records from a prisoner's home practice will only be requested if the prison doctor thinks there is a good reason for requesting them and the prisoner needs to sign to consent to it.[80]

Exit examination

Prisoners are examined by the medical officer just before discharge – in most cases this will be the previous day. If the prisoner is seriously unwell he can ask to stay in prison until he feels better, but this decision is up to the medical officer and the Governor.[80] The Reed Committee recommended that prisoners should be subject to discharge planning as much as patients being discharged from hospital.[81]

When prisoners leave custody at the end of sentence or after a period on remand, transfer back to the NHS can pose problems. After a long sentence, the prisoner may no longer be registered with a GP. Registration in his home area is difficult when he may be detained many miles away. Since the NHS assumes responsibility on the basis of area of residence, it is a particular problem that some prisoners have no home address when they are released and it may not be clear which health authority should assume responsibility for their care. In the past problems were made worse by the structural disjunction between the NHS and the Prison Health Care Service, which meant that prison health care notes did not get transferred to the GP in the community.

Medical reports

Health care personnel are also required to prepare parole reports, custody reports, psychiatric reports and court orders. The numbers of reports prepared over the last five years are listed in **Table 68.**

Table 68: Numbers of medical reports.

Type of report	Number of reports prepared in that year				
	1993/94	1994/95	1995/96	1996/97	1997/98
Parole reports	6,636	5,151	4,970	3,885	2,879
Full psychiatric reports other than to court	450	1,492	1,834	2,111	1,975
Custody reports by MO to court – psychiatric	2,880	2,481	2,490	2,199	1,613
Custody reports by MO to court – physical health	780	197	376	437	264
Voluntary reports by MO to court – psychiatric	621	265	480	252	196
Voluntary reports by MO to court – health only	102	85	157	214	105
Court orders arising from MO (excluding S47 & S48)	–	–	316	265	224

Source: Annual Report of the Director of Health Care 1997–98.[48]

Health care services available in prisons for specific health problems

This remainder of this section considers the health services that are available to address the health problems discussed in the earlier section on the incidence and prevalence of health problems in prisons.

Services for minor illnesses

Self-care and informal care

Patient information

The range of patient information available to the public comes from multiple sources: leaflets, books, websites and internet resources. General practitioners are also obliged to produce practice leaflets explaining how to access their services. The contents of these leaflets vary from the minimum required information to comprehensive explanations of practice policy and advice on how to deal with common health problems.

In prison, information is much less easy to obtain. Many prisons produce some information on how to access and make use of health services. Some also give basic advice on the management of minor illness. Leaflets are available on a number of prison related health topics such as hepatitis and drug misuse. However, these tend not to be directed towards encouraging self-care.

Over the counter medication

In general prisoners are not able to buy over the counter medications.

Resources within the prisoner community

As part of their strategy to prevent suicide and self-harm, many prisons have developed listener schemes. These use prisoners as lay counsellors. Some prisoners have undertaken training in First Aid and of those who have not, many express an interest when asked.[79]

Semi-formal care

Access to voluntary and self-help organisations

Prisoners have some access to voluntary and self-help organisations. For example, some prisons encourage contact with the Samaritans or groups such as Narcotics Anonymous.

Pharmacy and supply of drugs to patients

Health Care Standard No 9[74] requires prisons to provide a safe, efficient and cost-effective pharmaceutical service to prisoners which complies with legal requirements, professional standards and ethical codes, and is at least commensurate with that in the NHS and ensures that a comprehensive range of medicinal products is available for the prevention, diagnosis and treatment of clinical conditions. The force of this is blunted by the fact that the prison service claims Crown Immunity in this area.[82]

Prisoners are not allowed to keep any medicines that they have been taking outside of prison, so all medicines must be issued from the prison pharmacy. In many prisons a range of medications are available from the pharmacy or dispensary, on the basis of a protocol, following consultation with a health care worker.

Prescribing formularies are recommended and are evident in some prisons. A formulary is a compilation of medicines approved for use within the prison establishment that reflects the current judgement of managing medical officers, clinical doctors and pharmacists, on the basis of efficiency, safety and cost.

Complementary medical services

Some prisons provide complementary medicine such as acupuncture or aromatherapy. Services are generally at the initiative of individual health care workers who have an interest in these areas.

A limited range of complementary therapies may be made available to individual prisoners on the recommendation of the prison doctor. The doctor must be satisfied that the therapy is in the interests of the inmate's health; that it will be given by an appropriately qualified and experienced practitioner; and that the therapy represents value for money and can be funded from the establishment's health care budget. This range of therapies includes acupuncture, osteopathy, chiropractic, yoga, meditation and movement therapies (T'ai Chi).

Primary care

Most minor illness is dealt with at the level of primary care. Following consultation with a health care worker or a doctor, patients are given advice, reassurance, specific treatment or are referred to a specialist.

Services for physical health problems

The scope of this report does not allow for a full description of all services that are available to address the physical health problems of prisoners. Essentially the services available to prisoners will mirror those available in the community although the way these services are delivered may be different. **Appendix 2** and **Appendix 3** include brief overviews of the management of physical health problems and drug or alcohol misuse in the community. Described below is some prison-specific information on the services available to address physical health problems.

Epilepsy

Most prisoners with epilepsy will have already been diagnosed prior to imprisonment. In this case, reception screening and liaison with the patient's GP are important in establishing the diagnosis and how epilepsy is currently being managed.

Attitudes to epilepsy by other prisoners, prison officers and other staff (such as those involved in prison education) are influenced by health education. This may also be important in the management of seizures when they do occur. In addition, patients themselves become informed through self-help groups, health care staff and other sources. This is important because many aspects of the management of epilepsy require the patient to engage in appropriate self-care.

Asthma

Most day-to-day management of asthma is by patients themselves. This involves the avoidance of known allergens, monitoring of symptoms and sometimes of peak expiratory flow and adjustment of medications.

A number of prisons provide respiratory care clinics. One example is the clinic which was established in HM Prison Wandsworth after a need was identified.[83] The clinic is set up to provide specialist respiratory care to inmates. Its purpose is to advise, treat and support inmates with respiratory disease. It also assesses inmates' respiratory function, establishes a baseline for those not on medication and monitors the progress of those on regular medication. It trains patients in the most effective use of the prescribed medicines, assesses those who are smokers and refers them to smoking cessation programmes. Finally it provides a resource base on smoking and respiratory diseases for the use of staff and inmates.

Diabetes

Again, self-care will be important in the management of diabetes. Patients with diabetes need to understand the importance of adhering to their diabetic diet, will need to monitor their own blood sugar and (in the case of insulin-dependent diabetes) may need to adjust their dose of insulin in response to this. They also need to be aware of the symptoms of impending hypoglycaemia so that they can take appropriate steps to avoid it. It may also be important for other prison officers and prisoners to recognise the signs of hypoglycaemia, so that they can act to prevent diabetic coma.

Control of diabetes is improved if the patient follows a regular routine in their daily activities and mealtimes. Good diabetic control can be achieved in the majority of patients in prison, probably due to the rigid dietary regime, no alcohol and compliance with treatment.[84]

A number of problems of prison diabetes care have been reported from both prisoners and a diabetes specialist's viewpoint. These included no access to dieticians and/or diabetes specialists, lack of self-monitoring facilities, suboptimal diabetes care, unrecognised metabolic decompensation and self-induced ketoacidosis in order to gain admission to outside hospitals.[84] In addition prison staff may misinterpret the symptoms of poorly controlled diabetes as 'acting-up' by prisoners and inappropriate care may be given.

It has been said that there is generally no specialist knowledge of diabetes amongst prison medical officers.[84] They usually manage diabetic prisoners themselves and only refer for further advice if and when they deem it necessary. In large prisons there is usually a visiting physician from the local NHS hospital who may or may not be a diabetes specialist. Prisoners may also be referred to a local NHS diabetes clinics but this can be expensive, as transport and an accompanying prison guard is required, as well as time-consuming.

At Walton Prison in Liverpool the local hospital diabetes team started to run a fortnightly diabetes clinic in response to problems with diabetic prisoners.[85] During a two-year period (1989–1991) 42 male diabetic prisoners (23 who were insulin-dependent) were assessed. The diabetic metabolic control of these patients was significantly improved after several months in prison and no serious diabetic instability occurred. In this example prison allowed the opportunity for screening for diabetic complications and reassessment of treatment of a number of young men who had defaulted from their home diabetic clinics.

The Scottish prison service in 1994 produced a protocol for diabetes management which included such issues as the establishment of a diabetes register, a system of call and recall, procedures for regular review, care management plans and a referral policy.[86]

Ischaemic heart disease and cardiovascular risk factors

Prisoners have some influence over their own cardiovascular risk through their choice of diet, smoking behaviour and exercise, although diet and exercise are largely controlled by the institution. By offering a diet low in saturated fat and salt but high in polyunsaturates, fruit and vegetables, prisons can influence cholesterol levels, blood pressure and risk of heart disease.

Many activities, such as smoking cessation programmes, aimed at preventing ischaemic heart disease are carried out in prisons. Some prisons offer Well Man Clinics, where cardiovascular risk factors are systematically investigated.[31]

There appears to be demand from prisoners for services addressing cardiovascular risk. In a survey of three women prisons, 34% of inmates identified 'Help/advice about giving up smoking' as a health need, 49% identified 'Help/advice about exercise' as a health need and 36% identified 'Help/advice about diet'.[24] A similar survey in a male prison indicated that 43% wanted help with addiction to smoking.[79]

Infectious diseases

Sexually transmitted diseases

The management of most sexually transmitted diseases in prisons is carried out by visiting specialists in genito-urinary medicine (GUM). In 1997/98, inmates were referred to a visiting GUM specialist on 16 378 occasions (262 per 1000 ADP), 2637 sessions were held, amounting to an average of 6 inmates seen per session.[48]

Table 69 illustrates activity rates in the genito urinary medicine service of a large women's prison. Not every new patient has a genito-urinary infection diagnosed, but among those who do the most frequent diagnoses were *Gardnerella* vaginosis, *Candida albicans*, *Trichomonas vaginalis*, non-specific urethritis, genital warts, *Chlamydia* infection and gonorrhoea.

Table 69: Genito-urinary medicine services in a large women's prison.

	Year		
	1996	**1997**	**1998**
New patients	1,118	961	1,242
Follow up	1,289	1,359	1,614
Total	2,407	2,320	2,856
ADP	294	527	N/A
New receptions	2,749	3,987	N/A
Clinical sessions	295	219	–

Source: Gabriel G. Women's Health Clinic. Audit of clinic sessions and patient turnover for 1996/97. HMP Holloway (personal communication 2/7/99).

Bloodborne viruses

Prevention

The risk of acquiring hepatitis B, hepatitis C and HIV infection can be reduced by adopting safer sexual practices (such as the use of condoms) and by avoiding unsafe practices such as sharing injecting equipment by drug abusers.

Sterilisation tablets to clean needles used to inject drugs were reintroduced to prisons in England and Wales in 1997 via a pilot scheme. Disinfecting tablets were introduced into the Scottish prison system in 1993 following a serious outbreak at HMP Glenochil, when 14 prisoners were infected with HIV and 8 with hepatitis B as a result of needle sharing. Condoms can be prescribed by the medical officer if there are clinical grounds to believe that it is in the best interests of the prisoner's health.

Hepatitis B immunisation

There is a specific vaccine against hepatitis B, a complete course of which requires three injections over a period of three months (see **Box 5**). HM Prison Service recommends immunisation against hepatitis B for all prisoners and staff as good practice. This view is upheld by the Department of Health, who recommends that all those at current or possible future risk should be. In 1996 a protocol was circulated to all Heads of Health Care in prisons (DDL (1996) 2) to advise on action that should be taken to ensure this recommendation was implemented (see **Box 5**). Immunisation courses are not always completed because prisoners on remand or short sentences may be released from custody or transferred. From March 1996 the cost of hepatitis B vaccine has been financed by individual prisons.

Box 5: Action points from the protocol sent to all heads of health care on immunisation against hepatitis B (not all action points have been included).

- Immunisation against hepatitis B should be offered to every prisoner on reception and given within one week of reception.
- Signed informed consent should be obtained for the patient and recorded in the IMR.
- Consenting patients will be offered the accelerated schedule of immunisation, involving three injections at 0, 1 and 2 months.
- In the case of prisoners serving a sentence of sufficient length, a booster injection should be offered at month 12.
- Prisoners returning on subsequent remand or sentence should be offered completion of a course or booster as relevant.
- Prisoners/patients for whom the extended course has already been initiated should complete the extended timetable of immunisation (0, 1 and 6 months).

In a survey carried out in 1997,[35] only a small minority of adult prisoners report having been immunised against hepatitis B, although a similar number reported being unsure as to whether they had been immunised (see **Figure** 11). Of this minority about half (slightly less than half of female prisoners and slightly more than half of male prisoners) reported having received a full course of immunisation. Almost no young offenders seem to have been immunised against hepatitis B.

Hepatitis B immunisation: prisoners' self-perceived needs

In a survey of male prisoners in two prisons, there were marked differences in the proportion of inmates immunised. In one prison over half had been immunised and half the remainder had been offered immunisation (about three-quarters offered or immunised). In the other, a third had been immunised and only one in twenty of the remainder had been offered immunisation (just over a third offered or immunised). Overall, two-thirds of those who had neither been immunised nor offered immunisation said they would like to be immunised.[79] This suggests that prisoners perceive a need for protection against hepatitis B, which is not always being met.

Testing, counselling and advice

Prisoners may request voluntary testing to establish their HIV or hepatitis status. The level of counselling before and following this procedure in prisons has, however, been reported as derisory.[80]

Tuberculosis

Prisons pose particular problems in relation to tuberculosis. Incarceration, transfer or discharge may disrupt treatment. Contact tracing is also rendered more difficult by movement of prisoners and the crowded conditions found in prisons mean that a single patient may have many contacts.

Dental health

In the community, the NHS contributes 20% of the cost of most dental services and the patient pays 80%. A number of categories of patients are exempt from the patient's contribution. These are pregnant women,

women during the first year after childbirth and young people under 18. The prison service pays the patient's contribution for those patients who are not exempted. This means that, in effect, dental services are available to prisoners free of charge. There is a variety of dental health service provision in prisons, the majority by General Dental Practitioners. A smaller proportion is provided by Community Dental Health services through contracts with individual prisons. The prison service also provides dental equipment. At least £1.8 million is spent annually on dental services.

In most prisons dental appointments are booked via the medical officer. Because demand exceeds the supply of dentists, there are waiting lists for all but emergency treatments. In a survey of sentenced adult male prisoners over half of the prisoners had seen a dentist since imprisonment.[23]

In 1997/98, inmates were referred to a visiting dentist on 104 718 occasions. Dentists held 10 753 sessions with an average of 10 inmates per session.[48] The rate of dental consultations was 0.4 per new reception into custody and 1.7 per prisoner year. Consultation rates are high in all types of prisons (**Table 70**).

Table 70: Consultations with dentists and the consultation rate among prisoners (1996/97).

Type of prison	Dentist consultations		
	Numbers	Per ADP	Per new reception
Closed training (F)	2,186	2.7	0.6
Local (F)	1,591	2.4	0.3
Open training (F)	829	1.8	0.4
YOI (F)	19	0.2	0.0
Closed training (M)	34,082	2.0	1.2
Local (M)	33,097	1.4	0.3
Open training (M)	7,740	2.4	0.7
YOI (M)	14,141	1.5	0.4
All prisons	93,751	1.7	0.5

Source: Directorate of Health Care, Prison Service (unpublished).

The King's Community Dental Institute provides dental services for one YOI and one high security prison. Their activities give an indication of the type of activities which would be expected in typical prisons of these categories[87,88] (see **Table 71**). The great majority of prisoners who consult the dentist are seen twice. In general terms, oral health advice, scale and polish, fillings, dressings and extractions are the most common procedures in young offenders. Half of young offenders have mild to moderate plaque. Older prisoners have a similar range of problems but prosthetics are also common.

The transfer of commissioning health services from the prison to PCTs included the commissioning of dental services.

Special senses and disability

Services for deaf prisoners

Provision of services for deaf prisoners, whether for practical or therapeutic assistance, are reported to be lacking in prisons.[89] Access to mini-coms or other specialised equipment, prison officers who can use British Sign Language or who can lip-read, and policies/guidelines on the problems and care of deaf prisoners are a rare commodity.

Table 71: Clinical activity by King's Community Dental Service in prisons (1998–99).

	YOI	High security
Emergency	32%	13%
Consultation	51%	49%
Radiographs	78%	3%
Type of treatment		
Oral health advice	55%	8%
Scale and polish	20%	1%
Periodontal	1%	No data
Conservative (fillings)	44%	2%
Crown and bridge	1%	0%
Endodontics (root canal therapy)	1%	4%
Prosthetics	0.4%	9%
Extractions	17%	21%
Minor oral surgery	1%	2%
Dressing	18%	14%
Trauma	1%	0%
Type of pathology		
No plaque	45%	
Mild plaque	37%	
Moderate plaque	17%	
Severe plaque	0.3%	

Source: Annual reports of clinical activity undertaken by King's Community Dental Service 1998–99.[87,88]

Optical services

Optical services are available to prisoners. However, there may be a charge to prisoners depending on how long the prisoner has been in prison or how much of their sentence they still have to serve, and the type of treatment they require. As with dental appointments, most appointments to see an optician are arranged via the medical officer.

In 1997/98 inmates were referred to an optician on 13 631 occasions, visiting opticians held 2000 sessions with an average number of 7 inmates seen per session[48]

Pregnancy, maternal health and postnatal care

In the community, responsibility for maternity care is often shared between the general practitioner, community-based midwives and a specialist obstetrician. Postnatal care is initially the responsibility of the midwife (for at least 10 days after the birth). A health visitor will then visit the mother and baby in a developmental role, providing advice, assistance and social support.

In prison, pregnant women will receive their antenatal care either in the prison or at a nearby hospital. However, in 1994, in a survey of women prisoners[55] the majority of expectant mothers (63%, n=39) had not attended antenatal classes since arriving at their current prison. A more recent review of women's prisons found that contracts for maternity care are being agreed between local NHS Trusts and the prisons concerned.[26]

If a prisoner is pregnant and likely to have the baby whilst in prison or has recently given birth to a baby, they may be able to go to one of seven prisons with mother and baby units.

Mother and baby units

The main principle of a mother and baby unit in a prison is to enable the mother/baby relationship to develop whilst safeguarding and promoting the child's welfare.[11]

The capacity of each mother and baby unit is listed in **Table 72**. In 1994 a survey of 93% of women prisoners in England[55] found that there were 122 women potentially eligible for a place, of whom 82 mothers wanted a place. This was at a time when there were only 48 mother and baby unit places available. The same survey also found that information about mother and baby units was not readily available to women on reception to prison.

Table 72: Mother and baby units in prisons in England and Wales.

Prison	Capacity of M&BU	Age limit of babies	Type of prison	Age of prisoners	Type of prisoners
Askham Grange	20	Aged up to 18 months	Open	Adult	Sentenced
Holloway	13	Aged up to 9 months	Closed	Adult	Remand and sentenced
New Hall	9	Aged up to 9 months	Closed	Adult & YOI	Remand and sentenced
Styal	22	Aged up to 18 months	Open	Adult & YOI	Remand and sentenced

Source: Report of a review of principles, policies and procedures on mothers and babies/children in prison.[11]

Although a mother and baby unit is not a health care service, some of the services provided to mothers and babies within the unit are health care services and these have associated costs. As at present no separate budget is allocated for the mother and baby units and the cost of running the units is met from individual prison's central budget[11] these health care services should be considered. A breakdown of costs generated by the care for babies provided by the four existing mother and baby units shows a wide variation in spending between the units (see **Table 73**).

Table 73: Cost per baby place in Prison Service mother and baby units for health care services.

Item	Askam Grange	Holloway	New Hall	Styal
Escorts to outside hospital (to treat the baby)	£72 (mother on licence)	£4,000	Nil	£8,000
GP for babies	£3,153	£18,500	£3,000	£4,014
Pharmaceuticals for babies	£1,044	£4,000	Nil	£2,400

Adapted from: *Report of a Review of Principles, Policies and Procedures on Mothers and Babies/Children in Prison.*[11]

A health visiting service is provided to each mother and baby unit but it is often limited in its range and influence.[11] There are, however, proposals for an enhanced role for health visitors[90] and the new health care standard for women will require babies living in prison to be registered with a local general practitioner. The implementation of the latter standard should allow babies to access the full range of services available in primary care from the most appropriate professionals.[11]

Services for mental disorders

Mental health problems accounted for 35% of total in-patient admissions to health care centres in 1996/97 and 30% in 1997/98.[48] Inmates were referred to a psychiatrist on 28 437 occasions in 1997/98, the number of sessions held being 9491, with an average number of three inmates seen per session.

However, like physical health problems, the majority of mental health problems are dealt with through informal care and primary care. This is particularly true of less serious problems such as neurotic symptoms, which are likely to be self-limiting. The main regime of the prison determines how prisoners are occupied during the day, which is likely to have an influence on mental health. This is also true of educational activity, which from the mental health point of view involves time spent productively and some degree of social interaction. When they do experience mental health or emotional problems, many prisoners deal with this by talking to other inmates, or trusted staff members (such as prison officers on their wings). Some prisons build on these informal networks by training prisoners as 'listeners' or by using cell sharing to help prisoners and as a means of controlling self-harm.[66]

A remand counselling programme is operated in some prisons. Counselling is usually offered on a weekly basis to help prisoners on remand with the stress they experience and to enable them to cope with imprisonment.[26]

Less serious mental health problems (neurotic disorders) are dealt with by the primary care team: health care workers and prison doctors. More serious problems (severe neurotic disorders and psychoses) are more commonly dealt with by visiting psychiatrists. The prisons inspectorate expects mental health care to be given by or under the direction of a doctor whose name is on a relevant specialist register.[82]

The Mental Health Act enables patients to be detained in a psychiatric hospital for assessment without his consent. Under a different section of the same act, patients with serious psychiatric illness who are under the care of a hospital can be treated without their consent. The conditions under which compulsory detention for assessment or treatment can be carried out are contained in Section 2 and Section 3 respectively of the Mental Health Act. In brief, it must be the opinion of two doctors, at least one of whom is experienced in psychiatry, that the patient is suffering from a psychiatric disorder which can be improved by treatment and that they are at risk of causing harm to themselves or to others. Prisoners cannot be treated under the Mental Health Act. While prisons usually have in-patient beds where psychiatric emergencies are assessed and treated, these are not included in the definition of a psychiatric hospital. In other words, prison inmates cannot be treated without their consent. If this is deemed necessary they must be transferred to the care of a psychiatric hospital.

Remand prisoners

Remand prisoners requiring urgent in-patient psychiatric treatment can be transferred from prison service custody to hospital under section 48 of the Mental Health Act 1983 (England and Wales). The power to direct a transfer lies with the Home Secretary following reports from two doctors. To qualify for section 48 transfer, a prisoner's mental disorder must fall within the Mental Health Act categories of either mental illness or severe mental impairment and be of a nature which necessitates urgent treatment in hospital. In a sample of unsentenced prisoners transferred in 1992 (n=370), nearly two-thirds had previously received in-patient psychiatric treatment, just over a third of whom had been detained under the Mental Health Act.[91] The most common type of mental illness of those transferred was schizophrenia (56%), followed by depression (10%) and manias/other affective disorders (10%).

There has been an increase in the number of unsentenced prisoners transferred, from 77 cases in 1987 to 494 in 1997, with a high of 536 cases in 1994 (see **Table 74**). Of the sample mentioned above, over half

(54%) were transferred to medium secure hospitals, 29% went to Interim Secure Units or locked wards, 8% were transferred to special hospitals and 9% went to open hospital wards.[91]

When it is felt that a patient no longer needs treatment or that no effective treatment can be given, patients can be returned to prison. In most cases when patients are readmitted to prison assessment in hospital has shown that the person was suffering from a personality disorder or substance abuse rather than a mental illness.[91]

Table 74: Numbers of patients transferred from prison establishment to psychiatric hospital (1987 to 1997).

| Year | Transfers from prison to psychiatric hospital | | |
	Sentenced	Unsentenced or untried	All transfers
1987	103	77	180
1988	94	82	176
1989	120	98	218
1990	145	180	325
1991	182	264	446
1992	227	378	605
1993	284	483	767
1994	249	536	785
1995	250	473	723
1996	264	481	745
1997	251	494	745

Source: Kershaw C and Renshaw D. *Statistics of Mentally Disordered Offenders in England and Wales 1997.* London: Home Office Research, Development and Statistics Directorate, 1998.

Sentenced prisoners

Following reports from two doctors, the Home Secretary may transfer a sentenced prisoner suffering from a severe mental disorder to hospital. This procedure is authorised under Section 47 of the Mental Health Act of 1983 (England and Wales) and is known as a 'transfer direction'.[92]

The grounds for making a transfer are listed in **Box 6**. The section lasts until the patient's earliest date of release from prison although they can be detained beyond this date if they remain mentally disordered, to a nature and degree to warrant in-patient treatment, under a notional Hospital Order. Similarly if their mental disorder responds to treatment they can be returned to prison to complete their sentence.

Box 6: Grounds for issuing a Section 47.

- The prisoner is suffering from mental illness, psychopathic disorder, mental impairment or severe mental impairment.
- The mental disorder is of a nature or degree which makes it appropriate for the patient to be detained in hospital for medical treatment.
- In the case of psychopathic disorder or mental impairment the treatment is likely to alleviate or prevent deterioration of the patient's condition.
- The Home Secretary is of the opinion, having regard to the public interest and all the circumstances, that the person's transfer is expedient.

Source: Huckle P.[92]

Table 74 and **Table 27** illustrate data released from the Home Office in 1998 on transfers to psychiatric hospital between 1987 and 1997. These indicate that there was a rapid rise in the number of transfers to psychiatric hospital between 1987 and 1994. This rise is most prominent among unsentenced and untried prisoners, which have risen more than six-fold. From 1994 to 1997 the number of transfers has been relatively constant.

In a survey of 29 prisoners transferred under Section 47, the most common type of mental illness was schizophrenia (50%), followed by recurrent depressive disorder (13%), personality disorder (7%), drug-induced psychosis (4%) and hypomania (4%).[92]

Prisoners who do not meet the criteria for detention receive treatment in prison, often as in-patients in the health care centre. Many have important health problems that outside of prison would be under the care of a consultant psychiatrist.

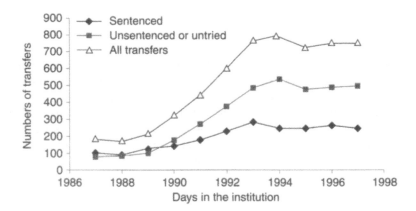

Source: Kershaw C and Renshaw D. *Statistics of Mentally Disordered Offenders in England and Wales 1997*. London: Home Office Research, Development and Statistics Directorate, 1998.

Figure 27: Patients transferred from prison establishment to psychiatric hospital (1987 to 1997).

Personality disorders

At present there are a number of specialist services for prisoners with psychopathic personality disorder. These include places in special hospitals (Broadmoor Hospital and Ashworth Hospital) and therapeutic communities such as those at HMP Grendon Underwood and the Max Glatt Centre within HMP Wormwood Scrubs. The prison service also intends to establish an additional therapeutic community with a further 250 places.[93]

The term 'therapeutic community' is used to refer to a residential, multi-modal treatment programme for people with a variety of mental health problems. Programmes typically include some formal therapeutic components such as group psychotherapy and art therapy, but the key and unique component of the approach involves the observation and analysis of daily interactions within the community. It is a contract-based regime – the prisoner needs to recognise they have a problem, be motivated to do something about it and be capable of entering into a therapeutic contract. Alternative treatment options for people with personality disorder include a range of outpatient based therapies, some of which will occur as part of a typical therapeutic community treatment programme, or an intense period of in-patient psychotherapy in an open ward.

Gunn et al. on looking at the treatment needs of male prisoners with psychiatric disorders found that approximately 6% of the men were judged to require treatment in a therapeutic community setting for personality disorders, substance misuse, or sexual disorder.[61] Maden et al.[94] suggest that 8% of sentenced women require therapeutic treatment. A review of women's prisons[26] found that many prisons have inadequate resources to help women with serious personality disorders.

Functional psychoses

The most common functional psychoses are schizophrenia and the delusional disorders. However, some patients suffer from severe depression or hypomania. These are all chronic disorders which are characterised by occasional episodes of mental disturbance interspersed with problem-free periods. Chronic mental illness is associated with a range of psychological, emotional, social and occupational problems. These can be addressed in a structured way known as a *care programme approach.*

The *care programme approach* is a standardised system which can incorporate statutory aftercare or other arrangements such as supervision orders or care management by social services. It is based on a multidisciplinary approach to care, but to avoid diffusion of responsibility a single *key worker* is identified as the lead person involved in care. The *key worker* has overall responsibility for overseeing and monitoring the services provided under the care plan. Alongside this a detailed and systematic assessment of the individual patient's needs is carried out, together with regular reviewing and recording of the care and support given. This should involve the patient and relevant informal carers wherever possible. Specific responsibilities are allocated to specific people (health and social services professionals and informal carers) involved in care. Care is planned on a proactive basis, in an attempt to anticipate problems, and is reviewed as circumstances change.

For most chronic mental illnesses an important role is played by the psychiatrist. The frequency and the duration of relapses can be significantly reduced with appropriate medications. In prisons chronic mental illnesses are generally managed by a psychiatrist. The more structured *care programme approach* is not widespread in prisons, often because of difficulties in co-ordinating care between prisons and outside agencies.

Neurotic disorders

Not all neurotic illness is detected in primary care, as patients also experience physical symptoms which may distract from the neurotic illness. Of those that are detected, the great majority are managed in a primary care setting.

The first step in the management of neurotic illness is often to validate the patient's experience and to reframe his or her symptoms as having a psychological element. Having diagnosed anxiety, depression or any of a range of neurotic symptoms (such as insomnia), general practitioners most commonly provide counselling or supportive care and arrange for subsequent follow-up. They may prescribe antidepressants or anxiolytic drugs or give specific advice with respect to neurotic symptoms. Supportive counselling, cognitive behaviour therapy or behaviour therapy or follow-up of patients with neurotic symptoms may also be carried out by another primary care professional such as a community psychiatric nurse, a social worker or a practice nurse trained in counselling or problem-solving.

In a minority of cases, patients are referred for specialist assessment by a clinical psychologist or psychiatrist. In the former case this may result in a psychotherapeutic intervention such as cognitive therapy or psychodynamic psychotherapy. In the latter case this usually results in prescription of medication (such as an antidepressant), but this may be combined with a psychotherapeutic approach.

Whether they are managed at a primary care or a secondary care level, patients with severe neurotic illness are managed using the care programme approach described above in functional psychoses. This essentially means that a systematic, multidisciplinary approach is taken to address all of their social, psychological and health needs.

Services for patients with neurotic disorders in prisons tend to parallel those in the community. However, at the primary care level, access to other primary care professionals such as counsellors or community psychiatric nurses may be limited in comparison to the situation in the community. At the secondary care level, psychiatric referral may be more common as access to clinical psychology is limited.

Help with emotional problems

A remand counselling programme is operated in some prisons. Counselling is usually offered on a weekly basis to help prisoners on remand with the stress they experience and to enable them to cope with imprisonment.[26]

Self-harm and suicide

The management of self-harm in the community

In the community deliberate self-harm is one of the top five causes of acute medical admissions for both men and women.[95] The usual management of persons who self-harm in the community is to treat the injury and then to assess the risk of mental illness or subsequent injury. Assessment may be carried out by a psychiatric social worker, a community psychiatric nurse or a doctor (either a psychiatric specialist or junior doctor specialising in psychiatry).

Specialist aftercare usually involves referral to psychiatric outpatients and social services. Around a quarter of hospitals have a dedicated self-harm team. About 5–10% of cases lead directly to a psychiatric admission.[96]

The management of self-harm in prisons

It is recognised that most prisoners who self-harm do not go on to kill themselves. There are however, links between self-harm and suicide: half of those who commit suicide in prison have previously injured themselves.[66]

It has been suggested that the Prison Service places a much greater emphasis on the prevention of the suicide than on tackling the problem of self-harm.[64] In August 1992 the Prison Service published an information paper entitled *The Way Forward*, as part of its work to develop a revised strategy towards the prevention of suicide. Following on from this, a piece of work looked at lists of risk behaviours which should alert staff to suicide vulnerability, and of triggers which may hasten the onset of suicidal feelings. This led to the Prison Service strategy *Caring for the Suicidal in Custody*, which was introduced in 1994. It provides a systematic approach to the identification, care and monitoring of those considered to be at risk of suicide. The main policy features of the strategy include the appointment of Suicide Awareness teams in each establishment, the introduction of a form for managing those considered as being at risk (F2052SH), involvement of the Samaritans and the development of listener schemes.

Assessment

Guidelines on assessment are included in *The Management of Deliberate Self-harm*, issued by the DHSS in 1984.[97] The guidelines recommend that every patient should have a specialist psychosocial assessment to identify factors associated with suicidal behaviour, to determine the motivation for the self-harm, to identify potentially treatable mental disorder and to assess continuing risk of suicidal behaviour. The DHSS guidelines recognise that assessment can be undertaken by staff other than psychiatrists providing they have had proper training. Social workers and psychiatric nurses are given as examples.

Interventions

A number of interventions are employed to address self-harm and suicide:

Informal and semi-formal care

Many prisons provide information to encourage use of informal and formal services when prisoners feel that they are in crisis. Some prisons provide *crisis cards*, which carry advice about seeking help in the event of future suicidal feelings.

Listener schemes were introduced to enable suitable prisoners to help other prisoners. The scheme operates according to the principles of the Samaritans. Most prisons have a listener scheme in operation and in a small number of establishments, listeners get paid for this service.[66]

A *self-help group* facilitated by staff at HMP Durham enables women with a history of self-injury to meet on a weekly basis and share their feelings and talk about their impulses to self injure.[66]

It may be appropriate to refer prisoners to *non-statutory agencies* or specialist services such as the Samaritans. The Samaritans visit 93% of prison establishments on a regular basis. However, a dedicated phone line to the Samaritans is only available in 40% of establishments.[66]

If a Prison Officer is confronted by a prisoner who has harmed themselves, or is talking about doing so, an *F2052SH booklet* is opened. This booklet is used by all staff to record the observations about the prisoner. It was designed to manage the measures to be taken to support an individual at a time of a suicidal crisis to the point where risk was reduced and the form could be closed. The booklet is intended as a framework not the answer to the problem.

Formal care

Prisoners who self-harm may also be managed by medical staff or other health care workers. The main approaches to self-harm are psychological and medical: either can be used alone or both in combination. Psychological approaches include problem-solving therapy and other behavioural approaches to self-harming behaviour. They also include the full range of psychological interventions for underlying neurotic disorders such as depression. Medical approaches include conventional psychiatric care, drug treatment for depression and specific drug treatments for impulsive behaviour.

Services for alcohol and drug misuse

Health Care Standard No 8[74] advises prisons to provide clinical services for the assessment, treatment and care of substance misusers comparable to those available in the community and appropriate to the prison setting. The Prison Service has also stated that it is committed to providing clinical services for substance misusers which are in line with the Department of Health guidelines. This includes a commitment that all prisons receiving remand prisoners should provide clinical detoxification services.

Drug abuse

Services for drug abuse in the community

In the community a minority of drug misusers come into contact with formal services. Those that do are dealt with by the primary care team, in drug-dependency clinics and sometimes by psychiatric services. A range of voluntary organisations also offer services for drug misusers.

Services for drug abuse in prisons

Drug strategies vary between prisons; in his 1996–97 Annual Report, the Chief Inspector of Prisons stated that, 'the employment of outside agencies, and the introduction of drug-free wings is very haphazard'. Some prisoners are aware of their needs with regard to drug misuse. In surveys 17% of male prisoners and 23% of female prisoners identified a need for help with addiction to illicit drugs.[24,79]

Between September 1995 and January 1997, 21 drug treatment and rehabilitation programmes were established in 19 prisons in England and Wales. These were intended to test a range of different drug treatment and rehabilitation services.[98]

The services included:

- counselling, advice and education services
- enhanced detoxification services
- 12-step programmes
- residential drug treatment programmes
- modified therapeutic communities
- therapeutic communities.

CARATs: Counselling, Assessment, Referral Advice and Throughcare

A support service for prisoners with drug problems was made available to all prisoners with drug problems from the end of October 1999. CARATs (Counselling, Assessment, Referral Advice and Throughcare) is a multi-agency approach to tackling drug abuse in prison. It co-ordinates approaches to tackling drug abuse in prison with support for prisoners after release. It aims to identify drug misusers as soon as possible, provide ongoing support and advice throughout their sentence, work in conjunction with other agencies (inside and outside prison) and provide links between the various departments and agencies dealing with prisoners in order to provide continuity. The multi-agency approach involves drug agency staff, prison officers, probation officers, health care staff and psychologists.

CARATs is part of the Prison Service's new drug treatment framework, which promised to deliver 31 new drug rehabilitation programmes by the end of 1999 (in addition to the existing 18). Four new therapeutic communities for prisoners with the most severe drug problems and related offending behaviour were planned doubling the number of centres available.

Detoxification and withdrawal

Detoxification courses are provided in all prisons with remand prisoners. The total number of prisoners completing drug detox courses increased from 13 932 prisoners in 1996/97 to 17 696 in 1997/98. The average number of prisoners on drug detox courses on 31 March 1998 was 480.[48]

Examples of initiatives to address drug abuse in prisons

Winchester Prison's substance misuse team was expanded in 1991 when two outside part-time drug workers were brought in to provide amongst other things group counselling.[99] The services had been provided by statutory drug agencies for the catchment areas and the funding for these posts was shared between the prison service and the local health authority. Through care is also operated at Winchester. A drug worker will follow the misuser through the criminal justice system and ensure contact with a suitable agency/drug worker when they return to the community.

Alcohol misuse

Services for alcohol abuse in the community

In the community a small minority of alcohol misusers come into contact with formal services. Those that do are dealt with by the primary care team, by the voluntary sector, or in alcohol dependency clinics run by psychiatric services.

Services for alcohol abuse in prison

Alcohol abuse should not present a serious problem inside prisons as it is difficult for prisoners to get access to sufficient quantities for prisoners to maintain a state of dependency. However, it is thought that paradoxically, absence of alcohol makes it difficult to address drink problems inside prison. Alcohol becomes a problem when the prisoner is released.[73]

However, on arrival in prison, some prisoners are alcohol-dependent and will undergo acute withdrawal *delerium tremens*. These need to be identified and managed appropriately.

Services that may be offered by a prison include detoxification for prisoners who are dependent on alcohol, education programmes on alcohol misuse, counselling and visits from outside agencies such as Alcoholics Anonymous.

The total number of prisoners completing alcohol detoxification courses increased from 2345 prisoners in 1996/97 to 3942 prisoners in 1997/98. The average number of inmates on alcohol detoxification courses on 31 March 1997/98 was 87.[48]

Prisoners' self-perceived needs

Many prisoners are aware of their needs with regard to alcohol misuse. In separate surveys, 29% of male prisoners and 15% of female prisoners identified a need for help with addiction to alcohol.[24,79]

Cost of services

The proportion of costs borne by the NHS and the prison service for health care services varies with different types of health care. In some cases there will be cost implications on different parts of the prison

Table 75: Costs of different approaches to the management of health care problems.

Type of health care	General population	Prisoners		
		Costs to the prison service		Costs to the NHS
	Costs to the NHS	Health care costs	Other costs	
Health promotion				
Occupational advice or advice on main prison regime	Yes	None	In some cases	None
Nutritional or other lifestyle advice	Yes	None	In some cases	None
Informal and semi-formal care				
Over the counter (OTC) medication and self-care	None	Not available	–	None
Advice from a pharmacist	None	Yes	–	None
Advice and care from family or friends	None	Not available	–	None
Voluntary organisations	None	None	–	None
Self-help groups, e.g. Alcoholics Anonymous	None	None	–	None
NHS Direct or other telephone advice line	Yes	None	–	Yes
Formal care: primary care team				
Consultation with a practice nurse	Yes	Yes	–	None
Consultation with a general practitioner	Yes	Yes	–	None
Optician	Yes	Yes	–	None
Dentist	20% of cost	80% of cost	–	None
Consultation with an NHS specialist	Yes	None	Escorting costs	Yes
Formal care: secondary care				
Consultation with a visiting NHS specialist	–	Yes	–	None
Consultation with an outside specialist service	Yes	None	Escorting costs	Yes
In-patient care in a health care centre bed	–	Yes	–	None
In-patient care in an NHS hospital bed	Yes	None	Escorting costs	Yes
Formal care: other forms of direct access				
Accident and emergency	Yes	None	Escorting costs	Yes
Alternative and complimentary medicine	Sometimes	Yes	–	None
Self-referral to specialist services, e.g. genito-urinary medicine	Yes	Not available	–	None
Private health care, e.g. BUPA, private dental care	None	Rarely available	–	None

budget. The precise costs will vary from one prison to another. **Table 75** illustrates where costs of different types of care may fall.

In 1996, it was estimated that the prison service spent around £1000 per prisoner per year on health care. However, this figure conceals wide variation in expenditure on health care, with some institutions spending as little as a few hundred pounds per inmate and others as much as £9000, or between 3% and 20% of their total budget on health care.[13] Over three-quarters of prison health care expenditure is on the salaries of health care staff. The remainder is divided between pharmaceutical costs and various contracted-in specialist services (see **Table 76**).

The total number of health care staff employed by the Prison Service at 31 March 1998 was 2031; of these 216 were part-time the remaining 1815 were full-time[48] (see **Table 77**).

Table 76: Breakdown of costs of health care provision in the prison service (1996/97).

Type of health care	Cost (millions)	Percentage
Staff pay	£44.417	73.9%
Other locums and consultants	£5.060	8.4%
Medical supplies (very largely pharmacy drugs)	£4.872	8.1%
Dental treatment	£1.855	3.1%
Visiting psychiatrists	£1.621	2.7%
Nurses	£1.040	1.7%
Contracted out services	£0.503	0.8%
Optical treatment	£0.500	0.8%
Occupational health	£0.215	0.4%
Total	£60.083	100%

Source: Home Office statistics for 1996/97.

Table 77: Health care staff.

	Number employed on 31 March		
	1995/96	1996/97	1997/98
Total health care staff	2,056	1,958	2,031
Part-time	180	176	216
Full-time	1,876	1,782	1,815
Total nursing grades	684	718	879
Part-time	59	60	92
Full-time	625	658	783
Total unified grades	1,001	880	774
Part-time	6	5	2
Full-time	995	875	772
Total medical grades	222	190	213
Part-time	89	66	87
Full-time	133	124	126
Total pharmacy grades	77	85	75
Part-time	11	20	18
Full-time	66	65	57
Total admin grades	72	85	90
Part-time	15	25	17
Full-time	57	60	73

Source: Annual Report of the Director of Health Care 1997–98.[48]

6 Effectiveness of services and interventions

There have been few well conducted, randomised controlled trials of health care interventions in prisoners. However, based on our knowledge of an illness and an intervention it may be reasonable to extrapolate based on studies which have been carried out in other settings. For example, there are no direct studies of the effectiveness of hepatitis B vaccination in the prison population, but we know it is effective in a wide variety of other settings and it is probably reasonable to assume that it is effective in prisons.

It is beyond the scope of this document to review the effectiveness of all possible treatments or interventions for the health problems experienced by prisoners. On the one hand there is little evidence on the effectiveness of health care interventions specific to prisoners. On the other hand, however, there is a great deal of evidence on the effectiveness of interventions in other settings. Although this too is far from complete, some of it is relevant to the prison population. Unfortunately, such a range of evidence is too extensive to be reviewed in detail in a document such as this. It will therefore consider in a little more detail some health problems that are most pertinent to the prison population. Where conclusions have been reached, these are drawn from information on the effectiveness of health care interventions in the community. This section should not be considered a substitute for a systematic appraisal of the available evidence.

Effectiveness of health care services

Table 78 summarises, in broad terms, the types of evidence available for the main categories of health problems. Where evidence is available it is often not directly relevant to the prison setting and this should be borne in mind when recommendations are being made or guidelines drawn up.

Effectiveness of health care services specific to the prison service

Health screening on arrival in prison

The effectiveness of screening prisoners at reception (using form F2169) has been questioned.[62,63,71] The conditions and time constraints under which reception health screening is carried out have been found to militate against the detection of clinically important information. The validity of the screening questionnaires used has also been doubted. More specifically, the screening is neither sensitive nor specific for detecting mental disorder.[63]

Health screening at reception is not sensitive at picking up mental disorder. In one research project reception screening identified only 23% of 148 mentally disordered remand prisoners (95% CI 16–30%). This included only 25% of 24 who were acutely psychotic (95% CI 8–42%). Another study found that 18 out of 43 young inmates had failed to report their mental health problems at reception.[14] A study on substance use in remand prisoners also concluded that prison reception health screening consistently underestimates drug and alcohol use.[71]

In a further study the findings of the prison reception health screening of 546 consecutive new remand prisoners were compared with independent assessments carried out by research psychiatrists.[100] The independent assessments took from 20 minutes to an hour. The study concluded that a considerable amount of morbidity remained undetected by routine screening. Initial health screening (by prison hospital officers) and subsequent health assessments (by the prison doctors) picked up the great majority of prisoners with a history of self-harm. However, they only detected about half of those with a current

Table 78: Evidence of effectiveness of interventions for health problems found in prisons.

Type of health problem	Level of evidence of effectiveness	Is evidence generalisable to prisons?
Health services specific to the prison population	Primary care screening procedures compared with 'gold standard'.	Some evaluation of current practice in regard to screening.
Minor illness	Some evidence from controlled trials and systematic reviews. Some expert recommendations.	Evidence not based on a prison setting, but probably generalisable.
Physical health problems		
Epilepsy	Controlled trials of specific drugs. Expert recommendations and guidelines for usual management.	Evidence not based on a prison setting, but probably generalisable.
Diabetes	Controlled trials of glycaemic control and blood pressure control. Little evaluation of service delivery.	Evidence not based on a prison setting, but probably generalisable.
Ischaemic heart disease and cardiovascular risk factors	Controlled trials and systematic reviews of the management of cardiovascular disease and risk factors. Has been synthesised into evidence-based guidelines.	Evidence not based on a prison setting. See below for modelling and recommendations based on expected prevalence of cardiovascular risk factors in prisoners.
Infectious diseases	Evidence for specific interventions (antibiotics, immunisation). Some evidence for preventive strategies based on behavioural change.	Evidence on specific interventions probably generalisable to prisons. Evidence on preventive strategies based on behavioural change unlikely to be applicable.
Special senses and disability	Limited evidence. Expert recommendations.	Probably applicable to prisons.
Pregnancy and maternity care	Extensive evidence on specific interventions from controlled trials and systematic reviews in Cochrane Library. Limited evidence on delivery of care.	Evidence not based on a prison setting. Not clear how generalisable this is to prisoners.
Mental disorders		
Personality disorders	Very limited evidence.	Not clear how generalisable this is to prisoners.
Functional psychoses	Extensive evidence from controlled trials and systematic reviews in Cochrane Library.	
Neurotic disorders	Extensive evidence from controlled trials and systematic reviews in Cochrane Library.	
Self-harm and suicide	Some evidence from randomised controlled trials and systematic reviews.	Not clear how applicable evidence is to the prison setting. There are prison-based expert recommendations.
Alcohol and drug misuse		
Alcohol misuse	Some evidence from controlled trials. Expert recommendations.	Not clear how applicable evidence is to the prison setting.
Drug misuse	Some evidence from controlled trials. Expert recommendations.	Not clear how applicable evidence is to the prison setting.
Health promotion	Very little direct evidence.	

history of illicit drug use or a past psychiatric history (see **Table 79**). Most of the problems were detected during the initial screen (i.e. by prison hospital officers): little was added to the process by the doctor's routine assessment.

Table 79: Percentage of mental health problems detected by routine screening at reception.

Mental health problem	Percentage detected following initial screening by Hospital Officer and subsequent health assessment by medical officer
Current illicit drug use	56% (95% CI: 50–61%)
Past psychiatric history	52% (95% CI: 45–58%)
History of self-harm	82% (95% CI: 75–88%)

Source: Birmingham *et al.*[100]

Exit screening prior to release

In order to draw conclusions about the effectiveness of exit screening we need a clear idea of its objectives. These could be the detection of previously hidden illness, informing and guiding discharge arrangements or ruling out specific health problems. There is no published evidence on the effectiveness of exit screening. Nor is it clear what the primary purpose of exit screening is. It is therefore difficult to draw conclusions about its effectiveness.

Effectiveness of services for minor illness

For the majority of the minor illnesses that are prevalent in the prison population, and that are the most common reasons for consultation with health care staff, there are means of self-care. However, the evidence on the effectiveness of the various types of self-care is variable. There is little direct evidence on which health professionals should deal with minor illnesses, but there is some evidence that for a range of problems, professions allied to medicine following guidelines can successfully substitute the role of physicians.[101]

Skin conditions

The effectiveness of over the counter preparations and pharmaceutical advice on the burden of skin disease in the community is unknown.[102]

Acne

Topical treatments are effective for mild to moderate acne.[103] These include benzoyl peroxide preparations, which are available without a prescription. Systemic antibiotics remain the mainstay of treatment for acne, and tetracycline is the treatment of first choice.[103]

Dandruff

Shampoos containing zinc pyrithione seem to be more effective at controlling dandruff than those without.[104] There is also some evidence that selenium-containing shampoos may be more effective than standard commercial antidandruff preparations.[105] There is also evidence that shampoos containing polytar and specific antifungals are effective in controlling dandruff.[106] Shampoos containing the active ingredients selenium sulphide, coal tar extract and zinc pyrithione are available without prescription.

Psoriasis

Mild cases of psoriasis may be treated with a variety of effective topical treatments such as coal tar, dithranol, topical corticosteroids and calcipotriol.[102]

Atopic eczema

The main treatment for mild to moderate atopic eczema is with emollients to moisturise the skin and mild to moderate potency corticosteroids.[102] A wide range of emollients and a small number of steroid-containing creams are available without a prescription. Severe atopic eczema is usually treated with potent topical corticosteroids[102] but these are only available with a prescription.

Other skin disorders

Many effective topical and systemic anti-fungal agents have been evaluated for the treatment of fungal infections of the skin, hair and nails. Controlled trials have shown that oral and topical antibiotics are effective in treating bacterial skin conditions such as impetigo. Herpes simplex infections may be treated effectively using specific anti-viral agents such as acyclovir, given topically or orally.[102]

Headache

Tension headache

Episodic tension headache can be treated with aspirin, paracetamol or ibuprofen. Combination treatments containing codeine or caffeine are best avoided because of the potential for dependence. Tension headaches which occur more than twice per week, are leading to medication misuse or are causing significant disability should be regarded as chronic tension headaches. There is some evidence that low dose amitriptyline (50–100 mg daily) is effective in reducing the frequency and duration of chronic headaches. Muscle relaxation, either with or without electromyographic biofeedback, may be effective in reducing the symptoms of chronic tension headache.[107] Behavioural treatments may also be effective when used by patients at home rather than in a clinic.[108] Spinal manipulation may be effective in reducing the frequency of tension headache.[109]

Migraine

Subcutaneous sumatriptan is probably the most effective treatment for acute migraine attacks. Oral sumatriptan, intranasal sumatriptan and any of a range of similar drugs (zolmitriptan and rizatriptan) are the next most effective treatments and oral aspirin with metoclopramide is of similar effectiveness. The cost per treatment of sumatriptan is approximately £21 for subcutaneous administration, £6 orally and £8 to £16 intranasally. Zolmitriptan and rizatriptan cost between £4 and £9 depending on the dose used. Aspirin 900 mg with metoclopramide 10 mg (issued as separate tablets) costs £0.03.[110,111]

Beta-blockers, in particular metoprolol, propranolol and alenolol; a range of non-steroidal anti-inflammatory drugs; amitryptyline; methylsergide, dihydroergotamine and pizotifen; and certain anti-convulsant drugs are effective in the prevention of migraine.[112] There is some evidence that feverfew may be effective in reducing the frequency of episodes of migraine.[113]

Upper respiratory infection

Common cold

Antibiotics are ineffective in treating the common cold.[114] However, there is evidence that suggests that some *Echinacea* preparations may be effective in the prevention and treatment of the common cold.[115] There also appears to be a modest benefit in reducing duration of cold symptoms from ingestion of relatively high doses of vitamin C although long-term daily supplementation with vitamin C in large doses does not appear to prevent colds.[116] The evidence for the effectiveness of zinc for treating the common cold is inconclusive.[117] Intranasal ipatropium bromide spray, and to a lesser extent topical oxymetalozine and some antihistamines, are probably effective for nasal symptoms only.[118]

Acute sinusitis

Current evidence is limited but supports penicillin or amoxicillin for 7 to 14 days for acute maxillary sinusitis confirmed radiographically or by aspiration. Clinicians should weigh the moderate benefits of antibiotic treatment against the potential for adverse effects.[119]

Sore throat

The benefits of treating a sore throat with antibiotics are small and may be outweighed by the disadvantages of antibiotics.[120] It also seems to be the case that patients who are prescribed antibiotics for sore throat are more likely than those who are managed without antibiotics to consult with the problem in the future.[121]

Acute cough

Patients with acute cough who are treated with antibiotics are twice as likely to suffer side effects as those treated with placebo: that is, about one in five suffer from side effects. Antibiotics do not significantly shorten the duration of the illness. This suggests that antibiotics offer no advantages over placebo in the treatment of acute cough.[122]

Acute bronchitis

Patients with acute bronchitis who are treated with antibiotics return to work or usual activities about one day sooner. Adverse effects such as nausea, vomiting, headache, skin rash or vaginitis were reported by 18% of patients treated with antibiotics, compared to 12% of those given placebo. The advantages and disadvantages of treatment are fairly evenly balanced.[123]

Musculoskeletal disorders

Back pain

In the care of patients with back pain, there is evidence that nurses following guidelines can provide superior outcomes to general practitioners.[124] Guidelines on acute back pain emphasise that bed rest should be avoided and pain treated with regular paracetamol or ibuprofen. They also emphasise the role of exercise to prevent recurrences or to treat chronic pain. It is recommended that physical activity is guided by setting goals (even if there is some discomfort) rather than to allow pain to restrict activities.[125] However, the recommendations of the guidelines with respect to clinical examination have been criticised as not evidence-based.[126] It is not clear whether acupuncture is effective in back pain.[127]

A needs assessment on low back pain in *Health Care Needs Assessment 2nd Series* provides a useful summary of effectiveness and cost-effectiveness material.[128]

Various musculoskeletal disorders

A range of rubefacients and simple analgesics are available without prescription for the relief of muscular pain. There is some evidence that ibuprofen may be more effective than opiates in the treatment of musculoskeletal pain.[129]

Naproxen 750 mg a day and aspirin 2000 mg a day seem to be of similar effectiveness in sports injuries.[130]

There is little evidence on the effectiveness of various interventions for shoulder pain.[131]

There is no evidence that patient education helps reduce pain in mechanical neck disorders.[132]

Menstrual disorders

A range of non-steroidal anti-inflammatory drugs (including ibuprofen) are effective in the treatment of dysmenorrhoea. Ibuprofen is thought to have the most favourable risk–benefit ratio. Paracetamol is probably less effective than the non-steroidal anti-inflammatory drugs.[133]

The progestagen-releasing intrauterine system (LNG IUS) is more effective at reducing menstrual blood loss than oral progestagen therapy administered from day 5 to 26 of the menstrual cycle. Oral progestagen therapy seems to offer no advantages over tranexamic acid or non-steroidal anti-inflammatory drugs.[134] Until recently, norethisterone was the most widely used treatment for menorrhagia and tranexamic acid the least widely used treatment, despite evidence suggesting the former to be ineffective and the latter effective.[135] Non-steroidal anti-inflammatory drugs (including ibuprofen) are more effective than placebo in the treatment of menorrhagia, although they seem to be less effective than tranexamic acid.[136]

There is insufficient evidence to be certain which treatments are effective in the premenstrual syndrome.[137]

A needs assessment on gynaecology in *The Health Care Needs Assessment 2nd Series* provides a useful summary of relevant effectiveness and cost-effectiveness material.[138]

Effectiveness of services for physical health problems

Reviewing the effectiveness data for all services available to address the physical health problems of prisoners would be an enormous task and is not within the scope of this review. Instead for each health problem appropriate reference material has been listed. The list of guidelines is by no means exhaustive and the guidelines themselves are constantly being updated and new ones being produced.

Epilepsy

Some indicators of sources of evidence are provided in **Appendix 4**.

Asthma

A number of widely accepted guidelines are available on the management of asthma. These are based on a mixture of evidence and expert recommendations. Further information on these is provided in **Appendix 4**.

Diabetes

There are a number of widely accepted guidelines, based on expert recommendations and some evidence, on the management of diabetes. Further information on these is provided in **Appendix 4**. In addition, the *Health Care Needs Assessment* series includes an epidemiological needs assessment of diabetes mellitus.

Ischaemic heart disease and cardiovascular risk factors

Raised blood pressure and raised cholesterol

Extensive evidence on the management of ischaemic heart disease and cardiovascular risk factors has been synthesised into a number of evidence-based guidelines. These have in common an increasing emphasis on estimation of the *absolute risk* of cardiovascular events and using this as a basis for the decision to treat. This can be summarised as follows.

Guidelines recommend that anyone whose systolic blood pressure exceeds 180 mmHg or whose diastolic blood pressure exceeds 105 mmHg should be treated irrespective of their estimated vascular risk. This is because in persons with very high blood pressure the estimated vascular risk may underestimate their true risk. In addition, any patient whose estimated annual risk of a vascular event is greater than 2% (10% five year risk), should be considered for treatment if their blood pressure is raised (i.e. over 140 mmHg systolic or 90 mmHg diastolic). There remains some doubt about whether lowering systolic blood pressure to below 140 mmHg (or diastolic to below 90 mmHg) confers any advantages.

The guidelines are similar for cholesterol-lowering drugs (statins). Guidelines recommend treating anyone whose estimated annual risk of a vascular event is greater than 3% (15% five year risk), provided their total cholesterol to HDL cholesterol ratio is average or above average. In addition, anyone with a total cholesterol to HDL cholesterol ratio of 8 or higher should be offered treatment, irrespective of their estimated vascular risk. This is because the estimated vascular risk may underestimate their true risk.

The approach that only patients in whom there is a reasonable chance that treatment may be offered should be screened has important implications for who should be screened for high blood pressure and raised serum lipids. The information in **Appendix 4** uses data on the prevalence of cardiovascular risk factors such as raised blood pressure and raised cholesterol to estimate the likelihood of encountering patients who need treatment in different age-groups. Among younger patients a very small proportion are at high risk of a cardiovascular event, whereas among older patients, a high proportion are at high risk. What this means in practical terms is that it is likely to be unproductive screening male or female prisoners under 40 for high blood pressure or raised cholesterol. Because a higher proportion of blacks have high blood pressure, it may be worthwhile screening black prisoners between the ages of 30 and 39.

Smoking cessation

Appendix 4 summarises some of the evidence for the benefits of interventions to assist smoking cessation.

Infectious diseases

Hepatitis B

Vaccination against hepatitis B is given as a course of three injections. Once completed it provides very effective protection against infection especially in younger people. Present Home Office recommendations are that this is offered to all prisoners (see **Box 5**).

Tuberculosis

On average, immunisation with BCG reduces the risk of tuberculosis by half.[139] Further sources of information on effective interventions for the control and treatment on tuberculosis are listed in **Appendix 4**.

Sexually transmitted diseases (STDs)

There is evidence that educational interventions targeting socially and economically disadvantaged women can, at least in the short-term, lead to reductions in risky sexual behaviour. The educational intervention included information provision and was complemented by sexual negotiation skill development. The focus of this research was reduction in the transmission of human papilloma virus to reduce the incidence of cervical carcinoma, however it has implications for the prevention of other sexually transmitted diseases.[140]

Special senses and disability

There is evidence that speech therapy is effective for treating stuttering and stammering.[141,142]

Pregnancy, maternity and postnatal care

There is evidence to suggest that women in custody may have better birth outcomes in terms of weight and risk of stillbirth.[143,144] This is thought to be because of lifestyle changes – improved diet, removal from domestic stresses, decreased consumption of alcohol and drugs and reduced smoking. In addition, another study has shown that women imprisoned for longer periods (over 120 days as opposed to fewer than 90 days) appear to benefit from better prenatal care, improved nutrition, and a structured environment and thus a more favourable perinatal outcome.[145]

Mother and baby units

A study by Catan in 1989[146] looked at the progress of babies in prison in mother and baby units. The development of unit babies was compared with babies separated from their imprisoned mothers and cared for in the community. Both groups of babies showed normal, healthy physical growth and their overall development fell within accepted norms. However, the babies who stayed in the units for four months or more showed a slight and gradual decline in locomotor and cognitive scores. When babies left the units, there was a significant increase in their general development scores, whereas the development of babies left outside remained stable over the follow up period.

Parent education

Outcomes of prison parenting programs in the US included improved self-esteem, behavioural expectations, empathy, discipline, family roles, relationships and a commitment to avoid substance use and reincarceration.[147]

Effectiveness of services for mental health problems

Personality disorders

An evaluation of the effectiveness of the therapeutic community approach for treating borderline personality disorder concluded that there has been a number of observational studies that showed potentially important clinical effects which may be associated with some savings to secondary care and prison services. However, the validity of the findings remained open to some doubt.[148]

Dialectical behaviour therapy may be of value to patients with personality disorders and judicious use of drug therapy (monoamine oxidase inhibitors, carbamazepine and neuroleptics) is likely to be beneficial.[149]

Functional psychoses

Schizophrenia

All antipsychotic medications are superior to placebo in the treatment of schizophrenia. They lessen positive symptoms and gradually diminish disturbed thought processes, but are not curative.[150] A group of drugs generally termed as atypical antipsychotic drugs (clozapine, risperidone, olanzapine and quetiapine) have a greater efficacy, especially for negative symptoms, and a better clinical response in patients than traditional antipsychotics.[150,151] At present beta-blockers as an adjunct to antipsychotic medication cannot be recommended in the treatment of schizophrenia.[152]

A review of the effects of cognitive behaviour therapy (CBT) for patients with schizophrenia found that for those who were willing to receive CBT, access to this treatment approach is associated with a substantially reduced risk of relapse.[153] However, the review highlighted that at present CBT is a rare commodity often provided by highly skilled and experienced therapists and therefore its application in day-to-day practice may be limited by the availability of suitable practitioners.

There is some evidence to support the use of electroconvulsive therapy (ECT) for patients with schizophrenia for short-term relief of symptoms. ECT may be advocated as an adjunct to antipsychotic medication for patients who show limited response to medication alone but the evidence for this is not strong.[154]

Neurotic disorders

As neurotic disorders are very common in the prison population, they have been addressed in some detail. Effective interventions for neurotic disorders are dealt with under three headings: prevention (mental health promotion), recognition (detection) and treatment. Since depression, or depression with anxiety, are by far the most common neurotic disorders, the focus has been on these. Mental health promotion consists of general measures to reduce the occurrence of a range of neurotic symptoms and neurotic disorders. Recognition of mental health problems focuses more on the identification of neurotic disorders, particularly depression. Treatment is partly dictated by the nature of the disorder itself and the patient's preferences. Nevertheless, there are some common elements, such as the need for a therapeutic alliance with a single key carer and the need to consider social and psychological aspects of the problem.

Prevention of neurotic disorders: mental health promotion

The national service framework for mental health[155] specifically identifies the value of promoting mental health in prisons. Strategies to achieve this include anti-bullying strategies, regular physical exercise and contact with family friends and the outside community.

Box 7: The three elements of crisis support.

- The presence of someone close in whom the person at risk may confide about the crisis event (e.g. conviction, sentencing or imprisonment).
- Active ongoing emotional support from the supporting person.
- During the period of support, no negative comments made by the supporting person about the person seeking help.

Adapted from: Brown (1992).[156]

Many prisoners' personal social circumstances and psychological histories mean that they are predisposed to depression prior to their arrival in prison. For most, imprisonment is a life event which has the potential to precipitate depression. There is evidence that in a situation where depression is likely, crisis support may be associated with a substantially reduced risk of depression.[156] There is also evidence that if crisis support is expected but not provided, patients are even more likely to become depressed than if it were not expected. The elements of crisis support are shown in **Box 7**.

Recognition of neurotic disorders

Recognition of depression is an essential prerequisite to establishing a therapeutic alliance between patient and carer. This therapeutic alliance is believed to be an important factor in aiding recovery.[157] It is also necessary to recognise depression before treatment can be initiated.

Depression is commonly missed, especially in patients with chronic physical disease, who are five times more likely to have their depression missed.[158,159] It is thought that up to 50% of patients with depression are missed.[160] It is therefore likely that this also holds true in the prison population. Detection and treatment of depression considerably improves the prognosis.[161,162]

The ability to detect emotional distress among patients is linked to specific interview skills. In brief these include making eye contact with the patient, clarifying the complaint, attention to verbal and non-verbal cues and asking specific psychiatric questions.[163] Recognition and diagnosis of depression can be carried out by all members of the primary health care team. It is possible to teach improved interview skills to primary care team members.[164]

Treatment of neurotic disorders

The great majority of neurotic disorders can be treated in a primary care setting. In the community this is usually the case. Drugs are the mainstay of treatment in the community despite some commonly used drugs having significant disadvantages (such as dependency). Where skills are available, psychological treatments (in particular cognitive behaviour therapy) and some effective pharmacological treatments (plant extracts) are available without prescription. There does not appear to be evidence that any particular professional is required for the recognition or treatment of neurotic disorders. It follows that appropriate skills may be more important than specific qualifications.

Depression

Both psychological and drug treatments are effective in the treatment of depression. **Table 80** illustrates the range of treatments and with their main advantages and disadvantages. The most effective approach to treating depression seems to be a combination of drug therapy and psychotherapy.[165]

There is good evidence that cognitive behaviour therapy is effective in the treatment of depression. It is of similar effectiveness to drug treatments or possibly more effective. There is also good evidence that interpersonal therapy is effective in the treatment of depression.[166-168] It is difficult to estimate the effectiveness of counselling services as many patients recover spontaneously. The best evidence of effectiveness comes from studies of counselling which incorporates modified versions of specific therapeutic models such as interpersonal counselling, exploratory therapy and behaviour therapy.

Antidepressant drugs are generally effective in treating depression and different types of antidepressants are equally efficacious[169,170] Antidepressant drugs are also effective in treating depressed patients who are physically ill.[171] In addition, extract of St. John's Wort (*Hypericum perforatum*) is more effective than placebo in the treatment of depression and patients report fewer side effects than with low dose antidepressants.[172,173] Because it is not classified as a drug, it can be sold over the counter and issued without a doctor's prescription.

Benzodiazepine drugs do not generally seem to be effective in treating depression.[174] In view of their addictive properties and potential for abuse it is recommended that they are not generally be used for depression.

A depressed patient is more likely to take treatment if he is educated about its potential side effects and the likelihood of success. If a treatment is going to be successful, the patient should have shown a 50% reduction in symptoms after a 4–6 week trial of medication or a 6–8 week trial of cognitive behaviour therapy or other therapy. The patient needs to be reassessed at this point: if there has been no response an alternative drug or therapy should be tried (i.e. a treatment from a different row in **Table 80**). If the patient does respond to treatment, it should be continued for a further 4–9 months.[166-168]

Dysthymia (chronic mild depression)

Antidepressant drugs are also effective in treating dysthymia (chronic mild depression). Again, there are no significant differences in effectiveness between different groups of drugs, such as tricyclic antidepressants, selective serotonin reuptake inhibitors (SSRIs) and monoamine oxidase inhibitors (MAOIs).[175]

It is not yet clear whether psychotherapy is effective in treating dysthymia and drug treatment has been recommended as the first line treatment.[166-168]

Generalised anxiety disorder and other neurotic disorders

There is evidence that generalised anxiety disorder, panic disorder (and dysthymia) can be effectively treated with tricyclic antidepressants, self-help or cognitive behaviour therapy. Benzodiazepines are less effective than these three approaches.[176,177] The self-help approach involves teaching procedures for managing somatic and cognitive symptoms and for dealing with avoidance and low self-confidence.[178] It may be relevant to the prison setting that there is some evidence that the self-help approach is less effective and antidepressants more effective in patients with personality disorders.[179]

Cognitive therapy is probably more effective in the long term than anxiety management training. However, treatment requires 8–10 individual sessions. Both cognitive therapy and anxiety management training seem to be more effective than psychodynamic (analytic) psychotherapy. Behaviourally based anxiety management can be carried out by health professionals after only brief instruction.[180] Anxiety

Table 80: The main types of effective treatments for depression.

Psychological treatments

Type of treatment	Advantages	Resource implications	Disadvantages
Therapeutic support: by GP or nurse	Beneficial effect in mild to moderate depression. Can be combined with drug treatment.	Individual counselling requires a lot of staff time and may not offer advantages over GP counselling or nurse follow-up. Requires minimal training and support for practitioners. Involves only small changes to usual practice.	May offer little advantage over therapeutic support by GP or nurse.
Non-directive counselling	Beneficial effect in mild to moderate depression. Can be combined with drug treatment.	Resource-intensive: ideally 8 to 12 one hour sessions. Can be carried out by clinical psychologists, nurses, doctors and other health professionals. Need to arrange for supervision of therapists.	
Cognitive behaviour therapy	Effective. Can be combined with drug treatment.		

Drug treatments

Type of treatment	Advantages	Resource implications	Disadvantages
Older tricyclic antidepressants (imipramine, amitriptyline, clomipramine etc.)	Effective.	Imipramine £2 a month. Amitriptyline £2 a month. Clomipramine £10 a month.	Side effects such as dry mouth, constipation and sedation. May be fatal in overdose. Often prescribed in inadequate doses.
Newer tricyclic antidepressants and similar (mianserin, lofepramine etc.)	Effective. Generally better tolerated than older tricyclic antidepressants.	Lofepramine £10 to £15 a month. Mianserin £10 to £15 a month.	Side effects such as dry mouth and constipation are less frequent than with older tricyclic antidepressants. Not commonly fatal in overdose. Sometimes prescribed in inadequate doses. Patients on mianserin require monthly blood counts.

Table 80: Continued.

Drug treatments

Type of treatment	Advantages	Resource implications	Disadvantages
SSRIs (fluoxetine, citalopram, fluvoxamine, paroxetine, sertraline etc.)	Effective. Adequate doses are generally prescribed. Generally better tolerated than older tricyclic antidepressants.	Fluoxetine £21 to £42 a month. Citalopram £21 to £42 a month. Fluvoxamine £19 a month. Paroxetine £21 to £31 a month. Sertraline £26 to £40 a month.	Side effects such as agitation, sleeplessness, nausea and diarrhoea. Dangerous interaction with MAOIs if one is prescribed at the same time as or within two weeks of stopping the other.
St. John's Wort (*Hypericum perforatum*)	Effective. Not legally classified as a drug: can be bought over the counter and could be issued without a doctor's prescription. Low incidence of side effects.	Cost varies with source, generally £10 to £20 per month.	Side effects are very infrequent, similar to SSRIs. Believed to be safe in overdose. Possibly similar dangerous interaction with MAOIs and SSRIs.
MAOIs (moclobemide, phenelzine)	Effective.	Phenelzine £6 a month. Moclobemide £16 to £32.	Dangerous interaction with SSRIs (see above). Dangerous interaction with decongestant medications and certain foods: cheese, pickled herring, yeast extract and broad bean pods. Dietary interactions less of a problem with moclobemide

management can also be effectively organised for groups of six to eight patients.[181] The advantages and disadvantages of different approaches to treating anxiety are summarised in **Table 81**.

Table 81: Treatments for neurotic disorders such as generalised anxiety disorder, panic disorder and dysthymia.

Intervention	Effectiveness	Resource implications	Personnel and training implications
Benzodiazepines	Effective, but less so than antidepressants. May lead to dependence. Commonly relapses after discontinuation.	Inexpensive. Drug costs are very low.	Requires prescription by medical practitioner.
Antidepressants	Effective. May be more effective in patients with personality disorder. Commonly relapses after discontinuation.	Depends on choice of drug: tricyclics are inexpensive, SSRI more expensive (£12 to £150 for 6 months' treatment).	Requires prescription by medical practitioner.
Cognitive behaviour therapy	Effective. In the long term this may be the most effective approach.	Individual therapy: 8–10 therapist hours (approximately £400 to £500) per patient. (One hour a week over 8–10 weeks.)	Following appropriate training can be carried out by various health professionals. Supervision arrangements are necessary.
Self-help (anxiety management training)	Effective. May be less effective in patients with personality disorder.	Group therapy possible: $1\frac{1}{2}$ therapist hours (approximately £75) per patient. (Six to eight patients per group, $1\frac{1}{2}$ hours a week for 6 weeks.)	Some therapist training is required.
Psychodynamic (analytic) therapy	Relatively ineffective.	Individual therapy: 8–10 therapist hours (approximately £400 to £500) per patient. (One hour a week over 8–10 weeks.)	Extensive training is required although this can be undertaken by various health professionals. Supervision arrangements are necessary.

Antidepressants (tricyclic antidepressants, SSRIs and MAOIs), benzodiazepines and cognitive-behavioural treatments all are more effective than control treatments. Cognitive-behavioural treatments seem to be the most effective. Benzodiazepines have the disadvantage of dependence.[182] For many anxiety-related conditions, the benefits of drug treatment may cease when medication is withdrawn. This means that psychological treatments may offer significant long-term advantages.[166]

Obsessive-compulsive disorder

Psychological treatments which include exposure to the trigger stimulus and prevention of the compulsive response are effective in the treatment of obsessive-compulsive disorder. This essentially means that treatment should include elements of behavioural therapy. Psychological treatments which do not include exposure and response prevention are not effective.[183,184] Improvements after behaviour therapy seem to be maintained in the long term.[185]

Obsessive-compulsive disorder can be effectively treated with clomipramine (a tricyclic antidepressant which has some effects on serotinin reuptake) and the selective serotinin reuptake inhibitors (SSRI). It is not clear whether there is a difference between these drugs on effectiveness grounds: they are either equally effective or clomipramine may be more effective.[186,187] A month's treatment with clomipramine is considerably less costly than a typical SSRI (£10 versus £21 to £63).

Relapse is common after discontinuation of drug therapy and long-term outcomes are clearly better with behaviour therapy (exposure and response prevention).[166]

Treatment of neurotic symptoms: insomnia

A number of effective non-drug treatments for insomnia are listed in **Box 8**. Stimulus control therapy consists of instructions designed to curtail sleep-incompatible behaviours and to regulate sleep-wake schedules. Sleep restriction therapy involves curtailing the amount of time spent in bed to time actually spent asleep (i.e. patients are encouraged to get up if they cannot sleep). Relaxation therapies include progressive muscle relaxation, biofeedback and meditation. They are intended to alleviate somatic or cognitive arousal. Paradoxical intention involves persuading the patient to engage in their most feared behaviour (staying awake) to induce sleep. Sleep hygiene education means the regulation of health and environmental factors that may be detrimental or beneficial to sleep.

Box 8: Non-drug treatments for insomnia.

- Relaxation approaches incorporating progressive muscle relaxation.
- Meditation.
- Desensitisation.
- Imagery.
- Hypnosis and autogenic training.
- Stimulus control.
- Paradoxical intervention.
- Sleep restriction therapy.
- Combination treatment: consisting largely of composites of stimulus control and relaxation.

One review concluded that psychological interventions were effective in reducing the time taken to fall asleep, increasing the length of time asleep, reducing awakenings and improving the quality of sleep. The improvements were both short-term and long-term. Insomniacs who were *not* using sleep medications seemed to benefit more from these approaches than those who were users.[188]

A second review of non-drug treatments for insomnia found that psychological interventions averaging 5 hours of therapy time produced reliable changes in two of the four sleep measures (sleep onset latency and for time awake after sleep onset). Stimulus control was the most effective single therapy procedure. The review concluded that although psychological treatment may be more expensive and time-consuming than pharmacotherapy, the current data indicate that it may prove more cost-effective in the long term.[189]

Hypnotic drugs and anxiolytics are effective in the short-term treatment of insomnia. Prescribing of these drugs is widespread but dependence and tolerance occurs. This may lead to difficulty in withdrawing the drug after the patient has been taking it regularly for more than a few weeks.[190]

Prevention and treatment of post-traumatic stress disorder

Although debriefing is widely practised, there is no current evidence that psychological debriefing is a useful treatment for the prevention of post traumatic stress disorder after traumatic incidents. The accumulated evidence to date suggests that psychological debriefing may increase the numbers who suffer from post-traumatic stress disorder one year after the event.[191]

There is some evidence that psychological and pharmacological treatments for post-traumatic stress disorder are more effective at reducing symptoms than placebo. Behaviour therapy and eye-movement desensitisation and reprocessing seem to be effective psychological treatments. There is no evidence that biofeedback-guided relaxation, dynamic psychotherapy or hypnotherapy are effective. Evidence for the effectiveness of pharmacological treatments is most convincing for SSRIs. These are used in relatively high doses (e.g. fluoxetine 60 mg). There is some evidence that carbamazepine may be effective. There is no evidence that tricyclic antidepressants, monoamine oxidase inhibitors or benzodiazepines are effective.[192]

Effectiveness of services for self-harm and suicide

A number of systematic reviews evaluating the effectiveness of interventions aimed at preventing suicide and self-harm have been published in recent years.[193–195] A review by Hawton *et al*[195] concluded that there remains considerable uncertainty about which forms of psychosocial and physical treatments of self-harm patients are the most effective.

An approach in the USA to preventing suicides among inmates has reduced suicides in New York City's jails to five or fewer each year. Prisoners, who are paid 23 pence an hour, act as monitors keeping an eye on fellow prisoners most at risk of suicide. Selected inmates are specially screened, trained and tested before they become observation aides. Prison officers also have suicide prevention training and mental health staff play a big role.[196]

Effectiveness of services for alcohol misuse

A report on the effectiveness of brief interventions in reducing harm associated with alcohol consumption[197] concluded that:

- simple screening instruments are available for the routine detection of people drinking harmful levels of alcohol which can easily be applied opportunistically in both primary and secondary care health settings. These include the validated AUDIT questionnaire which initial estimates indicated detection levels of 92% of harmful or hazardous drinkers (sensitivity) and identification of 94% of people who consume below the harmful levels (specificity)[198]
- brief interventions consisting of assessment of intake and provision of information and advice are effective in reducing alcohol consumption by over 20% in the large group of people with raised alcohol consumption. However, it is not clear how this translates into changes in health status
- evidence from clinical trials suggests that brief interventions are as effective as more specialist treatments (counselling/therapy sessions, skills training etc.)

Pharmacotherapy for alcohol dependence

A review of the evidence for the efficacy of pharmacotherapy for alcohol dependence found the following:[199]

- **Disulfiram:** There is little evidence that disulfiram enhances abstinence, but there is evidence that it reduces drinking days. Studies of disulfiram implants are methodologically weak and generally without good evidence of bioavailability.
- **Naltrexone:** There is good evidence that naltrexone reduces relapse and number of drinking days in alcohol dependent subjects. There is some evidence that it reduces craving and enhances abstinence and there is good evidence that it has a favourable harms profile.
- **Acamprosate:** There is good evidence that acamprosate enhances abstinence and reduces drinking days in alcohol dependent subjects, there is minimal evidence on its effects on craving or rates of severe relapse and there is good evidence that it is well tolerated and without serious harms.
- **Serotonergic agents:** There is minimal evidence on the efficacy of serotonergic agents for treatment of the core symptoms of alcohol dependence but there is some evidence for the treatment of alcohol-dependent symptoms in patients with co-morbid mood or anxiety disorders, although data are limited.
- **Lithium:** There is evidence that lithium is not efficacious in the treatment of the core symptoms of alcohol dependence. There is minimal evidence for efficacy of lithium for the treatment of alcohol-dependent symptoms in co-morbid depression.

A Health Care Needs Assessment on Alcohol Misuse in the *Health Care Needs Assessment series* summarises the effectiveness of services available to address alcohol misuse.[200]

Effectiveness of services for drug misuse

The Department of Health has published evidence based guidelines on the Clinical Management of Drug Misuse and Dependence in 1999.[201] The guidelines have been written with a particular focus on generalist practitioners.

A Health Care Needs Assessment on Drug Abuse in the *Health Care Needs Assessment series* summarises the effectiveness of services available to address drug misuse.[202]

Effectiveness of health promotion

There is very little evidence on the effectiveness of health promotion interventions in a prison setting. Some published research literature does exist, much of it related to HIV and drug education. Useful unpublished reports of individual initiatives can also sometimes be accessed, but many – like most of those described in the Directorate of Health Care's 1998 *Good Practice Guide to Health Promotion in Prisons* – have not been rigorously evaluated.

Looking to the literature of a more general nature which could be drawn upon, a majority of health promotion initiatives which have been evaluated/written up are based on poorly designed research and evaluation, and are in the main descriptive. Indeed, health promotion in general does not routinely have access to the funding and expertise for comprehensive evaluative research. Nevertheless, research-based knowledge is available, such as meta-analyses produced by the NHS Centre fore Reviews and Dissemination at the University of York on various topics of relevance to prisons, e.g. 'Smoking Cessation: what the Health Service Can Do', with advice on what works best in the wider community, and which could be adapted to the prison setting.[203] Similarly there is more general research which could be adapted in publications such as the *Health Education Journal* and specialist journals such as *Addiction*. A King's Fund literature search carried out in 1998 and going back five years found 45 references for 'prisons and health promotion', the majority about HIV and drug use. However, a further search 'evaluation/effectiveness of health promotion' was so extensive it needed to be restricted to 1998 to be manageable, covering a variety of topics as well as evaluation in general (carried out by Paul Hayton).

A literature review[204] commissioned by the Directorate of Health Care in 1998 recorded that, 'Common characteristics have emerged from this review that appear to increase the effectiveness of health promotion. Their transferability to the prison setting have not been adequately demonstrated through existing identified research.' Nevertheless, the same factors that characterise effective health promotion interventions in other settings were considered likely to render health promotion in prisons more effective. The main features of effective health promotion interventions are described in **Box 9**.

Box 9: Features of effective health promotion interventions.

Effective health promotion interventions:

- are strategic and comprehensive with multiple rather that individual initiatives
- occur in a supportive environment through addressing organisational, policy and structural issues
- are needs-based
- are appropriate to the target group
- actively involve participants
- use peer support or are peer-led
- give basic information relevant to the needs and concerns of the target group, although giving information alone is rarely sufficient to change behaviour
- address self-esteem, values and life-skills training
- are ongoing: effectiveness appears to decline over time once the intervention ceased.

---

7 Models of care and recommendations

The role of health care needs assessment

The need for health care should be the central consideration when planning health care services in prisons. By need we mean the prison populations' ability to benefit from health care. Planning on the basis of need requires assessment of the health care needs of the prison population and because different prisons have different problems, these should be *local* assessments of need. In the short term, it may seem easier to simply adapt services which are currently available in the light of present demands. However, this does not constitute needs-based planning and where possible should be avoided.

The range of health problems experienced by prisoners

The prison population, on the whole, is a population of young adults. Many of the needs of prisoners are the same as those of any population of young adults. Prisoners therefore need access to the full range of services, ranging from informal care and primary care through to highly specialised interventions, which are available to young adults in the community.

Special circumstances of the prison setting

A number of special circumstances affect the delivery of health care in a prison setting and should be considered in addressing the health care needs of prisoners. Ethnic minorities are over-represented in prisons and many prisoners have had little formal education. Services need to be sensitive to the special needs of patients from these groups. Prisons isolate inmates from their families and social networks. This has important implications for the degree of informal support available to prisoners. Self-harm and suicide are not uncommon among prisoners. Because of this and because of the occurrence of drug misuse on the prison wings, prisoners cannot be given open access to medications which are freely available in the community. The culture which prisoners are drawn from and indeed the culture of prisons themselves does not always place a high priority on health concerns. There are a range of problems related to the primacy of security in a prison setting and the high turnover of the prison population.

Co-operating with the NHS also presents a range of problems. The transfer of patient records from NHS to prisons and from prisons to the NHS is by no means easy. Finally, there can be considerable problems transferring patients from prison to NHS facilities during or at the end of their sentences. Many problems are attributable to issues related to areas of residence. In addition, NHS facilities are responsible for residents within defined geographical areas, but the district of residence of prisoners can be difficult to pin down.

Incidence and prevalence of health problems

Prisoners are heavy users of primary care. Although direct data on the reasons for primary care consultations among prisoners is lacking, it is likely that the commonest reasons for consultation are similar to those among young adults in the community. This suggests that minor illnesses and other problems dealt with at the level of primary care are the commonest reasons for prisoners using health care. In the terminology of needs assessment, minor illnesses and other primary care problems are the largest *demands* on the health care services. However, most minor illnesses are (by definition) self-limiting. In some cases, medical treatment is as likely to do harm as to improve the outcome. In those cases where there is effective treatment, this is often available without a doctor's prescription. In needs assessment terminology, there is little *need* for health care for minor illnesses and in those cases where there is need it may be most cost-effective for patients to access it themselves.

In the prison setting mental health problems are very common. Of these, neurotic disorders such as depression and anxiety are by far the most prevalent. There are effective interventions for all the common neurotic disorders. In other words, the greatest health care *needs* among prisoners are services for mental health, whereas the greatest health care *demands* are for the treatment of minor illness.

Health services

Where evidence of effectiveness for services is available, those services that are provided should be those that are effective. Services which are known to be ineffective should not be provided. In addition, where there is cost effectiveness information, the most cost-effective services should be chosen. In many cases there is no direct evidence of the effectiveness or cost-effectiveness of health care services in prisons. In all cases, it is reasonable to try to provide effective services equivalent to those found in the community.

The relationship between informal and formal health care

Male and female prisoners respectively consult primary health care workers 77 and 197 times more frequently and prison doctors three times more frequently than young adults in the community. However, since prisoners do not suffer from over 70 times as much minor illness as young adults in the community, it follows that community populations deal with much minor illness without using the formal health services. This difference is not surprising: prisoners have good access to primary health care and face a number of barriers to informal care. Lack of access to informal care diverts prisoners into the formal health care system. **Figure 28** illustrates this problem. To address this, specific efforts should be made to identify barriers to informal methods of care and strategies should be developed to promote informal care and to encourage prisoners to make use of it. Alongside this it is probably reasonable to use an appointments system to regulate access to the formal health care system. Approaches to the problem of informal care are discussed in **Appendix 6**.

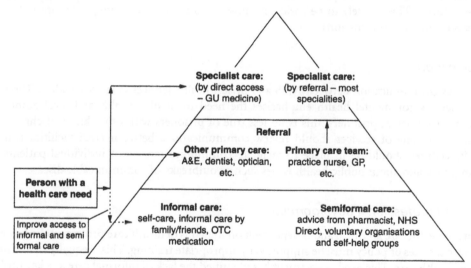

Figure 28: Providing services to prisoners similar to those available to a person in the community.

The use of in-patient beds

Prisoners have access to the full range of NHS beds. Their admission rates to NHS beds are slightly lower than admission rates for young adults in the community. This is not surprising, since imprisonment makes access to NHS hospital beds more difficult and health care staff are likely to have a higher threshold for hospital admission. It is likely that the pattern of admissions differs to that in the community, since some health problems (traumatic injuries and road accidents) are less common in prisoners and others (mental health problems) are more common.

Prisoners also have access to a large number of health care centre beds in prisons. These amount to 29 hospital beds per 1000 inmates, i.e. around six times the per capita number of hospital beds available to the UK population as a whole. Because prisoners have easy access to such a large number of hospital beds, admission rates are very high. Women prisoners are admitted 16 times more frequently to health care centre beds than young women in the community; inmates in local prisons are admitted 14 times more frequently; young offenders nine times more frequently; and inmates in training prisons twice as frequently. These are very high admission rates. A small proportion of admissions are for reasons which are not frequently encountered in the community. These include sanctuary (to avoid bullying) and for supervision following self-harm.

While there is no doubt that there is *demand* for health care centre beds, it is not clear whether this is always the most appropriate or cost-effective way of meeting health care *needs*. For example, there does not seem to be a need for 'cottage hospital' facilities for young adults in the community. Young adults with physical and mental health problems are managed either in NHS hospitals or at home. Relying on in-patient health care also inhibits the development of community-based health care. If the management of prisoners with health care problems includes removing them from the prison wings, this means that health care may be seen as solely the responsibility of the health care centre. This is inimical to fostering a prison culture which puts a concern for health at the centre of all prison life.

It is difficult to make specific recommendations with regard to the provision of health care centre beds. Undoubtedly the provision of in-patient beds in prisons should be reviewed. It is likely that provision should be reduced. This is likely to be easiest in those prisons were occupancy rates are not high (see **Appendix 5** for further information).

Communication

In many cases communication between NHS and prison health services is far from ideal. The national service framework for mental health emphasises the need to involve health and local authorities in preparation for release of prisoners: this is no less true of prisoners with other kinds of chronic health problems. Any review of services should review communications between NHS facilities and prison services. Procedures should be in place to facilitate communication about individual patients, about changes in policy and about public health issues such as outbreaks of communicable disease.

Training and professional development

The quality of health care is critical and is dependent on the skills of health care professionals. Any changes in health care services or policy must be supported by appropriate training. This is equally true of informal as of formal health care. This needs assessment has identified the lack of informal care as a key problem in the delivery of prison health care. This needs to be addressed by the provision of training and information for prison inmates. While it may not be realistic to provide training for prisoners, it is entirely possible to provide information on the more common minor illnesses, guidelines on how to manage them and guidelines on how to make use of the prison health services.

As there is evidence that professions allied to medicine can successfully manage a range of conditions by following guidelines, there is also a case for developing locally agreed guidelines for the management of minor illness. These can also encourage consistency in the management of minor illness. If brief outlines of the guidelines were included in the information provided to prisoners, they could also promote individual responsibility and shared care.

This document has also identified neurotic disorders as a particularly great health care need among prison inmates. The identification and management of neurotic disorders can be improved with training. This suggests that training in the management of neurotic disorders should be given a high priority for all prison health care staff.

8 Outcome measures

A number of health problems are common in all prisons and some general recommendations can be made about the provision of health care services to meet the health care needs created by these problems. However, since many health care problems of prisoners vary from one prison to another it is not possible to make recommendations about the total provision of health care services in all prisons.

Health promotion

A 'settings' or 'whole institution' approach to health promotion should be adopted and developed with support of local NHS health promotion specialists, considering the needs of both staff and prisoners. Links should be made to initiatives and documents of the Prison Health Promotion Development Project and the WHO (Europe) Health in Prisons Project – both of which can be contacted through the Directorate of Health Care or via the Project website (www.euro.who.int/prisons).

Prisons have a unique ability to control the occupational and dietary regimes of their inmates. Advice should be sought from appropriate specialists (in particular occupational therapists and dieticians) on how to organise the prisons main regime to optimise prisoners' health.

Primary care trusts and public health departments who have experience in promoting health and well-being should be contacted. Health promotion is not just the concern of health care staff, other prison workers should also be encouraged to be actively involved in providing a 'health promoting' environment. Health promotion should concentrate on areas appropriate to the prison population. In addition, efforts should be made to encourage prisoners to adopt healthy lifestyles by means of health promotion and illness prevention initiatives.

Physical health problems

A system should be in place to allow all prisoners with chronic illnesses such as epilepsy, asthma and ischaemic heart disease to be identified. In most cases it will be helpful to contact their general practitioners to confirm the diagnosis and any other related problems and to establish what medications they are taking. All prisoners with chronic illnesses should be reviewed by appropriate specialists and treated following evidence-based guidelines.

Cardiovascular risk factors

In the absence of specific indications (such as diabetes or pre-existing ischaemic heart disease), prisoners under 45 should not routinely have their cholesterol levels checked. Few will be at sufficiently high risk to be treated. In the absence of specific indications (such as diabetes or pre-existing ischaemic heart disease), white prisoners under 45 should not routinely have their blood pressure checked. Although a small number will have raised blood pressure, few will be at sufficiently high risk to be treated.

Black prisoners are an exception to this rule. Black prisoners over 30 should have their blood pressure checked because of the high prevalence of raised blood pressure in the black population.

Infectious diseases

Immunisation against hepatitis B should be offered to all prisoners and uptake should be actively encouraged.

Patients consulting with suspected sexually transmitted diseases should be seen by a genito-urinary medicine specialist and should be offered health education (either by video or face to face) on risk factors for sexually transmitted diseases.

Special senses and disability

A system should be in place to identify prisoners with disabilities including speech and language difficulties. They should be offered appropriate advice and support.

Mental disorders

In 2001, Prison Health (the Department of Health) published *Changing the Outlook: a strategy for developing and modernising mental health services in prison.* This document sets out a 3–5-year vision for prison mental health services.

The underlying ethos of the prison mental health programme has always been that NHS services should be 'mainstreamed' into prisons, in other words, the same standards of care should be available to prisoners as to people living in the community. Reflecting this mainstream approach, responsibility for implementing the prison mental health programme passed from the Department of Health to the National Institute for Mental Health in England (NIMHE) in 2003. Just as NIMHE is supporting NHS Trusts and PCTs to implement the National Service Framework for Mental Health, so it will support the prison service.

Functional psychoses

An improved system should be developed for the identification of patients with serious mental illness. All such patients should be managed using a care programme approach. If necessary, staff should undergo training in the care programme approach to mental health care.

Neurotic disorders

The primary health care team should undergo systematic training in the detection and management of depression. This should be repeated on a regular basis to allow for turnover of staff.

Psychological therapies are very underused in prisons. Prisons should get access to these skills either by contracting in a clinical psychologist or by nominating and training existing staff in the use of behaviour therapy, cognitive behaviour therapy and anxiety management training.

Creating some supportive social networks within the prison community is likely to be important in the prevention of mental health problems. In the first place the health service should have a register of all those prisoners at risk of mental health problems. This includes all prisoners in the first four weeks after reception (and in some cases after sentencing), all young prisoners and all prisoners whose mental health continues to be a concern. It is unrealistic to expect health care staff to have time to build up relationships with these prisoners. However, each could be allocated to and encouraged (at least once) to meet with a named prisoner in a 'befriending' or 'listening' scheme.

Prisoners at high risk of mental health problems should be offered crisis support. Those at high risk are those with known mental health problems who are considered a suicide risk and any others who become known to the health services or 'befriending' scheme. In theory crisis support can be provided by a health professional or prison officer, but as 24-hour access is required it may be more practical for this to be provided as an extension of a 'befriending' or 'listening' scheme. The Ranby Care Support Scheme combines 'befriending' with 'shared accommodation'. However, if this is not practical, it may be possible to use alternative approaches. These include providing wing staff with 24-hour access to a list of prisoners and their befrienders or during periods of personal crisis, providing a mobile phone with access to the befrienders pager or mobile phone (and access to other numbers blocked).

The Prison Service has produced guidelines on how to set up and monitor such schemes in the document *Caring for the Suicidal in Custody: involving prisoners*. Further advice is available from the Suicide Awareness Support Unit or the Samaritans' Prison Liaison Officer. Not every prisoner will be able or willing to use a 'befriending' scheme or crisis support. Alternatives should also be made available, such as access to the Samaritans.

Prisons should run group courses in anxiety management training and behavioural interventions for insomnia. These should be led by prison staff who have themselves undergone training in behaviour therapy for groups.

Self-harm and suicide

An Effective Health Care Bulletin[96] builds on the review by Hawton *et al.*[195] evaluating the effectiveness of interventions following deliberate self-harm. This review also considers the research evidence on the characteristics of an effective clinical service for the assessment and aftercare of people who present following an episode of deliberate self-harm. The authors note that most research has been conducted on deliberate self-poisoning rather than other forms of self-harm such as cutting. The Effective Health Care bulletin suggests a number of recommendations for practice. These are listed in **Box 10**.

Box 10: Recommendations for the management of self-harm.

Assessment
- All hospital attendance following deliberate self-harm should lead to a psychosocial assessment. This should aim to identify motives for the act and associated problems which are potentially amenable to intervention such as psychological or social problems, mental disorder and alcohol and substance misuse.
- Staff who undertake assessments should receive specialist training and have supervision available.

Intervention
- There is insufficient evidence to recommend a specific clinical intervention after deliberate self-harm.
- Brief psychological therapies such as interpersonal therapy and problem solving therapy are effective in the treatment of depression in similar clinical settings, and the latter has been shown to have benefits after self-harm.

Aftercare

- Direct discharge from A&E should only be contemplated if a psychosocial assessment and aftercare plan can be arranged in A&E prior to discharge.
- Aftercare arrangements should include the provision of verbal and written information on services available for people who are contemplating self-harm.

General

- GPs should have ready access to training and advice about the assessment and management of self-harm patients.
- Accessible and comprehensive services will need a mechanism for engaging people who do not attend routine clinic appointments. Access to follow-up needs to be rapid.
- Service providers should work to improve attitudes towards self-harming patients.

Source: Effective Health Care Bulletin, *Deliberate Self-harm*, Dec 1998, Vol 4, No. 6, NHS Centre for Reviews & Dissemination.

Alcohol and drug misuse

Alcohol misuse

Primary care staff should be trained in the use of screening tools for the identification of prisoners with alcohol problems. Protocols should be in place for the management of acute alcohol withdrawal and for referral of prisoners with alcohol problems to appropriate services prior to discharge.

Drug misuse

Protocols should be in place for the management of acute drug withdrawal and for referral of prisoners with drug problems to appropriate services prior to discharge. A framework for the provision of a drug treatment service has been drawn up by PDM Consulting Limited after a comprehensive evaluation of drug treatment in prisons (see **Table 82**).[98] These are in line with treatment guidelines issued by the Department of Health.

Table 82: Framework for provision of Drug Treatment Service (*Source:* PDM Consulting Ltd, 1998).[98]

Service type	Location	Time in sentence	Intensity	Threshold	Supervision	Tolerance
Voluntary testing unit	All prisons B, C, D, including Women's, YOI and high security	Any time	Low	Medium	High	Low
Drug worker offering: time-limited, sessional, group and individual counselling, education and advice; assistance with assessments and applications for treatment in prison and in community; aftercare; and release planning		Any time	Low	low	Low	High
Basic detoxification services and longer-term prescribing	Local/remand prisons	Early	Low	Low	High	High
Drug and HIV/hepatitis awareness and education for all prisoners		Early	Low	Low	Low	High
Detoxification centres with NHS specialist input methadone maintenance	Local/remand on area basis	Early	Low	Low	High	High
8–12 week programmes, using group work. Participants located either on a residual unit or on a VTU. Models include 12-step and cognitive-behavioural programmes	Area basis Category B and C. Including Women's, YOI & High Security	Early or late*	Medium	Medium	High	Medium
12 month rehabilitation programmes – therapeutic communities	National basis Category B & C, Women's, YOI	Late	High	High	Medium	Low

* Some programmes should aim at harm minimisation and relapse prevention in the prison setting; these should be targeted at prisoners early in their sentence. Other programmes should be aimed at pre-release planning, living without drugs, personal relationships etc. These would be best suited to prisoners in the last year of their sentence.
Notes:
Intensity: intensity of the programme content, the demands placed on participants and the period of time spent in therapeutic contact.
Threshold: the lower the threshold, the lower the requirements for entry. High threshold programmes have strict criteria for admission.
Supervision: frequency of urine testing degree of segregation from other prisoners. A high level of supervision consists of weekly urine testing and strict segregation. A medium level may be monthly testing and strict segregation; or more frequent testing and a lesser degree of segregation.
Tolerance: action taken on a urine test positive for drugs. A programme with a low tolerance would dismiss prisoners instantly. A programme with a high tolerance may operate a policy of dismissal after three positive test, for example.

9 Information and research requirements

There are a number of areas where research is a priority.

Higher primary-care consultation rates

Prisoners make much greater use of primary care services than equivalent populations in the community. One important area for research is to determine what the main reasons for these higher consultation rates. This requires collection of routine data on the reasons for prisoners' consultations.

Following this, research should be directed at finding interventions to address prisoners' high demand for primary health care. This might involve greater use of informal care; greater access to over the counter medications; or use of primary care staff other than physicians.

Management of chronic diseases

A number of chronic diseases (mental health problems, epilepsy, asthma, diabetes) are common within the prison population. Research should be directed towards improving the identification and systematic management of these patients. Current models for chronic disease management in primary care emphasise the need for disease registers and active case management.

Co-ordination of care within and outside the prison sector

Research should investigate ways of improving communication of health information between prisons and from within to outside prison sector. This may involve shared records or the use of information technology.

Monitoring the prevalence of risky behaviour and bloodborne viral infections

There should be continuing monitoring of the prevalence of bloodborne viral infections in the prison population.

Assessment of the prevalence of disorders of the special senses

The prevalence of hearing, speech and language problems should be assessed in the prison population.

Appendix 1: The Initial Interview Questionnaire: a screening tool for speech and language problems

Initial interview questionnaire

1   The client is seen individually.
2   Social greetings are exchanged.
3   The client is asked for his name and number and these are recorded on the Assessment Sheet.
4   Throughout the interview he is called by his first name.
5   The Speech and Language Therapist introduces herself and describes her role, in terms of total communication.
6   The client is asked if he is willing to answer any questions about speech, language and communication.
7   If this is agreed, the following questions are asked:
   (a) Do you have any problems with hearing?
   (b) Do you lack any rhythm in speech, do you stammer or stutter over words?
   (c) Do you have any problems understanding what is said to you?
   (d) Do other people understand what you say?
   (e) Do you think you have any memory loss associated with drug abuse or accident, which has affected your ability to think, speak and communicate?
   (f) Have you ever had an accident to the face, head or throat which has affected your speech and communication?
   (g) Can you read, write and spell easily?
   (h) Do you think you have any problems with:
       speech
       language
       communicating with other people?

If any question evokes a response which needs expansion, these are elaborated and discussed as the questionnaire is administered.

(Time taken: 3–5 minutes)

Source: A Review of Communication Therapy with Young Male Offenders: internal report.[54]

Appendix 2: Services available for the management of physical health problems in the community

Epilepsy

Diagnosis

The diagnosis of epilepsy is usually made by a neurologist on the basis of a history of more than one epileptic seizure. A number of investigations – electroencephalograms (EEG), brain imaging scans (computerised tomography or magnetic resonance imaging) – may also be carried out.

Self-management

Many aspects of the management of epilepsy require the patient to engage in appropriate self-care. This includes avoiding situations which they know may bring on a seizure, for example, lack of sleep, too much alcohol, emotional upsets or non-compliance with medication. It also involves an awareness of the hazards of seizures and recognition of the pre-ictal aura (which gives warning of a seizure). Occupational activities and general education are also important because of the effects of epilepsy on self-confidence and because of the occurrence of mental retardation in some patients with epilepsy.

Treatment

The mainstay of epilepsy management is drug treatment, usually with one of the first-line drugs such as sodium valproate, carbamazepine, phenytoin or ethosuximide. Some patients require more than one medication. Patients also receive education about the side effects and interactions of these drugs (such as their interaction with the oral contraceptive pill), regular follow-up and monitoring of drug levels. This follow-up may be provided either by a neurologist, a specialist epilepsy nurse or a general practitioner.

Patients with epilepsy are also frequently referred to a psychiatrist for assessment, in particular if they are also affected by mental retardation.

Emergency treatment

In cases where seizures become very prolonged or repeated seizures occur, patients require intravenous diazepam, followed by transfer to hospital.

Other treatments

The National Society for Epilepsy report that complementary therapies such as relaxation, aromatherapy, acupuncture, bio-feedback and ketogenic diets have been used to help people with epilepsy to complement drug treatment. Vagal nerve stimulation (mild electrical stimulation of the vagus nerve) has received some interest in the UK for the treatment of epilepsy. In addition a small minority of patients with epilepsy are helped by neurosurgery.

Asthma

Self care

Most day-to-day management of asthma is by patients themselves. This involves the avoidance of known allergens (such as grass pollen), monitoring of symptoms and sometimes of peak expiratory flow rate (using a Wright's peak expiratory flow meter) and adjustment of medications. For this to be successful, patients need knowledge of the uses of their medications and the distinction between those inhalers which relieve symptoms (mainly salbutamol) and those which prevent the occurrence of symptoms (inhaled steroids such as beclomethasone). They also need training in inhaler technique. Patients who smoke should be offered support to give up smoking, such as smoking cessation programmes or nicotine replacement therapy.

Primary care management of asthma

Asthma is normally diagnosed, treated and followed-up in a primary care setting. The most widely followed guidelines for asthma advocate a stepped care programme. Initially patients are treated only with inhaled salbutamol as required. If this is needed once a day or more, patients are prescribed regular corticosteroid (beclomethasone) inhalers to reduce the frequency of attacks. This can be increased or decreased as the situation demands. If corticosteroid (beclomethasone) at high doses is considered insufficient, oral medications (such as aminophylline) can be added. At this stage, it is often considered appropriate to seek specialist advice. In practice, a minority of patients with asthma will require referral and assessment by specialist physicians.

Prevention of complications

Patients with asthma may be immunised against influenza and pneumococcal infection, to prevent the occurrence of these infections.

Diabetes

Self-care and informal care

Self care is important in the management of diabetes for a number of reasons. Patients with diabetes need to understand the importance of adhering to their diabetic diet. They need to monitor their own blood sugar and (in the case of insulin-dependent diabetes) may need to adjust their dose of insulin in response to this. They also need to be aware of the symptoms of impending hypoglycaemia so that they can take appropriate steps to avoid it.

Control of diabetes is improved if the patient follows a regular routine in their daily activities and mealtimes.

Primary and secondary care

In the community the main components of diabetes services are the hospital-based diabetes team or teams (usually one or more consultant diabetologist, other specialist physicians, specialist nurse, dietician and podiatrist, with suitable junior, medical, laboratory and administrative support), the primary care team (general practitioner, practice nurse and administrative support) and other community support (podiatrist, dietician and community nurse). Diabetes centres often provide the hub of the local diabetes service.[205]

Diabetics are normally reviewed in clinic twice a year. The main purpose of the review is to ensure that blood sugar control is adequate and detect the complications of diabetes before they become serious. Diabetic control is monitored by blood tests (glycosylated haemoglobin and glucose). Complications are detected by examination of the feet and injection sites, analysis of urine for protein, blood tests for creatinine and fundoscopy. In addition the review is an opportunity to identify and treat risk factors for cardiovascular disease (which is more common in diabetics) and to discuss other problems associated with the condition.

These six monthly reviews may be carried out by a GP with an interest in diabetes (usually supported by a nurse), a specialist diabetic nurse or by a diabetologist. In particular it is important that the person who undertakes fundoscopy is experienced in the examination of eyes. In 1992 the British Diabetic Association produced a 'Patients' Charter' on the diabetic care patients should expect (see **Box A2.1**). This gives an indication of the services that would be expected to be available to a person with diabetes in the general population.

Box A2.1: 'What diabetic care to expect' The British Diabetic Association Patients' Charter.

When you have been diagnosed, you should have:

- a full medical examination
- a talk with a registered nurse who has a specialist interest in diabetes. They will explain what diabetes is and talk to you about individual treatment
- a talk with a state registered dietician who will want to know what you are used to eating and will give you basic advice on what to eat in the future. A follow up-meeting should be arranged for more detailed advice
- a discussion on the implications of diabetes on your job, driving insurance prescription charges etc. and whether you need to inform the DVLA and your insurance company if you are a driver
- information about the BDA's services and details of your local BDA group
- ongoing education about your diabetes and the beneficial effects of exercise, and assessments of your control.

Plus
If you are treated by insulin:

- frequent sessions for basic instruction in injection technique, looking after insulin and syringes, blood glucose and ketone testing and what the results mean
- supplies of relevant equipment
- discussions about hypoglycaemia (hypos): when and why it may happen and how to deal with it.

If you are treated by tablets:

- a discussion about the possibility of hypoglycaemia (hypos) and how to deal with it
- instruction on blood or urine testing and what the results mean, and supplies of relevant equipment.

If you are treated by diet alone:

- instruction on blood or urine testing and what the results mean, and supplies of relevant equipment.

Once your diabetes is reasonably controlled, you should:

- have access to the diabetes team at regular intervals – annually if necessary. These meetings should give time for discussion as well as assessing diabetes control

- be able to contact any member of the health care team for specialist advice when you need it
- have more education sessions as you are ready for them
- have a formal medical review once a year by a doctor experienced in diabetes.

At this review:

- your weight should be recorded
- your urine should be tested for protein
- your blood should be tested to measure long-term control
- you should discuss control, including your home monitoring results
- your blood pressure should be checked
- your vision should be checked and the back of your eyes examined
- your legs and feet should be examined to check your circulation and nerve supply
- if you are on insulin, your injection sites should be examined
- you should have the opportunity to discuss how you are coping at home and at work.

Your role:
- you are an important member of the care team so it is essential that you understand your own diabetes to enable you to be in control of your condition
- you should ensure you receive the described care from your local diabetes clinic, practice or hospital. If these services are not available to you, you should:
    - contact your GP to discuss the diabetes care available in your area
    - contact your local community health council
    - contact the BDA or your local branch.

Source: British Diabetic Association. *Diabetes Care: what you should expect.* London: BDA, 1992.

Ischaemic heart disease and cardiovascular risk factors

Primary prevention

Patients have some influence over their own cardiovascular risk through their choice of diet, smoking behaviour and exercise. In prisons, diet and exercise are largely controlled by the institution. By offering a diet low in saturated fat and salt but high in polyunsaturates, fruit and vegetables, prisons can influence cholesterol levels, blood pressure and risk of heart disease.

Primary care management of cardiovascular risk factors

Patients often have their blood pressure and other cardiovascular risk factors monitored in a primary care setting. This may be carried out by GPs or other primary care workers. If their blood pressure is found to be raised, patients are usually monitored on an ongoing basis and treated with anti-hypertensive drugs. If their cholesterol levels are found to be raised or they are overweight, patients are often referred to a dietician. They may also be prescribed a cholesterol-lowering drug. Patients who smoke are usually advised to give up and may be referred to a smoking cessation programme. Some of these programmes incorporate nicotine replacement therapy, such as nicotine containing gum or patches.

Management of patients with cardiovascular disease

GPs are expected to be able to identify all of their patients with cardiovascular disease. These patients require regular follow-up, monitoring of their condition and management of their cardiovascular risk factors. In the period immediately after diagnosis this may be done by a specialist physician, but later on it can be carried out by the GP and other members of the primary care team.

In 1998, the British Cardiac Society, the British Hyperlipidaemia Association and the British Hypertension Society published national guidelines for the prevention of coronary heart disease in clinical practice. A summary their of their recommendations is given in **Box A2.2**.

Box A2.2: Summary of Joint British recommendations on prevention of CHD in clinical practice.

Lifestyle
- Discontinue smoking, make healthier food choices, increase aerobic exercise and moderate alcohol consumption.

Other risk factors
- Body Mass Index <25 kg/m^2 is desirable with no central obesity.
- Blood pressure <140 mmHg systolic and <85 mmHg diastolic.
- Total cholesterol <5.0 mmol/l (LDL cholesterol <3.0 mmol/l).
- Optimal control of diabetes mellitus and BP reduced to <130 mmHg systolic and <80 mmHg diastolic (and where there is proteinuria BP <125 mmHg systolic and <75 mmHg).

Cardioprotective drug therapy
- Aspirin for all coronary patients and those with other major atherosclerotic disease, and for healthy individuals who are older than 50 years and are either well-controlled hypertensive patients or men at risk of CHD.
- Beta-blockers at the doses prescribed in the clinical trials following MI, particularly in high-risk patients, and for at least 3 years.
- Cholesterol-lowering therapy (statins) at the doses prescribed in the clinical trials.
- ACE inhibitors at the doses prescribed in the clinical trials for patients with symptoms or signs of heart failure at the time of MI, or for those with persistent left ventricular systolic dysfunction (ejection fraction <40%).
- Anticoagulants for patients at risk of systemic embolisation.

Screening of first-degree blood relatives
- Screening of first-degree blood relatives of patients with premature CHD or other athersclerotic disease is encouraged, and in the context of familial dyslipidaemias is essential.

Infectious diseases

Sexually transmitted diseases

The management of most sexually transmitted diseases is carried out by specialists in genito-urinary (GU) clinics. These investigate, diagnose and treat patients as appropriate. Patients may be referred to GU clinics by their GPs but the public also enjoy direct access and more commonly patients self-refer. GU clinics also arrange follow-up and trace the sexual contacts of patients so that they too can be offered investigation and treatment. This is an important part of the control of sexually transmitted diseases because disease is often asymptomatic and contacts would not otherwise seek medical advice. In some sexually transmitted disease clinics all new patients are offered individual personal sexual health counselling in order to promote safer sexual practices.

Bloodborne viruses

Prevention

The risk of acquiring hepatitis B, hepatitis C and HIV infection can be reduced by adopting safer sexual practices (such as the use of condoms) and by avoiding unsafe practices such as drug abusers sharing injecting equipment.

Because staff may come into contact with infectious material of patients, it is routine practice in the health service to require all staff involved in patient care to show evidence of vaccination against hepatitis B. This is considered good risk management in the health service.

Testing, counselling and advice

Chronic HIV infection and chronic hepatitis are diagnosed by blood tests. If they feel they are at risk, patients may request voluntary testing to establish their HIV or hepatitis status. Patients so doing are often referred to a specialist service such as a GU clinic to ensure that they receive appropriate counselling about the implications of both testing and viral infection. In the community there is a wide range of advice and support available for those who are concerned about HIV, e.g. National AIDS Helpline.

Treatment

Patients with chronic hepatitis B or hepatitis C infection may develop chronic liver disease. Because of this they require management by an appropriate medical specialist. There is no specific treatment for chronic hepatitis B infection, but interferon is used in the treatment of hepatitis C infection. Chronic HIV infection also requires specialist referral and treatment. Patients are usually treated with combination therapy (simultaneous treatment with several anti-retroviral therapies) to delay the onset of immunodeficiency problems.

Tuberculosis

The risk of tuberculosis infection can be reduced by administration of the live BCG vaccination, which requires only one injection. BCG vaccination is contraindicated in patients with impaired cell-mediated immunity, for example those with HIV infection.

Patients can be screened for possible tuberculosis by Heaf testing. This is a skin-prick test which separates patients into those likely and those who are unlikely to be infected. Diagnosis is confirmed by chest x-ray and by microbiological examination of sputum. Because many of the symptoms of tuberculosis (persistent cough and weight loss) are common, diagnosis of tuberculosis depends on vigilance by the primary care team. Tuberculosis is treated with a combination of specific anti-tubercular antibiotics, for a period of four to six months. Treatment is usually initiated and monitored by a specialist. To avoid the emergence of multi-drug-resistant tuberculosis, it is important to ensure that treatment is completed. Contacts of patients should be are traced and screened for possible infection. This is usually undertaken by the public health department of the local health authority.

Dental health

Persons receiving income support, pregnant women and women who are in the postnatal period are entitled to free dental care from NHS general dental practitioners. NHS general dental practitioners provide most dental procedures to all other persons at 80% of the cost. Private dental practitioners provide dental care at full cost. In practice, access to an NHS general dental practitioner may be difficult as all NHS dentists in an area may be oversubscribed. In addition, because there is a fee for dental care, many patients attend their dentists infrequently.

General dental practitioners provide preventive care and treatment of dental problems.

Appendix 3: Services for drug and alcohol misuse in the community

Drug abuse

Services for drug abuse in the community

In the community a minority of drug misusers come into contact with formal services. Those that do are dealt with by the primary care team, in drug-dependency clinics and sometimes by psychiatric services. A range of voluntary organisations also offer services for drug misusers.

There are two main approaches to managing drug abuse; services designed to minimise harm and services intended to help users to abstain from drugs. Harm minimisation services include information and advice on drugs misuse, free access to injecting or sterilisation equipment and in some cases methadone maintenance. Because some drug misusers are not registered with a general practitioner, they may also be offered general medical services and other preventive measures such as contraceptive advice and hepatitis B immunisation. When methadone is provided it is part of an agreed programme with clearly defined rules. If drug misusers deviate from these rules, methadone maintenance is withdrawn.

Those drug misusers who are deemed suitable are offered services designed to help them abstain from drugs. These are generally organised on an outpatient basis but some services are residential. Some of these services are organised by the voluntary sector. Such programmes operate on the basis of a contract, where participation is dependent on the client not misusing drugs. The main features of such programmes are psychotherapeutic support individually or as a group exercise and monitoring of participants to ensure that they do not misuse drugs. Some programmes offer detoxification, i.e. short reducing courses of medication to attenuate the symptoms of withdrawal during the initial stages of the programme. Some emphasise behavioural interventions to promote abstinence. Others are based on a psychodynamic approach to drug misuse.

Alcohol misuse

Services for alcohol abuse in the community

In the community a small minority of alcohol misusers come into contact with formal services. Those that do are dealt with by the primary care team, by the voluntary sector, or in alcohol dependency clinics run by psychiatric services.

The simplest intervention in primary care is for general practitioners to give clear advice to reduce intake of alcohol. This may be backed up by liver function tests to demonstrate liver damage. Those alcohol misusers who are supported by voluntary agencies or formal psychiatric services are usually offered either psychological or pharmacological support to help reduce consumption or to promote abstention. Psychological support may involve group therapy, skills training to promote abstinence, counselling or psychodynamic psychotherapy. Pharmacological support may involve the use of drugs to promote abstinence such as disulphiram (which causes unpleasant symptoms if alcohol is consumed). Patients take this once a day under supervision to act as a disincentive to consumption of alcohol.

Unlike drug withdrawal, *delerium tremens* is a potentially dangerous medical condition. Patients withdrawing from alcohol need to be nursed in a well-lit room. They also need to be given appropriate doses of chlormethiazole or a benzodiazepine to replace alcohol consumption. This medication is then gradually withdrawn.

Appendix 4: Sources of information, guidelines and effectiveness material of health care interventions for physical health problems

Epilepsy

- The Scottish Intercollegiate Guidelines Network (SIGN) has produced evidence-based guidelines on the diagnosis and management of epilepsy in adults (*Diagnosis and Management of Epilepsy in Adults: A Quick Reference Guide*, SIGN Publication No. 21, November 1997).
- The Royal College of Physicians, the Institute of Neurology and the National Society for Epilepsy funded by the NHS Executive have produced evidence-based guidelines on *Adults with Poorly Controlled Epilepsy*. The guidelines are in two parts. Part 1 is *Clinical Guidelines for Treatment* whilst Part 2 is *Practical Tools for Aiding Epilepsy Management*, comprising various checklists and protocols to provide information to assist GPs, specialists, other health professionals and providers in the care and management of epilepsy patients. The guidelines have been appraised by the Health Care Evaluation Unit at St George's Hospital Medical School (www.sghms.ac.uk/phs/hceu//report01.htm).

Asthma

- The North of England Asthma Guideline Group has produced evidence-based guidelines for the primary care management of asthma in adults (North of England Asthma Guideline Development Group. *North of England Evidence Based Guideline Development Project: evidence based guideline for the primary care management of recurrent wheeze in adults*. Newcastle upon Tyne: Centre for Health services Research, 1995). These give guidance on diagnosis, management, drug treatment, non-drug treatment and referral and have been commended by the NHS Executive.
- The British Thoracic Society has produced guidelines on the management of asthma. The guideline comprises two journal articles (*Thorax* 1997; **52**(Suppl 1): S1–S21 and *Thorax* 1993; **48**(2): S1–S24). It is recommended that the papers are viewed as one complete document.
- The Scottish Intercollegiate Guidelines Network (SIGN) has produced evidence-based guidelines on the management of asthma in primary care (*Primary Care Management of Asthma: a quick reference guide*. SIGN Publication No. 33, December 1998).
- A systematic review assessing education programmes that teach people with asthma how to self-manage their medication concluded that training in asthma self-management which involves self-monitoring by either peak expiratory flow or symptoms, coupled with regular medical review and a written action plan appears to improve health outcomes for adults with asthma.[206]

Diabetes

- The British Diabetic Association has produced guidelines on *Recommendations for the Management of Diabetes in Primary Care* in 1997. These have been commended by the NHS Executive.
- The NHS Executive in England has produced health service guidelines that outline the key features of a good diabetes service (NHS Executive. *Key Features of a Good Diabetes Service*. HSG (97)45, October 1997).

- The European NIDDM policy group has produced *A Desktop Guide for the Management of Non-insulin-dependent Diabetes Mellitus*. This is available from the International Diabetes Federation (1 rue Defaqz, B-1000 Brussels, Belgium).
- A health care needs assessment on diabetes in the *Health Care Needs Assessment* series also provides a useful summary of effectiveness and cost-effectiveness material.[207]

Ischaemic heart disease and cardiovascular risk factors

The most recent international and UK guidelines on the management of cardiovascular risk factors[208,209] emphasise the identification of patients by their cardiovascular risk rather than simply by the presence or absence of particular risk factors. The rationale for this is that those at highest risk of future cardiovasular or cerebrovascular events are those who benefit most from preventive treatment.

However, in order to calculate patients' risk of future vascular events, it is necessary to know the patients blood pressure and cholesterol in addition to their age, sex, smoking status and medical history. Checking of blood pressure and cholesterol is not routinely carried out on every patient in primary care or in prisons. It is therefore important to consider which patients it might be useful to investigate either by measuring their blood pressure or their cholesterol level. Logically it is only useful to investigate if there is a possibility that the patient may be found to be at sufficiently high risk to benefit from treatment. This question is discussed below.

High risk groups

Patients with ischaemic heart disease or cardiovascular disease

Patients who already suffer from ischaemic heart disease or have previously suffered from a stroke or a myocardial infarction are at high risk of subsequent vascular events. Since they are at highest risk these patients benefit most from treatment. These patients should all be offered aspirin, beta-blockers and cholesterol-lowering therapy (statins). Those who have suffered myocardial infarction or who have a reduced ejection fraction should be offered angiotensin-converting enzyme inhibitors.[209] Because the prison population is young, few will have a diagnosis of ischaemic heart disease. However, it is important to be able to identify these patients and to provide them with appropriate treatment.

Patients with diabetes

Patients with diabetes are at a higher risk of vascular events than non-diabetics. This risk can be reduced by the treatment of raised blood pressure.[210] Part of the routine follow-up of diabetics should therefore involve assessing and managing cardiovascular risk.

Low risk groups: blood pressure testing and treatment

The objective of treating high blood pressure is to reduce the risk of ischaemic heart disease and stroke (vascular events). The benefits of treatment are greatest in those at greatest initial risk. The risk of a vascular event increases with age and in the presence of specific risk factors: cigarette smoking, diabetes, raised blood pressure, male sex and raised cholesterol levels. Typically, drug treatment lowers systolic blood pressure by about 10 to 12 mmHg and reduces risk by about 30%. This means that we would have to treat 33 persons who were at 10% risk of a vascular event in the next five years in order to prevent one of them from suffering from a vascular event. In other words, 32 out of the 33 would not benefit from the treatment; 30 would not suffer a vascular event anyway and 2 would suffer a vascular event whether or not they were treated. Since treatment carries its own drawbacks, such as the effects of labelling, side effects and medicalisation, it has been suggested that it is probably only worth considering drug treatment of high blood pressure in two groups:

- those whose systolic blood pressure exceeds 140 (or diastolic >90) *and* whose risk of a vascular event is more than 10% in the next five years
- those with very high blood pressures (systolic >180 or diastolic >110) should be treated, irrespective of their vascular risk (because of the risk of accelerated hypertension).

Using data on the distribution of blood pressures and total cholesterol to high density cholesterol ratios in the UK population it is possible to estimate the age-sex specific percentage of the population who might benefit from anti-hypertensive treatment. From this we can estimate the number of prisoners who will have to have their blood pressure treated in order to find one who might benefit from treatment (see **Table A4.1**). The blood pressure data has been taken from the Health Survey for England[29] and the data on total cholesterol to high density cholesterol ratios were provided by the University of Newcastle.

Despite the fact that most smoke, very few inmates are at greater than 10% risk of a vascular event: this is largely because the prison population is young. Among those aged 35–44, only one in 39 men and one in 99 women might benefit from anti-hypertensive treatment. The implication of this is that it is only worthwhile checking the blood pressure of men and women over 45.

Table A4.1: Age-sex specific prevalence of need for blood pressure treatment: UK population.

Age band	What percentage need an antihypertensive?		How many prisoners' blood pressure need to be checked to find one needing an antihypertensive?	
	Males	Females	Males	Females
16–24	0%	0%	∞	∞
25–34	1%	0%	100	∞
35–44	3%	1%	39	99
45–54	36%	21%	3	5
55–64	59%	56%	2	2
65–74	68%	68%	1	1
75+	72%	79%	1	1

All those with >10% 5-year risk and a bp of at least 140/90 need treatment *and* all those with a bp of at least 180/110, irrespective of the risk. Vascular risk is calculated on the assumption that all prisoners are smokers.

High blood pressure is more prevalent among blacks than whites. As it is difficult to obtain data on the distribution of blood pressure in UK blacks, data on the distribution of blood pressures in US blacks have been used instead. These originate from the US National Health Survey (quoted in Baba *et al.*[211]). The number of prisoners who will need blood pressure treated in order to find one who might benefit from treatment is shown in **Table A4.2**. Based on this estimate, one in 18 black men aged 30–39 and one in 30 black women would benefit from blood pressure treatment.

Table A4.2: Age-sex specific prevalence of need for blood pressure treatment: US blacks.

Age band	What percentage need an antihypertensive?		How many prisoners' blood pressure needs to be checked to find one needing an antihypertensive?	
	Males	Females	Males	Females
30–39	6%	3%	18	30
40–49	31%	18%	3	6
50–59	51%	64%	2	2
60–69	74%	71%	1	1
70–75	67%	72%	1	1

All those with >10% 5-year risk and a bp of at least 140/90 need treatment *and* all those with a bp of at least 180/110, irrespective of the risk. Vascular risk is calculated on the assumption that all prisoners are smokers.

Cholesterol testing and drug treatment

It has already been noted that blood cholesterol alone is a relatively poor predictor of individual cardiovascular risk. The majority of cardiovascular events occur in people with average or low blood cholesterol levels. Therefore cholesterol screening is unlikely to reduce mortality and can be misleading.[212]

A similar analysis to that for treating raised blood pressure can be applied to the percentage of persons who need treatment for raised cholesterol levels. Drug treatment to lower cholesterol levels reduces the risk of a vascular event by about 30%. Those at highest risk therefore benefit most. Current guidelines recommend treatment for patients whose risk of a cardiovascular event is more than 15% in the next five years (>3% annual risk), provided their cholesterol is average or higher. The calculated risk of patients with very high cholesterol ratios may underestimate their true risk. The *Joint British Recommendations on the Prevention of CHD in Clinical Practice*[209] do not provide clear guidance on whether some patients should be treated irrespective of their estimated vascular risk. The recommendations of the New Zealand guidelines have therefore been followed in this report. These suggest that patients with a total cholesterol to high density lipoprotein cholesterol ratio of 8 or more should also be treated.[213]

Table A4.3 and **Table A4.4** show the estimated age-specific prevalence of patients who need statin treatment. Before the age of 45, very few patients are at sufficiently high risk to warrant treatment. In addition, many of those who are at high risk will also be candidates for blood pressure lowering: which should lower their risk. This suggests that it is probably not worth carrying out cholesterol testing on any prisoners under the age of 45. The estimated appropriate age threshold for cholesterol estimation in blacks is similar to that for the general UK population (see **Table A4.4**).

Table A4.3: Age-sex specific prevalence of need for statins: UK population.

Age band	What percentage need a statin?		How many prisoners' lipids need to be checked to find one needing a statin?	
	Males	Females	Males	Females
16–24	4%	0%	23	82,807
25–34	4%	0%	23	83,643
35–44	2%	0%	53	3,778
45–54	19%	3%	5	29
55–64	59%	43%	2	2
65–74	67%	51%	1	2
75+	68%	48%	1	2

Those who need treatment are all those at greater than 15% 5-year risk with a total cholesterol to HDL cholesterol of at least 4. In addition all those whose total cholesterol to HDL cholesterol is 8 or greater need treatment, irrespective of the estimated risk.

Table A4.4: Age-sex specific prevalence of need for lipid-lowering treatment: US blacks.

Age band	What percentage need a statin?		How many prisoners' lipids need to be checked to find one needing a statin?	
	Males	Females	Males	Females
30–39	0%	0%	453	217,927
40–49	2%	0%	41	430
50–59	16%	16%	6	6
60–69	55%	41%	2	2
70–75	69%	55%	1	2

Smoking cessation

The risks of diseases such as lung cancer and heart disease are reduced following smoking cessation and those smokers who stop before middle age can avoid most of the excess risk they would have suffered.[214]

A number of smoking cessation interventions seem to be ineffective. These include acupuncture, aversive smoking, hypnotherapy and the drug lobeline.[215–218]

Clonidine seems to be effective at helping smokers to quit, but side effects limit its usefulness.[219]

However, there are also a number of practical smoking cessation interventions which are effective. These are: advice and counselling given by nurses, brief advice from a physician, the use of nicotine replacement therapy and individual behavioural counselling.[220–223]

There is also evidence that group behaviour therapy programmes for smoking cessation are better than self-help and other less intensive interventions.[224] The provision of self-help materials is more effective than no intervention and training health professionals in smoking cessation has a modest effect on patient cessation rates.[225,226]

Advice and support to pregnant women also increases rates of smoking cessation.[227]

Much of this evidence is summarised in the NHS Centre for Reviews and Dissemination bulletin on smoking cessation.[203]

Infectious diseases

Hepatitis B

Vaccination against hepatitis B is given as a course of three injections. Once completed it provides very effective protection against infection especially in younger people. Present Home Office recommendations are that this is offered to all prisoners (see **Box 5**).

Tuberculosis

General guidance on tuberculosis control and detailed guidance on the drug treatment of tuberculosis can be obtained from the following publications.

- The Interdepartmental Working group on Tuberculosis. *The Prevention and Control of Tuberculosis in the United Kingdom: recommendations for the prevention and control of tuberculosis at local level.* Department of Health and the Welsh Office, 1996.
- Joint Tuberculosis Committee of the British Thoracic Society. Control and prevention of tuberculosis in the UK: code of practice 1994. *Thorax* 1994; **49**: 1193–1200.
- Joint Tuberculosis Committee of the British Thoracic Society. Chemotherapy and management of tuberculosis in the United Kingdom: recommendations 1998. *Thorax* 1998; **53**: 536–48.

Guidance on the prevention and control of transmission of HIV-related Tuberculosis and drug-resistant, including multiple-drug-resistant, tuberculosis has also been published by the Department of Health.

- The Interdepartmental Working Group on Tuberculosis. *The Prevention and Control of Tuberculosis in the United Kingdom: UK guidance on the prevention and control of transmission of HIV-related tuberculosis and drug resistant, including multiple drug-resistant, tuberculosis.* London: Department of Health, 1998.

Sexually transmitted diseases (STDs)

There is evidence that health education by video in the setting of a genito-urinary medicine clinic has an effect on knowledge and attitudes about STDs and condoms.[228]

There are a limited number of evidence-based guidelines on the management of common sexually transmitted diseases. These are listed below.

- Herpes Viruses Association. *Management Guidelines for Herpes Simplex.*
- Stokes T. *Leicestershire Genital Chlamydia Guidelines.* Leicestershire Health Authority, 1997.

A health care needs assessment of Genito-urinary Services in the *Health Care Needs Assessment 2nd Series* provides a useful summary of other relevant effectiveness and cost effectiveness material.[39]

Appendix 5: Recommendations on the provision of health care centre beds

Health care centre beds

In all health care systems, the use of in-patient beds is at least partly driven by the supply of beds. If beds are available, the threshold for admitting a patient tends to be lower and the threshold for discharge higher. This means that more patients are admitted for longer periods of time if more beds are available. In the community this may be an inefficient approach to dealing with illness, as hospital admission is expensive compared to community-based treatment. The fact that hospital admission is possible can inhibit the development of community-based services, which may in turn make it difficult to manage problems in the community or reduce length of stay.

The situation in prisons differs in some respects. Health care centre beds are not as intensively staffed as hospital beds and caring for prisoners on the wings has its own costs. Because of this, in-patient care in health care centre beds may cost little more than care in the main prison. In other respects, the situation is similar to that in the community. Access to hospital beds may inhibit the development of health care in the main prison and this in turn makes it difficult to manage health problems without admission to health care centre beds. This is particularly likely to be the case when hospital beds are available within the prison site. This is an important consideration, given that in addition to access to NHS beds, prisons have five times as many health care centre beds per prisoner as the general population has hospital beds.

Appendix 6: Promoting self-care in prisons

Recommendations for promoting self-care of minor illness

A systematic attempt should be made to reduce the rate of primary care consultation and to substitute consultations with other health care workers for medical consultations with doctors. One strategy would be to provide all prisoners with information on common minor illness and how to manage them. This could be supported by guidance on how to make appropriate use of the health care services. To ensure consistency, this guidance should be consistent with guidelines used by primary health care staff.

Access to self-care

Supply of pharmaceuticals and safety

A policy should be developed to give prisoners better access to over the counter medications. This will necessitate setting up a group of interested stakeholders (the pharmacist, medical officer, prison governor, health care officers and nurses) to draw up a list of medications and the conditions under which they can be made available to prisoners. It is important that any change in policy on medications should command widespread support in the prison.

Table A6.1 illustrates some of the more common over the counter medications, the potential hazards of improved access and suggested solutions. Some medications have a low potential for misuse. Where these can be legally sold to the public it may be possible to provide prisoners with more or less free access. To introduce a small element of control, prisoners might be obliged to bring their prisoners' health booklet and state the indication for the medication. If some medications (such as emollients and shampoos) are to be made available to prisoners through the prison shop, it may be necessary to provide them at reduced cost or at no cost. Otherwise, prisoners will continue to consult health care workers in order to obtain medications for free. If this seems inequitable to staff (who have to pay for similar medications in the community), these preparations could be made available to staff at the same low cost.

Other medications are legally available from pharmacists. In these cases, medications would have to be made available from health care workers following the guidance of a pharmacy protocol. Medications with a low potential for misuse include certain treatments for dyspepsia such as aluminium hydroxide, magnesium trisilicate and cimetidine; a wide range of skin preparations for acne, dandruff, eczema, psoriasis and fungal infections; clotrimazole pessaries and cream for vaginal candidiasis.

Some useful medications have a potential for misuse or overdose. This could be addressed by making available only a limited supply on a named-patient basis. Paracetamol is particularly dangerous in overdose. Methionine is an antidote to paracetamol overdose reducing the incidence of hepatic damage and death. In one study methionine given within ten hours of overdose reduced hepatic damage from 18% (with 1.5% mortality) to 7% (with no mortality), compared to patients given methionine up to 24 hours after ingestion.[229] In animal studies the combined preparation has been shown to be less toxic in overdose.[230] A preparation of paracetamol containing methionine (co-methiamol) is available in the UK. The risk of overdose could be minimised by only providing co-methiamol and by restricting access to 2 g of paracetamol (4 tablets) a week per named-patient.

Because aspirin and ibuprofen could potentially be dangerous in overdose, the quantity available could be restricted to 2.4 g aspirin per prisoner per week and 1.6 g ibuprofen per prisoner per week. By switching from one painkiller to another, three or four days of analgesia could be provided without a medical consultation.

Table A6.1: Medications for minor illnesses: factors relevant to custodial setting and suggested availability in prisons.

Medication	Cost (NHS prices)	Potential hazards and factors relevant to a custodial setting	Legal limits on availability	Suggested availability
Analgesics and antipyretics				
Aspirin 300 mg	£0.08 for 20 tablets	>20 tablets potentially dangerous in overdose.	Up to 16 tablets can be sold from any retailer. Greater number from pharmacist.	Up to 4 tablets a week to each prisoner. More could be made available on the basis of pharmacy protocol.
Co-methiamol 500 mg	£2.77 for 96 tablets	>20 paracetamol tablets potentially dangerous in overdose. Co-methiamol less toxic than paracetamol alone.		
Ibuprofen 200 mg	£0.14 for 20 tablets	>25 tablets potentially dangerous in overdose.		
Skin preparations				
Hydrous ointment	£0.30 for 100g	Low potential for misuse.	Unrestricted sale.	Unrestricted. Could keep supply in cell.
White soft paraffin	£0.31 for 100g		Unrestricted sale.	
Hydrocortisone 1%	£0.27 for 15g		From pharmacist.	On the basis of pharmacy protocol. Could keep supply in cell.
Coal tar (Alphosyl)	£2.44 for 100g		From pharmacist.	
Benzoyl peroxide 5%	£3.00 for 60g		From pharmacist.	
Drugs for dyspepsia				
Aluminium hydroxide	£0.41 for 200ml	Low potential for misuse.	Unrestricted sale.	Unrestricted. Could keep supply in cell.
Magnesium carbonate	£0.59 per 200ml		Unrestricted sale.	Unrestricted. Could keep supply in cell.
Antispasmodics				
Hyoscine butylbromide	£2.59 for 56 tablets	Potentially toxic in overdose. Possible misuse.	From pharmacist.	Up to 80 mg a week on the basis of pharmacy protocol
Antihistamines				
Chlorpheniramine	£0.20 for 20 tablets	Sedating. Possibility of misuse.	From pharmacist.	
Cetirizine	£8.73 for 30 tablets	Low potential for misuse.	Up to 10 from pharmacist.	
Preparations which may be useful in the common cold	Prices vary with preparation.			
Echinacea		Low potential for misuse.	Unrestricted sale.	Unrestricted. Could keep supply in cell.
Zinc lozenges			Unrestricted sale.	
Vitamin C			Unrestricted sale.	
Preparations for neurotic disorders				
Hypericum perforatum	£10 to £20 for 900 mg daily for one month	Low potential for misuse.	Unrestricted sale.	Supplied by nurses with mental training.

This list is not intended to be exhaustive.

Information

It is recommended that prisoners are provided with information on how to access and make best use of the prison health services. This should include what services they can expect (e.g. 'all medical consultations are regarded as confidential') and what they cannot expect (e.g. 'it is policy not to offer medications to relieve the symptoms of amphetamine withdrawal'; 'it is the policy of the health care centre not to prescribe sleeping tablets').

Prisoners could, where appropriate, also be provided with information on the self-care of many common minor illnesses. The simplest way to provide this would be in the form of a booklet issued to all prisoners on arrival in prison. Such a booklet could be produced centrally with local adaptations to suit each prison. It could be developed from a range of pre-existing sources of patient information. While it is probably unrealistic to expect more than a minority of prisoners to use a booklet, even use by a minority could have a significant impact on consultations.

A general plan of the type of information provided in such a booklet is listed in **Table A6.2**. Essentially it would consist of an alphabetic list of common conditions with a few lines explaining what this condition is. It would also include a list of simple self-care measures to help the condition. It would then explain what medications or remedies were available for each problem. It would indicate which of these were available to prisoners without prescription and how these could be obtained. The rules (such as the number of tablets per week) under which these could be made available would also be spelled out. Finally it would explain when it was appropriate to seek medical advice about these conditions.

In order to be consistent and to ensure that the booklet was used, it would be important for health care staff and others to be aware of the booklet and to follow its recommendations. Appointment cards to see the prison medical officer would include a line asking prisoners whether they had previously consulted the booklet. Alternatively, the appointment cards could be printed as part of the booklet, so prisoners were obliged at least to open the booklet before making an appointment.

Table A6.2: Common symptoms and minor illnesses, information needs and appropriate care.

Minor illness or symptom	Information needs	Appropriate self-care	Appropriate use of formal health care
Headache: tension headache migraine	Explanation of the causes of tension headache and that it is self-limiting. Self-care and the use of simple painkillers. The causes of migraine and appropriate self-care.	Anxiety management training and other self-help approaches. Paracetamol with methionine, aspirin, ibuprofen.	Diagnosis of mental health problems (depression) presenting with physical symptoms. Management of chronic tension headache; management of migraine; diagnosis of rare causes of headache.
Skin conditions: acne, dandruff dermatitis/eczema psoriasis tinea infections	Recognition and self-care of common skin conditions.	Benzoyl peroxide, shampoos, emollients and topical hydrocortisone, coal tar preparations, clotrimazole and other anti-fungals.	Management of severe psoriasis; eczema needing potent steriods; acne needing tetracyclines.
Upper respiratory infections: cough cold sore-throat	Recognition and self-care of upper respiratory infections and their usually benign prognosis.	Echinacea, ephedrine, zinc, oxymetalozine, vitamin C, paracetamol with methionine, aspirin and ibuprofen.	Diagnosis of chest infection or exacerbation of lung disease (antibiotics rarely indicated).
Gastro-intestinal problems: constipation diarrhoea dyspepsia (indigestion)	Recognition and self-care of gastro-intestinal problems and their usually benign prognosis.	Magnesium sulphate, loperamide, co-magaldrox suspension and cimetidine 100 mg.	Diagnosis of infectious diarrhoea. Diagnosis of rare causes of diarrhoea such as inflammatory bowel disease and, in older prisoners, colorectal cancer. Diagnosis of ulcers.
Allergies: hayfever/allergic rhinitis	Recognition and self-care of allergies.	Antihistamines.	Management of severe allergies. Referral for allergen desensitisation.
Psychological symptoms: insomnia/sleep problems anxiety	Recognition and self-care of common psychological symptoms.	Self-help approaches to insomnia.	Diagnosis and treatment of mental health problems (depression) presenting with physical symptoms.
Musculoskeletal problems: low back pain minor injuries	Recognition and self-care of minor injuries and low back pain.	Rubifacients. Access to gymnasium.	Diagnosis and treatment of mental health problems (depression) presenting with physical symptoms. Diagnosis and referral of rare causes of low back pain (e.g. disc prolapse). Diagnosis and referral of serious injuries.

Table A6.2: Continued.

Menstrual disorders: menstrual mood changes dysmenorrhoea menorrhagia menstrual irregularities	Recognition and self-care of menstrual disorders.	Ibuprofen, paracetamol with methionine, aspirin. Hyoscine butylbromide.	Diagnosis of mental health problems (depression) presenting with physical symptoms. Prescription of tranexamic acid for menorrhagia; antidepressants for mood changes; combined oral contraceptive for menstrual irregularities etc.
Genito-urinary infections: candidiasis (thrush) cystitis	Recognition and self-care of genito-urinary infections.	Clotrimazole, additional fluid consumption.	Diagnosis and prescription of appropriate antifungal or antibiotics. Diagnosis and management of STDs

References

1 Reed J, Lyne M. The quality of health care in prison: results of a year's programme of semistructured inspections. *BMJ* 1997; **315**: 1420–4.

2 Smith R. Prisoners: an end to second class health care? *BMJ* 1999; **318**: 954–5.

3 Health Advisory Committee for the Prison Service. *The Provision of Mental Health Care in Prisons.* London: Prison Service, 1997.

4 HM Inspectorate of Prisons. *Patient or Prisoner? A new strategy for health care in prisons.* London: Home Office, 1996.

5 Joint Prison Service and National Health Service Executive Working Group. *The Future Organisation of Prison Health Care.* London: Department of Health, 1999.

6 Willmott Y. Prison nursing: the tension between custody and care. *British Journal of Nursing* 1997; **6**: 333–6.

7 www.hmprisonservice.gov.uk/resourcecentre/estate_map (last accessed 21 March 2005).

8 www.publications.parliament.uk/pa/cm200405/cmhansrd/cm050307/debtext (last accessed 21 March 2005).

9 HM Inspectorate of Prisons. *Patient or Prisoner? A new strategy for health care in prisons.* London: Home Office, 1996.

10 HM Inspectorates of Prisons and Probation. *Lifers: A joint thematic review by Her Majesty's inspectorates of prisons and probation.* London: Home Office, 1999.

11 Women's Policy Group. *Report of a Review of Principles, Policies and Procedures on Mothers and Babies/Children in Prison.* London: Home Office, 1999.

12 www.hmprisonservice.gov.uk/resourcecentre/publicationsdocuments/index.asp?cat=85 (last accessed 21 March 2005).

13 Joint Prison Service and National Health Service Executive Working Group. *The Future Organisation of Prison Health Care.* London: Department of Health, 1999.

14 HM Chief Inspector of Prisons. *Young Prisoners: A thematic review by HM Chief Inspector of Prisons for England and Wales.* London: Home Office, 1997.

15 White P. *The Prison Population in 1997: A statistical review.* London: Home Office Research and Statistics Directorate, 1998.

16 White P, Park I, Butler P. *Prison Population Brief, England and Wales: March 1999.* London: Home Office, 1999.

17 Walmsley R. *World Prison Population List, Research Findings No.88.* London: Home Office Research, Development and Statistics Directorate, 1999.

18 www.hmprisonservice.gov.uk/assets/documents/10000442HMPS_Annual_Report_2004_Part_1.pdf (last accessed 21 March 2005).

19 Bell P, Fisher J, Loomis A. *Environmental Psychology.* London: Harcourt Brace and College, 1978.

20 DHC/Paul Hayton. *Promoting Health in Prisons in England and Wales: a strategy.* Draft and unpublished document from DHC, 1999.

21 McCallum A. Healthy prisons: oxymoron or opportunity? The role of public health in the care of the medically compromised offender. *Critical Public Health* 1995; **6**(4): 4–15.

22 McCormick A, Fleming D, Charlton J. *Morbidity Statistics from General Practice. Fourth national study, 1991–1992.* London: HMSO, 1995.

23 Bridgwood A, Malbon G. *Survey of the Physical Health of Prisoners 1994. A survey of sentenced male prisoners in England and Wales, carried out by the Social Survey Division of OPCS on behalf of the Prison Service Health Care Directorate.* London: HMSO, 1995.

24 Smith C. Assessing health needs in women's prisons. *Prison Service Journal* 1998; **118**: 22–4.

25 Baker G. A brief introductory survey of health care needs, Glen Parva YOI, Personal Communication. In: HM Chief Inspector of Prisons (ed) *Thematic Review of Young Offender Institutions.* London: Home Office, 1997.

26 HM Chief Inspector of Prisons. *Women in Prison: a thematic review by HM Chief Inspector of Prisons.* London: Home Office, 1997.

27 Gunn J. The prevalence of epilepsy among prisoners. *Proceedings of the Royal Society of Medicine* 1969; **62:** 60–3.

28 Whitman S, Coleman T, Patmon C, Desai B, Cohen R, King LN *et al.* Epilepsy in prison: elevated prevalence and no relationship to violence. *Neurology* 1984; **34:** 775–82.

29 Prescott-Clarke P, Primatesta P. Joint Health Surveys Unit of Social and Community Planning Research (SCPR) and University College London. *Health Survey for England 1996.* London: The Stationery Office, 1998.

30 Office for National Statistics. *Key Health Statistics from General Practice 1996.* London: Office for National Statistics, 1998.

31 Biswas S, Chalmers C, Woodland A. risk assessment of coronary heart disease in a male prison population and prison staff. *Prison Service Journal* 1997; **110:** 19–21.

32 Colhoun H, Prescott-Clarke P. *Health Survey for England 1994: a survey carried out on behalf of the Department of Health.* London: HMSO, 1996.

33 Dong W, Erens B (eds). *Scottish Health Survey 1995: a survey carried out on behalf of The Scottish Office Department of Health.* Edinburgh: The Stationery Office, 1997.

34 Singleton N, Meltzer H, Gatward R, Coid J, Deasy D. *Psychiatric Morbidity Among Prisoners in England and Wales: The report of a survey carried out in 1997 by Social Survey Division Of the Office for National Statistics on behalf of the Department of Health.* London: The Stationery Office, 1998.

35 Public Health Laboratory Service. *Prevalence of HIV in England and Wales in 1997: Annual Report of the Unlinked Anonymous Prevalence Monitoring Programme.* London: Department of Health, 1998.

36 Edwards A, Curtis S, Sherrard J. Survey of risk behaviour and HIV prevalence in an English prison. *International Journal of STD & AIDS* 1999; **10:** 464–6.

37 Strang J, Heuston J, Gossop M, Green J, Maden T. *HIV/AIDS Risk Behaviour Among Adult Male Prisoners.* London: Home Office Research, Development and Statistics Directorate, 1998.

38 David N, Tang A. Sexually transmitted infections in a young offenders institution in the UK. *International Journal of STD & AIDS* 2003; **14:** 511–3.

39 Renton A, Hawkes S, Hickman M, Claydon E, Ward H, Taylor-Robinson D. Genitourinary medicine. In: Stevens A, Raftery J (eds). *Health Care Needs Assessment: the epidemiologically based needs assessment reviews.* Oxford: Radcliffe Medical Press, 1997.

40 Public Health Laboratory Service. Public Health Laboratory Service – Facts and figures: genital Chlamydia trachomatis infection. www.phls.co.uk/facts/chla-inf.htm. 1999.

41 Public Health Laboratory Service. Public Health Laboratory Service – Facts and figures: Genital Herpes Simplex. www.phls.co.uk/facts/herp-inf.htm. 1999.

42 Sridhar M, Ross-Plummer R. The prevention of tuberculosis in prison staff. *Occupational Medicine (Oxford)* 2000; **50:** 614–5.

43 Mangtani P, Jolley D, Watson J, Rodriguez L. Socio-economic deprivation and notification rates for tuberculosis in London during 1982–1991. *BMJ* 1995; **310:** 963–6.

44 Kumar D, Citrom K, Leese J, Watson J. Tuberculosis among the homeless at a temporary shelter in London: report of a chest x-ray screening programme. *Journal of Epidemiology and Community Health* 1995; **49:** 629–33.

45 Kumar D, Watson J, Charlett A, Darbyshire J, Public Health Laboratory Service, British Thoracic Society *et al.* Tuberculosis in England and Wales in 1993: results of a national survey. *Thorax* 1997; **52:** 1060–7.

46 Jochem K, Tannenbaum T, Menzies D. Prevalence of tuberculin skin test reactions among prison workers. *Canadian Journal of Public Health* 1997; **88**: 202–6.

47 Steenland K, Levine A, Sieber K, Schulte P, Aziz D. Incidence of tuberculosis infection among New York State prison employees. *American Journal of Public Health* 1997; **87**: 2012–4.

48 Longfield M. *Annual Report of the Director of Health Care 1997–1998.* London: The Stationery Office Group Ltd, 1999.

49 Todd JE, Lader A. *The Adult Dental Health Survey.* London: HMSO, 1991.

50 Todd JE. *Adult Dental Health 1988: United Kingdom: a survey conducted by the Social Survey Division of the Office of Population Censuses and Surveys.* London: HMSO, 1991.

51 Jones CM, McCann N, Nungent Z. Scottish Prisons' Dental Health Survey 2002. www.scotland.gov.uk/library5/health/spdhs-00.asp. 2003.

52 Mixson JM, Eplee HC, Feil PH, Jones JJ, Rico M. Oral health status of a federal prison population. *Journal of Public Health Dentistry* 1990; **50**: 257–61.

53 Ackerman N. 'Deaf prisoners'. Oxford Brookes University. Unpublished dissertation cited in: Gibbs A, Ackerman N. Deaf prisoners: needs, services and training issues. *Prison Service Journal* 1998; **122**: 32–3.

54 Johnson S. *A Review of Communication Therapy with Young Male Offenders: internal report.* Scottish Prison Service, 1994.

55 Caddle D, Crisp D. *Imprisoned Women and Mothers: Home Office Research Study 162.* London: Home Office, 1997.

56 BMRB International. *Women Prisoners: work experience and intentions.* London: HM Prison Service, 1999.

57 Edens JF, Peters RH, Hills HA. Treating prison inmates with co-occurring disorders: an integrative review of existing programs. *Behavioral Sciences and the Law* 1997; **15**: 439–57.

58 American Psychiatric Association. *Diagnostic and Statistical Manual of Mental Disorders (4e) (DSM IV).* Washington DC: APA, 1994.

59 Meltzer H, Gill B, Petticrew M, Hinds K. *OPCS Surveys of Psychiatric Morbidity in Great Britain, Report 1: the prevalence of psychiatric morbidity among adults living in private households.* London: HMSO, 1995.

60 World Health Organization. *The ICD-10 Classification of Mental and Behavioural Disorders: clinical descriptions and diagnostic guidelines.* Geneva: World Health Organization, 1992.

61 Gunn J, Maden A, Swinton M. Treatment needs of prisoners with psychiatric disorders. *BMJ* 1991; **303**: 338–41.

62 Brooke D, Taylor C, Gunn J, Maden A. Point prevalence of mental disorder in unconvicted male prisoners in England and Wales. *BMJ* 1996; **313**: 1524–7.

63 Birmingham L, Mason D, Grubin D. Prevalence of mental disorder in remand prisoners: consecutive case study. *BMJ* 1996; **313**: 1521–4.

64 Dolan J. Self harm in the prison environment. *Prison Service Journal* 1998; **118**: 11–3.

65 OPCS. *Population Trends 92.* London: The Stationery Office, 1998.

66 HM Chief Inspector of Prisons. *Suicide is Everyone's Concern: a thematic review.* London: Home Office, 1999.

67 Hales H, Davison S, Misch P, Taylor P. Young male prisoners in a Young Offenders' Institution: their contact with suicidal behaviour by others. *Journal of Adolescence* 2003; **26**: 667–85.

68 Swann R, James P. The effect of the prison environment on inmate drug taking behaviour. *The Howard Journal* 1998; **37**: 252–65.

69 Bird S, Hutchinson SJ. Male drugs-related deaths in the fortnight after release from prison: Scotland, 1996–99. *Addiction* 2003; **98**: 185–90.

70 Gore SM, Hutchinson SJ, Cassidy J, Bird G, Biswas S. How many drug rehabilitation places are needed in prisons to reduce the risk of bloodborne virus infection? *Communicable Disease and Public Health* 1999; **2**: 193–5.

71 Mason D, Birmingham L, Grubin D. Substance use in remand prisoners: a consecutive case study. *BMJ* 1997; **315**: 18–21.

72 Keene J. Drug misuse in prison: views from inside; a qualitative study of prison staff and inmates. *The Howard Journal* 1997; **36**: 28–41.

73 Smith R. *Prison Health Care.* London: British Medical Association, 1984.

74 HM Prison Service. *Health Care Standards for Prisons in England and Wales.* London: Home Office, 1994.

75 OECD. *Organization for Economic Cooperation and Development Statistical Compendium.* Paris: OECD, 1996.

76 World Health Organization. *Health in Prisons Project: a European network for promoting health in prisons (project description).* London: DHC, 1996.

77 Greenwood N, Amor S, Boswell J, Joliffe D, Middleton B. *Scottish Needs Assessment Programme: Health Promotion in Prisons.* Glasgow, Office for Public Health in Scotland, 1999.

78 Airey N, Marriott J. Measuring therapeutic attitudes in the prison environment: development of the Prison Attitude to Drugs scale. *Addiction* 2003; **98**: 179–84.

79 Cassidy J, Biswas S, Hutchinson SJ, Gore SM, Williams O. Assessing prisoners' health needs. *Prison Service Journal* 1999; **122**: 35–8.

80 Leech M. *The Prison Handbook.* Winchester: Waterside Press, 1999.

81 Hardie T, Bhui K, Brown PM, Watson JP, Parrott JM. Unmet needs of remand prisoners. *Medical Science Law* 1998; **38**: 233–6.

82 Reed J, Lyne M. The quality of health care in prison: results of a year's programme of semistructured inspections. *BMJ* 1997; **315**: 1420–4.

83 Robbins C. Respiratory care in prison. *Prison Service Journal* 1998; **118**: 8–10.

84 MacFarlane IA. The development of healthcare services for diabetic prisoners. *Postgraduate Medical Journal* 1996; **72**: 214–7.

85 MacFarlane IA, Gill GV, Masson E, Tucker NH. Diabetes in prison: can good diabetic care be achieved? *BMJ* 1992; **304**: 152–5.

86 Scott MM. Diabetes in Scottish prisons. *Diabetic Nursing* 1998; **28**: 2–4.

87 Zoitopoulos L et al. *Annual Report of Clinical Activity Undertaken by King's Community Dental Service to the Young Offenders of Feltham Prison 1998–1999.* 1999 (personal communication).

88 Zoitopoulos L et al. *Clinical Activity Undertaken by King's Community Dental Service to the Inmates of Belmarsh Prison June–October 1999.* 1999 (personal communication).

89 Gibbs A, Ackerman N. Deaf Prisoners: Needs, services and training issues. *Prison Service Journal* 1999; **122**: 32–3.

90 Home Office. *Supporting Families: a consultation document.* London: Home Office, 1998.

91 Mackay R, Machin D. *Transfers from Prison to Hospital: the operation of section 48 of the Mental Health Act 1983.* London: Home Office Research, Development and Statistics Directorate, 1998.

92 Huckle PL. A survey of sentenced prisoners transferred to hospital for urgent psychiatric treatment over a three-year period in one region. *Medicine, Science and the Law* 1997; **37**: 37–40.

93 Roberts J. Therapeutic communities in prisons. *Prison Service Journal* 1997; **111**: 3.

94 Maden A. A criminological and psychiatric survey of women serving a prison sentence. *British Journal of Criminology* 1994; **34**: 172–91.

95 Hawton K, Fagg J. Trends in deliberate self poisoning and self injury in Oxford, 1976–1990. *BMJ* 1992; **304**: 1409–11.

96 House A, Owens D, Patchett L. Deliberate self-harm. *Effective Health Care Bulletins* 1998; **4**(6).

97 Department of Health and Social Security. *The Management of Deliberate Self-harm.* HN (84): 25. 1984.

98 Mason P, Farrell M, Clarke D. *Care and Control: towards quality drug treatment services in prisons.* HM Prison Service. Prison service health care conference, 1998.

99 Grummit C. *Through Care for Drug Users in the Criminal Justice System.* HM Prison Service, Prison service health care conference, 1998.

100 Birmingham L, Mason D, Grubin D. Health screening at first reception into prison. *The Journal of Forensic Psychiatry* 1997; **8**: 435–9.

101 Thomas L, Cullum N, McColl E, Rousseau N, Soutter J, Steen N. Guidelines in professions allied to medicine (Cochrane Review). Issue 3. *The Cochrane Library.* Oxford: Update Software, 1999.

102 Williams HC. Dermatology. In: Stevens A, Raftery J (eds). *Health Care Needs Assessment: the epidemiologically based needs assessment series. Second series.* Oxford: Radcliffe Medical Press, 1997.

103 Healy E, Simpson N. Acne vulgaris. *BMJ* 1994; **308**: 831–3.

104 Marks R, Pearse AD, Walker A. The effects of a shampoo containing zinc pyrithione on the control of dandruff. *British Journal of Dermatology* 1985; **112**: 415–22.

105 Rapaport M. A randomized, controlled clinical trial of four anti-dandruff shampoos. *Journal of International Medical Research* 1981; **9**: 152–6.

106 Amos HE, MacLennan A, Boorman GC. Clinical efficacy of Polytar AF (Fongitar) and Nizoral scalp treatments in patients with dandruff/seborrhoeic dermatitis. *Journal of Dermatological Treatment* 1994; **5**: 127–30.

107 Management of tension-type headache. *Drugs and Therapeutics Bulletin* 1999; **37**: 41–4.

108 Haddock C, Rowan A, Andrasik F, Wilson P, Talcott G, Stein R. Home-based behavioral treatments for chronic benign headache: a meta- analysis of controlled trials. *Cephalalgia* 1997; **17**: 113–8.

109 Vernon HT. The effectiveness of chiropractic manipulation in the treatment of headache: an exploration in the literature. *Journal of Manipulative and Physiological Therapeutics* 1995; **18**: 611–7.

110 Moore A, McQuay H, Muir Gray J (eds). Drug treatments for migraine. *Bandolier* 1996; 3.

111 Moore A, McQuay H, Muir Gray J (eds). Making sense of migraine treatments? *Bandolier* 1999; **6**: 1–4.

112 Ramadan NM, Schultz LL, Gilkey SJ. Migraine prophylactic drugs: proof of efficacy, utilization and cost. *Cephalalgia* 1997; **17**: 73–80.

113 Vogler B, Pittler M, Ernst E. Feverfew as a preventive treatment for migraine: a systematic review. *Cephalalgia* 1998; **18**: 704–8.

114 Arroll B, Kenealy T. Antibiotics versus placebo for the common cold (Cochrane Review). Issue 2. *The Cochrane Library.* Oxford: Update Software, 1999.

115 Melchart D, Linde K, Fischer P, Kaesmayr J. Echinacea for preventing and treating the common cold. *The Cochrane Library.* Oxford: Update Software, 1999.

116 Douglas RM, Chalker EB, Treacy B. Vitamin C for preventing and treating the common cold (Cochrane Review). Issue 2. *The Cochrane Library.* Oxford: Update Software, 1999.

117 Marshall I. Zinc for the common cold (Cochrane Review). Issue 2. *The Cochrane Library.* Oxford: Update Software, 1999.

118 Young J. *The Treatment and Prevention of the Common Cold.* Birmingham: Aggressive Research Intelligence Facility, 1999 (unpublished work).

119 Williams Jr JW, Aguilar C, Makela M, Cornell J, Hollman DR, Chiquette E, Simel DL. Antimicrobial Therapy for Acute Maxillary Sinusitis (Cochrane Review). Issue 3. *The Cochrane Library.* Oxford: Update Software, 1999.

120 Del Mar CB, Glasziou PP. Antibiotics for sore throat. Issue 2. *The Cochrane Library.* Oxford: Update Software, 1999.

121 Little P *et al.* Open randomised trial of prescribing strategies in managing sore throat. *BMJ* 1997; **314:** 722–7.

122 Fahey T, Stocks N, Thomas T. Quantitative systematic review of randomised controlled trials comparing antibiotic with placebo for acute cough in adults. *BMJ* 1998; **316:** 906–10.

123 Becker L, Glazier R, McIsaac W, Smucny J. Antibiotics for acute bronchitis (Cochrane Review). Issue 3. *The Cochrane Library.* Oxford: Update Software, 1999.

124 Thomas L, Cullum N, McColl E, Rousseau N, Soutter J, Steen N. Clinical guidelines in nursing, midwifery and other professions allied to medicine (Cochrane Review). Issue 2. *The Cochrane Library.* Oxford: Update Software, 1999.

125 Waddell G, Feder G, McIntosh A, Lewis M, Hutchinson A. *Low Back Pain Evidence Review.* London: Royal College of General Practitioners, 1996.

126 Little P, Smith L, Cantrell T, Chapman J, Langridge J, Pickering R. General practitioners' management of acute back pain: a survey of reported practice compared with clinical guidelines. *BMJ* 1996; **312:** 485–8.

127 Tulder MW van, Cherkin DC, Berman B, Lao L, Koes BW. The effectiveness of acupuncture in the treatment of low back pain (Cochrane Review). Issue 2. *The Cochrane Library.* Oxford: Update Software, 1999.

128 Croft P, Papageorgious A, McNally R. Low back pain. In: Stevens A, Raftery J (eds). *Health Care Needs Assessment: the epidemiologically based needs assessment reviews. Second series.* Oxford: Radcliffe Medical Press, 1997.

129 Goswick C Jr. Ibuprofen versus propoxyphene hydrochloride and placebo in acute musculoskeletal trauma. *Current Therapeutic Research, Clinical & Experimental* 1983; **34:** 685–92.

130 Andersen LA, Gotzsche PC. Naproxen and aspirin in acute musculoskeletal disorders: A double-blind, parallel study in patients with sports injuries. *Pharmatherapeutica* 1984; **3:** 531–7.

131 Green S, Buchbinder R, Glazier R, Forbes A. Interventions for shoulder pain (Cochrane Review). Issue 3. *The Cochrane Library.* Oxford: Update Software, 1999.

132 Gross AR, Aker PD, Goldsmith CH, Peloso P. Patient education for mechanical neck disorders (Cochrane Review). Issue 3. *The Cochrane Library.* Oxford: Update Software, 1999.

133 Zhang WY, Li Wan Po A. Efficacy of minor analgesics in primary dysmenorrhoea: a systematic review. *British Journal of Obstetrics and Gynaecology* 1998; **105:** 780–9.

134 Lethaby A, Irvine G, Cameron I. Cyclical progestogens for heavy menstrual bleeding (Cochrane Review). Issue 2. *The Cochrane Library.* Oxford: Update Software, 1999.

135 Coulter A, Kelland J, Peto V, Rees MCP. Treating menorrhagia in primary care: an overview of drug trials and a survey of prescribing practice. *International Journal of Technology Assessment in Health Care* 1995; **11:** 456–71.

136 Lethaby A, Augood C, Duckitt K. Nonsteroidal anti-inflammatory drugs for heavy menstrual bleeding (Cochrane Review). Issue 2. *The Cochrane Library.* Oxford: Update Software, 1999.

137 Carter J, Verhoef MJ. Efficacy of self-help and alternative treatments of premenstrual syndrome. *Womens Health Issues* 1994; **4:** 130–7.

138 Wolfe C. Gynaecology. In: Stevens A, Raftery J (eds). *Health Care Needs Assessment: the epidemiologically based needs assessment series.* Oxford: Radcliffe Medical Press Ltd, 1997.

139 Colditz G, Brewer T, Berkey C *et al.* Efficacy of BCG vaccine in the prevention of tuberculosis: meta-analysis of the published literature. *Journal of the American Medical Association* 1994; **271:** 698–702.

140 Shepherd J, Weston R, Peersman G, Napuli IZ. Interventions for encouraging sexual lifestyles and behaviours intended to prevent cervical cancer (Cochrane Review). *The Cochrane Library.* Oxford: Update Software, 1999.

141 Waterloo K, Gotestam K. The regulated-breathing method for stuttering: an experimental evaluation. *Journal of Behavior Therapy & Experimental Psychiatry* 1988; **19:** 11–9.

142 Rustin L, Kuhr A, Cook P, James I. Controlled trial of speech therapy versus oxprenolol for stammering. *British Medical Journal Clinical Research Edition* 1981; **283**: 517–9.

143 Martin S, Kim H, Kupper LL, Meyer RE, Hays M. Is incarceration during pregnancy associated with infant birthweight? *American Journal of Public Health* 1997; **87**: 1526–31.

144 Egley CC, Miller DE, Granados JL, Ingram-Fogel C. Outcome of pregnancy during imprisonment. *Journal of Reproductive Medicine* 1992; **37**: 131–4.

145 Cordeo L, Hines S, Shibley KA, Landon MB. Duration of incarceration and perinatal outcome. *Obstetrics & Gynecology* 1991; **78**: 641–5.

146 Catan L. *The Development of Young Children in Prison Mother and Baby Units.* University of Sussex. Working Papers in Psychology Series – No. 1, 1989.

147 Thompson PJ, Harm NJ. Parent education for mothers in prison. *Paediatric Nursing* 1995; **21**: 552–5.

148 Cornah D, Stein K, Stevens A. *The Therapeutic Community Method of Treatment for Borderline Personality Disorder.* Southampton, Wessex Institute for Health Research and Development, 1997.

149 Harris L. Personality disorders. In: Health Evidence Bulletins Wales. http://hebw.uwcm.ac.uk/mental/chap1.html, 1998.

150 Schultz S, Andreasen NC. Schizophrenia. *The Lancet* 1999; **353**: 1425–30.

151 Wahlbeck K, Cheine M, Essali MA. Clozapine versus typical neuroleptic medication for schizophrenia. Issue 2. *The Cochrane Library.* Oxford: Update Software, 1999.

152 Cheine M, Ahonen J, Wahlbeck K. Beta-blockers supplementation of standard drug treatment for schizophrenia. Issue 2. *The Cochrane Library.* Oxford: Update Software, 1999.

153 Jones C, Cormac I, Mota J, Campbell C. Cognitive behaviour therapy for schizophrenia. Issue 2. *The Cochrane Library.* Oxford: Update Software, 1999.

154 Tharyan P. Electroconvulsive therapy for schizophrenia. Issue 2. *The Cochrane Library.* Oxford: Update Software, 1999.

155 Department of Health. *A National Service Framework for Mental Health.* London: Department of Health, 1999.

156 Brown G. Life events and social support: possibilities for primary prevention. In: Jenkins R *et al.* (eds). *The Prevention of Depression and Anxiety.* London: HMSO, 1992.

157 Weiss M, Gaston L, Propst A, Wisebord S, Sicnerman V. The role of the alliance in the pharmacological treatment of depression. *Journal of Clinical Psychiatry* 1997; **58**: 196–204.

158 Tylee A, Freeling P, Kerry S. Why do GPs recognise major depression in one woman patient yet miss it in another? *British Journal of General Practice* 1993; **43**: 327–30.

159 Tylee A. How does the content of consultations affect the recognition by GPs of major depression in women? *British Journal of General Practice* 1995; **45**: 575–8.

160 Oxfordshire Health Authority & the Centre for Evidence Based Mental Health. A systematic guide for the management of depression in primary care. www.psychiatry.ox.ac.uk/cebmh/guidelines/depression/detection.html, 1998.

161 Zung W, Magill M, Moore J, George D. Recognition and treatment of depression in a family medicine practice. *Journal of Clinical Psychiatry* 1983; **44**: 3–6.

162 Paykel E, Priest R. Recognition and management of depression in general practice: consensus statement. *BMJ* 1992; **305**: 1198–202.

163 Goldberg D. Early Diagnosis and Secondary Prevention. In: Jenkins R *et al.* (eds). *The Prevention of Depression and Anxiety.* London: HMSO, 1992.

164 Standart S, Drinkwater C, Scott J. Multidisciplinary training in the detection, assessment and management of depression in primary care. *Primary Care Psychiatry* 1997; **3**: 89–93.

165 Churchill R, Wessely S, Lewis G. Pharmacotherapy and psychotherapy for depression (Protocol for a Cochrane Review). Issue 1. *The Cochrane Library.* Oxford: Update Software, 1999.

166 Roth A, Fonagy P. *What Works for Whom? A critical review of psychotherapy research.* New York: Guilford Press, 1996.

167 American Psychiatric Association. *American Psychiatric Association Practice Guidelines.* Washington DC: American Psychiatric Association, 1996.

168 Agency for Health Care Policy and Research. *Depression in Primary Care. Volumes I and II. Clinical Practice Guidelines No. 5.* Rockville, Maryland: US Departments of Health and Human Services, 1993.

169 NHS Centre for Reviews and Dissemination. The treatment of depression in primary care. *Effective Health Care Bulletin* 1993; **1**.

170 Joffe R, Sokolov S, Streiner D. Antidepressant treatment of depression: a meta-analysis. *Canadian Journal of Psychiatry* 1996; **41**: 613–6.

171 Gill D, Hatcher S. A systematic review of the treatment of depression with antidepressant drugs in patients who also have a physical illness (Cochrane Review). Issue 1. *The Cochrane Library.* Oxford: Update Software, 1999.

172 Mulrow CD, Linde K, Ramirez G, Pauls A, Weidenhammer W, Melchart D. St John's wort for depression – an overview and meta-analysis of randomised clinical trials. *BMJ* 1996; **313**: 253–8.

173 Linde K, Mulrow CD. St John's Wort for depression (Cochrane Review). *The Cochrane Library.* Oxford: Update Software, 1999.

174 Birkenhager TK, Moleman P, Nolen WA. Benzodiazepines for depression? a review of the literature. *International Clinical Psychopharmacology* 1995; **10**(3): 181–95.

175 Lima MS, Moncrieff J. Drugs versus placebo for dysthymia (Cochrane Review). Issue 2. *The Cochrane Library.* Oxford: Update Software, 1999.

176 Tyrer P, Seivewright N, Murphy S, Ferguson B, Kingdon D, Barczak P *et al.* The Nottingham study of neurotic disorder: comparison of drug and psychological treatments. *The Lancet* 1988; **2**(8605): 235–40.

177 Power K, Simpson R, Swanson V, Wallace L, Feistner A, Sharp D. A controlled comparison of cognitive behaviour therapy, diazepam, and placebo, alone and in combination, for the treatment of generalised anxiety disorder. *Anxiety Disorders* 1990; **4**: 267–92.

178 Butler G, Cullington A, Hibbert G, Klimes I, Gelder M. Anxiety management for persistent generalised anxiety. *British Journal of Psychiatry* 1987; **151**: 535–42.

179 Tyrer P, Seivewright N, Ferguson B, Murphy S, Johnson AL. The Nottingham study of neurotic disorder. Effect of personality status on response to drug treatment, cognitive therapy and self help over two years. *British Journal of Psychiatry* 1993; **162**: 219–26.

180 Durham R, Murphy T, Allan T, Richard K, Treliving L, Fenton G. Cognitive therapy, analytic psychotherapy and anxiety management training for generalised anxiety disorder. *British Journal of Psychiatry* 1994; **165**: 315–23.

181 Kennerley H. *Managing Anxiety: a training manual.* Oxford: Oxford University Press, 1990.

182 Gould RA, Otto MW, Pollack MH. A meta-analysis of treatment outcome for panic disorder. *Clinical Psychology Review* 1999; **15**: 819–44.

183 Cox BJ, Swinson RP, Morrison B, Lee PS. Clomipramine, fluoxetine, and behaviour therapy in the treatment of obsessive-compulsive disorder: a meta-analysis. *Journal of Behavioural Therapy and Psychiatry* 1993; **24**: 149–53.

184 van Balkom AJ, van Oppen P, Vermeulen AW *et al.* A meta-analysis on the treatment of obsessive compulsive disorder: a comparison of antidepressants, behavior, and cognitive therapy. *Clinical Psychology Review* 1994; **14**: 359–81.

185 O'Sullivan G, Noshirvani H, Marks I, Monteiro W, Lelliott P. Six-year follow-up after exposure and clomipramine therapy for obsessive compulsive disorder. *Journal of Clinical Psychiatry* 1991; **52**: 150–5.

186 Piccinelli M, Pini S, Bellantuono C, Wilkinson G. Efficacy of drug treatment in obsessive compulsive disorder: a meta analytic review. *British Journal of Psychiatry* 1995; **166**: 424–43.

187 Stein DJ, Spadaccini E, Hollander E. Meta-analysis of pharmacotherapy trials for obsessive-compulsive disorder. *International Clinical Psychopharmacology* 1995; **10**: 11–8.

188 Murtagh DR, Greenwood KM. Identifying effective psychological treatments for insomnia: a meta-analysis. *Journal of Consulting & Clinical Psychology* 1995; **63**: 79–89.

189 Morin CM, Culbert JP, Schwartz SM. Non-pharmacological interventions for insomnia: a meta-analysis of treatment efficacy. *American Journal of Psychiatry* 1994; **151**: 1172–80.

190 British Medical Association & The Royal Pharmaceutical Society of Great Britain. *British National Formulary*. London: Pharmaceutical Press, 1999.

191 Wessely S, Rose S, Bisson J. A systematic review of brief psychological interventions ('debriefing') for the treatment of immediate trauma related symptoms and the prevention of post traumatic stress disorder (Cochrane Review). Issue 3. *The Cochrane Library*. Oxford: Update Software, 1999.

192 van Etten ML, Taylor S. Comparative efficacy of treatments for post-traumatic stress disorder: a meta-analysis. *Clinical Psychology and Psychotherapy* 1998; **5**: 126–44.

193 Gunnell D. The potential for preventing suicide. A review of the literature on the effectiveness of interventions aimed at preventing suicide. Bristol: HCEU University of Bristol Department of Epidemiology and Public Health, 1994.

194 Van der Sande R, Buskens E, Allart E. Psychosocial intervention following suicide attempt: a systematic review of treatment interventions. *Acta Psychiatrica Scandinavica* 1997; **96**: 43–50.

195 Hawton K, Arensman E, Townsend E *et al.* Deliberate self-harm: systematic review of efficacy of psychosocial and pharmacological treatments in preventing repetition. *BMJ* 1998; **317**: 441–7.

196 BBC News Online. Preventing prison suicides. http://news.bbc.co.uk/2/low/americas/312676.stm, 10 May 1999.

197 Freemantle N, Gill P, Godfrey C, Long A, Richards C, Sheldon T *et al.* Brief interventions and alcohol use. *Effective Health Care Bulletin* 1993; **1**.

198 Saunders JB, Aasland OG, abor TF *et al.* Development of the alcohol use disorders identification test (AUDIT): WHO Collaborative Project on early detection of persons with harmful alcohol consumption – II. *Addiction* 1993; **88**: 791–804.

199 Garbutt JC, West SL, Carey T, Lohr K, Crews FT. Pharmacological treatment of alcohol dependence. *JAMA* 1999; **281**: 1318–25.

200 Edwards G, Unnithal S. Alcohol misuse. In: Stevens A, Raftery J (eds). *Health Care Needs Assessment: the epidemiologically based needs assessment reviews*, pp. 341–75. Oxford: Radcliffe Medical Press, 1994.

201 Department of Health. *Drug Misuse and Dependence: guidelines on clinical management*. London: The Stationery Office, 1999.

202 Strang J. Drug Abuse. In: Stevens A, Raftery J (eds). *Health Care Needs Assessment: the epidemiologically based needs assessment reviews*. Oxford: Radcliffe Medical Press Ltd, 1994.

203 NHS Centre for Reviews and Dissemination. Smoking cessation: what the health services can do. *Effectiveness Matters* 1998; **3**.

204 McBride A. *Literature Review of Health Promotion Policies and Practice of Relevance to Prison Service Establishments in England and Wales*. Oxford: University of Oxford, Health Promotion in Professional Practice, Research and Development Unit, 1998.

205 British Diabetes Association. *Diabetes Centres in the United Kingdom. Results of a survey of UK diabetes centres*. London: BDA, 1998.

206 Gibson PG, Coughlan J, Wilson AJ, Abramson M, Bauman A, Hensley MJ, Walters, EH. Self-management education and regular practitioner review for adults with asthma (Cochrane Review). Issue 2. *The Cochrane Library*. Oxford: Update Software, 1999.

207 Williams R, Farrar H. Diabetes Mellitus. In: Stevens A, Raftery J, Mant J, Simpson S (eds). *Health Care Needs Assessment: the epidemiologically based needs assessment reviews, First Series.* Second Edition. Oxford: Radcliffe Publishing, 2004.

208 Wood DA, De Backer G, Faergeman O, Graham I. Recommendations of the Second Joint task Force of European and other societies on coronary prevention. *European Heart Journal* 1998; **19**: 1434–503.

209 Wood DA, Durrington P, McInnes G, Poulter N, Rees A, Wray R. Joint recommendations on prevention of coronary heart disease in clinical practice. *Heart* 1998; **80 (Suppl. 2)**: 1–28.

210 Fuller J, Stevens LK, Chaturvedi N, Holloway, JF. Antihypertensive therapy in diabetes mellitus (Cochrane Review). Issue 3. *The Cochrane Library.* Oxford: Update Software, 1999.

211 Baba S *et al.* Blood pressure levels, related factors, and hypertension control status of Japanese and Americans. *Journal of Human Hypertension* 1991; **5**: 317–32.

212 NHS Centre for Reviews and Dissemination. Cholesterol and coronary heart disease: screening and treatment. *Effective Health Care Bulletin* 1998; **4**.

213 Sharpe N *et al. Core Services Committee: Guidelines for the management of mildly raised blood pressure in New Zealand.* Wellington: Royal New Zealand College of General Practitioners, 1995.

214 Doll R, Peto R, Wheatley K *et al.* Mortality in relation to smoking: 40 years' observations on male British doctors. *BMJ* 1994; **309**: 901–11.

215 White AR, Rampes H. Acupuncture for smoking cessation (Cochrane Review). Issue 3. *The Cochrane Library.* Oxford: Update Software, 1999.

216 Hajek P, Stead, LF. Aversive smoking for smoking cessation (Cochrane Review). Issue 3. *The Cochrane Library.* Oxford: Update Software, 1999.

217 Abbot NC, Stead LF, White AR, Barnes J, Ernst E. Hypnotherapy for smoking cessation (Cochrane Review). Issue 3. *The Cochrane Library.* Oxford: Update Software, 1999.

218 Stead LF, Hughes JR. Lobeline for smoking cessation (Cochrane Review). Issue 3. Oxford: Update software. *The Cochrane Library*, 1999.

219 Gourlay SG, Stead LF, Benowitz NL. Clonidine for smoking cessation (Cochrane Review). Issue 3. Oxford: Update Software. Cochrane Library, 1999.

220 Rice VH, Stead LF. Nursing interventions for smoking cessation (Cochrane Review). Issue 3. *The Cochrane Library.* Oxford: Update Software, 1999.

221 Silagy C, Ketteridge S. Physician advice for smoking cessation (Cochrane Review). Issue 3. *The Cochrane Library.* Oxford: Update Software, 1999.

222 Silagy C, Mant D, Fowler G, Lancaster T. Nicotine replacement therapy for smoking cessation (Cochrane Review). Issue 3. Oxford, Update Software. *The Cochrane Library*, 1999.

223 Lancaster T, Stead LF. Individual behavioural counselling for smoking cessation (Cochrane Review). Issue 3. *The Cochrane Library.* Oxford: Update Software, 1999.

224 Stead LF, Lancaster T. Group behaviour therapy programmes for smoking cessation. Issue 2. *The Cochrane Library.* Oxford: Update Software, 1999.

225 Lancaster T, Stead LF. Self-help interventions for smoking cessation (Cochrane Review). Issue 3. Oxford: Update software. *The Cochrane Library*, 1999.

226 Lancaster T, Silagy C, Fowler G, Spiers I. Training health professionals in smoking cessation (Cochrane Review). Issue 3. *The Cochrane Library.* Oxford: Update Software, 1999.

227 Dolan-Mullen P, Ramirez G, Groff J. A meta-analysis of randomized trials of prenatal smoking cessation interventions. *American Journal of Obstetrics and Gynaecology* 1994; **171**: 1328–34.

228 Healton CG, Messeri P. The effect of video interventions on improving knowledge and treatment compliance in the sexually transmitted disease clinic setting. Lesson for HIV health education. *Sexually Transmitted Diseases* 1993; **20**: 70–6.

229 Vale J, Proudfoot AT. Paracetamol (acetaminophen) poisoning. *The Lancet* 1995; **346**: 547–52.

230 Neuvonen P, Tokola O, Toivonen M, Simell O. Methionine in paracetamol tablets, a tool to reduce paracetamol toxicity. *International Journal of Clinical Pharmacology, Therapeutics and Toxicology* 1985; **23**: 497–500.

231 Jenkins R. Depression and anxiety: an overview of preventive strategies. In: Jenkins R *et al.* (ed). *The Prevention of Depression and Anxiety.* London: HMSO, 1992.

Index

Printed and bound by CPI Group (UK) Ltd, Croydon, CR0 4YY

23/10/2024

01778246-0011